EMBOLIZATION THERAPY

EMBOLIZATION THERAPY

Principles and Clinical Applications

MARCELO GUIMARAES, MD, FSIR

Associate Professor of Radiology and Surgery
Division of Vascular & Interventional Radiology
Medical University of South Carolina
Charleston, South Carolina

RICCARDO LENCIONI, MD, FSIR, EBIR

Professor and Division Director
Diagnostic Imaging and Intervention
Pisa University School of Medicine
Pisa, Italy

GARY P. SISKIN, MD, FSIR

Professor and Chairman
Department of Radiology
Albany Medical College
Albany, New York

Wolters Kluwer
Health

Philadelphia • Baltimore • New York • London
Buenos Aires • Hong Kong • Sydney • Tokyo

Acquisitions Editor: Ryan Shaw
Product Development Editor: Amy G. Dinkel
Marketing Manager: Dan Dressler
Production Project Manager: Bridgett Dougherty
Design Coordinator: Stephen Druding
Manufacturing Coordinator: Beth Welsh
Prepress Vendor: Absolute Service, Inc.

9 8 7 6 5 4 3 2 1

Printed in China

Library of Congress Cataloging-in-Publication Data

Embolization therapy : principles and clinical applications / [edited by] Marcelo Guimaraes, Riccardo Lencioni, Gary P. Siskin.
p. ; cm.
Includes bibliographical references and index.
ISBN 978-1-4511-9144-8 (alk. paper)
I. Guimaraes, Marcelo, editor. II. Lencioni, R. (Riccardo), 1961- , editor. III. Siskin, Gary P., editor.
[DNLM: 1. Embolization, Therapeutic. WH 310]
RD33.55
617'.05—dc23

2014039792

LWW.com

RRS1410

I dedicate this work to Mateus and Julia: In your pursuit of happiness,
include passion, persistence, and patience daily.
Rossana, thank you for your incredible perseverance and support.
Love all of you.

M.G.

To Dania and Elisabetta
Life is forever: don't let anyone or anything "embolize" your joy!
I love you

R.L.

I wish to thank my family for their constant support of my professional endeavors and my partners for their ongoing patience with me.
Both have provided me with an enviable amount of personal and professional fulfillment.

G.S.

CONTRIBUTORS

Carlos Abath, MD
Chief
Department of Interventional Radiology
Instituto de Medicina Integral de Pernambuco
Recife, Brazil

Ashley Adamovich, MD
Resident in Radiology
Albany Medical Center
Albany, New York

Joshua D. Adams, MD
Assistant Professor
Department of Surgery and Radiology
Medical University of South Carolina
Charleston, South Carolina

Jaime All, MD
Division of Vascular and Interventional Radiology
Department of Radiology and Medical Imaging
University of Virginia Health System
Charlottesville, Virginia

Matthew E. Anderson, MD
Assistant Professor of Radiology
Interventional Radiology
University of Texas Southwestern Medical Center
Dallas, Texas

Michael Bret Anderson, MD
Assistant Professor
Division of Vascular and Interventional Radiology
Department of Radiology and Radiological Science
Medical University of South Carolina
Charleston, South Carolina

John F. Angle, MD
Professor of Radiology
Director, Division of Interventional Radiology
Department of Radiology and Medical Imaging
University of Virginia Health System
Charlottesville, Virginia

Yasuaki Arai, MD
Director, National Cancer Center Hospital
Chair, Department of Diagnostic Radiology
Tokyo, Japan

Bulent Arslan, MD
Associate Professor of Radiology
Department of Interventional Radiology
Rush University Medical Center
Chicago, Illinois

Raj Ayyagari, MD
Assistant Professor
Department of Radiology
Yale School of Medicine
Interventional Radiologist
Yale-New Haven Hospital
New Haven, Connecticut

Marcos Barbosa de Souza Júnior, MD
Specialization in Vascular Surgery by IMIP
Resident in Radiology Vascular and Interventional—Angiorad
Recife, Brazil

James F. Benenati, MD
Clinical Associate Professor
Miami Cardiac and Vascular Institute
Miami, Florida

Goetz Benndorf, MD, PhD
Section Chief, Interventional Neuroradiology
Ben Taub General Hospital
Associate Professor
Department of Radiology
Baylor College of Medicine
Houston, Texas

Alan D. Birney, MD
Resident in Radiology
Albany Medical Center
Albany, New York

Pierre E. Bize, MD
Associate Physician
Clinical Sciences
University of Lausanne
Associate Physician
Radiodiagnostic Interventional Radiology
University Hospital of Lausanne CHUV
Lausanne, Switzerland

Austin Bourgeois, MD
Resident in Radiology
Department of Radiology
The University of Tennessee Graduate School of Medicine
Knoxville, Tennessee

Daniel B. Brown, MD
Professor of Radiology and Radiological Sciences
Director, Division of Interventional Oncology
Vanderbilt-Ingram Cancer Center
Nashville, Tenesee

Daniel C. Brown, MD
Department of Radiology and Radiological Sciences
Vanderbilt University
Nashville, Tennessee

Karen T. Brown, MD
Professor of Clinical Radiology
Department of Radiology
Weill Cornell Medical College
Attending Radiologist
Memorial Sloan Kettering Cancer Center
New York, New York

Patricia E. Burrows, MD
Professor of Radiology
Medical College of Wisconsin
Children's Hospital of Wisconsin
Milwaukee, Wisconsin

Theresa M. Caridi, MD
Assistant Professor of Vascular and Interventional Radiology
MedStar Georgetown University Hospital
Washington, DC

Francisco Cesar Carnevale, MD
Professor
Chief of Interventional Radiology
University of São Paulo Medical School
São Paulo, Brazil

Julius Chapiro, MD
Research Fellow
The Russell H. Morgan Department of Radiology and Radiological Science
Division of Vascular and Interventional Radiology
The Johns Hopkins Hospital
Baltimore, Maryland

M. Imran Chaudry, MD
Associate Professor
Department of Radiology
Medical University of South Carolina
Charleston, South Carolina

Long Chen, MD, PhD
Department of Interventional Radiology
The First Affiliated Hospital of Soochow University
Suzhou, Jiangsu Province, China

John C. Dalfino, MD
Assistant Professor of Surgery
Albany Medical College
Albany, New York

Michael Darcy, MD
Professor of Radiology
Chief, Interventional Radiology
Mallinckrodt Institute of Radiology
Washington University in St. Louis
St. Louis, Missouri

Miguel A. De Gregorio, MD
Full Professor and Chairman of Radiology
University of Zaragoza
Chief of Interventional Radiology
Hospital Clínico Universitario Lozano Blesa
Zaragoza, Spain

Alban Denys, MD, Msc
Department of Radiology and Interventional Radiology
University Hospital of Lausanne CHUV
Lausanne, Switzerland

Ajita Deodhar, MD
Fellow, Interventional Radiology
Dotter Interventional Institute
Oregon Health & Science University Hospital
Portland, Oregon

Daniel Do, MD
Assistant Professor
Vascular & Interventional Radiology
University of Kentucky
Lexington, Kentucky

Rafael Duran, MD
The Russell H. Morgan Department of Radiology and Radiological Science
Division of Vascular and Interventional Radiology
The Johns Hopkins Hospital
Baltimore, Maryland

Moneeb Ehtesham, MD
Department of Neurological Surgery
Vanderbilt University Medical Center
Nashville, Tennessee

Brian Funaki, MD, FSIR, FAHA, FCIRCE
Professor of Radiology
Chief, Section of Vascular and Interventional Radiology
The University of Chicago Medicine
Chicago, Illinois

Eric J. Gandras, MD, FSIR
Assistant Professor of Radiology
Hofstra North Shore-LIJ School of Medicine
Associate Chief
Division of Interventional Radiology
North Shore University Hospital at Manhasset
Manhasset, New York

John R. Gaughen, Jr, MD
Assistant Professor
Department of Radiology and Medical Imaging
University of Virginia Health System
Charlottesville, Virginia

Jean-François H. Geschwind
Professor of Radiology, Surgery, and Oncology
The Russell H. Morgan Department of Radiology and Radiological Science
Division of Vascular and Interventional Radiology
The Johns Hopkins Hospital
Baltimore, Maryland

Craig R. Greben, MD, FSIR
Chief, Vascular and Interventional Radiology
North Shore University Hospital
North Shore-LIJ Medical Group
Associate Professor of Radiology and Surgery
Hofstra North Shore-LIJ School of Medicine
Manhasset, New York

Marcelo Guimaraes, MD, FSIR
Associate Professor of Radiology and Surgery
Division of Vascular & Interventional Radiology
Medical University of South Carolina
Charleston, South Carolina

Christopher Hannegan, MD
Assistant Professor of Radiology
Attending Physician
Director of the Interventional Radiology Fellowship Program
Medical University of South Carolina
Charleston, South Carolina

Harris Hawk, MD
Fellow
Neuroendovascular Surgery
Medical University of South Carolina
Charleston, South Carolina

Ali Akber Hazari
Student
Royal College of Surgeons
Dublin, Ireland

Ryan M. Hickey, MD
Health Systems Clinician
Northwestern University Feinberg School of Medicine
Chicago, Illinois

Shinichi Hori, MD, PhD
Director and Chief Physician
Department of Radiology
Gate Tower Institute for Image Guided Therapy
Izumisano, Osaka, Japan

Mark D. Iafrati, MD, FACS
Chief of Vascular Surgery
Associate Professor of Surgery
Tufts Medical Center
Boston, Massachusetts

Robert F. James, MD
Associate Professor
Director, Vascular Neurosurgery
Department of Neurosurgery
University of Louisville School of Medicine
Louisville, Kentucky

Sanjeeva P. Kalva, MD, FSIR
Chief, Interventional Radiology
Associate Professor of Radiology
University of Texas Southwestern Medical Center
Dallas, Texas

Krishna Kandarpa, MD, PhD
Chief Scientific Officer
Executive Vice President, Research and Development
Delcath Systems, Inc.
New York, New York

John A. Kaufman, MD, MS
Director, Dotter Interventional Institute
Frederick S. Keller Professor of Interventional Radiology
Oregon Health & Science University Hospital
Portland, Oregon

Lawrence J. Keating, MD
Assistant Professor of Radiology
Albany Medical Center
Albany, New York

Imad S. Khan, MD
Department of Neurological Surgery
Vanderbilt University Medical Center
Nashville, Tennessee

Omid Kohannim, MD, PhD
Resident Physician
David Geffen School of Medicine at UCLA
Los Angeles, California

Alicia Laborda, DVM, PhD
Assistant Professor
University of Zaragoza
Senior Researcher
Group of Research in Minimally Invasive Techniques, Government of Aragon
Zaragoza, Spain

Yann Lachenal, MD, EBIR
Senior Registrar
Interventional Radiology Unit
Radiodiagnostic and Interventional Radiology Department
University Hospital of Lausanne
Lausanne, Switzerland

Jonathan R. Lena, MD
Department of Neurosciences
Division of Neurosurgery
Medical University of South Carolina
Charleston, South Carolina

Riccardo Lencioni, MD, FSIR, EBIR
Professor and Division Director
Diagnostic Imaging and Intervention
Pisa University School of Medicine
Pisa, Italy

Robert J. Lewandowski, MD, FSIR
Associate Professor of Radiology
Section of Interventional Radiology
Northwestern University Feinberg School of Medicine
Chicago, Illinois

David Li MD, PhD
Assistant Professor
Weill Cornell Medical College
New York Presbyterian Hospital
New York, New York

Romaric Loffroy, MD, PhD
Professor
E2i Laboratory
Burgundy University
Chief, Department of Vascular and Interventional Radiology
Bocage Teaching Hospital
Dijon, France

Paul N. M. Lohle MD, PhD
Department of Radiology
St. Elisabeth Ziekenhuis
Tilburg, The Netherlands

William J. Mack, MD, MS
Assistant Professor of Neurosurgery
Keck School of Medicine
University of Southern California
Los Angeles, California

Laura MacNeil
Student
Biomedical Engineering
University of Guelph
Ontario, Canada

David C. Madoff, MD
Professor of Radiology
Chief, Division of Interventional Radiology
New York-Presbyterian Hospital/Weill Cornell Medical Center
New York, New York

Romero Marques, MD
Interventional Radiologist
Angiorad—Interventional Radiology Group
Instituto de Medicina Integral Prof. Fernando Figueira
Recife, Brazil

Richard H. Marshall, MD
Division of Interventional Radiology
New York-Presbyterian Hospital/Weill Cornell Medical Center
New York, New York

Lacey B. Martin, BS
Medical Student
Division of Neurosurgery, Department of Surgery
Brody School of Medicine at East Carolina University
Greenville, North Carolina

Justin McWilliams, MD
Assistant Professor
UCLA Interventional Radiology
Los Angeles, California

James C. Meek, DO
Interventional Radiologist
Department of Radiology
University of Arkansas for Medical Sciences
Little Rock, Arkansas

Mary E. Meek, MD
Director, HHT Center of Excellence
Director, Interventional Radiology
University of Arkansas for Medical Sciences
Little Rock, Arkansas

J Mocco, MD, MS
Associate Professor of Neurological Surgery
Department of Neurological Surgery
Vanderbilt University Medical Center
Nashville, Tennessee

Airton Mota Moreira, MD, PhD
Assistant of Interventional Radiology Section
University of Sao Paulo Medical School
Hospital Sírio Libanês
Sao Paulo, Brazil

Kieran Murphy, MB, FRCPC, FSIR
Professor of Radiology
Toronto Western Hospital
University Health Network
Toronto, Ontario, Canada

Tara Murray, EdM, RN, CCRN, CES
Albany Medical Center
Albany, New York

Gregory Nadolski, MD
Assistant Professor of Radiology
Interventional Radiology
Hospital of the University of Pennsylvania
Philadelphia, Pennsylvania

Jason J. Naidich, MD, MBA
Chairman, Department of Radiology
Hofstra North Shore-LIJ School of Medicine
Chairman, Department of Radiology
North Shore University Hospital at Manhasset
Manhasset, New York
Long Island Jewish Medical Center
New Hyde Park, New York

Rakesh C. Navuluri, MD
Assistant Professor of Radiology
Section of Vascular and Interventional Radiology
The University of Chicago Medicine
Chicago, Illinois

Bruno C. Odisio, MD
Assistant Professor
Division of Interventional Radiology
Department of Diagnostic Radiology
The University of Texas MD Anderson Cancer Center
Houston, Texas

Jose Luiz Orlando, MD
Department of Vascular and Interventional Radiology
A.C. Camargo Cancer Center
Sao Paulo, Brazil

Keigo Osuga, MD, PhD
Associate Professor
Department of Diagnostic and Interventional Radiology
Osaka University Graduate School of Medicine
Osaka, Japan

Jae Hyung Park, MD
Professor of Radiology
Gachon University Gil Medical Center
Professor Emeritus
Seoul National University
Seoul, South Korea

Sang Joon Park, MD
Professor
Intervention Chief
Department of Radiology
International St. Mary's Hospital
Catholic Kwandong University
Incheon, South Korea

Susie J. Park, MD
Resident in Radiology
Albany Medical Center
Albany, New York

Constantino S. Peña, MD
Interventional Radiologist
Miami Cardiac and Vascular Institute
Miami, Florida

Elena N. Petre, MD
Senior Research Scientist
Department of Radiology
Memorial Sloan Kettering Cancer Center
New York, New York

Jeffrey S. Pollak, MD
Robert I. White, Jr. MD Professor of Interventional Radiology
Co-Section Chief
Vascular and Interventional Radiology
Yale University School of Medicine
New Haven, Connecticut

Marcus Presley, MD
Resident in Radiology
Department of Radiology and Radiological Sciences
Vanderbilt University
Nashville, Tennessee

Dheeraj K. Rajan, MD, FRCPC, FSIR
Head and Associate Professor
Division of Vascular and Interventional Radiology
Department of Medical Imaging
University of Toronto
University Health Network
Toronto, Ontario, Canada

Francisco Ramos, MD
Attending Physician
Hemangiomas and Vascular Malformations Center
A.C. Camargo Cancer Center
Sao Paulo, Brazil

Howard Richard, MD
Associate Professor
Department of Diagnostic Radiology and Nuclear Medicine
University of Maryland School of Medicine
University of Maryland Medical Center
Baltimore, Maryland

William S. Rilling, MD, FSIR
Professor of Radiology and Surgery
Division of Vascular Interventional Radiology
Medical College of Wisconsin
Director, Vascular Interventional Radiology
Froedtert Hospital
Milwaukee, Wisconsin

Wael E. Saad, MD, FSIR
Professor of Radiology
Director, Vascular and Interventional Radiology
University of Michigan Medical Center
Ann Arbor, Michigan

Riad Salem, MD, FSIR
Professor of Radiology, Medicine-Hematology/Oncology, and Surgery-Organ Transplantation
Northwestern University Feinberg School of Medicine
Chicago, Illinois

Claudio J. Schönholz, MD
Professor of Radiology
Department of Radiology and Radiological Science
Medical University of South Carolina
Charleston, South Carolina

J. Bayne Selby, MD
Professor of Radiology
Director of Interventional Radiology
Department of Radiology and Radiological Science
Medical University of South Carolina
Charleston, South Carolina

Richard Shlansky-Goldberg, MD
Professor of Radiology, Surgery, and Obstetrics/Gynecology
Department of Radiology/Division of Interventional Radiology
Perelman School of Medicine at the University of Pennsylvania
Philadelphia, Pennsylvania

P. Sideras, MD, PhD
Research Fellow
Department of Radiology
Memorial Sloan Kettering Cancer Center
New York, New York

Sergio Sierre, MD, FSIR
Director Department of Interventional Radiology
Hospital de Pediatría "Prof. JP Garrahan"
Buenos Aires, Argentina

Gary P. Siskin, MD, FSIR
Professor and Chairman
Department of Radiology
Albany Medical College
Albany, New York

C. T. Sofocleous, MD, PhD, FSIR, FCIRSE
Professor of Radiology
Weill Cornell Medical College
Attending Physician, Interventional Radiology
MH Member; Memorial Sloan Kettering Cancer Center
New York, New York

Miyuki Sone, MD
Consultant Radiologist
Department of Diagnostic Radiology
National Cancer Center Hospital
Tokyo, Japan

James B. Spies, MD, MPH
Professor and Chair
Department of Radiology
Medstar Georgetown University Hospital
Washington, DC

Alejandro Spiotta, MD
Adjunct Professor
Department of Neurosurgery
Medical University of South Carolina
Charleston, South Carolina

S. William Stavropoulos, MD
Associate Professor of Radiology and Surgery
Vice Chair of Clinical Operation
Interventional Radiology Fellowship Program Director
Department of Radiology
Perelman School of Medicine at the University of Pennsylvania
Philadelphia, Pennsylvania

Jordan C. Tasse, MD
Assistant Professor of Radiology
Department of Interventional Radiology
Rush University Medical Center
Chicago, Illinois

Ulku Cenk Turba, MD
Associate Professor of Radiology
Department of Interventional Radiology
Rush University Medical Center
Chicago, Illinois

Aquilla Turk, DO
Professor
Departments of Radiology and Neurosurgery
Medical University of South Carolina
Charleston, South Carolina

Raymond Turner, MD
Associate Professor
Department of Radiology
Medical University of South Carolina
Charleston, South Carolina

Andre Uflacker, MD
Resident Physician
Division of Vascular and Interventional Radiology
Department of Radiology and Medical Imaging
University of Virginia Health System
Charlottesville, Virginia

Luke R. Wilkins, MD
Assistant Professor
Department of Radiology and Medical Imaging
Division of Angiography and Interventional Radiology
University of Virginia School of Medicine
Charlottesville, Virginia

Ricardo Yamada, MD
Interventional Radiology Fellow
Medical University of South Carolina
Charleston, South Carolina

Chang Jin Yoon, MD, PhD
Associate Professor
Department of Radiology
Seoul National University College of Medicine
Seoul, South Korea
Seoul National University Bundang Hospital
Seongnam, Gyeonggi-do, South Korea

Joseph J. Zechlinski, MD
Department of Radiology
Froedtert and the Medical College of Wisconsin
Milwaukee, Wisconsin

Joseph Zuniga, MD
Vascular Surgery Fellow
Tufts Medical Center
Boston, Massachusetts

FOREWORD

It is a great personal pleasure for me to write the Foreword to *Embolization Therapy*, the first book of its type dedicated to an important area of endovascular therapy and vascular intervention.

Although the field of embolotherapy has been continually growing since its early descriptions in the late 1960s and 1970s, it has truly exploded in importance and diversity in the past decade. In the early years of interventional therapy, vascular radiologists began to explore the use of the catheter as a therapeutic instrument not only to make diagnoses but also to deliver methods of therapy. These initially included drug therapy and then ultimately material to actually occlude blood vessels.

As with the entire field of interventional radiology, embolization therapy has had dramatic growth in the past 10 to 15 years, as the value of devascularization has grown. Additionally, technology available for embolization therapy has dramatically increased. The endovascular therapist today has the option of occluding vessels of every size from the microcirculation using liquid and/or microparticles to large vessels using dedicated vessel occluders, and any option of occluding blood flow is available.

The field of embolization therapy has also become associated with higher levels of scientific study to prove efficacy. Clever and innovative ideas have been substantiated in value by clinical studies providing high-quality data to support change in practice and convince colleagues from other disciplines of the value of embolization. The role in treating diseases as remote as hemorrhage and active bleeding to benign diseases such as uterine fibroids and angiomyolipomas as well as more complex diseases such as cancer and arteriovenous malformations has become undeniable.

As the world has become a smaller place, and the medical and interventional community has been able to communicate in ways never before possible, *Embolization Therapy* represents the greatest accumulation of authors from throughout the world to bring their experience in treating various diseases and using a great variety of embolic materials. The text is organized in a very practical way, by anatomic area as well as clinical activity, all of which represent increasing clinical importance in daily practice.

I'm certain this will be an extremely valuable text and reference for anyone practicing embolization therapy and is an important addition to the body of interventional literature.

My hardy congratulations to the three editors who brought together the most distinguished interventionalists in the world from multiple disciplines to contribute to this text.

Barry T. Katzen, MD

PREFACE

Embolization procedures have evolved tremendously in the last two decades and are among the most common procedures performed by vascular and interventional radiologists. Embolization, although previously limited to patients with hemorrhagic conditions, has expended to areas such as the treatment of hepatic malignancies, vascular malformations, uterine fibroids, and neurovascular conditions among others. In other words, it has become a commonly used primary or adjunctive procedure for a growing number of indications.

Despite the fact that there are several excellent books about vascular and interventional radiology procedures, the editors felt it was time to provide comprehensive and dedicated material on embolization procedures.

Embolization Therapy: Principles and Clinical Applications aims to provide basic and advanced concepts in embolization. The core of this textbook contains updated and comprehensive reviews on the most commonly performed embolization procedures. In addition, we have made sure that less commonly performed procedures are discussed in similar detail so that interventionalists can expand their portfolio of services that they are able to offer their patients. We are pleased that we are able to cover the breadth of this topic in a single source, which would not have been possible without contributions from dozens of experienced and recognized interventionalists from around the world. This book truly presents a global look at embolization, which has become the core of many interventional practices.

The Editors

ACKNOWLEDGMENTS

The editors would like to thank all of our vascular and interventional radiology, neurointerventional radiology, and vascular surgery colleagues who dedicated time to work on the chapters within this text. They have not only updated standard of care techniques but also have shared personal experiences which are summarized in the "Tips and Tricks" sections of each chapter. It is our hope that this textbook will prove be a useful tool to introduce new interventionalists to embolotherapy to serve as an updated source of information for our more experienced physicians.

The editors are very thankful to Sandra Stringer's efforts, suggestions, and help in the review process. The editors also would like to thank and recognize the work of Grace Caputo, development editor; Harold Medina from Absolute Service, Inc.; and Amy Dinkel from WKH, who each tenaciously helped to make this project a reality.

CONTENTS

I

Embolic Materials

1

Brief History and Classification of Embolic Agents

Gary P. Siskin • Tara Murray • Marcelo Guimaraes

PRINCIPLES OF EMBOLIZATION THERAPY

Embolization is defined as the intentional endovascular occlusion of an artery or vein.[1] Presently, this procedure has been applied to almost every organ of the body for various indications. The procedure is performed by percutaneously delivering embolic agents into a target vascular system either through selective catheterization or direct puncture of the target organ/vessel. The correct use of embolization techniques require an in-depth knowledge of the clinical condition being treated, the available and appropriate embolic agents and delivery systems (catheters, microcatheters, and guiding catheters), the anticipated postprocedure patient care, and the potential complications of the procedure.

As a general rule for the practice of any percutaneous interventional therapy, every clinical situation must be thoroughly reviewed to help determine how and when to proceed with the embolization procedure. Review of any available imaging is paramount to plan the procedure approach and technique to be used. In general, an embolization procedure should be able to resolve the clinical problem in a single procedure because repeat procedures may not be possible. This is often the case in emergency situations, when alternatives may be limited and rapid decisions need to be made to use embolic therapy sooner rather than later. Ultimately, the final decision to perform an embolization procedure lies with the physician responsible for performing the procedure after an appropriate risk–benefit analysis has been made.

HISTORY

From a historical perspective, the initial agents used for embolization and the procedural indications have significantly changed over time.

The concept of therapeutic vascular occlusion actually began in 1933 when Hamby and Gardener treated a carotid cavernous fistula at surgery by embolizing the fistula with small fragments of muscle via arteriotomy.[2] Doppman and Newton have been credited with performing the first percutaneous therapeutic embolization procedures.[3,4] In 1968, these early interventionalists published separate case reports describing their independent experience with percutaneous embolization of spinal cord arteriovenous malformations. Doppman et al.[3] used 3-mm stainless steel pellets for embolization, and Newton and Adams[4] used lead pellets and small fragments of muscle.

In the early 1970s, experience with peripheral embolization was initially gained as a treatment option for acute gastrointestinal bleeding.[5] During that time, the indications expanded into the treatment of gastroesophageal varices, arteriovenous fistulas and malformations, control of hemoptysis, treatment of varicocele, and ablation of tumors or organs.[6] Initially, autologous clot was used as the embolic agent for these indications, but other agents were introduced during this time. The use of gelfoam for endovascular occlusion grew in popularity but was actually first reported as an embolic agent by Speakman[7] in 1964. In 1974, Tadavarthy et al.[8] reported the first use of polyvinyl alcohol (PVA) as an embolic agent, and Serbinenko[9] reported on the use of detachable balloons to treat intracerebral aneurysms. In 1975, Gianturco et al.[10] reported on the development and use of the first coils: the cotton-tail device consisting of eight cotton threads attached to a 3-mm body of steel and the wool-tail device consisting of four wool fibers attached to a 5-cm length of guidewire. The wool-tail device design eventually transformed into the stainless steel coil in 1976, and in time, the thrombogenic wool fibers were replaced with nonantigenic synthetic fibers.[11]

Since that time, the basic tools of embolization have undergone significant development and improvement. New coil configurations, including detachable coils and vascular plugs, have been developed to increase the safety and effectiveness of coil embolization for both neurovascular and peripheral vascular applications.[12,13] In addition, experience grew with liquid embolic agents such as cyanoacrylate and Onyx (Covidien, Irvine, California).[14] For years, irregularly shaped PVA particles have been the particulate agent of choice. With the maturation of procedures such as chemoembolization and uterine fibroid embolization, new particulate agents were developed, including spherical embolic agents,[15] drug-eluting beads,[16] yttrium 90 microspheres,[17] and soon, bioresorbable spheres.[18,19]

CLASSIFICATION OF EMBOLIC AGENTS

When looking at all of the available agents for embolization, it is often helpful to classify these agents from a clinical perspective, allowing a particular class or type of embolic agent to be an option for a specific indication or procedure. However, this is easier said than done because it can be difficult to define the terms that are traditionally used for this type of classification system. In addition, there is a significant amount of potential overlap between agents in different categories.

Historically, embolic materials have been grouped in several ways: by physical characteristics (type of material), longevity of vascular occlusion (temporary or permanent), level of occlusion (proximal or distal), pathology being treated, type of delivery technique, cost, and many other alternatives. When attempting to classify these materials clinically, consider that not all materials are available in every angiography suite due to local supply constraints and cost concerns or to marketing and regulatory issues. The availability of various embolic agents to allow for the appropriate performance of embolization procedures for various indications is a requirement for any interventionalist and hospital offering this service.

Traditional Classification System

The most common way to classify embolic agents has been to define them as being either temporary or permanent.[1] This is helpful when selecting an embolic agent because some applications of embolization, such as trauma, may only require the use of a temporary agent, whereas in other applications, a permanent agent may be more appropriate. When this system is used, the temporary category is small and consists of only gelfoam, collagen, thrombin, and new biodegradable microspheres that are being developed but are not commercially available at this time.[18,19] The remaining available agents are considered to be permanent.

When using this classification system, however, the question needs to be asked regarding what one is referring to when using the terms *temporary* and *permanent*. This classification system refers to temporary and permanent as terms used to describe the biodegradability of the actual embolic agent. It does not refer to the occlusion caused by the embolic agent because if it does, the group assignment might change for several agents. This can be exemplified with PVA particles. These particles have been classically described as permanent because they are not biodegradable and can be found in embolized tissue years after embolization.[20] However, the occlusion caused by PVA particles is not always permanent. Recanalization has been demonstrated, with proposed mechanisms including angiogenesis and capillary regrowth caused by vascular proliferation inside organized thrombus and resorption of the thrombus in between PVA particles found in the vessel lumen after resolution of the initial inflammatory response.[21–24] Similarly, gelatin sponge particles are considered to be a temporary embolic agent.[25] This has historically been based on the work of Light and Prentice[26] in 1945. Later studies have demonstrated the temporary nature of the occlusion induced by gelfoam,[27,28] supporting its classification as a temporary embolic agent. However, permanent occlusion after gelfoam embolization has also been described and attributed to dense packing[29] and to fibrotic or necrotic changes induced by the gelfoam.[30,31] These examples demonstrate the difficulty in using the "temporary versus permanent" classification system unless a clear distinction is made between the temporary and permanent nature of the embolic agent or of the vascular occlusion induced by the embolic agent.

Classification of embolic agents based on the size of the vessel being embolized has also been described.[32,33] Although this system can be useful in guiding interventionalists toward the use of appropriate agents, it becomes clear that overlap can exist between these categories. For example, coils are available in various sizes, making them appropriate to use for certain indications in both large and small vessels.

Present Classification System

Various pathologies are treated today by embolization. In general, these can be divided into focal abnormalities (i.e., aneurysms, traumatic injury, arteriovenous fistulae) and more diffuse abnormalities that are treating abnormal vascular beds in part or in their entirety. Focal abnormalities

Table 1.1 Classification of Embolic Agents

Category	Indication	Embolic Agent
Mechanical embolic agents	Treatment of focal vascular abnormalities (e.g., aneurysm, hemorrhage, trauma)	Coils (pushable, detachable) Plugs Gelfoam (pledgets, torpedoes)
Flow-directed embolic agents	Treatment of diffuse vascular abnormalities (e.g., AVM, tumors, solid organ pathology)	
Particulate embolic agents		PVA particles Spherical embolic agents Drug-eluting beads Resorbable microspheres
Liquid embolic agents		*N*-butyl cyanoacrylate Onyx Sclerosants
Gelfoam		Gelfoam (slurry, particles)

AVM, arteriovenous malformation; PVA, polyvinyl alcohol.

are typically treated by the insertion of mechanical embolic agents at or in close proximity to the abnormality being treated. Diffuse abnormalities, such as tumors and vascular malformations, are typically treated by placing a catheter proximal to the abnormal vascular bed and using a flow-directed embolic agent to embolize the abnormal vasculature. Therefore, it seems useful to classify agents as either mechanical (delivered at the site of a focal vascular abnormality) or flow-directed (delivered by flow from a catheter position proximal to a vascular abnormality (Table 1.1).

Mechanical Agents

Various mechanical agents are available to treat focal vascular abnormalities. The most common agents include coils and plugs. Detachable balloons, which are available in most of the world outside of the United States, can also be used as a mechanical agent to treat focal vascular abnormalities. In theory, they can be used to quickly occlude a vessel at a precise position and have the ability to be repeatedly repositioned as needed. However, they were recalled in the United States due to manufacturing and placement issues and have essentially been replaced with new, detachable coils.

Pushable and detachable coils are available, and both are manufactured in sizes that can be delivered through standard 4-Fr or 5-Fr angiographic catheters or microcatheters. Synthetic fibers are often attached to these coils to increase their thrombogenicity (Fig. 1.1). Pushable coils require a guidewire or dedicated coil pusher to advance the coil through and out of the delivery catheter to the site of the vascular abnormality. Detachable coils are attached to the coil pusher and are released either mechanically or electrically when they are appropriately positioned (Fig. 1.2). Typically, multiple coils are required for embolization, although the hydrogel-coated coils may decrease the number of coils required for occlusion.

Plugs are larger than coils and are able to create a focal occlusion in larger vessels with a single device. Amplatzer Vascular Plugs (St. Jude Medical, Inc., St. Paul, Minnesota) are the most commonly used device in this category (Fig. 1.3).[13] Newer products have also recently become available and include the Medusa Vascular Plug (EndoShape, Inc., Boulder, Colorado) and the MVP Micro Vascular Plug System (Reverse Medical Corporation, Irvine, California) (Fig. 1.4). Both of these plugs have received U.S. Food and Drug Administration (FDA) approval in 2013 for use in the peripheral vasculature. The MVP Micro Vascular Plug is a smaller system and is delivered through a microcatheter to occlude small vessels.

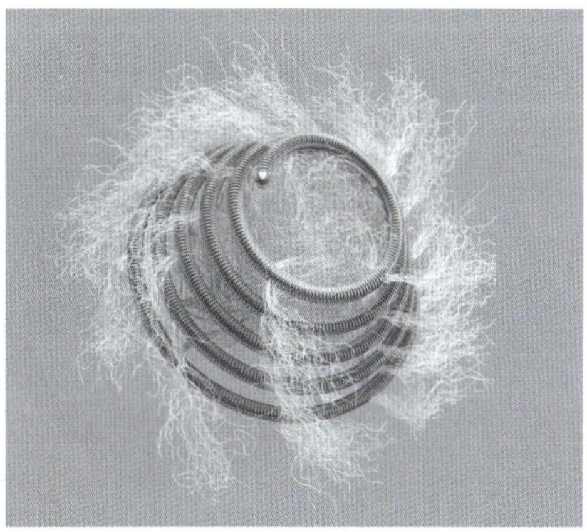

Figure 1.1 Tornado coil demonstrating the platinum coil and synthetic fibers. (Courtesy of Cook Medical, Inc., Bloomington, Indiana.)

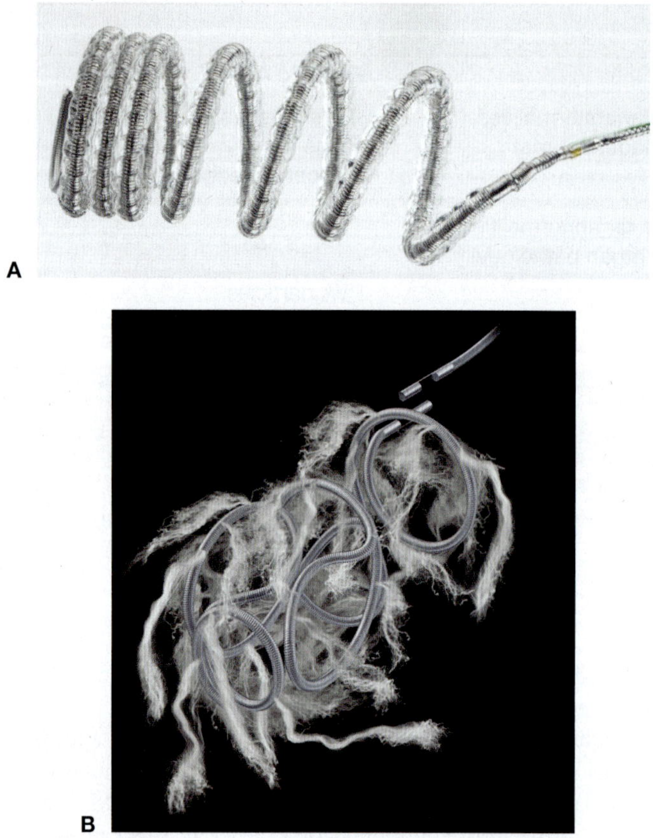

Figure 1.2 Two examples of detachable peripheral coils. **A:** AZUR Peripheral HydroCoil Embolization System. (Courtesy of Terumo Medical Corporation, Somerset, New Jersey). **B:** Interlock Fibered IDC Occlusion System. (Courtesy of Boston Scientific Corporation, Natick, Massachusetts.)

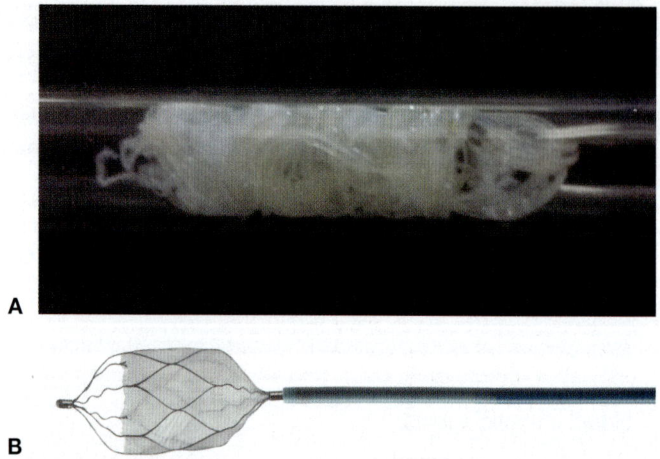

Figure 1.4 Two new vascular plugs. **A:** Medusa Vascular Plug. (Courtesy of EndoShape, Inc., Boulder, Colorado.) **B:** MVP Micro Vascular Plug System. (Courtesy of Reverse Medical Corporation, Irvine, California.)

Gelfoam is one agent that can straddle the line between mechanical agents and flow-directed agents. Where it becomes assigned is often due to the technique used for preparation. When cut as pledgets or larger torpedoes, it can be considered as a mechanical device because it is often staying in close proximity to the tip of the catheter used for delivery. When gelfoam is cut in smaller pieces or prepared as a slurry by passing it between two syringes through a stopcock, it can become flow directed and travel distal beyond the tip of the catheter.

Flow-Directed Agents

This category consists of agents that are delivered through a catheter and are then directed beyond the tip of the catheter into an abnormal vascular bed by normal arterial flow.

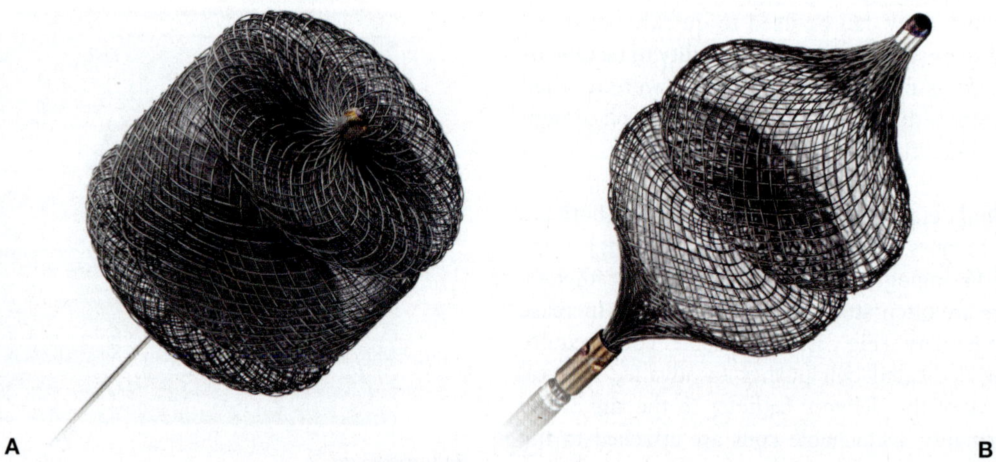

Figure 1.3 Amplatzer Vascular Plug: AVP II **(A)** and AVP 4 **(B)**. (Courtesy of St. Jude Medical, Inc., St. Paul, Minnesota.)

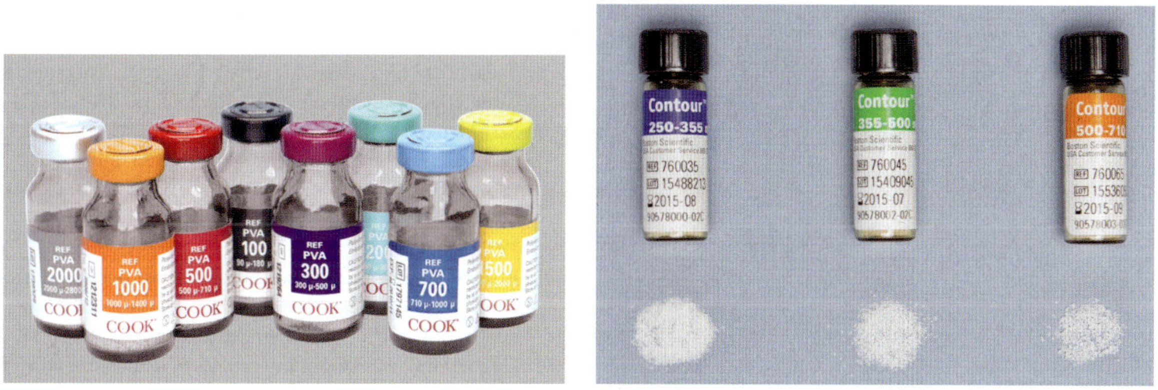

A B

Figure 1.5 Particulate PVA. **A:** PVA Foam Embolization Particles. (Courtesy of Cook Medical, Inc., Bloomington, Indiana.) **B:** Contour PVA Embolization Particles. (Courtesy of Boston Scientific Corporation, Natick, Massachusetts.)

In addition to small gelfoam particles or a gelfoam slurry, the agents in this category include particulate and liquid embolic agents. Because these agents are using normal flow to carry an agent distally, close attention must be paid during their administration to be certain that delivery ceases when forward flow into the abnormal vascular bed is no longer recognized.

Irregularly shaped PVA particles were the initial particulate embolic agent and still remain the standard particulate agent used by most interventionalists (Fig. 1.5). There are disadvantages that are inherent to the use of particulate PVA, including size variability, particle aggregation, and microcatheter occlusion during delivery. This prompted the development of spherical embolic agents, allowing for significant growth in this area during the last two decades.[34] Calibrated spherical agents are now available, including PVA-based microspheres, trisacryl gelatin microspheres, and Polyzene-F–based microspheres. These agents are used commonly for procedures such as uterine fibroid embolization and other tumor and organ-based indications. Drug-eluting microspheres (Fig. 1.6) and yttrium 90 microspheres have helped develop an entire subspecialty of interventional oncology. Resorbable microspheres represent a significant future advance in this area, potentially allowing for the creation of temporary, reproducible arterial occlusion with embolization.[19,35]

Liquid embolic agents are also classified in the category of flow-directed agents, although this can be somewhat variable based on the agent and the amount of dilution used during administration. Sclerosants such as ethanol have been used successfully as an embolic agent for certain tumors and vascular malformations, whereas more mild agents such as sodium tetradecyl sulfate have been used for venous applications such as varicose veins, varicoceles, and pelvic congestion syndrome. Other sclerosants include hypertonic glucose, doxycycline, and OK-432. Agents such as *N*-butyl

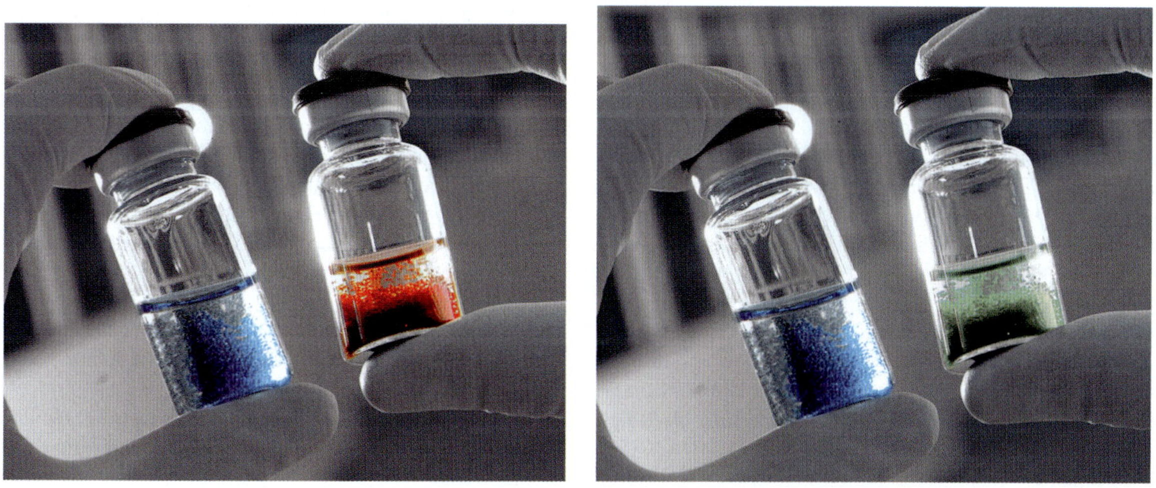

A B

Figure 1.6 Drug-eluting DC Bead before and after loading with doxorubicin **(A)** and irinotecan **(B)**. (Courtesy of Biocompatibles, Inc., Oxford, Connecticut.)

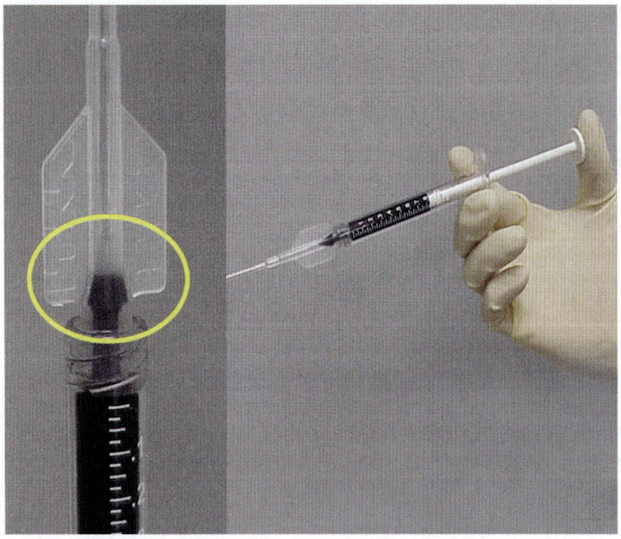

Figure 1.7 Onyx Liquid Embolic System within a syringe before delivery. (Courtesy of Covidien, Irvine, California.)

cyanoacrylate and Onyx (Fig. 1.7) are playing a growing role in the treatment of cerebral and peripheral arteriovenous malformations.

In conclusion, embolotherapy has gone through significant changes since its development in the late 1960s and early 1970s. The indications for these procedures have greatly expanded, as have the agents available for us. Although classifying these agents does not necessarily change the way they are used, it is important to understand how they work and when they should potentially be used. As new agents are introduced and new indications are established, modern interventional radiology will continue to evolve, resulting in the reorganization of the classification schemes used for embolization.

REFERENCES

1. Vaidya S, Tozer KR, Chen J. An overview of embolic agents. *Semin Intervent Radiol.* 2008;25:204–215.
2. Vitek JJ, Smith MJ. The myth of the Brooks method of embolization: a brief history of the endovascular treatment of carotid-cavernous sinus fistula. *J Neurointerv Surg.* 2009;1:108–111.
3. Doppman JL, Di Chiro G, Ommaya A. Obliteration of spinal-cord arteriovenous malformation by percutaneous embolization. *Lancet.* 1968;1:477.
4. Newton TH, Adams JE. Angiographic demonstration and nonsurgical embolization of spinal cord angioma. *Radiology.* 1968;91:873–876.
5. Rosch J, Dotter CT, Brown MJ. Selective arterial embolization. A new method for control of acute gastrointestinal bleeding. *Radiology.* 1972;102:303–306.
6. Rosch J, Keller FS. Historical account: cardiovascular interventional radiology. In: Lanzer P, ed. *Catheter-Based Cardiovascular Interventions: A Knowledge-Based Approach.* Berlin, Germany: Springer-Verlag; 2013:15–26.
7. Speakman TJ. Internal occlusion of a carotid-cavernous fistula. *J Neurosurg.* 1964;21:303–315.
8. Tadavarthy SM, Knight L, Ovitt TW, et al. Therapeutic transcatheter arterial embolization. *Radiology.* 1974;111:13–16.
9. Serbinenko FA. Balloon catheterization and occlusion of major cerebral vessels. *J Neurosurg.* 1974; 41:125–145.
10. Gianturco C, Anderson JH, Wallace S. Mechanical devices for arterial occlusion. *Am J Roentgenol Radium Ther Nucl Med.* 1975;124:428–438.
11. Rose SC. Mechanical devices for arterial occlusion and therapeutic vascular occlusion utilizing steel coil technique: clinical applications. *AJR Am J Roentgenol.* 2009;192:321–324.
12. Guglielmi G. History of the genesis of detachable coils. *J Neurosurg.* 2009;111:1–8.
13. Wang W, Li H, Tam MD, et al. The Amplatzer Vascular Plug: a review of the device and its clinical applications. *Cardiovasc Intervent Radiol.* 2012;35:725–740.
14. Guimaraes M, Wooster M. Onyx (ethylene-vinyl alcohol copolymer) in peripheral applications. *Semin Intervent Radiol.* 2011;28:350–356.
15. Laurent A, Beaujeux R, Wassef M, et al. Trisacryl gelatin microspheres for therapeutic embolization, I: development and in vitro evaluation. *AJNR Am J Neuroradiol.* 1996;17:533–540.
16. Lewis AL, Gonzalez MV, Lloyd AW, et al. DC Bead: in-vitro characterization of a drug-delivery device for transarterial chemoembolization. *J Vasc Interv Radiol.* 2006;17:335–342.
17. Yan ZP, Lin G, Zhao HY, et al. An experimental study and clinical pilot trials on yttrium-90 glass microspheres through the hepatic artery for treatment of primary liver cancer. *Cancer.* 1993;72:3210–3215.
18. Weng L, Rostambeigi N, Zantek ND, et al. An in situ forming biodegradable hydrogel-based embolic agent for interventional therapies. *Acta Biomater.* 2013;9:8182–8191.
19. Owen RJ, Nation PN, Polakowski R, et al. A preclinical study of the safety and efficacy of Occlusin™ 500 artificial embolization device in sheep. *Cardiovasc Intervent Radiol.* 2012;35:636–644.
20. Davidson GS, Terbrugge KG. Histopathologic long-term follow-up after embolization with polyvinyl alcohol particles. *Am J Neuroradiol.* 1995;16:843–846.
21. Germano IM, Davis RL, Wilson CB, et al. Histopathological follow-up study of 66 cerebral arteriovenous malformations after therapeutic embolization with polyvinyl alcohol. *J Neurosurg.* 1992;76:607–614.
22. Tomashefski JF, Cohen AM, Doershuk CF. Long-term histopathological follow-up of bronchial arteries after therapeutic embolization with polyvinyl alcohol (Ivalon) in patients with cystic fibrosis. *Hum Pathol.* 1988;19:555–561.
23. Link DP, Strandberg JD, Virmani R, et al. Histopathologic appearance of arterial occlusions with hydrogel and polyvinyl alcohol embolic material in domestic swine. *J Vasc Interv Radiol.* 1996;7:897–905.
24. Siskin GP, Englander M, Stainken BF, et al. Embolic agents used for uterine fibroid embolization. *AJR Am J Roentgenol.* 2000;175:767–773.
25. Abada HT, Golzarian J. Gelatin sponge particles: handling characteristics for endovascular use. *Tech Vasc Interv Radiol.* 2007;10:257–260.
26. Light RU, Prentice HR. Surgical investigation of new absorbable sponge derived from gelatin for use in hemostasis. *J Neurosurg.* 1945;2:435–455.

27. Barth KH, Strandberg JD, White RI. Long-term follow-up of transcatheter embolization with autologous clot, oxycel, and gelfoam in domestic swine. *Invest Radiol.* 1977;12: 273–280.
28. Gold RE, Grace DM. Gelfoam embolization of the left gastric artery for bleeding ulcer: experimental considerations. *Radiology.* 1975;116:575–580.
29. Jander HP, Russinovich NA. Transcatheter gelfoam embolization in abdominal, retroperitoneal, and pelvic hemorrhage. *Radiology.* 1980;136:337–344.
30. Tabata Y, Ikada Y. Synthesis of gelatin microspheres containing interferon. *Pharm Res.* 1989;6:422–427.
31. Maeda N, Verret V, Eng LM, et al. Targeting and recanalization after embolization with calibrated resorbable microspheres versus hand-cut gelatin sponge particles in a porcine kidney model. *J Vasc Interv Radiol.* 2013;24:1391–1398.
32. Lubarsky M, Ray CE, Funaki B. Embolization agents—which one should be used when? Part 1: large-vessel embolization. *Semin Intervent Radiol.* 2009;26:352–357.
33. Lubarsky M, Ray CE, Funaki B. Embolization agents—which one should be used when? Part 2: small-vessel embolization. *Semin Intervent Radiol.* 2010;27:99–194.
34. Laurent A. Microspheres and nonspherical particles for embolization. *Tech Vasc Interv Radiol.* 2007;10:248–256.
35. Weng L, Rusten M, Talaie R, et al. Calibrated bioresorbable microspheres: a preliminary study on the level of occlusion and arterial distribution in a rabbit kidney model. *J Vasc Interv Radiol.* 2013;24:1567–1575.

Section B Coils and Plugs

2

Pushable Coils

Keigo Osuga

Pushable coils have been widely used for mechanical occlusion of peripheral and visceral vessels because they are relatively inexpensive, easily available, and simple to handle. Since the original stainless steel coils were developed in the mid-1970s,[1] refinements have been made in the materials and designs used for pushable coils, including the recent addition of hydrogel coating technology.[2] Similarly, detachable microcoils, although they are expensive, have been also increasingly indicated in peripheral vessels because they can be repositioned and offer more precise coil deployment. However, pushable coils still remain the standard tool for indications requiring mechanical embolic agents and can save both cost and procedure time.

DEVICE DESCRIPTION

Pushable fibered coils are composed of metallic springs with inert synthetic fibers, such as polyester or nylon, attached to the spring to induce thrombosis around the coil. Pushable coils are supplied in a straight cartridge and are typically loaded into the catheter using a guidewire or the provided mandrel. The loop sizes, lengths, thickness, and configurations vary among pushable coil designs (Fig. 2.1). Two major options are 0.035-in coils for delivery through 4-Fr to 5-Fr catheters and 0.018-in microcoils for delivery through microcatheters for more selective embolization.[3] Platinum coils are softer and more radiopaque than stainless steel or Inconel alloy coils. Because stainless steel is responsible for severe local artifacts on magnetic resonance (MR) imaging, MR conditional coils made of platinum and Inconel alloy are currently preferred. Long pushable platinum coils or microcoils with an extended lengths are pliable and pack easily into a dense coil mass.[4] Most recently, hydrogel-coated pushable coils (AZUR Pushable 35 and 18; Terumo Medical Corporation, Somerset, New Jersey) have become available, and they have the advantage of greater filling volume, independent of thrombus formation.[2]

TECHNIQUE

As a rule, the coil delivery process should be carefully monitored under fluoroscopy. The coil should be appropriately sized according to the vessel size and anatomy. The first coil should be approximately 20% larger in size than the vessel diameter to minimize the risk of coil migration. The delivery catheter should be accurately positioned within the target vessel. The coaxial technique, using a guide catheter and a coaxial delivery catheter, gives stability and control for coil deployment. A standard catheter can also serve as a guide catheter to deploy microcoils through a microcatheter. There are two methods for delivery of pushable coils. The first method is the "push" technique, in which the coil is pushed by a floppy guidewire or designated pusher wire. The other method is the "flush" technique, in which the coil is forced out of the catheter by saline flush. Although this technique can speed up the delivery process, it should be avoided when precise coil placement is critical and when coil dislodgement is a concern, especially for the first or last coil.

Clinical Application

Pushable coils are mechanical embolic agents used both in arteries and veins for various indications: to control

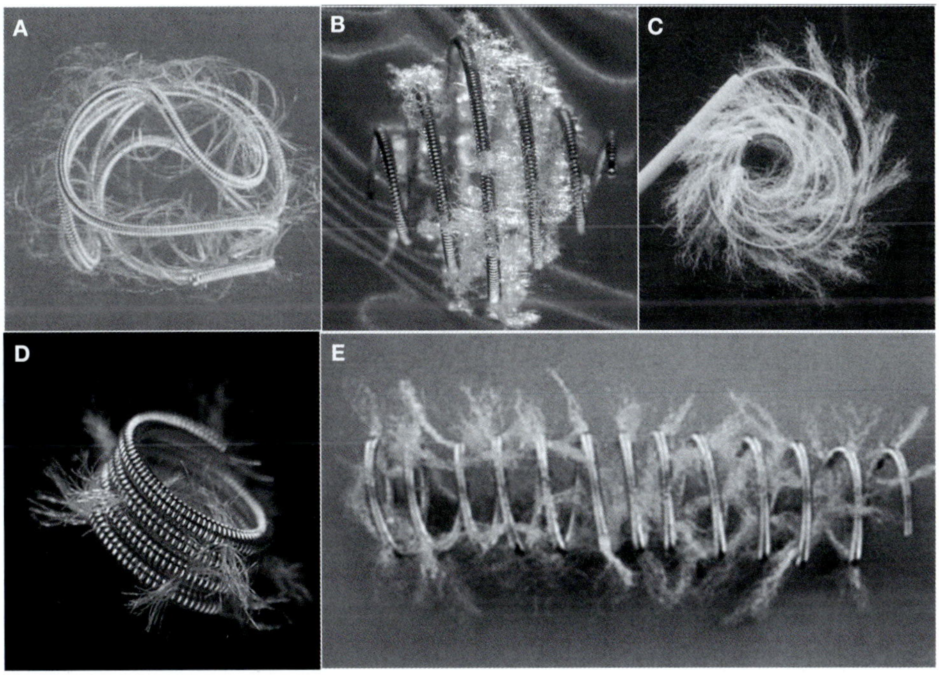

Figure 2.1 Examples of pushable fibered microcoils: Trufill (**A**; courtesy of Codman & Shurtleff, Raynham, Massachusetts); VortX-18 Diamond (**B**; courtesy of Boston Scientific Corporation, Natick, Massachusetts.); and Tornado **(C)**, Hilal **(D)**, and MicroNester (**E**; all courtesy of Cook Medical, Inc., Bloomington, Indiana).

bleeding; to occlude vascular lesions such as aneurysms, varices, and arteriovenous fistulas (AVFs); and to redistribute blood flow to protect nontarget vessels. The details for each indication will be described in later chapters. In general, to occlude a terminal artery that is unlikely to have associated collateral circulation, coils are simply pushed out at, or just before, the site to be occluded. In a larger vessel, proximal coil occlusion may allow persistent flow distal to the site of occlusion via collaterals but at a lower pressure than before embolization. For example, proximal splenic artery embolization is an accepted technique in the setting of traumatic splenic injury to control bleeding. If significant retrograde filling of an embolized vessel(s) is likely via collaterals, the sandwich technique is effective; that is, coils should be placed both proximal and distal to arterial pathology such as a wide-necked aneurysm or pseudoaneurysm (Fig. 2.2). Proximal coil embolization is not effective for arteriovenous malformations (AVMs), as it not only results in persistent flow to the nidus of the AVM via collaterals but also sacrifices the main arterial access for subsequent interventions. For pulmonary AVMs, pushable coils are often used to occlude the distal feeding artery as close to the venous sac as possible.[5] Finally, for the purpose of protective embolization, the right gastric and gastroduodenal arteries are often occluded with coils before liver-directed therapy such as arterial infusion chemotherapy or radioembolization for liver tumors.[2]

Potential Complications

Technical failures and complications can occur during or after coil embolization, although few are specific to pushable coils. First, the coil thickness, lumen of the delivery catheter, and size of the pusher wire should be properly matched, or else the coil can become stuck inside the catheter. Catheters with a side hole should not be used for delivery because the coil can get caught in the side hole. Sizing coils is important because inappropriately sized coils may migrate distally into nontarget vessels if too small or deployed in a straight, poorly controlled manner if too large. Coils can potentially migrate upon catheter removal if the proximal end of the coil remains inside the catheter. Reversal of blood flow can also cause migration of a short straight coil placed in an arterial arcade. Retrieval devices such as a loop snare and basket should be always available to retrieve migrated coils. Rarely, coils can cause vessel wall rupture when the coil is oversized or if the vessel wall is very fragile due to severe inflammation near a pseudoaneurysm. Late recanalization can occur through the coils when the target vessel is inadequately packed or if the patient is coagulopathic. Clinically, ischemic adverse events can occur as a result of intended or nontarget embolization. When adequate perfusion distal to the site of occlusion does not remain via collaterals, organ infarction may occur in the corresponding territory, such as the kidney and lower intestinal tracts.[6]

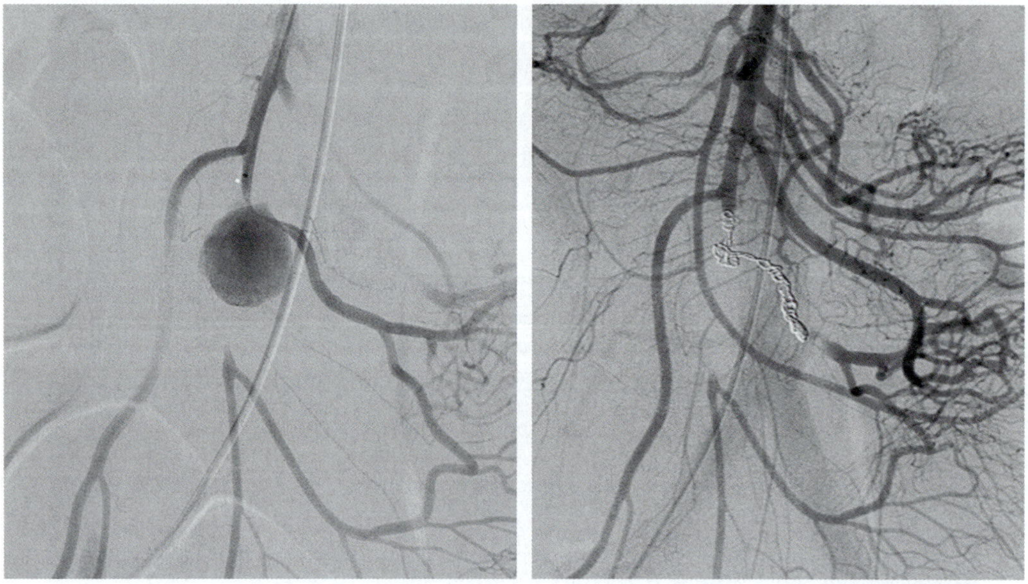

A B

Figure 2.2 **A:** Diagnostic superior mesenteric angiogram demonstrating a 15-mm pseudoaneurysm in the ileal artery, which resulted from infectious endocarditis. **B:** Platinum-fibered microcoils 0.018 in (3 to 4 mm Tornado; Cook Medical, Inc., Bloomington, Indiana) were deployed through a microcatheter from distal to proximal to the pseudoaneurysm (sandwich technique). After embolization, the pseudoaneurysm was excluded with adequate collateral flow distal to the site of occlusion.

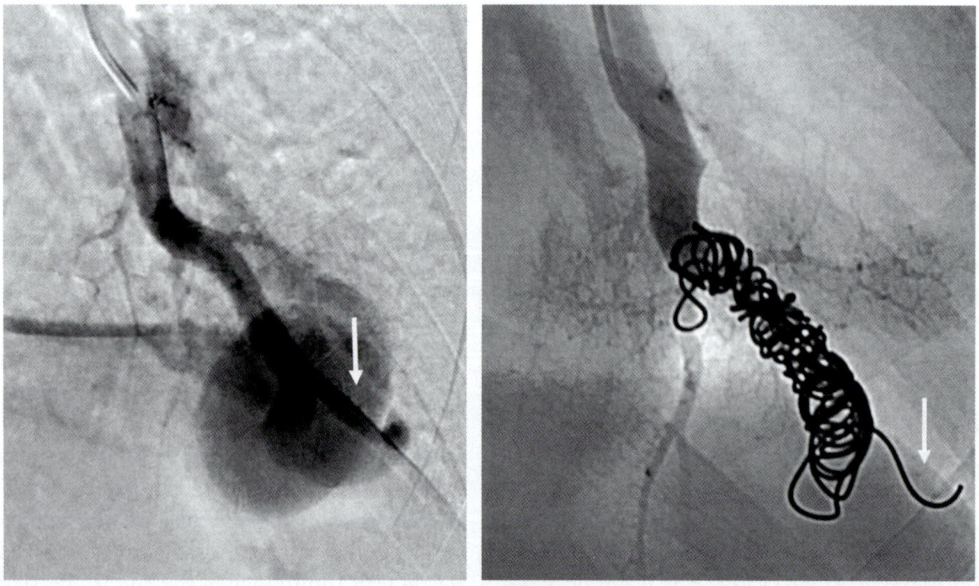

A B

Figure 2.3 **A:** Left pulmonary angiogram demonstrating a simple AVM in the left lower lobe. The feeding vessel bifurcates before entering the venous sac. The smaller branch (*arrow*) was selected for anchoring the first coil. **B:** After embolization of the feeding vessels to the left lower lobe AVM. A 6-Fr guide catheter was placed in the segmental artery, and a 4-Fr coaxial catheter was selectively advanced into the anchor branch. Once the initial 2 cm of the first 0.035-in long pushable coil (8 mm × 14 cm Nester; Cook Medical, Inc., Bloomington, Indiana) was placed in the anchor branch (*arrow*), the 4-Fr catheter was withdrawn to the main feeding artery to deploy the rest of the coil. Subsequently, four 0.035-in long pushable coils (6 to 4 mm × 14 cm Nester) were tightly packed to achieve cross-sectional occlusion (anchor technique).

TIPS AND TRICKS

- It is critical to find suitable anatomy and adequate vessel length for safe coil deployment.
- The catheter chosen for coil delivery is as important as the coils selected for embolization. A coaxial technique helps to control coil delivery and prevent coil elongation.
- Adjunctive techniques may be necessary to prevent coil migration, especially in a large high-flow vessel. If there is a side branch close to the target vessel, the initial part of the first coil can be anchored into the side branch and then deployed in the target vessel as the delivery catheter is withdrawn[7] (Fig. 2.3). When there is no suitable anchor branch, oversized high-radial force coils can be initially deployed to provide a scaffold for subsequent softer platinum coils (scaffold technique).[7]
- Proximal balloon occlusion is useful for temporary blood flow arrest that will reduce the risk of coil migration.
- In suitable vessels, Amplatzer Vascular Plugs (St. Jude Medical, Inc., St. Paul, Minnesota) can be deployed initially with coils added proximally to the plug. In this case, the plug will help prevent coil migration.[8]

REFERENCES

1. Gianturco C, Anderson JH, Wallace S. Mechanical devices for arterial occlusion. *Am J Roentgenol Radium Ther Nucl Med.* 1975;124:428–435.
2. Maleux G, Deroose C, Fieuws S, et al. Prospective comparison of hydrogel-coated microcoils versus fibered platinum microcoils in the prophylactic embolization of the gastroduodenal artery before yttrium-90 radioembolization. *J Vasc Interv Radiol.* 2013;24:797–803.
3. Morse SS, Clark RA, Puffenbarger A. Platinum microcoils for therapeutic embolization: nonneuroradiologic applications. *AJR Am J Roentgenol.* 1990;155:401–403.
4. Osuga K, White RI Jr. Micronester: a new pushable fibered microcoil for embolotherapy. *Cardiovasc Intervent Radiol.* 2003;26:554–556.
5. Pollak JS, White RI Jr. Distal cross-sectional occlusion is the "key" to treating pulmonary arteriovenous malformations. *J Vasc Interv Radiol.* 2012;23:1578–1580.
6. Funaki B, Kostelic JK, Lorenz J, et al. Superselective microcoil embolization of colonic hemorrhage. *AJR Am J Roentgenol.* 2001;177:829–836.
7. White RI Jr, Pollak JS. Controlled delivery of pushable fibered coils for large vessel embolotherapy. In: Golzarian J, Sun S, Sharafuddin MJ, eds. *Vascular Embolotherapy. A Comprehensive Approach.* Vol 1. New York, NY: Springer; 2006:35–42.
8. Trerotola SO, Pyeritz RE. PAVM embolization: an update. *AJR Am J Roentgenol.* 2010;195:837–845.

3

Detachable Coils

Craig R. Greben • Eric J. Gandras • Jason J. Naidich

Guido Guglielmi, the father of the detachable coil, stated that the development of this device was the result of the merging of three arts: electronics, neurosurgery, and interventional neuroradiology.[1] The Guglielmi detachable coil (GDC) was invented in 1990 and revolutionized the field of neurointerventional radiology by allowing endovascular procedures to replace neurosurgical treatment in several cases over time. The ability to manipulate the coil and reposition it precisely into small, delicate aneurysms via an endovascular approach before deployment confers a significant advantage over pushable coils, which behave less predictably. The ability to pack coils densely into an aneurysm and successfully exclude it from the circulation represented a paradigm shift in the field of neurosurgery that has changed the way these lesions are managed.[2]

The success of the detachable coil in the field of neurointerventions led to the spread and cross-fertilization of this technology into the domain of peripheral embolization. Although the GDC was invented in 1990 and was used largely in the intracranial circulation, reports of its use for extracranial pathologies appeared shortly thereafter.[3]

GDCs detach from their delivery wire following the administration of an electric current. As a result, they can be fully pushed out of their delivery catheter but retracted completely if their position is unsatisfactory. In recent years, newer coil designs with different detachment mechanisms have been developed (Fig. 3.1). For example, the Interlock detachable coil (IDC) (Interlock Fibered IDC Occlusion System; Boston Scientific Corporation, Natick, Massachusetts) appeared on the market in the 1990s, and its early use for peripheral interventions was first described by Reidy and Qureshi[4] in 1996. In contradistinction to the GDC, the IDC detaches through a mechanical release between the interlocking proximal end of the coil and the distal end of the pusher wire. As a result, the IDC can only be retracted if this interlocking domain remains within the delivery catheter. This can limit the precision of deployment and lead to inadvertent embolization requiring retrieval, as outlined by Reidy and Qureshi.[4]

DEVICE DESCRIPTION

The success of the GDC drove the development of other types of detachable coils, all of which remain attached to a wire until a release mechanism is used to achieve deployment. Electrical, mechanical, and hydraulic detachment mechanisms have all been used. This precise detachment allows for manipulation until a satisfactory position is achieved and minimizes the risk of migration or nontarget embolization. The physical properties that have been considered important in coil design include the stiffness and configuration of the device. Most current coil designs include a platinum alloy because it is biologically inert and has an optimal strength and rigidity to allow for conformational changes required for use in packing (Table 3.1). Because of the delicate nature of neurointerventional work, these coils have to be relatively soft to minimize complications. The design and configuration of the coil will determine its softness. These coils are manufactured with a stock wire wrapped around a mandril to produce a secondary structure, which usually has a helical configuration. A tertiary configuration can be constructed into the coil, which can include spherical and complex three-dimensional designs to optimize coil packing.[5] These three-dimensional "framing" coils provide stability to the aneurysm wall. Softer two-dimensional "finishing" or "packing" coils can be placed within the framing coil to obliterate the space within the aneurysm with a safer margin during packing. These coils have historically ranged in size from 0.010 to 0.018 in in diameter and are meant to be deployed through a microcatheter, which serves to constrain the coil before deployment.

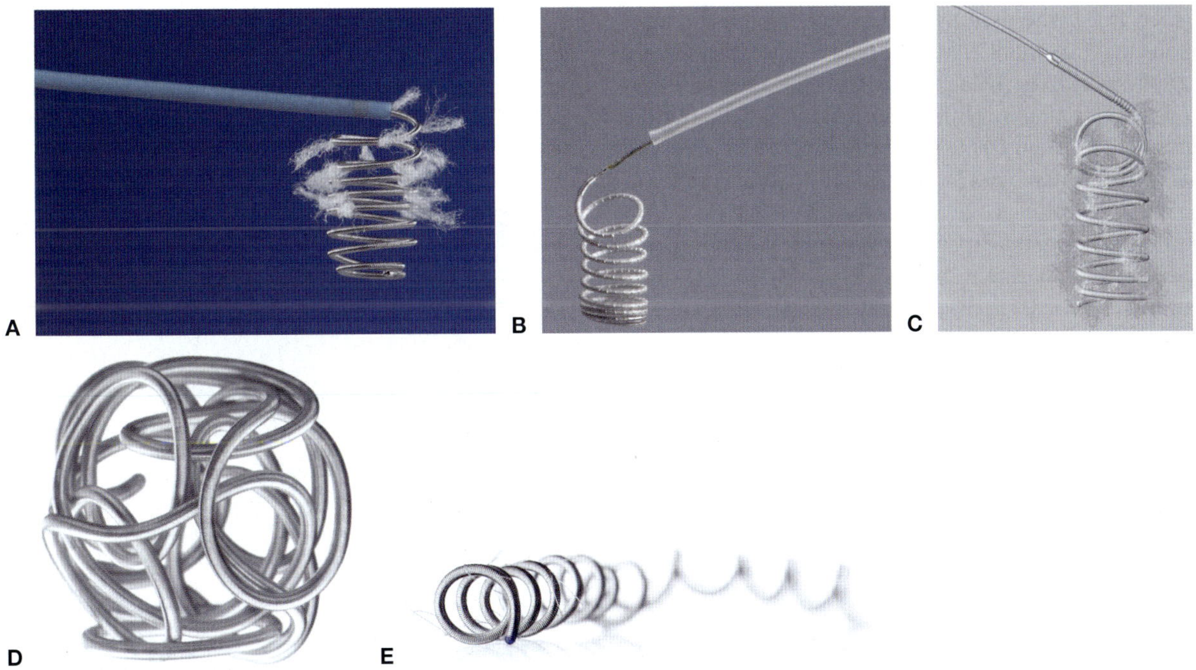

Figure 3.1 Currently available detachable coils. **A:** Interlock Fibered IDC Occlusion System (Boston Scientific Corporation, Natick, Massachusetts). **B:** AZUR Peripheral HydroCoil Embolization System (Terumo Medical Corporation, Somerset, New Jersey). **C:** Retracta Detachable Embolization Coil (Cook Medical, Inc., Bloomington, Indiana). **D:** Ruby Coil (Penumbra, Inc., Alameda, California). **E:** Axium Detachable Coil System (Covidien, Irvine, California).

As with pushable coils, detachable coils work by encouraging stasis of flow and inducing thrombosis. Bare coils can fulfill this role, but blood can continue to flow through them, especially in high-flow regions or in the setting of coagulopathy. This is particularly true if the coils are loosely packed.[6] Fibered coils have been developed to promote thrombosis, and the IDC is an example of this category of device. Other materials used to coat coils and promote thrombosis include polyglycolic acid (PGA) and nylon. Bioactive coils containing polylactic acid (PLA) have been developed to promote endothelialization and wound healing over the coil neck and mass.[7] A further development in coil design has been the coating of platinum coils with a hydrogel polymer. These coils increase the density of packing by expanding in diameter once the gel is exposed to an ionic solution such as blood. The coils can swell between four and seven times the original diameter and thus increase packing density for the same length of coil deployed. This, theoretically, can lead to fewer coils required to exclude aneurysms, but this advantage is difficult to quantify in clinical practice.[7,8] These hydrogel coils were first employed for peripheral interventions

Table 3.1 Detachable Coils Available for Peripheral Embolization

Peripheral Detachable Coils Manufacturer	Name	Size	Fibered	Bioactive Coating	Detachment Mechanism
Terumo/MicroVention	AZUR HydroCoil	0.018 in 0.035 in	No	Yes Hydrogel	Electrical
Terumo/MicroVention	AZUR Framing	0.018 in	No	No	Electrical
Boston Scientific	Interlock (IDC)	0.018 in 0.035 in	Yes	No	Mechanical
Covidien	Axium Covidien	0.0115–0.0145 in 0.0165–0.021 in.	No Yes	No No	Mechanical Mechanical
Penumbra	Ruby	0.020 in	No	No	Mechanical
Cook	Retracta	0.035 in	Yes	No	Mechanical

by Greben et al.[9] who used them to exclude pulmonary arteriovenous malformations (AVMs) in 2005. The development of a peripheral hydrogel detachable coil (AZUR Peripheral HydroCoil Embolization System; Terumo Medical Corporation, Somerset, New Jersey) has led to further reports of their use for extracranial pathologies.[10–12] These hydrocoils are predominantly used as finishing coils, as they must be detached within 3 to 5 minutes or else the expanded gel cannot be withdrawn or retracted back into the microcatheter delivery system. A 0.035-in hydrogel coil has been developed as well, which is considerably stiffer than the 0.018-in coils, with a larger volume of hydrogel associated with them. As with any detachable coil, the haptic experience of the stiffness is appreciated greatest at the junction of the coil and the delivery wire, or detachment zone, and this must be considered when attempting to place this segment of the coil into a confined, delicate space to avoid complications such as perforation.

TECHNIQUE

The ability to withdraw and reposition detachable coils before deployment affords a level of precision that may not be reliably achieved with pushable coils. This precision becomes more important in high-flow areas such as renal arteriovenous fistulas or aneurysms, pulmonary AVMs, and visceral aneurysms and pseudoaneurysms when the neck is close to the aorta or visceral branches. Detachable coils allow these challenging lesions to be treated safely while minimizing coil migration or inadvertent thrombosis of the native artery. There is also a risk of reperfusion from collateral circulation if lesions such as fistulas are closed too proximally. Occlusion at the level of the arteriovenous communication is necessary to prevent this from occurring. For larger high-flow fistulas, additional treatment strategies may be necessary such as balloon occlusion or double microcatheter, single guiding catheter technique that facilitates the building of a stable coil mass with the use of detachable coils.[13] These techniques can also be employed in the treatment of wide-necked aneurysms, where detachable coils are safer to use than pushable coils in these challenging lesions. The risk of coil compaction and reperfusion or migration of the entire coil mass into the native vessel can be minimized with the addition of a stent to cage the mass.

CLINICAL APPLICATIONS

In general, detachable coils can be used for any indication where pushable coils are used. They are particularly useful for embolization when the delivery catheters are in tenuous positions or when the risk of coil migration is felt to be particularly high based on the pathology being treated (Figs. 3.2 and 3.3). However, they are significantly more expensive than pushable coils, which means that for more routine indications, the operator must consider the justification of the added cost. The time spent retrieving a migrated coil and the potential morbidity of this complication are intangibles that need to be weighed by the interventionalist. One method we employ to reduce cost is to use a combination of pushable and detachable coils; for the initial and completion coils, we use detachable coils with pushable coils in between. This permits precision during the procedure when the risk of coil migration is greatest.

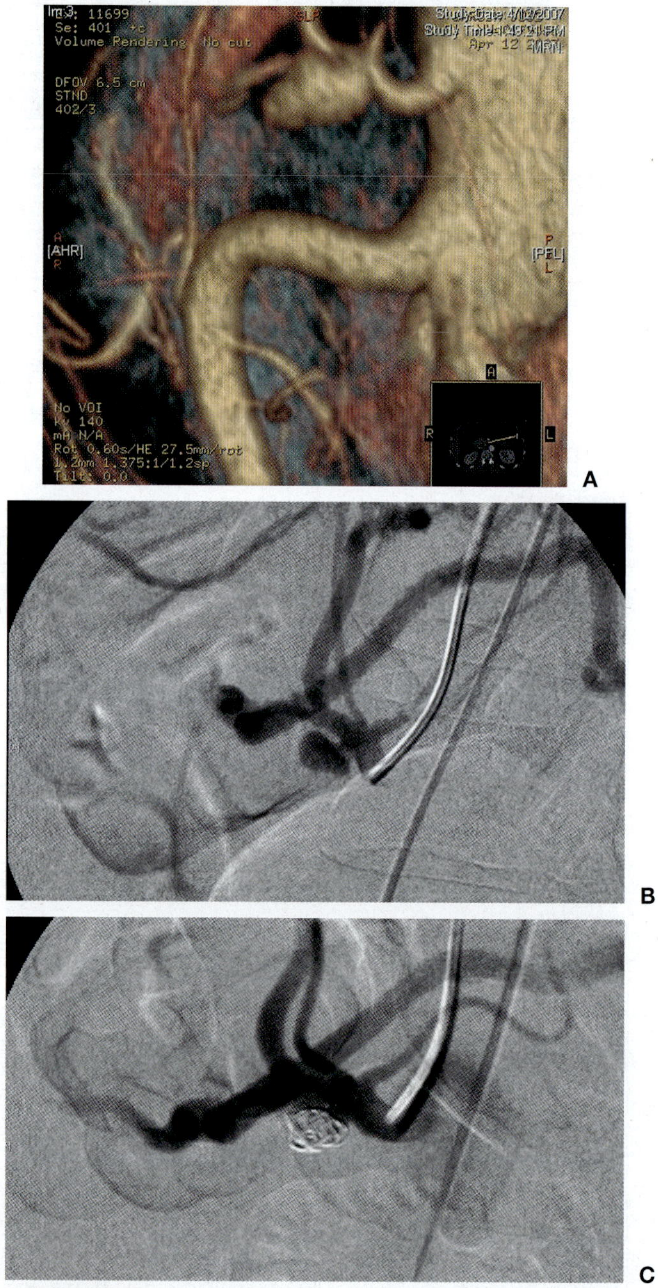

Figure 3.2 Images obtained before and after treatment of a celiac aneurysm in a 41-year-old male patient. **A:** Sagittal image from a computed tomography (CT) angiogram demonstrating an aneurysm arising from the celiac axis. **B:** Diagnostic angiographic image confirming the origin of this aneurysm from the celiac axis. **C:** Single angiographic image after embolization of the aneurysm with detachable coils.

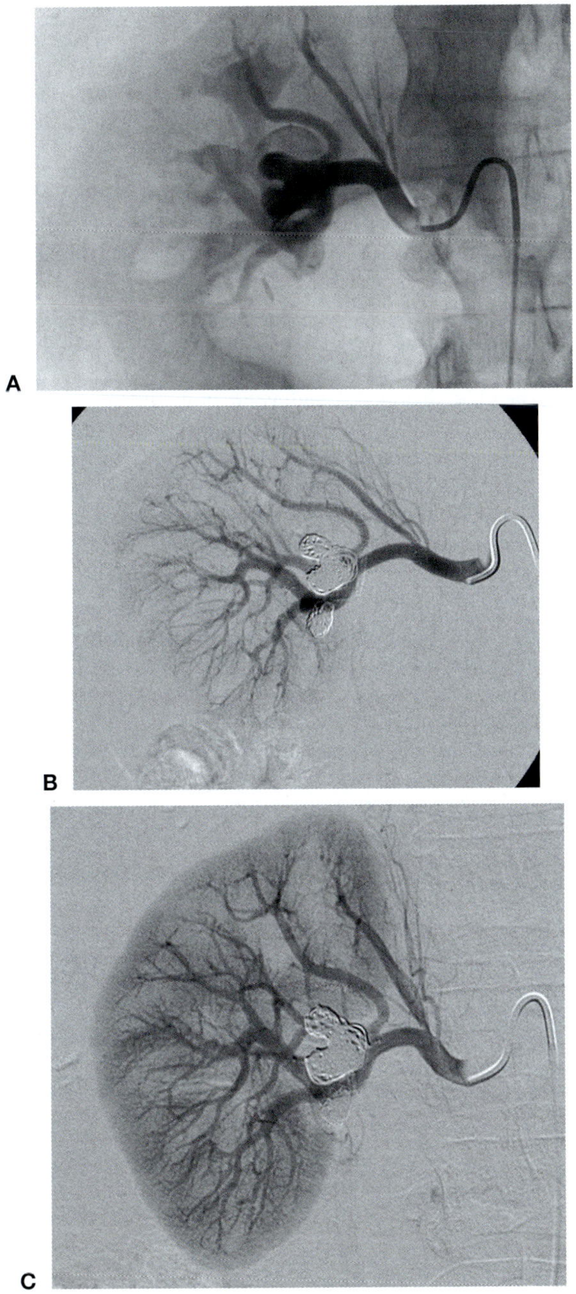

Figure 3.3 Images obtained before and after treatment of renal artery aneurysms in a 46-year-old patient presenting with abdominal pain. **A:** Single angiographic image demonstrating multiple aneurysms arising from several branches of the right renal artery. **B,C:** Early and late-phase image from an angiogram performed after stent-assisted embolization of these renal aneurysms with detachable coils.

POTENTIAL COMPLICATIONS

In addition to the types of complications encountered with pushable coils such as migration, perforation, and thromboembolic events in the native vessel, there are potential complications that are only encountered with the use of detachable coils. Detachable coils can fail to detach or can detach prematurely. Most manufacturers have incorporated a secondary mechanism of detachment in the event that the primary method fails. Prematurely detached coils may still carefully be pushed out of the catheter with the delivery wire, but there is a risk that the wire can wedge astride the coil within the catheter. A stretched coil can pose an extremely challenging situation as the coil can unwind and neither be pushed into the lesion nor withdrawn from the catheter. Snaring of the coil may be attempted, or the use of a balloon or stent to tack the stretched coil to the vessel wall may be considered in this situation. Knotting, interlocking, and fracture of coils can all potentially occur because attempts at repositioning can create excessive forces on the coil, particularly at the detachment zone.[14] These complications can lead to movement of the entire coil mass while it is being created. Fortunately, these complications are rare and can generally be avoided with careful attention to technique.

TIPS AND TRICKS

Peripheral Detachable Coil	Tips and Tricks
AZUR Peripheral HydroCoil Embolization System (Terumo Medical Corporation, Somerset, New Jersey)	Check detachment integrity by inserting pusher wire into handle and noting green light before introducing coil; detach within 3–5 min (AZUR only), otherwise hydrogel may swell too much to permit retrieval; no detachment time limit for framing coil
Interlock Fibered IDC Occlusion System (Boston Scientific Corporation, Natick, Massachusetts)	Interlocking arm mechanism positioned just beyond catheter tip to prevent snaring other coils; not retractable once interlocking arm exits catheter tip
Axium Detachable Coil System (Covidien, Irvine, California)	Very soft coils; minimal catheter kick out at detachment link
Ruby Coil (Penumbra, Inc., Alameda, California)	Long coil lengths and graded softness allow for tight coil packing (from the manufacturer)
Retracta Detachable Embolization Coils (Cook Medical, Inc., Bloomington, Indiana)	Detaches from pusher wire with 8–10 counterclockwise twists; keep detachment juncture zone just inside catheter tip to assure detachment

CONCLUSIONS

The use of detachable coils for extracranial indications has increased over the past several years and should continue to do so as more operators become comfortable with these devices and appreciate the level of safety and precision that they add to patient care. This newer technology can facilitate endovascular treatment of lesions that historically have required open surgery. The limit to more widespread use is cost because detachable coils can be 5 to 10 times more expensive than pushable coils. Future directions may include development of novel materials used to engineer and coat these coils and advances in delivery wire and detachment zone technology.

REFERENCES

1. Guglielmi G. History of the genesis of detachable coils. A review. *J Neurosurg.* 2009;111(1):1–8.
2. Molyneux A, Kerr R, Stratton I, et al; International Subarachnoid Aneurysm Trial (ISAT) Collaborative Group. International Subarachnoid Aneurysm Trial (ISAT) of neurosurgical clipping versus endovascular coiling in 2143 patients with ruptured intracranial aneurysms: a randomized trial. *Lancet.* 2002; 360(9342):1267–1274.
3. Klein GE, Szolar DH, Breinl E, et al. Endovascular treatment of renal artery aneurysms with conventional non-detachable microcoils and Guglielmi detachable coils. *Br J Urol.* 1997; 79(6):852–860.
4. Reidy JF, Qureshi SA. Interlocking detachable platinum coils, a controlled embolization device: early clinical experience. *Cardiovasc Intervent Radiol.* 1996;19(2):85–90.
5. White JB, Ken CGM, Cloft HJ, et al. Coils in a nutshell: a review of coil physical properties. *AJNR Am J Neuroradiol.* 2008;29(7):1242–1246.
6. Milic A, Chan RP, Cohen JH, et al. Reperfusion of pulmonary arteriovenous malformations after embolotherapy. *J Vasc Interv Radiol.* 2005;16(12):1675–1683.
7. Hui FK, Fiorella D, Masaryk TJ, et al. A history of detachable coils: 1987-2012. *J Neurointerv Surg.* 2014;6(2):134–138.
8. White PM, Lewis SC, Gholkar A, et al; for the HELPS Trial Collaborators. Hydrogel-coated versus bare platinum coils for the endovascular treatment of intracranial aneurysm (HELPS): a randomized controlled trial. *Lancet.* 2011; 377(9778):1655–1662.
9. Greben CR, Setton A, Gandras EJ, et al. The use of hydrogel detachable coils in the treatment of pulmonary fistulas. Presented at: SIR Annual Meeting; March 2006; Toronto, Canada.
10. Bui JT, West DL, Pai R, et al. Use of a hydrogel-coated self-expandable coil to salvage a failed transcatheter embolization of a mesenteric hemorrhage. *Cardiovasc Intervent Radiol.* 2006; 29(6):1121–1124.
11. Greben CR, Axelrod DJ, Charles H, et al. Treatment of post-traumatic aortic pseudoaneurysms using detachable hydrogel-coated coils. *J Trauma.* 2009;66(6):1735–1738.
12. Nambiar AP, Bozlar U, Angle JF, et al. Initial clinical experience with biopolymer-coated detachable coils (HydroCoil) in peripheral embolization procedures. *J Vasc Interv Radiol.* 2008; 19(7):995–1001.
13. Greben CR, Setton A, Putterman D, et al. Double microcatheter single vascular access embolization technique for complex peripheral vascular pathology. *Vasc Endovascular Surg.* 2010; 44(3):217–222.
14. Eddleman CS, Welch BG, Vance AZ, et al. Endovascular coils: properties, technical complications and salvage techniques. *J Neurointerv Surg.* 2013;5(2):104–109.

4

Vascular Plugs

Sang Joon Park

Percutaneous embolization has become a common procedure to treat acute bleeding and vascular abnormalities. A permanent occlusion can be created with an embolization procedure with various embolic materials, including polyvinyl alcohol (PVA) particles, embolic microspheres, glue, coils, and occlusion balloons; coils are the most commonly used device.[1] The major disadvantages of coils are that multiple coils are often required for the complete occlusion of the targeted vessel and that accurate placement can be challenging depending on the vessel size and blood flow rate. Moreover, the chance of coil migration is always high when embolizing large feeding vessels with a high flow rate. To overcome this shortcoming of coils, the Amplatzer Vascular Plug (AVP; St. Jude Medical, Inc., St. Paul, Minnesota) was introduced and approved by the U.S. Food and Drug Administration (FDA) in 2004 for peripheral embolization. The first report on the successful use of the AVP was published by Hill et al.[2] in December 2004. Since then, numerous reports have been published in various medical journals. The device has shown an excellent technical success rate for an expanding number of indications,[3] and no significant contraindication to embolization using this device has been recognized.[4] As described in Chapter 1, new plugs such as the Medusa Vascular Plug (EndoShape Inc., Boulder, Colorado) and the MVP Micro Vascular Plug System (Reverse Medical Corporation, Irvine, California) have been recently introduced. This chapter will focus on use of the AVP given the extensive experience with this device.

DEVICE DESCRIPTION

The original AVP was derived from the Amplatzer septal occluder and the Amplatzer duct occluder. The AVPs consist of a self-expanding cylindrical nitinol mesh that can be deployed both rapidly and accurately. The elasticity of the nitinol allows the device to become firmly anchored to the vessel wall due to its outward radial force.[5] There are radiopaque platinum marker bands at both ends for high visibility under fluoroscopy. The plug is attached to a delivery wire with a stainless steel screw on one of the platinum marker bands.[6] One significant advantage of the AVP as an embolic device is that it can be repositioned before final release, which is performed by rotating the delivery wire.

After the introduction of the first AVP, the AVP family has grown to four types: AVP I, AVP II, AVP III, and AVP IV (Fig. 4.1). Each type has a unique design and features making it suitable for different vascular anatomies, hemodynamics, and clinical situations. Subsequently, a newer generation does not mean that it can replace the older type. In appearance, the AVP I has a single lobe, the AVP II has three lobes, and the AVP III and IV have two lobes. In addition, the AVP I and IV have single-layered braids, whereas the AVP II and III have a multiple-layered design, except for the 3-mm AVP II. The characteristics of the AVPs are described in Table 4.1.

The AVP I was the first product of the AVP family. Most of the published case reports have been performed with this device.[7] The diameters of the AVP I range from 4 to 16 mm with increases in 2-mm increments. This device is well suited for landing zones that are limited in length.[8]

The AVP II is the second-generation product in the AVP family; it received FDA approval in 2007. It has been used in various clinical settings,[9–13] but no randomized trials comparing the AVP II with well-established embolization devices has been reported to date. This device is multiple layered and made of more densely woven nitinol mesh than the AVP I, except for the 3-mm device, which is single layered. It consists of three segments with a central lobe and two discs on each side of the lobe. Compared to the AVP I, the AVP II exerts greater radial force, over four axes, and may thus be expected to migrate less and cause more rapid occlusion.[14]

The AVP III has a unique, oblong, cross-sectional shape and multiple nitinol mesh layers. It also has rims that extended

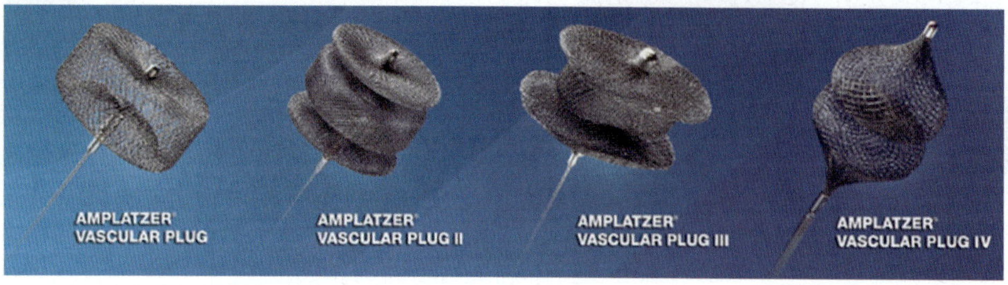

Figure 4.1 Four generations of the AVP family. (Courtesy of St. Jude Medical, Inc., St. Paul, Minnesota.)

beyond the device body, which may enhance stability. There are only few reports on the clinical application of this device.[15] This device received CE mark approval of Europe in 2008.

The AVP IV has a double-cone shape and is mounted on a fixed-core wire guide with a 20-cm floppy distal tip. Unlike other AVPs, it can be delivered through a 4-Fr or 5-Fr diagnostic catheter with a 0.038-in inner lumen without the need to exchange for a sheath or a guiding catheter. This feature enables this device to be used in smaller and tortuous vessels in the arterial or venous vasculature.[16,17] This is the biggest advantage of this device over other generations of the AVPs. Like other plugs, the AVP IV can be recaptured and repositioned if necessary. It received CE mark approval in 2009 for Europe and was cleared by the FDA in 2012.

TECHNIQUE

When treating vascular pathology with the AVP, the size of the target vessel and the length of the landing zone for the device must be determined to choose the most appropriate AVP for use. It is currently suggested that the AVP be oversized by 30% to 50% relative to the diameter of the target vessel. The elasticity of nitinol allows the plug to fully expand within the vessel for adequate wall apposition.

Once the device has been selected, the initial consideration for its placement is the determination regarding what catheter will be used to deliver the plug to the site of deployment. A 4-Fr sheath or 5-Fr guiding catheter is required for the AVP I and AVP II, whereas a 4-Fr sheath or 6-Fr guiding catheter is required for the AVP III. Therefore, a relatively straight segment of target vessel with a relatively constant diameter is needed for deployment for the AVP I, AVP II, and AVP III.[3]

The newest device, the AVP IV, can be delivered through a 4-Fr or 5-Fr diagnostic catheter without an additional sheath or guiding catheter. The combination of low profile and flexible delivery wire tip makes it possible for this device to be used in smaller vessels such as the splenic, lumbar, and gluteal arteries.[16] The size of this device is limited, covering vessels with diameters of 2.6 to 6.2 mm, providing the requirement for at least 30% oversizing.

The delivery catheter is not the only part of the system that needs to be advanced to the anticipated site of deployment. The plug and delivery wire must be advanced through the delivery catheter or sheath, and this can be problematic in some cases. The delivery wire is stiff and may be difficult to advance through the delivery catheter. This is especially the case when the target vessels are tortuous. To overcome the tortuosity of the artery, two methods can be used. One is to use a guiding catheter within the sheath to increase the stability and ease of deployment according to Zhu et al.,[18] and the other is the use of a larger introducing system to gain access to the landing zone.[19]

When the desired position of the device is reached, the device can be easily deployed by rotating the cable counterclockwise to complete implantation. Subsequently, repositioning the device is possible before release. Moreover, a test injection of contrast medium is possible through the delivery catheter to verify the location of the device before deployment.[5]

Table 4.1 Characteristics of the Amplatzer Vascular Plug Family

AVP Type	Device Size (mm)	Landing Zone	Occlusion Time	Radial Force	Delivery Method	Flow Type
AVP I	4–18	Shortest	Fast	High	Guide catheter Sheath	Low to medium
AVP II	3–22	Medium or long	Faster	High	Guide catheter Sheath	Medium to high
AVP III	2.8–8.4	Long	Fastest	Highest	Guide catheter Sheath	High
AVP IV	4–8	Short	Faster	Medium to high	Diagnostic catheter	Low to medium

AVP, Amplatzer Vascular Plug.

CLINICAL APPLICATIONS

The AVP has been used successfully for various indications suitable for the use of a mechanical embolic agent. Often, the limiting factors in determining whether a plug would be appropriate to use include the size of the target vessel, the tortuosity of the vessels leading to the site targeted for occlusion, the length of the landing zone, and the nature of the pathology being treated.

Several arterial indications for the AVP have been described. These devices have been used successfully in the internal iliac artery for endoleak prevention before endovascular aneurysm repair (EVAR)[20] as well as to treat pseudoaneurysms.[21] They have also been used successfully for embolization of the gastroduodenal artery before radioembolization with yttrium 90 microspheres. Both the AVP II and IV have been used successfully for this indication.[14,22,23] Additional indications include embolization of the proximal splenic artery as treatment for portal hypertension and splenic artery syndrome after orthotopic liver transplantation,[18] splenic artery aneurysms,[24] and splenic trauma to avoid splenectomy.[25,26]

The use of the AVPs in the venous circulation has also been reported. These devices have been used successfully in combination with coils and gelatin sponge for portal vein embolization.[27,28] In addition, these plugs have been used for the treatment of gonadal vein embolization for varicoceles and pelvic congestion syndrome either alone or in combination with coils or liquid embolic agents.[29,30]

These devices essentially began in the cardiac setting, treating conditions such as a patent ductus arteriosus (PDA) and patent ductus venosus (PDV).[7] Now, other congenital arteriovenous communication can often be effectively treated with these plugs. For example, pulmonary arteriovenous malformations can be treated with the AVP (Fig. 4.2), which can be advantageous due to the low risk of migration into the pulmonary venous outflow after deployment.[19,31-33] Other potential applications in this area include splenorenal shunts,[34] renal arteriovenous fistulae,[35] mesocaval shunts,[36] and the rerouting of a scimitar vein to the left atrium.[37] Acquired lesions can also be treated with the AVP. This includes the treatment of hemodialysis arteriovenous fistulae that require closure for steal syndrome or enlarging aneurysms[38] as well as for either occlusion of a transjugular intrahepatic portosystemic shunt (TIPS)

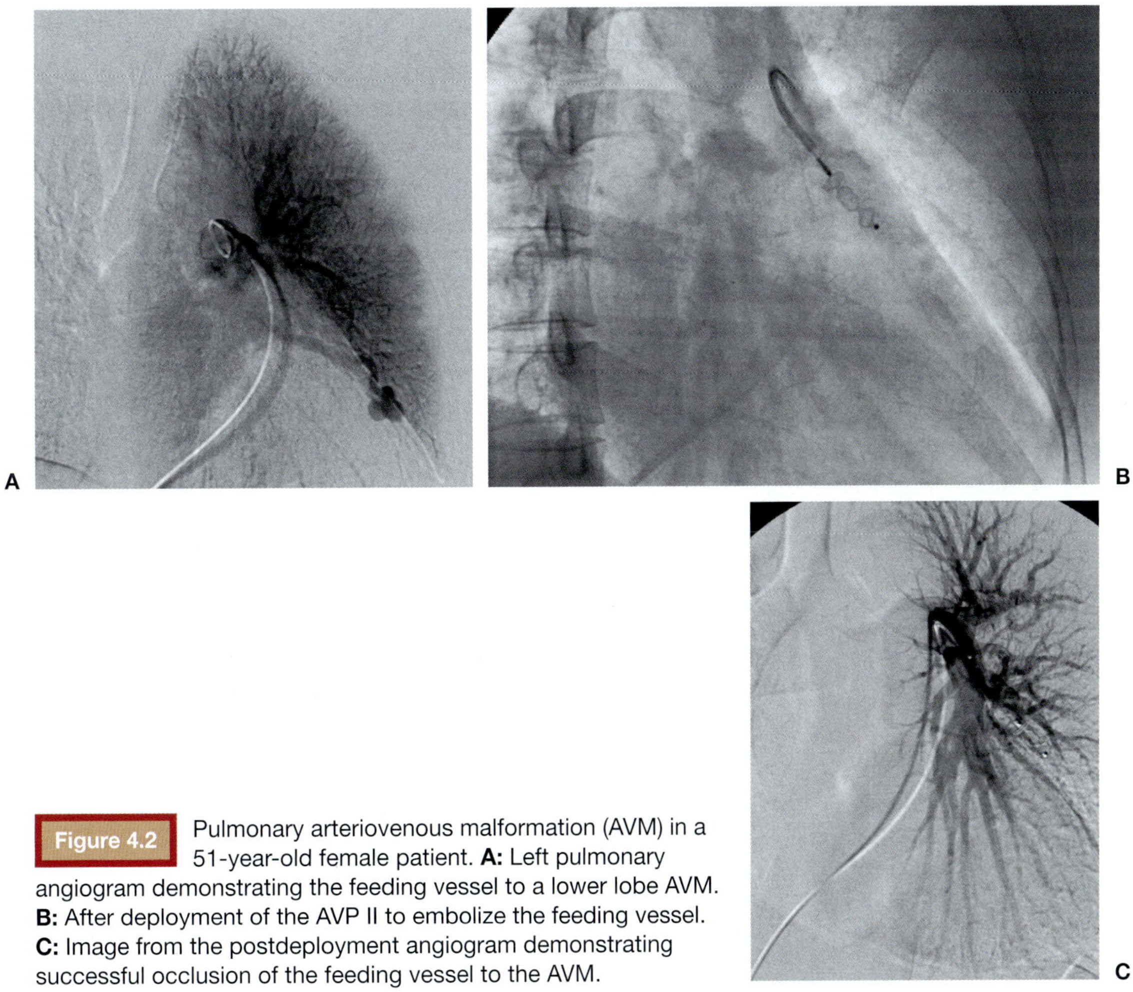

Figure 4.2 Pulmonary arteriovenous malformation (AVM) in a 51-year-old female patient. **A:** Left pulmonary angiogram demonstrating the feeding vessel to a lower lobe AVM. **B:** After deployment of the AVP II to embolize the feeding vessel. **C:** Image from the postdeployment angiogram demonstrating successful occlusion of the feeding vessel to the AVM.

in the setting of refractory postprocedure encephalopathy or for embolization of varices during TIPS creation.[39]

There are also potential nonvascular uses of the AVP that have been reported. These include the closure of bronchopulmonary[40] and esophagopleural[41] fistulae. In addition, the AVP can be used for ureteral occlusion in patients with vesicovaginal, vesicointestinal or ureterointestinal, or uterocutaneous fistulae secondary to pelvic cancers.[42]

POSSIBLE COMPLICATIONS

The AVP has been shown to be a safe and effective embolic; complications associated directly with the AVP are rare. Persistent patency after deployment is one area of concern associated with these plugs. This can be particularly seen after embolization of large-diameter, high-flow vessels in coagulopathic patients. It is important to understand that occlusion takes time after deployment of the AVP. When a rapid occlusion is unnecessary, time can be taken for the vessel to occlude after deployment. However, when embolization is being performed for more urgent indications, a supplemental embolic agent may be required for a more rapid occlusion. In these cases, agents such as coils, gelfoam, glue, and additional AVPs can be used as adjuncts for the complete occlusion. Once occlusion occurs, recanalization is rare due to the space-occupying nature of the AVP, but it can occur in approximately 1% of cases compared to 8% to 15% with coil embolization.[43,44] Migration is also possible[45] but rare due to the radial force seen when the plugs are oversized relative to the size of the target vessel.

TIPS AND TRICKS

- Oversizing of the AVPs at least 30%–50% is crucial.
- AVP I, II, and III require either a sheath or guiding catheter, whereas AVP 4 only requires a standard 0.038-in diagnostic catheter for the deployment. However, be aware of the fact that the maximal diameter of the AVP IV is 8 mm.
- To overcome the tortuosity of the target vessel, the use of a guiding catheter within the sheath can be useful to increase the stability and ease of deployment.

REFERENCES

1. Ferro C, Petrocelli F, Rossi UG, et al. Vascular percutaneous transcatheter embolization with a new device: Amplatzer Vascular Plug. *Radiol Med.* 2007;112:239–251.
2. Hill SL, Hijazi ZM, Hellenbrand WE, et al. Evaluation of the Amplatzer Vascular Plug for embolization of peripheral vascular malformations associated with congenital heart disease. *Catheter Cardiovasc Interv.* 2006;67:113–119.
3. Mangini M, Lagana D, Fontana F, et al. Use of Amplatzer Vascular Plug (AVP) in emergency embolisation: preliminary experience and review of literature. *Emerg Radiol.* 2008;14:153–160.
4. Hijazi ZM. New device for percutaneous closure of aortopulmonary collaterals. *Catheter Cardiovasc Interv.* 2004;63:482–485.
5. Lagana D, Carrafiello G, Mangini, et al. Indications for the use of the Amplatzer Vascular Plug in interventional radiology. *Radiol Med.* 2008;113:707–718.
6. Schwartz M, Glatz AC, Rome JJ, et al. The Amplatzer Vascular Plug and Amplatzer Vascular Plug II for vascular occlusion procedures in 50 patients with congenital cardiovascular disease. *Catheter Cardiovasc Interv.* 2010;76:411–417.
7. Wang W, Li H, Tam MD, et al. The Amplatzer Vascular Plug: a review of the device and its clinical applications. *Cardiovasc Intervent Radiol.* 2012;35:725–740.
8. Farra H, Balzer DT. Transcatheter occlusion of a large pulmonary arteriovenous malformation using the Amplatzer Vascular Plug. *Pediatr Cardiol.* 2005;26:683–685.
9. Tabori NE, Love BA. Transcatheter occlusion of pulmonary arteriovenous malformation using the Amplatzer Vascular Plug II. *Catheter Cardiovasc Interv.* 2008;71:940–943.
10. Tuite DJ, Kessel DO, Nicholson AA, et al. Initial clinical experience using the Amplatzer Vascular Plug. *Cardiovasc Intervent Radiol.* 2007;30:650–654.
11. Taneja M, Lath N, Soo TB, et al. Renal artery stump to inferior vena cava fistula: unusual clinical presentation and transcatheter embolization with the Amplatzer Vascular Plug. *Cardiovasc Intervent Radio*l. 2008;31(suppl 2):S92–S95.
12. Ringe KI, Weidemann J, Rosenthal H, et al. Transhepatic preoperative portal vein embolization using the Amplatzer Vascular Plug: report of four cases. *Cardiovasc Intervent Radiol.* 2007;30:1245–1247.
13. Brountzos EN, Ptohis N, Grammenou-Pomoni M, et al. High-flow renal arteriovenous fistula treated with the Amplatzer Vascular Plug: implementation of an arterial and venous approach. *Cardiovasc Intervent Radiol.* 2009;32:543–547.
14. Pech M, Kraetsch A, Wieners G, et al. Embolization of the gastroduodenal artery before selective internal radiotherapy: a prospectively randomized trial comparing platinum-fibered microcoils with the Amplatzer Vascular Plug II. *Cardiovasc Intervent Radiol.* 2009;32:455–461.
15. Swaans M, Post M, van der Ven H, et al. Transapical treatment of paravalvular leaks in patients with a logistic EuroSCORE of more than 15%: acute and 3-month outcomes of a "proof of concept" study. *Catheter Cardiovasc Interv.* 2012;79:741–747.
16. Gu X, Qian Z, Zhao C, et al. A new class of Amplatzer Vascular Plug (AVP-IV) delivered through diagnostic catheters: bench testing and in-vivo assessment (ab). *J Vasc Interv Radiol.* 2009;20(2)(suppl):S109.
17. Ferro C, Rossi UG, Bovio G, et al. The Amplatzer Vascular Plug 4: preliminary experience. *Cardiovasc Intervent Radiol.* 2010;33:844–848.
18. Zhu X, Tam MD, Pierce G, et al. Utility of the Amplatzer Vascular Plug in splenic artery embolization: a comparison study with conventional coil technique. *Cardiovasc Intervent Radiol.* 2011;34:522–531.
19. Abdel Aal AK, Hamed MF, Biosca RF, et al. Occlusion time for Amplatzer Vascular Plug in the management of pulmonary arteriovenous malformations. *AJR Am J Roentgenol.* 2009;192: 793–799.
20. Vandy F, Criado E, Upchurch GR Jr, et al. Transluminal hypogastric artery occlusion with an Amplatzer Vascular Plug during

endovascular aortic aneurysm repair. *J Vasc Surg.* 2008;48: 1121–1124.
21. Uberoi R, Chung D. Endovascular solutions for the management of visceral aneurysms. *J Cardiovasc Surg.* 2011;52:323–331.
22. Bulla K, Hubich S, Pech M, et al. Superiority of proximal embolization of the gastroduodenal artery with the Amplatzer Vascular Plug 4 before yttrium-90 radioembolization: a retrospective comparison with coils in 134 patients. *Cardiovasc Intervent Radiol.* 2014;37:396–404.
23. Pech M, Mohnike K, Wieners G, et al. Advantages and disadvantages of the Amplatzer Vascular Plug IV in visceral embolization: report of 50 placements. *Cardiovasc Intervent Radiol.* 2011;34:1069–1073.
24. Carrafiello G, Lagana D, Dizonno M, et al. Endovascular ligature of splenic artery aneurysm with Amplatzer Vascular Plug: a case report. *Cardiovasc Revasc Med.* 2007;8:203–206.
25. Widlus DM, Moeslein FM, Richard HM III. Evaluation of the Amplatzer Vascular Plug for proximal splenic artery embolization. *J Vasc Interv Radiol.* 2008;19(5):652–656.
26. Puppala S, Wood A. Re: initial clinical experience using the Amplatzer Vascular Plug. *Cardiovasc Intervent Radiol.* 2008;31: 444–445.
27. Libicher M, Herbrik M, Stippel D, et al. Portal vein embolization using the Amplatzer Vascular Plug II: preliminary results [in German]. *Rofo.* 2010;182:501–506.
28. Yoo H, Ko GY, Gwon DI, et al. Preoperative portal vein embolization using an Amplatzer Vascular Plug. *Eur Radiol.* 2009;19: 1054–1061.
29. Cil B, Peynircioglu B, Canyigit M, et al. Peripheral vascular application of the Amplatzer Vascular Plug. *Diagn Interv Radiol.* 2008;14(1):35–39.
30. Basile A, Marletta G, Tsetis D, et al. The Amplatzer Vascular Plug also for ovarian vein embolization. *Cardiovasc Intervent Radiol.* 2008;31(2):446–447.
31. Tapping CR, Ettles DF, Robinson GJ. Long-term follow-up of treatment of pulmonary arteriovenous malformations with Amplatzer Vascular Plug and Amplatzer Vascular Plug II devices. *J Vasc Interv Radiol.* 2011;22:1740–1746.
32. Letorneau-Guillon L, Faughnan ME, Soulez G, et al. Embolization of pulmonary arteriovenous malformations with Amplatzer vascular plugs: safety and midterm effectiveness. *J Vasc Interv Radiol.* 2010;21:649–656.
33. Lee DW, White RI Jr, Egglin TK, et al. Embolotherapy of large pulmonary arteriovenous malformations: long-term results. *Ann Thorac Surg.* 1997;64:930–940.
34. Wang MQ, Liu FY, Feng D. Management of surgical splenorenal shunt-related hepatic myelopathy with endovascular interventional techniques. *World J Gastroenterol.* 2012;18:7104–7108.
35. Shih CH, Liang PC, Chiang FT, et al. Transcatheter embolization of a huge renal arteriovenous fistula with Amplatzer Vascular Plug. *Heart Vessels.* 2010;25:356–358.
36. Boixadera H, Tomasello A, Quiroga S, et al. Successful embolization of a spontaneous mesocaval shunt using the Amplatzer Vascular Plug II. *Cardiovasc Intervent Radiol.* 2009;33:1044–1048.
37. Singh H, Luthra M, Bharadwaj P, et al. Interventional rerouting of scimitar vein to left atrium using an Amplatzer Vascular Plug. *Congenit Heart Dis.* 2007;2:265–269.
38. Powell S, Narlawar R, Odetoyinbo T, et al. Early experience with the Amplatzer Vascular Plug II for occlusive purposes in arteriovenous hemodialysis access. *Cardiovasc Intervent Radiol.* 2010;33:150–156.
39. Pattynama PM, Wils A, van der Linden E, et al. Embolization with the Amplatzer Vascular Plug in TIPS patients. *Cardiovasc Intervent Radiol.* 2007;30:1218–1221.
40. Boudoulas KD, Elinoff J, Resar JR. Bronchopulmonary fistula closure with an Amplatzer multi-fenestrated septal occluder. *Catheter Cardiovasc Interv.* 2010;75:455–458.
41. Koo JH, Park KB, Choo SW, et al. Embolization of postsurgical esophagopleural fistula with Amplatzer Vascular Plug, coils, and Histoacryl glue. *J Vasc Interv Radiol.* 2010;12:1905–1910.
42. Pieper CC, Meyer C, Hauser S, et al. Transrenal ureteral occlusion using the Amplatzer Vascular Plug II: a new interventional treatment option for lower urinary tract fistulas. *Cardiovasc Intervent Radiol.* 2014;37:451–457. doi:10.1007/s00270-013-0662-7.
43. Trerotola SO, Pyeritz RE. Does use of coils in addition to Amplatzer Vascular Plugs prevent recanalization? *AJR Am J Roentgenol.* 2010;195:766–771.
44. Milic A, Chan RP, Cohen JH, et al. Reperfusions of pulmonary arteriovenous malformations after embolotherapy. *J Vasc Interv Radiol.* 2005;16:1675–1683.
45. Maleux G, Rega F, Heye S, et al. Asymptomatic migration of a first-generation Amplatzer Vascular Plug into the abdominal aorta: conservative management may be an option. *J Vasc Interv Radiol.* 2011;22:569–570.

5

Gelatin Sponge

Miyuki Sone • Yasuaki Arai

Gelatin sponge (GS) has been used worldwide for more than 40 years for various embolization procedures. Although it was originally developed as a surgical hemostatic material in 1945,[1,2] Ishimori et al.[3] reported the first case of vascular embolization with GS for a carotid-cavernous fistula in 1967. Since then, GS has been a basic embolic material that is used in various disease entities such as hypervascular tumors, bleeding, and preoperative embolization.

DEVICE DESCRIPTION

General Characteristics

GS is prepared from purified porcine or bovine skin gelatin or collagen and processed with nitrogen to obtain a porous structure. It is biodegradable and insoluble in water. Although the commercially available products vary between countries, they are classified into two types based on their shape: preshaped and sheet-shaped. Preshaped GS (GELITA-SPON IR [Gelita Medical, Eberbach, Germany], Gelpart [Nippon Kayaku, Tokyo, Japan]) is a ready-to-use, 1- to 4-mm diameter dry product. Sheet-shaped dry GS (Gelfoam [Pharmacia & Upjohn, New York, USA], Sponzel [Astellas Pharma Inc., Tokyo, Japan], GELITA-SPON [Gelita Medical, Eberbach, Germany], Serescue [Nippon Kayaku, Tokyo, Japan]) requires manual preparation but is flexible in size and shape and can be used to treat various target vessels.

Mechanisms of Vessel Occlusion

Vessel occlusion with GS occurs mainly by mechanical obstruction caused by filling of the vascular lumen with GS and subsequent thrombus formation.[4,5] Additionally, GS has hemostatic properties, which shorten coagulation time and accelerate thrombus formation.[6]

Recanalization and Resorption

GS is categorized as a temporary, degradable embolic material because of its unique features of resorption and vessel recanalization. The advantages of using degradable embolic materials are the preclusion of retaining foreign materials and recovery of blood flow in the target vessels. As a result, repeated embolization can be performed if required in the setting of various disease entities such as hepatocellular carcinoma or hemoptysis and for preserving fertility when embolization is used for the control of postpartum hemorrhage.

Because GS is insoluble in water, it is removed by phagocytosis, as a foreign body reaction usually occurs within 2 to 6 weeks.[7] In animal studies, the time to vessel recanalization varies between a few days to several months.[8,9] Louail et al.[9] demonstrated that the recanalization rate of the porcine renal artery was 63% at 7 days and 100% at 14 days after GS embolization. In a similar study by Maeda et al.,[10] the recanalization rate was 79% at 7 days after GS embolization. In a clinical study of uterine artery embolization (UAE) with GS by Katsumori et al.,[11] magnetic resonance angiography performed at 4 months after UAE demonstrated recanalization of the ascending uterine artery in 88% of patients. However, there are several reports of recanalization failure in cases of preoperative embolization or embolization performed to control bleeding.[12,13] Possible causes of inconsistency in the timing of recanalization after embolization include the amount of GS used, the inflammatory reactions induced, and the tissue necrosis that occurs after embolization. When the amount of GS is larger than the target vessel diameter, dense accumulation in the lumen may lead to an irreversible interruption of blood flow. An inflammatory reaction is also prominent after GS embolization.[4,10,14] The inflammatory cells infiltrate the vessel wall, resulting in stenosis of the vessel because of the proliferation of fibroblasts, vasculitis, and acceleration of thrombosis.[4,14,15] Furthermore, possible tissue necrosis after embolization may affect vessel patency[10] because necrotic areas need fewer vessels than intact areas.

TECHNIQUE

Preparation of Sheet-Shaped Gelatin Sponge

To use sheet-shaped GS in vascular embolization, manual preparation is required to obtain the specific characteristics of the embolic material. Commonly used techniques include hand-cut, pumping, and torpedo.

Hand-Cut Method

With this technique, sheet-shaped GS is sliced into four thin sections with a scalpel (Fig. 5.1A,B). Each section is pressed with the fingers or a Petri dish to make it thinner (Fig. 5.1C). The section is cut in half with a small straight scissors, which is then cut, starting from one side, into approximately 1-mm wide columns without cutting the end (Fig. 5.1D). Subsequently, every column is cut perpendicularly into small square particles and placed in a Petri dish filled with contrast material (Fig. 5.1E). The particles are aspirated with a syringe and transferred to a 1-mm syringe if a microcatheter is being used for embolization (Fig. 5.1F).

Pumping Method

Thin sections are prepared as described previously in the hand-cut technique. A section is then cut into 2- to 3-mm wide columns (Fig. 5.2A) and placed in a 2.5-mL or 5-mL syringe and another syringe is filled with contrast material (Fig. 5.2B,C). Subsequently, GS is agitated and mixed with contrast material through a three-way stopcock for 10 to 30 times (Fig. 5.2D).

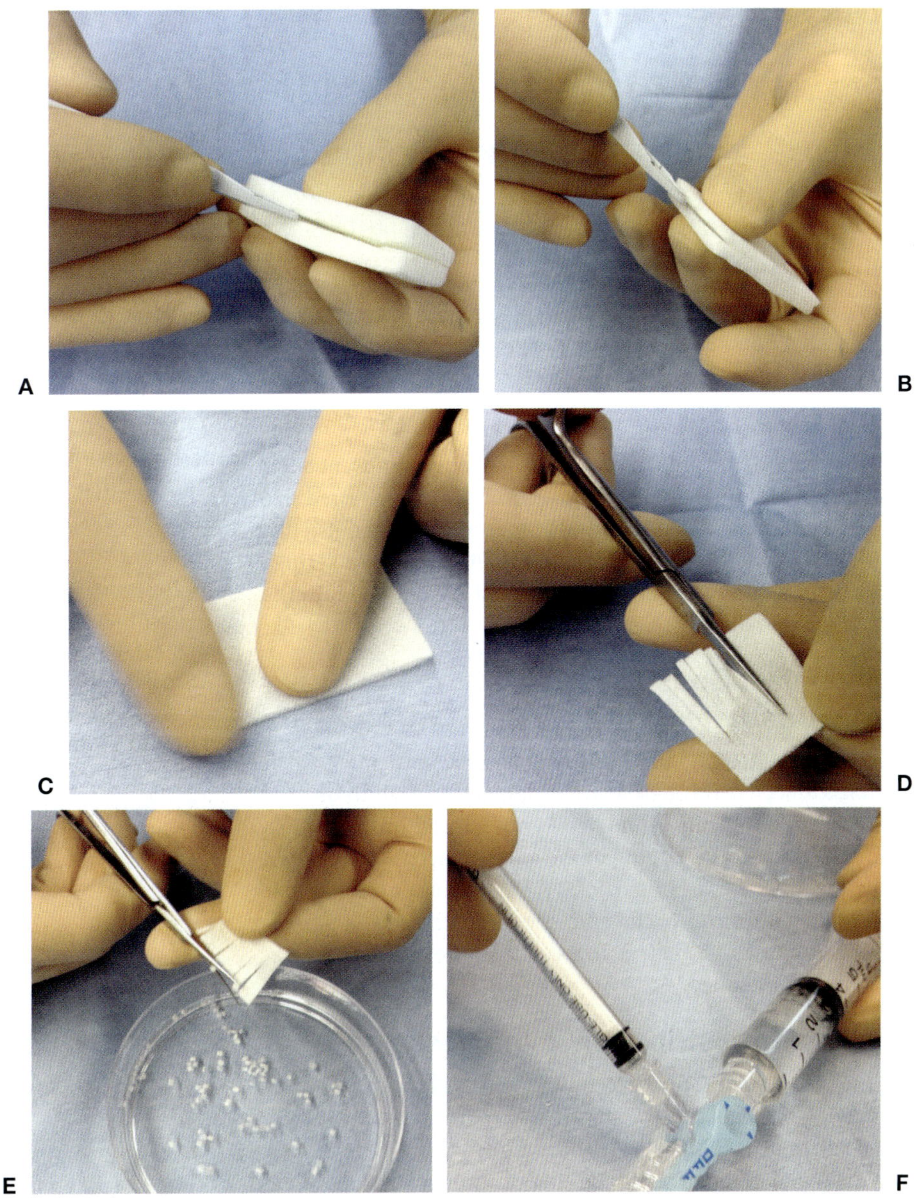

Figure 5.1 Hand-cut method. **A,B:** A sheet-shaped GS is sliced into four thin sections with a scalpel. **C:** Each section is pressed with the fingers. **D:** The section is cut from one side into approximately 1-mm wide columns. **E:** The columns are cut perpendicularly into small square particles. **F:** The particles are aspirated with a syringe and transferred to a 1-mm syringe.

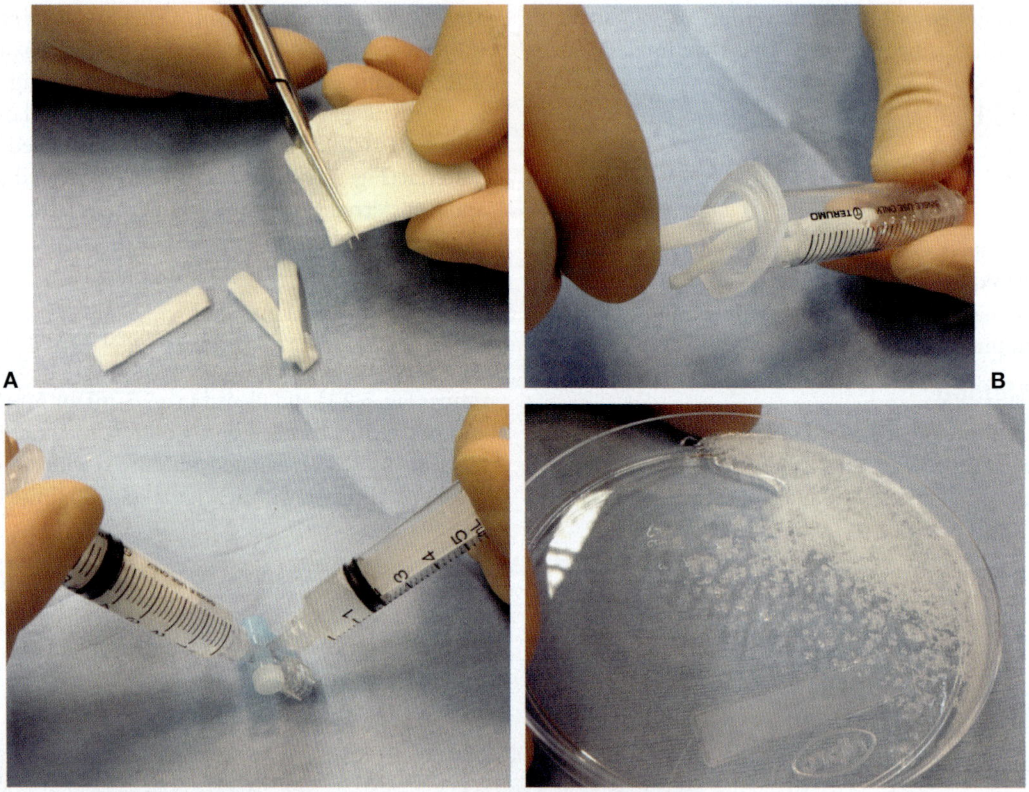

Figure 5.2 Pumping method. **A:** A section is cut into 2-3mm-width columns. **B:** Columns are placed in a 2.5-ml or 5-ml syringe and another syringe is filled with contrast material. **C:** Mix and agitate through GS with contrast material through a 3-way stopcock for 10-30 times. **D:** Small, ununiform particles are prepared with pumping method.

Torpedo Method

Thin sections are prepared as described in the hand-cut technique. A section is then cut into columns of the preferred size and a column is twisted with the fingers to sharpen its edge (Fig. 5.3A,B). These torpedoes are then placed in a syringe through its tip (Fig. 5.3C), and contrast is aspirated into the syringe as well.

Technical Considerations for Microcatheter Use

A 1-mL or 2.5-mL Luer Lock syringe is recommended when GS is injected through a microcatheter.[16] In addition, the injection of normal saline between GS injections is recommended to avoid clogging of the microcatheter. Care should be taken when larger particles (>2 mm) are used because fragmentation can occur after the microcatheter is passed, resulting in very small particles and a more distal embolization than intended.[17]

Size and Distribution in the Vessels

The size of the GS is not uniform in both manually prepared GS sheets and preshaped GS.[14,17,18] Specifically for the sheet-shaped GS, the size and uniformity of the particles largely depend on the preparation technique. Hand-cut GS is uniform in size, whereas the pumping technique produces particles with various sizes.[18] Katsumori and Kasahara[18] reported that cutting produced lower rates of smaller particles (≤500 μm) and larger particles (>2,000 μm) than pumping (8.5% vs. 20.4% and 0% vs. 48.1%, respectively) when Gelfoam was used.

Similar to other embolic materials, the vessel distribution after GS embolization depends on the size of GS. Although GS is deformable, it has the tendency to embolize vessels that are smaller than its size. Moreover, calibrating the size of GS particles is difficult not only for manually prepared sheet-shaped GS but also for preshaped 1-mm and 2-mm diameter GS.[19] In theory, this represents the disadvantages of GS use, as the level of embolization is difficult to control. In animal studies, when 1- to 2-mm hand-cut and preshaped GS were used, the mean diameter of the occluded vessels was approximately 500 μm.[14,20] In an animal study by Miyamoto,[21] GS particles prepared by pumping were distributed in a wide range of porcine uterine arteries, including vessels less than 100 μm in diameter.

CLINICAL APPLICATIONS

GS has been used extensively in various disease entities (Table 5.1). It has been used as antitumor treatment for

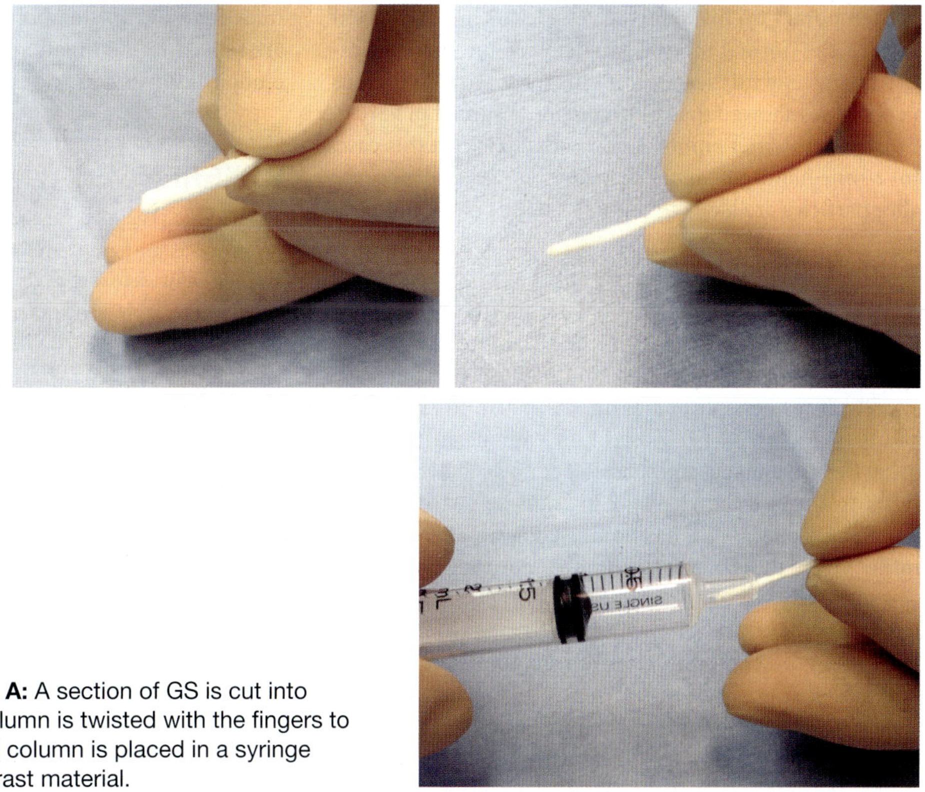

A B C

Figure 5.3 Torpedo method. **A:** A section of GS is cut into columns. **B:** A column is twisted with the fingers to sharpen its edge. **C:** The twisted column is placed in a syringe through its tip and aspirate contrast material.

hypervascular tumors and to control bleeding in various types of hemorrhages. Although data from randomized controlled comparative trials with newer spherical embolic materials are limited, the use of GS as a standard embolic material is supported by wide clinical experience and various clinical reports.

Table 5.1 Clinical Applications of Gelatin Sponge Embolization

Hypervascular tumor
Malignant tumor
Hepatocellular carcinoma
Presurgical embolization (renal cell carcinoma, bone tumor, etc.)
Benign tumor
Uterine fibroid
Juvenile angiofibroma
Presurgical embolization
Bleeding
Trauma
Postpartum hemorrhage
Gastrointestinal bleeding
Epistaxis
Hemoptysis
Tumor bleeding
Presurgical portal vein embolization
Partial splenic embolization for hypersplenism
Nonvascular embolization
Tract of biopsy or transhepatic puncture

Hepatocellular Carcinoma

Transarterial chemoembolization (TACE) for intermediate stage hepatocellular carcinoma (HCC) using GS has led to improved clinical outcome by prolonging survival in randomized controlled trials[22,23] and meta-analyses.[24–26] The use of GS as a temporary agent in HCC is preferred because of the necessity to repeat TACE for residual, recurrent, and newly developed tumors.

Although the use of spherical embolic materials and drug-eluting beads is emerging in many countries, the use of TACE as a standard procedure remains controversial because its use is not fully evidence-based. TACE with iodized oil (Lipiodol, Ethiodol) and anthracycline agents followed by embolization with GS was developed in Japan in the 1980s.[27–29] This is still a standard technique of performing TACE for HCC in Asian countries, and a recent prospective study by Ikeda et al.[30] demonstrated a favorable 2-year survival rate of 75.0%. Key features of this technique include super selective TACE and use of iodized oil to block the draining route and surrounding portal blood flow of the tumor.[30,31]

Postpartum Hemorrhage

Brown et al.[32] first reported a case of embolization with GS for postpartum hemorrhage (PPH) in 1979. Arterial embolization is now widely used for PPH, with a reported clinical efficacy of 72% to 100%.[33–35] For arterial embolization of PPH, the main embolic material has been GS because it causes temporary occlusion of the vessel, which may prevent damage to the normal uterine parenchyma and may be sufficient to prevent further bleeding in most cases. Previous clinical studies showed that menstruation resumed in 93% to 100% of patients after embolization with GS.[35–37] In this case, 1- to 2-mm hand-cut or preshaped GS was used because smaller particles are likely to cause ischemic complications.

Uterine Fibroid Embolization

UAE for the treatment of symptomatic uterine fibroid was first described by Ravina et al.[38] in 1995. Over the past decade, UAE has been increasingly used, and because of its efficacy and safety, it was established as an alternative to surgery as standard treatment.[39–42] The use of an embolic material for UAE has been evaluated, and spherical embolic materials such as Embosphere are the standard in countries where access to them is feasible.[43,44] GS has been used as an alternative in countries where these materials are either not accessible or not preferred for cost-saving reasons. Katsumori et al.[45,46] first described a large case series of UAE with GS with favorable mid- and long-term outcomes in terms of symptom improvement in 96% of patients at 1 year, 94.5% at 2 years, and 89.5% at 5 years. A prospective multicenter study by Sone et al.[47] demonstrated a similar outcome at 1 year with an improvement in menorrhagia in 90% of patients, bulk symptom in 76%, and pelvic pain in 96%. Depending on the situation, the use of GS as an alternative embolic material for UAE can be considered.

TIPS AND TRICKS

- GS is applicable to a wide range of disease entities.
- GS is flexible in size depending on the preparation technique. Ultimately, this will determine the level of occlusion with the target vasculature.

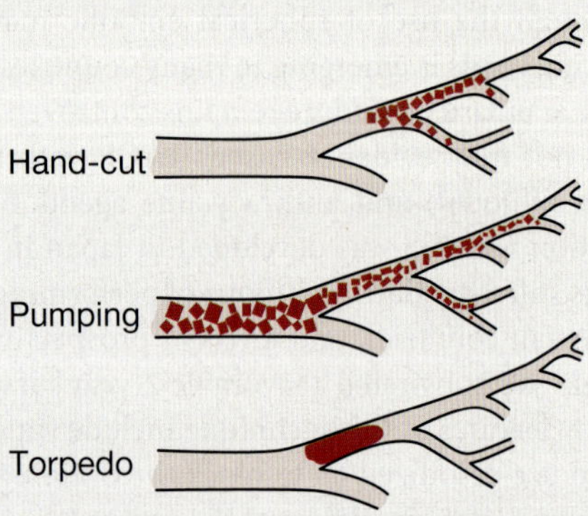

POTENTIAL COMPLICATIONS

There have been two reports of rare anaphylactic reactions during surgical use of GS.[48,49] To date, only one study demonstrated anaphylaxis presumably caused by GS during TACE with cisplatin and GS, without contrast material.[50] Additional complications include nontarget embolization, ischemia, infection, and postembolization syndrome; however, these are related to the organ and vascular bed being targeted for embolization and are not specific to GS.

REFERENCES

1. Jenkins HP, Janda R. Studies on the use of gelatin sponge or foam as an hemostatic agent in experimental liver resections and injuries to large veins. *Ann Surg*. 1946;124:952–961.
2. Jenkins HP, Janda R, Clarke J. Clinical and experimental observations on the use of gelatin sponge or foam. *Surgery*. 1946;20:124–132.
3. Ishimori S, Hattori M, Shibata Y, et al. Treatment of carotid-cavernous fistula by gelfoam embolization. *J Neurosurg*. 1967;27:315–319.
4. Sato M, Yamada R. Experimental and clinical studies on the hepatic artery embolization for treatment of hepatoma. *J Jpn Radiol Soc*. 1983;43:977–1005.
5. Loffroy R, Guiu B, Cercueil JP, et al. Endovascular therapeutic embolisation: an overview of occluding agents and their effects on embolised tissues. *Curr Vasc Pharmacol*. 2009;7:250–263.
6. Blaine G. Absorbable gelatin sponge in experimental surgery. *Lancet*. 1951;2:427–429.
7. Kawano H, Arakawa S, Satoh O, et al. Foreign body granulomatous change from absorbable gelatin sponge and microcoil embolization after a guidewire-induced perforation in the distal coronary artery. *Intern Med*. 2010;49:1871–1874.
8. Barth KH, Strandberg JD, White RI Jr. Long term follow-up of transcatheter embolization with autologous clot, oxycel and gelfoam in domestic swine. *Invest Radiol*. 1977;12:273–280.
9. Louail B, Sapoval M, Bonneau M, et al. A new porcine sponge material for temporary embolization: an experimental short-term pilot study in swine. *Cardiovasc Intervent Radiol*. 2006;29:826–831.
10. Maeda N, Verret V, Moine L, et al. Targeting and recanalization after embolization with calibrated resorbable microspheres versus hand-cut gelatin sponge particles in a porcine kidney model. *J Vasc Interv Radiol*. 2013;24:1391–1398.
11. Katsumori T, Kasahara T, Kin Y, et al. Magnetic resonance angiography of uterine artery: changes with embolization using gelatin sponge particles alone for fibroids. *Cardiovasc Intervent Radiol*. 2007;30:398–404.
12. Bracken RB, Johnson DE, Goldstein HM, et al. Percutaneous transfemoral renal artery occlusion in patients with renal carcinoma. Preliminary report. *Urology*. 1975;6:6–10.
13. Jander HP, Russinovich NA. Transcatheter gelfoam embolization in abdominal, retroperitoneal, and pelvic hemorrhage. *Radiology*. 1980;136:337–344.
14. Sone M, Osuga K, Shimazu K, et al. Porous gelatin particles for uterine artery embolization: an experimental study of intra-arterial distribution, uterine necrosis, and inflammation in a porcine model. *Cardiovasc Intervent Radiol*. 2010;33:1001–1008.
15. Ishikura H, Sotozaki Y, Adachi H, et al. Granulomatous arteritis with massive eosinophilic leukocyte infiltration and transient peripheral eosinophilia subsequent to transarterial embolization therapy with a gelatin sponge. *Acta Pathol Jpn*. 1991;41:618–622.
16. Osuga K, Miyayama S, Yamagami T, et al. New porous gelatin particles for hepatic arterial embolization—investigation of passage through current microcatheters [in Japanese]. *Gan To Kagaku Ryoho*. 2007;34:59–64.

17. Osuga K, Anai H, Takahashi M, et al. Porous gelatin particles for hepatic arterial embolization; investigation of the size distribution and fragmentation before and after microcatheter passage [in Japanese]. *Gan To Kagaku Ryoho*. 2009;36:437–442.
18. Katsumori T, Kasahara T. The size of gelatin sponge particles: differences with preparation method. *Cardiovasc Intervent Radiol*. 2006;29:1077–1083.
19. Katsumori T. The size distribution of porous gelatin particles (GelpartR). *IVR: Intervent Radiol*. 2007;22:469–471.
20. Sonomura T, Yamada R, Kishi K, et al. Dependency of tissue necrosis on gelatin sponge particle size after canine hepatic artery embolization. *Cardiovasc Intervent Radiol*. 1997;20:50–53.
21. Miyamoto S. Uterine artery embolization using gelatin sponge in a miniature pig: a study of arterial size and the distribution of embolic materials [in Japanese]. *Nihon Igaku Hoshasen Gakkai Zasshi*. 2005;65:452–454.
22. Lo CM, Ngan H, Tso WK, et al. Randomized controlled trial of transarterial lipiodol chemoembolization for unresectable hepatocellular carcinoma. *Hepatology*. 2002;35:1164–1171.
23. Llovet JM, Real MI, Montana X, et al. Arterial embolisation or chemoembolisation versus symptomatic treatment in patients with unresectable hepatocellular carcinoma: a randomised controlled trial. *Lancet*. 2002;359:1734–1739.
24. Marelli L, Stigliano R, Triantos C, et al. Transarterial therapy for hepatocellular carcinoma: which technique is more effective? A systematic review of cohort and randomized studies. *Cardiovasc Intervent Radiol*. 2007;30:6–25.
25. Llovet JM, Bruix J. Systematic review of randomized trials for unresectable hepatocellular carcinoma: chemoembolization improves survival. *Hepatology*. 2003;37:429–442.
26. Camma C, Schepis F, Orlando A, et al. Transarterial chemoembolization for unresectable hepatocellular carcinoma: meta-analysis of randomized controlled trials. *Radiology*. 2002;224:47–54.
27. Yamada R, Sato M, Kawabata M, et al. Hepatic artery embolization in 120 patients with unresectable hepatoma. *Radiology*. 1983;148:397–401.
28. Nakamura H, Hashimoto T, Oi H, et al. Transcatheter oily chemoembolization of hepatocellular carcinoma. *Radiology*. 1989; 170:783–786.
29. Uchida H, Ohishi H, Matsuo N, et al. Transcatheter hepatic segmental arterial embolization using lipiodol mixed with an anticancer drug and Gelfoam particles for hepatocellular carcinoma. *Cardiovasc Intervent Radiol*. 1990;13:140–145.
30. Ikeda M, Arai Y, Park SJ, et al. Prospective study of transcatheter arterial chemoembolization for unresectable hepatocellular carcinoma: an Asian cooperative study between Japan and Korea. *J Vasc Interv Radiol*. 2013;24:490–500.
31. Matsui O, Miyayama S, Sanada J, et al. Interventional oncology: new options for interstitial treatments and intravascular approaches: superselective TACE using iodized oil for HCC: rationale, technique and outcome. *J Hepatobiliary Pancreat Sci*. 2010;17:407–409.
32. Brown BJ, Heaston DK, Poulson AM, et al. Uncontrollable postpartum bleeding: a new approach to hemostasis through angiographic arterial embolization. *Obstet Gynecol*. 1979;54:361–365.
33. Touboul C, Badiou W, Saada J, et al. Efficacy of selective arterial embolisation for the treatment of life-threatening post-partum haemorrhage in a large population. *PloS One*. 2008;3:e3819.
34. Mathe ML, Morau E, Vernhet-Kovacsik H, et al. Impact of the new French clinical practice recommendations in embolization in postpartum and post-abortion hemorrhage: study of 48 cases. *J Perinat Med*. 2007;35:532–537.
35. Thabet A, Kalva SP, Liu B, et al. Interventional radiology in pregnancy complications: indications, technique, and methods for minimizing radiation exposure. *Radiographics*. 2012;32:255–274.
36. Boulleret C, Chahid T, Gallot D, et al. Hypogastric arterial selective and superselective embolization for severe postpartum hemorrhage: a retrospective review of 36 cases. *Cardiovasc Intervent Radiol*. 2004;27:344–348.
37. Yamashita Y, Takahashi M, Ito M, et al. Transcatheter arterial embolization in the management of postpartum hemorrhage due to genital tract injury. *Obstet Gynecol*. 1991;77:160–163.
38. Ravina JH, Herbreteau D, Ciraru-Vigneron N, et al. Arterial embolisation to treat uterine myomata. *Lancet*. 1995;346:671–672.
39. Jun F, Yamin L, Xinli X, et al. Uterine artery embolization versus surgery for symptomatic uterine fibroids: a randomized controlled trial and a meta-analysis of the literature. *Arch Gynecol Obstet*. 2012;285:1407–1413.
40. van der Kooij SM, Hehenkamp WJ, Volkers NA, et al. Uterine artery embolization vs hysterectomy in the treatment of symptomatic uterine fibroids: 5-year outcome from the randomized EMMY trial. *Am J Obstet Gynecol*. 2010;203:105.e1–105.e13.
41. Hehenkamp WJ, Volkers NA, Birnie E, et al. Symptomatic uterine fibroids: treatment with uterine artery embolization or hysterectomy—results from the randomized clinical Embolisation versus Hysterectomy (EMMY) Trial. *Radiology*. 2008;246: 823–832.
42. Gupta JK, Sinha A, Lumsden MA, et al. Uterine artery embolization for symptomatic uterine fibroids. *Cochrane Database Syst Rev*. 2012;5:CD005073.
43. Spies JB, Allison S, Flick P, et al. Spherical polyvinyl alcohol versus tris-acryl gelatin microspheres for uterine artery embolization for leiomyomas: results of a limited randomized comparative study. *J Vasc Interv Radiol*. 2005;16:1431–1437.
44. Spies JB, Allison S, Flick P, et al. Polyvinyl alcohol particles and tris-acryl gelatin microspheres for uterine artery embolization for leiomyomas: results of a randomized comparative study. *J Vasc Interv Radiol*. 2004;15:793–800.
45. Katsumori T, Nakajima K, Mihara T, et al. Uterine artery embolization using gelatin sponge particles alone for symptomatic uterine fibroids: midterm results. *AJR Am J Roentgenol*. 2002;178:135–139.
46. Katsumori T, Kasahara T, Akazawa K. Long-term outcomes of uterine artery embolization using gelatin sponge particles alone for symptomatic fibroids. *AJR Am J Roentgenol*. 2006;186:848–854.
47. Sone M, Arai Y, Shimizu T, et al. Phase I/II multiinstitutional study of uterine artery embolization with gelatin sponge for symptomatic uterine leiomyomata: Japan Interventional Radiology in Oncology Study Group study. *J Vasc Interv Radiol*. 2010;21:1665–1671.
48. Spencer HT, Hsu JT, McDonald DR, et al. Intraoperative anaphylaxis to gelatin in topical hemostatic agents during anterior spinal fusion: a case report. *Spine J*. 2012;12:e1–e6.
49. Khoriaty E, McClain CD, Permaul P, et al. Intraoperative anaphylaxis induced by the gelatin component of thrombin-soaked gelfoam in a pediatric patient. *Ann Allergy Asthma Immunol*. 2012;108:209–210.
50. Kawakura K, Imai S, Miura Y, et al. A case of anaphylactic shock due to porous gelatin sponge during transarterial chemoembolization. *Fukushima J IVR*. 2013;17:24.

6

Polyvinyl Alcohol Particles

Ajita Deodhar • John A. Kaufman

Polyvinyl alcohol (PVA) is one of the oldest, particulate embolic materials providing inexpensive, permanent occlusion of blood vessels. It is a water-soluble, colorless synthetic polymer made from polyvinyl acetate through partial or full hydrolysis to remove the acetate groups. The extent of hydroxylation determines the physical, chemical, and mechanical properties of the PVA.[1] Typically, PVA is highly soluble in water but resistant to most organic solvents, which allows it to be used for many applications, including paper manufacturing, cosmetics, household sponges, food packaging, and medical devices.[2] The first ever medical use of PVA was reported by Grindlay[3] in 1949 at the Mayo Clinic as a prosthesis after pneumonectomy. Since then, it has found multiple medical applications such as cardiac surgery, skin grafting, embolic material, artificial cartilage, artificial tear replacement, etc.[2] Its nontoxic, inert properties have been well established over the last several decades. Tadavarthy et al.[4,5] was the first to report the use of PVA as an embolic material in the mid-1970s. It was used to treat patients with cervical carcinoma, hemangiosarcoma of the liver, hemangioendothelioma of the neck and forehead, and an arteriovenous malformation of the spine.

DEVICE/MATERIAL DESCRIPTION

PVA is most commonly available as an intrinsically nonvisible occlusive agent that is typically used in combination with contrast to be radiographically visible. The preparation of PVA particles first involves its conversion into a foam that can absorb water and become readily compressible. Historically, sheets or blocks of dried foam were shaved to yield irregular particles of varying sizes. The resulting shavings or particles were then passed through sieves with sequentially smaller holes to separate them into various sizes.[6] Given the irregular configuration of each individual particle, it was possible for larger particles to pass through small holes depending on its orientation as it passes through the sieve. This explains why there was variability in early particle preparations.[7] Today, PVA is supplied as a preparation of irregular or spherical particles within a standardized size range (Fig. 6.1), although the potential for size variability still exists within the nonspherical preparations. This is a potential issue when using particulate PVA because the presence of smaller particles than anticipated may lead to uncontrolled distal embolization (with tissue infarction), whereas the presence of larger particles than anticipated may lead to proximal embolization (with potential recanalization).

PVA is extremely resilient and compressible with excellent memory, allowing it to regain its shape and size once it comes in contact with body fluids.[7] In fact, due to its inherent memory, PVA particles have the potential to expand approximately 4 to 15 times once they come in contact with solution and can therefore occlude blood vessels slightly larger than the internal diameter of the catheter.[7] In addition, the particles have a tendency to clump together when suspended in saline. Therefore, the effective size of this agent is often larger than that of the individual dried particles, which can contribute to a more proximal occlusion than intended.[8] This property can also increase the risk of microcatheter occlusion during delivery.

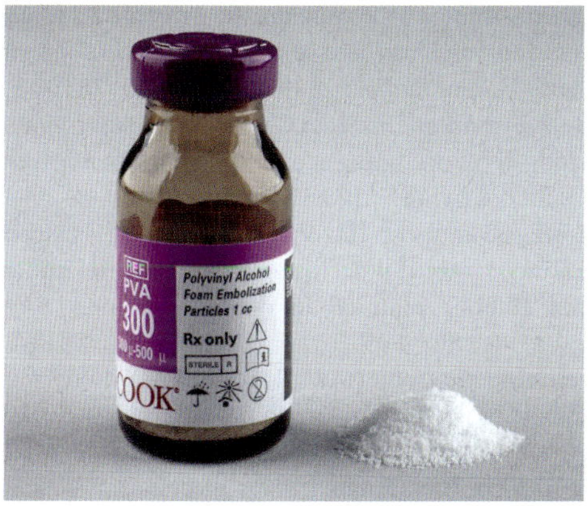

Figure 6.1 PVA preparation.

MECHANISM OF ACTION

The administration of PVA particles initially leads to slow flow due to adherence of the particles to the vessel wall.[9] This ultimately leads to an inflammatory reaction, a foreign body reaction, and thrombosis.[10–12] PVA is a nonbiodegradable embolic agent that has traditionally been thought to lead to a permanent vascular occlusion.[7] This occurs with organization of thrombus, disappearance of the inflammatory infiltrate, and ingrowth of connective tissue resulting in fibrosis. However, luminal recanalization after embolization with PVA has been reported as well, which may be due to resorption of thrombus and/or angiogenesis and capillary regrowth caused by vascular proliferation inside the organized thrombus.[9,12,13]

TECHNIQUE

Before using PVA as an embolic material, particulate PVA should be reconstituted to allow for radiographic visualization during delivery. This can be achieved by adding contrast, barium sulfate 60% or tantalum powder. To decrease particle clumping, albumin, dextran, absolute alcohol, or absorbable gelatin foam may be added to the saline suspension.[2]

PVA embolization uses a flow-directed technique and is performed under fluoroscopic guidance. During embolization, it is therefore necessary to monitor the administration at all times to quickly recognize when antegrade flow is slowing and vascular occlusion has taken place. Failure to recognize the slowing and changing direction of flow can increase the possibility of nontarget embolization due to particle reflux out of the target vessel. Given the tendencies of these particles to clump, arterial occlusion may occur faster than anticipated. In addition, frequent catheter flushing is recommended to minimize the possibility of catheter occlusion.

CLINICAL APPLICATIONS

PVA finds application wherever particulate embolization of a permanent nature is required. In general, this includes gastrointestinal or internal hemorrhage secondary to trauma, anticoagulation, etc.; therapeutic or presurgical tumor embolization; and embolization of uterine fibroids (uterine artery embolization).

POTENTIAL COMPLICATIONS

The complications reported in association with embolization using PVA particles have typically been related to the organ and pathology being embolized as opposed to the embolic agent itself. However, complications related to the characteristics of PVA can occur and are typically a function of flow. As described, the characteristics of PVA particles can lead to particle clumping, leading to proximal embolization with a potential for subsequent recanalization and procedural failure. Avoiding particle clumping and nontarget embolization requires attention to detail while preparing and delivering PVA.

TIPS AND TRICKS

- PVA particles should be matched to the size of the arteries to be occluded.
- The particles should be delivered in small aliquots with a 1-mL Luer lock syringe using road map imaging to monitor for flow and reflux.
- After reaching the desired end point, it is prudent to wait for 5 min and then perform another angiogram to check for return of flow due to distal migration of clumped PVA.
- Adding a little 25% albumin to the contrast/saline dilutant (1:20) minimizes clumping in the syringe. If the delivery catheter is blocked with particles, it can be cleared with a 1-mL Luer lock saline syringe.

REFERENCES

1. Tubbs RK. Sequence distribution of partially hydrolyzed polyvinyl acetate. *J Polym Sci Part A-1: Polym Chem*. 1968;4:623–629.
2. Baker MI, Walsh SP, Schwartz Z, et al. A review of polyvinyl alcohol and its uses in cartilage and orthopedic applications. *J Biomed Mater Res B Appl Biomater*. 2012;100:1451–1457.
3. Grindlay JH, Clagett OT. A plastic sponge prosthesis for use after pneumonectomy; preliminary report of an experimental study. *Proc Staff Meet Mayo Clin*. 1949;24:538.
4. Tadavarthy SM, Knight L, Ovitt TW, et al. Therapeutic transcatheter arterial embolization. *Radiology*. 1974;111:13–16.
5. Tadavarthy SM, Moller JH, Amplatz K. Polyvinyl alcohol (Ivalon): a new embolic material. *Am J Roentgenol Radium Ther Nucl Med*. 1975;125:609–616.

6. Siskin GP, Englander M, Stainken BF, et al. Embolic agents used for uterine fibroid embolization. *AJR Am J Roentgenol.* 2000;175:767–773.
7. Derdeyn CP, Moran CJ, Cross DT, et al. Polyvinyl alcohol particle size and suspension characteristics. *Am J Neuroradiol.* 1995;16:1335–1343.
8. Choe DH, Moon HH, Gyeong HK, et al. An experimental study of embolic effect according to infusion rate and concentration of suspension in transarterial particulate embolization. *Invest Radiol.* 1997;32:260–267.
9. Germano IM, Davis RL, Wilson CB, et al. Histopathological follow-up study of 66 cerebral arteriovenous malformations after therapeutic embolization with polyvinyl alcohol. *J Neurosurg.* 1992;76:607–614.
10. Castaneda-Zuniga WR, Sanchez R, Amplatz K. Experimental observations on short and long-term effects of arterial occlusion with Ivalon. *Radiology.* 1978;126(3):783–785.
11. White R, Stranberg JV, Gross G, et al. Therapeutic embolization with long-term occluding agents and their effects on embolized tissue. *Radiology.* 1977;125:677–687.
12. Link DP, Strandberg JD, Virmani R, et al. Histopathologic appearance of arterial occlusions with hydrogel and polyvinyl alcohol embolic material in domestic swine. *J Vasc Interv Radiol.* 1996;7:897–905.
13. Tomashefski JF, Cohen AM, Doershuk CF. Long-term histopathologic follow-up of bronchial arteries after therapeutic embolization with polyvinyl alcohol (Ivalon) in patients with cystic fibrosis. *Hum Pathol.* 1988;19:555–561.

7

Spherical Embolic Agents

Alan D. Birney • Gary P. Siskin

Since 1974, polyvinyl alcohol (PVA) particles have been used as a particulate agent for embolization procedures.[1] However, as experience was gained with this agent, its inherent limitations and disadvantages were recognized. These include size variability in a given preparation of particles due to the manufacturing process, particle aggregation, and microcatheter occlusion during delivery. Spherical embolic agents were developed in response to these limitations and become increasingly popular since their introduction.[2]

DEVICE DESCRIPTION

Trisacryl Gelatin Microspheres

In 1996, Laurent et al.[3] reported on the development of a spherical, nonresorbable embolization agent. These microspheres (Embosphere Microspheres; Merit Medical Systems, Inc., South Jordan, Utah) consist of a trisacryl polymer that is impregnated and embedded with gelatin (Fig. 7.1A). Trisacryl gelatin microspheres had been initially manufactured in the mid-1980s for use as a microcarrier for cell cultures.[4] These microspheres are biocompatible, hydrophilic, and deformable. In addition, cellular adhesion to these microspheres is supported by the presence of denatured collagen on their surface.[3,4]

Interventionalists instantly accepted these microspheres once they became commercially available because they successfully addressed the limitations of particulate PVA. The manufacturing process of these microspheres enabled a more narrow and reliable range of particles to be produced.[2,3] In addition, these microspheres did not aggregate, possibly due to their spherical configuration, the presence of a positive surface charge on the microspheres, and their hydrophilic nature.[2,5,6] In addition, a more predictable target occlusion could be achieved due to the fact that these microspheres did not aggregate. Derdeyn et al.[5] demonstrated that trisacryl gelatin microspheres occlude more distally than PVA particles of matched size, supporting the absence of aggregation when these microspheres are used. In fact, the level of vascular occlusion appears to correlate closely with the diameter of the microspheres used for embolization.[6–8] The narrow size range of microspheres, their lack of aggregation, and their deformability minimize the risk of microcatheter occlusion and contribute to the ease of delivery during administration.

The cellular response to embolization with trisacryl gelatin microspheres has been described. Macrophages, polymorphonuclear cells, and sparse lymphocytes have all been described after embolization with these microspheres, as has vessel recanalization.[3,9–11] Interestingly, these microspheres often undergo transvascular migration and can be found within the vessel lumen, within the vessel wall, or completely outside of the vessel after embolization[11]; PVA particles are less likely to be found outside of the vessel. This has been attributed to the inflammatory reaction induced by these microspheres.

Polyvinyl Alcohol Microspheres

Given the decades of success seen with embolization procedures performed with particulate PVA, it seems logical that a PVA-based microsphere (Contour SE Microspheres; Boston Scientific Corporation, Natick, Massachusetts) would be developed as a next generation embolic agent (Fig. 7.1B). PVA microspheres appear to generate a milder inflammatory response than both particulate PVA and trisacryl gelatin microspheres.[9] After embolization, neutrophils are acutely seen, but these are ultimately replaced by macrophages and occasional lymphocytes.

PVA microspheres, like trisacryl gelatin microspheres, address the disadvantages of particulate PVA with better

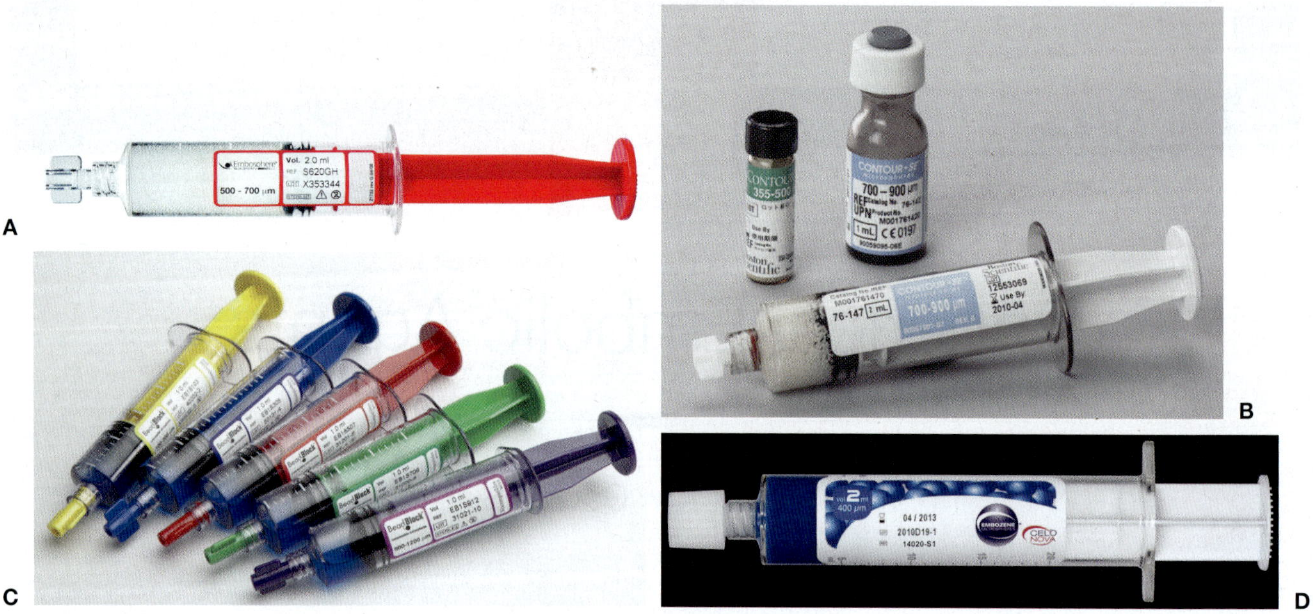

Figure 7.1 Images of commercially available embolic microspheres in the United States. **A:** Trisacryl gelatin microspheres (Embosphere Microspheres). (Courtesy of Merit Medical Systems, Inc., South Jordan, Utah.) **B:** PVA microspheres (Contour SE Microspheres). (Courtesy of Boston Scientific Corporation, Natick, Massachusetts.) **C:** Acrylamido PVA microspheres (Bead Block microspheres). (Courtesy of Biocompatibles, Inc., Oxford, Connecticut). **D:** Polyphosphazene-coated PMMA microspheres (Embozene Microspheres). (Courtesy of CeloNova BioSciences, Inc., San Antonio, Texas.)

size uniformity, less aggregation, and ease of administration. However, many of the inherent properties differ between these microspheres, including compressibility and elastic recovery.[10] PVA microspheres have been shown to be highly compressible with a delayed and incomplete elastic recovery, leading to a more distal embolization when compared to other spherical embolic agents.[7,8] This is felt to be due to change in shape of the particle with compression during delivery, which allows them to deform and occlude more distally than intended.

Acrylamido PVA microspheres (Bead Block microspheres; Biocompatibles, Inc., Oxford, Connecticut) consist of a PVA-based hydrogel polymer (Fig. 7.1C). Its properties have been shown to be intermediate between spherical PVA microspheres and trisacryl gelatin microspheres, with similar compression and nearly immediate subsequent reexpansion when compared with trisacryl gelatin microspheres.[2] These microspheres have been found to occlude slightly more distal than trisacryl gelatin microspheres, which is likely due to the slight differences in force required to compress the microspheres.

Polyphosphazene-Coated PMMA Microspheres

Polyphosphazene-coated polymethylmethacrylate (PMMA) microspheres (Embozene Microspheres; CeloNova BioSciences, Inc., San Antonio, Texas) consist of a Polyzene-F shell surrounding a hydrogel core of PMMA (Fig. 7.1D). When PMMA undergoes an alkaline hydrolysis, its structural flexibility increase, making it an appropriate material to use for an embolic agent.[12] This was theorized as early as 1989 by Jayakrishnan et al.[13] Polyzene-F is a proprietary, biocompatible, and nonresorbable version of the poly(bis[trifluoroethoxy]phosphazene) (PTFEP) polymer class and is applied as a thin coating on the PMMA core.[14] Polyzene-F has previously been used in vascular stents where it was found to have an absence of a significant inflammatory reaction.[15] A preclinical evaluation by Stampfl et al.[14] demonstrated similar findings, with only a minimal lymphocyte-mediated inflammatory reaction noted after embolization in a renal artery model. This is different from the findings of Verret et al.,[12] which noted early recruitment of phagocytic cells in a uterine artery model. In terms of the distribution of these microspheres within embolized vasculature, Verret et al.[16] demonstrated that they occlude more distal vessels than similarly sized trisacryl gelatin microspheres. They attributed this finding to their compressibility and deformability, enabling them to conclude that deformability determines the size of the vessel occluded as opposed to the actual particle size, which potentially makes the level of occlusion unpredictable with these microspheres.

TECHNIQUE

In general, spherical microspheres are packaged in a syringe consisting of a defined volume of embolic and normal saline. For administration, contrast material is added to make the solution radiopaque. A maximum saline-to-contrast ratio of 1:1 is recommended. Typically, gentle swirling of the solution is recommended before delivery; this and time will allow for the microspheres to be adequately suspended in the saline and contrast solution. To-and-fro aspiration between two syringes connected via a three-way stopcock is both unnecessary and not recommended as it may damage the microspheres.

Once the microspheres have been prepared, they are typically administered through a microcatheter under fluoroscopic guidance. Although the catheter selection can be based on the size of the microspheres being used for any given procedure, these microspheres tend to be more easily administered with microcatheters having an inner diameter of 0.027 to 0.028 in as opposed to smaller microcatheters.

One limitation of the trisacryl gelatin microspheres is that they are clear, which can make preparation difficult and visual confirmation of delivery from the syringe challenging. A subsequent product used elemental gold to stain the microspheres, which improved visualization. However, the addition of elemental gold resulted in a greater degree of inflammation after embolization, which ultimately led to the discontinuation of this product.[17]

CLINICAL APPLICATIONS

Beaujeux et al.[10] reported the initial clinical success of using trisacryl gelatin microspheres on 105 patients with tumors or arteriovenous malformations in the head, neck, or spine. Since this initial report, all of the available embolic microspheres have been rapidly incorporated into present-day embolization procedures and have been used successfully for various indications that are suitable for a particulate embolic agent.

These microspheres have had particularly notable success when used for uterine artery embolization (UAE) to treat symptomatic uterine fibroids. Although the success seen with the use of trisacryl gelatin microspheres has set the standard for subsequent comparative clinical trials,[18] each of the available embolic microspheres have demonstrated high clinical success and fibroid infarction rates in association with this procedure.[19,20] However, all of the attention paid to this procedure has brought to light how the different characteristics of these embolic microspheres can affect clinical outcomes and as a result has improved our understanding of these agents. For example, Contour SE Microspheres have been shown to be less effective for this procedure than other agents.[21,22] This is felt to be due to the differences in compressibility, deformability, and elasticity of this particular product when compared to the other available embolic microspheres, which was previously not appreciated until the differences in clinical outcomes were recognized.

NEXT GENERATION MICROSPHERES

Resorbable Microspheres

In theory, there is an inherent appeal to the concept of resorbable microspheres. All embolization procedures are being performed for certain indications, and if the goal of the procedure can be accomplished without implanting a permanent foreign body into the patient, then why would not that be preferred? In 2007, Laurent[2] suggested that the ideal resorbable microsphere would have four characteristics: it would have controlled resorption time, it would cause only a limited local inflammatory response, it would be associated with a complete functionality of the target vascular bed, and it would be loadable. If these expectations could be met, then one could be assured that the target pathology would be definitively and appropriately treated while leaving open the possibility that the target organ would fully recover and suffer no long-term effects from the embolization procedure.

There has been significant effort to develop bioresorbable microspheres in recent years. Nowadays, degradable starch microspheres have been evaluated for several years[23] and are commercially available (EmboCept S; PharmaCept, Berlin, Germany). These microspheres have been used for liver-directed tumor therapy.[24,25] The problem is that the starch microspheres are only available in a 50-μm diameter size and have a very short half-life, limiting their acceptance for the more common applications requiring particulate embolization.

Weng et al.[26] have done much work with bioresorbable hydrogel microspheres prepared from carboxymethylcellulose and chitosan. Chitosan (*N*-acetylglucosamine) is a linear polysaccharide derived from chitin after deacetylation.[27] Introducing carboxymethyl groups into the chitosan produces chitosan derivatives that are readily soluble in a physiologic pH.[28] The carboxymethyl chitosan can then be cross-linked with oxidized carboxymethylcellulose to form microspheres through an inverse emulsion method. These microspheres are degraded by lysozyme into glucosamine, which can be absorbed completely by the body. The degradation time appears to depend on the parameters of microsphere preparation, specifically on the degree of cross-linking density. These microspheres do not aggregate due to low coefficient of surface friction. In vivo evaluation comparing these microspheres with trisacryl gelatin microspheres has been performed with renal embolization in a rabbit model.[29] The performance of the two agents was similar in terms of the mean size of the vessels occluded with the two microspheres. These microspheres were biocompatible and well tolerated, with a mild tissue reaction and no evidence of vessel wall disruption. The authors did demonstrate that preparing the resorbable microspheres with a higher cross-linking density makes the spheres more rigid, which subsequently causes a more proximal embolization. Of note, the carboxylic groups in the microsphere matrix and their highly porous internal structure may allow for loading and release of positively charged drugs such as doxorubicin hydrochloride.[28]

Microspheres consisting of poly(lactic-co-glycolic acid) (PLGA) coated with type I bovine fibrillar collagen have also been evaluated (Occlusin 500 Artificial Embolization Device; IMBiotechnologies Ltd., Edmonton, Alberta, Canada). These noncompressible microspheres create a vascular occlusion mechanically and by binding platelets. An in vivo evaluation of these microspheres has been performed with UAE in a sheep model.[30] In this study, the effects of embolization with 150- to 212-μm PLGA microspheres were compared with the effects after embolization with trisacryl gelatin microspheres. At 6 months, none of the embolic material in the animals embolized with PLGA microspheres was detectable. At 12 months, all uterine arteries treated with the PLGA microspheres were recanalized or in the process of being recanalized; recanalized vessels were histologically indistinguishable from untreated vessels. The arteries treated with trisacryl gelatin microspheres remained occluded at 12 months.

There are other agents in various stages of development. Water-soluble PVA microspheres have been developed and evaluated in a pig kidney model.[31] The duration of arterial occlusion using these microspheres is possibly related to the degree of saponification of PVA. Microspheres manufactured from hydrophilic methacrylate monomer copolymerized with degradable cross-linkers have been evaluated as well.[32]

Visible Microspheres

An additional point of development for embolic microspheres is in the area of radiographic visibility. Nowadays, microspheres used for embolization are not radiographically visible and must therefore be mixed with contrast to be seen under fluoroscopy during delivery. An agent that could be visualized under fluoroscopy as well as under computed tomography (CT) or magnetic resonance (MR) imaging would be helpful to assess particle distribution during embolization and to assess nontarget embolization.[33] Work has been done in this area by Sharma et al.[34] who demonstrated that PVA hydrogel microspheres (LC Beads; Biocompatibles UK Ltd., Farnham, Surrey, United Kingdom) loaded with Lipiodol are visible on fluoroscopy and CT. Bartling et al.[35] developed an embolization particle that consists of an x-ray visible, iodine-containing core and an MRI-visible, paramagnetic iron oxide–based coating. Stampfl et al.[33] have modified a Polyzene-F–coated embolic microsphere with barium sulfate and iodine as well as with iron oxide, making them visible on radiography, CT, and MRI. This continues to be an ongoing area for development.

TIPS AND TRICKS

- All spherical embolic agents are not the same. Compressibility and other characteristics may significantly impact the clinical results achieved with each agent.
- The use of larger inner diameter microcatheters (≥0.027 in) is recommended to ease administration of embolic microspheres.
- The best way to obtain an optimal suspension of embolic microspheres after the addition of contrast to the saline and microsphere mix is with time; to-and-fro aspiration between two syringes via a three-way stopcock may damage the microspheres.

CONCLUSION

The popularity of embolic microspheres has increased significantly in recent years, becoming a category of embolic agent that is safely and effectively used for various clinical applications. During this time, significant research has been done in the area of embolic microspheres, enabling us to obtain a good understanding of their characteristic and of their clinical strengths and limitations. This has all resulted in continuing development of new spherical products that are not limited to drug elution. In time, the attention being paid to this area will inevitably enhance the drug-eluting abilities of new and existing microspheres and lead to the development of both resorbable and visible microspheres. Each of these new characteristics will improve our ability to treat a growing number of patients using spherical embolic agents.

REFERENCES

1. Tadavarthy SM, Knight L, Ovitt TW, et al. Therapeutic transcatheter arterial embolization. *Radiology*. 1974;111:13–16.
2. Laurent A. Microspheres and nonspherical particles for embolization. *Tech Vasc Interv Radiol*. 2007;10:248–256.
3. Laurent A, Beaujeux R, Wasset M, et al. Trisacryl gelatin microspheres for therapeutic embolization, I: development and in vitro evaluation. *Am J Neuroradiol*. 1996;17:533–540.
4. Obrenovitch A, Maintier C, Sene C, et al. Microcarrier culture of fibroblastic cells on modified trisacryl beads. *Biol Cell*. 1982;46:249–256.
5. Derdeyn CP, Graves VG, Salamant MS, et al. Collagen-coated acrylic microspheres for embolotherapy: in vivo and in vitro characteristics. *Am J Neuroradiol*. 1997;18:647–653.
6. Andrews RT, Binket CA. Relative rates of blood flow reduction during transcatheter arterial embolization with tris-acryl gelatin microspheres or polyvinyl alcohol: quantitative comparison in a swine model. *J Vasc Interv Radiol*. 2003;14:1311–1313.
7. Laurent A, Wassef M, Saint Maurice JP, et al. Arterial distribution of calibrated tris-acryl gelatin and polyvinyl alcohol microspheres in a sheet kidney model. *Invest Radiol*. 2006;41:8–14.
8. Laurent A, Wassef M, Namur J, et al. Arterial distribution of calibrated tris-acryl gelatin and polyvinyl alcohol embolization microspheres in sheep uterus. *Cardiovasc Intervent Radiol*. 2010;33:995–1000.
9. Siskin GP, Dowling K, Virmani R, et al. Pathologic evaluation of a spherical polyvinyl alcohol embolic agent in a porcine model. *J Vasc Interv Radiol*. 2003;14:89–98.
10. Beaujeux R, Laurent A, Wassef M, et al. Trisacryl gelatin microspheres for therapeutic embolization, II: preliminary clinical evaluation in tumors and arteriovenous malformations. *Am J Neuroradiol*. 1996;17:541–548.
11. Laurent A, Wassef M, Namur J, et al. Recanalization and particle exclusion after embolization of uterine arteries in sheep: a long-term study. *Fertil Steril*. 2009;91:884–892.
12. Verret V, Wassef M, Pelage JP, et al. Influence of degradation on inflammatory profile of polyphosphazine coated PMMA and trisacryl gelatin microspheres in a sheep uterine artery embolization model. *Biomaterials*. 2011;32:339–351.

13. Jayakrishnan A, Chittambara Thanoo B, Rathinam K, et al. Hydrogel microspheres from crosslinked poly (methylmethacrylate): synthesis and biocompatibility study. *Bull Mater Sci.* 1989;12:17–25.
14. Stampfl S, Stampfl U, Bellemann N, et al. Biocompatibility and recanalization characteristics of hydrogel microspheres with Polyzene-F as polymer coating. *Cardiovasc Intervent Radiol.* 2008;31:799–806.
15. Richter GM, Stampfl U, Stampfl S, et al. A new polymer concept for coating of vascular stents using PTFEP (poly(bis(trifluoroethoxy)phosphazene)) to reduce thrombogenicity and late in-stent stenosis. *Invest Radiol.* 2005;40:210–218.
16. Verret V, Homayra Ghegediban S, Wassef M, et al. The arterial distribution of Embozene and Embosphere microspheres in sheep kidney and uterine embolization models. *J Vasc Interv Radiol.* 2011;22:220–228.
17. Richard HM, Siskin GP, Stainken BF. Endometritis after uterine artery embolization with gold-colored gelatin microspheres. *J Vasc Interv Radiol.* 2004;15:406–407.
18. Spies JB, Cornell C, Worthington-Kirsch R, et al. Long-term outcome from uterine fibroid embolization with tris-acryl gelatin microspheres: results of a multicenter study. *J Vasc Interv Radiol.* 2007;18:203–207.
19. Worthington-Kirsch RL, Siskin GP, Hegener P, et al. Comparison of the efficacy of the embolic agents acrylamido polyvinyl alcohol microspheres and tris-acryl gelatin microspheres for uterine artery embolization for leiomyomas: a prospective randomized controlled trial. *Cardiovasc Intervent Radiol.* 2011;34:493–501.
20. Smeets AJ, Nijenhuis RJ, Jan van Rooij W, et al. Embolization of uterine leiomyomas with Polyzene F-coated hydrogel microspheres: initial experience. *J Vasc Interv Radiol.* 2010;21:1830–1834.
21. Siskin GP, Beck A, Schuster M, et al. Leiomyoma infarction after uterine artery embolization: a prospective randomized study comparing tris-acryl gelatin microspheres versus polyvinyl alcohol microspheres. *J Vasc Interv Radiol.* 2008;19:58–65.
22. Yu SC, Lok I, Ho SS, et al. Comparison of clinical outcomes of tris-acryl microspheres versus polyvinyl alcohol microspheres for uterine artery embolization for leiomyomas: results of a randomized trial. *J Vasc Interv Radiol.* 2011;22:1229–1235.
23. Forsberg JO. Transient blood flow reduction induced by intra-arterial injection of degradable starch microspheres. Experiments on rats. *Acta Chir Scand.* 1978;144:275–281.
24. Nishiofuku H, Tanaka T, Matsuoka M, et al. Transcatheter arterial chemoembolization using cisplatin powder mixed with degradable starch microspheres for colorectal liver metastases after FOLFOX failure: results of a phase I/II study. *J Vasc Interv Radiol.* 2013;24:56–65.
25. Yamasaki T, Saeki I, Harima Y, et al. Effect of transcatheter arterial infusion chemotherapy using iodized oil and degradable starch microspheres for hepatocellular carcinoma. *J Gastroenterol.* 2012;47:715–722.
26. Weng L, Le HC, Talaie R, et al. Bioresorbable hydrogel microspheres for transcatheter embolization: preparation and in vitro evaluation. *J Vasc Interv Radiol.* 2011;22:1454–1470.
27. Alves da Silva ML, Crawford A, Mundy JM, et al. Chitosan/polyester-based scaffolds for cartilage tissue engineering: assessment of extracellular matrix formation. *Acta Biomater.* 2010;6:1149–1157.
28. Weng L, Rostamzadeh P, Nooryshokry N, et al. In vitro and in vivo evaluation of biodegradable embolic microspheres with tunable anticancer drug release. *Acta Biomaterialia.* 2013;9:6823–6833.
29. Weng L, Rusten M, Talaie R, et al. Calibrated bioresorbable microspheres: a preliminary study on the level of occlusion and arterial distribution in a rabbit kidney model. *J Vasc Interv Radiol.* 2013;24:1567–1575.
30. Owen RJ, Nation PN, Polakowski R, et al. A preclinical study of the safety and efficacy of Occlusin™ 500 Artificial Embolization Device in sheep. *Cardiovasc Intervent Radiol.* 2012;35:636–644.
31. Shomura Y, Tanigawa N, Shibutani M, et al. Water-soluble polyvinyl alcohol microspheres for temporary embolization: development and in vivo characteristics in a pig kidney model. *J Vasc Interv Radiol.* 2011;22:212–219.
32. Louguet S, Verret V, Bédouet L, et al. Poly(ethylene glycol) methacrylate hydrolyzable microspheres for transient vascular embolization. *Acta Biomater.* 2014;10:1194–1205.
33. Stampfl U, Sommer CM, Bellemann N, et al. Multimodal visibility of a modified Polyzene-F coated spherical embolic agent for liver embolization: feasibility study in a porcine model. *J Vasc Interv Radiol.* 2012;23:1225–1231.
34. Sharma KV, Dreher MR, Tang Y, et al. Development of "imageable" beads for transcatheter embolotherapy. *J Vasc Interv Radiol.* 2010;21:865–876.
35. Bartling SH, Budjan J, Aviv H, et al. First multimodal embolization particles visible on x-ray/computed tomography and magnetic resonance imaging. *Invest Radiol.* 2011;46:178–186.

8

Drug-Eluting Beads

Matthew E. Anderson • Sanjeeva P. Kalva

The introduction of drug-eluting beads represents a shift in the principal way in which chemotherapeutic agents are delivered, concentrated, and maintained within tumor during transarterial chemoembolization. Rather than using particles and/or Ethiodol to occlude the arterial flow in an attempt to keep the chemotherapy in the neoplasm, the particle (the bead) itself is the carrier of the chemotherapeutic agent. Once the particle is trapped within the neoplasm, it serves as the depot, allowing for sustained release of the drug with reduced systemic drug concentrations. This also reduces associated side effects while sustaining high chemotherapeutic concentrations within tumor. The concept of drug delivery through microparticles using various nondegradable and degradable synthetic polymers (such as polyglycolic acid, polyhydroxybutyrate, or ethylene vinyl acetate) or natural materials (albumin, gelatin, chitosan, or alginate) for carrying drugs such as doxorubicin, mitomycin C, cisplatin, methotrexate, and paclitaxel was described as early as 1983.[1] However, commercially available drug-capable beads were not developed until 2004.[2]

DEVICE/MATERIALS

Currently, there are three commercially available drug-eluting beads. These are U.S. Food and Drug Administration (FDA) approved for the treatment of hypervascular tumors and arteriovenous malformations. The drug-loading feature is not yet FDA-approved. However, all these beads carry CE mark approval status for drug loading in Europe. These include LC Beads (DC Beads in Europe) manufactured by Biocompatibles UK, Ltd. (Farnham, Surrey, United Kingdom), QuadraSphere (HepaSphere in Europe) manufactured by Merit Medical Systems, Inc. (South Jordan, Utah), and Oncozene beads (Embozene Tandem in Europe) manufactured by CeloNova BioSciences, Inc. (San Antonio, Texas). Although the drug loading and drug elution of these beads are based on ion exchange mechanism, the differing physical and chemical properties of the beads lead to variable drug-loading and drug-eluting characteristics, embolic effect, and intratumoral distribution.

LC Beads

LC beads (LC = low compression), also known as *DC beads* in Europe (DC = drug capable), are biocompatible, hydrophilic, nonresorbable, deformable polyvinyl alcohol acrylic polymer hydrogel microspheres produced by inverse polymerization with 2-acrylamido-2-methylpropane sulfonate.[3] The negatively charged sulfonate groups allow interaction with positively charged drugs such as doxorubicin and irinotecan, which bind reversibly by an ion exchange mechanism, allowing for a high loading efficiency. The beads are available in various sizes ranging from 100 to 900 μm (100 to 300 μm, 300 to 500 μm, 700 to 900 μm). They are distributed in a 2-mL aliquot and delivered in a 10-mL vial. There are approximately 200,000 beads per vial of 100- to 300-μm beads; 38,000 beads per vial of 300- to 500-μm beads; and 10,000 beads per vial of 500- to 700-μm beads. Recently, smaller 70- to 150-μm beads known as the *LC BeadM1* are marketed for more distal intratumoral penetration. There are approximately 1,300,000 beads in a 2-mL aliquot of LC BeadM1.

The time required to load the LC beads with doxorubicin depends on the size of the beads (which affects the available surface area of the beads for drug loading), drug concentration within the medium, and absence of any other positively charged particles in the medium. Smaller diameter beads load quickly. When loading 25 mg of doxorubicin per 1 mL of beads, greater than 99% is loaded on to the 100- to 300-μm beads in less than 10 minutes, whereas it requires closer to 2 hours to completely load the 700- to 900-μm beads to the same concentration. No significant difference in maximum loading capacity is seen for LC beads of sizes between 100 and 900 μm, with an average maximum loading capacity of 39 mg doxorubicin per milliliter observed.[4] The loading characteristics of irinotecan parallel those of doxorubicin. At 2 hours, 100- to 300-μm beads load 98.1% of 50 mg/mL of irinotecan, whereas 700- to 900-μm beads load 93.5% of the drug. The maximum loading capacity is 50 mg of irinotecan per 1 mL of beads, irrespective of the size of the beads.[5]

Drug loading leads to loss of water in the hydrogel and results in a decrease in the diameter of the bead (an average of 35% diameter reduction of the beads with doxorubicin and 20% to 40% decrease with irinotecan) and reduction in the compressibility of the bead.[5,6] These physical changes do not affect delivery of the beads through microcatheters of appropriate size (2.4-Fr for 100 to 500 μm, 2.7-Fr for 500 to 700 μm, and 3-Fr for 700 to 900 μm). The manufacturer does not recommend mixing LC beads with Lipiodol.

The elution of chemotherapeutic drugs from LC beads appears to be a function of bead size (smaller beads elute faster) and ionic strength and composition of elution media (no drug elution in pure water but increasing rates of elution with increasing concentration of ionic solution) and is influenced by drug–bead interactions (irinotecan elutes faster than doxorubicin due to weak ionic bond) and drug–drug interactions.[7] Rapid elution of irinotecan (burst) from LC beads of up to 10% has been observed with mixing of the beads with certain contrast materials.[8] Therefore, premixing contrast material with the beads during preparation in the pharmacy has been discouraged.[8]

Preclinical and clinical studies have shown elevated and sustained retention of doxorubicin within the tumor after chemoembolization with drug-eluting beads and decreased systemic doxorubicin plasma levels (both peak drug concentration and area under the curve) compared to conventional chemoembolization.[9,10] The location of vascular occlusion appears to parallel the size of the beads: 100- to 300-μm beads block vessels with a mean diameter of 237-μm penetrating tumor at a mean distance of 3.8 mm. Explanted livers following chemoembolization with drug-eluting beads demonstrated 42% of the beads occluding intratumoral vessels. Sustained cytotoxic levels of drug at the vascular occlusion sites were observed for at least 1 month. Tumor necrosis was associated with deeper penetration of the beads and higher concentration of the drug.[11]

QuadraSpheres

QuadraSpheres are polyvinyl alcohol–acrylic acid superabsorbent copolymer beads, which swell up to 64 times their dry volume when hydrated. The microspheres are shipped dehydrated and are available in 30 to 60 μm, 50 to 100 μm, 100 to 150 μm, and 150 to 200 μm dry diameter corresponding to 120 to 240 μm, 200 to 400 μm, 400 to 600 μm, and 600 to 800 μm hydrated diameters, respectively. Each 10-mL glass vial contains 25 mg of dry spheres corresponding to 815,000; 139,000; 28,100; and 9,400 spheres per vial, respectively. Up to 75 mg doxorubicin can be loaded into each vial of QuadraSpheres with a 60-minute loading time when loading with reconstituted powdered doxorubicin and a 120-minute loading time when loading with presolubilized doxorubicin. QuadraSpheres demonstrate a 10% diameter reduction when loaded with doxorubicin and less homogenous loading with both doxorubicin and irinotecan when compared to LC beads and show comparable doxorubicin release kinetics to LC beads in vitro. A 7-minute burst release of nearly 75% of bound irinotecan from the spheres is reported due to weaker drug–bead interaction. When loaded with doxorubicin, HepaSpheres become more fragile and prone to fracturing.[12]

Oncozene Beads

Oncozene beads are biocompatible, nonresorbable hydrogel microspheres, which are coated with an inorganic polyphosphazene polymer (Polyzene-F). These tightly calibrated beads are available in 40 ± 10-μm, 75 ± 15-μm, and 100 ± 25-μm diameter sizes and are supplied in 2- or 3-mL aliquots. The anionic sodium methacrylate backbone of the microsphere structure provides a site for loading of the positively charged doxorubicin or irinotecan molecule. Each milliliter of Oncozene beads can load 50 mg of doxorubicin or irinotecan and can be loaded in 60 minutes when loading with powdered doxorubicin and in 30 minutes when loading with irinotecan solution (20 mg/mL) with a 98% loading efficiency. When loaded with drug, Oncozene beads shrink in diameter by less than 5%. Both doxorubicin and irinotecan elute more slowly from Oncozene beads when compared to DC bead in vitro, which may further mitigate side effects of systemic drug exposure, especially with irinotecan, although further investigation is warranted.[13]

TECHNIQUE

To maximize loading of the chemotherapeutic drug onto the carrier bead, the corresponding manufacturer's guidelines ("instructions for use") must be followed. In general, a total of 25 mg of doxorubicin per milliliter of beads or 50 mg of irinotecan per milliliter of beads is loaded irrespective of the type of carrier bead, given the common indications for their use.

Loading of Drug-Eluting Beads

LC Beads

When loading LC beads with powdered doxorubicin, a 50-mg vial of doxorubicin is reconstituted with 2 mL of sterile water. After removing saline from the LC bead vial, the 2 mL of reconstituted doxorubicin is then added to the LC bead vial and the vial is occasionally agitated to encourage mixing. Loading time is up to 120 minutes for the largest LC bead size. When loading LC bead with irinotecan, solution (20 mg/mL) only should be used. After removing as much saline as possible from the LC bead vial, 5 mL of irinotecan solution is added to the vial and the vial is gently agitated to encourage mixing. A minimum 2-hour loading time is required for all bead sizes.

QuadraSpheres

QuadraSpheres may be loaded with powdered (lyophilized) or presolubilized doxorubicin. When loading with powdered doxorubicin, the 50 mg doxorubicin needs to be reconstituted with preservative-free 0.9% sodium chloride (not sterile water) and drawn into a 30-mL syringe. After rolling the QuadraSphere vial several times to disperse the microspheres, 10 mL of the reconstituted doxorubicin is injected into the vial, and the vial is rotated and inverted 5 to 10 times and then let stand for 10 minutes. The entire contents of the vial are then withdrawn into the remaining 10 mL of doxorubicin solution in the syringe and gently agitated to disperse the contents. The syringe is recapped and intermittently agitated, requiring an additional 60 minutes to complete loading of the drug onto the beads. After the 60 minutes, the supernatant can be discarded. A minimum of 20 mL of nonionic contrast is then added to the beads before delivery. If presolubilized doxorubicin (50 mg/25 mL) is being used to load the QuadraSpheres, the 25 mL of doxorubicin solution is drawn into a 30-mL syringe. After rolling the vial several times to disperse the microspheres, 10 mL of the doxorubicin solution is injected into the vial, and the vial is rotated and inverted 5 to 10 times and then let stand for 10 minutes. The entire contents of the vial is then withdrawn into the remaining 15 mL of doxorubicin solution in the syringe and gently mixed and agitated to disperse the contents. The syringe is recapped and intermittently agitated, requiring an additional 120 minutes to complete loading of the drug onto the beads. After the 120 minutes, the supernatant can be discarded. A minimum of 20 mL of nonionic contrast material is then added to the beads before delivery.

Oncozene Beads

When loading Oncozene beads with powdered doxorubicin, the desired amount of powdered doxorubicin is reconstituted in 5.0 mL of sterile water if preparing 2 mL of beads and in 7.5 mL of sterile water if preparing 3 mL of beads. After removing excess transport solution from the syringe of Oncozene beads using a filter needle, the drug is drawn into the microsphere syringe via sterile needle. The syringe is then inverted every 5 minutes for the first 30 minutes. Loading time is 30 minutes for irinotecan and 60 minutes for doxorubicin and epirubicin. Maximum dose is 50 mg/1 mL for each drug.

Delivery of Drug-Eluting Beads

Drug-eluting beads are routinely mixed with nonionic contrast material (10 to 20 mL per 1 mL of beads) for visualization of delivery of the beads to determine bead distribution and to monitor for change in flow dynamics as distal arterioles become occluded. There is no consensus on the end point of embolization. Some operators advocate complete stasis of tumor-feeding vessels (while preserving segmental and lobar arterial flow) during chemoembolization with drug-eluting beads (and supplementing with bland embolization to achieve stasis if drug-eluting beads fail to achieve complete stasis), whereas others avoid achieving complete stasis to prevent thrombosis of the feeding artery (in this method, drug-eluting beads are used as a method of drug delivery), thereby allowing for future repeat transarterial interventions. Efforts are typically made to be as selective as possible when performing chemoembolization for oligofocal hepatocellular carcinoma to maximize delivery of chemotherapy to the tumor while sparing uninvolved liver parenchyma. When diffuse multifocal disease is present, a lobar approach can be employed if liver function is preserved. In patients with metastatic disease, a lobar approach is commonly used given the widespread multifocal nature of metastases.

CLINICAL APPLICATIONS

Chemoembolization with drug-eluting beads loaded with doxorubicin (DEBDOX) are used for treatment of hepatocellular carcinoma, whereas the irinotecan beads (DEBIRI) are used for metastatic colon cancer. Other cancers such as intrahepatic cholangiocarcinoma, neuroendocrine metastases, and metastases from breast, choroid (uveal) melanoma, and pancreatic cancer are treated either with DEBDOX or DEBIRI.

Overall, DEBDOX is well tolerated, with significantly decreased incidence and severity of transaminitis and doxorubicin-related side effects compared to conventional chemoembolization. DEBDOX appears to be more efficacious and safer compared to conventional chemoembolization in patients with advanced disease (bilobar disease, recurrent disease, and in patients with Eastern Cooperative Oncology Group [ECOG] performance status of 1) (Table 8.1).[10,14–28] The reported objective response rates ranged from 50% to 100% (Fig. 8.1).[10,14–28] Except for one retrospective study that reported survival advantage of DEBDOX over conventional transarterial chemoembolization (cTACE),[17] DEBDOX appears to offer similar overall survival rates compared to that of cTACE. However, survival advantage, if any, of DEBDOX in advanced stage hepatocellular carcinoma is yet to be explored.

DEBIRI is well suited for treatment of colorectal metastases given the high sensitivity of colorectal carcinoma to irinotecan. The reported median survival following DEBIRI for colorectal hepatic metastases ranges from 15.2 months to 25 months (Table 8.2).[29–33] Drug-eluting beads loaded with oxaliplatin in combination with systemic chemotherapy have been used for treatment of intrahepatic cholangiocarcinoma with significantly better overall survival (30 months vs. 12.7 months) when compared to systemic chemotherapy alone.[34]

Nonhepatic applications of drug-eluting beads are being tested for treatment of peritoneal carcinomatosis through intraperitoneal delivery, for treatment of recurrent

Table 8.1 Clinical Results of DEBDOX for Hepatocellular Carcinoma

Publication	Type of Therapy	Patients	Efficacy	Safety
Prospective Randomized Controlled Studies				
Lammer et al.[14]	DEBDOX versus cTACE	93 (child A/B: 77/16) received DEBDOX and 108 (child A/B: 89/19) received cTACE	No difference in overall rates of objective response (51.6% vs. 43.5%), disease control (52.4% vs. 51.9%), and complete response (25.9% vs. 22.2%). Significantly better response in patients with child B, ECOG 1, and bilobar or recurrent disease.	Significantly lower elevation of AST and ALT with DEBDOX. Significantly lower incidence of doxorubicin-related liver toxicity with DEBDOX. Decreased incidence of serious adverse events with DEBDOX in sicker patients.
Sacco et al.[15]	DEBDOX versus cTACE	33 (child A/B: 29/4) received DEBDOX and 34 (child A/B: 25/9) received cTACE	100% tumor response (CR + PR) in both groups. No difference in PFS and OS.	Significantly higher elevation of ALT with cTACE
Malagari et al.[16]	DEBDOX versus TAE	41 (child A/B: 23/18) received DEBDOX and 43 (child A/B: 26/17) received TAE with Bead Block particles (Terumo, Tokyo, Japan)	EASL response rates (CR + PR) at 6 mo: 73% versus 56%; significantly longer TTP with DEBDOX (10.6 mo vs. 9.05 mo) and lower rates of recurrence at 12 mo (46% vs. 78%). Similar survival rates (85% vs. 86%) at 12 mo.	Similar rates of postembolization syndrome (80% vs. 81%)
Case Control Studies				
Dhanasekaran et al.[17]	DEBDOX versus cTACE	45 (child A/B/C: 22/11/12) received DEBDOX and 26 (child A/B/C: 11/11/4) received cTACE	Significantly better survival with DEBDOX. 1-y and 2-y survival: 58% and 48% versus 31% and 12%	Similar grade 5 clinical toxicities and death: 6.6% versus 7.8%
Ferrer Puchol et al.[18]	DEBDOX versus cTACE	47 received DEBDOX and 25 received cTACE	Similar median survival: 672 d versus 709 d	Significantly fewer immediate complications with DEBDOX
Nicolini et al.[19]	DEBDOX versus TAE	8 (child A/B: 5/3) received DEBDOX and 8 received TAE (child A/B: 6/2) with Embospheres (Merit Medical Systems, Inc., South Jordan, Utah)	100% radiologic necrosis: 89% versus 45%; 100% histologic necrosis: 77% versus 27%; no difference in tumor recurrence rates	No difference in complications
Guiu et al.[20]	DEBDOX versus cTACE	59 (142 sessions of DEBDOX) versus 29 (56 sessions of cTACE) patients		Biliary duct injury: 18% versus 2%; portal vein narrowing: 7.1 % versus 1.4%
DEBDOX Single Cohort Studies				
Varela et al.[10]	DEBDOX	27 patients, child A/B/C: 27/0/0	EASL response at 6 mo: 75%; 89% survival at 2 y	Hepatic abscess: 7%; death: 3.5%
Reyes et al.[21]	DEBDOX	20 patients, child A/B/C: 15/5/0	EASL response at 6 mo: 60%; 55% survival at 2 y	Postembolization syndrome: 6%; grade 3 transaminitis: 6%
Poon et al.[22]	DEBDOX	35 patients, child A/B/C: 35/0/0	EASL response at 6 mo: 70%	Treatment-related complications: 11.4%

Continued

Table 8.1 Clinical Results of DEBDOX for Hepatocellular Carcinoma *(continued)*				
Publication	Type of Therapy	Patients	Efficacy	Safety
DEBDOX Single Cohort Studies				
Malagari et al.[23]	DEBDOX	62 patients	EASL response at 6 mo: 81%; 91% survival at 2 y	Severe procedure-related complications: 3.2% (cholecystitis, n = 1; liver abscess, n = 1)
Martin et al.[24]	DEBDOX	118 patients, child A/B: 83/32	EASL response at 6 mo: 58%; 75% survival at 1 y	Liver dysfunction: 4% of treatments
Kalva et al.[25]	DEBDOX	54 patients, child A/B/C: 27/25/2	EASL response at 6 mo: 35%; 59% survival at 1 y	10% grade 3 transaminitis at 1 mo
Sousa et al.[26]	DEBDOX	47 patients	EASL response at 6 mo: 50%; 54% survival at 1 y	
Burrel et al.[27]	DEBDOX	104 patients, child A/B: 99/4	66% survival at 3 y	
Malagari et al.[28]	DEBDOX	237 patients		30-d mortality: 1.3%; abscess: 2.5%; irreversible liver failure: 1.7%; ascites/encephalopathy: 4.2%; cholecystitis 5.5%

DEBDOX, chemoembolization with drug-eluting beads loaded with doxorubicin; cTACE, conventional transarterial chemoembolization with lipoid and chemotherapeutic agents; ECOG, Eastern Cooperative Oncology Group; AST, aspartate aminotransferase; ALT, alanine aminotransferase; CR, complete response; PR, partial response; PFS, progression-free survival; OS, overall survival; TAE, transarterial embolization with bland particles; EASL, European Association of Study of Liver; TTP, time to tumor progression.

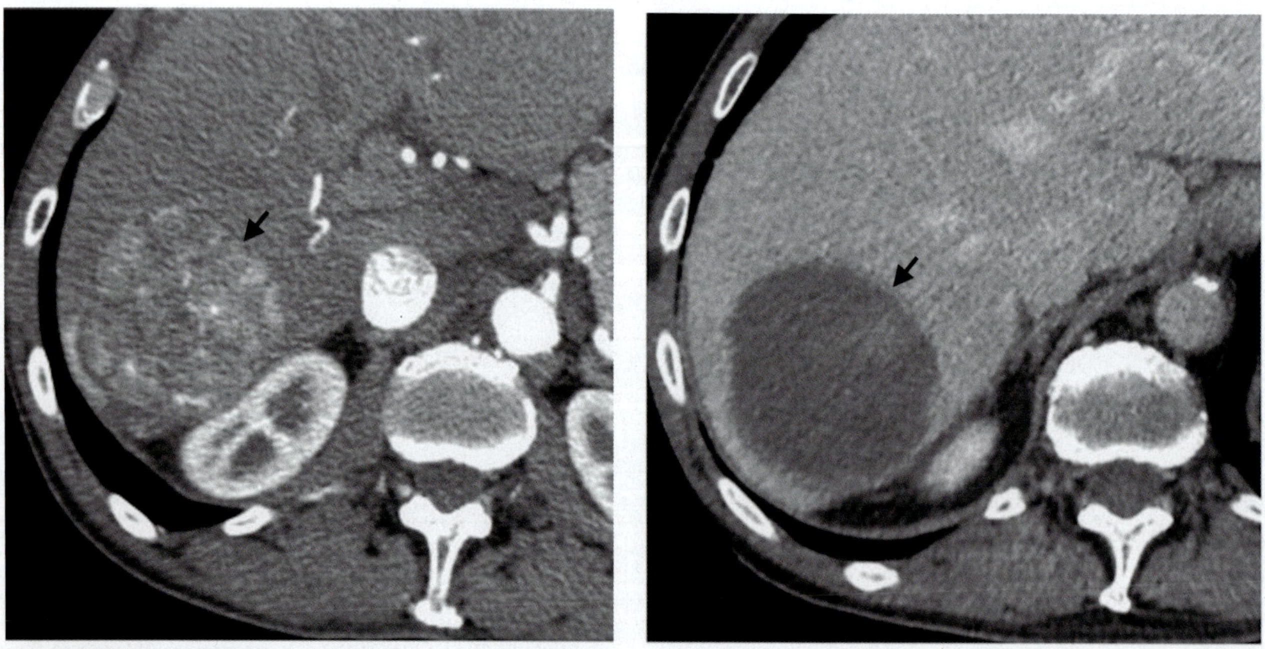

A B

Figure 8.1 **A:** Contrast-enhanced computed tomography demonstrates a hypervascular hepatocellular carcinoma (*arrow*) in the right lobe of the liver. **B:** Following chemoembolization with drug-eluting beads loaded with doxorubicin, there is near total necrosis (*arrow*) of the tumor with no enhancing residual tumor.

Table 8.2 DEBIRI for Colorectal Hepatic Metastases

Publication	Treatment	Patients	Efficacy	Safety
Martin et al.[29]	DEBIRI with LC beads	10 patients, no prior chemotherapy	Median survival: 15.2 mo	1 grade 3 hypertension
Vogl et al.[30]	Starch microspheres with irinotecan and mitomycin	77 patients, all received prior systemic oxaliplatin	Median survival: 22.5 mo	No grade 3/4 toxicities
Martin et al.[31]	DEBIRI with LC beads	55 patients; 17 patients received FOLFOX + bevacizumab alone, 14 received FOLFOX and bevacizumab, FOLFIRI cetuximab	Median survival: 19 mo	Grade 3 or more toxicities in 7 patients
Aliberti et al.[32]	DEBIRI with LC beads	82 patients, all received ≥2 systemic chemotherapy regimens	Median survival: 25 mo	Grade 3 pain in 20 patients
Fiorentini et al.[33]	DEBIRI with LC beads	36 patients, all received ≥2/3 systemic chemotherapy regimens		Grade 2/3 pain in 30%; vomiting: 25%; asthenia: 20%

DEBIRI, chemoembolization with drug-eluting beads loaded with irinotecan; FOLFOX, 5-fluorouracil, leucovorin, oxaliplatin; FOLFIRI, 5-fluorouracil, leucovorin, irinotecan.

glioblastoma by direct injections of drug-eluting beads suspension in to the resection cavity, and transarterial therapy of pancreatic cancer.[3]

POTENTIAL COMPLICATIONS

Complications associated with DEBDOX and DEBIRI are similar to those encountered with conventional chemoembolization. Many studies have reported a lower incidence of transaminitis following DEBDOX.[10,14–25] One study reported a higher incidence of biliary complications with the use of drug-eluting beads.[20] The incidence of liver failure, abscess, cholecystitis, and nontarget embolization are similar to those encountered with conventional chemoembolization.[28] Intraprocedural pain and hypertension appear to be very common with DEBIRI, possibly related to burst release of 10% to 20% of the drug during delivery of the beads.[30–34]

TIPS AND TRICKS

Tips

- Smaller beads are more effective in causing tumor necrosis.
- Preparation of beads: Authors mix 1 mL of beads with 20 mL of contrast material and saline mixture (50:50 dilution) and embolize the tumor using 0.5–1 mL aliquots of this mixture per 30 s.
- A well-demarcated contrast material accumulation in the tumor on fluoroscopy is a good end point of embolization.
- Superselective embolization is key to achieve good tumor necrosis and to avoid liver dysfunction.
- Concomitant use of biologic agents is not a contraindication for chemoembolization.

Tricks

- All drug-eluting beads do not behave the same way. Follow the manufacturer's guidelines when loading drugs. Some beads have more favorable pharmacokinetic profile than others with certain drugs.
- Use appropriate-sized microcatheters for delivery of the beads.

CONCLUSIONS

Drug-eluting beads represent a new paradigm shift in the way transarterial drug delivery and vascular occlusion is applied for treatment of hepatic tumors. Therapy with drug-eluting beads appears to be safe and superior to conventional chemoembolization for hepatocellular carcinoma in sicker patients and in patients with advanced disease. The role of drug-eluting beads in the management of hepatic metastases is still evolving.

REFERENCES

1. Lewis AL. Drug eluting beads in the treatment of liver cancer. In: Lewis AL, ed. *Drug-Device Combination Products Delivery Technologies and Applications*. Cambridge, United Kingdom: Woodhead Publishing; 2010:154–189.
2. Lewis AL, Gonzalez MV, Lloyd AW, et al. DC bead: in vitro and in vivo characterization of a drug-delivery device for transarterial chemoembolization. *J Vasc Interv Radiol*. 2006;17:335–342.
3. Lewis AL, Dreher MR. Locoregional drug delivery using image-guided intra-arterial drug eluting bead therapy. *J Control Release*. 2012;16:338–350.

4. Lewis AL, Gonzalez MV, Leppard SW, et al. Doxorubicin eluting beads -1: effects of drug loading on bead characteristics and drug distribution. *J Mater Sci Mater Med.* 2007;18:1691–1699.
5. Taylor RR, Tang Y, Gonzalez MV, et al. Irinotecan drug eluting beads for use in chemoembolization: in vitro and in vivo evaluation of drug release properties. *Eur J Phram Sci.* 2007;30:7–14.
6. Liapi E, Lee KH, Georgiades CC, et al. Drug-eluting particles for interventional pharmacology. *Tech Vasc Interv Radiol.* 2007;10:261–269.
7. Gonzales MV, Tang Y, Phillips GJ, et al. Doxorubicin eluting beads 2: methods for evaluating drug elution and in vitro:in vivo correlation. *J Mater Sci Mater Med.* 2008;19:767–775.
8. Kaiser J, Thiesen J, Kramer I. Stability of irinotecan-loaded drug eluting beads (DC bead) used for trans-arterial chemoembolization. *J Oncol Pharm Pract.* 2010;16:53–61.
9. Hong K, Khwaja A, Liapi E, et al. New intra-arterial drug delivery system for the treatment of liver cancer: preclinical assessment in a rabbit model of liver cancer. *Clin Cancer Res.* 2006;12:2563–2567.
10. Varela M, Real MI, Burrel M, et al. Chemoembolization of hepatocellular carcinoma with drug eluting beads: efficacy and doxorubicin pharmacokinetics. *J Hepatol.* 2007;46:474–481.
11. Namur J, Citron SJ, Sellers MT, et al. Embolization of hepatocellular carcinoma with drug-eluting beads: doxorubicin tissue concentration and distribution in patient liver explants. *J Hepatol.* 2011;55:1332–1338.
12. Jordan O, Denys A, De Baere T, et al. Comparative study of chemoembolization loadable beads: in vitro drug release and physical properties of DC bead and hepasphere loaded with doxorubicin and irinotecan. *J Vasc Interv Radiol.* 2010;21:1084–1090.
13. Blummel J, Reinhardt S, Schäfer M, et al. Drug-eluting beads in the treatment of hepatocellular carcinoma and colorectal cancer metastases to the liver. *Eur Oncol Haematol.* 2012;8:162–166.
14. Lammer J, Malagari K, Vogl T, et al; PRECISION V Investigators. Prospective randomized study of doxorubicin-eluting-bead embolization in the treatment of hepatocellular carcinoma: results of the PRECISION V study. *Cardiovasc Intervent Radiol.* 2010;33:41–52.
15. Sacco R, Bargellini I, Bertini M, et al. Conventional versus doxorubicin-eluting bead transarterial chemoembolization for hepatocellular carcinoma. *J Vasc Interv Radiol.* 2011;22: 1545–1552.
16. Malagari K, Pomoni M, Kelekis A, et al. Prospective randomized comparison of chemoembolization with doxorubicin-eluting beads and bland embolization with BeadBlock for hepatocellular carcinoma. *Cardiovasc Intervent Radiol.* 2010;33:541–551.
17. Dhanasekaran R, Kooby DA, Staley CA, et al. Comparison of conventional transarterial chemoembolization (TACE) and chemoembolization with doxorubicin drug eluting beads (DEB) for unresectable hepatocelluar carcinoma (HCC). *J Surg Oncol.* 2010;101:476–480.
18. Ferrer Puchol MD, la Parra C, Esteban E, et al. Comparison of doxorubicin-eluting bead transarterial chemoembolization (DEB-TACE) with conventional transarterial chemoembolization (TACE) for the treatment of hepatocellular carcinoma [in Spanish]. *Radiologia.* 2011;53:246–253.
19. Nicolini A, Martinetti L, Crespi S, et al. Transarterial chemoembolization with epirubicin-eluting beads versus transarterial embolization before liver transplantation for hepatocellular carcinoma. *J Vasc Interv Radiol.* 2010;21:327–332.
20. Guiu B, Deschamps F, Aho S, et al. Liver/biliary injuries following chemoembolisation of endocrine tumours and hepatocellular carcinoma: lipiodol vs. drug-eluting beads. *J Hepatol.* 2012;56:609–617.
21. Reyes DK, Vossen JA, Kamel IR, et al. Single-center phase II trial of transarterial chemoembolization with drug-eluting beads for patients with unresectable hepatocellular carcinoma: initial experience in the United States. *Cancer J.* 2009;15:526–532.
22. Poon RT, Tso WK, Pang RW, et al. A phase I/II trial of chemoembolization for hepatocellular carcinoma using a novel intra-arterial drug-eluting bead. *Clin Gastroenterol Hepatol.* 2007;5:1100–1108.
23. Malagari K, Chatzimichael K, Alexopoulou E, et al. Transarterial chemoembolization of unresectable hepatocellular carcinoma with drug eluting beads: results of an open-label study of 62 patients. *Cardiovasc Intervent Radiol.* 2008;31:269–280.
24. Martin RC II, Rustein L, Pin L, et al. Hepatic arterial infusion of doxorubicin-loaded microsphere for treatment of hepatocellular cancer: a multi-institutional registry. *J Am Coll Surg.* 2011;213:493–500.
25. Kalva SP, Iqbal SI, Yeddula K, et al. Transarterial chemoembolization with doxorubicin-eluting microspheres for inoperable hepatocellular carcinoma. *Gastrointest Cancer Res.* 2011;4:2–8.
26. Sousa PF, Preto AS, Leão D, et al. Transcatheter arterial chemoembolization with doxorubicin eluting beads in the treatment of hepatocellular carcinoma. *Acta Med Port.* 2011;24:29–36.
27. Burrel M, Reig M, Forner A, et al. Survival of patients with hepatocellular carcinoma treated by transarterial chemoembolisation (TACE) using drug eluting beads. Implications for clinical practice and trial design. *J Hepatol.* 2012;56:1330–1335.
28. Malagari K, Pomoni M, Spyridopoulos TN, et al. Safety profile of sequential transcatheter chemoembolization with DC Bead™: results of 237 hepatocellular carcinoma (HCC) patients. *Cardiovasc Intervent Radiol.* 2011;34:774–785.
29. Martin RC II, Scoggins CR, Tomalty D, et al. Irinotecan drug-eluting colorectal liver metastasis with concomitant systemic fluorouracil and oxaliplatin: results of pharmacokinetics and phase I trial. *J Gastrointest Surg.* 2012;16:1531–1538.
30. Vogl TJ, Jost A, Nour-Eldin NA, et al. Repeated transarterial chemoembolisation using different chemotherapeutic drug combinations followed by MR-guided laser-induced thermotherapy in patients with liver metastases of colorectal carcinoma. *Br J Cancer.* 2012;106:1274–1279.
31. Martin RC, Joshi J, Robbins K, et al. Hepatic intra-arterial injection of drug-eluting bead, irinotecan (DEBIRI) in unresectable colorectal liver metastases refractory to systemic chemotherapy: results of multi-institutional study. *Ann Surg Oncol.* 2011;18:192–198.
32. Aliberti C, Fiorentini G, Muzzio PC, et al. Trans-arterial chemoembolization of metastatic colorectal carcinoma to the liver adopting DC Bead®, drug-eluting bead loaded with irinotecan: results of a phase II clinical study. *Anticancer Res.* 2011;31(12):4581–4587.
33. Fiorentini G, Aliberti C, Tilli M, et al. Intra-arterial infusion of irinotecan-loaded drug-eluting beads (DEBIRI) versus intravenous therapy (FOLFIRI) for hepatic metastases from colorectal cancer: final results of a phase III study. *Anticancer Res.* 2012;32: 1387–1395.
34. Poggi G, Amatu A, Montagna B, et al. OEM-TACE: a new therapeutic approach in unresectable intrahepatic cholangiocarcinoma. *Cardiovasc Intervent Radiol.* 2009;32:1187–1192.

Section D Liquid Agents

9

Glue

Yasuaki Arai

Ardis first described the synthesis of cyanoacrylates in 1949,[1] and since that time, its use for applications such as wound closure, skin grafts, and organ anastomoses has been investigated.[2,3] *N*-butyl cyanoacrylate (NBCA) has been used since the 1980s as a liquid embolic material, mainly for neurointerventional indications; it was approved in the United States by the U.S. Food and Drug Administration for use in cerebral arteriovenous malformations in 2000. Since that time, its use in the periphery has grown significantly. Presently, glue is one of the most important and indispensable embolic materials in interventional radiology. NBCA is approved as a medical device in most countries, but its approval for embolization varies from country to country. Therefore, it is often used off-label for embolization.

DEVICE DESCRIPTION

NBCA is a liquid embolic agent that consists of a two-carbon ethylene molecule with a cyano group and an ester (carbonyl group) attached to one of the carbons; the ester in NBCA is attached to an *N*-butyl hydrocarbon.[4,5] Polymerization occurs upon contact with any ionic substances (e.g., blood, saline, ionic contrast media, and vessel endothelium) due to bonding of the ethylene units after exposure to an anion (such as a hydroxyl group).[1] Because of this mechanism, NBCA is able to flow through the vasculature to the target lesion as a liquid but leads to embolization once it polymerizes and becomes solid.

Once administered, the polymerization process causes the release of formaldehyde, which can contribute to the toxicity of NBCA. The extent of the toxicity depends on the size of the side chain ester; NBCA is less toxic than methyl and ethyl cyanoacrylates.[6] Embolization with NBCA leads to an acute inflammatory response in the vessel wall and surrounding tissue.[1] With time, this leads to a chronic granulomatous inflammatory process.[7–9]

TECHNIQUE

To use NBCA appropriately as an embolic agent in interventional procedures, there are two points to keep in mind: visualization under image guidance and control of the polymerization time. Both of these points can be addressed with the use of iodized oil (Lipiodol), which can be mixed with NBCA at any ratio to make it visible under fluoroscopy and to increase its polymerization time and viscosity (Figs. 9.1 and 9.2).[10] The dilution rate is usually 10% to 50% (NBCA/Lipiodol) for most clinical indications.

The viscosity of the NBCA–Lipiodol mixture becomes higher upon contact with blood and endothelium in vessels. This ultimately leads to vascular occlusion once blood flow cannot push the mixture due to its high viscosity. This mechanism of embolization is different when compared with materials such as microspheres, polyvinyl alcohol (PVA), and gelatin sponge, which typically occlude vessels at a level within the vasculature, which matches the size of the embolic agent. An NBCA–Lipiodol mixture also stops at the point of branching vessels once the mixture cannot get into smaller vessels due to its high viscosity. Therefore, high-concentration NBCA–Lipiodol mixtures with a dilution rate of 40% to 50% can be used for proximal embolization. Dilution rates of 10% to 20% can be used to embolize

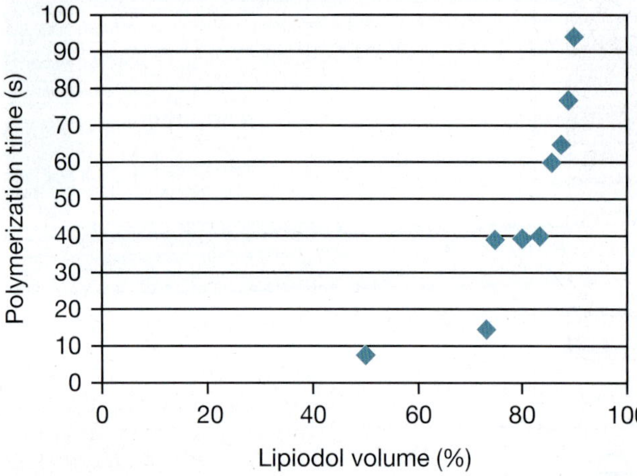

Figure 9.1 The polymerization time of NBCA–Lipiodol increases with the Lipiodol volume. Polymerization times were similar between ratios 1:1 and 1:2 and also between ratios 1:3 and 1:5. The times increased exponentially, however, in ratios 1:6 and 1:9. (Courtesy of Prof. Yasuao Nakajima, St. Marianna University School of Medicine, Kawasaki, Kanagawa, Japan.)

long and branching vessels (Fig. 9.3). However, when compared with particles measuring 100 to 500 μm in diameter, an NBCA–Lipiodol mixture leads to a more proximal embolization.

When preparing the mixture of NBCA and Lipiodol, attention is required to avoid any contact between NBCA and Lipiodol and any ionic substance.[5] The author always aspirates NBCA from the NBCA ampule directly into a new syringe with a new needle and then aspirates the desired volume of Lipiodol into the same syringe. If a high-diluted NBCA–Lipiodol is to be prepared, a second Lipiodol-containing syringe should be prepared, and both should be mixed to obtain the target dilution rate for the NBCA–Lipiodol mixture (Fig. 9.4). To avoid polymerization, the NBCA–Lipiodol mixture should not be allowed to be in contact with room air for long period. The syringe containing the NBCA–Lipiodol mixture should therefore be capped at all times. The author usually uses the mixture within 10 minutes after preparation.

When injecting the NBCA–Lipiodol mixture, a coaxial catheter system must be used because it is difficult to control the injection with a larger lumen catheter. When the coaxial microcatheter tip reaches the target point, a test injection of contrast is performed to confirm the position of catheter tip and to assess blood flow. The catheter is then flushed with a 5% glucose solution to clear all contrast from the inner lumen.[5,11] This is an important step in the use of NBCA because it is difficult to distinguish the NBCA–Lipiodol

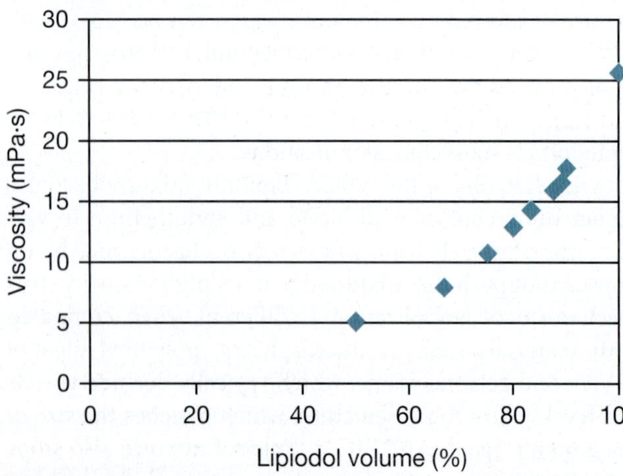

Figure 9.2 There is a linear correlation between the NBCA–Lipiodol viscosity in relation with Lipiodol volume. (Courtesy of Prof. Yasuao Nakajima, St. Marianna University School of Medicine, Kawasaki, Kanagawa, Japan.)

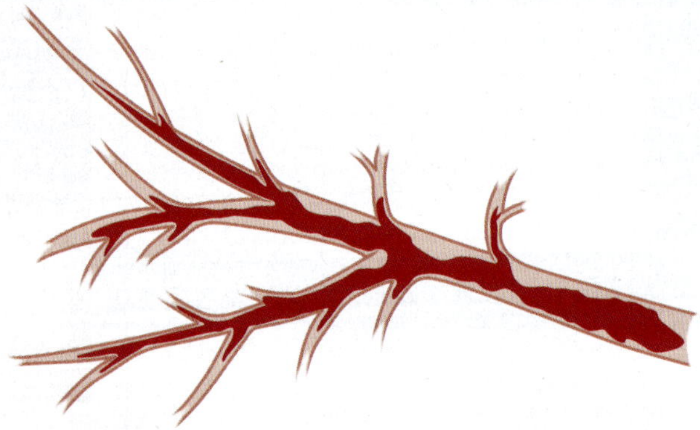

Figure 9.3 Schema of embolization with low-concentration NBCA–Lipiodol mixture.

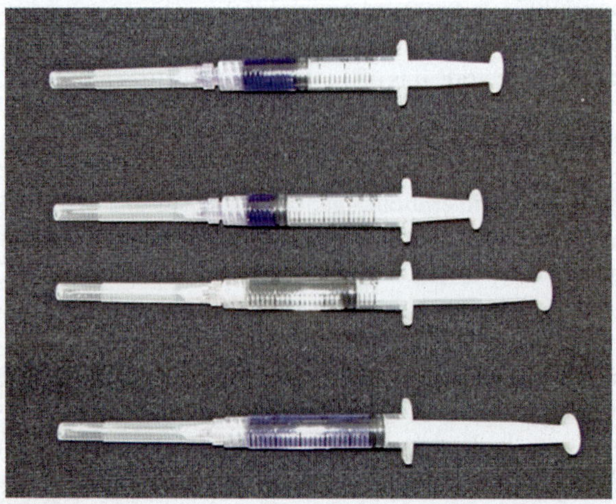

Figure 9.4 Preparation of NBCA–Lipiodol mixture. *Top:* 50% NBCA–Lipiodol mixture 1 mL (0.5 mL NBCA + 0.5 mL Lipiodol). *Center:* 50% NBCA–Lipiodol mixture 0.5 mL and Lipiodol 2 mL (before mixture). *Bottom:* 10% NBCA–Lipiodol mixture 2.5 mL.

mixture from contrast under fluoroscopy. Clearing the contrast from the catheter after the test injection allows the operator to confirm when NBCA is being administered. Three seconds after an optimal amount of NBCA–Lipiodol has been injected, the microcatheter should be removed to minimize the risk that the tip of the catheter will adhere to the vessel wall. A small amount of time is needed because if the catheter is removed too quickly, the risk of backflow of unpolymerized NBCA can occur due to the negative pressure caused by catheter removal. If the intent of the procedure is to inject a fixed amount of NBCA–Lipiodol mixture, it is possible to push the mixture with 5% glucose. Following embolization, the microcatheter should be disposed of immediately because the polymerized NBCA–Lipiodol mixture may remain in the lumen of the catheter. It may be possible to flush the catheter with sufficient volume of Lipiodol and 5% glucose if necessary.[11] If a guidewire can be passed without any resistance after flushing, the author sometimes uses the same microcatheter system.

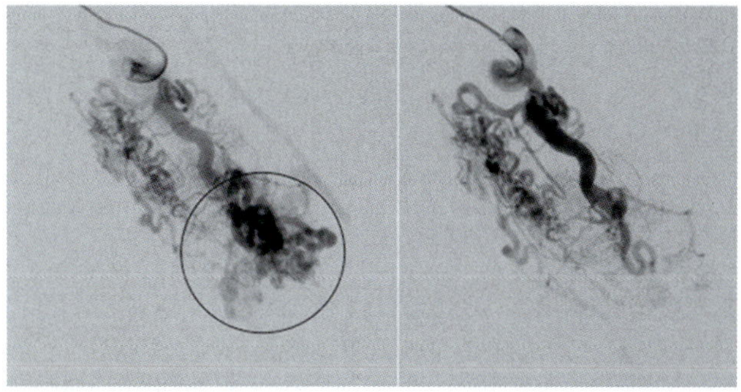

Figure 9.6 Embolization of arteriovenous malformation (AVM) (*circle* in **A**) with NBCA–Lipiodol mixture. Digital Subtraction Angiography (DSA) was supplied via the intercostal artery. **B:** After embolization, AVM findings have disappeared. (Courtesy of Dr. Keigo Osuga, Osaka University, Japan.)

CLINICAL APPLICATIONS

Based on its special features, the use of NBCA as an embolic agent is theoretically indicated for the following three situations. First, it is optimal to occlude a vessel with multiple branches or communications to other vessels. For example, NBCA can be used to embolize atypical vessels responsible for the arterial supply to liver tumors, such as the inferior phrenic artery. The inferior phrenic artery is rather long and has many communications with other arteries (e.g., intercostal arteries, internal mammary artery, etc.). Given the potential territory supplied by this vessel, NBCA is an effective agent to use for embolization in this situation (Fig. 9.5). For this reason, NBCA is a commonly used agent for the treatment of arteriovenous malformations (Fig. 9.6).[12] Second, NBCA is used to occlude target vessels when the catheter position is unstable. Catheter stability is very important when using coils for embolization because catheters are under tension when coils are being introduced. If a coil is inserted through a catheter with an unstable position, the catheter tip may move back and forth, which can lead to coil migration into an unexpected or undesired location. Instead of coils, NBCA–Lipiodol mixture can be used in this scenario because it comes out of the catheter in a few seconds. This may often be the case when embolizing a right gastric artery for the purpose of redistribution for hepatic infusion chemotherapy and yttrium 90 infusion (Fig. 9.7),[13] portal vein branches for preoperative portal vein

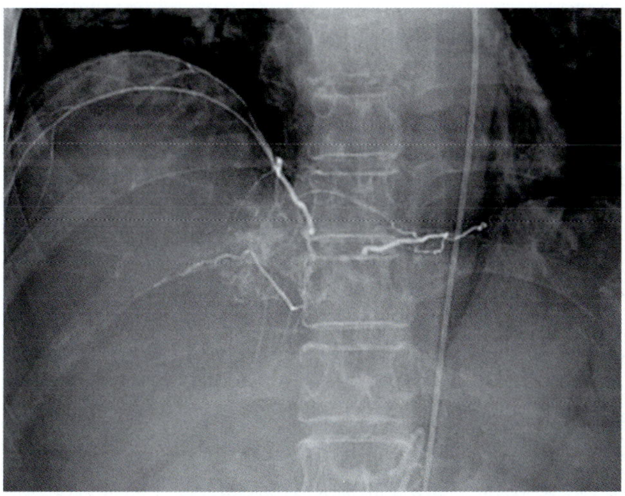

Figure 9.5 Embolization of right inferior phrenic artery with low-concentration (10%) NBCA–Lipiodol mixture.

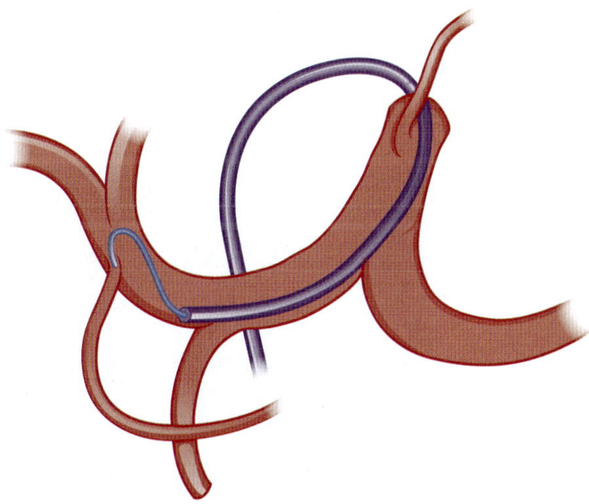

Figure 9.7 Embolization of the right gastric artery with NBCA–Lipiodol mixture via an unstable microcatheter tip. When embolization with coils is impossible because of unstable catheter tip, embolization with NBCA–Lipiodol mixture is possible.

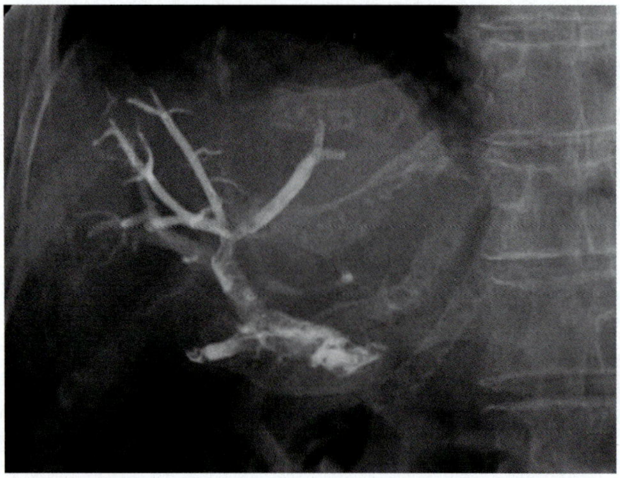

Figure 9.8 Portal vein embolization with NBCA–Lipiodol mixture.

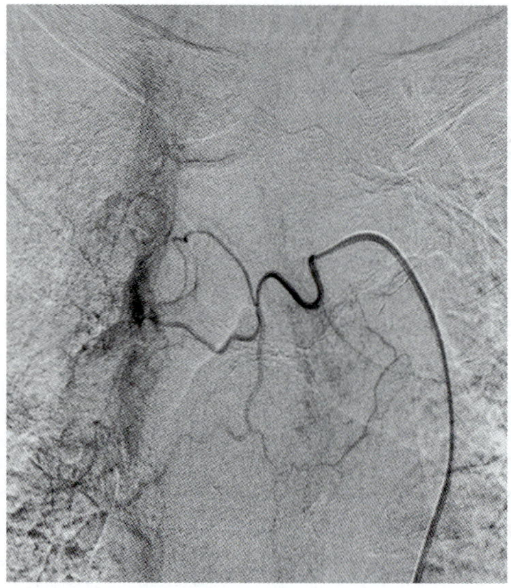

Figure 9.9 Embolization with NBCA–Lipiodol mixture via unstable catheter. The right bronchial arteriogram in a case with hemoptysis. However, the catheter tip was very unstable, and only the tip of the microcatheter could be inserted into the orifice of the right brachial artery. Fifteen percent NBCA–Lipiodol mixture was infused via this unstable microcatheter, and this artery was successfully embolized.

embolization (Fig. 9.8),[14–16] or a bronchial artery in patients with hemoptysis (Fig. 9.9).[17] NBCA has also been shown to be an effective agent to treat gastrointestinal bleeding.[18] Third, NBCA–Lipiodol can potentially be a more effective embolic agent than coils or particles in coagulopathic patients.[19,20] Coils and particles rely on normal coagulation for vessel occlusion. Therefore, if a patient with bleeding is coagulopathic, coils or particles may not help to stop the bleeding. However, NBCA mixture can mechanically occupy the intravascular lumen and stop blood flow regardless of blood coagulability.

An NBCA–Lipiodol mixture can be also used for nonvascular applications. This mixture is suitable for tract embolization to avoid bleeding from the tract of blood-rich organ. This may be done in association with percutaneous biopsy or ablation procedures. The author usually uses NBCA–Lipiodol mixture after the transsplenic interventions to prevent bleeding from the spleen (Fig. 9.10).

POTENTIAL COMPLICATIONS

Rosen and Contractor[1] defined the complications of NBCA administration as either being associated with the actual administration of the liquid agent or being associated with the anatomy of the target vasculature. More specifically, this can include occlusion of normal territory due to misinterpretation of anatomy, distal migration or reflux of embolic material, or artery-to-artery anastomoses; migration of embolic material to the venous side of the target vascular bed; and catheter gluing.[21]

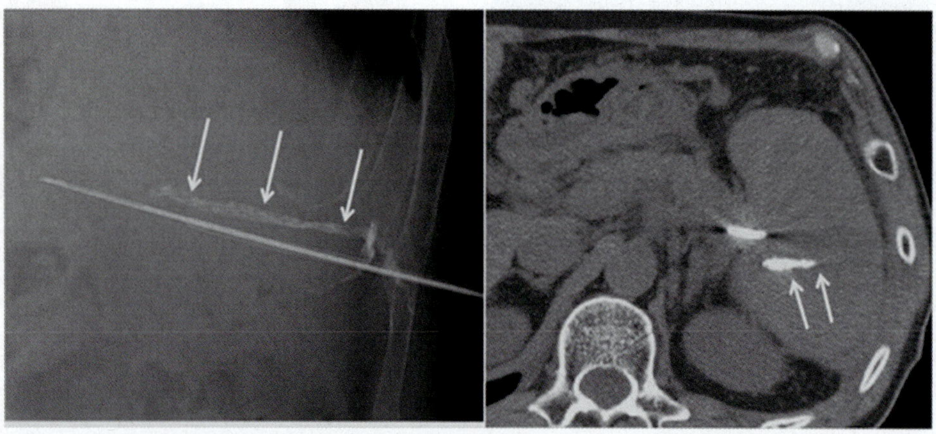

A B

Figure 9.10 **A,B:** Tract embolization with NBCA–Lipiodol mixture to avoid bleeding in transsplenic biopsy to the pancreas tumor. NBCA–Lipiodol mixture with a dilution rate of 40% was used (*arrows*) for this tract embolization.

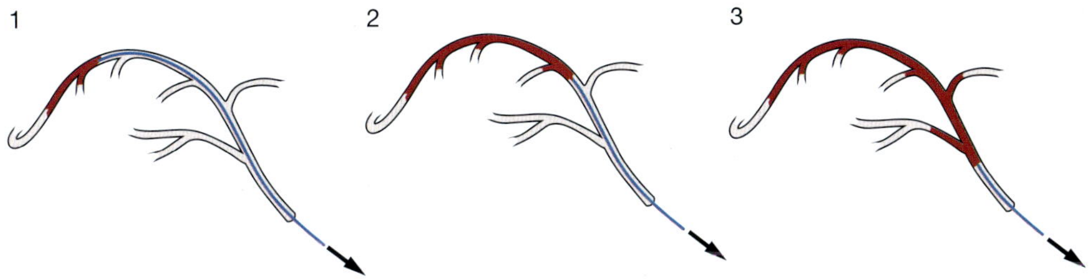

Figure 9.11 Technique to embolize the entire vessel with multiple branches or communications with other vessels. Inject low-concentration NBCA–Lipiodol mixture (10% to 15%) while pulling back the microcatheter from the distal portion to the proximal portion.

Migration of embolic material to the venous side of a malformation can potentially lead to venous hypertension or pulmonary emboli. Given the fact that close fluoroscopic monitoring is typically employed during an NBCA embolization, the likelihood of a large volume of material passing into the pulmonary circulation is low. Therefore, this complication is not typically clinically significant.[22]

The gluing of the delivery catheter to the vessel wall is a rare phenomenon that can be minimized with the use of hydrophilic microcatheters and NBCA at lower concentrations. It is often due to reflux of NBCA during embolization, early polymerization, or a failure to retract the microcatheter in an appropriate amount of time.[5] In general, a quick tug on the microcatheter is often able to separate a microcatheter from a glue cast due to the relatively low tensile strength of the polymerized NBCA.[1]

TIPS AND TRICKS

- There are two colors of NBCA available. One is blue and the other is clear. When using the clear NBCA, it is important to label the syringe to prevent it from being confused with contrast or saline.
- To avoid undesirable distribution of an NBCA–Lipiodol mixture, coils can be deployed in vessels which require protection before NBCA administration (see Fig. 9.10).
- To embolize a long vessel with NBCA, optimal embolization can be obtained by pulling back the microcatheter from the distal to the proximal portion of the vessel during injection (Fig. 9.11). Using this technique, a vessel with multiple branches or communications to other vessels can be entirely occluded.

SUMMARY

NBCA is a very useful embolic agent for interventional radiologists in various clinical applications. Its mechanism of embolization is different from that of other materials, and there are many technical steps required for the appropriate handling and administration of NBCA. Acquiring sufficient knowledge and skills of controlling this unique embolic agent will allow for its successful use.

REFERENCES

1. Rosen RJ, Contractor S. The use of cyanoacrylate adhesives in the management of congenital vascular malformations. *Semin Intervent Radiol.* 2004;21:59–66.
2. Galil KA, Schonfield ID, Wright GZ. Effect of butyl 2-cyanoacrylate on the healing of skin wounds. *J Can Dent Assoc.* 1984;50:565–569.
3. Petrella E, Orlandini G, Poisetti P, et al. A new end to side anastomosis formed without sutures for hemodialysis fistulas. *Nephron.* 1975;14:398–400.
4. Kerber CW, Wong W. Liquid acrylic adhesive agents in interventional neuroradiology. *Neurosurg Clin N Am.* 2000;11:85–99.
5. Pollak JS, White RI. The use of cyanoacrylate adhesives in peripheral embolization. *J Vasc Interv Radiol.* 2001;12:907–913.
6. Schweitzer JS, Chang BS, Madsen P, et al. The pathology of arteriovenous malformations of the brain treated by embolotherapy. *Neuroradiology.* 1993;35:468–474.
7. Brothers MF, Kaufman JC, Fox AJ, et al. N-butyl 2-cyanoacrylate substitute for IBCA in interventional neuroradiology: histopathological and polymerization time studies. *Am J Neuroradiol.* 1989;10:777–786.
8. White RI, Strandberg JV, Gross GS, et al. Therapeutic embolization with long-term occluding agents and their effects on embolized tissues. *Radiology.* 1977;125:677–687.
9. Vinters HV, Galil KA, Lundie MJ, et al. The histotoxicity of cyanoacrylates: a selective review. *Neuroradiology.* 1985;27:279–291.
10. Takasawa C, Seiji K, Matsunaga K, et al. Properties of N-butyl cyanoacrylate-iodized oil mixtures for arterial embolization: in vitro and in vivo experiments. *J Vasc Interv Radiol.* 2012;23:1215–1221.
11. Moore C, Murphy K, Gailloud P. Improved distal distribution of n-butyl cyanoacrylate glue by simultaneous injection of dextrose 5% through the guiding catheter: technical note. *Neuroradiology.* 2006;48:327–332.
12. Lee BB, Do YS, Yakes W, et al. Management of arteriovenous malformations: a multidisciplinary approach. *J Vasc Surg.* 2004;39:590–600.

13. Arai Y, Takeuchi Y, Inaba Y, et al. Percutaneous catheter placement for hepatic arterial infusion chemotherapy. *Tech Vasc Interv Radiol.* 2007;10:30–37.
14. De Baere T, Denys A, Paradis V. Comparison of four embolic materials for portal vein embolization: experimental study in pigs. *Eur Radiol.* 2009;19:1435–1442.
15. Denys A, Lacombe C, Schneider F, et al. Portal vein embolization with N-butyl cyanoacrylate before partial hepatectomy in patients with hepatocellular carcinoma and underlying cirrhosis or advanced fibrosis. *J Vasc Interv Radiol.* 2005;16(12):1667–1674.
16. Guiu B, Bize P, Gunthern D, et al. Portal vein embolization before right hepatectomy: improved results using n-butyl-cyanoacrylate compared to microparticles plus coils. *Cardiovasc Intervent Radiol.* 2013;36:1306–1312.
17. Razavi MK, Murphy K. Embolization of bronchial arteries with n-butyl cyanoacrylate for management of massive hemoptysis: a technical review. *Tech Vasc Interv Radiol.* 2007;10:276–282.
18. Yata S, Ihava T, Kaminou T, et al. Transcatheter arterial embolization of acute arterial bleeding in the upper and lower gastrointestinal tract with n-butyl 2-cyanoacrylate. *J Vasc Interv Radiol.* 2013;24:422–431.
19. Yonemitsu T, Kawai N, Sato M, et al. Comparison of hemostatic durability between n-butyl cyanoacrylate and gelatin sponge particles in transcatheter arterial embolization for acute arterial hemorrhage in a coagulopathic condition in a swine model. *Cardiovasc Intervent Radiol.* 2010;33;1192–1197.
20. Yonemitsu T, Kawai N, Sato M, et al. Evaluation of transcatheter arterial embolization with gelatin sponge particles, microcoils, and n-butyl cyanoacrylate for acute arterial bleeding in a coagulopathic condition. *J Vasc Interv Radiol.* 2009;20:1176–1187.
21. Niimi Y, Berenstein A, Setton A. Complications and their management during NBCA embolization of craniospinal lesions. *Int Neuroradiol.* 2003;9(suppl 1):157–164.
22. Pelz DM, Lownie SP, Fox AJ, et al. Symptomatic pulmonary complications from liquid acrylate embolization of brain arteriovenous malformations. *Am J Neuroradiol.* 1997;16:19–26.

10

EVOH/DMSO in Peripheral Application

Ricardo Yamada • Andre Uflacker • Austin Bourgeois
Joshua D. Adams • Marcelo Guimaraes

Onyx (Covidien, Irvine, California) was initially manufactured as a dialysis matrix for separating immunoglobulin from albumin and then as a matrix for controlled release of chemotherapeutics.[1] However, it was also found to have embolic properties, and its clinical use for this purpose was first described in 1990 for embolization of intracranial arteriovenous malformation (AVM).[2]

At that time, Onyx showed promising results, overcoming the drawbacks of cyanoacrylate, a well-known embolic liquid agent commonly used for the same purpose. The lack of adhesiveness and slow copolymerization rate permit more distal nidus embolization, sometimes including the proximal venous outflow, without significant risk of microcatheter entrapment. After several studies, including a multicenter randomized trial comparing Onyx and cyanoacrylate, in July 2005, the U.S. Food and Drug Administration approved its use for intracranial AVM embolization.[3] European device approval (CE marking) preceded that in the United States by approximately 5 years for embolization of AVMs and intracranial aneurysms as well. Since then, given the safety and effectiveness of Onyx in the intracranial vasculature, use on peripheral organs has been described and successfully applied. Nowadays, it has been used mainly for the treatment of peripheral AVMs and abdominal aorta stent graft–related endoleaks.[4–7] In addition, Adamus et al.[8] published a series of cases describing 23 patients in whom Onyx embolization was successfully performed, including treatment of the renal, hepatic, iliac, and bronchial arteries and esophageal varices. The authors concluded that Onyx offers advantages over other embolic agents due to good controllability and faster vessel occlusion.[8]

DEVICE/MATERIAL DESCRIPTION

Onyx is a liquid permanent embolic agent composed of ethylene vinyl alcohol (EVOH) copolymer dissolved in dimethyl sulfoxide (DMSO) and micronized tantalum powder. The latter provides contrast for fluoroscopic visualization. The nonadhesive and viscous properties make it a unique agent, mostly differing from the other two known liquid embolic agents—glue and dehydrated alcohol. Its nonadhesive characteristic significantly decreases the risk of microcatheter entrapment, compared to glue (Table 10.1). The higher viscosity allows controlled deployment, which is extremely difficult to achieve with dehydrated alcohol.

The Onyx package includes three 1-mL delivery syringes, two labeled for Onyx use (white plunger) and one for DMSO (yellow plunger); one 1.5-mL vial of Onyx; and one 1.5-mL vial of DMSO (Fig. 10.1). The Onyx white plunger syringe has lower friction compared to the DMSO yellow one, which gives better control while the agent is being injected. DMSO is a solvent and is used to wash out the microcatheter and prevent immediate direct contact between Onyx and the bloodstream, which ultimately triggers the solidification. Because of the theoretical risk of melting down non–DMSO-compatible microcatheters, it is recommended using only pretested microcatheters, including Marathon, Rebar, Echelon, and UltraFlow (Covidien, Irvine, California). They have been extensively tested regarding their compatibility with DMSO, which is outlined further in Chapter 12. In addition, their dead space volume is provided in the microcatheter package (dead space: volume necessary to fill up the lumen of the microcatheter completely).

Three different Onyx viscosities are available with different EVOH concentrations: Onyx 18 (with 6% of EVOH),

Table 10.1 Comparison between Onyx and Cyanoacrylate (Glue) Regarding Mechanism of Action, Preparation, and Administration

	Onyx	Glue
Time to solidification	4–5 min	Typically in seconds[a]
Injection time	Several minutes	Few seconds
Adhesiveness	Low	High
Final consistency	Foamlike substance	Rocky formation
Microcatheter compatibility	Restricted	Universal
Preparation	20-min shaking	Immediate use
Solidification process	Copolymerization	Polymerization
Preembolization flushing	DMSO	D5%

[a]It will depend on the glue concentration.
DMSO, dimethyl sulfoxide.
From Guimaraes M, Wooster M. Onyx (ethylene-vinyl alcohol copolymer) in peripheral applications. *Semin Intervent Radiol*. 2011;28(3):350–356.

Onyx 34 (with 8% of EVOH), and Onyx 500 (recommended for giant intracranial aneurysms). The second formulation is almost twice as viscous as the first one. Higher viscosity (Onyx 34) offers better control while the embolic agent is injected, but as the copolymerization process is faster, agent delivery in areas too distal to the microcatheter tip is more difficult. Therefore, this formulation is best suited for very high-flow lesion, with important vascular branches that must be preserved, and when the microcatheter tip is close or within the target lesion. On the other hand, a lower viscosity formulation (Onyx 18) is preferred when the microcatheter cannot be advanced any closer to the lesion and the target area is still too far away from the microcatheter tip. The lower viscosity and slower copolymerization time allow the liquid embolic agent to flow deeper, reaching more distal areas of the lesion. As one can note, it is usually a trade-off between a more controlled delivery but with less chance of full lesion embolization or complete lesion embolization with higher risk of occlusion of nontarget vessels.

Another unique Onyx characteristic is the "outside-in" solidification process. First, the outer layer forms a solid cast while a spongy or foamlike consistency is created inside, similar to what happens to the volcano lava when it cools off. The solidification process, also called *copolymerization*, starts once Onyx comes in contact with ionic fluids, such as blood, iodine contrast material, and saline solution, and usually takes 5 minutes to reach a solid and stable consistency. In contrast to dehydrated alcohol that causes an acute and severe endothelitis, Onyx induces a mild inflammatory reaction in the adjacent vessel walls, and as a nonabsorbable embolic agent, recanalization of the embolized area is nonexistent.[9]

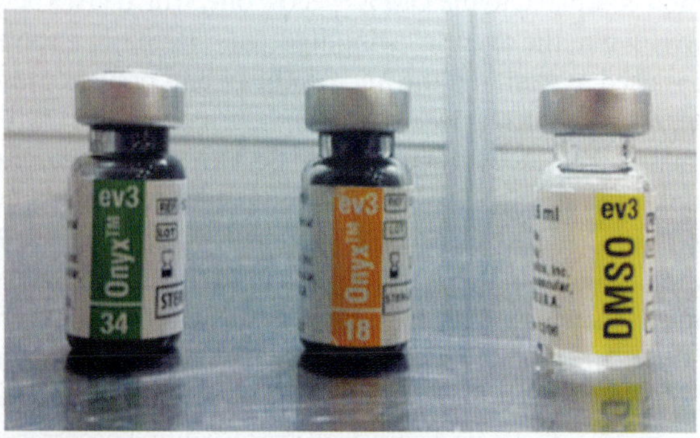

Figure 10.1 Picture of the two most used solutions, Onyx 34 (*green vial*) and Onyx 18 (*orange vial*), and the solvent, DMSO (*yellow vial*). Each vial contains 1.5 mL of agent.

CLINICAL APPLICATIONS IN PERIPHERAL EMBOLIZATIONS

Early report on peripheral Onyx application date back to 2001, when Martin and colleagues[6] reported Onyx embolization of endoleak types II and Ia. All patients presented with decreased aneurysmal sac diameter after a mean follow-up of 19.2 weeks.[6] Since then, multiple reports have been published, describing successful Onyx embolization for different pathologies among different peripheral vascular territories, including visceral aneurysm; pseudoaneurysm; hemoptysis; gastrointestinal bleeding; and abdominal, pulmonary, and upper and lower extremity AVMs.[4,5,10–13] For all these entities, Onyx has been shown to be as useful as other conventional embolic agents or sometimes even more effective due to faster vessel occlusion and good delivery control.[8] Moreover, Onyx can be considered the embolic agent of choice for peripheral AVMs and type II endoleak embolization.[14]

Typically, AVMs are challenging lesions to be treated due to the combination of potential high-flow environment and the need for distal intranidus embolization. As a liquid embolic agent, Onyx can reach small vessels deep within the nidus, sometimes far away from the delivery microcatheter. At the same time, different predictable viscosities allow safe agent delivery, with low risk of distal nontarget embolization (Fig. 10.2).

With a similar flow dynamics, type II endoleaks can behave like AVMs, having the aneurysmal sac as a functional "nidus," associated with multiple inflow and outflow vessels. In this scenario, Onyx has been shown as an extremely efficient embolic agent, achieving complete filling of the open channels within the aneurysmal sac and also proximal occlusion of the involved vessels (Fig. 10.3).

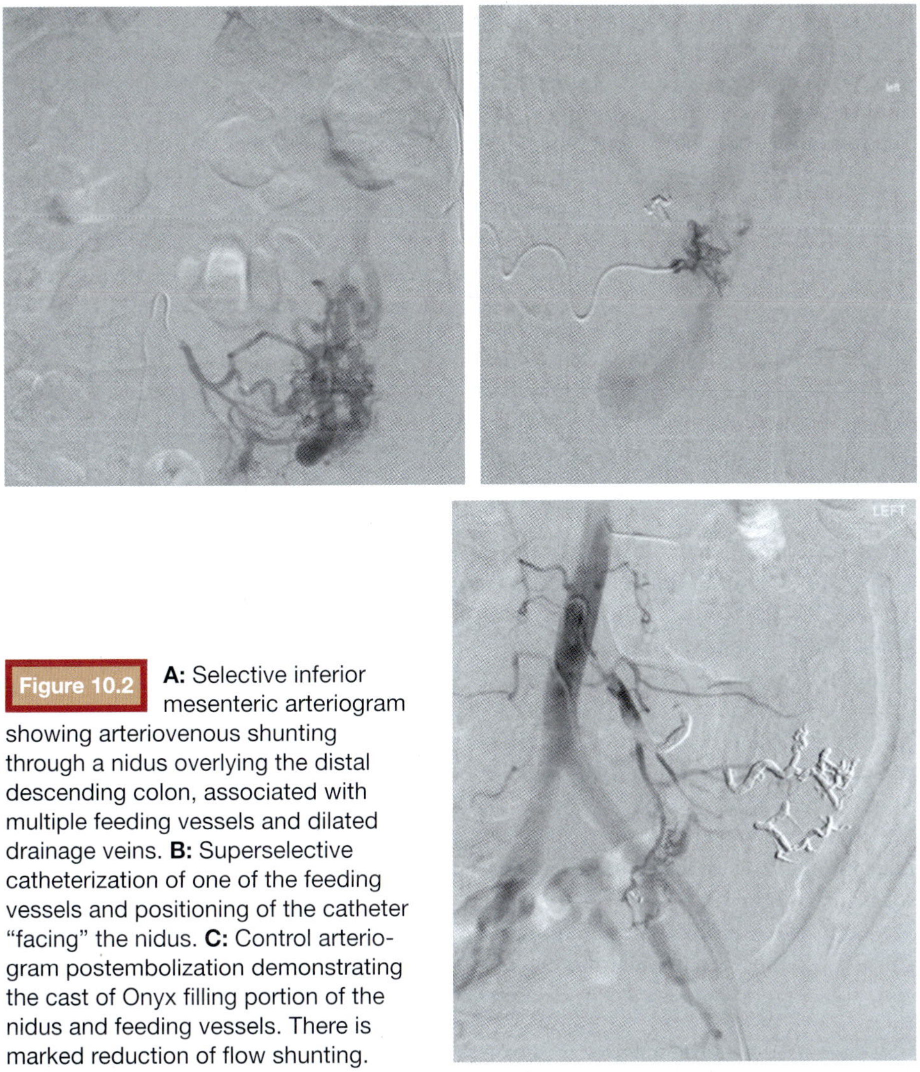

A B C

Figure 10.2 **A:** Selective inferior mesenteric arteriogram showing arteriovenous shunting through a nidus overlying the distal descending colon, associated with multiple feeding vessels and dilated drainage veins. **B:** Superselective catheterization of one of the feeding vessels and positioning of the catheter "facing" the nidus. **C:** Control arteriogram postembolization demonstrating the cast of Onyx filling portion of the nidus and feeding vessels. There is marked reduction of flow shunting.

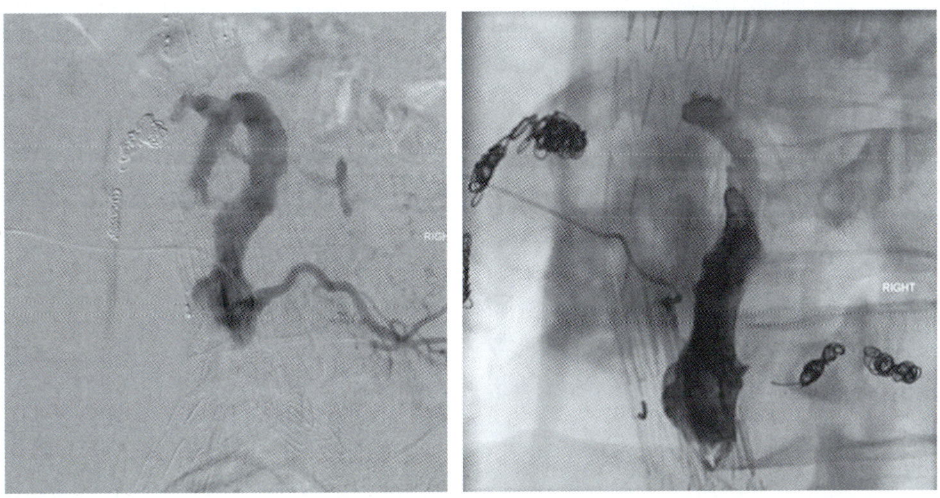

A B

Figure 10.3 **A:** After obtaining translumbar access to the abdominal aortic aneurysmal sac under computed tomography guidance, the patient was brought to the angiography room and an initial image was acquired with hand contrast injection through a KMP catheter. Note the filling of the aneurysmal sac and retrograde opacification of hypertrophied lumbar arteries. **B:** Completion image after occlusion of the lumbar artery with coils and Onyx embolization of the aneurysmal sac. Note the extensive embolization achieved with Onyx due to its spreadability, making possible occlusion of gaps away from the delivery catheter.

As noted, Onyx is a versatile embolic agent with a broad clinical application, therefore it should be part of any interventionalist's armamentarium. Comprehensive knowledge of agent properties and delivery technique are essential for an efficient and safe embolization. Peripheral use of Onyx is a field yet to be fully explored, and for that, familiarity with the technique is fundamental.

TECHNIQUE

To obtain a homogeneous Onyx solution, ensuring easy delivery and good opacification, the vial of Onyx has to be shaken for at least 20 minutes before the Onyx is aspirated into the delivery syringe. Therefore, to avoid delay, shaking process using an automatic system should start while access to the target lesion is obtained (Fig. 10.4). After proper positioning of the diagnostic catheter, a Tuohy Borst adapter (Cook Medical) is connected to the catheter hub, and coaxially, a microcatheter is advanced up to the target zone.

Hand iodine contrast injection is performed to check the working position and system stability. Ideally, the microcatheter should be as distal as possible, "facing" the lesion (see Fig. 10.2B). In situations where the microcatheter cannot be advanced closer to the lesion, which might be 1 or 2 cm away from the tip, a less viscous solution (Onyx 18) should be selected, as explained earlier.

Again, according to the manufacturer, only DMSO-compatible microcatheters should be used, and these include the Marathon, Rebar, Echelon, and UltraFlow. It is import to notice that the Marathon and UltraFlow microcatheters are flow-directed catheters with very small inner diameters, allowing maximum 0.010-in guidewires. This implies less maneuverability, which can impose difficulty when dealing with complex anatomy, with increased tortuosity and multiple branching vessels.

When in proper position, the microcatheter is washed out with normal saline and slowly filled up with DMSO. The microcatheter dead space volume is available on the package label. DMSO in high concentration can cause acute irritation to the endothelium, leading to painful sensation. So, if the patient experiences pain at this point, it means too much DMSO has been injected, above the dead space limit, or it has been injected too fast, not allowing enough time for the DMSO to mix with the blood. Because DMSO is not radiopaque, fluoroscopy is not necessary during catheter filling. Overwashing the microcatheter hub with residual amount of DMSO will prevent triggering of the copolymerization process while the Onyx solution is still inside the catheter, avoiding its occlusion. At this point, the Onyx syringe should be already filled.

Aspiration of the microcatheter before Onyx injection is not permitted. Therefore, to avoid presence of air bubble within the catheter, connection of the Onyx syringe to the microcatheter hub should be done in a vertical position, and a drop of Onyx may be necessary to fill up a residual gap within the microcatheter hub (Fig. 10.5). Onyx must always be injected slowly, since the very first time, allowing

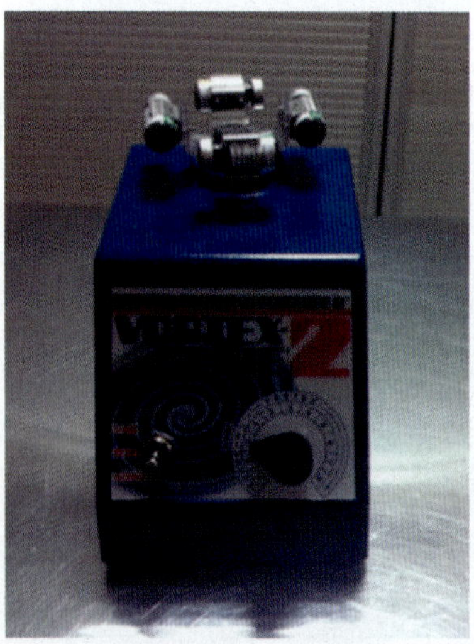

Figure 10.4 Picture of the automatic shaker used to obtain a homogenous Onyx solution before aspiration into the delivery syringe. The vials are placed on top of the machine, and the shaking process should last at least 20 minutes. To avoid time wasting, shaking process should start while access to the lesion is being obtained.

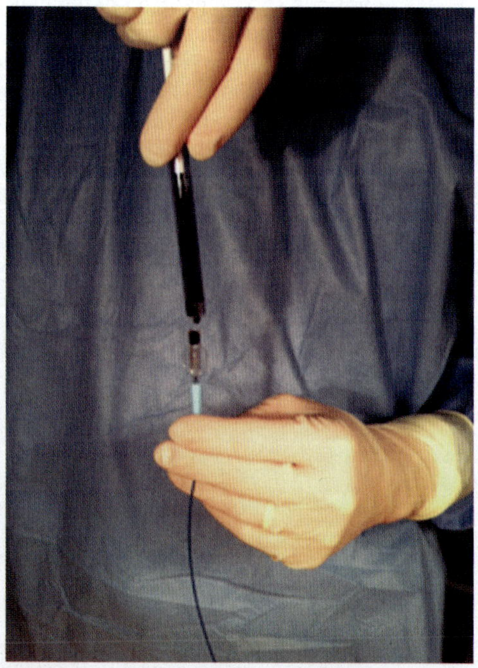

Figure 10.5 Note the vertical position of the microcatheter and the Onyx syringe when both are being attached. At this time, a small amount of Onyx is dropped into the catheter hub to fill any air gap, avoiding bubbles within the system.

adequate and asymptomatic dilution of the DMSO column within the bloodstream. If the patient complains of pain, the injection rate should be slowed down because Onyx is displacing DMSO too fast into the blood vessel, leading to endothelium irritation as mentioned earlier.

Usually, a cast of Onyx in front of the microcatheter forms fast, with a tendency of retrograde flow toward the body of the microcatheter. Although Onyx is not an adhesive agent, the catheter can get stuck within the vessel due to increased extrinsic compression by the "plug" around the microcatheter. For this reason, excessive retrograde flow along the microcatheter body should be avoided. Also, small arteries have low compliance, leading to higher pressure around the catheter and therefore increasing the risk of having the microcatheter entrenched within the vessel.

However, a stable plug around the catheter tip is very useful as it prevents any further retrograde Onyx flow. Therefore, the goal is to create a plug around the tip of the microcatheter, with sufficient amount of Onyx that can prevent retrograde flow but not too much that can increase the risk of catheter entrapment. Hence, no more than 1 to 1.5 cm of Onyx is allowed to move back along the tract of the microcatheter. If too much vessel tortuosity is present, that length should not exceed 0.5 cm (Fig. 10.6). Once the plug is well organized, it will prevent further backflow of the embolic agent, and the Onyx is then delivered only forward in relation to the microcatheter tip. This is called the *plug technique*, and for obvious reasons, it is unnecessary when there is free anterograde flow in the vessels, such as in portal vein embolization.

Depending on the capacity of the target lesion, large amount of Onyx may be required. The syringes should be simply exchanged, avoiding gaps and without additional DMSO injection. Several minutes or multiple Onyx injections might be required to obtain satisfactory embolization. Rate of infusion is defined by careful observation of Onyx behavior within the target area, which depends on the blood flow and vessel capacity. The gap between injections should be minimal to keep a continuous column of Onyx, with constant forward flow toward the target zone. This will achieve a larger embolized area with less risk of nontarget embolization as flow redirection by solidified Onyx is less likely to occur.

Due to Onyx radiopacity and complex configuration of most of the lesions, it may be difficult to visualize in which direction the agent is being delivered in a posteroanterior or even in oblique views as the previously injected Onyx might obscure the microcatheter. At this point, road mapping should be used to subtract from the image the Onyx that has been already delivered, allowing visualization of the Onyx that is being currently injected. In that way, it is possible to obtain full control and visualization during injection. Successive road mappings may be performed repeatedly every time there is a compromise in Onyx delivery visualization. However, the most important limitation of this technique is the respiratory-dependent artifact, which blurs the road mapping image. Thus, although this technique is extremely helpful when treating intracranial or extremity lesions, its use is limited when working in the abdomen or chest.

After satisfactory embolization of the target area, the entry point of the lesion may be blocked by slow retraction of the microcatheter while Onyx is gently injected, leaving a "tail." In theory, this technique helps isolate the lesion and prevents further inflow from that particular feeding vessel. This can be applied in endoleaks type I or II and pedicles of AVM nidus. Any inadvertent microcatheter pulling may lead to loss of delivery control and possible nontarget embolization.

Microcatheter removal should be done by applying negative pressure through the delivery syringe and without much effort, giving the nonadhesive nature of Onyx. If resistance is present due to excessive external compression, continuous small increments in the traction intensity should be

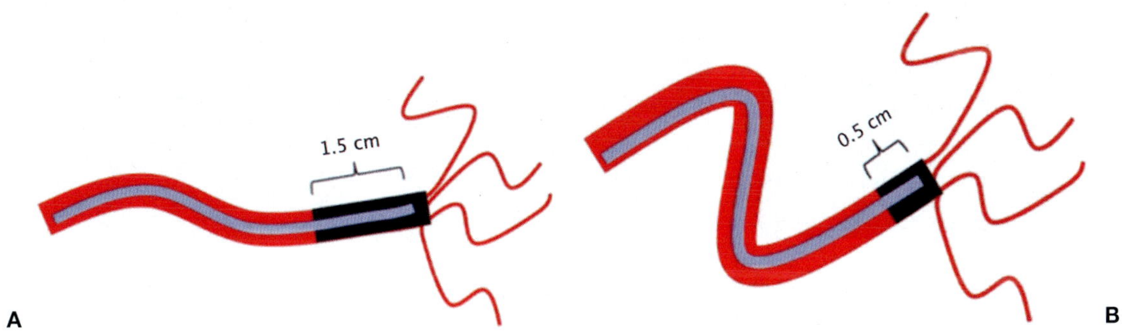

Figure 10.6 **A:** Schematic drawing demonstrating selective catheterization of straight feeding vessel (*red*) and the microcatheter facing the target lesion. In this situation, the Onyx plug (*black*) can be as long as 1.5 cm along the catheter's tip (*blue*). **B:** Schematic drawing of a different situation where the feeding vessel (*red*) has significant tortuosity. Again, the microcatheter is facing the lesion, and at this time, the Onyx plug (*black*) should not exceed 0.5 cm along the microcatheter's tip (*blue*).

applied to the microcatheter. Never pull the microcatheter abruptly as there is a risk of fracture. Once the catheter is out and filled with embolic agent, it cannot be reused. This is a major drawback as a lot of times, more than one catheterization is required even in a single session, increasing the cost of the procedure as multiple microcatheters may be necessary.

Finally, one useful application for Onyx, through a special technique, is aneurysmal sac embolization using the concepts of the "remodeling technique." This technique was first described in 1997 by Moret et al.[15] for coil embolization of large-neck intracranial aneurysms. For this, temporary occlusion of the aneurysm neck is achieved by inflating a balloon during each coil deployment, preventing coil migration. Instead of coils, Onyx can be applied to occlude the aneurysmal sac while an inflated balloon is protecting the neck (Fig. 10.7). It can also be applied to treat abdominal aortic aneurysm type I endoleaks.

The balloon diameter must match the diameter of the target vessel, without overdistention, to avoid endothelium damage. The microcatheter may be advanced coaxially through an occlusion balloon or in parallel to an angioplasty balloon catheter. If the latter is selected, a low-profile 0.014- to 0.018-in balloon is preferable to accommodate both the balloon catheter and the microcatheter through a single guiding catheter or introducer sheath. DMSO injection should be performed while the balloon is deflated to avoid accumulation of DMSO within the sac, which can dilute the Onyx solution, leading to a longer or unpredictable copolymerization time. Therefore, the balloon should be inflated just before Onyx delivery and with a very diluted iodine contrast solution to avoid obscuring the area of interest. Usually, 4 or 5 minutes are enough to complete the solidification process, allowing safe balloon deflation.

POTENTIAL COMPLICATIONS

Onyx embolization has the same complications as embolization with other embolic agents, which is basically nontarget embolization. To avoid that, superselective catheterization, appropriate application of the plug technique, and correct choice of agent viscosity are key factors. Despite the nonadhesive characteristic, there is potential risk of having the catheter stuck within the vessel due to excessive external compression around the catheter's tip. As described earlier, to prevent that, the plug should not exceed 1.5 cm in length, and if a lot of tortuosity is present, 0.5 cm should be the maximum plug extension. A common side effect is the garlic-like smell that the patient presents the day after the procedure. That is related to DMSO metabolization and usually resolves after 2 days.

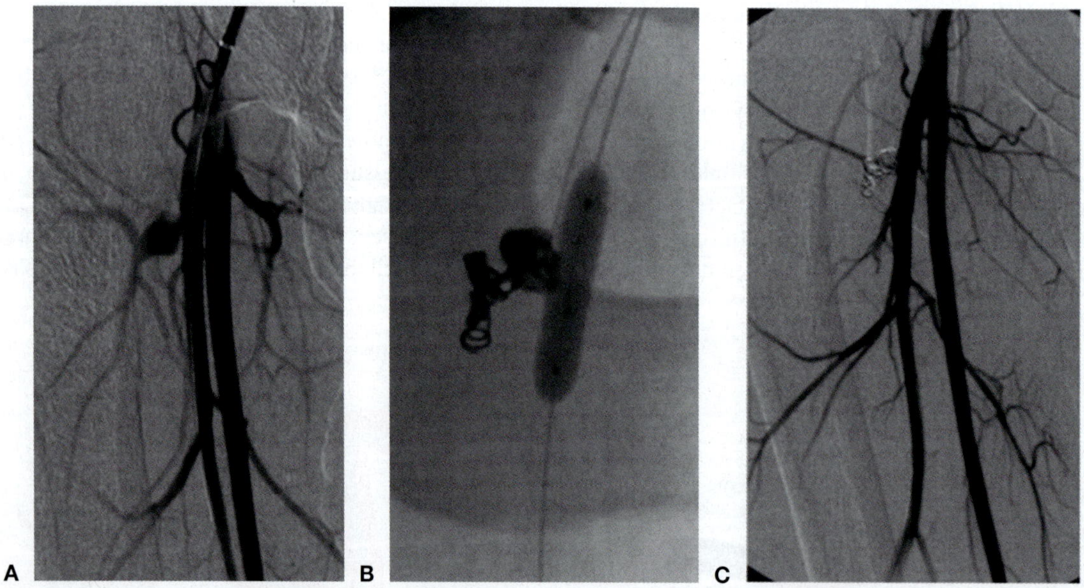

Figure 10.7 **A:** Right femoral arteriogram demonstrates pseudoaneurysm originating from a branch of the profunda femoral artery. Note the two small branches coming off the lesion itself. **B:** After coil embolization of the two small branches coming off the pseudoaneurysm, the sac and parent vessel were occluded with Onyx, whereas protection of the profound femoral artery was accomplished with an inflated angioplasty balloon. Note the parallel disposition of the microcatheter used to deliver the embolic agent and the angioplasty balloon. **C:** Completion arteriogram demonstrating complete exclusion of the pseudoaneurysm from the circulation and preserved flow in the profound femoral artery. (From Guimaraes M, Wooster M. Onyx [ethylene-vinyl alcohol copolymer] in peripheral applications. *Semin Intervent Radiol.* 2011;28[3]:350–356.)

TIPS AND TRICKS

- Onyx needs to be shaken for at least 20 min. It is important to start the shaking process while access to the lesion is being obtained.
- Use only DMSO-compatible microcatheters. DMSO will not affect the microcatheter structure. Also, the microcatheter dead space volume is available in the package label.
- DMSO should be injected slowly. If the patient complaints of pain during the injection, either the dead space volume was overestimated or the hand injection rate is too high (inadequate time for dilution with blood).
- The residual DMSO volume, after the dead space injection, should be used to overwash the hub to avoid any air bubble at the back of the syringe.
- If the microcatheter tip is far away from the nidus (in AVMs) or from target lesion, consider Onyx 18. If it is close to the target or if it is desired to have better control during the injection, consider Onyx 34. Onyx 500 is typically used for giant aneurysms.
- Once Onyx is injected through the microcatheter tip, attention should be paid on the reflux toward the hub of the microcatheter. It is desired to form a short plug around the tip that will allow further injection of Onyx to be pushed forward.
- Differently than glue, Onyx may be slowly injected for several minutes as long as adequate plug is formed and there is no interruption in the column of Onyx injection.
- Onyx occupies free space by sedimentation; it does not polymerize like glue. However, microcatheter tip still can get trapped if the plug created around the tip gets too long (>2 cm).
- In case the microcatheter tip gets trapped, it typically will come out if a gentle, continuous pullback is applied from the hub of the microcatheter. Avoid sudden and intense pullback.

REFERENCES

1. Kayashima K, Sueoka A, Smith JW, et al. Development of new hollow fiber membrane macromolecular filters. *Trans Am Soc Artif Intern Organs.* 1982;28:66–70.
2. Taki W, Yonekawa Y, Iwata H, et al. A new liquid material for embolization of arteriovenous malformations. *AJNR Am J Neuroradiol.* 1990;1(1):163–168.
3. *U.S. Multicenter, Randomized Controlled Study Comparing the Performance of Onyx (EVOH) and TRUFILL (n-BCA) in the Presurgical Embolization of Brain Arteriovenous Malformations (BAVMs).* Washington, DC: Georgetown University Hospital; 2003.
4. Castaneda F, Goodwin SC, Swischuk JL, et al. Treatment of pelvic arteriovenous malformations with ethylene vinyl alcohol copolymer (Onyx). *J Vasc Interv Radiol.* 2002;13(5):513–516.
5. Numan F, Omeroglu A, Kara B, et al. Embolization of peripheral vascular malformations with ethylene vinyl alcohol copolymer (Onyx). *J Vasc Interv Radiol.* 2004;15(9):939–946.
6. Martin ML, Dolmatch BL, Fry PD, et al. Treatment of type II endoleaks with Onyx. *J Vasc Interv Radiol.* 2001;12(5): 629–632.
7. Nevala T, Biancari F, Manninen H, et al. Type II endoleak after endovascular repair of abdominal aortic aneurysm: effectiveness of embolization. *Cardiovasc Intervent Radiol.* 2010;33(2): 278–284.
8. Adamus Nurnberg R, Uder Erlangen M, Kleinschmidt T, et al. Embolization of acute abdominal and thoracic hemorrhages with ethylene vinyl alcohol copolymer (Onyx): initial experiences with arteries of the body trunk [in German]. *Rofo.* 2010;182(10):900–904.
9. Jahan R, Murayama Y, Gobin YP, et al. Embolization of arteriovenous malformations with Onyx: clinicopathological experience in 23 patients. *Neurosurgery.* 2001;48(5):984–995.
10. Bratby MJ, Lehmann ED, Bottomley J, et al. Endovascular embolization of visceral artery aneurysms with ethylene-vinyl alcohol (Onyx): a case series. *Cardiovasc Intervent Radiol.* 2006; 29(6):1125–1128.
11. Vanninen RL, Manninen I. Onyx, a new liquid embolic material for peripheral interventions: preliminary experience in aneurysm, pseudoaneurysm, and pulmonary arteriovenous malformation embolization. *Cardiovasc Intervent Radiol.* 2007; 30(2):196–200.
12. Lenhart M, Paetzel C, Sackmann M, et al. Superselective arterial embolisation with a liquid polyvinyl alcohol copolymer in patients with acute gastrointestinal haemorrhage. *Eur Radiol.* 2010;20(8):1994–1999.
13. Guimaraes M, Wooster M. Onyx (ethylene-vinyl alcohol copolymer) in peripheral applications. *Semin Intervent Radiol.* 2011; 28(3):350–356.
14. Massis K, Carson WG III, Rozas A, et al. Treatment of type II endoleaks with ethylene-vinyl-alcohol copolymer (Onyx). *Vasc Endovascular Surg.* 2012;46(3):251–257.
15. Moret J, Cognard C, Weill A, et al. Reconstruction technic in the treatment of wide-neck intracranial aneurysms. Long-term angiographic and clinical results. Apropos of 56 cases [in French]. *J Neuroradiol.* 1997;24(1):30–44.

11

Sclerosing Agents

Jordan C. Tasse • Bulent Arslan • Ulku Cenk Turba

Sclerosing agents represent another category of liquid embolic agents. They act by damaging endothelial cells, leading to an inflammatory fibrosis and irreversible vascular thrombosis. The sclerosant effect typically depends on the strength of the particular agent being used and the amount of time that it is in contact with the endothelial lining of the vessel.

ABSOLUTE ALCOHOL (ETHANOL)

Alcohol is one of the most potent of the liquid embolic agents. It can be injected using a catheter-based intravascular approach or using a direct percutaneous approach. Absolute alcohol is an effective permanent embolization agent that has been used in various scenarios. Some of the applications of absolute alcohol include percutaneous tumor ablation/treatment, presurgical embolization of renal cell carcinoma, and treatment of vascular malformations. Direct alcohol injection has been used for treatment of small (<2 cm) hepatocellular carcinomas and for sclerotherapy of painful abdominal cysts and postsurgical seromas.

Alcohol acts by denaturing endothelial proteins, leading to activation of the coagulation cascade inducing subsequent thrombosis.[1] Ethanol also induces vasospasm. Occlusion is typically seen within seconds after injection and progresses for several days. The effect depends on ethanol concentration, time of exposure, and injection rate; rapid injection rates produce more endothelial damage and parenchymal necrosis with less thrombosis, whereas slower injection rates produce more thrombosis but less endothelial damage and necrosis.[2] The use of alcohol as an embolic agent is not without risk. The disadvantages of alcohol include the risk of damage to surrounding tissues including nerves, skin, and mucosa due to its penetrative properties. Patients may experience severe procedural pain. Monitoring for systemic toxicity is also crucial when the dose of alcohol is greater than 1 mL/kg or if the total volume exceeds 60 mL. The side effects may include central nervous system depression, hemolysis, and cardiac arrest.

Given these possible effects, it is important to minimize the incidence of nontarget embolization. The techniques used to reduce this risk include slow injection, use of balloon occlusion of the arterial inflow, or balloon occlusion of the draining vein.

ETHANOLAMINE OLEATE

Ethamolin (QOL Medical, LLC, Kirkland, Washington)

Ethanolamine oleate is a salt of a fatty acid with excellent thrombogenic properties. It is typically injected as a mixture consisting of 5% ethanolamine oleate and nonionic contrast material or iodized oil (5:1 ratio) for radiopacity. It combines its inherent thrombogenic properties with an inflammatory response to oleic acid that occurs in the vascular wall. When compared to ethanol, ethanolamine oleate has a less penetrating effect in comparison and is therefore considered safer to use in vascular structures with close proximity to nerves, skin, and mucosa.

Ethanolamine oleate has most commonly been used for sclerosis of gastroesophageal varices, venous malformations, and sclerotherapy of cyst, seromas, etc. Some risks associated with ethanolamine oleate include renal failure, pulmonary edema, and anaphylaxis. Although it is considered experimental, haptoglobin can be administered with ethanolamine oleate to bind free hemoglobin and albumin before injection to prevent hemolysis-induced renal insufficiency.[3]

SODIUM TETRADECYL SULFATE

Sotradecol (AngioDynamics, Queensbury, New York), FibroVein (STD Pharmaceuticals Ltd., Hereford, United Kingdom), Trombovar (Aventis Pharma, Le Trait, France), Tromboject (Omega Laboratories Ltd., Montreal, Quebec, Canada)

Sodium tetradecyl sulfate (STS; Sotradecol) is a long-chain fatty acid salt with detergent properties. It is an effective sclerosing agent that acts by inducing endothelial damage and dissolution of the endothelial cell membrane, which causes cell overhydration. Sotradecol is U.S. Food and Drug Administration (FDA) approved for distribution in 1% and 3% concentrations. It is typically mixed with a water-soluble contrast agent to provide radiopacity. It can also be mixed with iodized poppy seed oil (i.e., Lipiodol) with air or carbon dioxide to create a foam.[4] Foamed detergent sclerosants have been reported to be more potent than their liquid counterpart.[5]

Sotradecol has been in use for more than 50 years and can be injected via an intravascular route or a direct percutaneous approach. Typical uses include the direct injection of varicose veins (0.1% to 3% concentration), sclerosis of gonadal veins in the management of varicoceles and pelvic congestion syndrome (1% to 3% concentration), sclerotherapy of peripheral venous malformation (1% to 3% concentration), as well as balloon-occluded retrograde transvenous obliteration (BRTO) procedures for bleeding gastric varices treatment (Fig. 11.1).

POLIDOCANOL

Asclera (Merz Aesthetics, San Mateo, California), Aethoxysclerol (Kreussler Pharma, Wiesbaden, Germany)

Polidocanol is the most widely used venous sclerosant in Europe and was recently approved by the FDA for use in the United States. It consists of 95% hydroxypolyethoxydodecane, a cationic detergent with anesthetic properties. Similar

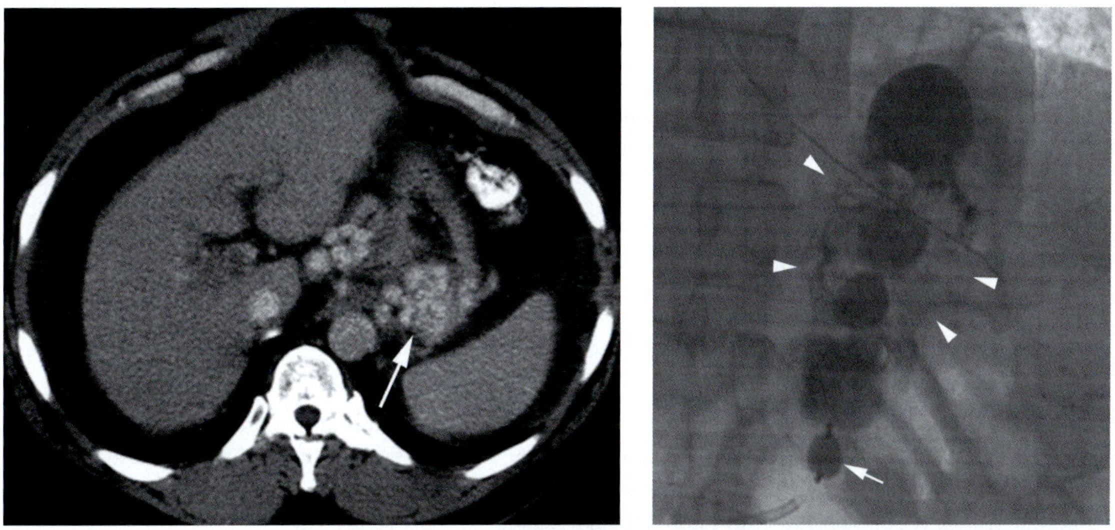

A B

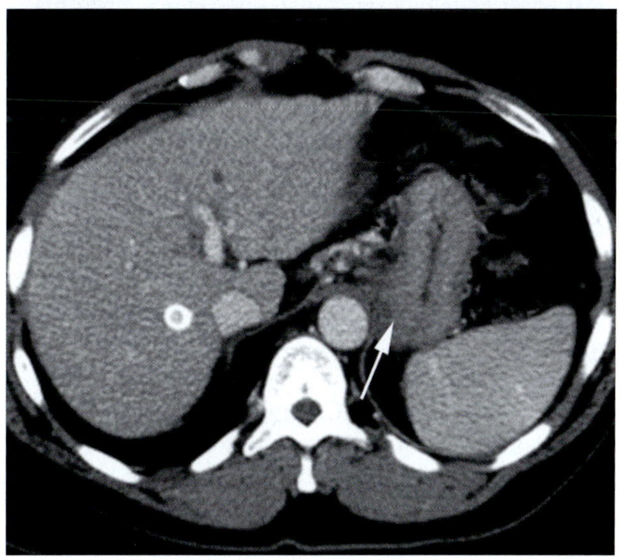

C

Figure 11.1 Three images from a patient who presented with an acute upper gastrointestinal bleed secondary to gastric varices. **A:** A single image from an abdominal computed tomography (CT) scan demonstrates numerous gastric varices at the stomach wall (*arrow*). **B:** Single image obtained during a BRTO procedure. This demonstrates balloon-occluded (*arrow*) retrograde transvenous obliteration with foam consisting of contrast agent, air, and Sotradecol. The foam used for sclerotherapy has a lacy, salt-and-pepper appearance on fluoroscopy images (*arrowheads*). **C:** Single image from a follow-up CT scan of the abdomen demonstrates complete disappearance of the gastric wall varices (*arrow*). (Courtesy of Warren Swee, MD.)

Table 11.1 Some Sclerosing Agents

Agent	Preparation	Uses	Advantages	Risks
Absolute alcohol	99% ethanol drawn up directly and mixed with nonionic contrast at 1:1 ratio	AVM Venous malformations Varicoceles Lymphatic malformations Solid organ embolization Tumor embolization Cyst/seroma sclerosis	Inexpensive Potent Highly effective	Damage to surrounding structures Nontarget embolization CNS depression Hemolysis Renal failure Pain
Ethanolamine oleate	5% ethanolamine oleate directly mixed with nonionic contrast or iodized oil at 5:1 ratio	Varices Venous malformations Cyst/seroma sclerosis	Effective Compared to ethanol: – Less severe and less frequent side effects – Less risk to surrounding structures	Hemolysis Renal failure Pulmonary edema Anaphylaxis
Sodium tetradecyl sulfate (STS)	1%–3% Sotradecol mixed directly with contrast or iodized oil and CO_2 or air at 1:1:4 ratio to create foam 0.1%–3% STS directly injected for varicose vein sclerosis	Venous malformations Varicocele/pelvic congestion syndrome BRTO AVM Hemangioma Varicose veins	Effective Safe Painless intravascular injection	Local tissue damage from extravasation Anaphylaxis
Polidocanol	0.5%–1% mixed directly with nonionic contrast or iodized oil and CO_2 or air at 1:1:4 ratio to create foam 0.3%–1% directly injected for varicose veins	Venous malformations Varicose veins	Painless injection	Cardiac depression Anaphylaxis

AVM, arteriovenous malformation; CNS, central nervous system; CO_2, carbon dioxide; BRTO, balloon-occluded retrograde transvenous obliteration.

to STS, its detergent action induces rapid overhydration of endothelial cells, leading to vascular injury. Polidocanol can be obtained in 1% and 3% concentrations, and its potency is approximately half of Sotradecol. Polidocanol has been used to treat lower extremity varicosities and venous malformations. Its anesthetic properties have been reported to significantly reduce procedure-related pain.[6]

The risks of polidocanol administration include anaphylaxis and cardiac depression. The cardiac effects are due to its anesthetic properties, which cause depression in the electrical excitability of and conduction rate through the heart and spontaneous pacemaker activity in the sinus node, resulting in sinus bradycardia and possible sinus arrest.[7]

Table 11.1 summarizes the aforementioned agents.

SODIUM MORRHUATE

Scleromate (Glenwood LLC, Englewood, New Jersey)

Sodium morrhuate is a sclerosing agent composed of a sodium salt of fatty acids in cod liver oil. The agent has been used in the treatment of varicose veins and venous malformations. It has been reported to be 1.5 to 4 times less effective than Sotradecol.[8] Additionally, high rates of anaphylaxis and complications from extravasation, including pain and tissue necrosis, have limited its use.

ETHIBLOC

Ethibloc (Ethicon, Norderstedt, Germany)

Ethibloc consists of a solution of zein, sodium amidotrizoate, oleum papaveris, and propylene glycol. It has been used effectively for the treatment of venous, lymphatic, and arteriovenous malformations. It requires approximately 15 minutes to solidify into a viscous solution, allowing it to remain static within the target lesion to cause intravascular thrombosis, necrosis, and fibrosis.

OTHERS

In general, there are various sclerosing agents. In addition to the aforementioned agents, any agent that has detergent properties, hyperosmolar agents, chemical irritants, and even antibiotics (doxycycline, erythromycin, etc.) may be used as sclerosing agents. The impact of the treatment is generally determined by the tissue/endothelium contact time and strength of the sclerosing agent.

TIPS AND TRICKS

Tips

- Ethanol injection is painful and anesthesia assistance should be considered.
- Always use a microcatheter coaxial to the diagnostic catheter or a triaxial system with elongated sheath to provide optimal stability.
- Be careful during diagnostic angiography for an arteriovenous malformation to identify high-flow versus low-flow lesion for potential alcohol injection.
- Perform thorough diagnostic angiography during BRTO to identify any complex outflow and ensure that occlusion balloon is above all outflow veins to maximize treatment and prevent nontarget embolization.

Tricks

- Contrast injection is helpful to estimate volume of sclerosant necessary in BRTO procedures.
- Ethanol should be mixed with nonionic contrast in a 1:1 ratio to allow optimal visualization.
- For limb lesions, use a tourniquet to decrease venous outflow and systemic effects of sclerosants.
- For small lesions, use small 1.7-Fr to 2.1-Fr microcatheters.
- Use vascular plugs to complement sclerosant for gonadal vein embolization to decrease coil use and procedure time and to maximize embolization effect.

CONCLUSION

Sclerosing agents can be used as an embolic agent for several different indications. Given their liquid form and mechanism of action, the potential does exist for unintended distal embolization and tissue effects not seen with other agents. Therefore, care must be taken when using these agents.

REFERENCES

1. Do YS, Yakes WF, Shin SW, et al. Ethanol embolization of arteriovenous malformations: interim results. *Radiology*. 2005;235(2):674–682.
2. Ellman BA, Parkhill BJ, Marcus PB, et al. Renal ablation with absolute ethanol: mechanism of action. *Invest Radiol.* 1984;19(5):416–423.
3. Kato GJ. Haptoglobin halts hemoglobin's havoc. *J Clin Invest.* 2009;119(8):2140–2142. doi:10.1172/JCI40258.
4. Sabri SS, Swee W, Turba UC, et al. Bleeding gastric varices obliteration with balloon-occluded retrograde transvenous obliteration using sodium tetradecyl sulfate foam. *J Vasc Interv Radiol.* 2011;22(3):309–316.
5. Cabrera J, Cabrera J Jr, Garcia-Olmedo MA, et al. Treatment of venous malformations with sclerosant in microfoam form. *Arch Dermatol.* 2003;139(11):1409–1416.
6. Mimura H, Kanazawa S, Yasui K, et al. Percutaneous sclerotherapy for venous malformations using polidocanol under fluoroscopy. *Acta Med Okayama.* 2003;57(5):227–234.
7. Marrocco-Trischitta MM, Guerrini P, Abeni D, et al. Reversible cardiac arrest after polidocanol sclerotherapy of peripheral venous malformation. *Dermatol Surg.* 2002;28(2):153–155.
8. Woods JE. Extended use of sodium tetradecyl sulfate in treatment of hemangiomas and other related conditions. *Plast Reconstr Surg.* 1987;79(4):542–549.

12

Catheters and Catheterization Techniques

Susie J. Park • Gary P. Siskin

Throughout this textbook, there are several chapters that focus on the embolic agents used for embolization and many more chapters focusing on the clinical indications being treated with embolization procedures. There is no doubt that these two broad areas of focus are essential for these procedures to be successfully performed. However, there is a third area of focus that requires attention as well: the catheters and the catheterization techniques used today for embolization. Many times, embolization procedures are either successful or unsuccessful based on the choices made by individual physicians regarding the materials and techniques used to deliver an agent to its intended target. This chapter will take a unique look at embolization from this perspective.

CATHETERS USED FOR EMBOLIZATION

Almost every available angiographic catheter can be used to deliver one or more of the many agents available today for embolization. Standard 4-Fr and 5-Fr angiographic catheters can be used to deliver coils, plugs, and particulate embolic agents. However, the expanded indications for embolization into smaller vessels that are increasingly located distally within a target vascular bed are requiring the use of microcatheters. Microcatheter characteristics that are favorable when it comes to the performance of embolization procedures include trackability, flexibility, kink resistance, and radiopacity; radiopacity is important to ensure that an embolic agent will be deployed exactly where deployment is intended to be. Many microcatheters are being manufactured with various tip configurations to facilitate catheterization of target vessels. In addition, microcatheters are now available with various inner and outer diameter sizes, so care must be taken to ensure that the microcatheter selected is compatible with the agent being planned for embolization. Selective catheterization in the setting of embolization can be challenging at times, and almost nothing can be more frustrating for an interventionalist than to find out that the microcatheter used cannot accommodate a particular coil or microsphere after it has been positioned appropriately within the target vasculature.

CATHETER AND EMBOLIC AGENT COMPATIBILITY

Every embolic agent reviewed in the previous chapters requires a catheter for delivery to the vascular bed being targeted for embolization. The actual catheter selected for delivery will, of course, depend on the embolic agent being used and the degree of selective catheterization required for the condition being treated. It will also depend on the inner diameter of the selected catheter because different agents either require or are more easily delivered through appropriately sized catheters. There are some specific issues surrounding catheter selection and the agent being used for embolization.

Coils

When using coils for embolization, the delivery catheter must have an inner diameter that constrains the coil as it is being delivered. If the inner diameter of the catheter is too large relative to the size of the coil, then the potential exists for the coil to begin forming within the catheter. This can result in the coils getting stuck within the catheter, forcing the catheter to be removed. If catheterization of the target vessel was technically challenging, then being forced to remove the delivery catheter could have significant implications in terms of the additional radiation dose, contrast volume, and physician time required to repeat that portion of the procedure. This is particularly the case with the use of microcatheters and newer detachable coils. For example, the hydrogel coating of an AZUR detachable coil (AZUR Peripheral HydroCoil Embolization System; Terumo Medical Corporation, Somerset, New Jersey) may make it better placed with a microcatheter with a 0.027-in inner diameter as compared with other coils that are easily placed through a microcatheter with a 0.021-in inner diameter. Therefore, attention must be paid to catheter selection to avoid this type of catheter–coil mismatch.

Coil passage through a catheter can be held up for other reasons as well. It can occur with retrograde blood flow into the catheter with subsequent thrombosis. This can be prevented with frequent flushing of the catheter or even the use of a continuous infusion of saline through the catheter via a Tuohy Borst adapter (Cook Incorporated, Bloomington, Indiana).[1] In addition, hydrophilic catheters can be softer than other catheters, which may cause fibered coils to get stuck in the catheter near a curve or the tip.[2] This can result in a failure to deliver the coil to its target and the need to prematurely remove the obstructed catheter.

Catheter stability is an important component of coil delivery to prevent incorrect positioning of the coil as it is being deployed. The use of a guide catheter or long sheath can assist with minimizing this potential technical complication. In addition, before the use of any pushable coil, it is good practice to test the stability of the delivery catheter by either injecting saline through the catheter or by advancing the coil pusher to the tip of the catheter before any coil is placed.[3]

Plugs

It is important to understand that the available plugs typically require larger catheters for delivery when compared with coils, and they cannot be delivered with a microcatheter. For example, depending on the exact configuration and size of an Amplatzer Vascular Plug (St. Jude Medical, Inc., St. Paul, Minnesota), either a 4-Fr to 5-Fr catheter or 4-Fr to 7-Fr guide catheter/sheath would be required for delivery.[4] Therefore, this understandably requires that the target vessel can accommodate a catheter or sheath of this size. It may or may not be possible for these catheters to track over a guidewire to an area of arterial pathology if the vessels leading to the pathology are small, tortuous, or diseased. This must be recognized before settling on the use of a plug for embolization.

Liquid Agents

Cyanoacrylates are one example of a liquid adhesive used for embolization procedures, and the main pathology treated with these agents are arteriovenous malformations. Glue embolization is typically performed through a microcatheter positioned as close as possible to the nidus.[5] Because polycarbonate can be destroyed by cyanoacrylate, polypropylene syringes should be used for these procedures.[5,6] Although attention to the technical details of administration is important to prevent catheter adhesion to intraluminal glue (e.g., dilution, catheter position, etc.), there is no specific microcatheter that is recommended for use with cyanoacrylates.

This is not the case with Onyx (Covidien, Irvine, California), which is another liquid embolic agent. Onyx is an ethylene vinyl alcohol copolymer used in conjunction with dimethyl sulfoxide (DMSO). Onyx is nonadhesive, which means that the delivery catheter is unlikely to become adhered to it after delivery. DMSO is necessary during Onyx administration because it inhibits the polymerization of Onyx, which begins after the diffusion of DMSO in the presence of aqueous media such as blood.[7] The problem is that DMSO can also potentially erode a delivery catheter. As a result, the microcatheters used in association with DMSO administration must be DMSO compatible, indicating that the catheter manufacturer has done the appropriate testing to ensure that the catheter will maintain its integrity during DMSO and Onyx administration. The manufacturer of Onyx has done their own internal testing leading to specific recommendations for which catheters should be used with DMSO. The testing they perform is extensive, including detachment force testing (to determine the amount of force required to detach a catheter from Onyx), dynamic pressure testing (to determine the required pressure to push Onyx through a patent catheter), precipitated Onyx testing (to determine the pressure required to dislodge precipitated Onyx from both sides of the catheter), fuse joint segment burst testing (to determine the pressure required to burst each catheter-fused joint segment and the distal segment with marker band[s]), and others including catheter tensile strength testing, static burst testing, pressure profile testing, and collapsed lumen (kink) testing (Covidien, Laci Costa, written personal communication). As a result of this testing, recommended catheters include the Apollo, Marathon, UltraFlow, Echelon, and Rebar catheters, all of which are manufactured by Covidien (Irvine, California). There are other manufacturers claiming DMSO compatibility with their microcatheters as well, but the manufacturer of Onyx has not tested these catheters.

Particles

Particulate polyvinyl alcohol (PVA) particles have historically been associated with microcatheter clogging. This is most likely due to particulate aggregation, making the effective size of the PVA particles larger than their actual size.[8]

Selecting a catheter with an appropriate inner diameter is essential to ensure that catheters do not become occluded while using PVA particles. Although 4-Fr and 5-Fr catheters can certainly be used to administer PVA particles, it is more common practice for microcatheters to be used for this purpose. This is due to the vascular beds or tumors and other pathology that are typically targeted with PVA particles. In general, microcatheters with inner diameters of 0.027 to 0.028 in are more appropriate and easier to use in association with particulate embolization than smaller inner diameter catheters. Although it is possible to use microcatheters with smaller inner diameters, more injection force and more frequent flushing are required to avoid catheter occlusion. From a delivery perspective, the development of spherical embolic agents in recent years, including bland and drug-eluting microspheres, has resulted in easier administration and a lower incidence of microcatheter occlusion due to the fact that these microspheres do not aggregate.

Gelfoam

Gelatin sponge particles are commonly used for embolization. Interventionalists often prepare these particles at the time of the embolization procedure with the use of a cutting method or pumping method.[9] Although gelfoam is most easily administered through a 4-Fr to 5-Fr angiographic catheter, it can be administered through a microcatheter as well. Administering gelfoam through a microcatheter can be done with the use of smaller syringes and higher injection pressures. However, concern has been raised that this can result in fragmentation of the gelfoam, leading to smaller particles being administered. Katsumori and Kashara[10] as well as Osuga et al.[11] have shown that this is not the case and that gelfoam can be safely delivered intact through a microcatheter.

CONSIDERATIONS FOR CATHETERIZATION DURING EMBOLOTHERAPY

Vascular Anatomy

During all embolization techniques, a thorough knowledge of vascular anatomy is required before embolization. Understanding the tissues and organs being supplied by individual vessels allows the interventionalist to increase the level of certainty that the target organ is being embolized and to gauge the risk of nontarget embolization. In addition, it is well established that there are various branching patterns of vessel origins all falling under the heading of "normal anatomy." Without understanding where anomalous vessels to particular organs may arise, it would be impossible to be certain that all of the vessels responsible for the arterial supply are accounted for and embolized as necessary. For example, it has been well established that branches of the internal mammary artery can supply lung parenchyma in a patient with hemoptysis, that branches of the ovarian artery can supply the uterus in a patient with uterine fibroids, and that branches of the superior mesenteric artery can supply the liver in a patient with hepatocellular carcinoma. Having this knowledge can enable the interventionalist to study all possible sources of arterial supply to a target organ before concluding that the procedure has been successfully completed.

Nonselective versus Selective Catheterization

As part of the angiographic assessment before embolization, a nonselective angiogram is often performed to gain an overview of the arterial supply to the specific part of the body being targeted for embolization. There are several potential benefits to performing nonselective angiography before selective catheterization and embolization. Nonselective angiography permits an assessment regarding which vessels are actually responsible for supplying a target organ, which can eliminate or greatly reduce the time spent catheterizing vessels that are ultimately found to not be involved in the pathology being treated. In addition, the variant anatomy described in the previous section can be quickly identified so as not to allow for time being spent on the catheterization of noncontributory vessels. Nonselective angiography also allows for an assessment of those vessels that do require selective catheterization and can provide information to simplify the process of selective catheterization. Abdominal aortography, for example, can identify the number of renal arteries before selective renal embolization and which vessels are contributing to the abnormal target vasculature (Fig. 12.1). It can also identify the angle at which a renal artery originates from the abdominal aorta and can allow for appropriate selection of a catheter configuration that closely mimics the patient's anatomy. This can reduce the time needed for selective catheterization, which in turn can limit the radiation dose and volume of contrast administered during this portion of an embolization procedure.

Proximal versus Distal Embolization

Once a particular vessel has been embolized, the development of collateral flow circumventing the point of vascular occlusion is a possibility that can undermine the initial intent of embolization. Therefore, this possibility should always be considered when determining the exact location within a target vessel for embolization. In some cases, such as distal embolization of an end organ such as the spleen or kidney, collateralization from one distinct territory to another is unlikely to occur. However, when performing a proximal embolization in the setting of trauma or aneurysmal disease, it is entirely possible that collateral vessels will continue perfusing the target vascular bed, effectively rendering the embolization ineffective. In these cases, embolizing a vessel both proximal and distal to an area of focal pathology would be appropriate to prevent this possibility from occurring.

The level of catheterization within a target vessel is also important because it will determine how much actual

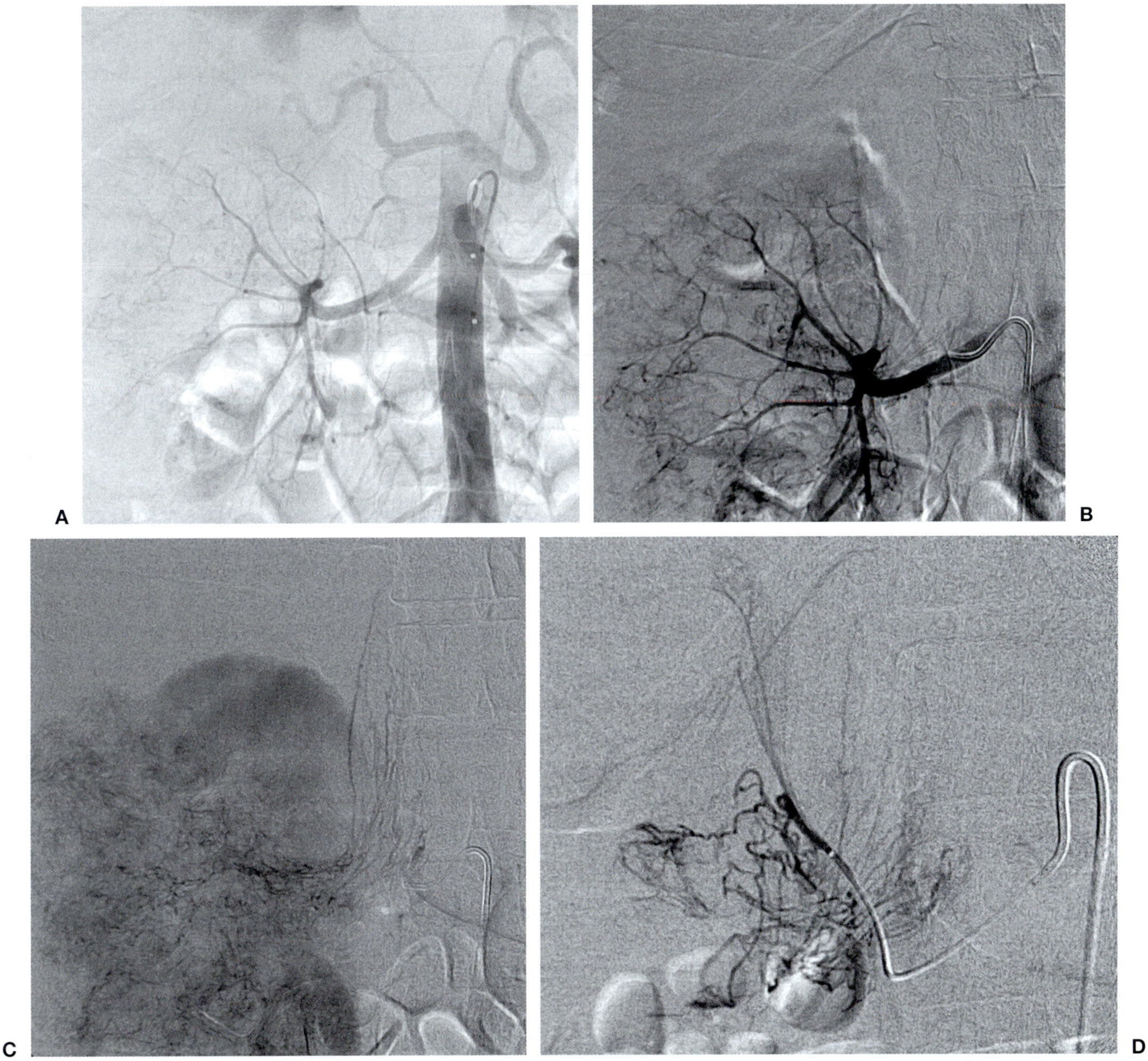

Figure 12.1 Multiple images from a preoperative right renal embolization procedure in a 34-year-old patient with renal cell carcinoma. **A:** Single image from a nonselective aortogram demonstrating a dominant right renal artery and a smaller caudal accessory renal artery. **B,C:** Two images from selective angiography of the main right renal artery demonstrating a markedly hypervascular mass with extension into the renal vein and inferior vena cava. **D:** Single image from a selective angiography of the smaller accessory right renal artery demonstrating that a significant contribution to the tumor vasculature comes from this vessel.

end organ ischemia will occur with embolization. As described earlier, a more proximal embolization can potentially fail due to collateral flow development, but at other times, a more proximal embolization with the development of collateral vessels can help prevent unwanted end organ ischemia.

Catheter position within the target vessel is particularly important when using a particulate or liquid embolic agent. Particulate or liquid embolic agents often require normal antegrade flow to pass alongside the delivery catheter within the target vessel to deliver the embolic agent into the pathologic vascular bed. If the delivery catheter is positioned in a vessel of similar size, minimizing flow around the catheter, then the delivery of a particulate or liquid embolic may be hampered by spasm or true arterial occlusion. This may lead to a less effective embolization. Therefore, an appropriate catheter position that limits the flow of these agents into unwanted side branches but still allows for flow-mediated delivery of the particles or liquid into the target vascular bed is ideal in this setting. This highlights the importance of thinking about the exact level of arterial occlusion selected for any embolization procedure.

Risk of Reflux

The risk of refluxing an embolic agent into a side branch of the target vessels or entirely out of the target vessel is a clearly unwanted occurrence during any embolization procedure. Nontarget embolization is often an entirely preventable complication of embolotherapy, but this requires both recognition of this possibility and steps taken toward prevention.

During the course of many embolization procedures, the identification of reflux during embolic agent administration is one sign used to determine if the end of the procedure is near. For example, during uterine artery embolization procedures to treat symptomatic fibroids, we allow for some controlled reflux to determine the residual rate of flow in the uterine artery as embolization progresses. For applications in which purposeful or nonpurposeful reflux is going to occur, it is important for the position of the delivery catheter to be well distal to any side branches that require protection from reflux and nontarget embolization. This of course also requires close and careful fluoroscopic monitoring during embolic agent delivery.

There are specific catheters that can be used as well when either the embolic agent being used or the catheter position required for embolic agent delivery is associated with significant risk for reflux and nontarget embolization. For example, when ethanol is used for embolization, many interventionalists will use a balloon catheter to prevent reflux. In this setting, inflating the balloon during embolization slows the balloon to protect against reflux and nontarget embolization by manually preventing backflow past the inflated balloon. The Surefire Infusion System (Surefire Medical, Inc., Westminster, Colorado) can also be helpful in many situations to reduce this risk. This catheter has an expandable cone-style tip that prevents reflux around the expanded tip during embolic agent delivery (Fig. 12.2). This expandable tip does collapse in the setting of forward flow, allowing for native flow to help deliver a particulate or liquid embolic agent distally into a target vascular bed. However, should reflux occur, the tip fully expands, allowing for apposition against the vessel wall and prevention of retrograde flow past the expandable tip. This particular catheter has been used more frequently in the setting of radioembolization to optimize the delivery of yttrium 90 microspheres and to prevent reflux into gastric and duodenal vessels and subsequent ulcer formation as a result of this procedure.[12]

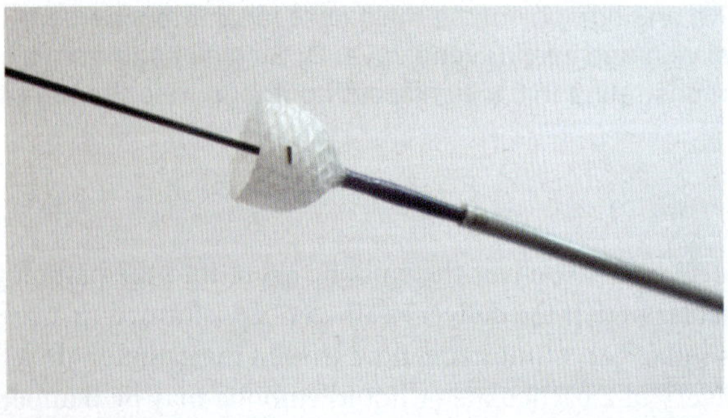

Figure 12.2 Single image of the Surefire Infusion System with a 0.018-in guidewire. The configuration helps to prevent reflux during particulate embolization procedures because the expandable tip becomes apposed to the vessel wall in the presence of reversed flow. (This image is courtesy of Surefire Medical, Inc., Westminster, Colorado.)

TIPS AND TRICKS

- A thorough knowledge of vascular anatomy is critical before the performance of any embolization procedure.
- For any embolization procedure, know what embolic agent is going to be used so that an appropriate catheter can be selected for delivery of that agent.
- Particulate embolic agents are best delivered through a microcatheter with an inner lumen of 0.027 in. Use of a catheter with a smaller inner diameter increases the risk for catheter occlusion.
- Nonselective angiography is recommended before selective catheterization to optimize the catheterization technique and to ensure that all involved vessels are embolized.
- When using a particulate embolic agent to embolize an abnormal vascular bed, controlled reflux may help identify the angiographic end point. Placing the catheter into a secondary branch within the target vascular bed allows for reflux to occur into a more proximal but still abnormal branch before the risk of nontarget embolization becomes significant.

CONCLUSION

The successful performance of embolization procedures requires a well-developed knowledge base regarding normal vascular anatomy, the indications for embolization, and the embolic agents used during these procedures. It is important to remember, though, that experience with various delivery catheters and catheterization techniques is just as important for ensuring success in this area of interventional radiology.

REFERENCES

1. Van Ha TG. Use of the Interlock Fibered IDC Occlusion System in clinical practice. *Semin Intervent Radiol.* 2008;25:3–10.
2. Arepally A, Osterman FA, Wakeman L. Pulmonary arteriovenous malformations. In: Savader SJ, Trerotola SO, eds. *Venous Interventional Radiology with Clinical Perspectives.* 2nd ed. New York, NY: Thieme Medical Publishers; 2000:163–176.

3. Coldwell DM, Stokes KR, Yakes WF. Embolotherapy: agents, clinical applications, and techniques. *Radiographics.* 1994;14:623–643.
4. Wang W, Li H, Tam MD. The Amplatzer Vascular Plug: a review of the device and its clinical applications. *Cardiovasc Intervent Radiol.* 2012;35:725–740.
5. Pollak JS, White RI. The use of cyanoacrylate adhesives in peripheral embolization. *J Vasc Interv Radiol.* 2001;12:907–913.
6. Kerber CW, Wong W. Liquid acrylic adhesive agents in interventional neuroradiology. *Neurosurg Clin N Am.* 2000;11: 85–99.
7. Guimaraes M, Wooster M. Onyx (ethylene-vinyl alcohol copolymer) in peripheral applications. *Semin Intervent Radiol.* 2011;28:350–356.
8. Choe DH, Moon HH, Gyeong HK, et al. An experimental study of embolic effect according to infusion rate and concentration of suspension in transarterial particulate embolization. *Invest Radiol.* 1997;32:260–267.
9. Abada HT, Golzarian J. Gelatin sponge particles: handling characteristics for endovascular use. *Tech Vasc Interv Radiol.* 2007;10:257–260.
10. Katsumori T, Kashara T. The size of gelatin sponge particles: differences with preparation method. *Cardiovasc Intervent Radiol.* 2006;29:1077–1083.
11. Osuga K, Miyayama S, Yamagami T, et al. Porous gelatin particles for hepatic arterial embolization—investigation of passage through current microcatheters [in Japanese]. *Gan To Kagaku Ryoho.* 2007;34:59–64.
12. Rose SC, Kikolski SG, Chomas JE. Downstream hepatic arterial blood pressure changes caused by deployment of the surefire antireflux expandable tip. *Cardiovasc Intervent Radiol.* 2013;36:1262–1269.

II

Clinical Applications

Section A Intracranial and Spine Embolization

13

Vascular Malformations

Moneeb Ehtesham • Imad S. Khan • J Mocco

Central nervous system arteriovenous malformations (AVMs) are congenital anomalies generally consisting of an abnormal tangle of thin-walled vessels (usually referred to as a *nidus*) located within the brain or spinal cord receiving inflow from one or more large- to medium-sized arterial pedicles with subsequent direct outflow to one or more large draining veins. Blood flowing through the nidus bypasses any normal intervening capillary bed, thereby creating a high-flow arteriovenous shunt which results in the presence of high-pressure arterialized blood in the draining veins.[1] When located intracranially, this pathologic state presents a significant risk for devastating intracranial hemorrhage.[2,3] Additional symptomatology can include seizures as well as cognitive or objective neurologic deficits related to either ischemia or venous hypertension and resultant cerebral or spinal cord edema.[4] The primary goal of treating these lesions is to eliminate the risk of hemorrhage. Furthermore, treatment can successfully address the localized dysfunction created by presence of the nidus by means of decreasing seizure frequency and/or preserving or improving current neurologic function.[5,6]

There are four main treatment approaches toward managing a patient with an intracranial AVM: expectant observation, microsurgical resection, endovascular embolization, and radiotherapy.[7] In reality, when pursuing treatment, many centers will use a combination of either embolization followed by surgery or embolization with subsequent radiotherapy. The evidence to support the efficacy of any specific combination of treatment modalities is currently limited to small retrospective series and remains a topic of controversy.[8–10] Regardless, the fundamental approach to any treatment plan centers on appropriate patient selection followed by defining an optimal plan for treatment for each specific patient.

PATIENT SELECTION

There is tremendous controversy regarding specific patient populations in whom treatment of intracranial AVMs should be undertaken. This is evidenced by the recently halted ARUBA (A Randomized Trial of Unruptured Brain AVMs) trial, which was a prospective randomized multicenter trial designed to compare outcomes in patients with unruptured intracranial AVMs treated expectantly with medical management versus surgical and/or endovascular intervention.[11–13] Early data reporting seems to indicate a significantly higher adverse event rate in the surgical/endovascular treatment group that led to early suspension of the study by the data safety monitoring board.[14] The full results of this study are still pending and will provide important insight into appropriate patient selection in patients who have not had a prior hemorrhage. In contrast, there is considerable (although not universal) agreement that patients who present with an AVM-related hemorrhage are generally candidates in whom therapy should be considered. Data suggest that the rebleeding rate after AVM rupture is approximately 2% to 4% per year and that each hemorrhage episode carries with it a 30% to 50% morbidity rate as well as a 10% risk for mortality.[15] Seizure control in patients with AVMs that have remained refractory to medical management can also be improved with treatment of AVMs.[16]

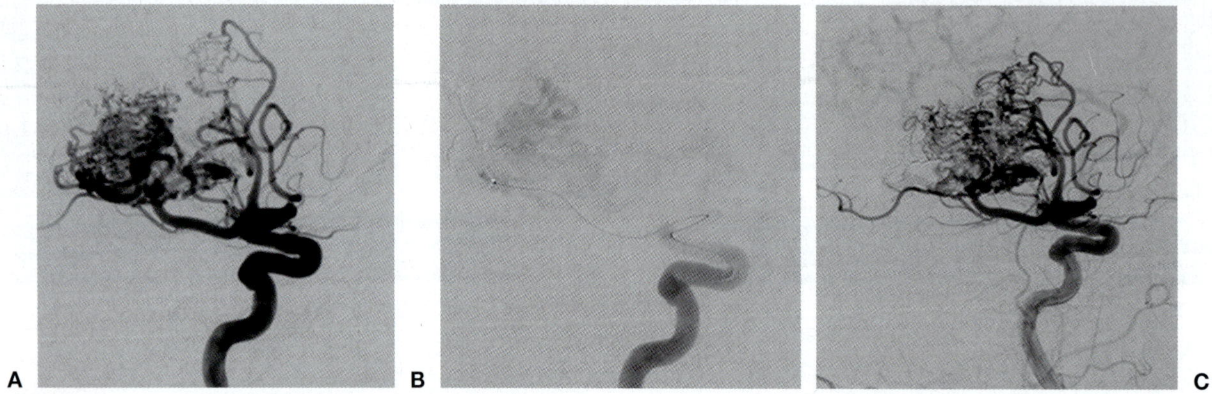

Figure 13.1 Representative digital subtraction angiography demonstrating intracranial AVMs. **A:** Lateral cranial projection of internal carotid artery injection demonstrating posterior temporal AVM being fed by multiple middle cerebral artery branches as well as a large tentorial branch off of the internal carotid artery. **B:** Lateral cranial projection of internal carotid artery injection demonstrating a parietal AVM fed by ACA and MCA pedicles. Shadow from previous embolic material in posterior aspect of nidus can also be seen. **C:** Anteroposterior cranial projection of internal carotid artery demonstrating a frontoparietal AVM being fed by ACA and MCA pedicles.

Assessment of the lesion's angioarchitecture forms a second critical arm when assessing a patient as part of the treatment planning process. To this end, it is highly recommended that all patients with newly diagnosed intracranial AVMs undergo a comprehensive cervicocerebral digital subtraction angiogram as this allows for clear delineation of the vascular anatomy of the AVM as well as its flow dynamics. The key aspects of an AVM's vascular anatomy include identifying all contributing arterial pedicles, draining veins, any associated aneurysms, as well as collateral circulation and any compensatory flow dynamics that are responsible for perfusing normal neural tissue[1] (Fig. 13.1). Furthermore, from the specific regard of suitability for endovascular treatment, it is also important to delineate potential impediments to accessing the nidus starting from aortic arch disease, carotid bifurcation disease, tortuous extracranial or intracranial carotid anatomy, as well as tortuous feeding pedicles. It is also critical to determine whether arterial feeders to the nidus are either "end pedicles" exclusively perfusing the lesion or, instead, are "en passage" with a component of supply to normal neural tissue. In the latter situation, endovascular embolization without sufficient superselective catheterization can significantly jeopardize unaffected tissue and present a prohibitive risk for treatment. Up to 50% of AVMs are associated with aneurysms.[17] These may either be intranidal or present on feeding arterial pedicles (flow-related). It is generally recognized that the presence of such aneurysms presents a higher risk of hemorrhage. More specifically, in patients presenting with hemorrhage, these aneurysmal lesions require urgent treatment if there is any suspicion based on anatomical distribution of the hemorrhage that they may be the contributory lesion.[18,19] Finally, the flow dynamics through the lesion also presents important considerations for treatment planning especially with regard to endovascular therapy. Specifically, high-flow AVMs may harbor fistulous connections between feeding arteries and draining veins, and it is important to recognize these as their extent will affect the choice of embolic material used and whether specific pedicles can be safely targeted for embolization or not.

GOALS OF ENDOVASCULAR EMBOLIZATION

As detailed earlier, endovascular therapy represents only one of several therapeutic modalities available for treating intracranial AVMs.[20] It is therefore critical that before deciding on a final treatment plan, a patient's history and angiographic anatomy (as delineated by a digital subtraction angiogram) should be reviewed by a multidisciplinary team consisting of neurointerventionalists, neurosurgeons, and radiation oncologists to allow for formulation of an optimal course of therapy best suited to that particular patient. In this regard, endovascular embolization can be incorporated as a potent tool to either decrease flow to an AVM as a precursor to planned surgical resection or as a means of decreasing nidus size to allow for more focused stereotactic radiation. Rarely, and usually only in cases of small nidal size, can embolization be used as a solitary curative modality. Therefore, the goals of embolization will be determined by which additional treatment methodologies are to be employed for that particular lesion. In the setting of preoperative embolization, the ideal embolization strategy centers on decreasing inflow into the nidus from the aspect of the lesion that will be most difficult to access from the planned surgical corridor. In this setting, a focused approach targeting catheterization via deep arterial pedicles that will not be directly visible to the surgeon can result in improved intraoperative visibility during microsurgical dissection and decreased blood loss.

Similarly, nidal penetration of embolic material helps to better delineate the nidus during microsurgical dissection, and knowledge of the angiographic pattern of embolization helps orient the surgeon particularly in the setting of large, complex nidal resections.[21] In certain situations, surgical resection may not be feasible given the presence of eloquent neural tissue in close proximity to the nidus. In these scenarios, targeted embolization of nidal segments adjacent to eloquent regions can help decrease radiation exposure to important functional neural tissue as stereotactic radiotherapy can be targeted to the residual lesion with increased dose step-off between the radiation field and adjacent eloquent tissue. If pursued, endovascular embolization can be performed in a "staged" technique wherein specific portions of the nidus are targeted (frequently via a distinct single feeding pedicle at each sitting). When used, staged embolizations are felt to be safer as they decrease the total radiation exposure in a single sitting and also minimize the likelihood of overaggressive nidal embolization.[22]

TECHNIQUES

Materials

Various materials have been used for embolotherapy in the setting of endovascular AVM treatment. Of historical interest is the previous use of liquid coils (essentially deliverable soft/coiled wires), detachable balloons for proximal arterial pedicle occlusion, silastic pellets, silk sutures, and absolute alcohol. The use of these diverse agents has now largely been supplanted by the development of new liquid embolic agents. Key among these is the cyanoacrylate polymer, Histoacryl Blue (*N*-butyl cyanoacrylate [NBCA]; Aesculap, Center Valley, Pennsylvania), and the DMSO-based liquid precipitate, Onyx (Covidien, Irvine, California).[20] NBCA is mixed with low-viscosity oil-based contrast medium (typically Ethiodol), and this mixture can be additionally supplemented with tantalum particles to enhance radiopacity. Given that NBCA precipitates nearly immediately upon contact with ionic solutes in blood, the delivery microcatheter has to be prerinsed with dextrose–water before administration. The flow rate and eventual penetration potential of the embolic agent as it emerges from the delivery catheter can be modulated by adjusting final viscosity based on concentration of Ethiodol as well as by adjusting the intensity and pace of the hand injection through the microcatheter. Given the significant adhesive properties of NBCA, it is imperative that the delivery catheter be removed immediately following delivery of agent as failure to do so can result in significant vascular injury as removal of a stuck microcatheter is attempted in a delicate intracranial vascular tree. Onyx is a newer liquid embolic agent that does not instantly precipitate, thereby theoretically allowing for greater downstream penetration. Furthermore, a developing Onyx cast does not demonstrate adhesion to the delivery catheter. As such, although it remains important to not allow excessive reflux along the microcatheter of Onyx precipitate, it is possible to build a small Onyx plug along the distal-most end of the microcatheter. This allows for enhanced proximal occlusion of the microcatheterized feeding pedicle, creating a "back pressure" that then permits subsequent Onyx injections to penetrate deep into downstream nidus.[23,24] Although a treatment session with Onyx can take significantly longer as compared to when using NBCA, in our experience, it allows for more controlled and targeted delivery of embolic agent.

Patient Preparation

The initial aspects of patient preparation include a detailed discussion with the patient and/or family regarding the goals of treatment. As discussed earlier, it is our recommendation that all patients being considered for treatment be initially evaluated with a digital subtraction cervicocerebral diagnostic angiogram. Review of the data provided by this study and correlation of the findings with each patient's specific clinical situation will allow the practitioner to formulate and present a comprehensive rationale for treatment. Following this, all patients should undergo an appropriate preoperative medical workup, including assessments of their medical comorbidities. The presence of significant medical conditions can significantly affect prognosis, and this should factor into discussions regarding the risks and benefits of therapy. Finally, renal function should be assessed as endovascular therapy of these lesions will often require a significant contrast load and those with impaired renal function should undergo appropriate preprocedure hydration. Following these steps, patients are brought to the angiography suite and placed under general anesthesia. Appropriate blood pressure monitoring in the form of invasive arterial transduction is established to allow for close blood pressure monitoring and titration.

Endovascular Treatment Platform

Arterial access for endovascular therapy is typically obtained via the transfemoral route and a 6-Fr short sheath. Alternative access can be established via a transradial route (if the aortic arch is significantly diseased or if a tortuous vertebral artery with unfavorable proximal anatomy is to be accessed). A longer sheath with its tip in the common carotid artery can be used if additional support is desired in the setting of a capacious descending aorta or aortic arch. In the absence of any recent intracranial hemorrhage, a loading bolus of 3,000 to 5,000 International Units of intravenous (IV) heparin is given and an activated clotting time goal of 200 to 260 seconds is set. If planning to use Onyx for embolization, it is imperative to use a DMSO-compatible microcatheter. Our current catheter of choice is the Marathon flow-directed catheter (Covidien, Irvine, California). Given the supple nature of this embolic delivery catheter, it is imperative to use an intermediate coaxial catheter system that will allow for distal navigation of the delivery microcatheter. For this purpose, we generally use a 6-Fr guide catheter (Neuron

0.70 in [Penumbra, Alameda, California] or Envoy MPD 0.70 in [DePuy Orthopaedics, Inc., Warsaw, Indiana]) along with a distal access catheter (DAC 0.38 in [Concentric Medical, Hertogenbosch, the Netherlands]). For the anterior cerebral circulation, the DAC is typically delivered into the proximal middle cerebral artery (MCA) or anterior cerebral artery (ACA), whereas for the posterior circulation, it is typically taken up to the level of the distal vertebral artery. Following this, the Marathon microcatheter is typically navigated over a 0.10-in microwire into a feeding arterial pedicle from which point onward the microwire is withdrawn into the microcatheter and the catheter tip is flow-directed to a point just proximal to entry into the nidus. The ability to navigate as close as possible to the nidus will allow for optimal penetration of delivered embolic material into the AVM nidus. This is critically important as embolization of feeding pedicles alone will not result in adequate treatment of the lesion as deafferented nidus will re-recruit additional arterial supply over time. Penetration of embolic material with resulting obliteration of the nidal lumen is critical for effective treatment of these lesions. It is therefore imperative that adequate effort be undertaken to navigate the microcatheter tip into as optimal a position as possible. The use of intermediate coaxial guide and delivery catheters (as detailed earlier) serves to assist with distal delivery of the microcatheter tip, particularly in the setting of tortuous vascular anatomy.

Embolization Technique

Once microcatheter delivery to an optimal location has been achieved, it is critical to study the relevant angiographic runs carefully before commencing embolization. These should consist first of an overall angiographic image of the vascular architecture of the relevant part of the brain, which is typically obtained by contrast injection into an upstream guide catheter. This should allow for complete visualization of the nidus and delineate all significant feeding arterial pedicles, draining veins, and blood flow patterns to the surrounding brain. Second, a microinjection through the microcatheter should be performed, and this will provide a focused overview of the angiographic anatomy downstream of the microcatheter tip.[23] Particular attention should be paid to the nidal penetration of injected contrast material, the presence of any *en passage* arterial supply to normal brain, and the location and timing of venous outflow. Only upon obtaining a clear understanding of the anatomy and flow dynamics of the lesion should embolization be undertaken. In preparation for use of Onyx, the microcatheter is prerinsed in situ with an appropriate volume of DMSO. This volume will be equivalent to the microcatheter dead space volume, which is available in the microcatheter package. It is imperative that the catheter be purged of ionic contents before Onyx injection as failure to do so will result in Onyx precipitation within the catheter itself. However, it is also important to note that DMSO injection into the catheter should be performed very slowly as this solvent is caustic and can induce vasospasm and angionecrosis in downstream vasculature. Once this has been performed, Onyx liquid embolic is gently injected under direct fluoroscopic visualization, and careful modulation of the hand injection intensity and pace is used to allow the injected stream to gradually progress down the catheterized arterial pedicle and into the nidus. It is essential that Onyx penetration into the draining venous system be avoided as venous compromise significantly increases the risk of hemorrhage and must be avoided. As the Onyx cast builds up proximally to the catheter tip, the initial injection is halted and the intravascular embolic cast is allowed to solidify. Subsequent injections are modulated very carefully to maximize distal penetration of embolic material and minimize proximal reflux. Although a small degree of Onyx reflux along the distal catheter can be tolerated, a significant cast should not be created along the microcatheter as this will impede its removal. Even though Onyx is not adhesive, its cohesive properties can cause microcatheters to get lodged, and attempted removal can result in significant traction on the intracranial vascular tree, significantly increasing the risk of hemorrhagic complications.[25,26] Once embolization through the pedicle of choice is completed, the microcatheter is gently disengaged from the Onyx cast. This will frequently require the progressive building of tension on the microcatheter tip. As this tension is built, the intermediate DAC catheter that was previously parked in the proximal vasculature can be brought into the proximal portion of the feeding pedicle, allowing for more direct force transmission to the microcatheter tip and less distortion of the intracranial vascular anatomy. Upon successful disengagement, the microcatheter is removed. Follow-up angiography is performed to assess the results of the embolization (Fig. 13.2). At this point, it is critical to look specifically for any signs of untoward occurrence including compromise of venous outflow, presence of embolic material in unintended locations, or any extravasation indicative of hemorrhage. In the absence of these conditions, a new microcatheter can then be navigated into the vascular tree for purposes of microcatheterizing additional feeding arterial pedicles if desired. Although there is debate regarding how much of the nidus can be safely embolized in a single treatment setting, in our practice, we generally limit ourselves to approximately one-third of the lesion. Embolizations that are more aggressive than this carry with them the risk of increasing hemorrhagic complications resulting from significantly increased transient flow through the remaining nonembolized nidus.[25,27] Therefore, it is important to emphasize tight blood pressure control following embolization. If there is inadvertent embolization of a significantly larger portion of nidus than was initially intended or any untoward sign concerning for venous outflow compromise, then strong consideration should be given to urgent same-day surgical resection of the remaining lesion. In case staged embolizations are deemed suitable, the patient is brought back for another embolization session 2 to 3 weeks after the previous session.

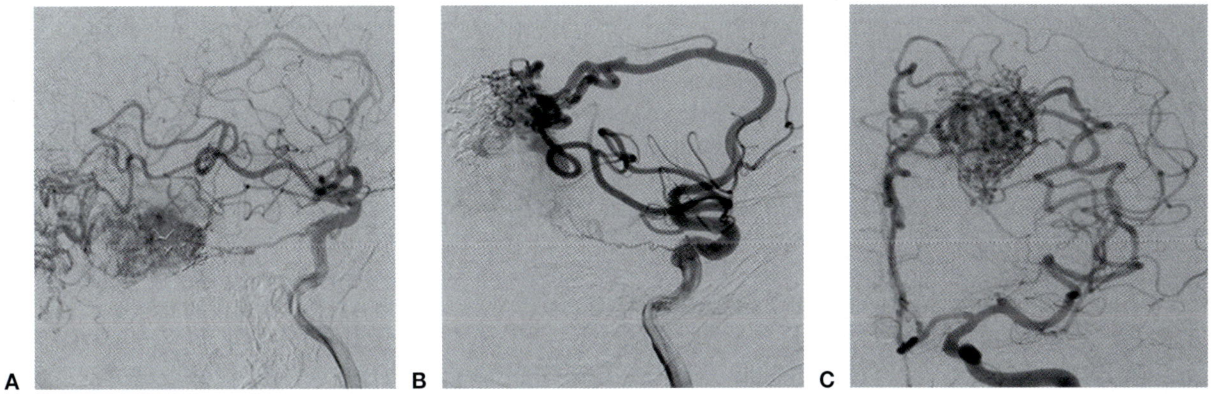

Figure 13.2 Partial endovascular embolization of posterior temporoparietal AVM. **A:** Preprocedure lateral projection view demonstrates large nidus being fed principally via large MCA pedicles. **B:** Microcatheter navigation into distal MCA pedicle with microcatheter injection demonstrating filling of nidus. **C:** Postembolization lateral projection of internal carotid artery injection demonstrating absence of filling in posterior aspect of embolized nidus.

POSTOPERATIVE MANAGEMENT

Upon completion of embolization and successful withdrawal of the microcatheter/DAC construct, a final set of angiographic images is obtained to assess the final results of the procedure. Specific attention is directed toward assessing the extent of final nidus embolization and ensuring that venous outflow patterns remain preserved. Additionally, the remaining hemispheric vasculature must be inspected carefully to ensure that there are no vascular cutoffs secondary to inadvertent distal embolization of embolic material or thromboembolism. The guide catheter should be withdrawn carefully from the cervical segment of the internal carotid or vertebral artery and a final cervical angiogram performed to confirm absence of inadvertent injury to the cervical segment. Finally, these terminal angiographic images can be closely scrutinized at the end of the case to determine the need (if any) for further staged embolization procedures and the potential vascular access route to be used if further endovascular intervention is to be pursued.

TIPS AND TRICKS

Complication and Potential Hazard	Avoiding Hazard	Addressing Complication
Large vessel dissection Distal placement of robust access platform frequently requires guide catheter placement in the high cervical internal carotid artery as well as intracranial navigation of intermediate-bore DACs. The stiffness of these catheters presents a risk of intimal dissection, particularly at areas of tortuosity.	• Place guide catheters/DACs either well proximal or distal to significant vascular anatomic "inflexion" points related to vessel tortuosity. This will minimize the risk of intimal injury by subsequent catheter movement during the procedure. • Maintain good visualization of guide catheter/DAC position on at least one plane during embolization procedure. • Use newer generation catheters that are better optimized to provide platform stability with enhanced catheter tip softness.	• Ensure thorough angiographic evaluation of vascular injury. • Load patient with dual antiplatelet agents. • If dissection is felt to be flow-compromising, stenting may be required.

Complication and Potential Hazard	Avoiding Hazard	Addressing Complication
Thromboembolism Formation of thrombus along or within guide catheters can lead to large vessel occlusion or (more frequently) embolism of thrombus into smaller, distal vasculature.	• Maintain all catheters on continuous heparinized saline flush. Ensure that all lines and connections remain air-free. • Pay close attention to all angiographic runs to detect any sign of vascular cutoff at earliest possible instant. • In the setting of nonruptured lesions, treat patient with IV heparin bolus before embolization and monitor serial activated clotting time (ACT).	• Ensure thorough angiographic evaluation of compromised vasculature as well as assessment of collateral supply. • In case of large vessel occlusion, consider mechanical clot retrieval/aspiration. • Consider treatment with intra-arterial antiplatelet agents (GpIIb/IIIa inhibitors) either via guide catheter or through targeted microcatheter delivery.
Inadvertent delivery of embolic material to unintended intracranial location Liquid embolic material (NBCA or Onyx) may embolize to locations other than the intended nidus, particularly if an *en passage* pedicle is being used as an access route or if embolization is being performed off a small branch originating from a large artery.	• Careful selection of arterial pedicle(s) for embolization with specific attention to presence of any *en passage* feeders that may be at risk in case of inadvertent embolization. • It is important to deliver the microcatheter to as distal a location as possible, particularly when the targeted pedicle is originating off of a large vessel (e.g., internal carotid artery or MCA). This will minimize the risk of embolic material refluxing into the large parent artery and then embolizing downstream. • It is critical that while embolic material is being delivered, it should be monitored with continuous live fluoroscopy to assess the exact location of the vascular tree where progressive embolization is occurring. If at *any* point visualization is compromised, embolization should be ceased immediately. • The radiopacity of Onyx derives from suspended tantalum particles. It is critical that when not in active use, Onyx should be continuously agitated to ensure that tantalum particles do not settle. Likewise, the radiopacity of NBCA can be supplemented by addition of tantalum particles.	• Ensure thorough angiographic evaluation of compromised vasculature as well as assessment of collateral supply. • If thrombus formation is felt to be accentuating vessel compromise at sites of inadvertent embolization, consider intra-arterial treatment with antiplatelet agents (GpIIb/IIIa inhibitors) to maintain flow across compromised vessels. • Consider raising blood pressure to help maintain perfusion via collateral vasculature.

REFERENCES

1. Achrol AS, Guzman R, Varga M, et al. Pathogenesis and radiobiology of brain arteriovenous malformations: implications for risk stratification in natural history and posttreatment course. *Neurosurg Focus*. 2009;26(5):E9.
2. Fullerton HJ, Achrol AS, Johnston SC, et al. Long-term hemorrhage risk in children versus adults with brain arteriovenous malformations. *Stroke*. 2005;36(10):2099–2104.
3. Brown RD Jr, Wiebers DO, Forbes G, et al. The natural history of unruptured intracranial arteriovenous malformations. *J Neurosurg*. 1988;68(3):352–357.
4. Buis DR, Van Den Berg R, Lagerwaard FJ, et al. Brain arteriovenous malformations: from diagnosis to treatment. *J Neurosurg Sci*. 2011;55(1):39–56.
5. Deruty R, Pelissou-Guyotat I, Morel C, et al. Reflections on the management of cerebral arteriovenous malformations. *Surg Neurol*. 1998;50(3):245–255.
6. Niazi TN, Klimo P Jr, Anderson RCE, et al. Diagnosis and management of arteriovenous malformations in children. *Neurosurg Clin N Am*. 2010;21(3):443–456.
7. Barr JC, Ogilvy CS. Selection of treatment modalities or observation of arteriovenous malformations. *Neurosurg Clin N Am*. 2012;23(1):63–75.

8. Monaco EA III, Niranjan A, Kano H, et al. Management of adverse radiation effects after radiosurgery for arteriovenous malformations. *Prog Neurol Surg.* 2013;27:107–118.
9. Reig AS, Rajaram R, Simon S, et al. Complete angiographic obliteration of intracranial AVMs with endovascular embolization: incomplete embolic nidal opacification is associated with AVM recurrence. *J Neurointerv Surg.* 2010;2(3):202–207.
10. Consoli A, Scarpini G, Rosi A, et al. Endovascular treatment of unruptured and ruptured brain arteriovenous malformations with Onyx18: a monocentric series of 84 patients [published online ahead of print October 14, 2013]. *J Neurointerv Surg.*
11. Fiehler J, Stapf C. ARUBA—beating natural history in unruptured brain AVMs by intervention. *Neuroradiology.* 2008;50(6): 465–467.
12. Mohr JP, Moskowitz AJ, Parides M, et al. Hull down on the horizon: A Randomized Trial of Unruptured Brain Arteriovenous Malformations (ARUBA) trial. *Stroke.* 2012;43(7):1744–1745.
13. Stapf C. The rationale behind "A Randomized Trial of Unruptured Brain AVMs" (ARUBA). *Acta Neurochir Suppl.* 2010;107: 83–85.
14. National Institute of Neurological Disorders and Stroke. A Randomized Trial of Unruptured Brain Arteriovenous Malformations (ARUBA). National Institute of Neurological Disorders and Stroke Web site. http://www.ninds.nih.gov/news_and_events/news_articles/ARUBA_trial_results.htm. Updated January 29, 214. Accessed October 31, 2013.
15. Ondra SL, Troupp H, George ED, et al. The natural history of symptomatic arteriovenous malformations of the brain: a 24-year follow-up assessment. *J Neurosurg.* 1990;73(3):387–391.
16. Englot DJ, Young WL, Han SJ, et al. Seizure predictors and control after microsurgical resection of supratentorial arteriovenous malformations in 440 patients. *Neurosurgery.* 2012;71(3): 572–580; discussion 580.
17. Elhammady MS, Aziz-Sultan MA, Heros RC. The management of cerebral arteriovenous malformations associated with aneurysms. *World Neurosurg.* 2013;80:e123–e129.
18. Ezura M, Takahashi A, Jokura H, et al. Endovascular treatment of aneurysms associated with cerebral arteriovenous malformations: experiences after the introduction of Guglielmi detachable coils. *J Clin Neurosci.* 2000;7(suppl 1):14–18.
19. Deruty R, Mottolese C, Soustiel JF, et al. Association of cerebral arteriovenous malformation and cerebral aneurysm: diagnosis and management. *Acta Neurochir (Wien).* 1990;107(3–4): 133–139.
20. Bristol RE, Albuquerque FC, McDougall CG. The evolution of endovascular treatment for intracranial arteriovenous malformations. *Neurosurg Focus.* 2006;20(6):E6.
21. Rodríguez-Boto G, Gutiérrez-González R, Gil A, et al. Combined staged therapy of complex arteriovenous malformations: initial experience. *Acta Neurol Scand.* 2013;127(4):260–267.
22. Kano H, Kondziolka D, Flickinger JC, et al. Stereotactic radiosurgery for arteriovenous malformations after embolization: a case-control study. *J Neurosurg.* 2012;117(2):265–275.
23. Weber W, Kis B, Siekmann R, et al. Endovascular treatment of intracranial arteriovenous malformations with onyx: technical aspects. *AJNR Am J Neuroradiol.* 2007;28(2):371–377.
24. Saatci I, Geyik S, Yavuz K, et al. Endovascular treatment of brain arteriovenous malformations with prolonged intranidal Onyx injection technique: long-term results in 350 consecutive patients with completed endovascular treatment course. *J Neurosurg.* 2011;115(1):78–88.
25. Ledezma CJ, Hoh BL, Carter BS, et al. Complications of cerebral arteriovenous malformation embolization: multivariate analysis of predictive factors. *Neurosurgery.* 2006;58(4): 602–611; discussion 602–611.
26. Sun Y, Lv X, Li Y, et al. Complications caused by cerebral arteriovenous malformation embolization. *Neuroradiol J.* 2012;25(5): 541–547.
27. Biondi A, Le Jean L, Capelle L, et al C. Fatal hemorrhagic complication following endovascular treatment of a cerebral arteriovenous malformation: case report and review of the literature. *J Neuroradiol.* 2006;33(2):96–104.

14

Intracranial Aneurysms

M. Imran Chaudry • Alejandro Spiotta • Raymond Turner
Harris Hawk • Jonathan R. Lena • Aquilla Turk

The International Symptomatic Aneurysm Trial (ISAT) and the Barrow Ruptured Aneurysm Trial (BRAT) firmly established endovascular therapy as a primary method for treating ruptured intracranial aneurysms. The development of new techniques has broadened the scope of practice to allow for the treatment of geometrically complex aneurysms.[1–6] Critical advances in coil technology and the development of novel flexible guide and intermediate catheters providing improved device stability and deliverability, intracranial stents, as well as the introduction of balloon remodeling and flow-diverting stent technology have expanded the indications of endovascular therapy to both wide-necked and fusiform aneurysms. The adoption of these devices has contributed to a larger proportion of aneurysms treated by endovascular means.[7]

DEVICE DESCRIPTIONS

Distal Access Guide Catheters

Fundamental to any endovascular intervention is the need for stable access to the target lesion. Proximal vessel tortuosity may limit the ability to deliver the guide catheter distally in the vessel of interest, thereby resulting in long distances that the working microcatheter must cover before addressing the target lesion. If the microcatheter and wire travel over redundant segments of a vessel or multiple acute-angled turns, the microcatheter and wire may respond unpredictably when manipulated. Erratic behavior of the microcatheter or microwire may result in technical complications, for example, aneurysm perforation during access for coil embolization and suboptimal stent placement during unsheathing if the microcatheter sails in either direction. The development of neurospecific guiding catheters has resulted in various access devices that offer various advantages with regard to trackability, distal and proximal support, and improved distal access. There is considerable crossover in the design of intermediary catheters and newer generation neurospecific guide catheters. The Neuron 0.053-in and 0.070-in in guide catheters, the 0.088-in Neuron Max sheath (Penumbra, Inc., Alameda, California), as well as the Chaperon 0.071-in guide catheter (MicroVention, Tustin, California) are designed to provide distal guide catheter access, often to the cavernous segment of the internal carotid artery, providing a large stable conduit for intracranial procedures (Fig. 14.1).

These devices have been shown to be safer than traditional axial guide catheters while providing distal access, often obviating the need for an intermediate catheter. The goal is to place the diagnostic insert into the petrous segment over a 0.038-in hydrophilic guidewire (Glidewire; Terumo Interventional Systems, Somerset, New Jersey) and then advance the guide or sheath over the diagnostic insert into at least the petrous carotid. These larger guide catheters and sheath allow for multiple devices (either balloon and coiling microcatheter or stent delivery catheter and coiling microcatheter) to be deployed simultaneously. The use of larger sheaths may allow for three devices to be deployed simultaneously when coiling with the aid of two balloons, for example.

Microcatheters and Microwires

Endosaccular coil embolization relies on the ability to safely access the aneurysmal sac with a microcatheter that can house a coil. Access to the aneurysm is safest with the microcatheter tracking over a microguidewire. Catheter and microguidewire technology has not significantly changed since the introduction of the 0.0165-in SL-10 (Boston Scientific Corporation, Natick, Massachusetts) microcatheter. To date, the SL-10

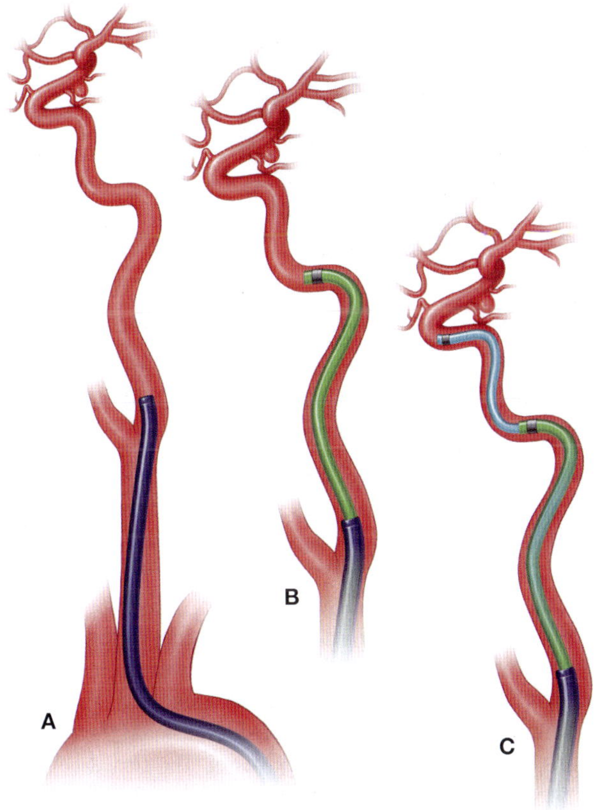

Figure 14.1 **A:** Traditional guide catheter placement in the internal carotid artery. **B,C:** New, distal access guide catheter placement in the petrous segment of the carotid artery. Frequently, these catheters can be placed into the vertical petrous segment or cavernous segment. This provides a stable platform and eliminates the axial excursions that occur with each heartbeat. This allows for safer microcatheter access for intracranial procedures.

remains our workhorse microcatheter as do the 0.014-in Transend Platinum (Stryker Corporation, Kalamazoo, Michigan) and Synchro-2 microwires (Boston Scientific Corporation, Natick, Massachusetts). These two wires deliver the adequate "softness" needed to negotiate tortuous anatomy without causing microperforations while providing sufficient support for over-the-wire microcatheter navigation. Note that intermittent reshaping of the microwire may be necessary during a procedure to navigate a patient's specific anatomy. We have found that the SL-10 microcatheter tracks favorably over an 0.014-in microwire even in acutely angled vessels. Microcatheters are available in straight and preshaped angled or curved variations, allowing more versatility. Slightly stiffer microcatheters such as the Echelon 10 (Covidien, Irvine, California) maybe used when there is concern for catheter prolapse out of the target aneurysm or when more support for coiling is required. Once access to the aneurysm is obtained, these flexible microcatheters will respond to the stress applied to it by superimposed curves by adopting the parent vessel curvature, which leads to their stability at the aneurysm during coil deployment. The introduction of large-volume coils (Penumbra PC 400; Penumbra, Inc., Alameda, California) has required the introduction of larger 0.025-in coiling microcatheters (Penumbra PX400 and Penumbra SLIM) to allow delivery of these coils. Catheter technology has improved to make these larger and inherently stiffer catheters extremely navigable. However, the main issue with these larger catheters is catching on the lip of the aneurysm neck that may limit catheter access. This may be overcome by advancing the microwire well into the aneurysm, loading the microcatheter and spinning the wire so as to raise the microcatheter from the aneurysm neck. Care must be taken not to load the microcatheter to a degree where it jumps forward into the aneurysm.

Coil Technology

The introduction of coils into an aneurysm provides a thrombogenic mechanical barrier to aneurysmal inflow, which immediately protects the dome while promoting intra-aneurysmal progressive thrombosis and occlusion. The coils furthermore provide a biologic scaffold to promote endothelial growth across the aneurysm neck and vessel healing, resulting in complete exclusion of the aneurysm from the circulation. The initial experience with aneurysm coil embolization did not involve any adjunctive devices such as balloons or stents ("unassisted" coil embolization). As such, the only factors that could be modified by the operator to achieve a successful embolization were the position of the microcatheter relative to the aneurysm neck and dome as well as the size, length, and shape of the coil selected. The introduction of complex coils that could adopt various geometric shapes once deployed resulted in a greater number of aneurysm morphologies considered suitable for coil embolization. The first commercially available detachable coils[8] were stiff by today's standards. Although the duration required for detachment ranged between 10–45 minutes, the detachment mechanism allowed for controlled deployment, repositioning, and removal. This was a significant improvement over detachable balloons used for vessel sacrifice. However, coil distribution of this two-dimensional design (helix) did not consistently allow for good neck coverage. The introduction of coils that adopt an intrinsic three-dimensional (3-D) spherical shape once deployed revolutionized the approach to coil embolization. These would become known as *framing coils*, thereby creating a robust frame covering the neck and dome of an aneurysm (Fig. 14.2).

Subsequently, the frame is filled with softer (filling) coils in a "Russian doll" manner. This technique allows for a greater safety margin as the framing coil restricts outward movement of subsequent coils away from the dome and parent vessel and directs filling towards the center of the aneurysm sac. Smaller and softer coils with irregular breakpoints were then introduced to act as "finishing coils" to fill in irregularly shaped neck remnants. The material of the coil greatly affects how it will behave in vivo. Although platinum, which is an inert metal with

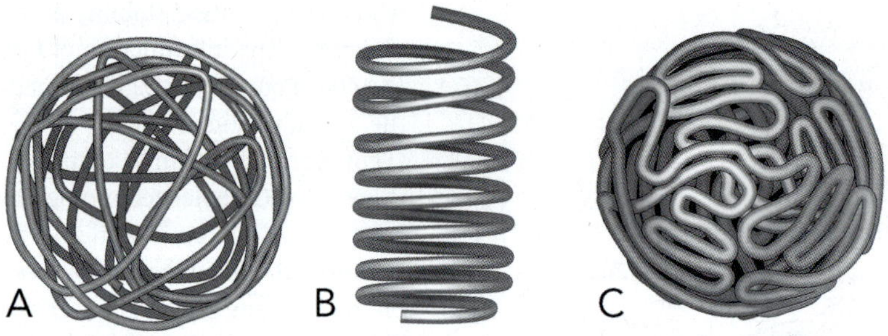

Figure 14.2 Diagram demonstrating the differences in complex coils, which intrinsically take a basket or 3-D shape **(A)**, helical coils **(B)**, and larger volume coils **(C)**.

material characteristics favorable for coil manufacturing, has emerged as the only material in clinical use, variations of coil composition have been introduced to impart additional biologic advantages. For example, a proinflammatory bioactive coil (Matrix; Boston Scientific Corporation, Natick, Massachusetts; Cerecyte; Micrus Endovascular Corporation, San Jose, California) may promote the wound healing cascade and cellular ingrowth into the coil mass and at the neck, whereas a gel–platinum hybrid coil (HydroCoil/HydroSoft; Terumo Interventional Systems, Somerset, New Jersey) that swells to a greater volume when in an aqueous solution such as blood may provide a higher packing density and thereby a lower recurrence rate. Recently, the Penumbra 400 (Penumbra, Inc., Alameda, California) represents another iteration of coil evolution. The Penumbra 400 has a much larger 0.020-in cross-sectional area, which is four times the cross-sectional area of a 0.010-in coil system. By using a nitinol core wire and an outer shell of platinum, the approach was to use a very high volume to length coil to rapidly fill aneurysms. Whatever coil system and strategy is employed, one factor remains constant: results from the Cerebral Aneurysm Rerupture After Treatment (CARAT) study[9] support aggressive coil embolization (packing density) as the likelihood of recurrence is related to the degree of initial occlusion.

Balloons

There are five commercially available neurovascular balloons. These are the HyperForm, HyperGlide (Covidien/EV3; Irvine, California), Scepter C, Scepter XC (Terumo/MicroVention, Inc., Tustin, California), and the Transform (Stryker Corporation, Kalamazoo, Michigan) balloons. The HyperGlide, Scepter C, and Transform balloons are compliant balloons intended for the treatment of sidewall aneurysms, whereas the HyperForm and Scepter XC are hypercompliant balloons intended for use in the treatment of wide-necked bifurcation aneurysms. These hypercompliant balloons tend to protrude well into the aneurysm neck and may be used to preserve vessels that arise within the neck of an aneurysm. To a large degree, we have found the compliance of the balloons to be somewhat similar and the balloons maybe used interchangeably. What sets the balloons apart is their ability to navigate tortuous, difficult anatomy as well as their stability at the aneurysm neck.

Stents

Currently, there are two commercially available nitinol self-expanding stents: an open-cell Neuroform stent (Stryker Corporation, Kalamazoo, Michigan) and a closed-cell Enterprise Vascular Reconstruction Device (VRD) (Cordis Corporation, Miami Lakes, Florida). Briefly, the open-cell design may have better wall apposition around sharp turns; however, it may create a shelflike extension into an aneurysm that arises around an acute bend or bifurcation (basilar apex). This shelf may be advantageous depending on its position but has the risk of coil loops prolapsing into the parent vessel. The closed-cell design of the Enterprise VRD may have suboptimal wall adherence around turns, but this can be reduced by more pushing of the stent as it is deployed rather than a true unsheathing. In theory, there is a lower chance of coil loops prolapsing into the parent vessel. On the other hand, newer, self-expanding braided stents are currently available as part of investigational device exemption (IDE) or 510(k) trials and should be commercially available within the next 2 to 3 years. Within the near future, we expect to see the commercial availability of braided stents such as the Low-Profile Visualized Intraluminal Support (LVIS) and LVIS Jr. (Terumo/MicroVention, Tustin, California). The advantage of these self-expanding braided stents is that there is better wall apposition around turns, and the braided structure allows for pore sized such that coil loop prolapse is highly unlikely.

Flow Diversion

Large and giant aneurysms and fusiform aneurysms remain a challenge to treat, whether from an endovascular or open standpoint. The Pipeline Embolization Device (PED) (Covidien/eV3, Irvine, California) is a novel flow-diverting stent that revolutionized the treatment paradigm for large and giant aneurysms from the petrous internal carotid artery to the ophthalmic segment. The PED is a high mesh braided stentlike device that allows for remodeling of the parent vessel wall and gradual occlusion of an aneurysm. The use of these devices may be technically less challenging than traditional treatments (open clipping, coiling, balloon, or stent coiling) of these aneurysms; however, the long-term durability and morbidity/mortality related to the use of these devices remain to be seen.

Currently, there is a randomized study (LARGE Aneurysm Randomized Trial: Flow Diversion versus Traditional Endovascular Coiling Therapy) that looks to evaluate the treatment of large and giant aneurysms with flow diversion versus traditional coiling methods. We eagerly await these results.

TECHNIQUES

Unassisted Coiling

The ISAT firmly established endovascular therapy as the primary method for treating ruptured aneurysms. With the considerable advances in coil technology, endovascular therapy is becoming the accepted treatment for ruptured and unruptured aneurysms. The introduction and development of complex framing coils, filling coils, and finishing coils have made many aneurysms previously considered uncoilable amenable to endovascular therapy.

The goal of any "coiling" procedure is the complete occlusion of the target aneurysm and the prevention of aneurysm rupture. The ideal aneurysm for unassisted coiling is one with a favorable neck (<4 mm) or dome-to-neck ratio greater than 2:1. Small-necked aneurysms are much more amenable to primary coiling, using the shoulders of the aneurysm neck to buttress the coils and keep them within the aneurysm sac. In smaller aneurysms (3 to 10 mm), the catheter is ideally positioned at the neck or within the proximal one-third of the base. In larger aneurysms, an "around the world" technique maybe used in which the coiling microcatheter is brought into the aneurysm and the tip placed approximately three-quarters of the way around the aneurysm sac in such a manner that the catheter is essentially pointing back at the neck. This allows the catheter to gradually migrate back to the neck, preventing early kick out of the catheter. Although there are many techniques in framing, filling, and finishing, we tend to use the "Russian doll technique." We frame with a framing coil with the goal of getting neck coverage and systematically stepping down in coil size to coil within the coil mass. Coil diameters are sized to the largest diameter in spherical aneurysms, and in irregular oblong or bilobed aneurysms, coil diameter size is often based on the average diameter ([Length × Width × Height]/3). Commonly, we will use multiple framing coils (decreasing in diameter and length) to frame and fill the aneurysm and subsequently switch to soft helical or complex finishing coils to pack both the aneurysm sac and neck. Our goal is always complete occlusion of the aneurysm (Fig. 14.3).

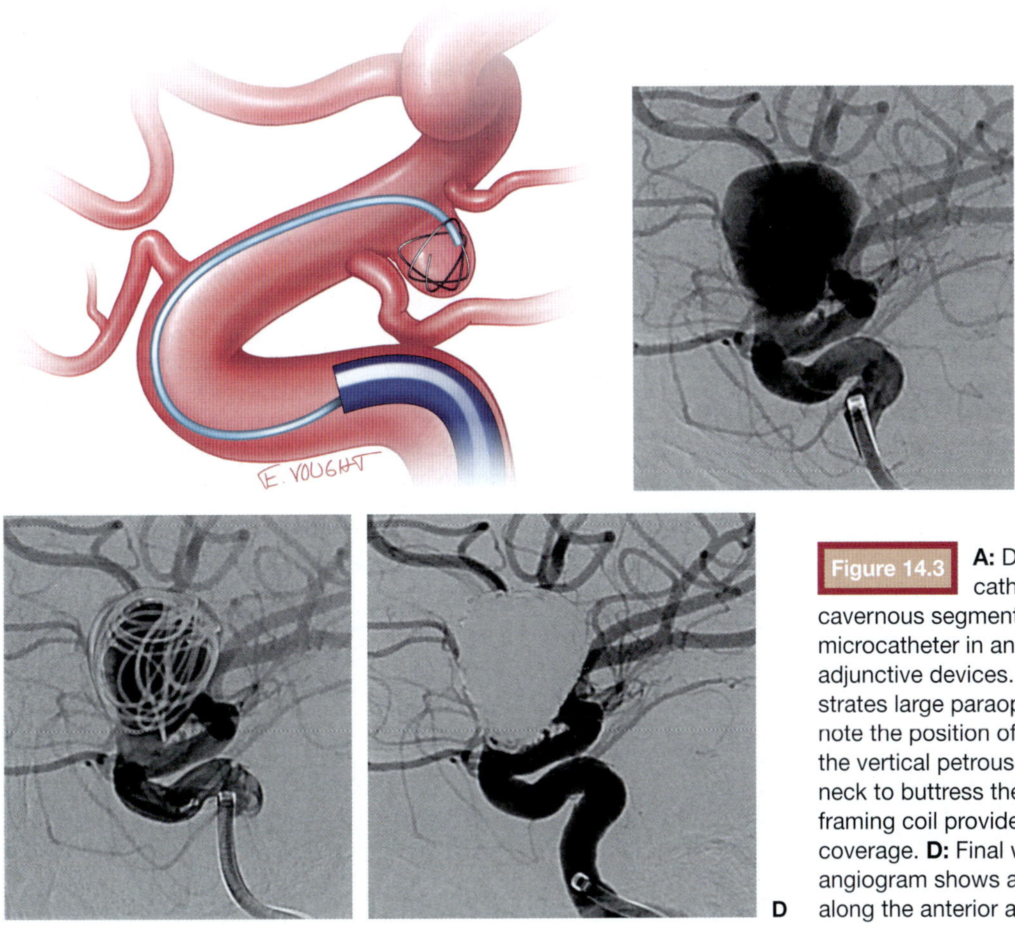

Figure 14.3 **A:** Diagram depicting guide catheter access into the cavernous segment of the carotid; single microcatheter in aneurysm without other adjunctive devices. **B:** Angiogram demonstrates large paraophthalmic aneurysm; note the position of the guide catheter in the vertical petrous segment. **C:** Using the neck to buttress the coils, the initial framing coil provides adequate neck coverage. **D:** Final working projection angiogram shows a very tiny neck remnant along the anterior aspect of the neck.

Dual Catheter Technique

The dual catheter technique was an earlier technique employed in the treatment of irregular wide-necked aneurysms before the availability of balloons and stents. It is still used occasionally in the setting of subarachnoid hemorrhage where stents (and antiplatelet therapy) is contraindicated and in tortuous small vessel anatomy where a balloon may not navigate. In this technique, two microcatheters are introduced into the aneurysm sac. The first is usually positioned at the neck through which a framing coil is delivered. The second catheter is placed into the aneurysm sac through which filling and finishing coils are introduced. The initial framing coil is not detached until the end in attempts to maintain its position and stability throughout the case. Commonly, the framing coil is undersized to prevent encroachment into the parent neck (Fig. 14.4).

Balloon Remodeling

The use of balloon remodeling, first described by Moret and colleagues[10] in 1997, involves the temporary inflation of a balloon across the neck of an aneurysm, allowing for coil deployment into aneurysms with unfavorable neck-to-dome ratios.[4] As coils are inserted, a stable 3-D coil structure forms, thereby holding the coil mass within the aneurysm in cases in which coil herniation into the parent vessel is a primary concern. An advantage of coil introduction with adjunctive balloon use is that the microcatheter is stabilized, preventing premature kickback and need to reaccess. However, there are two drawbacks: first, as the microcatheter is firmly pinned within the aneurysm, it prevents recoil when excessive pressure is applied on a deployed coil, thereby directing the pressure to the aneurysm dome, potentially contributing to perforation; and second, balloon inflation leads to cessation of antegrade flow, potentially risking ischemia. Balloon inflation leads to local anterograde flow arrest in the territory involved. The other well-described risks of balloon remodeling include perforator occlusion, parent vessel dissection or rupture, and promotion of thromboemboli.[3,11–13] The available evidence is conflicting with respect to use of balloon remodeling in aneurysm coil embolization and rates of ischemic complications, with some studies reporting a higher incidence[4,12,14–16] and others reporting an equal or decreased incidence compared

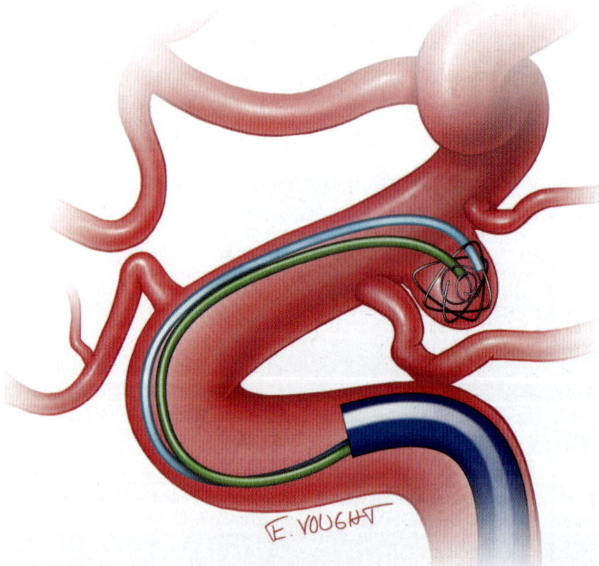

A

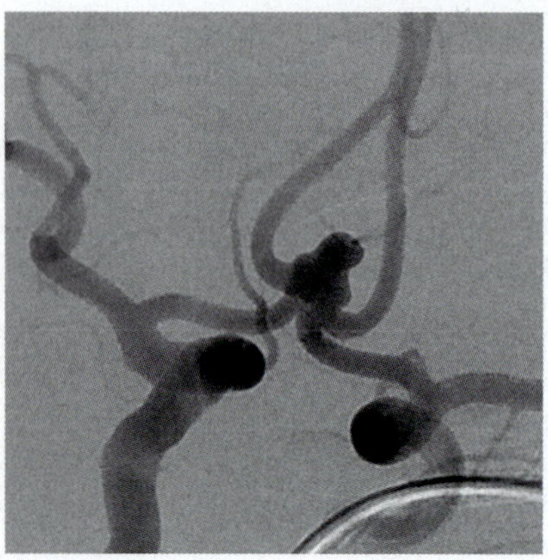

B

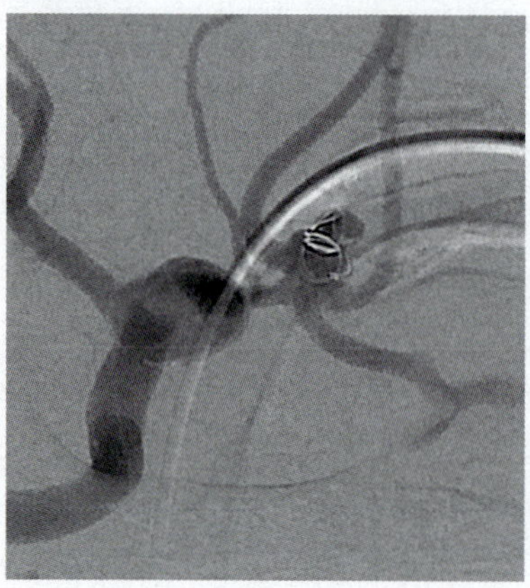

C

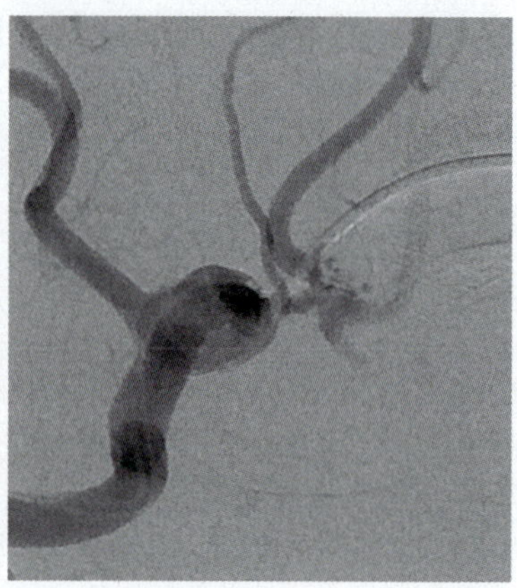

D

Figure 14.4 **A:** Diagram depicting a posterior communicating artery aneurysm with two microcatheters. The first catheter positions the framing coil and remains attached until the end of the procedure. The second catheter is used to fill the remainder of the aneurysm. This method is effective for wide-necked aneurysm where a balloon or stent may not be feasible. **B:** Anterior communicating artery (ACOM) aneurysm. The neck involves the right AI–A2 junction, a balloon was not able to cross into the A2, and a dual catheter technique was used. **C:** Shows placement of framing coil through first microcatheter. **D:** Angiogram demonstrating near-complete occlusion of ACOM aneurysm and preservation of the right A1–A2 junction. The framing coil is still attached to the first microcatheter and the aneurysm has been progressively occluded through a second microcatheter. This allows the framing coil to remain stable.

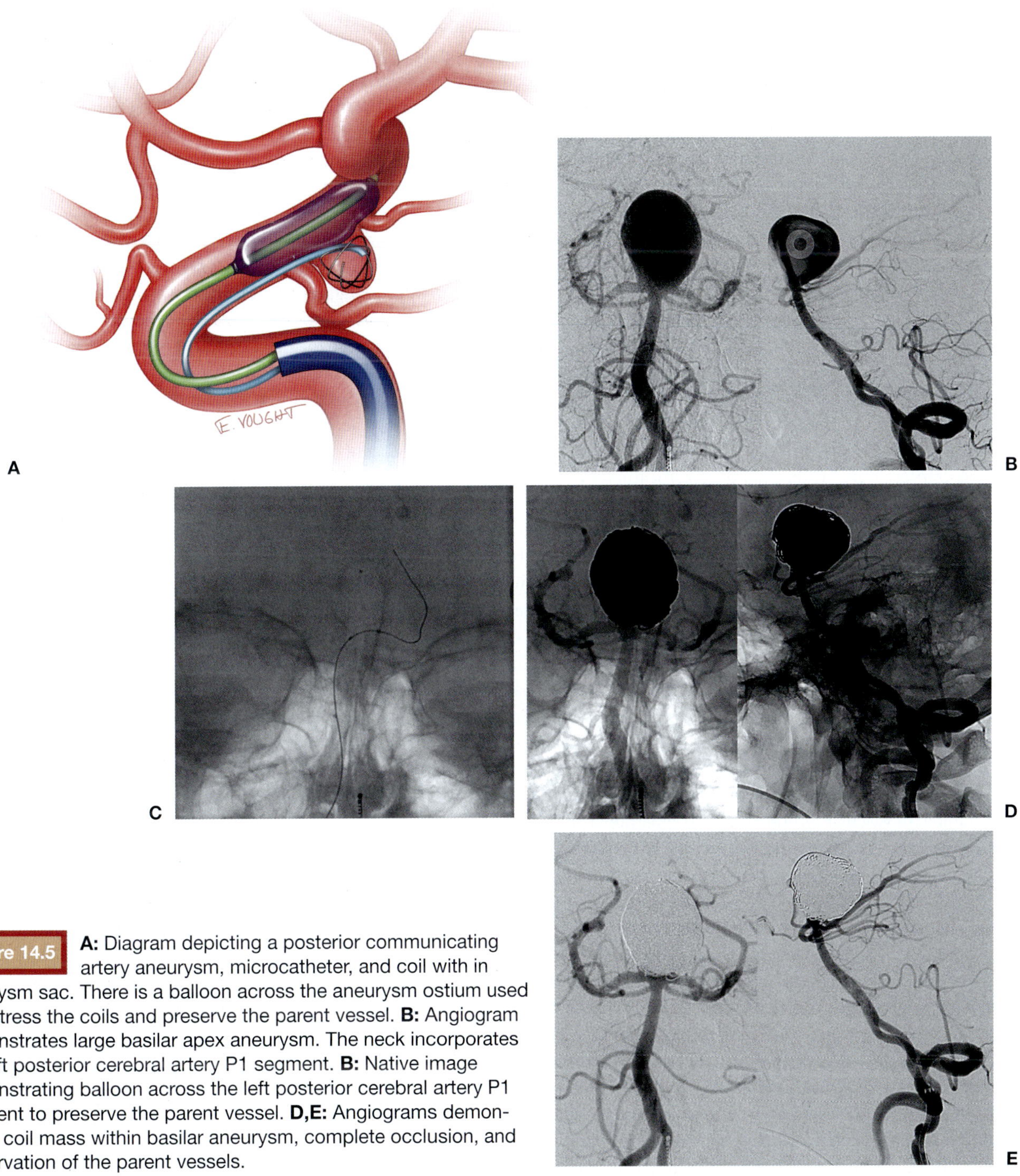

Figure 14.5 **A:** Diagram depicting a posterior communicating artery aneurysm, microcatheter, and coil with in aneurysm sac. There is a balloon across the aneurysm ostium used to buttress the coils and preserve the parent vessel. **B:** Angiogram demonstrates large basilar apex aneurysm. The neck incorporates the left posterior cerebral artery P1 segment. **B:** Native image demonstrating balloon across the left posterior cerebral artery P1 segment to preserve the parent vessel. **D,E:** Angiograms demonstrate coil mass within basilar aneurysm, complete occlusion, and preservation of the parent vessels.

to unassisted coiling.[13,17–20] Balloon inflation can be performed intermittently, allowing reperfusion of the distal vascular territory in addition to unconstrained manipulation of the microcatheter within the aneurysm itself, even after coiling has been initiated. Although there are risks to the use of balloons, the most dreaded is aneurysm perforation; the benefit of having a balloon ready and available to achieve immediate flow arrest and to continue coiling to aneurysm occlusion in a controlled fashion is a significant advantage. Balloon remodeling is a very useful adjunct in the hands of an experienced operator but should be employed cautiously in the uninitiated (Fig. 14.5).

Stent-Assisted Coiling

The technique of stent-assisted coiling in the clinical setting was first described in 1997.[21] Soon after, the availability of new flexible, self-expanding intracranial stents allowed for increasing application of this technique and observation of its benefits. Stents have been quickly adopted as promising adjuncts with potential mechanical, hemodynamic, and biologic properties, imparting an advantage over coil embolization alone.[22] Stent deployment provides mechanical support to prevent coil prolapse, and it may serve as a conduit to divert flow and provide a scaffold for endothelial growth and vessel healing.[22–24] In addition, an implanted stent may incur subtle changes in the parent vessel–aneurysm geometry, imparting significant hemodynamic alterations which change the inflow substantially.

A stent may be deployed across the aneurysm neck followed by microcatheter selection of the aneurysm through the twines of the stent, or the aneurysm can be selected first with the microcatheter and the stent deployed across the neck and microcatheter (jailing technique). The jailing strategy has the advantage of affixing or "pinning" the microcatheter between the outer confines of the stent and the lining of the parent vessel. This achieves a more stable, although somewhat locked-in, microcatheter position within the aneurysm and minimizes the risk of premature kickback of the microcatheter out of the aneurysm during coil deployment. A second strategy is the "coil through," in which a stent is first fully deployed across the aneurysm neck and then the aneurysm is catheterized by navigating through the tines of the stent. This method allows for relatively unrestricted movement of the microcatheter, allowing it to paint back and forth with the introduction of coils; however, at times, depending on anatomy, it may be difficult to traverse a newly deployed stent. The microcatheter may get caught up on the stent tines and there is risk of the stent migrating distally. Third, the "coil–stent" technique involves an unassisted coil embolization to completion, immediately followed by stent deployment, potentially to capitalize on the biologic benefit of vascular remodeling or to constrain a prolapsed coil loop. Last, the "balloon stent" method involves a stent placement after completion of a balloon-assisted embolization.

The advantage of employing a stent to bridge the neck of an aneurysm, as opposed to balloon remodeling, is that it does not involve flow arrest in the parent vessel. A disadvantage is that it requires permanent placement of the device and a minimum antiplatelet regimen of at least 3 months. Most aneurysms treated with stent-assisted coiling are geometrically complex and pose a technical challenge. Since the first clinical applications in the late 1990s, several studies have proven stent-assisted coiling to be a feasible, safe, and effective method of embolization[25–34] of aneurysms previously believed to be not amenable to coiling (Fig. 14.6).

Stent Reconstruction

Despite all these device advancements and the refinement of technical nuances by experienced operators, broad-necked aneurysms arising at bifurcations that incorporate the daughter vessel origins remain a formidable challenge to endovascular treatment. This is perhaps best exemplified by the difficulty in treating middle cerebral artery bifurcation aneurysms but also those at the basilar apex and carotid terminus. At vascular bifurcations, a stent can be used to stabilize a coil mass within an aneurysm while protecting the parent vessel and the daughter vessel at greatest risk. When the aneurysm neck incorporates the origins of both daughter vessels and there is a significant risk of coil herniation into either vessel, a single stent, even with balloon remodeling as an adjunct, may not be sufficient.

The "Y-stent" technique[35–40] involves the passage of a second stent through the interstices of the first deployed stent. Y-stent reconstruction enables the endovascular management of otherwise complex, wide-necked cerebral aneurysms by providing two critical functions: support for the coil mass and preservation of the daughter vessels. The open-cell design of the Neuroform stent as the initial placed stent allows this construct to be possible because the first stent deployed can expand at its interstices to accommodate the second self-expanding stent. Y-stent using a closed-cell design stent at the first stent, although technically feasible, results in undesirable synching of the second deployed stent because of its constrained interstices. The initial short- and midterm results using the Y-configuration technique are promising.[39,40] Although many of the aneurysms displayed residual filling at initial treatment, some were found to have spontaneous thrombosis on angiographic follow-up. These results have been considered satisfactory because the technique addresses aneurysms for which there are otherwise no viable treatment options. However, there are several concerns regarding the long-term effects in patients harboring the Y-configured reconstruction. The longer term effects of having two overlapping stents in the distal basilar as well as the junction of the Y in which there is considerable intraluminal stent overlap not amenable to endothelization without the scaffolding provided by adjacent intima are unknown. In addition, this reconstruction is technically demanding. Navigating through the first stent with either a 0.021-in (closed-cell) or 0.027-in (open-cell) microcatheter to prepare to deliver the second stent of the construct can be difficult and result in stent migration. Initial microcatheter selection and reaccessing of the aneurysm during coiling following Y stenting can also pose a challenge. Indeed, there are many steps required to successfully achieve Y-stent reconstruction, each with possibility of technical complications.

Stent Delivery through Balloon Catheter

Balloon-remodeling and stent assistance techniques may be used in combination to capitalize on the benefits that each affords. This "balloon–stent" method involves stent placement after completion of a balloon-assisted embolization. The drawback to this sequential technique is that employing currently available stent delivery systems requires either a 0.021-in or a 0.027-in microcatheter system; the coil mass achieved during balloon remodeling must be crossed before stent deployment. This additional maneuver introduces the potential risk of coil disruption, especially when there is coil loop prolapse or herniation into the parent vessel, which may lead to thromboembolic or ischemic complications. In addition, this step may add fluoroscopy and procedure time, especially when access to the lesion is challenging.

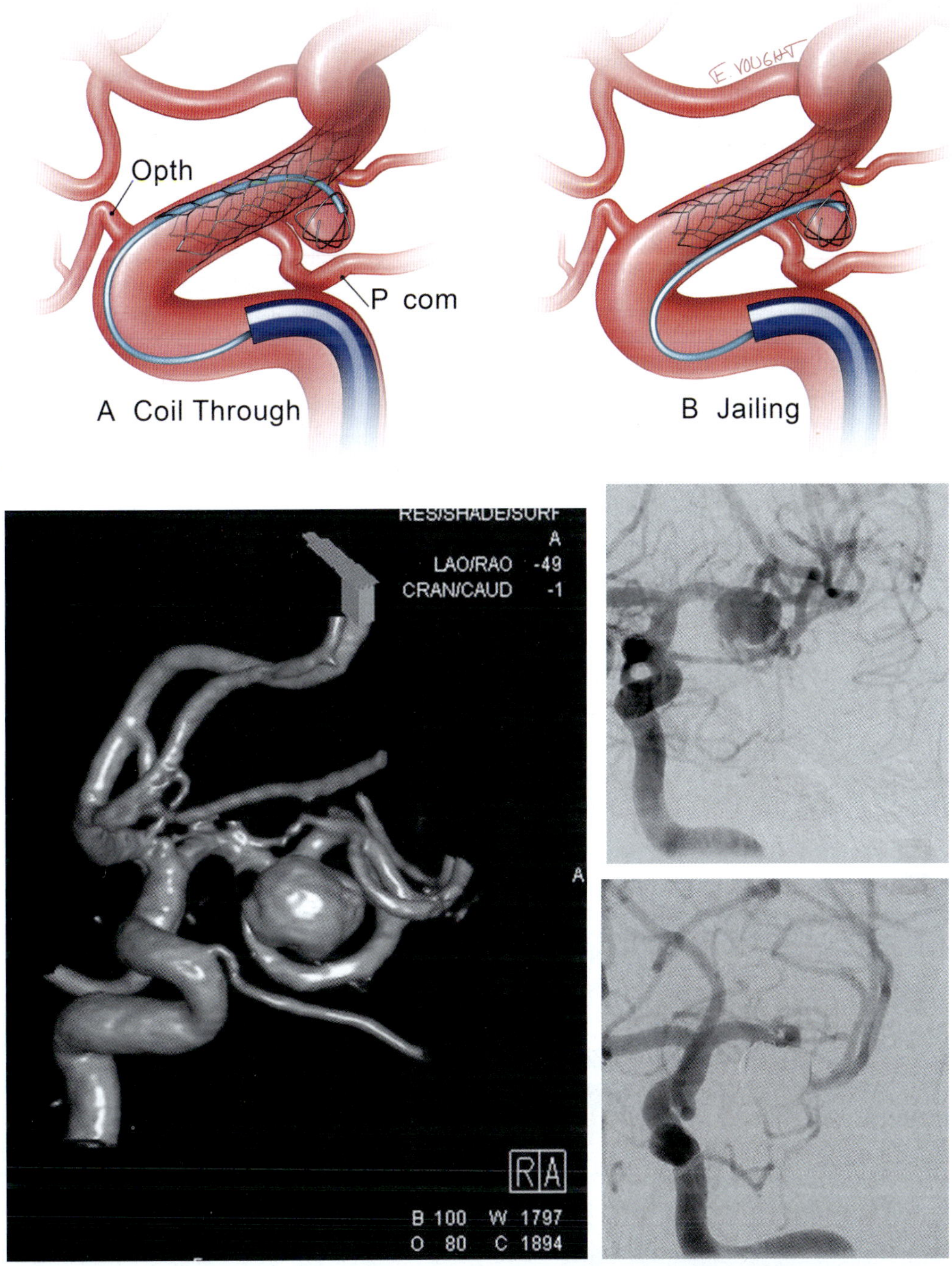

A

B

C

D

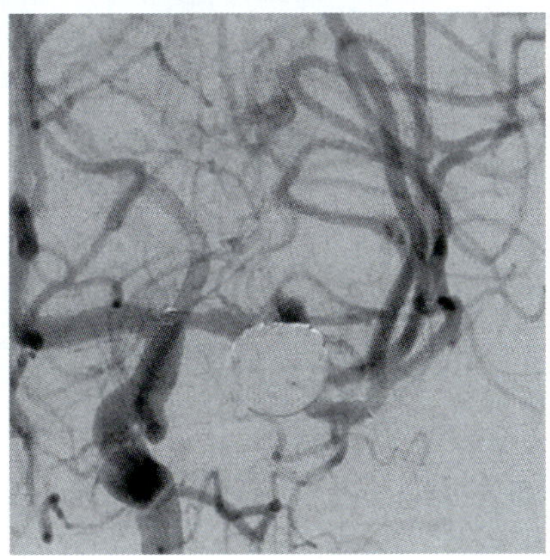

E

Figure 14.6 Diagram depicting stent coiling. There are two methods: **(A.a)** reaccess aneurysm after stent deployment and **(A.b)** jailing the microcatheter in the aneurysm with the stent. This method pins the microcatheter and may limit catheter movement; however, there is no need to reaccess across a freshly deployed stent, which may be challenging. **B:** 3-D angiogram demonstrates large complex middle cerebral artery (MCA) bifurcation aneurysm; the origin of the posterior division is incorporated into the neck. **C:** Working projection angiogram demonstrates right MCA aneurysm with poor visualization of the inferior division origin. **D:** Control arteriogram shows loss of the posterior division due to coil encroachment into posterior division. **E:** After stenting of the posterior division, arteriogram shows preservation of all vessels.

We described the first report of a novel technique for "balloon stenting," which incorporates the use of two novel devices.[41] The Scepter C is a new temporary occlusion balloon system that has a dual coaxial lumen catheter attached to a low-inflation pressure compliant balloon. The design accommodates a steerable 0.014-in guidewire through a 0.0165-in inner lumen. The LVIS is a novel neurovascular self-expanding retrievable stent system which is composed of a single nitinol round braided wire and double helix tantalum strands in addition to radiopaque tantalum proximal and distal markers to assist full-length visualization. It is a compliant, closed-cell system which is retrievable up to 80% deployment and provides 15% surface area coverage. The commercially available LVIS stent is 0.021-in microcatheter compatible. However, the LVIS Jr. stent is 0.017-in microcatheter compatible, allowing it to be delivered by the Scepter C balloon catheter system. We have found this technique to be safe and feasible, reducing both the number of steps involved in this technique and the opportunities for mechanical coil-related complications.

Flow Diversion

Stents were recognized to impart flow diversion properties on aneurysm inflow, spurring the introduction of flow diversion stents. Flow-diverting stents are constructed of lower porosity with higher device surface area coverage at the aneurysm neck. By shunting flow preferentially down the parent vessel and away from the aneurysm, it promotes conditions leading to progressive aneurysm thrombosis and eventual vessel remodeling (Fig. 14.7).

Theoretically, even small-caliber perforating vessels, which are covered by the flow diverter, will remain patent due to the siphoning effect of the distal territory they irrigate. Aneurysms have no such downstream outflow and will thrombose. Flow diversion has been used effectively in the treatment of fusiform and giant aneurysms. Disadvantages include the inability to cross the stent with a microcatheter for treatment of recurrences, reports of perforator occlusions leading to strokes, as well as reported cases of delayed aneurysmal rupture and subacute and remote intracerebral hemorrhage.

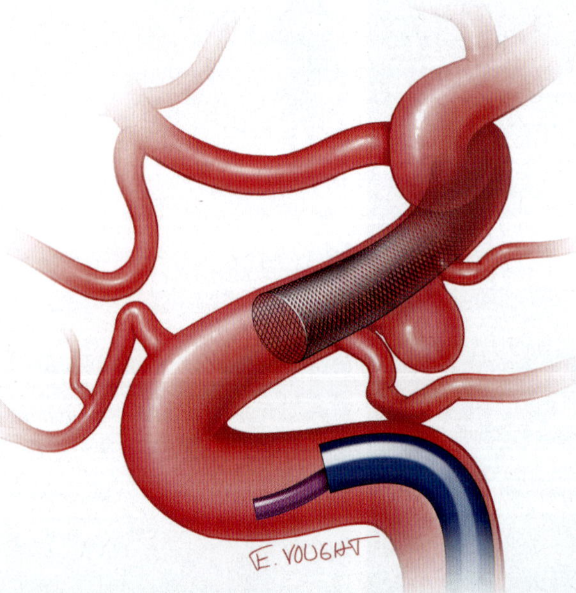

A

Figure 14.7 **A:** Diagram depicting a high mesh flow-diverting stent within the parent vessel. The advantage of this treatment is that the aneurysm does not need to be accessed and that procedures are often quicker. **B:** Angiogram demonstrates large fusiform cavernous carotid aneurysm. **C:** Six months follow-up angiogram demonstrates patent PED. There is complete occlusion of the aneurysm.

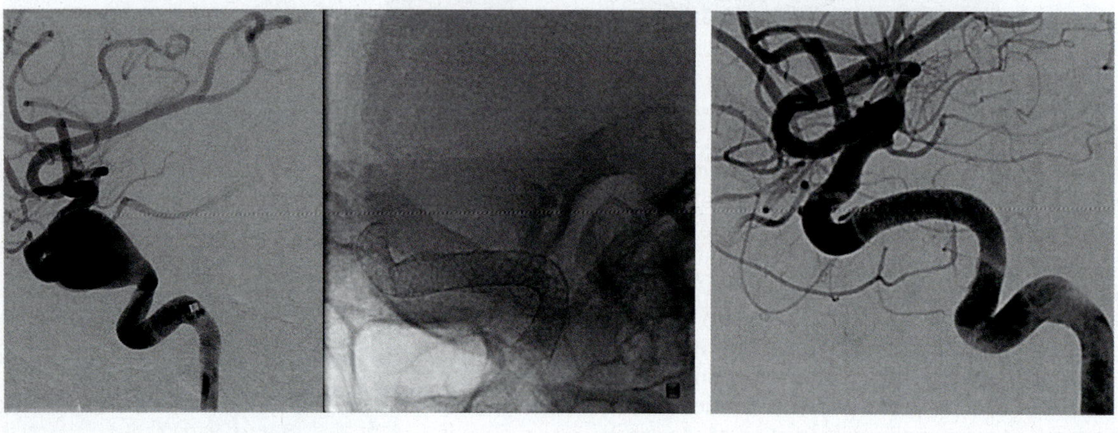

B

C

Pushing the Envelope

Despite these technologic advances, broad-based aneurysms continue to pose a formidable challenge for endovascular treatment, which requires creative solutions.[41–46] As long as there are complex aneurysms that require treatment and highly skilled neurointerventionalists who are knowledgeable about the devices available and motivated to treat them, devices will be used in an off-label fashion in an attempt to address the unmet needs of adjuncts. Retrievable, closed-cell design stents can be partially deployed across an aneurysm neck and then recaptured following stent-assisted coil embolization, thereby incorporating the benefits of balloon remodeling without the drawbacks of parent vessel occlusion and without permanent stent implantation. A stent may also be deployed with its distal extent aimed at the aperture of the aneurysm to support a coil mass rather than across the neck along the long axis of the parent vessel, the so-called waffle cone technique.[47,48] In the treatment of a fusiform aneurysm, stents can be deployed in parallel in the so-called double-barrel technique.[47] Aneurysms incorporating two daughter vessels have been addressed, employing two simultaneously inflated balloons after selecting the aneurysm with a microcatheter ("kissing balloon" technique). Last, to promote thrombosis and occlusion of fusiform aneurysms, some operators advocate jailing a microcatheter with a flow-diverting stent to capture the benefits of flow diversion and coil embolization in one strategy.

CLINICAL APPLICATIONS

At our institution, we tend to use a fair amount of primary coiling and balloon remodeling. We prefer the use of the balloon as an adjunctive device over stents as balloons are temporary implants, obviating the need for long-term dual antiplatelet therapy. Also, in the setting of subarachnoid hemorrhage where antiplatelet therapy is contraindicated, balloons allow for the treatment of complex, wide-necked aneurysms without the use of stents. Ultimately, the choice of how to coil, balloon remodel, or perform a stent-assisted coiling is up to the primary operator. The risks/benefits of each technique must be weighed against not only the anatomy and geometry of the aneurysm but also the operator's comfort level with each technique.

Preoperative Planning

Elective patients are pretreated with dual antiplatelet therapy regardless if stenting is planned to mitigate the risk of thromboembolic complications. Ideally, patients are given a 600 mg clopidogrel and 650 mg acetylsalicylic acid (ASA) load the night before a coiling procedure. Alternatively, a 5-day loading regiment may be used: 75 mg clopidogrel and 325 mg ASA daily starting 5 days before the procedure. For patients where a stent or endoluminal device is planned, clopidogrel and ASA response assays may be performed. At this time, a decision should be made regarding how to approach the aneurysm. Will primary coiling suffice? Will there be a need for an adjunctive device or will newer technologies such as flow-diverting stents or newer intrasaccular devices be used? These decisions will determine access devices and microcatheter selection on the day of operation.

We perform all embolization procedures under general anesthesia. All patients are systemically anticoagulated: Elective patients receive a bolus dose of 5,000 units of heparin, whereas subarachnoid hemorrhage patients receive 3,000 units bolus dose. After placement of the first coil, patients are titrated to an activated clotting time (ACT) of 2 to 2.5 times their ACT baseline.

Procedure

1. Femoral access: Depending on the devices used, either a 6-Fr or 8-Fr sheath is placed in the groin.
2. Guiding catheter: We commonly use the 0.070-in Neuron and 0.071-in Chaperon guiding catheters and the 0.088-in Neuron Max sheath. Our goal is safe distal access, ideally to at least the petrous segment of the internal carotid artery.
3. Working views: Orthogonal views that demonstrate the aneurysm neck and dome are ideal. When balloon remodeling, views may be modified with the balloon inflated and the first coil partially deployed to achieve a "down the barrel" view and an orthogonal view that lays out the dome.
4. Adjunctive device access: If an adjunctive device is used, it is advanced first before the coiling microcatheter across the aneurysm ostium.
5. Coiling microcatheter access: The coiling microcatheter is advanced into the aneurysm sac.
6. Control angiograms in working and anteroposterior (AP) and lateral projections are performed. Working to determine residual filling of aneurysm and AP and lateral to demonstrate patency of all vessels unchanged from the initial angiograms.

COMPLICATIONS

Potential complications can be divided into two main types: hemorrhagic and ischemic. Ischemic complications are more common and can be caused by vasospasm from guide catheter access, cessation of antegrade flow with use of a balloon catheter, and thromboembolic events from clot formation along the coil mass, which tends to occur when there is a large coil mass/parent vessel interface. Many of these issues can be avoided by preprocedure prophylactic antiplatelet therapy and systemic anticoagulation during the procedure. Hemorrhagic complications are uncommon but feared as they tend to result in major morbidity and mortality. Most commonly, this is a result of aneurysm perforation either from coil or microcatheter herniation through the wall of the aneurysm. Less common, microguidewire perforations can occur either during access of the parent vessel, distal wire access for balloons or other adjunctive devices, and wire perforation of the aneurysm dome.

TIPS AND TRICKS

	Tips	Tricks
Guiding catheter	The more distal access is obtained, the more stability is provided to the working devices (microcatheter, balloon, stent, etc.). The delivery of newer generation, flexible tip guiding catheters to the level of either the vertical petrous or proximal cavernous segment of the carotid artery results in improved control and a more true 1:1 control of the working device, thereby improving safety.	• Heparin should be administered before guiding catheter introduction to prevent thromboembolic complications. • Preadvancement vasodilator administration (verapamil, nicardipine) decreases the likelihood of catheter-related vasospasm that may cause flow arrest around the guide catheter. • Flexible tip newer generation guide catheters can be delivered distally in a coaxial fashion over its accompanying insert and a 0.038-in Glidewire. First, the insert should be navigated over the wire past the petrous segment curve, then the guiding catheter can be navigated over the insert and Glidewire.
Microwires	Microwires ranging from 0.010 to 0.016-in in size may be selected to provide appropriate degree of softness to negotiate tortuous anatomy without causing microperforations while providing support for over-the-wire microcatheter navigation.	• Reshaping of the microwire may be necessary to optimize navigation to a patient's specific anatomy. • Purposeful "J-ing" of the microwire tip so that it forms a recursive loop as the wire is advanced to lead with a curve rather than a wire tip point is a safe option to both navigate past perforator vessels while avoiding engaging their origins and aneurysm selection.
Microcatheters	Microcatheters ranging from 0.016 to 0.027-in in size may be used to navigate over an appropriate microwire for coil embolization and stent delivery.	• Aneurysm microcatheter selection is ideally performed via single operator control of both the microcatheter and microwire simultaneously in a "push and pull" technique. • Once access to the aneurysm is obtained, these flexible microcatheters will respond to the stress applied to it by superimposed curves by adopting the parent vessel curvature, which leads to their stability at the aneurysm during coil deployment.
Coils	Coils are available in various shapes, lengths, and diameters. Experience is required to optimize coil occlusion of an aneurysm, especially in those with irregular shapes.	• In a spherical aneurysm, select an appropriately sized spherical coil to form a framing "basket," then place additional coils within it in a Russian doll technique. • For bilobed or complex aneurysms, select complex 360-degree coils to frame the aneurysm. • Ensure that coil loops remain within the aneurysm without prolapse into the parent vessel.
Balloons	Useful for treatment of broad-necked aneurysms and does not involve a permanent implant. Involves the temporary inflation of a balloon catheter across the neck of an aneurysm. Critical technique in the event of intraprocedural aneurysmal perforation, allowing coil embolization to proceed with cessation of aneurysmal hemorrhage. The downside of this technique is that balloon inflation leads to arrest of anterograde flow across the parent vessel.	• Ensure optimal anticoagulation with heparin before balloon inflation. • Position the deflated balloon catheter across the aneurysm neck first, then select the aneurysm with the working microcatheter to minimize any potentially dangerous catheter interactions as one is advanced alongside the other. • Minimize balloon inflation times and allow reperfusion between repeat inflations to avoid infarctions. • During balloon inflation, create a negative road map control image to "cast a shadow" outlining the boundaries of the previously inflated balloon to enhance the identification of coil migration or prolapse into the parent vessel.

	Tips	Tricks
Stents	Useful for treatment of broad-necked aneurysms, stent deployment provides mechanical support to prevent coil prolapse, may serve as a conduit to divert flow, and provides a scaffold for endothelial growth and vessel healing.[22–24] In addition, an implanted stent may incur subtle changes in the parent vessel–aneurysm geometry, imparting significant hemodynamic alterations which change the inflow substantially. Downside is that it requires antiplatelet therapy and entails a permanent implant.	• Coil through technique involves deploying a stent across the aneurysm neck followed by microcatheter selection of the aneurysm through the tines of the stent. • The jailing technique involves first accessing the aneurysm with the microcatheter, followed by stent deployment across the neck and microcatheter. The jailing strategy has the advantage of affixing or pinning the microcatheter between the outer confines of the stent and the lining of the parent vessel. This achieves a more stable microcatheter position within the aneurysm and minimizes the risk of premature kickback of the microcatheter out of the aneurysm during coil deployment. • The coil–stent technique involves unassisted coil embolization followed by stent deployment. • The balloon–stent method involves stent placement after completion of a balloon-assisted embolization.
Flow diversion	Shunting flow preferentially down the parent vessel and away from the aneurysm promotes progressive aneurysm thrombosis. The stent itself acts as a scaffold for vessel reconstruction. Flow diversion has been used effectively in the treatment of fusiform and giant aneurysms. Disadvantages include the inability to cross the stent with a microcatheter for treatment of recurrences.	• Delivery of the device can be challenging due to its relative stiffness, so adequate proximal support with a larger guiding catheter and the use of an intermediate catheter is beneficial. • Minimize the number of small perforating vessels, which are covered by the stent to prevent ischemic complications.

REFERENCES

1. Aletich VA, Debrun GM, Misra M, et al. The remodeling technique of balloon-assisted Guglielmi detachable coil placement in wide-necked aneurysms: experience at the University of Illinois at Chicago. *J Neurosurg.* 2000;93(3):388–396.
2. Fiorella D, Albuquerque FC, Han P, et al. Preliminary experience using the Neuroform stent for the treatment of cerebral aneurysms. *Neurosurgery.* 2004;54(1):6–16.
3. Lefkowitz MA, Gobin YP, Akiba Y, et al. Balloon-assisted Guglielmi detachable coiling of wide-necked aneurysm: part II—clinical results. *Neurosurgery.* 1999;45(3):531–537.
4. Malek AM, Halbach VV, Phatouros CC, et al. Balloon-assisted technique for endovascular coil embolization of geometrically difficult intracranial aneurysms. *Neurosurgery.* 2000;46(6):1397–1406.
5. Moret J, Cognard C, Weill A, et al. Reconstruction technic in the treatment of wide-neck intracranial aneurysms. Long-term angiographic and clinical results. Apropos of 56 cases [in French]. *J Neuroradiol.* 1997;24(1):30–44.
6. Raymond J, Guilbert F, Roy D. Neck-bridge device for endovascular treatment of wide-neck bifurcation aneurysms: initial experience. *Radiology.* 2001;221(2):318–326.
7. Spiotta AM, Hui FK, Moskowitz SI. Trends in device-assisted aneurysm treatment at a single high-volume tertiary care center. *J NeuroInterv Surg.* 2013;5(2):117–120.
8. Guglielmi G, Vinuela F, Dion J, et al. Electrothrombosis of saccular aneurysms via endovascular approach. Part 2: preliminary clinical experience. *J Neurosurg.* 1991;75(1):8–14.
9. Johnston SC, Dowd CF, Higashida RT, et al. Predictors of rehemorrhage after treatment of ruptured intracranial aneurysms: the Cerebral Aneurysm Rerupture After Treatment (CARAT) study. *Stroke.* 2008;39(1):120–125.
10. Moret J, Cognard C, Weill A, et al. The "remodelling technique" in the treatment of wide neck intracranial aneurysms. Angiographic results and clinical follow-up in 56 cases. *Interv Neuroradiol.* 1997;3(1):21–35.
11. Cottier JP, Pasco A, Gallas S, et al. Utility of balloon-assisted Guglielmi detachable coiling in the treatment of 49 cerebral aneurysms: a retrospective, multicenter study. *AJNR Am J Neuroradiol.* 2001;22(2):345–351.

12. Qureshi AI, Luft AR, Sharma M, et al. Prevention and treatment of thromboembolic and ischemic complications associated with endovascular procedures. Part II—clinical aspects and recommendations. *Neurosurgery*. 2000;46(6): 1360–1375.
13. Shapiro M, Babb J, Becske T, et al. Safety and efficacy of adjunctive balloon remodeling during endovascular treatment of intracranial aneurysms: a literature review. *AJNR Am J Neuroradiol*. 2008;29(9):1777–1781.
14. Nelson PK, Levy DI. Balloon-assisted coil embolization of wide-necked aneurysms of the internal carotid artery: medium-term angiographic and clinical follow-up in 22 patients. *AJNR Am J Neuroradiol*. 2001;22(1):19–26.
15. Rordorf G, Bellon RJ, Budzik RE Jr, et al. Silent thromboembolic events associated with the treatment of unruptured cerebral aneurysms by use of Guglielmi detachable coils: prospective study applying diffusion-weighted imaging. *AJNR Am J Neuroradiol*. 2001;22(1):5–10.
16. Soeda A, Sakai N, Murao K, et al. Thromboembolic events associated with Guglielmi detachable coil embolization with use of diffusion-weighted MR imaging. Part II. Detection of the microemboli proximal to cerebral aneurysm. *AJNR Am J Neuroradiol*. 2003;24(10):2035–2038.
17. Brooks NP, Turk AS, Niemann DB, et al. Frequency of thromboembolic events associated with endovascular aneurysm treatment: retrospective case series. *J Neurosurg*. 2008;108(6): 1095–1100.
18. Lubicz B, Lefranc F, Bruneau M, et al. Balloon-assisted coiling of intracranial aneurysms is not associated with a higher complication rate. *Neuroradiology*. 2008;50(9):769–776.
19. Ross IB, Dhillon GS. Complications of endovascular treatment of cerebral aneurysms. *Surg Neurol*. 2005;64(1):12–18.
20. Spiotta AM, Bhalla T, Hussain MS, et al. An analysis of inflation times during balloon-assisted aneurysm coil embolization and ischemic complications. *Stroke*. 2011;42(4):1051–1055.
21. Higashida RT, Smith W, Gress D, et al. Intravascular stent and endovascular coil placement for a ruptured fusiform aneurysm of the basilar artery. Case report and review of the literature. *J Neurosurg*. 1997;87(6):944–949.
22. Wanke I, Forsting M. Stents for intracranial wide-necked aneurysms: more than mechanical protection. *Neuroradiology*. 2008;50(12):991–998.
23. Aenis M, Stancampiano AP, Wakhloo AK, et al. Modeling of flow in a straight stented and nonstented side wall aneurysm model. *J Biomech Eng*. 1997;119(2):206–212.
24. Phatouros CC, Sasaki TY, Higashida RT, et al. Stent-supported coil embolization: the treatment of fusiform and wide-neck aneurysms and pseudoaneurysms. *Neurosurgery*. 2000;47(1): 107–113.
25. Benitez RP, Silva MT, Klem J, et al. Endovascular occlusion of wide-necked aneurysms with a new intracranial microstent (Neuroform) and detachable coils. *Neurosurgery*. 2004; 54(6):1359–1367.
26. Biondi A, Janardhan V, Katz JM, et al. Neuroform stent-assisted coil embolization of wide-neck intracranial aneurysms: strategies in stent deployment and midterm follow-up. *Neurosurgery*. 2007;61(3):460–468.
27. Fiorella D, Albuquerque FC, Deshmukh VR, et al. Usefulness of the Neuroform stent for the treatment of cerebral aneurysms: results at initial 3-6 months follow-up. *Neurosurgery*. 2005;56(6):1191–1201.
28. Lee YJ, Kim DJ, Suh SH, et al. Stent-assisted coil embolization of intracranial wide-necked aneurysms. *Neuroradiology*. 2005; 47(9):680–689.
29. Liang G, Gao X, Li Z, et al. Neuroform stent-assisted coiling of intracranial aneurysms: a 5-year single-center experience and follow-up. *Neurol Res*. 2010;32(7):721–727.
30. Mocco J, Snyder KV, Albuquerque FC, et al. Treatment of intracranial aneurysms with the Enterprise stent: a multicenter registry. *J Neurosurg*. 2009;110(1):35–39.
31. Ogilvy CS, Natarajan SK, Jahshan S, et al. Stent-assisted coiling of paraclinoid aneurysms: risks and effectiveness. *J Neurointerv Surg*. 2011;3(1):14–20.
32. Piotin M, Blanc R, Spelle L, et al. Stent-assisted coiling of intracranial aneurysms: clinical and angiographic results in 216 consecutive aneurysms. *Stroke*. 2010;41(1):110–115.
33. Raslan AM, Oztaskin M, Thompson EM, et al. Neuroform stent-assisted embolization of incidental anterior communicating artery aneurysms: long-term clinical and angiographic follow-up. *Neurosurgery*. 2011;69(1):27–37.
34. Sedat J, Chau Y, Mondot L, et al. Endovascular occlusion of intracranial wide-necked aneurysms with stenting (Neuroform) and coiling: mid-term and long-term results. *Neuroradiology*. 2009;51(6):401–409.
35. Akpek S, Morsi H, Benndorf G, et al. Reconstruction of the basilar tip with T stent configuration for treatment of a wide-neck aneurysm. *J Vasc Interv Radiol*. 2004;15(9): 1024–1026.
36. Chow MM, Woo HH, Masaryk TJ, et al. A novel endovascular treatment of a wide-necked basilar apex aneurysm by using a Y-configuration, double-stent technique. *AJNR Am J Neuroradiol*. 2004;25(3):509–512.
37. Perez-Arjona E, Fessler RD. Basilar artery to bilateral posterior cerebral artery "Y stenting" for endovascular reconstruction of wide-necked basilar apex aneurysms: report of three cases. *Neurol Res*. 2004;26(3):276–281.
38. Sani S, Lopes DK. Treatment of a middle cerebral artery bifurcation aneurysm using a double Neuroform stent "Y" configuration and coil embolization: technical case report. *Neurosurgery*. 2005;57(1)(suppl):E209.
39. Spiotta AM, Gupta R, Fiorella D, et al. Mid-term results of endovascular coiling of wide-necked aneurysms using double stents in a Y configuration. *Neurosurgery*. 2011;69(2): 421–429.
40. Thorell WE, Chow MM, Woo HH, et al. Y-configured dual intracranial stent-assisted coil embolization for the treatment of wide-necked basilar tip aneurysms. *Neurosurgery*. 2005;56(5):1035–1040.
41. Spiotta AM, Miranpuri A, Chaudry MI, et al. Combined balloon stent technique with the Scepter C balloon and low-profile visualized intraluminal stent for the treatment of intracranial aneurysms. *J Neurointerv Surg*. 2013;5(suppl 3): iii79–iii82.
42. Benndorf G, Klucznik RP, Meyer D, et al. "Cross-over" technique for horizontal stenting of an internal carotid bifurcation aneurysm using a new self-expandable stent: technical case report. *Neurosurgery*. 2006;58(1)(suppl): ONS–E172.

43. Cross DT, Moran CJ, Derdeyn CP, et al. Neuroform stent deployment for treatment of a basilar tip aneurysm via a posterior communicating artery route. *AJNR Am J Neuroradiol.* 2005;26(10):2578–2581.
44. Fiorella D, Albuquerque FC, Masaryk TJ, et al. Balloon-in-stent technique for the constructive endovascular treatment of "ultra-wide necked" circumferential aneurysms. *Neurosurgery.* 2005;57(6):1218–1227.
45. Kelly ME, Turner R, Gonugunta V, et al. Stent reconstruction of wide-necked aneurysms across the circle of Willis. *Neurosurgery.* 2007;61(5)(suppl 2):249–254.
46. Moret J, Ross IB, Weill A, et al. The retrograde approach: a consideration for the endovascular treatment of aneurysms. *AJNR Am J Neuroradiol.* 2000;21(2):262–268.
47. Gruber TJ, Ogilvy CS, Hauck EF, et al. Endovascular treatment of a large aneurysm arising from a basilar trunk fenestration using the waffle-cone technique. *Neurosurgery.* 2010;67(3)(suppl):140–144.
48. Padalino DJ, Singla A, Jacobsen W, et al. Enterprise stent for waffle-cone stent-assisted coil embolization of large wide-necked arterial bifurcation aneurysms. *Surg Neurol Int.* 2013;4:9.

Section B Head and Neck Embolization

15

Epistaxis

Long Chen • Ali Akber Hazari • Laura MacNeil • Kieran Murphy

Epistaxis, commonly known as a *nosebleed*, is the most common otolaryngologic emergency.[1] It is estimated that 60% of people have experienced at least one episode of epistaxis, with 6% requiring medical attention.[2] Although this medical condition is not always recognized as life-threatening, there have been incidences where epistaxis has led to serious complications, and if not treated effectively, it can be fatal. Therefore, it is crucial that the techniques and treatments used in prevention are well understood.

Many studies indicate that the severity of the epistaxis depends on where the bleed originates. Clinically, anterior bleeds are usually less severe than posterior bleeds, and in about 80% of cases, epistaxis originates from the anterior septal area.[1,3] Kiesselbach plexus, an "anastomosis with branches from both the internal and external carotid artery systems," is responsible for most anterior septal nosebleeds, for example, those which children experience in the winter time.[3] Anterior septal nosebleeds would also include epistaxis resulting from trauma, digital irritation, and dryness.[3] The posterior septal area is where epistaxis can be severe, more specifically the Woodruff area where the "anastomoses of the sphenopalatine and pharyngeal arteries is found."[3]

In a case of epistaxis, the aim of treatment is to do at least one of the following: reduce bleeding through decreasing arterial inflow pressure, reduce mucosal irritation, or reduce blood flow by inducing clot formation. The initial treatment of epistaxis is based on nasal packing and chemical or electrocautery.[4] This is usually successful for the anterior septal area and is also a first-line therapy for posterior epistaxis.[4,5] However, the posterior nasal vault is located in an inaccessible region, causing this method to prove ineffective 25% to 50% of times.[6,7] Nasal packing can also be painful for the patient.[6] Patients with preexisting pulmonary or cardiac problems are at serious risk for hypoxia, cardiac arrhythmias, or sepsis when treated with nasal packing.[8] This is a particular risk in patients with heart disease where the mucosal absorption of epinephrine can result in ischemia.

If the prior proves unsuccessful, patients are treated with nasal packing along with transantral maxillary artery and ethmoid artery ligation.[8] The aim of this treatment is to surgically achieve homeostasis at the affected area by decreasing arterial blood flow so epithelial repair and clotting may occur.[8] However, this procedure is not always successful in achieving the desired homeostatic result and also puts the patient at risk for anesthetic problems, septal perforation, infraorbital nerve dysfunction, ophthalmoplegia, blindness, or myocardial infarction.[8] Rarely, postsurgical pseudoaneurysms develop.

Therefore, both these methods have been proven to carry a relatively high number of risks and possible complications, making alternative therapies more favorable for patients with severe cases of epistaxis.

One such alternative therapy, which has proven to be very effective, is endovascular embolization. Embolization is the process of inducing blood clots or embolus to occlude blood flow. In 1974, Sokoloff et al.[9] reported the first successful percutaneous embolization of the internal maxillary artery causing nasal hemorrhage. A later study conducted in 1995 by Elahi et al.[7] demonstrated a 96% success rate in treating patients with intractable epistaxis using embolization. Embolization is a relatively short procedure, which increases both safety and accuracy.[7] Moreover, a patient who has undergone embolization is able to remove his or her posterior nasal pack earlier, which allows for a reduced hospital stay and increased patient comfort.[7] The technique has since then been widely accepted and its efficacy confirmed.[10] Nevertheless, in some institutions and in case the of conservative treatment failure, angiographic embolization remains the procedure of first choice.[11]

DEVICE/MATERIAL DESCRIPTION

Once a year, our group is asked to review strokes that occur during epistaxis embolizations. Usually, this happens in a procedure performed by a well-intentioned interventional radiologist who uses a 5-Fr glide catheter to close the internal maxillary. This is a recipe for disaster. Strict guiding catheter and microcatheter technique must be used. Embolization is a procedure that can be conducted using various techniques or materials, for example, microcoils, gelfoam, glue, and polyvinyl alcohol (PVA) foam. Microcoils are overused by inexperienced practitioners and are a major problem in patients with recurrent bleeding as they recanalize, allowing reperfusion but obstructing embolization access. In transarterial embolization, physicians will use 6-Fr guiding catheters, microcatheters, and microwires to access the sphenopalatine branch of the internal maxillary artery.[12] As it is difficult to reach areas in the nasal cavity, microcatheters are often preshaped in a 30- to 45-degree angle.[12] The materials mentioned earlier are sometimes used in combination with one another. Patients should be heparinized during procedures to decrease the risk of periprocedural stroke.

PVA particles with a diameter of 300 to 500 μm are used for embolization of epistaxis.[13] Particles with a smaller diameter should be avoided as they can navigate through the skull base extracranial–intracranial dangerous anastomosis and cause stroke. On the other hand, a larger diameter can clump and block the microcatheter. To balance the benefit of embolization therapy and the risk of complications, it is recommended that the range in diameter is between 300 and 500 μm.[4,14]

N-butyl cyanoacrylate (NBCA), detachable balloons, and microcoil embolization should be reserved for massive bleeding, when it is necessary to sacrifice internal carotid artery for epistaxis caused by internal carotid artery lesion such as a gunshot wound.[15] For arteriovenous malformation (AVM) or dural arteriovenous fistula (DAVF), NBCA or Onyx (Covidien, Irvine, California) can be employed for embolization.[16–18]

TECHNIQUE

Transarterial embolization therapy should be conducted under conscious sedation, but in an agitated patient, general anesthesia (GA) should be used.[19,20] Embolization under GA is recommended for patients with major blood loss, especially for cases of epistaxis caused by trauma, which are usually accompanied with a major blood loss and of higher risk for aspiration. Confused patients move and you lose your road map guidance. In that situation, it is harder to detect excessive reflux of embolic material retrograde from the catheter tip and potentially into the carotid bifurcation and hence internal carotid artery and cause stroke.

Complete common carotid and bilateral internal and external carotid arterial angiography should be conducted before embolization[19,21] (Fig. 15.1). Preembolization angiography should be performed to indentify lesions such as AVMs, DAVF, and pseudoaneurysms. Preembolization diagnostic angiography can identify if extracranial–intracranial dangerous anastomosis exist. The key dangerous anastomosis exists between the middle meningeal artery and the ophthalmic artery. Due to anatomical variation, dangerous anastomoses exist between external and internal carotid arteries and their ophthalmic artery branches. Even if there is no extracranial–intracranial dangerous anastomosis detected by conventional angiography, potentially dangerous anastomosis will still open with an increase in the injection pressure during the embolization process. Internal and external carotid artery anastomoses can occur with vidian artery, artery of the foramen rotundum, the ascending pharyngeal artery, branches of middle meningeal artery and accessory meningeal artery, sphenopalatine artery, and branches between sphenopalatine artery and ophthalmic artery (Fig. 15.2).[4,19] If embolic materials traverse through these anastomosis from external carotid artery to internal carotid artery or ophthalmic artery, it may cause cranial nerve palsy, loss of vision from retinal artery embolization, or even stroke.[19,22]

The internal carotid artery angiography could directly reveal if the ophthalmic artery branches out from the internal carotid artery and if there is development of choroidal blush. The blood supply to the ophthalmic artery from the branches of the middle meningeal artery should be closely watched for. The recommended sequence for performing angiography is to start from the common carotid and internal carotid artery, followed by external carotid artery of the diseased side. Then the same procedure is repeated on the other side.[19]

The main blood supply to the nasal cavity is from the sphenopalatine artery, which is branched from the internal maxillary artery. The normal embolization method is through a superselective microcatheter to the distal end of internal maxillary artery for angiography before embolization. In some cases, it can be difficult to place a catheter into the distal end of the internal maxillary artery or the inside of sphenopalatine artery or if the parent artery is extremely tortuous.

The operator should always bear in mind that the purpose of treating epistaxis is not to devascularize the nose but rather to reduce the blood flow pressure in certain areas so as to facilitate the formation of local thrombus and self-healing of the hemorrhage area. Thus, it is recommended that the diameter of embolization particles should not be less than 150 μm to avoid the possibility that a smaller particle could go intracranial through dangerous anastomosis and cause

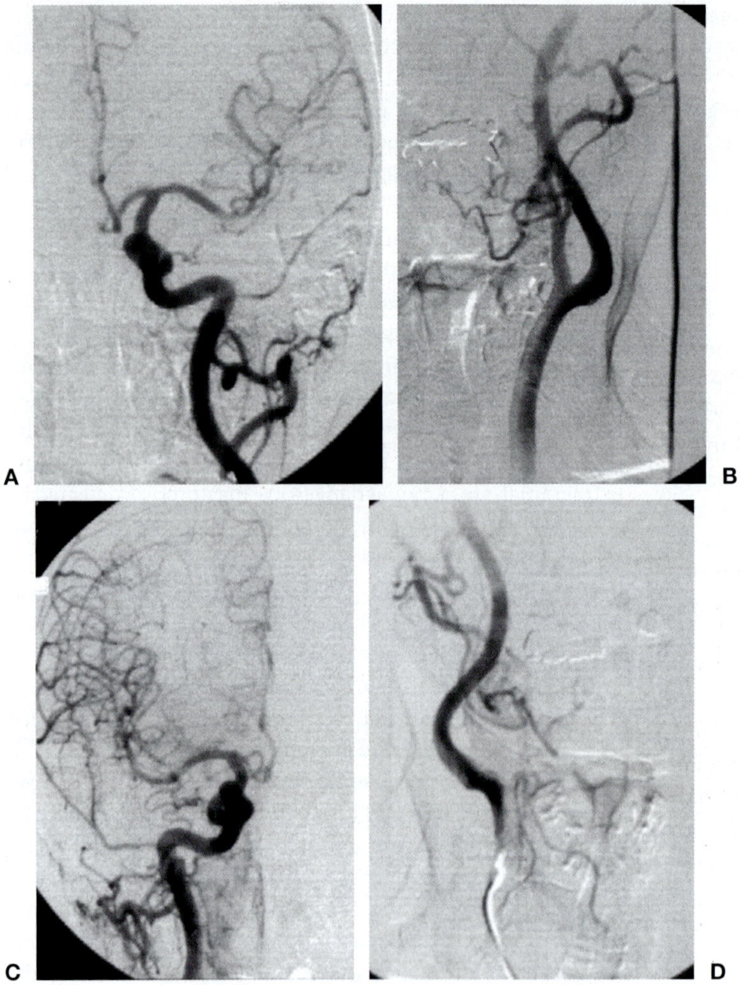

Figure 15.1 **A-D:** Always do a proper diagnostic angiogram with a 5-Fr glide catheter to understand the carotid bifurcation and the patient's anatomy. This will also diagnose unexpected findings such as HHT or coils from a previous embolization that now obstruct your access.

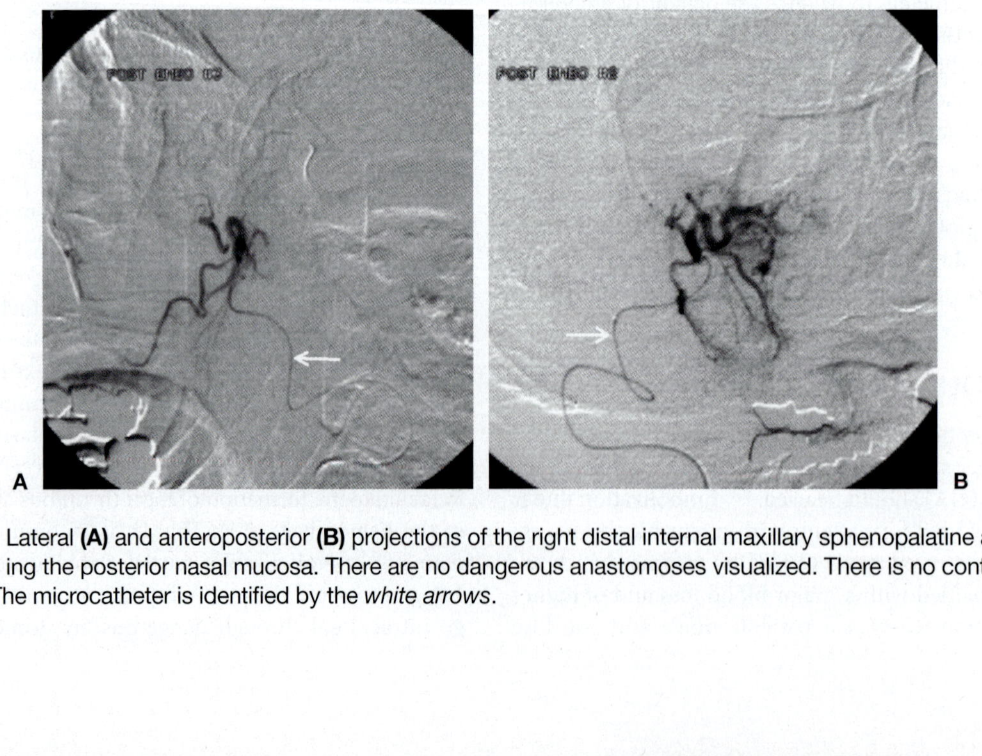

Figure 15.2 Lateral **(A)** and anteroposterior **(B)** projections of the right distal internal maxillary sphenopalatine arteries perfusing the posterior nasal mucosa. There are no dangerous anastomoses visualized. There is no contraindication to embolization. The microcatheter is identified by the *white arrows*.

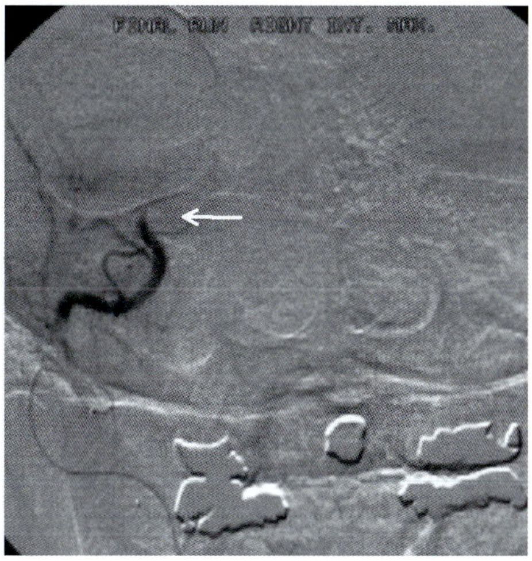

Figure 15.3 Final right internal maxillary angiogram postembolization. Final image postembolization. The *white arrow* indicates the occluded sphenopalatine artery.

catastrophic consequences. Before embolization, it is important that a wedged catheter position is avoided and there is still forward blood flow in the distal end of the microcatheter. If a wedged catheter position and complete cutoff of forward blood flow occurs, the injection pressure can increase during the embolization process, incurring the risk of opening potential extracranial–intracranial dangerous anastomosis. It would also increase the risk of reflux of embolic materials into nontargeted vessels. In addition, it is very important to keep the microcatheter stable during the embolization process. This is especially true in the later stages of the process to avoid displacement of the microcatheter, which can be caused by increased injection pressure. During the embolization, a suspension of embolic and contrast material is subsequently injected under fluoroscopic control until significant flow reduction is noted in the target vessel (Figs. 15.3 to 15.5).[19]

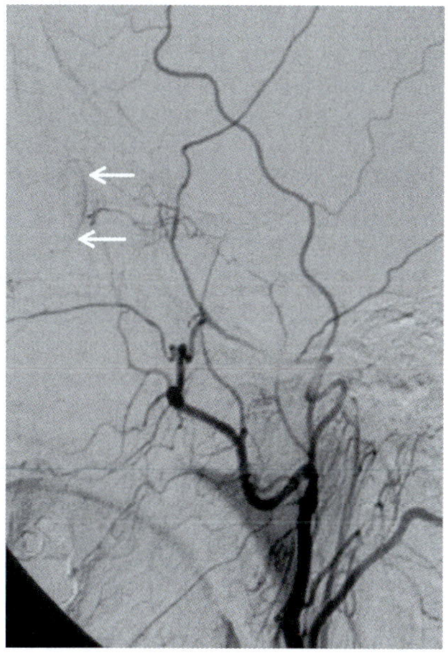

Figure 15.5 This lateral external injection demonstrates the middle meningeal collateral to the ophthalmic artery and filling of the retinal arteries with a beautiful semilunar retinal blush (*arrows*). These shunts open during procedures as pressure changes in occluding vessels cause more reflux along a microcatheter. The negative road map is critical to finding these. Listen to any report from the patient about vision change.

CLINICAL INDICATIONS

Idiopathic Epistaxis

At least 70% of epistaxis cases are idiopathic.[10,23] In this situation, there is often no characteristic angiography manifestations, and even otolaryngologist are unsure which side is the cause of bleeding. There is an extensive branch anastomosis among blood vessels of the two sides of nasal cavity, and thus the bilateral sphenopalatine artery may sometimes need to be

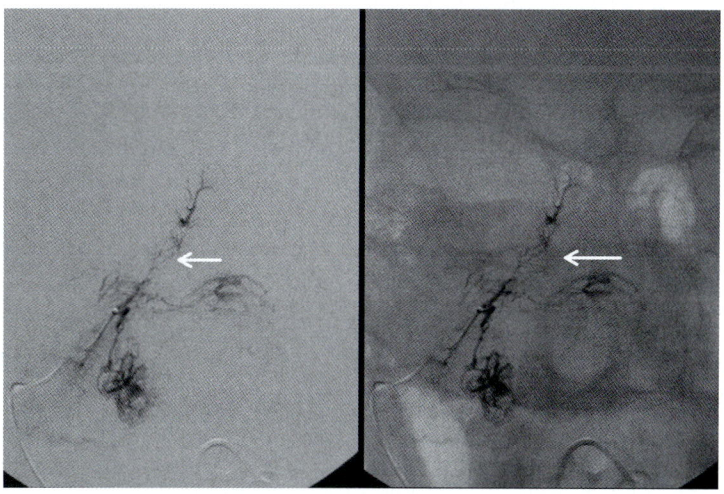

Figure 15.4 The dangerous anastomoses are potential collateral pathways that can open as the pressure changes in the arterial bed, creating potential paths by which embolic material can get into the intracranial carotid and cause stroke. These AP subtracted and unsubtracted images show the inferolateral trunk anastomosis between the internal maxillary and the inferolateral trunk of the cavernous carotid (*arrows*).

embolized. Normally, successful hemostasis is achieved with internal maxillary route embolization alone, although rarely, it is necessary to embolize both facial artery branches. This has an additional risk of minor complications such as skin or mucosal necrosis, particularly if very small embolic material is used (50 to 199 μm).[4,20,24] PVA particles with sizes 300 to 500 μm are the material of choice. It is not recommended to use microcoils to occlude main vessels as these become road blocks if a reembolization is needed in the future. Compared with other cases of epistaxis, the success rate of embolization therapy for idiopathic epistaxis is higher, and the long-term success rates could reach as high as 93.5%.[20]

Trauma or Iatrogenic Injury

For epistaxis caused by trauma or iatrogenic injury, bleeding usually occur immediately after the injury or medical procedure but can be delayed.[15] Most would happen within 3 weeks after injury.[15] For epistaxis caused by trauma or iatrogenic injury, diagnostic angiography may reveal a pseudoaneurysm of internal or external carotid artery, and in an active situation, you may see contrast media extravasation. For epistaxis caused by external carotid artery injury, the treatment method is similar to that for spontaneous epistaxis. However, trauma patients in shock may have injured vessels that are constricted or in spasm. Although bleeding can be controlled temporarily with embolization, blood pressure will increase once bleeding has stopped, the peripheral vascular bed will reopen, and the chances of bleeding reoccurring can be high. Using particles for embolizing diseased vessels, gelfoam pledgets, or microcoil for embolizing main branches of diseased vessels could be considered to consolidate the embolization effect and reduce the rate of bleeding. In urgent cases, NBCA is an excellent tool to achieve instant closure of a rapidly bleeding vessel. NBCA is, however, a complex material to use and should not be used by the inexperienced.

Pseudoaneurysm induced by injury of the internal maxillary or proximal external carotid can be difficult to handle. This is usually either traumatic or a complication of an endoscopic approach.[25] Permanent vessel occlusion is the best solution.

Infectious Aneurysm

The wall of infectious aneurysm is thin; direct embolization of an aneurysm could possibly cause rerupture due to the fragile nature of the aneurysmal wall. Principally, treating infectious aneurysm of branches of external carotid artery is done to embolize the parent artery. The operational procedure is the same as previously described. For treatments of infectious aneurysm of the internal carotid artery, the principle is similar to that for traumatic pseudoaneurysm. In cases where a balloon occlusion test is tolerated, sacrificing the internal carotid artery of the diseased side can be considered for treatment. Another alternative therapy is a stent graft.

Hereditary Hemorrhagic Telangiectasia

The treatment of epistaxis in patients with hereditary hemorrhagic telangiectasia (HHT) is initially conservative. The success rate of embolization for treating HHT-induced epistaxis is only 20% to 25%, whereas the rate is as high as 90% for idiopathic epistaxis.[20,26] It is difficult for embolization therapy to achieve radical treatment of HHT, and the purpose of the treatment is mainly to reduce the frequency of epistaxis occurrence and lessen the severity of each episode.[27] Due to the fact that abnormal angiogenesis constantly exists, it is very difficult to conduct permanent embolization therapy for diseased vessels caused by HHT.[26] In considering the refractory nature and high rate of recurrence for epistaxis induced by HHT, it is not recommended to use such permanent embolic materials as microcoil to embolize the main branches of diseased vessels so as to preserve the interventional approach for future treatment.[27]

POTENTIAL COMPLICATIONS

The complication of embolism therapy for epistaxis fall into two categories: minor transient adverse event and major complications. Major complications can be further categorized as major transient or persistent.[19] Patients with minor transient adverse event such as headache, facial pain, jaw pain, trismus, facial edema, or facial numbness are able to recover quickly without any disturbing aftereffects. Major transient complications include skin slough, temporary hemiparesis, temporary monocular visual field loss, and mucosal necrosis.[19] Persistent complications include facial scarring following ischemia, monocular blindness, peripheral facial nerve paralysis, cerebral infarction, and ischemic sialadenitis requiring surgery.[19] Larger series report minor transient complications in 25% to 59%, major transient in 0% to 1%, and persistent in 2% of cases.[19] Smith[4] retrospectively analyzed 15 clinical studies on embolism therapy for epistaxis and found that the occurrence rate of serious complication was 0% to 8% and the average rate was 3%.

TIPS AND TRICKS

- Create a separate table for the embolization materials and keep the bowls with the PVA, the contrast used for control injections, and all other equipment that have contact with embolic material. Do not cross-contaminate your diagnostic equipment.
- Do not do a final control injection with the guiding catheter in a common carotid ever. Most strokes occur from clot in the guide around the microcatheter.
- Use a negative road map. Foot on road map. Inject nothing, then use that image as the guide for the embolization. It allows you see dangerous anastomosis easier.
- Some of our patients have been elderly women with left-sided nosebleeds and a horrible ecstatic aortic arch. Keep a few Simmons 2 (Cook Medical Inc., Blooming-

ton, Indiana) Envoy guide catheters on your shelf for this situation. If that is not working for you, look at some of the cardiology internal mammary guide catheters.

- Control the patient's blood pressure.
- Heparinize the patient for the embolization. You can always give blood. You cannot give gray cells if you have a procedural stroke. The last thing you want to do is to give recombinant tissue plasminogen activator to someone with epistaxis.
- With a diagnostic catheter, do a complete preembolization angiography, common carotid to look for atheroma, then internal and external carotid arteries to identify extracranial–intracranial dangerous anastomosis.
- Appropriate range for diameter of PVA particles is 300–500 μm. Smaller particles increase the risk of skin necrosis and stroke.
- Do not wedge the catheter in the vessel and always maintain the forward flow of blood during embolization process; pay attention to the change of injection pressure or increase in resistance.
- If you block the microcatheter with PVA delivered by a 3-mL syringe, carefully unblock it using a contrast-filled 1-mL syringe or consider pulling the microcatheter out and recanalize it on the procedure table.
- Have a system to identify the syringes used in the embolization. We use 3-mL Luer lock syringes. We use Steri-Strips (3M, St. Paul, Minnesota) to identify the three different syringes, and they draw up from three different bowls. The syringes used for saline are bare, that is, no Steri-Strip; the contrast syringes have one Steri-Strip; and the PVA syringes have two Steri-Strips. The bowls have Steri-Strips that match this. The embolization space is self-sufficient. You never ever draw up saline or contrast from your diagnostic system with any syringe that came from the embolization table as a PVA particle can contaminate the clean system and cause a stroke.

REFERENCES

1. Shukla PA, Chan N, Duffis EJ, et al. Current treatment strategies for epistaxis: a multidisciplinary approach. *J Neurointerv Surg*. 2013;5(2):151–156.
2. Small M, Murray JA, Maran AG. A study of patients with epistaxis requiring admission to hospital. *Health Bull (Edinb)*. 1982;40(1):20–29.
3. Fatakia A, Winters R, Amedee RG. Epistaxis: a common problem. *Ochsner J*. 2010;10(3):176–178.
4. Smith TP. Embolization in the external carotid artery. *J Vasc Interv Radiol*. 2006;17(12):1897–1912; quiz 1913.
5. Schlosser RJ. Clinical practice: epistaxis. *N Engl J Med*. 2009; 360(8):784–789.
6. Breda SD, Choi IS, Persky MS, et al. Embolization in the treatment of epistaxis after failure of internal maxillary artery ligation. *Laryngoscope*. 1989;99(8, pt 1):809–813.
7. Elahi MM, Parnes LS, Fox AJ, et al. Therapeutic embolization in the treatment of intractable epistaxis. *Arch Otolaryngol Head Neck Surg*. 1995;121(1):65–69.
8. Schaitkin B, Strauss M, Houck JR. Epistaxis: medical versus surgical therapy: a comparison of efficacy, complications, and economic considerations. *Laryngoscope*. 1987;97(12):1392–1396.
9. Sokoloff J, Wickbom I, McDonald D, et al. Therapeutic percutaneous embolization in intractable epistaxis. *Radiology*. 1974; 111(2):285–287.
10. Tseng EY, Narducci CA, Willing SJ, et al. Angiographic embolization for epistaxis: a review of 114 cases. *Laryngoscope*. 1998;108(4, pt 1):615–619.
11. Asanau A, Timoshenko AP, Prades JM. Strategy of modern epistaxis management. *Cardiovasc Intervent Radiol*. 2012;35(3): 709–710.
12. Mahadevia AA, Murphy KJ, Obray R, et al. Embolization for intractable epistaxis. *Tech Vasc Interv Radiol*. 2005;8(3):134–138.
13. Koh E, Frazzini VI, Kagetsu NJ. Epistaxis: vascular anatomy, origins, and endovascular treatment. *AJR Am J Roentgenol*. 2000; 174(3):845–851.
14. Christensen NP, Smith DS, Barnwell SL, et al. Arterial embolization in the management of posterior epistaxis. *Otolaryngol Head Neck Surg*. 2005;133(5):748–753.
15. Chen D, Concus AP, Halbach VV, et al. Epistaxis originating from traumatic pseudoaneurysm of the internal carotid artery: diagnosis and endovascular therapy. *Laryngoscope*. 1998;108(3):326–331.
16. Friedlander RM. Clinical practice: arteriovenous malformations of the brain. *N Engl J Med*. 2007;356(26):2704–2712.
17. Agid R, Terbrugge K, Rodesch G, et al. Management strategies for anterior cranial fossa (ethmoidal) dural arteriovenous fistulas with an emphasis on endovascular treatment. *J Neurosurg*. 2009;110(1):79–84.
18. Thiex R, Wu I, Mulliken JB, et al. Safety and clinical efficacy of Onyx for embolization of extracranial head and neck vascular anomalies. *AJNR Am J Neuroradiol*. 2011;32(6):1082–1086.
19. Willems PW, Farb RI, Agid R. Endovascular treatment of epistaxis. *AJNR Am J Neuroradiol*. 2009;30(9):1637–1645.
20. Strach K, Schrock A, Wilhelm K, et al. Endovascular treatment of epistaxis: indications, management, and outcome. *Cardiovasc Intervent Radiol*. 2011;34(6):1190–1198.
21. Lasjaunias P. Nasopharyngeal angiofibromas: hazards of embolization. *Radiology*. 1980;136(1):119–123.
22. Geibprasert S, Pongpech S, Armstrong D, et al. Dangerous extracranial-intracranial anastomoses and supply to the cranial nerves: vessels the neurointerventionalist needs to know. *AJNR Am J Neuroradiol*. 2009;30(8):1459–1468.
23. Elden L, Montanera W, Terbrugge K, et al. Angiographic embolization for the treatment of epistaxis: a review of 108 cases. *Otolaryngol Head Neck Surg*. 1994;111(1):44–50.
24. Fukutsuji K, Nishiike S, Aihara T, et al. Superselective angiographic embolization for intractable epistaxis. *Acta Otolaryngol*. 2008;128(5):556–560.
25. Redekop G, Marotta T, Weill A. Treatment of traumatic aneurysms and arteriovenous fistulas of the skull base by using endovascular stents. *J Neurosurg*. 2001;95(3):412–419.
26. Risley J, Mann K, Jones NS. The role of embolisation in ENT: an update. *J Laryngol Otol*. 2012;126(3):228–235.
27. Layton KF, Kallmes DF, Gray LA, et al. Endovascular treatment of epistaxis in patients with hereditary hemorrhagic telangiectasia. *AJNR Am J Neuroradiol*. 2007;28(5):885–888.

16

Vascular Tumors

Robert F. James • Lacey B. Martin • John R. Gaughen, Jr • William J. Mack

Highly vascular tumors of the head and neck often pose significant surgical challenges. Bleeding can result in decreased operative visibility and inadvertent injury to adjacent vital structures. Significant blood loss and volume depletion can lead to major morbidities. Embolization of vascular head and neck tumors before surgical resection may help to minimize blood loss, reduce operative time, and facilitate surgical resection. However, the additional endovascular procedure is not without risk to the patient. Multiple anastomotic connections exist between the arteries of the head and neck. Aberrant embolization through these channels can lead to neurologic injuries such as visual loss, paralysis, or ischemic injury to the cranial nerves. It is imperative that the interventionalist and the operating surgeon discuss the goals of embolization and the overall treatment plan before the endovascular procedure. The most common vascular tumors of the head and neck region suitable for preoperative embolization include meningiomas, paragangliomas, juvenile nasopharyngeal angiofibromas, hemangiopericytomas, and hemangioblastomas. Here we will discuss the relevant procedure-related devices and materials, techniques, clinical applications, and potential complications. Most discussion focuses on meningiomas as they are the most frequently encountered of the vascular head and neck tumors. Subsections are devoted to specific concerns for the other tumor types. Table 16.1 details important dangerous anastomoses with the cranial nerve blood supply.

DEVICE/MATERIAL DESCRIPTION

Catheters

A coaxial system of an outer guide catheter and an inner microcatheter is usually employed for transarterial endovascular embolization. We typically use guide catheters with a 0.053-in or 0.070-in inner diameter. The 6-Fr 070 Neuron guide catheter (0.070-in inner diameter; Penumbra, Inc., Alameda, California) can be used for the internal carotid artery (ICA) access, the 053 Neuron guide catheter for the external carotid artery (ECA) (0.053-in inner diameter), and either the 053 or 070 Neuron guide catheter for the vertebral artery (VA), depending on vessel diameter.

There are various-sized microcatheters with multiple features that are beyond the scope of this chapter. The Echelon-10 and Marathon (Covidien, Irvine, California) microcatheters can be used for routine embolizations. The Scepter C balloon catheter (MicroVention, Inc., Tustin, California) enables a new balloon-augmented embolization technique through a single microcatheter.[1,2] Typically, 0.014-in diameter guidewires are used to help navigate the microcatheter because of their superior steering and trackability. However, smaller guidewires such as the 0.008-in Mirage (Covidien, Irvine, California) may be safer in small, distal cerebral vasculature (Note: the 0.008-in guidewires are essentially unsteerable and navigating bifurcations is often an exercise in persistence of the trial and error technique and/or uncanny tip reshaping proficiency). The size and angioarchitecture of the feeding vessel may require altering or modifying the microcatheter, often necessitating very small and "floppy" catheters for difficult-to-reach anatomy. In these situations, the Marathon flow-directed microcatheter could be advantageous. Unfortunately, guidewires 0.012 in or smaller are necessary when using the Marathon microcatheter due to its 0.013-in distal lumen diameter. However, the catheter is surprisingly compatible with the 0.014-in Traxcess guidewire (MicroVention, Inc., Tustin, California), as both the catheter and wire taper in a similar fashion. Preference is given to use the 0.014-in Traxcess guidewire when the Marathon microcatheter is required, as the Traxcess wire has superior steerability and provides a more rigid tracking platform compared to the other compatible guidewires.

Table 16.1 Major Cervico–Cerebral Arteries with Associated Cranial Nerve Supply and Common Dangerous Anastomoses

Major Artery	Branch	Cranial Nerve at Risk	Dangerous Anastomoses
ECA – IMA	MMA (proximal IMA)	VII (via petrous branch)	
		II	OA: second portion of OA via proximal lacrimal artery (superficial recurrent meningeal artery) and anterior falcine artery
		II	OA: second or third portion of OA via septal arteries, sphenopalatine artery, and greater palatine artery via anterior and posterior ethmoidal arteries
			ICA: anteromedial branch of ILT via superior orbital fissure along orbital branches of MMA
			ICA: superior or tentorial branch of ILT via cavernous branches along roof of cavernous sinus
	MMA – petrosal branch	VII (geniculate ganglion)	
	MMA – meningo-ophthalmic artery via primitive stapedial artery	II	OA: (may no longer arise from ICA in some cases)
	AMA – superior division via proximal IMA	V_3 (foramen ovale)	ICA: posteromedial branch of ILT via artery of foramen ovale
	Vidian artery (distal IMA)		ICA: petrous portion
	Artery of foramen rotundum	V_2 (foramen rotundum)	ICA: anterolateral branch of ILT
	Infraorbital artery	II	OA: second portion of OA via inferior branch of the distal lacrimal artery
			Terminal branch of OA via dorsal nasal artery
	Anterior deep temporal artery (distal IMA)	II	OA: second portion of OA via inferior branch of the distal lacrimal artery
ECA – STA	Frontal branch	II	OA: third portion of OA via supraorbital artery
ECA – posterior auricular artery	Stylomastoid branch	VII (geniculate ganglion)	Meningeal anastomoses to MMA and asc pha
ECA – occipital artery	Stylomastoid branch	VII (geniculate ganglion)	VA: muscular branches
			Transosseous direct supply to cerebellum – posterior fossa
			Direct origin via anatomical variants
ECA – facial artery	Angular artery	II	OA: terminal branch of OA via dorsal nasal artery
			Lingual artery (rare)
			Asc pha (rare)

Continued

Table 16.1 Major Cervico–Cerebral Arteries with Associated Cranial Nerve Supply and Common Dangerous Anastomoses *(continued)*

Major Artery	Branch	Cranial Nerve at Risk	Dangerous Anastomoses
ECA – lingual artery		XII (extracranial segments)	Contralateral lingual artery Superior thyroid artery
ECA – asc pha	Musculospinal branch Carotid branch Pharyngeal trunk – superior pharyngeal artery Neuromeningeal trunk – odontoid arch Neuromeningeal trunk – hypoglossal branch Neuromeningeal trunk – jugular branch	XI (spinal root) V (Meckel cave) XII (via cisternal and hypoglossal canal) VI (dorsum sella), IX, X, XI (cranial root); via jugular foramen	 ICA: via lateral clival artery, carotid branch within foramen lacerum VA: (adjacent to C1)
ECA – superior thyroid artery	Superior laryngeal artery	X (Superior laryngeal nerve)	Contralateral superior thyroid and inferior thyroid arteries
ECA	Proatlantal artery (persistent fetal): type 2		VA
Ascending and deep cervical arteries		XI (Spinal root)	VA (adjacent to C3–C7)
Vertebrobasilar system (VA, BA)	Mesencephalic perforating arteries Basilar vestige of trigeminal artery (arises from BA between SCA and AICA) AICA – internal auditory artery	III (common trunk), IV, VI (cisternal components) V (cisternal portion) VII, VIII (cisternal and IAC portions)	 ICA: cavernous portion via MHT or ILT
ICA	MHT – marginal tentorial artery (Bernasconi and Cassinari) MHT – lateral clival artery, medial branch ILT – anteromedial branch via superior orbital fissure Posterior communicating artery Proatlantal artery (persistent fetal): type 1 also known as *proatlantal intersegmental artery*	IV (tentorial edge and cavernous portions), VI (dorsum sella) Cavernous portions of III, IV, VI, V_2, V_3 III, IV, VI	 PCA VA

ECA, external carotid artery; IMA, internal maxillary artery; MMA, middle meningeal artery; OA, ophthalmic artery; ICA, internal carotid artery; ILT, inferolateral trunk; AMA, anterior meningeal artery; STA, superficial temporal artery; asc pha, ascending pharyngeal artery; VA, vertebral artery; BA, basilar artery; MHT, meningohypophyseal trunk; SCA, superior cerebellar artery; AICA, anterior inferior cerebellar artery; PCA, posterior cerebellar artery.

Based on data from Geibprasert S, Pongpech S, Armstrong D, et al. Dangerous extracranial-intracranial anastomoses and supply to the cranial nerves: vessels the neurointerventionalist needs to know. *AJNR Am J Neuroradiol*. 2009;30:1459–1468; Lazzaro MA, Badruddin A, Zaidat OO, et al. Endovascular embolization of head and neck tumors. *Front Neurol*. 2011;2:64.

Particles

The most common agent used for embolization of meningiomas and other head and neck tumors is a suspension of particles mixed with a contrast agent. Particles are small substrates that aggregate to obstruct the vessel. The choices of particle material and size impact results and potential complications associated with embolization. As differences in the granulometric distribution of particles exist, they may not match exactly with their advertised size range. Compressibility, elastic recovery, aggregation, and visualization of particles can all affect performance.

Polyvinyl alcohol (PVA) particles are nonspherical and are available in preparations of varying size ranges. Limitations with PVA embolization include difficulty with aggregation and microcatheter obstruction, leading to premature termination of the embolization or microcatheter exchange. Injection under increased pressure to clear the catheter should *never* be performed. This maneuver increases the risk of forcing particles into undesired territories once they are released.

Smaller particles allow deeper penetration into the tumor bed for more complete devascularization and increased tumor necrosis; however, they have a higher likelihood of reaching potentially dangerous or disabling arteries.[3] Larger particles are safer but may not fully penetrate and devascularize the tumor bed and, therefore, may be less efficient at reducing surgical blood loss. Maintaining particle size greater than 150 μm is thought to reduce the risk of damaging the vasa nervorum of the cranial nerves.[4,5] A large study of 201 embolized meningiomas found small particle size (45 to 150 μm) to be the sole risk factor for complications, hemorrhagic or otherwise.[5] In high-flow situations, increasing particle size to greater than 500 μm may be beneficial, or an alternate class of embolic agent can be considered. Size selection of the PVA particles is a balance between desired tumor penetration and unwanted target embolization. In most situations, selecting particles with a diameter between 150 and 350 μm will provide optimal results.[6]

Trisacryl Microspheres

Calibrated spherical particles made of trisacryl and cellulose porous beads were developed to address the disadvantages of PVA particles, specifically their irregular size and nonspherical nature. Trisacryl microspheres are partially compressible and, as a result, allow for easier transit through the delivery catheter.[7,8] Microspheres are thought to redistribute after initial clumping and delayed control angiography is therefore warranted. A study of 60 patients comparing trisacryl particles to nonspherical PVA particles found lower surgical blood loss with trisacryl embolization.[9]

Gelfoam

Gelfoam should be delivered via the transarterial embolization approach. For head and neck tumors, powder and sponge forms can be used.[10] Gelfoam persists for 3 to 6 weeks before recanalization begins.

Liquid Embolics

The two most common liquid embolic agents are *N*-butyl cyanoacrylate (NBCA: Trufill; Codman & Shurtleff, Inc., Raynham, Massachusetts) and ethylene vinyl alcohol (Onyx; Covidien, Irvine, California). The choice of liquid embolic is a matter of preference, with each having advantages and disadvantages. Onyx offers a decreased theoretical risk of catheter retention, whereas NBCA has more versatility by altering the rate of polymerization with dilution strategies.

Advantages of liquid embolic agents include decreased peritumoral edema and the prevention of delayed recanalization (sometimes seen after particle embolization). They can be used with transarterial or direct puncture embolization techniques. Potential disadvantages include an inability to select the size of vessels that the liquid embolic will enter (compared to particle embolization). There is risk that the liquid embolic agent will occlude vessels prematurely without deep penetration into the tumor.[11] Further, liquid embolics are more expensive than particles.

NBCA is a liquid embolic that is injected as a mixture with Ethiodol. The safety of tumor embolization with NBCA has been studied. Kim et al.[12] examined 35 consecutive tumor patients embolized with NBCA (17% meningiomas). The authors suggest that NBCA had better fluoroscopic visibility than PVA particles, enabling precise identification of embolized vessels and tumor mass. Disadvantages include quicker polymerization and risk of catheter retention. Proper embolization with NBCA requires greater technical skill than PVA administration. NBCA is also considered more permanent than PVA particles. When dangerous anastomoses are encountered, coils can be used to obstruct their origins and prevent distal embolization of the liquid embolic agent into unwanted territories.[12]

Onyx is an effective embolic agent that can penetrate into tumor capillaries. A small case series reported no increased postembolization tumor edema and no hemorrhagic complications following Onyx embolization.[11] The Onyx mixture is radiopaque and highly visible during angiography.[13] Care must be taken to create a meniscus between the dimethyl sulfoxide (DMSO) and the Onyx. Mixing of Onyx and DMSO in the catheter hub can dilute the Onyx, rendering it less radiopaque and more difficult to visualize. This can increase the risk of embolization to unwanted vascular territories. Onyx can be injected over a longer time frame than NBCA, which makes it more controllable and therefore may result in more uniform lesion penetration.[14]

Coils

Coils are shaped (curled) pieces of metal, usually platinum, that are released into a vessel for occlusion. Detachable and pushable coils can serve as an alternative to particle and liquid embolization methods. Some debate exists regarding the appropriateness and use of coils in the setting of head and neck tumors. Coils may be suitable for masses with large feeding vessels, greater than 1.5 mm in diameter.[15] However, some argue that proximal coil occlusion may not only create collaterals but may also prevent repeat access in case of tumor recurrences.[16] Coils can be an excellent adjunct to liquid embolization, preventing penetration of the liquid embolic into unwanted territories without causing ischemia.

Other Embolic Agents

Additional agents that have been used in embolization of vascular head and neck tumors include fibrin glue, ethyl alcohol (ETOH), hydroxyapatite ceramics, phenytoin, hyperosmolar mannitol, and Lipiodol.[17–22]

TECHNIQUE

Preembolization Workup and Considerations

A complete medical history and physical examination is required before any embolization procedure. A review of noninvasive imaging is critical; findings on computed tomography (CT) and magnetic resonance imaging (MRI) studies can help guide the treatment. A complete angiographic evaluation of the tumor is recommended. For intracranial meningiomas, a comprehensive study includes a six-vessel intracranial and extracranial angiogram (bilateral ECA, ICA, and VA). Large vessel sacrifice may be warranted when paragangliomas encase the carotid artery. In these cases, angiography can be combined with balloon test occlusion to assess the feasibility of vessel sacrifice.[23]

Subsequently, superselective angiography of individual arterial pedicles, with specific attention to dangerous anastomoses and the at-risk blood supply of cranial nerves, is necessary to plan the embolization procedure (Table 16.1).[24] Blood supply to most meningiomas is derived from the dural arterial vasculature (middle meningeal artery, posterior meningeal artery, tentorial artery of Bernasconi and Cassinari, etc.), arising from the ECA, VA, or ICA. A typical finding on superselective angiography is an intense vascular tumor blush from the arterial phase through the late venous phase, often with a "sunburst" type pattern.[25] Tumors located in specific anatomical locations such as the orbital, parasellar, petroclival, and cervicomedullary regions will have associated, and predictable, patterns of these dangerous anastomoses or at-risk cranial nerve blood supply relative to their location.[24] Careful study of the superselective angiographic images with a strong understanding of the usual dangerous anatomy is imperative for the avoidance of complications.

Procedural Considerations

Timing and Adjunctive Medications

Preoperative embolization is typically performed within several days of surgical resection. Delaying surgical resection at least 24 hours after embolization may be beneficial.[26] One study suggests the optimal latency for meningioma resection following embolization may be 7 to 9 days, allowing for maximal tumor softening, decreased operative times, and lower Simpson grades.[27] However, in tumors that have been embolized with excellent tumor bed penetration (especially with smaller particle size such as 60 to 150 μm), delay of surgical resection may lead to significant increases in peritumoral edema and mass effect.[6] Most interventionalists advocate high-dose intravenous steroids during and after meningioma embolization procedures where the tumor is large or there is already a significant amount of edema present.[5,6] Provocative testing with injection of Amytal and/or lidocaine with simultaneous neuromonitoring or immediate neurologic examination can help predict the risk of embolization to dangerous territories.[28] ECA vasospasm may occur during the embolization procedure. Prophylactic application of a transdermal nitroglycerin patch or sublingual calcium channel antagonists may reduce the occurrence of vasospasm. Administration of papaverine (30 to 60 mg), nitroglycerin (100 to 300 μg), or verapamil (5 to 20 mg) through the catheter system may reduce vasospasm and allow more predictable results.

Endovascular Technique

Embolization should be performed by a well-trained neurointerventionalist in a biplane digital subtraction fluoroscopy suite. Intravenous sedation, monitored anesthesia care (MAC), or general endotracheal anesthesia should be provided according to the specific goals and challenges of the procedure. Arterial endovascular access is obtained most often by puncture of the common femoral artery and insertion of a 5-Fr or 6-Fr short sheath using the modified Seldinger technique. Alternatively, embolization may be performed using a direct puncture technique (DPT).

The patient should be given a bolus of intravenous heparin with a goal of 2 to 2.5 times the baseline activated clotting time (ACT) to help prevent thromboembolic complications. If not performed previously, a detailed angiographic study of the tumor blood supply is then performed via superselective angiography using microcatheters.

After the decision to proceed with embolization is made, a suitable guide catheter is selected to allow for a working platform within the major artery supplying the tumor. The ICA, ECA, or the distal V4 segment of the VA may be accessed by a 90-cm guide catheter in most patients. However, vessel tortuosity or patient height may dictate the use of a longer guide catheter. The outer diameter of the guide catheter is usually 5-Fr or 6-Fr, and the inner diameter should easily accommodate the desired microcatheter(s).

After the microcatheter is in position within the target arterial pedicle and the interventionalist is confident that safe embolization can be performed, the embolic material is selected and prepared. The embolic material is injected slowly with simultaneous biplane fluoroscopy to identify flow into the feeding artery and tumor bed. Reduction of tumor blush by 80% or more following embolization should be the goal, as reaching this threshold may be necessary to impart a beneficial effect.[23] Injection should stop when the embolic agent no longer reaches the tumor or, in the case

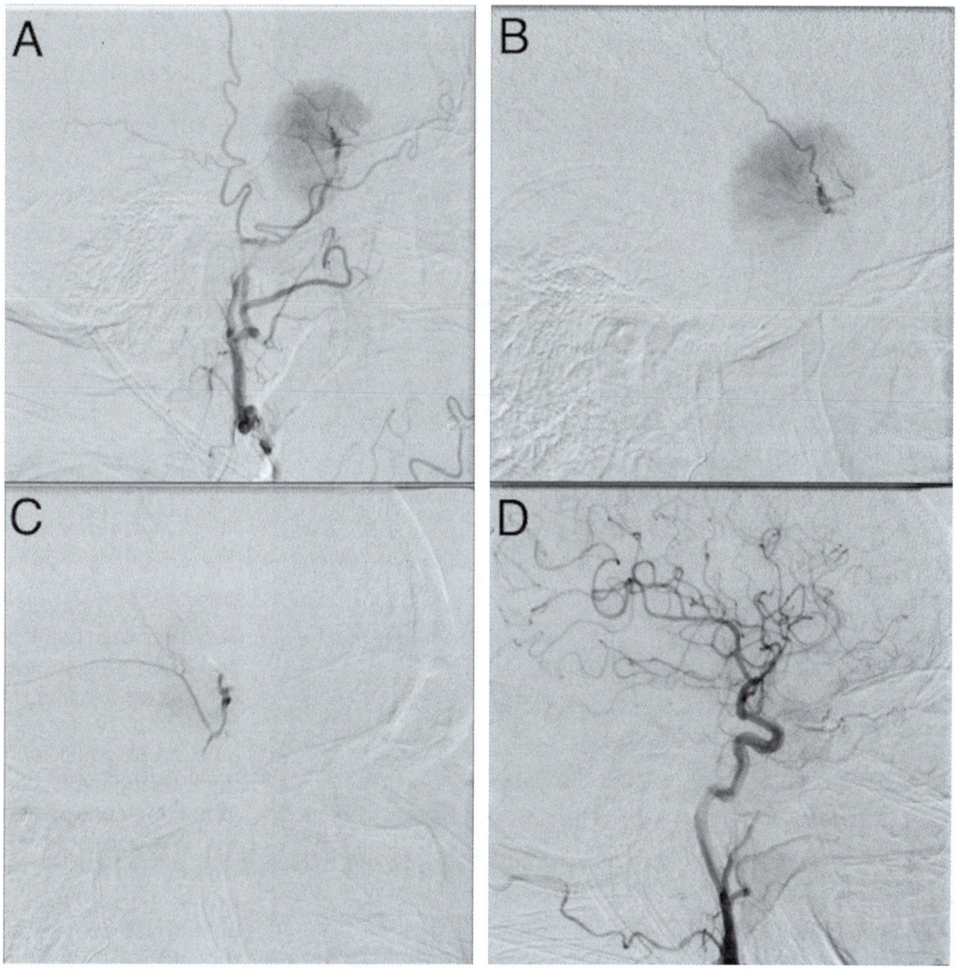

Figure 16.1 Right sphenoid wing meningioma. **A:** Right ECA and **(B)** selective right middle meningeal artery digital subtraction angiograms (DSAs) demonstrate the characteristic vascular blush of a right sphenoid wing meningioma, deriving arterial supply predominantly from branches of the right middle meningeal artery. Note: No choroidal blush from these injections. **C:** Selective right middle meningeal artery DSA following transarterial embolization of the tumor using PVA 150- to 250-μm and 250- to 355-μm particles, resulting in significant devascularization of the meningioma. **D:** Right common carotid artery DSA following subsequent coil embolization of the distal right middle meningeal artery trunk demonstrates near-complete devascularization of the tumor and truncation of the right middle meningeal artery. Note a small amount of residual vascular tumor blush arising from branches of the right inferolateral trunk off the cavernous segment of the right ICA.

of particle embolization, when there is contrast stagnation of the feeding artery (Fig. 16.1). If there is any identification of embolic material tracking into undesired territories, or reflux along the microcatheter, the injection should cease immediately. Deep penetration of embolic agent into the tumor bed may result in complete devascularization of the tumor, often without embolization of all of the feeding arteries. In other circumstances, selection of additional pedicles may be necessary to obtain adequate embolization results. This typically requires obtaining a fresh microcatheter. After completion of the embolization, a thorough neurologic examination is performed to assess for ischemic or hemorrhagic complications. Close clinical surveillance is indicated over the following hours as delayed complications such as intratumoral hemorrhage, increased edema, and mass effect may develop. These complications can usually be quickly and reliably treated if recognized in a timely manner.[4,5]

Route of Embolization

The approach to head and neck tumor embolization varies based on different factors including, but not limited to, the material chosen, the location of the tumor, and the comfort level of the operator. The traditional transarterial route has been used in most meningioma embolization procedures. Rarely, vascular anatomy prevents appropriate endovascular access to the tumor and, therefore, prevents intra-arterial treatment. In these situations, a percutaneous (or transmucosal) DPT may be the only available route for embolization.[23] Occasionally, a previous craniotomy can allow DPT access for the embolization of intracranial meningiomas (Fig. 16.2). Typically, liquid agents

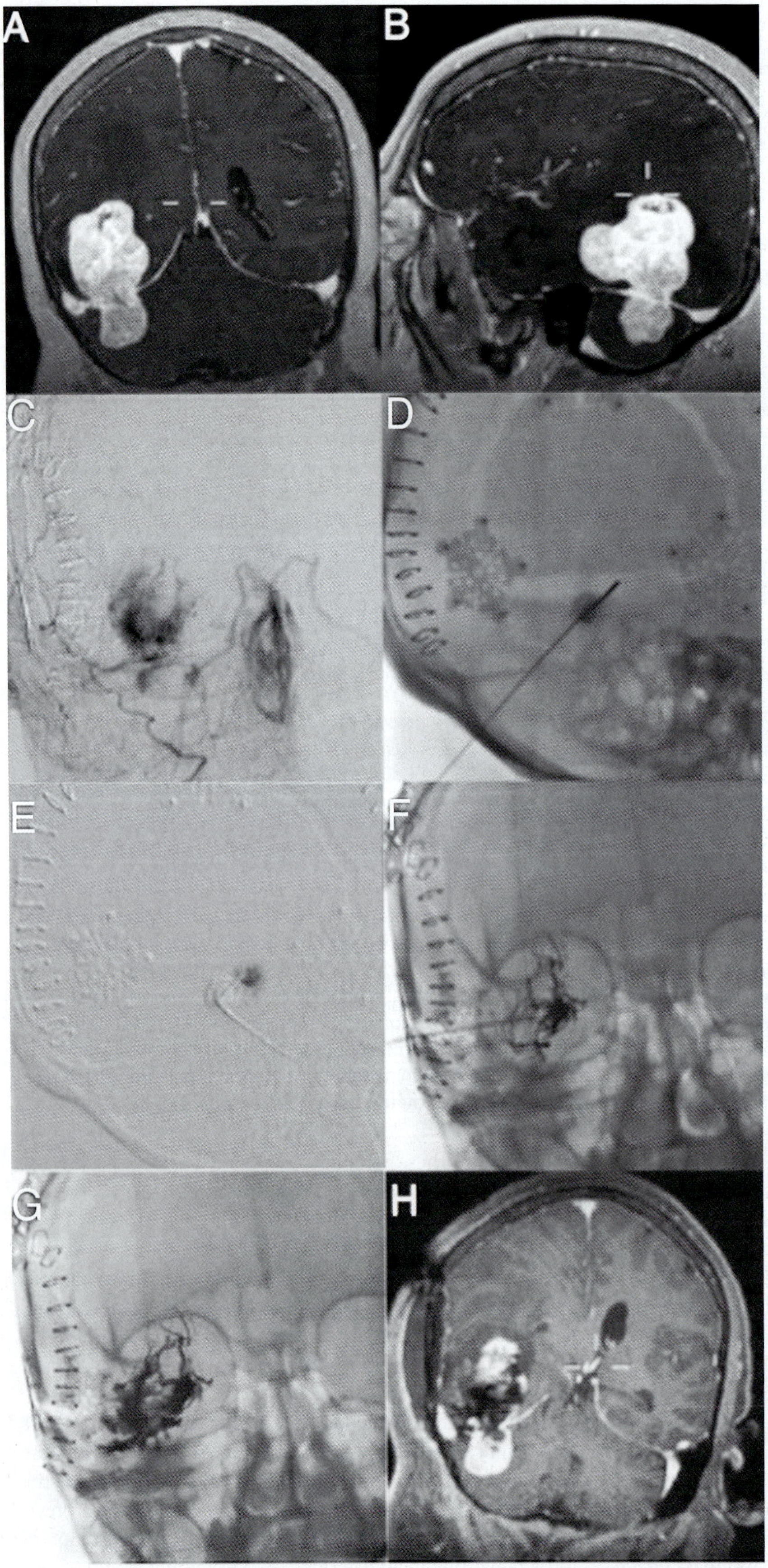

Figure 16.2 Bilobed right tentorial meningioma. **A:** Coronal and **(B)** sagittal contrast-enhanced (T1 weighted image [T1WI]) MRI performed preprocedurally demonstrate a heterogeneously enhancing bilobed dural-based mass along the right tentorium, consistent with meningioma, with components projecting infra- and supratentorially. **C:** DSA imaging performed from the right ECA in the anteroposterior (AP) projection shows a robustly vascular tumor blush corresponding to the earlier described tumor, supplied by numerous tiny branches arising from the right middle meningeal artery. Note changes of recent prior craniotomy. **D:** Digital fluoroscopic spot film (DFSF) in the lateral projection performed periprocedurally during percutaneous embolization of the tumor shows the needle traversing the craniotomy defect, and **(E)** DSA in the same projection during percutaneous contrast injection shows tumor blush, confirming appropriate needle position. **F:** DFSF in the AP projection performed periprocedurally during percutaneous embolization of the tumor shows partial embolization of the central component of the tumor with Onyx. **G:** DFSF in the AP projection performed following removal of the percutaneous needle shows dense embolization of the central tumor component. **H:** Coronal contrast-enhanced (T1WI) MRI performed postprocedurally shows significant devascularization of the supratentorial portion of the tumor.

with 18- to 20-gauge needles are employed for DPT alone or in combination with the transarterial approach. Although DPT may yield increased tumor penetration,[14] systematic comparisons of transarterial and DPT embolizations have not been performed. DPT does eliminate the issue of catheter obstruction. DPT is not without risk of major complications.[29] Care must be taken during DPT as the embolic material is driven by pressure and it may be pushed through physiologic collaterals into undesired territories because of the pressure gradient that is created.[30] Pain from tumor necrosis may occur during the DPT procedure. The patient should be aware of this possibility and may require general anesthesia.[31]

CLINICAL APPLICATIONS

Meningiomas

Meningiomas represent approximately 20% of all intracranial tumors.[11,25,28] They usually display benign histopathology and are typically extra-axial or intraventricular in location. Despite their typical benign pathology, they may cause seizures and/or neurologic deterioration as a result of their space-occupying nature. Tumors that are small and asymptomatic can be followed with periodic imaging monitoring for enlargement or development of neurologic dysfunction.[32,33] Symptomatic tumors often require surgical resection, which is typically curative and results in resolution of symptoms.[28]

Angiographic evaluation of meningiomas should be performed with catheterization of the bilateral external carotid, internal carotid, and vertebral arteries before embolization. Blood supply to meningiomas can be bilateral and may be derived from the intracerebral vessels (ICA and VA). On angiography, meningiomas typically appear as circumscribed areas of contrast staining that persists well into the venous phase. Large feeders may show the classic "sunburst" pattern.[15]

Surgical resection of meningiomas can result in significant morbidity and mortality. Chan and Thompson[34] reported on the surgical morbidity and mortality of meningioma resection in a series of 257 patients. The authors noted a surgical morbidity and a mortality of 30% and 4%, respectively.[34] Advanced age appears to be a significant surgical risk factor. A series of meningioma resections in an elderly patient population documented a 6.6% mortality rate and a 48% rate of surgical morbidity.[35]

Embolization of arteries supplying the tumor that are not anatomically accessible during surgery may help to reduce surgical morbidity and mortality by minimizing intraoperative bleeding or softening of the tumor.[26,28] A nonrandomized prospective study compared 30 patients who underwent preoperative embolization in one center with 30 patients in a second center who were not embolized. Those patients with greater than 90% tumor embolization had decreased blood loss but no other identified benefit. No differences in surgical morbidity and mortality were demonstrated between the two groups.[36] This study is limited by inherent selection bias and potential systematic differences in administration of care between the two centers. Other studies comparing patients who had preoperative embolization to those who did not undergo embolization have similar limitations. Macpherson[37] describes a personal series of 52 meningioma patients of whom 28 patients were embolized and 24 patients were not. The study reported decreases in surgical difficulty with bleeding, blood transfusions, surgical complications, and poor outcomes for the patients who were embolized. This study is influenced by the subjective scoring methods employed for determination of surgical bleeding difficulties. The operating surgeon generated scores by comparing the technical difficulty of each surgery to previous experiences of resecting tumors of comparable size situated in similar anatomic locations.[37] Similarly, in a retrospective matched-pair analysis of 18 meningioma patients treated with embolization and 18 patients without embolization, embolized patients had significant decreases in estimated blood loss and transfusions. This study is limited by a lack of sufficient detail reported for the methods of determining estimated blood loss and extent of devascularization achieved.[38]

Evidence of postembolization tumor necrosis can be documented via diminished perfusion on proton spectroscopy, contrast-enhanced CT, and contrast-enhanced MRI studies.[39–41] Embolization of meningiomas without subsequent surgical resection has been shown to be beneficial as palliative therapy in several cases.[39,42]

Decisions regarding preoperative meningioma embolization should be made on a case-by-case basis, considering both the risks and benefits associated with the procedure. Tumor location, size, overall vascularity, and specific angiographic features are key factors. Large convexity meningiomas are often ideal for presurgical embolization. In such cases, significant blood loss can result during the initial craniotomy before surgical control of the tumor. The convexity location renders embolization via the middle meningeal artery relatively low risk. Likewise, surgical resection of skull base meningiomas, and other vascular tumors, can be challenging due typically to narrow surgical corridors and firm tumor consistency. Tumor softening and necrosis can make surgical resection easier by minimizing the need for brain retraction and/or reducing mechanical injury to adjacent cranial nerves. Unfortunately, skull base meningiomas often have higher embolization risks as feeding arteries are often associated with the cranial nerve blood supply and dangerous anastomoses.

Paragangliomas

Paragangliomas are rare tumors of neural crest cell origin that typically arise from the temporal bone, carotid body, or nodose ganglion (i.e., glomus tympanicum, glomus jugulare, carotid body tumor, intravagal paraganglioma). Because these tumors develop where neural crest cells are located, the anatomical pattern of the feeding arteries may be predicted by the tumor size and location. Frequently involved arteries include the ascending pharyngeal, lingual, posterior auricular, stylohyoid, and occipital. In addition, the deep cervical artery and the thyrocervical trunk may contribute blood supply.[43] Advanced paragangliomas can seize blood supply from the anterior tympanic (branch of internal maxillary), caroticotympanic (branch of internal carotid), and superior tympanic (branch of middle meningeal) arteries.[30] When visualized on angiography, these hypervascular tumors are characterized by an intense blush.

For larger paragangliomas, the benefits of preoperative embolization appear to outweigh the associated risks. Perioperative blood loss can be reduced and surgical time decreased.[44] It may be prudent to limit preoperative embolization to those paragangliomas greater than 3 cm in diameter as smaller tumors can often be resected with less intraoperative risk. Small tumors are typically more difficult to embolize. They are associated with smaller feeding arteries that render injection of embolic material more difficult without reflux into the parent vessel. In select cases, the DPT can overcome this challenge.[30,45] In the case of carotid body tumors, balloon protection of the ICA during embolization is often helpful.

Paragangliomas may be effectively embolized with various materials (Fig. 16.3). Embolization is most commonly performed transarterially with PVA particles or liquid embolic agents.[30] DPT with NBCA or Onyx has yielded good results and appears to be effective and safe.[31,46,47] In one report, the DPT resulted in some degree of devascularization in more than 90% of patients without permanent complications.[48]

Juvenile Nasopharyngeal Angiofibromas

Juvenile nasopharyngeal angiofibromas (JNAs) are benign, yet highly aggressive and infiltrating, neoplasms that are almost exclusively seen in adolescent males. These tumors contain vessels that do not have a normal smooth muscle wall. JNAs are commonly supplied by the internal maxillary, ascending palatine, ascending pharyngeal, accessory meningeal, and internal carotid arteries.[49] JNAs have significantly larger shunts than most other head and neck tumors, which may limit the achievable extent of devascularization.[50] Characteristically, angiography demonstrates a reticulated pattern in the arterial phase and a dense tumor blush that continues into the venous phase.

The advantages of preoperative embolization for JNAs are compelling. Studies show diminished intraoperative blood loss, less blood transfusion needs, more complete resection, and fewer tumor recurrences.[51,52] Blood loss reduction during postembolization resection is considerable compared to the other head and neck tumors. JNAs are less likely to recur when the entire tumor is removed en bloc. Complete devascularization makes this type of removal easier. DPT may be a useful method for devascularization if all branches cannot be embolized through the transarterial route (Fig. 16.4).[31]

Similar to paragangliomas, multiple embolic materials can be used to treat JNAs. As JNAs tend to have large arterial shunts, particles greater than 150 μm may be advantageous. Larger particles may be needed if significantly larger shunts are discovered during angiography. The operator should, therefore, be prepared to make rapid intraoperative adjustments if necessary. Particles that travel through a large shunt may cause pulmonary complications. One potential solution to these high-flow shunts is to use balloon-augmented embolization to decrease the flow through the target vessels at the time of embolization.[1,2]

Hemangiopericytoma

Previously termed *angioblastic meningiomas*, hemangiopericytomas are rare, smooth muscle pericyte cell–derived tumors found around meningeal capillaries. Angiographically, these tumors are characterized by large arterial pedicles with many tiny corkscrew-like feeding vessels entering the tumor. The vascular stain is intense and fluffy with lingering contrast

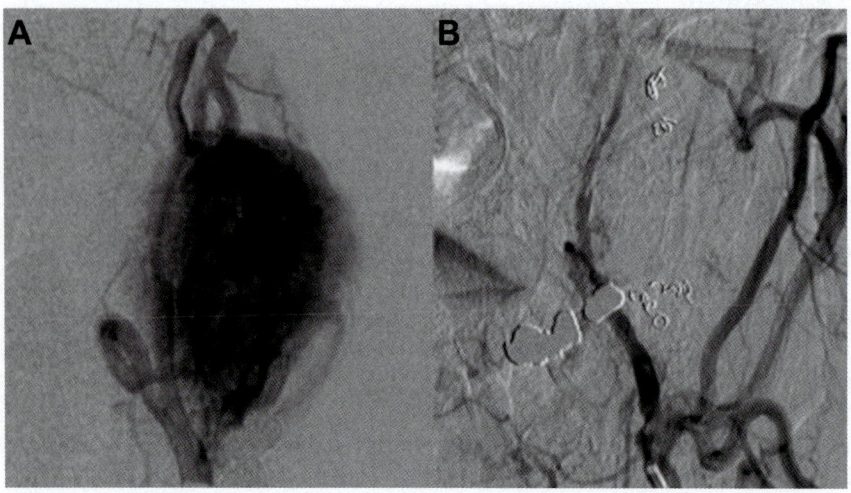

Figure 16.3 Left carotid body tumor (paraganglioma). **A:** Preoperative DSA from a left ECA injection demonstrates a highly vascular tumor situated in the crotch of the left common carotid artery bifurcation splaying the imaged branches of the left ECA. **B:** Postoperative DSA from a left ECA injection following transarterial embolization of the tumor using PVA 150- to 250-μm and 250- to 355-μm particles and platinum coils, resulting in complete tumor devascularization.

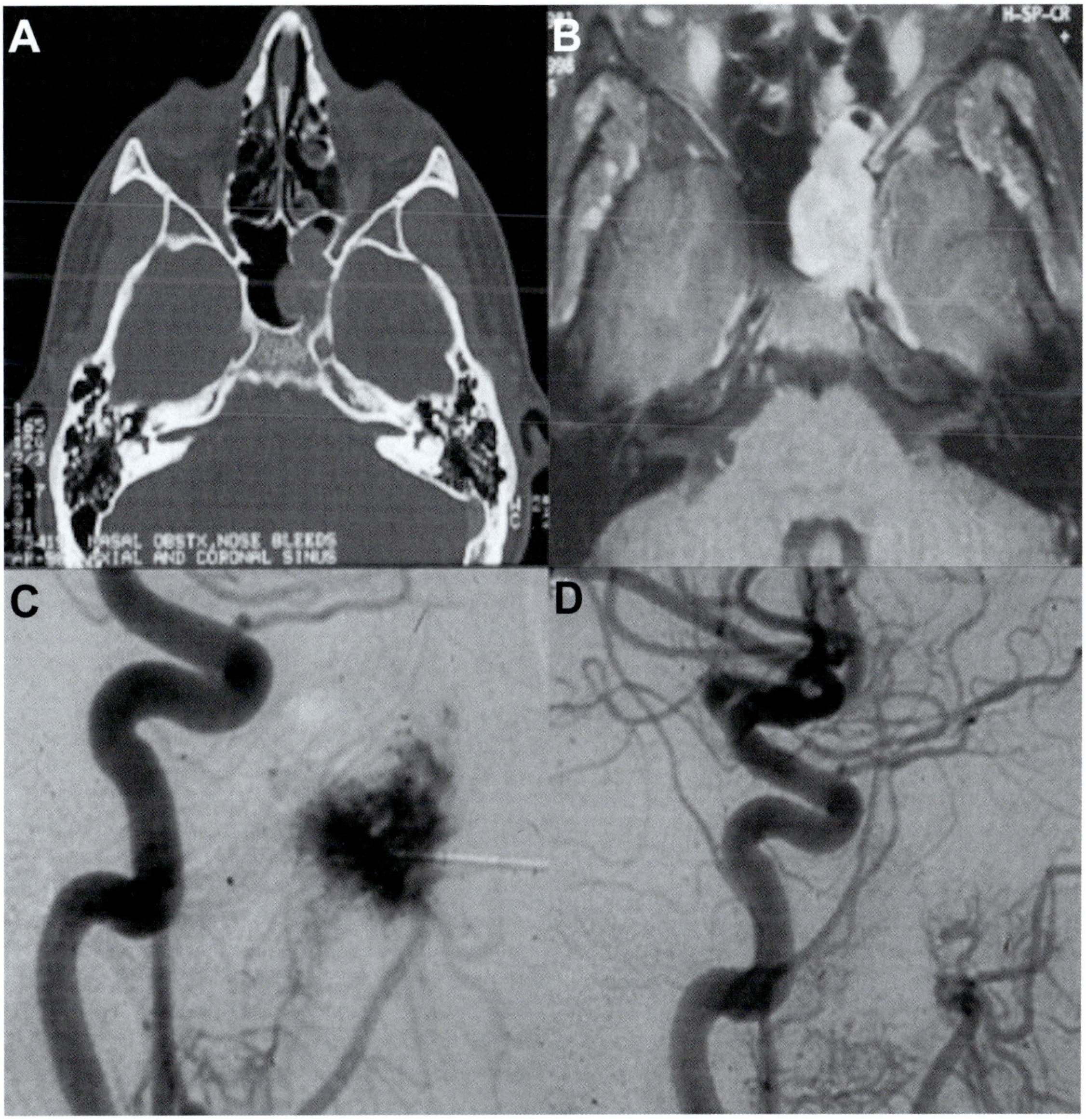

Figure 16.4 Juvenile nasopharyngeal angiofibroma. **A:** Axial CT image through the level of the sphenoid sinus demonstrates a polypoid, exophytic mass projecting into the left lateral aspect of the sphenoid sinus. **B:** Axial contrast-enhanced MRI (T1WI) through the same level demonstrates a homogeneously and avidly enhancing mass with both exophytic and infiltrative components, projecting into the sphenoid sinus and infiltrating the subjacent clivus and left middle cranial fossa. **C:** Percutaneous embolization of the tumor was performed. Perioperative DSA from a left common carotid artery injection demonstrates a highly vascular infiltrative left nasopharyngeal mass supplied by branches of the left ECA. This image also shows appropriate position of the percutaneous needle with the mass. **D:** Postoperative DSA from a left common carotid artery injection following percutaneous tumor embolization using Onyx liquid embolic agent demonstrates complete tumor devascularization.

in venous channels. The techniques for the embolization of hemangiopericytomas parallel those of meningiomas.[53]

Hemangioblastoma

Hemangioblastomas are benign vascular tumors typically found during infancy that occur predominantly in the spinal cord and cerebellum. Cerebellar hemangioblastomas are also one of the most common posterior fossa primary central nervous system tumors found in adults. Cerebellar hemangioblastomas derive most of their blood supply from the cerebellar arteries (as opposed to the external carotid circulation) as they are intra-axial in location. Meningeal, tentorial, and vertebral arteries may supply additional blood.[53] Hemangioblastomas typically display irregular vessels with intensely staining nodules exhibiting homogeneous or mottled appearance on angiography.

Preoperative embolization has been very successful in reducing intraoperative blood loss during hemangioblastoma surgery.[54] Reduced blood loss and improved outcomes were reported in tumors that had almost complete embolization. However, partial embolization resulted in increased transfusions and more operative complications in some cases.[55] Hemangioblastomas less than or equal to 1.5 cm do not typically warrant preoperative embolization as the procedural risks can outweigh those of bleeding during the surgical resection.[56] Embolization with particles greater than 150 μm or liquid NBCA may be safest.[57]

POTENTIAL COMPLICATIONS

Both major and minor complications can occur during embolization of vascular tumors of the head and neck. Major complications may include cranial nerve palsy, skin or mucosal tissue necrosis, stroke, intracranial hemorrhage, death, inadvertent embolization of pulmonary vasculature, and contrast-induced nephropathy.[23]

A recent meningioma embolization literature review identified 36 reports published between 1990 and 2011, including 459 patients who underwent meningioma embolization. Of these, 21 patients (4.6%) had complications related to embolization and 3 experienced a major complication or death (0.7%).[58] Several studies demonstrating even higher complication rates were eliminated from the analysis due to strict exclusion criteria. One excluded study evaluated 167 patients with skull base meningiomas. The authors documented an immediate postembolization complication rate of 21.6%, with 9% of patients sustaining permanent disability.[59]

Hemorrhagic complications may occur due to mechanical injury of the feeding artery by the microcatheter and wires or upon catheter retrieval when using liquid embolics. Hemorrhagic complications are also thought to occur in higher frequency when substantial devascularization of the tumor results in significant necrosis. This risk may be exacerbated by using very small particles that penetrate deep into the tumor bed.[5] Other theories suggest that compromised venous outflow may increase the risk of hemorrhage in high-flow tumors.[25,60,61]

Complication Avoidance

Reflux of small particles or liquid material may occur even during the most precise and careful procedure. Several steps may be taken to reduce this risk. Catheters should be placed distal to the origin of vessels that need to be preserved. Particle size should be considered carefully for controlled infusion as smaller particles are more likely to flow around the catheter. Balloon catheters may be deployed before delivery of embolic material to prevent or reduce the amount of refluxed substance.[15] Additionally, care should be taken to avoid proximal rupture of the microcatheter. Proximal rupture may allow particles to enter and occlude vessels not intended for embolization.[6]

Ischemia of the vasa nervorum and resultant cranial nerve palsies can occur due to reflux of embolic material or penetration of unknown anastomoses. For example, delivery of embolic material into the stylomastoid branch of the occipital artery may result in facial nerve palsy. This happens most frequently with liquid agents but has occurred with PVA particles as well.[30] Careful and thorough angiography of targeted, contralateral, and nearby vessels before embolic infusion can reveal possible unexpected anastomoses and aberrant vascular architecture. If a concern for losing blood supply to cranial nerves exists, provocative testing using lidocaine may be used.[62] The appearance of a new neurologic deficit during testing indicates the possibility of cranial nerve palsy following embolization. Repositioning of the microcatheter, as close to the tumor bed as possible, will decrease the likelihood of obstructing the blood supply to normal tissues.[15]

Minor Complications

Common minor complications include arterial access site issues such as hematoma formation, localized pain, and fever. Transient headache or temporofacial pain is the most common complication observed after embolization.[16] This can be caused by tumor swelling or, in the case of intracranial tumors, irritation of the meninges.[3] Pain is typically managed with analgesics.[15] Preoperative steroids may limit edema and reduce the likelihood of resultant complications.[30] Dexamethasone 10 mg can be given intravenously during preoperative assessment before the embolization procedure. If the tumor is large and a significant amount of embolization has been achieved, then continuing the dexamethasone at 4 mg every 6 to 8 hours (intravenous or oral) is advisable. A relatively rapid taper over the next 10 to 14 days is then prescribed. Bradycardia can develop after manipulation of the branches of the ECA, and sometimes the internal maxillary artery, which can evoke the trigeminocardiac reflex.[63]

Tumor-Specific Complications

One important potential complication specific to catecholamine-secreting paragangliomas is a life-threatening vasomotor attack.[64] If a paraganglioma of this type is discovered, α-antagonist agents should be used instead of β-antagonists, which are contraindicated.[6] Carotid sinus syndrome is another serious complication that can occur after carotid body tumor embolization.[65] In addition, embolization of a jugular paraganglioma has reportedly caused hypoglossal nerve palsy.[66] Accurate preoperative diagnosis and assessment of paragangliomas can help in preparing for and anticipating potential hemodynamic instability.

TIPS AND TRICKS

- In addition to bilateral selective catheter angiography of the external and internal carotid arteries, superselective catheterization of the external carotid branches is useful to reveal dangerous anastomoses.
- Balloon occlusion testing during catheter angiography can determine if carotid sacrifice is an option during surgical resection of some tumors.
- DPT for embolization may be the only option for vascular tumors with impossible endovascular access.
- Eighty percent reduction of tumor blush following embolization should be the minimum goal.
- Provocative testing of targeted vasculature with Amytal (grey matter) and lidocaine (white matter) can help predict cranial nerve palsy and other neurologic deficit that could be at risk during embolization. As a result, embolization under conscious sedation where neurologic examination can be performed should be considered.
- The goals of preoperative embolization should be discussed extensively with the surgeon.
- Balloon-augmented or protected embolization can help prevent complications and negate the risks associated with high-flow shunting.
- Great care should be taken in selecting the embolic agent. The experience of the operator with the agent may be the most critical factor.
- Particles should always be mixed with contrast agent to allow for visualization at the time of injection.
- Sizing of particles during particle embolization is extremely important. Small particles (45–150-μm diameter) may pose an increased risk of complications. Particle diameters ranging from 150 to 350 μm may be optimal, except in high-flow shunting where larger particles may be necessary.
- Particles should be injected with the flow of the blood and not pushed against resistance. This will help avoid traversing through dangerous anastomoses or reaching small terminal vessels that supply cranial nerves.
- If Onyx is used for embolization, the tumor surgeon should be notified that sparks can be generated with use of the Bovie monopolar cautery.
- Coils can be used to occlude a dangerous anastomotic channel, allowing preferential embolization of the target vessel without reflux into the dangerous anastomosis.
- The embolization catheter should be placed as distal as possible in the vessel feeding the tumor and must be distal to the origin of vessels that need preservation.
- Close clinical surveillance postembolization is important to rapidly identify any major procedure-related complications. Rapid identification and treatment of these types of complications can drastically improve patient outcome.

CONCLUSION

In conclusion, the outcome of preoperative embolization for vascular tumors of the head and neck depends on many factors, including the type and characteristics of the tumor, the location of the tumor, the vascular architecture of the patient, the technique implemented, the embolic material chosen, and the knowledge and experience of the operator. Careful consideration of all of these factors along with a thorough and thoughtful workup ensures the best chance of success.

REFERENCES

1. Spiotta AM, Miranpuri AS, Vargas J, et al. Balloon augmented Onyx embolization utilizing a dual lumen balloon catheter: utility in the treatment of a variety of head and neck lesions [published online ahead of print September 11, 2013]. *J Neurointerv Surg*. doi:10.1136/neurintsurg-2013-010833.
2. Jagadeesan BD, Grigoryan M, Hassan AE, et al. Endovascular balloon-assisted embolization of intracranial and cervical arteriovenous malformations using dual-lumen coaxial balloon microcatheters and Onyx: initial experience. *Neurosurgery*. 2013;73:238–243.
3. Wakhloo AK, Juengling FD, Van Velthoven V, et al. Extended preoperative polyvinyl alcohol microembolization of intracranial meningiomas: assessment of two embolization techniques. *AJNR Am J Neuroradiol*. 1993;14:571–582.
4. Bendszus M, Monoranu CM, Schütz A, et al. Neurologic complications after particle embolization of intracranial meningiomas. *AJNR Am J Neuroradiol*. 2005;26:1413–1419.
5. Carli DF, Sluzewski M, Beute GN, et al. Complications of particle embolization of meningiomas: frequency, risk factors, and outcome. *AJNR Am J Neuroradiol*. 2010;31:152–154.
6. Morris P. *Interventional and Endovascular Therapy of the Nervous System: A Practical Guide*. New York, NY: Springer-Verlag; 2002.
7. Hamada J, Ushio Y, Kazekawa K, et al. Embolization with cellulose porous beads, I: an experimental study. *AJNR Am J Neuroradiol*. 1996;17:1895–1899.
8. Kai Y, Hamada JI, Morioka M, et al. Clinical evaluation of cellulose porous beads for the therapeutic embolization of meningiomas. *AJNR Am J Neuroradiol*. 2006;27:1146–1150.
9. Bendszus M, Klein R, Burger R, et al. Efficacy of trisacryl gelatin microspheres versus polyvinyl alcohol particles in the preoperative embolization of meningiomas. *AJNR Am J Neuroradiol*. 2000;21:255–261.
10. Rutka J, Muller PJ, Chui M. Preoperative Gelfoam embolization of supratentorial meningiomas. *Can J Surg*. 1985;28:441–443.
11. Shi ZS, Feng L, Jiang XB, et al. Therapeutic embolization of meningiomas with Onyx for delayed surgical resection. *Surg Neurol*. 2008;70:478–481.
12. Kim LJ, Albuquerque FC, Aziz-Sultan A, et al. Low morbidity associated with use of n-butyl cyanoacrylate liquid adhesive for preoperative transarterial embolization of central nervous system tumors. *Neurosurgery*. 2006;59:98–104.
13. Gobin YP, Murayama Y, Milanese K, et al. Head and neck hypervascular lesions: embolization with ethylene vinyl alcohol copolymer—laboratory evaluation in Swine and clinical evaluation in humans. *Radiology*. 2001;221:309–317.

14. Gemmete JJ, Chaudhary N, Pandey A, et al. Usefulness of percutaneously injected ethylene-vinyl alcohol copolymer in conjunction with standard endovascular embolization techniques for preoperative devascularization of hypervascular head and neck tumors: technique, initial experience, and correlation with surgical observations. *AJNR Am J Neuroradiol.* 2010;31:961–966.
15. Lazzaro MA, Badruddin A, Zaidat OO, et al. Endovascular embolization of head and neck tumors. *Front Neurol.* 2011;2:64.
16. Bilbao JI, Martinez-Cuesta A, Urtasun F, et al. Complications of embolization. *Semin Intervent Radiol.* 2006;23:126–142.
17. Feng L, Kienitz BA, Matsumoto C, et al. Feasibility of using hyperosmolar mannitol as a liquid tumor embolization agent. *AJNR Am J Neuroradiol.* 2005;26:1405–1412.
18. Jungreis CA. Skull-base tumors: ethanol embolization of the cavernous carotid artery. *Radiology.* 1991;181:741–743.
19. Kubo M, Kuwayama N, Hirashima Y, et al. Hydroxyapatite ceramics as a particulate embolic material: report of the physical properties of the hydroxyapatite particles and the animal study. *AJNR Am J Neuroradiol.* 2003;24:1540–1544.
20. Kubo M, Kuwayama N, Hirashima Y, et al. Hydroxyapatite ceramics as a particulate embolic material: report of the clinical experience. *AJNR Am J Neuroradiol.* 2003;24:1545–1547.
21. Probst EN, Grzyska U, Westphal M, et al. Preoperative embolization of intracranial meningiomas with a fibrin glue preparation. *AJNR Am J Neuroradiol.* 1999;20:1695–1702.
22. Yasui K, Shoda Y, Suyama T, et al. Preoperative embolization for meningioma using lipiodol. *Interv Neuroradiol.* 1998;4(suppl 1):63–66.
23. Duffis EJ, Gandhi CD, Prestigiacomo CJ, et al. Head, neck, and brain tumor embolization guidelines. *J Neurointerv Surg.* 2012;4:251–255.
24. Geibprasert S, Pongpech S, Armstrong D, et al. Dangerous extracranial-intracranial anastomoses and supply to the cranial nerves: vessels the neurointerventionalist needs to know. *AJNR Am J Neuroradiol.* 2009;30:1459–1468.
25. Mack W, Vinuela F. Diagnostic evaluation and embolization of meningiomas. In: DeMonte F, McDermott MW, Al-Mefty O, eds. *Al-Mefty's Meningiomas.* New York, NY: Thieme Medical Publishers; 2011.
26. Chun JY, McDermott MW, Lamborn KR, et al. Delayed surgical resection reduces intraoperative blood loss for embolized meningiomas. *Neurosurgery.* 2002;50:1231–1235.
27. Kai Y, Hamada J, Morioka M, et al. Appropriate interval between embolization and surgery in patients with meningioma. *AJNR Am J Neuroradiol.* 2002;23:139–142.
28. Dowd CF, Halbach VV, Higashida RT. Meningiomas: the role of preoperative angiography and embolization. *Neurosurg Focus.* 2003;15:E10.
29. Casasco A, Houdart E, Biondi A, et al. Major complications of percutaneous embolization of skull-base tumors. *AJNR Am J Neuroradiol.* 1999;20:179–181.
30. Willing SJ. Transarterial embolization of vascular tumors in the head and neck. *Semin Interv Radiol.* 2003;20:3–12.
31. Casasco A, Herbreteau D, Houdart E, et al. Devascularization of craniofacial tumors by percutaneous tumor puncture. *AJNR Am J Neuroradiol.* 1994;15:1233–1239.
32. Nakamura M, Roser F, Michel J, et al. The natural history of incidental meningiomas. *Neurosurgery.* 2003;53:62–70.
33. Yano S, Kuratsu J; Kumamoto Brain Tumor Research Group. Indications for surgery in patients with asymptomatic meningiomas based on an extensive experience. *J Neurosurg.* 2006;105:538–543. doi:10.3171/jns.2006.105.4.538.
34. Chan RC, Thompson GB. Morbidity, mortality, and quality of life following surgery for intracranial meningiomas. A retrospective study in 257 cases. *J Neurosurg.* 1984;60:52–60.
35. Awad IA, Kalfas I, Hahn JF, et al. Intracranial meningiomas in the aged: surgical outcome in the era of computed tomography. *Neurosurgery.* 1989;24:557–560.
36. Bendszus M, Rao G, Burger R, et al. Is there a benefit of preoperative meningioma embolization? *Neurosurgery.* 2000;47:1306–1311.
37. Macpherson P. The value of pre-operative embolisation of meningioma estimated subjectively and objectively. *Neuroradiology.* 1991;33:334–337.
38. Dean BL, Flom RA, Wallace RC, et al. Efficacy of endovascular treatment of meningiomas: evaluation with matched samples. *AJNR Am J Neuroradiol.* 1994;15:1675–1680.
39. Bendszus M, Martin-Schrader I, Warmuth-Metz M, et al. MR imaging- and MR spectroscopy-revealed changes in meningiomas for which embolization was performed without subsequent surgery. *AJNR Am J Neuroradiol.* 2000;21:666–669.
40. Grand C, Bank WO, Balériaux D, et al. Gadolinium-enhanced MR in the evaluation of preoperative meningioma embolization. *AJNR Am J Neuroradiol.* 1993;14:563–569.
41. Jungling FD, Wakhloo AK, Hennig J. In vivo proton spectroscopy of meningioma after preoperative embolization. *Magn Reson Med.* 1993;30:155–160.
42. Koike T, Sasaki O, Tanaka R, et al. Long-term results in a case of meningioma treated by embolization alone—case report. *Neurol Med Chir (Tokyo).* 1990;30:173–177.
43. van den Berg R, Wasser M, van Gils A, et al. Vascularization of head and neck paragangliomas: comparison of three MR angiographic techniques with digital subtraction angiography. *AJNR Am J Neuroradiol.* 2000;21:162–170.
44. Westerband A, Hunter GC, Cintora I, et al. Current trends in the detection and management of carotid body tumors. *J Vasc Surg.* 1998;28:84–92.
45. Tikkakoski T, Luotonen J, Leinonen S, et al. Preoperative embolization in the management of neck paragangliomas. *Laryngoscope.* 1997;107:821–826.
46. Wanke I, Jäckel MC, Goericke S, et al. Percutaneous embolization of carotid paragangliomas using solely Onyx. *AJNR Am J Neuroradiol.* 2009;30:1594–1597.
47. Chaloupka JC, Mangla S, Huddle D, et al. Evolving experience with direct puncture therapeutic embolization for adjunctive and palliative management of head and neck hypervascular neoplasms. *Laryngoscope.* 1999;109:1864–1872.
48. Abud DG, Mounayer C, Benndorf G, et al. Intratumoral injection of cyanoacrylate glue in head and neck paragangliomas. *AJNR Am J Neuroradiol.* 2004;25:1457–1462.
49. Wilms G, Peene P, Baert AL, et al. Pre-operative embolization of juvenile nasopharyngeal angiofibromas. *J Belge Radiol.* 1989;72:465–470.
50. Schroth G, Haldemann AR, Mariani L, et al. Preoperative embolization of paragangliomas and angiofibromas. Measurement of intratumoral arteriovenous shunts. *Arch Otolaryngol Head Neck Surg.* 1996;122:1320–1325.

51. Roberson GH, Price AC, Davis JM, et al. Therapeutic embolization of juvenile angiofibroma. *AJR Am J Roentgenol.* 1979; 133:657–663.
52. Siniluoto TM, Luotonen JP, Tikkakoski TA, et al. Value of preoperative embolization in surgery for nasopharyngeal angiofibroma. *J Laryngol Otol.* 1993;107:514–521.
53. Krajina A, Cesak T, Zelenak K, et al. Therapeutic embolization of cranial tumors. In: Abujamra AL, ed. *Diagnostic Techniques and Surgical Management of Brain Tumors.* Rijeka, Croatia: InTech; 2011.
54. Eskridge JM, McAuliffe W, Harris B, et al. Preoperative endovascular embolization of craniospinal hemangioblastomas. *AJNR Am J Neuroradiol.* 1996;17:525–531.
55. Shigekazu T, Ruichi T, Yukihiko F, et al. Surgical treatment of hemangioblastomas with presurgical endovascular embolization. *Neurologic Med Chir (Tokyo).* 2001;41:246–252.
56. Glasker S, Van Velthoven V. Risk of hemorrhage in hemangioblastomas of the central nervous system. *Neurosurgery.* 2005;57:71–76.
57. Cornelius JF, Saint-Maurice JP, Bresson D, et al. Hemorrhage after particle embolization of hemangioblastomas: comparison of outcomes in spinal and cerebellar lesions. *J Neurosurg.* 2007;106:994–998. doi:10.3171/jns.2007.106.6.994.
58. Shah AH, Patel N, Raper DM, et al. The role of preoperative embolization for intracranial meningiomas. *J Neurosurg.* 2013;119:364–372.
59. Rosen CL. Ammerman JM, Sekhar LN, et al. Outcome analysis of preoperative embolization in cranial base surgery. *Acta Neurochir (Wien).* 2002;144:1157–1164. doi:10.1007/s00701-002-0965-y.
60. Kallmes DF, Evans AJ, Kaptain GJ, et al. Hemorrhagic complications in embolization of a meningioma: case report and review of the literature. *Neuroradiology.* 1997;39:877–880.
61. Yu SC, Boet R, Wong GK, et al. Postembolization hemorrhage of a large and necrotic meningioma. *AJNR Am J Neuroradiol.* 2004;25:506–508.
62. Barr JD, Mathis JM, Horton JA. Provocative pharmacologic testing during arterial embolization. *Neurosurg Clin N Am.* 1994;5:403–411.
63. Lv X, Li Y, Lv M, et al. Trigeminocardiac reflex in embolization of intracranial dural arteriovenous fistula. *AJNR Am J Neuroradiol.* 2007;28:1769–1770.
64. Kremer R, Michel RP, Posner B, et al. Catecholamine-secreting paraganglioma of glomus jugulare region. *Am J Med Sci.* 1989; 297:46–48.
65. Eskridge JM, Harris AB, Finch L, et al. Carotid sinus syndrome and embolization procedures. *AJNR Am J Neuroradiol.* 1993;14:818–820.
66. Maier W, Marangos N, Laszig R. Paraganglioma as a systemic syndrome: pitfalls and strategies. *J Laryngol Otol.* 1999;113: 978–982.

17

Carotid Blowout Syndrome

Daniel Do • Claudio J. Schönholz

Carotid blowout syndrome (CBS), first described in 1962, is a severe clinical condition that usually presents in the setting of patients with underlying head and neck cancer, specifically those with prior radiation treatments.[1–4] Its reported incidence is 3% to 4% in patients with neck dissection, with a 7.6-fold increased risk in the setting of additional radiation therapy.[5,6] CBS involves compromise of the carotid artery and/or its branches and can present as transoral or transcervical hemorrhage. When associated with open surgical treatment, high mortality (40%) and neurologic morbidity (60%) have been reported.[2,3] As such, multiple endovascular options have been developed and are divided into either deconstructive or reconstructive techniques. Deconstructive techniques have been described involving permanent occlusion of carotid vasculature through use of coils, liquid embolic agents, detachable balloons, and Amplatzer Vascular Plugs (St. Jude Medical, Inc., St. Paul, Minnesota).[2–5,7,8] Deconstructive techniques are typically used when the external carotid artery (ECA) is involved as neurologic sequelae would be unusual and unexpected (Fig. 17.1). In the setting of common carotid artery (CCA) or internal carotid artery (ICA) involvement, a balloon occlusion test (BOT) is typically performed for clinical assessment of adequate contralateral cerebral circulation. If the patient tolerates BOT without transitional neurologic deficit, then permanent vessel occlusion may be pursued. On the other hand, reconstructive techniques maintain vascular patency through use of covered stent. Depending on the institution, this may or may not represent first-line treatment in the setting of CBS. Generally, it is the preferred treatment option in those patients who either fail BOT, are unable to clinically undergo BOT, or demonstrate incomplete collateral circulation through the circle of Willis. CBS has been described to represent a clinical spectrum and categorized into multiple groups: threatened (group 1), sentinel hemorrhage/impending rupture (group 2), acute rupture (group 3), and recurrent CBS.[3,4] Group 1 involves patients with exposed carotid arterial segments either identified by physical examination or imaging whose natural course is likely rupture. Group 2 involves patients who have experienced a hemorrhagic event, which was either self-resolved or limited with simple surgical packing. Group 3 involves patients with active, large-volume hemorrhage that cannot be controlled with surgical packing alone. Recurrent CBS refers to the subset of patients who have undergone initial treatment and subsequently rebleed.

CLINICAL APPLICATIONS

Timing of intervention is primarily dictated by clinical presentation. By definition, threatened CBS patients are likely stable, whereas acute rupture would be actively exsanguinating, necessitating immediate intervention. In unstable patients, adequate resuscitation efforts with dedicated anesthesia monitoring and appropriate inotrope usage are necessary before intervention. If the patient is clinically stable, preprocedural cross-sectional imaging is recommended. Neck computed tomographic angiography (CTA), including the aortic arch, may be able to identify the causative lesion and assist in prediction of vessel size and tortuosity, preprocedural supplies, expedite methods of action and execution, and management. Pertinent CTA findings in CBS involve necrosis, artery exposure, viable tumor, pseudoaneurysm, and contrast extravasation.[9] If the clinical presentation precludes a CTA, the patient should be taken directly for a diagnostic arteriogram. If the CCA or ICA is found to contain the offending lesion, reconstructive therapy is preferred in cases where the patient fails BOT and if BOT or contralateral collateral examination cannot be performed secondary to

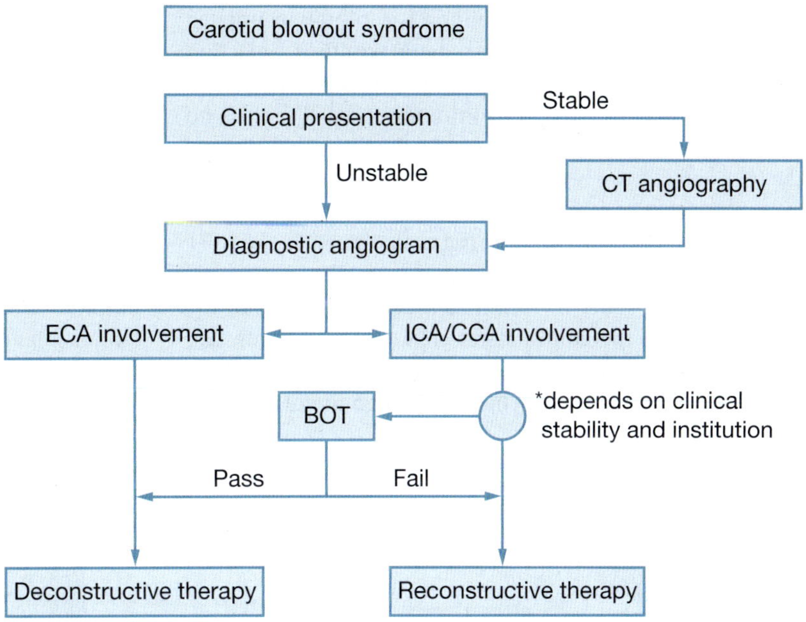

Figure 17.1 Management algorithm for CBS. CT, computed tomography; ECA, external carotid artery; ICA, internal carotid artery; CCA, common carotid artery; BOT, balloon occlusion test.

patient sedation, intubation, or fragile clinical status. Additionally, reconstructive management may be the primary treatment modality in all technically feasible cases dependent on institution given the ability to achieve hemostasis and preserve vascular patency. In cases of contralateral carotid occlusion, carotid reconstruction may be the only endovascular option. Deconstructive management is the preferred treatment option in cases involving the ECA as neurologic sequelae from permanent vessel occlusion is minimal. Regarding ICA and CCA lesions, if the patient has an uneventful BOT or angiographically demonstrates adequate contralateral collateral circulation through an intact circle of Willis, embolization may be performed. The selection of primary treatment modality is institution dependent. Deconstructive therapy may be a preferred option in the treatment of patients with preexisting carotid occlusion or when vessel tortuosity precludes adequate stent placement.

TECHNIQUE

When performing the diagnostic angiography, it is important to remember that most patients in either group 2 or 3 will likely have complex intubations or tracheostomies.[8] Performing the study under local anesthetic and moderate sedation is ideal, particularly in the setting of BOT. Typical standard femoral artery access and angiographic techniques are used. If the angiogram is the initial imaging modality, diagnostic interrogation of the entire carotid circulation is performed, which includes an aortic arch and selective bilateral common carotid and vertebral arteriograms. Identification of endoluminal irregularity, pseudoaneurysm formation, disruption, or frank extravasation within the CCA, ICA, or ECA should warrant definitive treatment. Evaluation of an intact circle of Willis and posterior collateral circulation via the vertebral arteries is mandatory if permanent CCA or ICA occlusion is considered. Additional interrogation of the subclavian artery, thyrocervical trunk, and costocervical branches should be considered in cases of lower neck hemorrhage.[8] Selection of the supra-aortic arch vessels can be performed with standard reverse curve (Simmons types 1 to 3) or angled tip catheters (Vertebral, Headhunter).

Deconstructive endovascular techniques involve the use of permanent arterial occlusion through coils, liquid embolic agents, and Amplatzer Vascular Plugs. Detachable balloons were previously used but are no longer available in North America. Embolization of the ECA is typically achieved through use of coils and/or liquid embolic agents. If used in conjunction, primary placement of coils followed by liquid embolic introduction is preferred for formation of a matrix.[8] Coverage distal and proximal to the hemorrhagic lesion is crucial in achieving hemostasis, eliminating the possibility of continued filling via collateralization. Particles can be used to achieve small vessel occlusion in distal ECA branches. Embolization of the ECA and the selection of the embolic agent should be done knowing that there are multiple collateral circulation pathways between branches of the ECA and ICA that could be the source of nontarget embolization leading to stroke complications.

If embolization of the CCA or ICA is considered, a BOT is performed to demonstrate patient's tolerance without increased neurologic sequelae. BOT is only used in a stable, cooperative patient. Following a baseline neurologic examination, a microcatheter with distal nondetachable Hyperform balloon (Covidien, Irvine, California) is placed proximally within the culprit vessel. After adequate systemic heparinization, the balloon is carefully insufflated with occlusion confirmed with hand contrast injection through the catheter. Continuous neurologic monitoring is then performed for a 15- to 20-minute period. If there is no change from the patient's neurologic baseline, occlusion of the ICA or CCA can be considered. If new neurologic symptoms are experienced, the balloon should immediately be deflated to prevent permanent ischemic injury. If the BOT cannot be performed due to patient instability or intubation and reconstructive techniques are unachievable, the examination of the contralateral collateral circulation can be performed during balloon insufflation for evaluation. The ICA occlusion can be achieved through use of coils and self-expandable occlusion devices. Optimally, embolization would begin intracranially, specifically at the level of the petrous or cavernous ICA segment. This reduces potential thromboembolic phenomenon often associated with proximal embolization caused by residual large-volume blood stagnation. Sparing of the ophthalmic segment is beneficial, allowing for reversed collateral supply into the remainder of the intracranial ICA.[8]

Endovascular reconstruction of the carotid artery employs use of covered stent placed across the offending lesion, achieving both hemostasis and preservation of blood flow (Fig. 17.2). However, as covered stents are known to serve as a thrombogenic nidus, an antiplatelet regimen

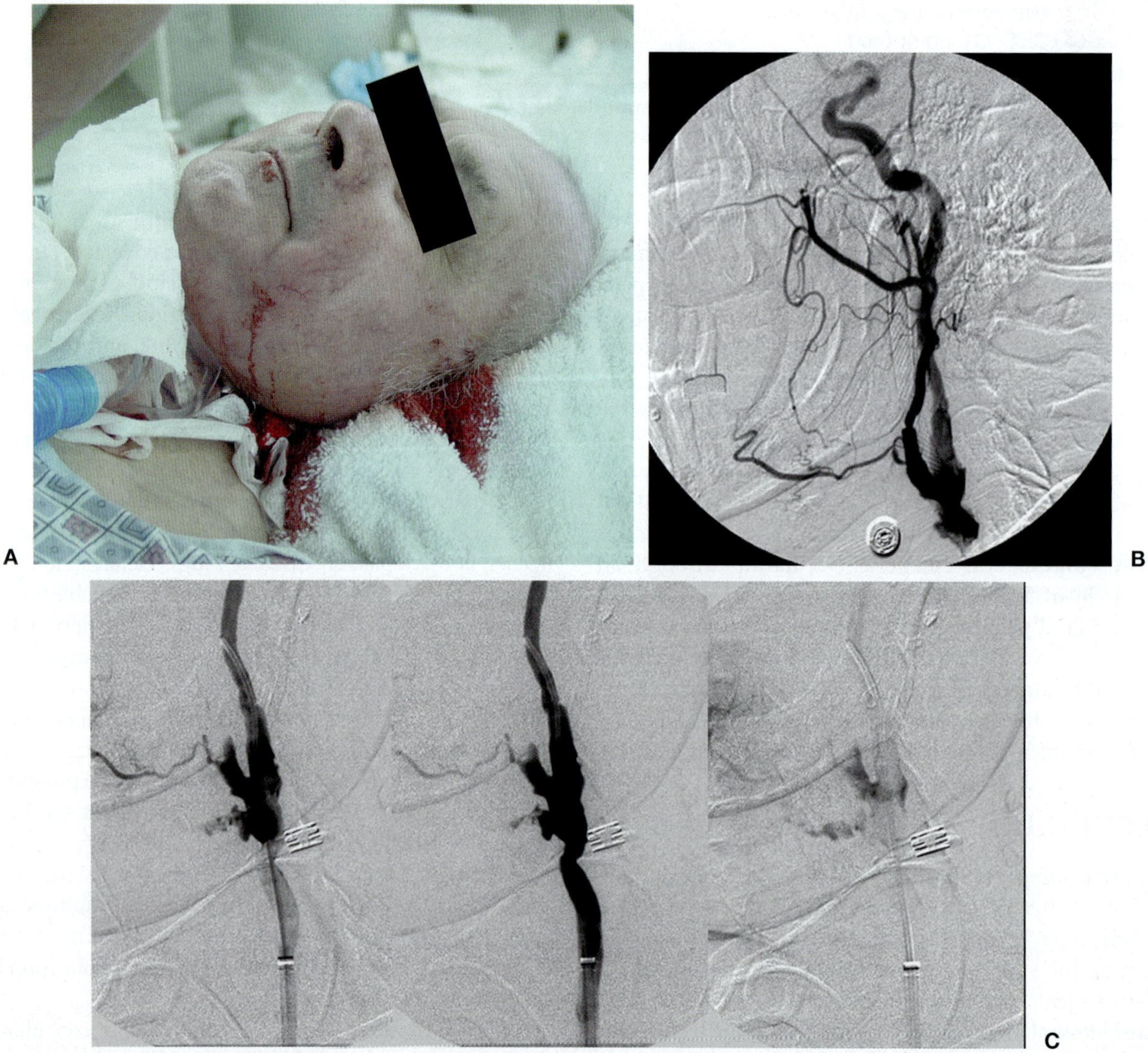

Figure 17.2 A 68-year-old man with squamous cell carcinoma of the neck treated with prior radiation, carotid endarterectomy, and right carotid stent placement presented with transoral and tracheostomy hemorrhage. **A:** Image of the patient at presentation. **B:** Left carotid angiogram demonstrating irregularity and pseudoaneurysm formation involving the distal CCA. **C:** Selective arteriogram of the left CCA demonstrating active arterial extravasation from the pseudoaneurysm. *(Continued)*

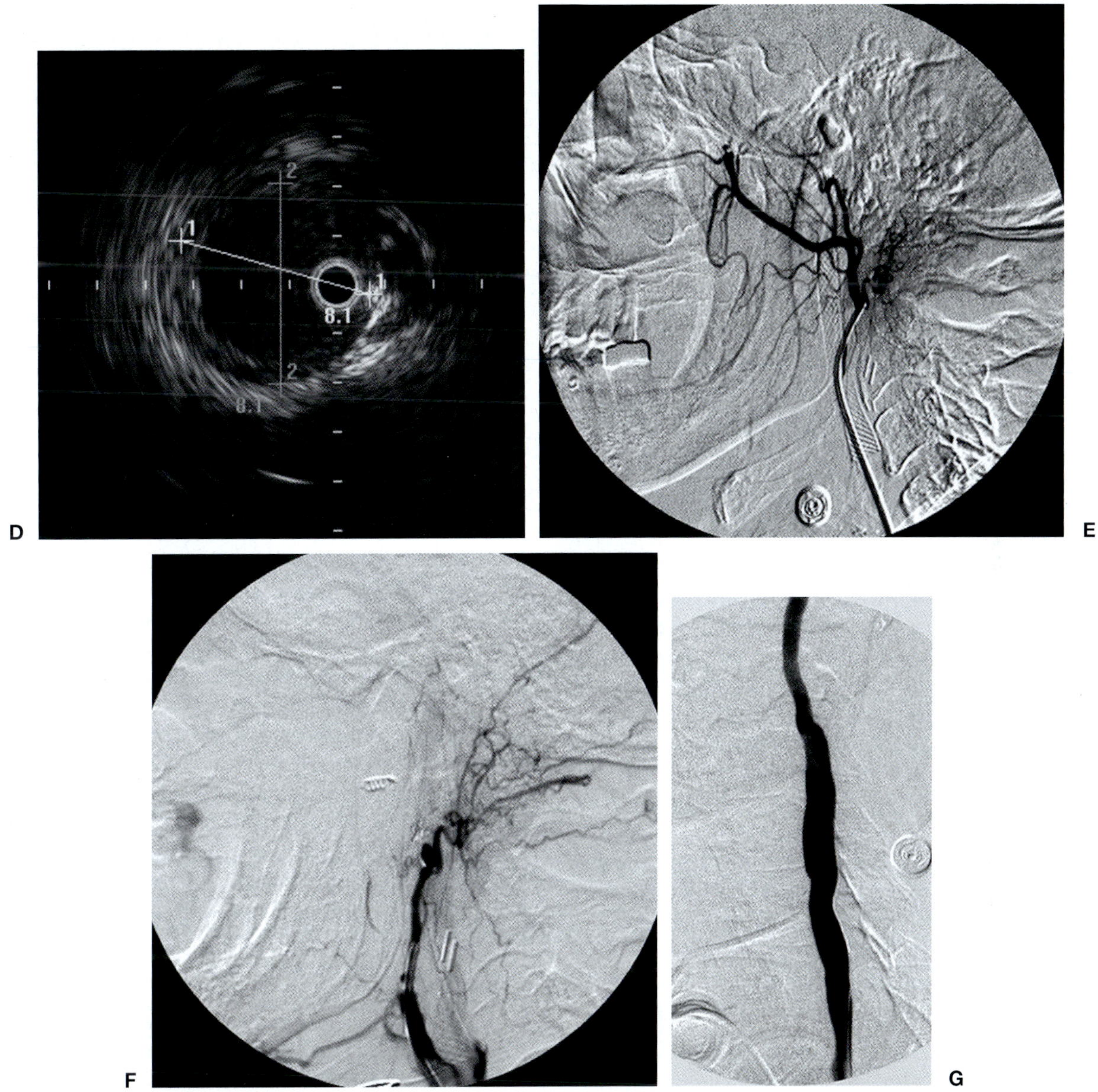

Figure 17.2 *(Continued)* **D:** Intravascular ultrasound of the CCA demonstrating size and extent of the pseudoaneurysm. **E,F:** Coil embolization of the ECA in preparation for stent graft placement. **G:** Completion angiogram demonstrating hemostasis and exclusion of the carotid pseudoaneurysm with use of an 8 mm × 5 cm Viabahn (W. L. Gore & Associates, Flagstaff, Arizona) stent graft.

with acetylsalicylic acid or clopidogrel should be incorporated.[10,11] Varying treatment patterns have been reported but commonly involve preprocedural antiplatelet administration and intraprocedural systemic heparinization, with the goal of having the activated clotting time two to three times the baseline. Again, antiplatelet regimen ad infinitum should follow the stent graft placement.[8,10,12–18] Additional use of intravenous glycoprotein IIb/IIIa inhibitors in conjunction with heparin has also been described, especially in cases where preprocedural antiplatelet treatment is not feasible.[13] If the anticipated stent placement crosses the carotid bifurcation, embolization of the ECA is recommended to prevent rebleeding through collateral filling. Due to the natural anatomic configuration of the carotid bulb, type I endoleaks may be encountered, producing a potential source for persistent or recurrent hemorrhage. Maldonado et al.[19] and Chen et al.[20] described the use of *N*-butyl cyanoacrylate (NBCA) to assist in sealing the endoleak. This is achieved through use of an additional access with placement of a microcatheter across the lesion before stent deployment. Following stent deployment, the microcatheter is positioned with NBCA administered in appropriate placement. Immediate microcatheter withdrawal is followed upon completion of injection. Embolization with liquid embolic agents like cyanoacrylate and Onyx (Covidien, Irvine, California) should be reserved for interventionists with extensive experience using these embolic agents. Additionally, broader stent graft coverage of the lesion has been suggested given natural disease progression in possible prevention of rebleeding complications.[21]

COMPLICATIONS

The results and complications involving the endovascular treatment of CBS have varied in the literature. Overall technical success rates with immediate hemostatic control have been reported to be very high. Zussman et al.[22] published a review of endovascular deconstructive management and showed that immediate hemostasis was achieved in 100% of the patients. Rebleeding rates for deconstructive management ranged from 13% to 27%. The overall pooled complication rate was reported as 12%, identified as significant unintentional morbidity unrelated to the primary disease process.[22] Delayed transient ischemia with neurologic sequelae related to the permanent vessel occlusion has been reported in 15% to 20% of cases with an immediate 0.4% occurrence of stroke.[3,14] Additionally, rates of complications associated with BOT have been reported as high as 3.2%, with potential cause of symptomatic vascular injury in underlying diseased vasculature.[2,3,17,23,24] Reported incidences of rebleeding involving reconstructive management are inconsistent with reports ranging from low, equal, to frequent rates of CBS recurrence when compared to deconstructive management.[10,14,15,22,25] Additional complications to varying degrees have been reported involving acute thromboembolism, delayed carotid stent occlusion, stent extrusion, and brain abscess formation.[10,12,21,22,24,26]

TIPS AND TRICKS

Reconstructive Therapy

- Preprocedural neck CTA (extending to the aortic arch) can help in identifying the culprit lesion, vessel tortuosity, and preexisting ipsilateral and contralateral occlusions, in addition to planning stent sizing.
- When placing a covered stent across the bifurcation, embolization of the ECA before stent deployment reduces risks of repeated/continued hemorrhage from collateral filling.
- Endoleaks are often encountered involving stent placement along the carotid bulb due to its anatomical curvature. Planned use of NBCA from a second access could be considered in these cases.
- Given the increased incidence of recurrent hemorrhages, consider closer imaging follow-up, aggressive reintervention, and broader stent graft coverage on initial placement.
- In cases with wound exposure, prophylactic and therapeutic antibiotics are suggested to decrease the risk of infection.
- As the patient's clinical condition allows, an antiplatelet regimen is recommended before and after covered stent placement due to the associated risk of thromboembolic phenomenon.

Deconstructive Therapy

- Preprocedural imaging can help define anatomy, identify the causative source, and assist in overall procedure planning.
- When embolizing the ECA and its branches, primary placement of coils followed by liquid embolic agents provide an effective combination to achieve hemostasis.
- Embolization should always be performed distal and proximal to exclude potential collateral filling.
- BOT or angiographic evaluation of adequate contralateral cerebral collateralization is crucial before ICA or CCA embolization to assess the risk of permanent neurologic sequelae.
- In cases of permanent ICA occlusion, embolization should begin at the petrous or cavernous segment if possible. This reduces potential dead space (with the potential formation of a column of clot above the occlusion site) and allows for the ophthalmic artery to fill the remainder of the ICA in a retrograde fashion.

General

- Many times, the patient will present with complicated airway management given the nature of the disease. Adequate resuscitation with appropriate inotrope usage is critical to help maintain cerebral perfusion in the setting of deconstructive therapy of the CCA/ICA.

REFERENCES

1. Borsany SJ. Rupture of the carotids following radical neck surgery in irradiated patients. *Eye Ear Nose Throat Mon.* 1962;41: 531–533.
2. Citardi MJ, Chaloupka JC, Son YH, et al. Management of carotid artery rupture by monitored endovascular therapeutic occlusion (1988–1994). *Laryngoscope.* 1995;1086–1092.
3. Chaloupka JC, Putman CM, Citardi MJ, et al. Endovascular therapy of carotid blowout syndrome in head and neck surgical patients: evolving diagnostic and management considerations. *AJNR Am J Neuroradiol.* 1996;17:843–852.

4. Chaloupka JC, Roth TC, Putman CM, et al. Recurrent carotid blowout syndrome: diagnostic and therapeutic challenges in a newly recognized subgroup of patients. *AJNR Am J Neuroradiol.* 1999;20:1069–1077.
5. Morrissey DD, Andersen PE, Nesbit GM, et al. Endovascular management of hemorrhage in patients with head and neck cancer. *Arch Otolaryngol Head Neck Surg.* 1997;123:15–19.
6. Maran AGD, Amin M, Wilson JA. Radical neck dissection: a 19-year experience. *J Laryngol Otol.* 1989;103:760–764.
7. Shankar JJ, Maloney WJ, Vandorpe R. Amplatzer vascular plug for occlusion of parent artery in carotid blowout with active extravasation. *Interv Neuroradiol.* 2011;17(2):224–227.
8. Patsalides A, Fraser JF, Smith MJ, et al. Endovascular treatment of carotid blowout syndrome: who and how to treat. *J Neurointerv Surg.* 2010;2(1):87–93.
9. Lee CW, Yang CY, Chen YF, et al. CT angiography findings in carotid blowout syndrome and its role as a predictor of 1-year survival. *AJNR Am J Neuroradiol.* 2014;35:562–567.
10. Chang FC, Lirng JF, Luo CB, et al. Carotid blowout syndrome in patients with head-and-neck cancers: reconstructive management by self-expandable stent-grafts. *Am J Neuroradiol.* 2007;28:181–188.
11. Sovik E, Klow NE, Brekke M, et al. Elective placement of covered stents in native coronary arteries. *Acta Radiol.* 2003; 44:294–301.
12. Chang FC, Luo CB, Lirng JF, et al. Complications of carotid blowout syndrome in patients with head and neck cancers treated by covered stents. *Interv Neuroradiol.* 2008;14(suppl 2): 29–33.
13. Chang FC, Lirng JF, Luo CB, et al. Patients with head and neck cancers and associated postirradiated carotid blowout syndrome: endovascular therapeutic methods and outcomes. *J Vasc Surg.* 2008;47(5):936–945.
14. Lesley WS, Chaloupka JC, Weigele JB, et al. Preliminary experience with endovascular reconstruction for the management of carotid blowout syndrome. *AJNR Am J Neuroradiol.* 2003;24(5):975–981.
15. Pyun HW, Lee DH, Yoo HM, et al. Placement of covered stents for carotid blowout in patients with head and neck cancer: follow-up results after rescue treatments. *AJNR Am J Neuroradiol.* 2007;28(8):1594–1598.
16. Zhao LB, Shi HB, Park S, et al. Acute bleeding in the head and neck: angiographic findings and endovascular management. *AJNR Am J Neuroradiol.* 2014;35:360–366.
17. Miller T, Burns J, Farinhas J, et al. Covered stents safely utilized to prevent catastrophic hemorrhage in patients with advanced head and neck malignancy. *J Neurointerv Surg.* 2012;4(6): 426–434.
18. Koutsimpelas D, Pitton M, Külkens C, et al. Endovascular carotid reconstruction in palliative head and neck cancer patients with threatened carotid blowout presents a beneficial supportive care measure. *J Palliat Med.* 2008;11(5):784–789.
19. Maldonado TS, Rosen RJ, Rockman CB, et al. Initial successful management of type I endoleak after endovascular aortic aneurysm repair with n-butyl cyanoacrylate adhesive. *J Vasc Surg.* 2003;38:664–670.
20. Chen YL, Wong HF, Ku YK, et al. Endovascular covered stent reconstruction improved the outcomes of acute carotid blowout syndrome. Experiences at a single institute. *Interv Neuroradiol.* 2008;14(suppl 2):23–27.
21. Sorial E, Valentino J, Given CA, et al. The emergency use of endografts in the carotid circulation to control hemorrhage in potentially contaminated fields. *J Vasc Surg.* 2007;46(4):792–798.
22. Zussman B, Gonzalez LF, Dumont A, et al. Endovascular management of carotid blowout. *World Neurosurg.* 2012;78-(1–2):109–114.
23. Mathis JM, Barr JD, Jungreis CA, et al. Temporary balloon test occlusion of the internal carotid artery: experience in 500 cases. *AJNR Am J Neuroradiol.* 1995;16:749–754.
24. Warren FM, Cohen JI, Nesbit GM, et al. Management of carotid "blowout" with endovascular stent grafts (case reports). *Laryngoscope.* 2002;112:428–433.
25. Hoppe H, Barnwell SL, Nesbit GM, et al. Stent-grafts in the treatment of emergent or urgent carotid artery disease: review of 25 cases. *J Vasc Interv Radiol.* 2008;19:31–41.
26. Wan WS, Lai V, Lau HY, et al. Endovascular treatment paradigm of carotid blowout syndrome: review of 8-years experience. *Eur J Radiol.* 2013;82(1):95–99.

18

Hemoptysis

Miguel A. De Gregorio • Alicia Laborda

Massive hemoptysis, also known as *life-threatening hemoptysis,* is a serious, critical condition that necessitates urgent assessment and treatment of the patient. Despite advances in the treatment of massive hemoptysis, it still imposes a high-risk condition. According to published data, in any given year, 28% of pulmonologists witness a case of death due to massive hemoptysis.[1]

The lungs receive blood from the pulmonary artery and bronchial systems under normal conditions. In pathologic situations, systemic arteries can penetrate into the lung and irrigate contained injuries. The low-pressure pulmonary system tends to produce small-volume hemoptysis, whereas bleeding from the bronchial system, which shares systemic pressure, tends to be profuse.[2]

Conservative medical treatment of patients with expectoration of 300 to 600 mL of blood per day is associated with mortality in 50% to 100% of the patients affected,[3] with asphyxia rather than hemorrhage commonly being the cause of death.[4] Although surgical treatment of massive hemoptysis is associated with mortality rates between 7.1% and 18.2%, it can reach up to 40% when surgery is performed urgently.[5]

Since embolization of the bronchial artery was first described by Remy et al.[6] in 1973, it has become the main option for the treatment of massive hemoptysis, either at first presentation or in case of recurrence. Various studies have demonstrated its effectiveness, safety, and usefulness.[7–15] However, surgery plays an important role in the treatment of massive hemoptysis caused by certain diseases, such as pulmonary hydatidosis, bronchial adenoma, and aspergilloma that is refractory to other treatments.[16] In such cases, prior urgent bronchial artery embolization facilitates surgical treatment and improves results because it allows scheduled rather than urgent surgery to be undertaken.[5] Surgery also represents the treatment of choice when bronchial artery embolization fails repeatedly or is insufficient to control massive life-threatening hemorrhage.[17]

Currently, when embolization of the bronchial artery fails, the use of endoscopically implanted thrombin preparations has been proposed on the basis of its high success rate.[18]

CLINICAL BACKGROUND AND PHYSICAL EXAMINATION

Most hemoptysis are generally small, do not require urgent action, and can be treated medically. It is crucial to differentiate hematemesis from hemoptysis. Before assuming a lower respiratory source of the bleeding, it is important to consider whether the blood may be coming from a nonpulmonary source, such as the upper airway or the gastrointestinal tract. Alkaline pH, foaminess, or the presence of pus may sometimes suggest the lungs as the primary source of bleeding rather than the stomach.

Other data such as age, nutritional status, and comorbidities may assist to the diagnosis and management of hemoptysis.

Epistaxis or expectoration without cough suggests that the source of bleeding is in the upper respiratory tract, whereas expectoration accompanied by cough indicates bleeding from the lower bronchial tree.[19]

It is difficult to quantify the amount of blood expectorated. In general, patients tend to overestimate, and besides, it is difficult to quantify the amount of blood retained in the alveolar space and the bronchial tree.

Clinical symptoms depend on several factors such as the underlying disease and causes of hemoptysis and the importance and amount of bleeding. Fever, hypoxia, tachycardia, and tachypnea are going to be the most important symptoms that may accompany a hemoptysis. The final cause of death in hemoptysis is not hypovolemia due to blood loss but asphyxiation by drowning.

ETIOLOGY

There are many causes of hemoptysis. Their frequency has varied with time. In the past, lung tuberculosis was the first and main cause, but the main cause nowadays is bronchiectasis. Salajka[20] has summarized the main hemoptysis causes in the acronym *BATTLE CAMP* (Table 18.1).

Hemoptysis, which can be life threatening, complicates the course of 50% to 85% of patients with an aspergilloma.[21] Tuberculosis can cause massive hemoptysis through multiple mechanisms: active cavitary or noncavitary lung disease can cause small or large amounts of bleeding. Active disease can cause sudden rupture of a Rasmussen aneurysm (aneurysm of the pulmonary artery that slowly expands into an adjacent cavity because of inflammatory erosion of the external vessel wall until it bursts).[21]

Many inflammatory or immune disorders can produce hemoptysis, such as Goodpasture syndrome, idiopathic pulmonary hemosiderosis, lupus pneumonitis, and Wegener granulomatosis. Other clinical situations can also explain a hemoptysis: coagulopathy, thrombocytopenia, or use of anticoagulants.

Iatrogenic etiology, especially due to either percutaneous or transbronchial lung biopsy, is a cause of hemoptysis, which is usually minor and transient and occurs in 5% to 10% of percutaneous lung biopsies, but massive hemorrhage and death have also been reported. Hemoptysis has been described in 6% of habitual smokers of free-base cocaine ("crack") and has been associated with diffuse alveolar hemorrhage.

When hemoptysis is recurrent and coincident with menstruation, it can be caused by intrathoracic endometriosis, usually involving the pulmonary parenchyma but occasionally affecting the airways.[21]

As it has already been commented previously, blood can come from the pulmonary artery. The main causes of pulmonary origin are as follows: pulmonary embolism; pulmonary arteriovenous malformation, either with or without underlying Rendu-Osler-Weber syndrome; and elevated pulmonary capillary pressure (mitral stenosis, significant left ventricular failure, congenital heart disease, severe pulmonary hypertension). Pulmonary artery perforation from a Swan-Ganz catheter can also produce hemoptysis.

Depending on the study, up to 30% of patients with hemoptysis have no cause identified even after careful evaluation. In a series of 67 patients with cryptogenic hemoptysis, prognosis was generally good, and most patients had resolution of bleeding within 6 months of evaluation.[22]

In our series[23] of 314 patients, the most frequent causes of massive hemoptysis were bronchiectasis (31.5%), followed by acute tuberculosis or scar tissue caused by tuberculosis (18.1%) and chronic bronchitis (14.9%). Other causes are shown in Table 18.2.

Table 18.1 Main Causes of Hemoptysis: BATTLE CAMP

Broncholitis	Coagulopathy
Bronchiectasis	Autoimmune disease
Aspergilloma	AV malformations
Tumor	Alveolar hemorrhage
Tuberculosis	Mitral stenosis
Lung abscess	Pneumonia
Emboli	

AV, arteriovenous.

Table 18.2 Causes of Massive Hemoptysis in 314 Patients

Causes	#	%
Bronchiectasis	99	31.52
Acute or residual tuberculosis	57	18.15
Chronic bronchitis	47	14.96
Suppurative processes	23	7.32
Lung carcinoma	12	3.82
Aspergillosis	9	2.86
Other cancers (pulmonary sarcoma, oncocytoma, metastasis)	8	2.54
Cyst fibrosis	8	2.54
Chronic pleural inflammation	6	1.91
Hydatid cyst	6	1.91
Pulmonary fibrosis	5	1.59
Pneumoconiosis	4	1.27
Pulmonary vasculature malformation	4	1.27
Behçet disease	3	0.95
Lung biopsy	3	0.95
Tracheal intubation	3	0.95
Ruptured aortic aneurysm	2	0.63
Bronchopulmonary sequestration	2	0.63
Rasmussen aneurysm	1	0.31
Swan-Ganz catheter manipulation	1	0.31
Aortobronchial fistula	1	0.31
Surgical revascularization of left coronary artery	1	0.31
Unknown	9	3.7

From de Gregorio MA, Medrano J, Mainar A, et al. Endovascular treatment of massive hemoptysis by bronchial artery embolization: short-term and long-term follow-up over a 15-year period. *Arch Bronconeumol*. 2006;42(2):49–56.

Multislice computed tomography (CT) represents the technique of choice for the etiologic diagnosis of nonmassive hemoptysis. Together with fiber bronchoscopy, they can settle down a very high percentage of the most important and severe causes of hemoptysis. Nevertheless, the use of the CT and the fiber bronchoscopy is discussed in acute massive hemoptysis, where arteriography can establish the diagnosis with good precision and, at the same time, contribute to its treatment.

BRONCHIAL ANATOMY

Bronchial arteries provide oxygen and nutritional elements to different pulmonary structures and also some adjacent mediastinal structures. They supply the trachea, bronchi, visceral pleura, and esophagus and the vasa vasorum of the aorta, pulmonary artery, and vein.[24]

Although there are many variations, there are usually two bronchial arteries that run in the right lung and one in the left lung. Bronchial arteries originally measure about 1 to 1.5 mm diameter. Above this diameter, they must be considered pathologic.[25] The most common source of hemoptysis is located in the bronchial arteries (90%), and only in 5% of cases the pulmonary circulation is the origin of the bleeding.[26]

The remaining 5% of pulmonary bleeding originates directly from the aorta or systemic intrathoracic or extrathoracic branches.[27–29] In over 70% of the general population, the bronchial arteries arise directly from the descending thoracic aorta, most commonly between the levels of T5 and T6.[30] When the bronchial arteries arise at these levels, they are called *orthotopic*, and when the source is outside these levels, their name is *ectopic* (8% to 35%). These ectopic bronchial arteries may originate from the aortic arch, brachiocephalic artery, subclavian artery, internal mammary artery, thyrocervical trunk, coronary arteries, costocervical trunk, pericardiacophrenic artery, inferior phrenic artery, or abdominal aorta[31] (Fig. 18.1).

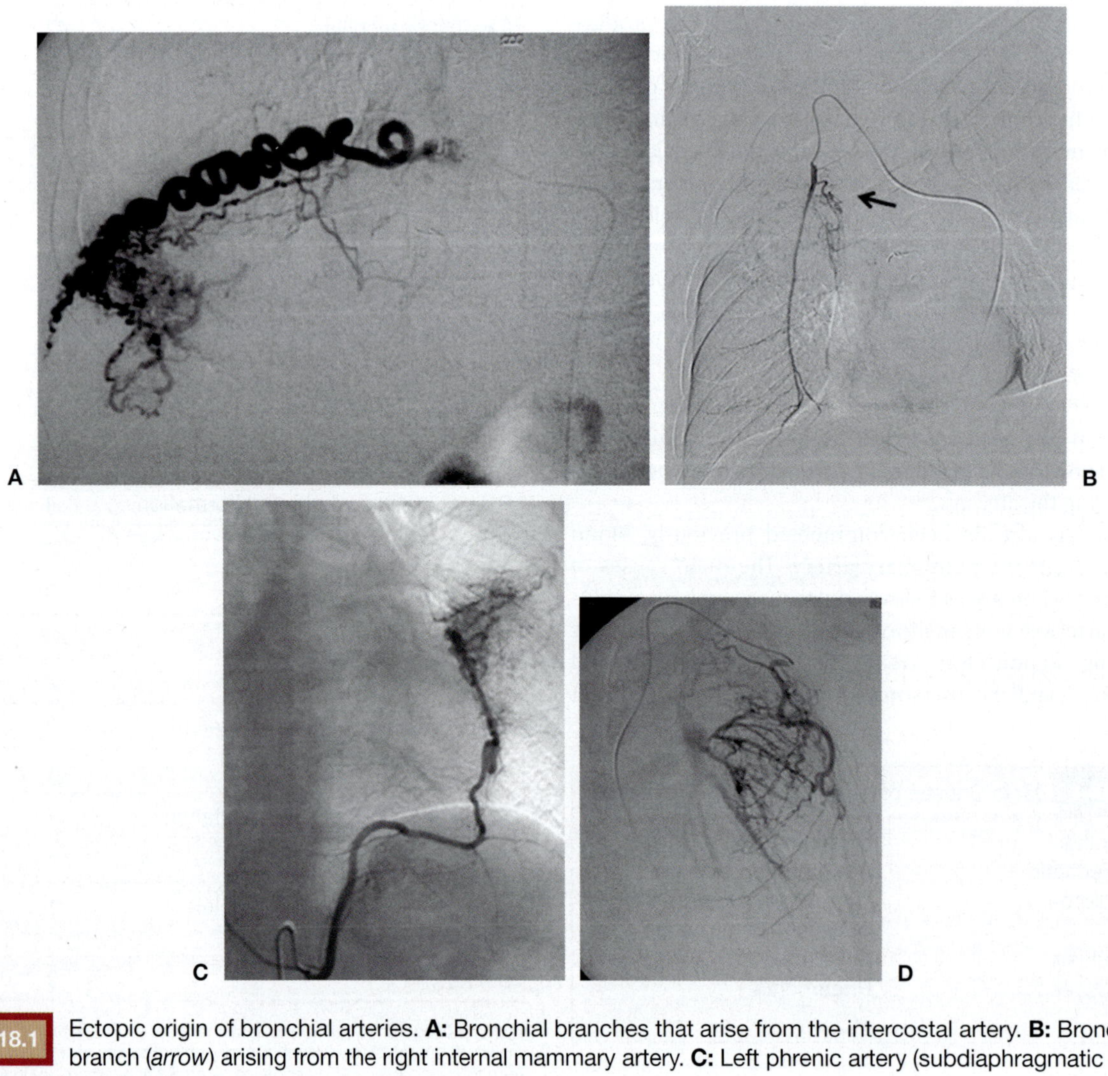

Figure 18.1 Ectopic origin of bronchial arteries. **A:** Bronchial branches that arise from the intercostal artery. **B:** Bronchial branch (*arrow*) arising from the right internal mammary artery. **C:** Left phrenic artery (subdiaphragmatic origin). **D:** Left lateral thoracic artery.

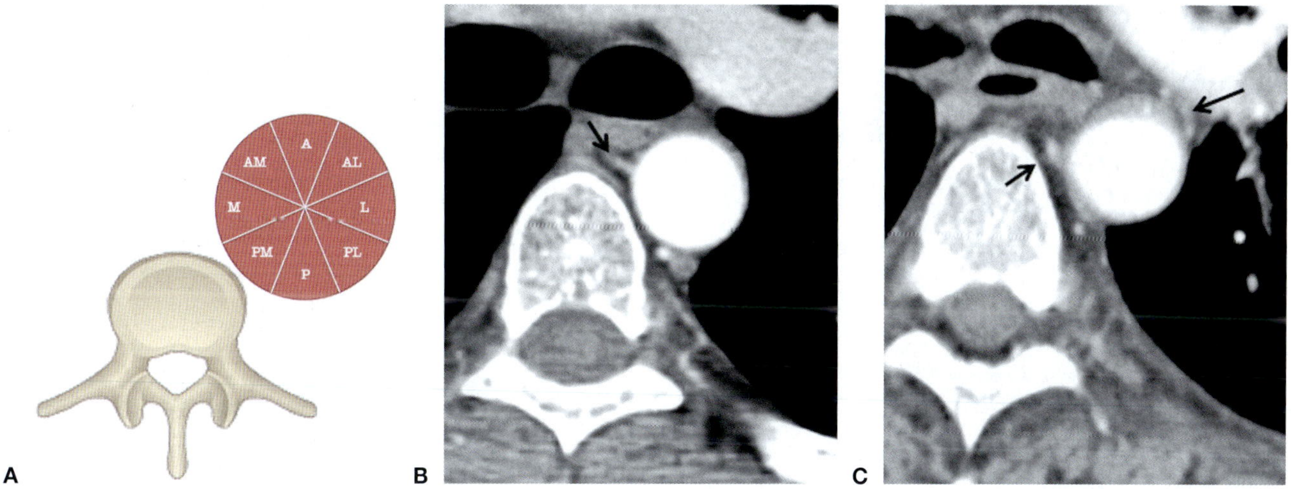

Figure 18.2 Anatomical origin of the bronchial arteries. **A:** Anatomical scheme. **B:** Right intercostobronchial artery usually arises from M or AM segment (*arrow*). **C:** Bronchial common trunk usually arises from AL segment (*arrows*). A, anterior; AL, anterolateral; L, lateral; PL, posterolateral; P, posterior; PM, posteromedial; M, medial; AM, anteromedial.

According to the classification of Morita et al.,[32] the main right bronchial artery arises from the intercostobronchial trunk in more than 50% of the cases, and in the rest, it comes from a common trunk (right and left bronchial arteries) from the subclavian artery or directly from the aorta. Left bronchial artery, on the other hand, arises from a bronchial common trunk (right-left) in over 95% of the cases. Referencing the axial division of the aorta into eight segments, the right intercostobronchial artery ostium is usually located in the medial segment or anteromedial, whereas the origin of the bronchial common trunk (right-left) arises from the anterolateral segment (>70%)[33] (Fig. 18.2).

Cauldwell et al.[34] reported four classic bronchial artery branching patterns: type I, one intercostobronchial trunk on the right and two bronchial arteries on the left (40%); type II, one intercostobronchial trunk on the right and one on the left (21%); type III, two branches on the right (one intercostobronchial trunk and one bronchial artery) and two bronchial arteries on the left (20%); and type IV, two on the right (one intercostobronchial trunk and one bronchial artery) and one bronchial artery on the left (9.7%) (Fig. 18.3).

The right intercostobronchial trunk is the most consistently seen vessel at angiography (80% of individuals) (Fig. 18.4). It usually arises from the right posterolateral aspect of the thoracic aorta, whereas the normal right and left bronchial arteries arise from the anterolateral aspect of the aorta. Right and left bronchial arteries that arise from the aorta as a common trunk are not uncommon at angiography (Fig. 18.5). The true prevalence of a common bronchial artery trunk is unknown.

Of particular relevance is the anatomy of the nearby spinal arteries. During bronchial angiography, we can

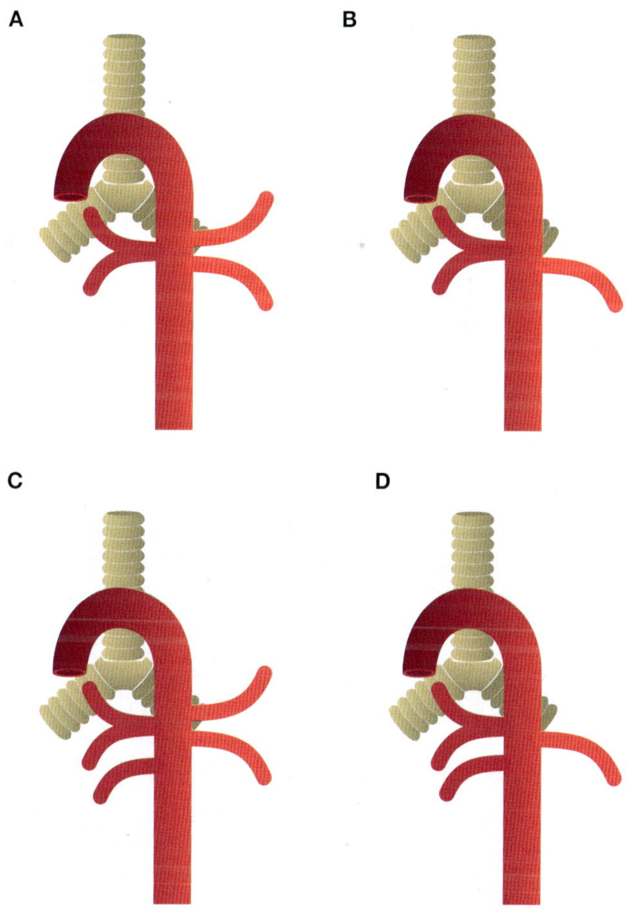

Figure 18.3 Anatomical origin of the bronchial arteries. (Modified from Cauldwell EW, Siekert RG, Lininger RE, et al. The bronchial arteries: an anatomic study of 105 human cadavers. *Surg Gynecol Obstet*. 1948;86:395–412.)

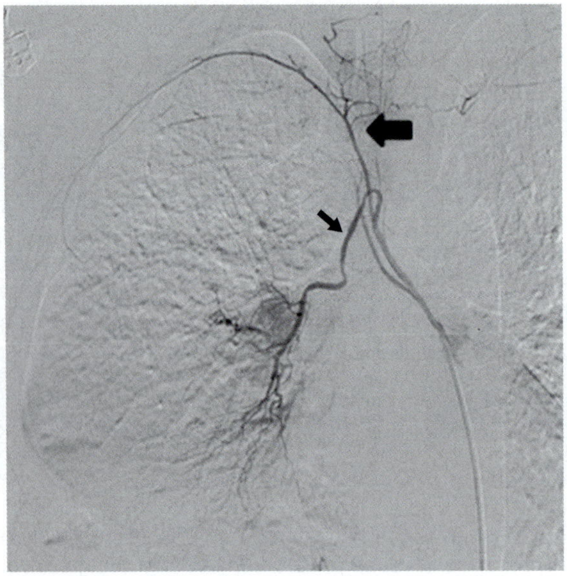

Figure 18.4 Right intercostobronchial trunk. *Arrows* point to bronchial artery (*small arrow*) and intercostal artery (*large arrow*).

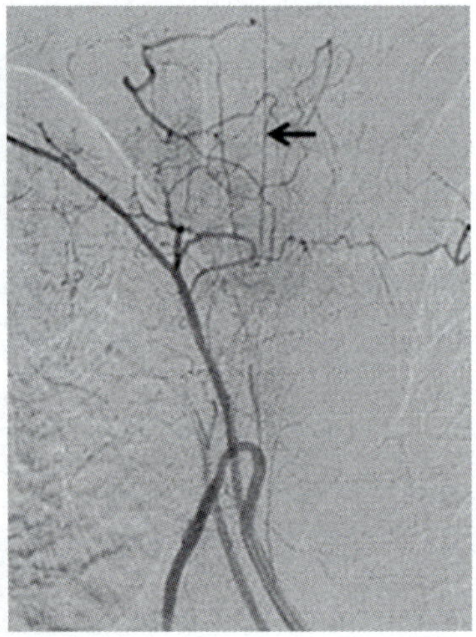

Figure 18.6 Right intercostobronchial artery. A small straight descendent branch can be observed (*arrow*), which is the medullary artery.

observe two types of spinal arteries that must always be avoided: the dorsal and ventral radicular arteries, which supply the dorsal and ventral nerve root and which emerge from the intercostal arteries, and the anterior medullary arteries. An average of eight arteries supply the spinal cord from its anterior side. In 5% to 10% of cases, they can be observed during bronchial angiography, usually arising from the intercostal artery of the right intercostobronchial trunk. Adamkiewicz artery or great anterior radiculomedullary artery is the most important artery in terms of medullary irrigation. This artery arises from the left side of the aorta, from T9 to L1, in 75% of cases. Anterior medullary arteries have a characteristic "hairpin" configuration at angiography[35] (Fig. 18.6).

Often, spinal arteries cannot be observed initially in the angiography. They only become visible when the distal vessels are embolized, as recalled by Brown and Ray[36] (Fig. 18.7).

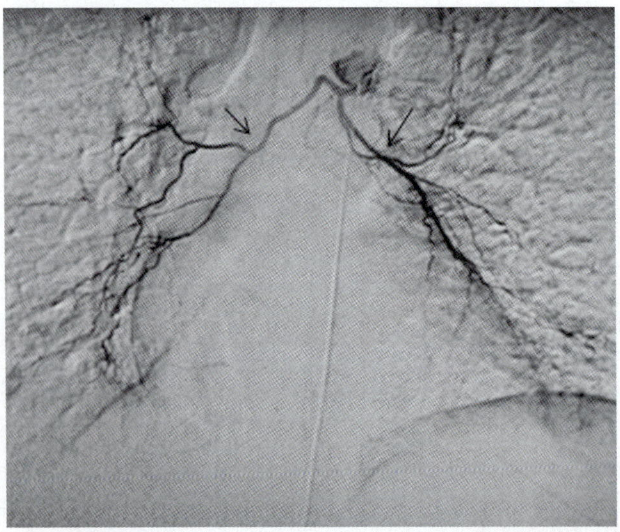

Figure 18.5 Right and left bronchial arteries common trunk (*arrows*).

WORKUP

Initial priorities are ensuring adequate airway protection, ventilation, and cardiovascular function. Patients with poor gas exchange, rapid ongoing hemoptysis, hemodynamic instability, or severe shortness of breath should be orally intubated with a large-bore endotracheal tube (size 8.0 or greater).[15,17] Coagulation disorders should be rapidly reversed.

If the location or site of bleeding is known, placing the bleeding lung in a dependent position may prevent blood spillage into the nonbleeding lung. An alternative strategy involves placement of a typical, single lumen endotracheal tube into either the right or the left mainstem bronchus. The approach of selective intubation is less practical when the right lung is bleeding because selective intubation of the left mainstem bronchus may be difficult. A third alternative is the placement of a double lumen endotracheal tube specially designed for selective intubation of the right or left mainstem bronchi.[21,37]

The evaluation should begin with the initial history and physical examination supplemented by chest radiograph.

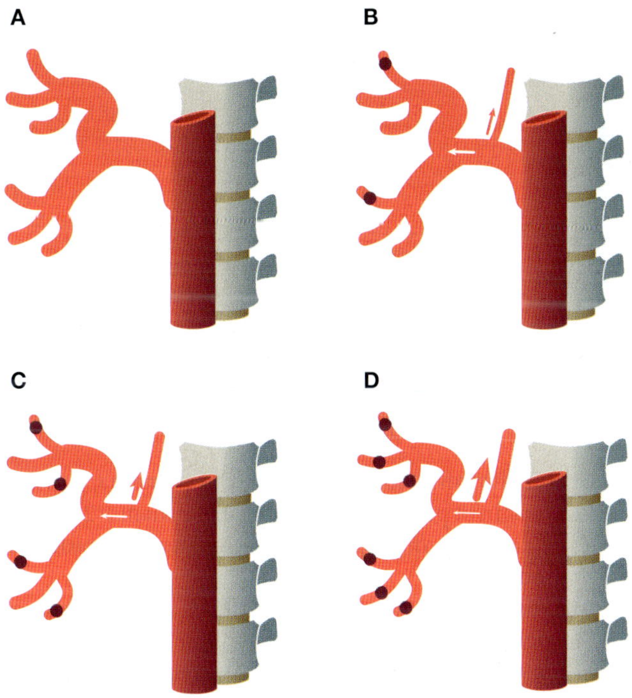

Figure 18.7 **A:** Angiography scheme previous to embolization. No spinal arteries are observed. **B–D:** When distal branches are embolized, a spinal artery becomes visible. (Modified from Brown AC, Ray CHE. Anterior spinal cord infarction following bronchial artery embolization. *Semin Intervent Radiol*. 2012; 29:241–244.)

Important features of the history include age, smoking history, duration of hemoptysis, and association with symptoms of acute bronchitis or an acute exacerbation of chronic bronchitis.[21]

Vital signs including pulse oximetry levels and blood gases, temperature, heart rate, and breathing should be recorded and fever, tachycardia, tachypnea, and hypoxia corrected.

In a survey of respiratory physicians during the 1998 American College of Chest Physicians (ACCP) Annual International Scientific Assembly, more than 50% of these clinicians favored the use of interventional angiography even in surgical patients, which was a substantial change from 1988 when only 23% had favored this approach.[1]

Location of Bleeding: Computed Tomography versus Bronchoscopy

Diagnostic examination in massive hemoptysis should focus on etiology and identification of the site of bleeding. Such examination commonly involves chest radiography, fiberoptic bronchoscopy, and chest CT.[38]

Despite the fact that chest radiography is a standard procedure and is always available, it rarely provides clear information on the site of bleeding.

Various studies have reported that fiberoptic bronchoscopy can help to locate the site of the hemorrhage in between 49% and 92.9% of cases.[21,23] Fiberoptic bronchoscopy is often considered in patients with hemoptysis and a normal or nonlocalizing chest X-ray to rule out endobronchial malignancy. Performed early in the evaluation, while the patient is actively bleeding, provides the highest performance for locating the bleeding site.[1]

Many experts advocate the use of fiberoptic bronchoscopy as the primary method of localizing the site of bleeding in massive hemoptysis,[39,40] but many studies have downplayed this technique and even set it aside just as an aid to the location of the bleeding before arterial embolization.[41]

Instead, an early chest CT has been advocated to help localize the bleeding site and diagnose the cause of hemoptysis.[42] The advantage of CT is that it may define one of several diagnoses such as bronchiectasis, lung abscess, and mass lesions, including cancer, mycetomas, and arteriovenous malformations. CT can localize the site of bleeding in 63% to 100% of cases. Specifically, CT can aid in diagnosing nonbronchial systemic supply in 80% of cases, with the lowest success in visualizing internal mammary supply.[43] Knowledge of nonbronchial supply in advance has the potential for increasing the success rate of initial embolization.[21,41] It may also help in acute cases to guide arteriography or bronchoscopy to the regions of highest yield.

Revel and coworkers[38] wondered if CT could replace bronchoscopy in the detection of the site and cause of bleeding in patients with large or massive hemoptysis. The disadvantage of chest CT is that it may require temporary movement of an unstable patient away from intensive care.

Nowadays with the availability of multislice CT, the use of the fibrobronchoscopy and the arteriography has been questioned for the location and diagnosis of the bleeding. Undoubtedly, the quality of the images, their precision, and the speed and readiness cause CT to play an important role in the diagnosis of the hemoptysis. It has several potential interests, including anatomic workup of bronchial and systemic arterial anatomy to the lung and diagnosis of uncommon sources of bleeding such as pulmonary artery[43,44] (Fig. 18.8).

Bronchial and Systemic Angiography

The main objective of a severe hemoptysis diagnosis is the design of an appropriate treatment approach. It is unquestionable that embolization stands out as the optimal treatment. Every embolization requires a previous

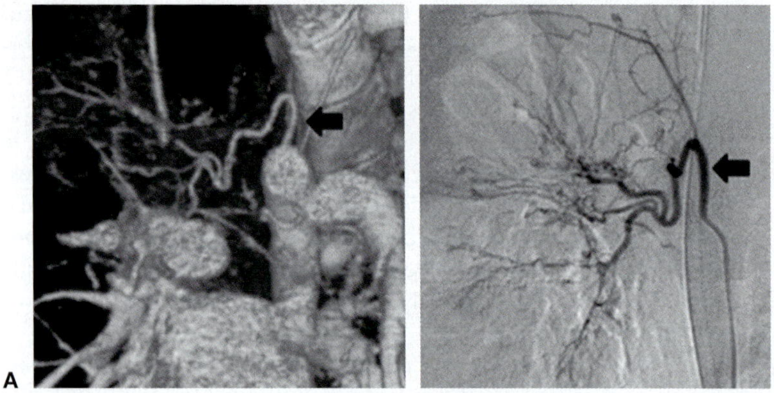

Figure 18.8 **A:** Volume rendering reconstruction of a bronchial artery CT angiography, right intercostobronchial trunk (*arrow*). **B:** Angiographic correspondence (*arrow*).

angiographic study, which is the gold standard for diagnosis of hemoptysis. However, although CT might delay the intervention, it may be very helpful to understand the etiology, the mechanism of bleeding, and the origin of aberrant bronchial or systemic arteries and to plan a successful procedure.[45]

If the patient continues bleeding and the source is still unknown, then arteriography should be performed next because it may be useful for therapy as well as for diagnosis. Because most massive bleedings arise from the bronchial circulation, bronchial arteriography has a higher performance than arteriography of the pulmonary or systemic arterial beds.

Knowledge of the anatomy of the bronchial arteries is crucial for their location and examination. The bronchial arteries exhibit several anatomic variations in terms of both their origin and their various branches.[32,34]

When the pulmonary arterial circulation is the source, the most common underlying conditions are pulmonary arteriovenous malformations, Rasmussen aneurysms, or iatrogenic pulmonary artery tears. A recent study observed that 8 (10.5%) in a series of 76 patients undergoing bronchial angiography for hemoptysis had visible pulmonary artery pseudoaneurysms.[46] In our series,[23] the pulmonary artery was the origin of pulmonary bleeding in 6 patients (2%) with different causes. In only one case a Rasmussen aneurysm was diagnosed (Fig. 18.9).

Occasionally, other systemic arteries of the chest or in the vicinity are the cause of bleeding or are involved together with the bronchial arteries. Nonbronchial systemic collateral arteries differ from anomalous bronchial arteries because they are not congenital but developed through several pulmonary diseases.[47]

Systemic collateral arteries may include a wide spectrum of arteries within or near the thorax, such as the thyrocervical trunk, intercostal, internal mammary, thoracodorsal, and lateral thoracic arteries and other branches from the subclavian artery. Intra-abdominal arteries, including the inferior phrenic arteries, may also provide nonbronchial collateral supplies for the lung lesions that cause hemoptysis[48–51] (see Fig. 18.1).

The nonbronchial systemic collateral arteries are common in the presence of pleural thickening and adhesion, in chronic inflammatory lung disease, or pulmonary malignancies, thereby facilitating transpleural systemic pulmonary anastomosis.[47]

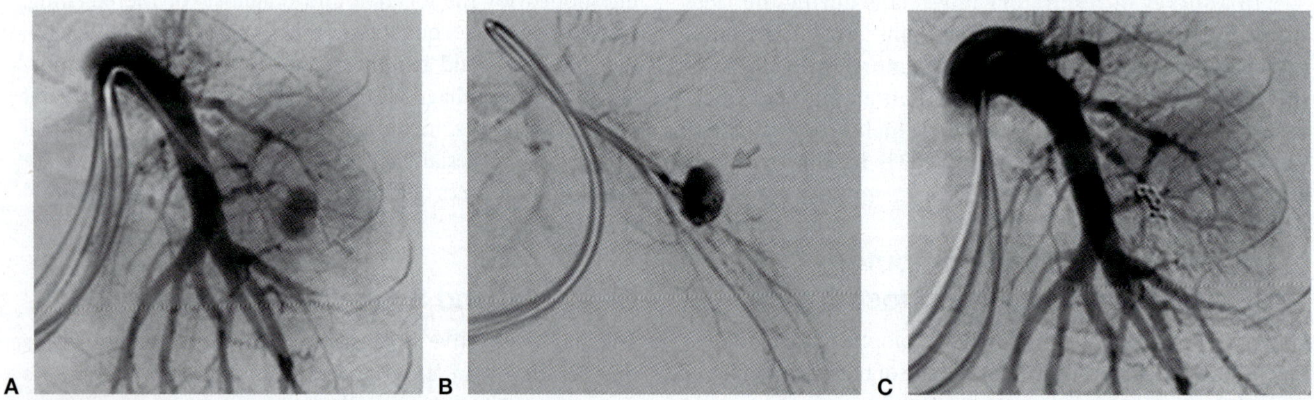

Figure 18.9 Rasmussen aneurysm, depending on a branch of left inferior lobar pulmonary artery. **A,B:** Diagnostic angiograms. **C:** Coil embolization. (Courtesy of Dr. César Ortega.)

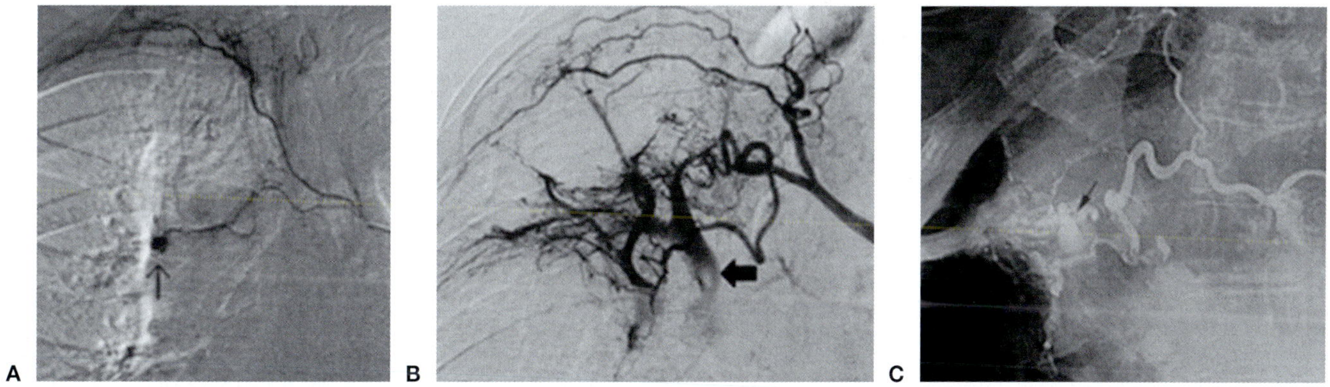

Figure 18.10 Direct bleeding signs. **A:** Contrast extravasation (*arrow*). **B:** Large bronchial artery–pulmonary vein fistula (*arrow*). **C:** Bronchial artery aneurysm (*arrow*) in a patient with cancer.

Angiographic Signs

The diagnosis of bleeding by arteriography is simple but controversial. When direct signs such as extravasation, aneurysms, or pseudoaneurysms are observed, diagnosis is easy and the cause of hemoptysis is clear. However, extravasation of contrast agent is observed in only 3.6% to 10.7% of cases[41] (Fig. 18.10).

Angiographic indirect findings in hemoptysis include hypertrophic and tortuous bronchial arteries, areas of hypervascularity and neovascularity, and shunting of blood into pulmonary artery or vein[52] (Fig. 18.11).

In our series,[23] bronchial angiography revealed abnormalities that would account for hemoptysis in 287 patients (91.4%).

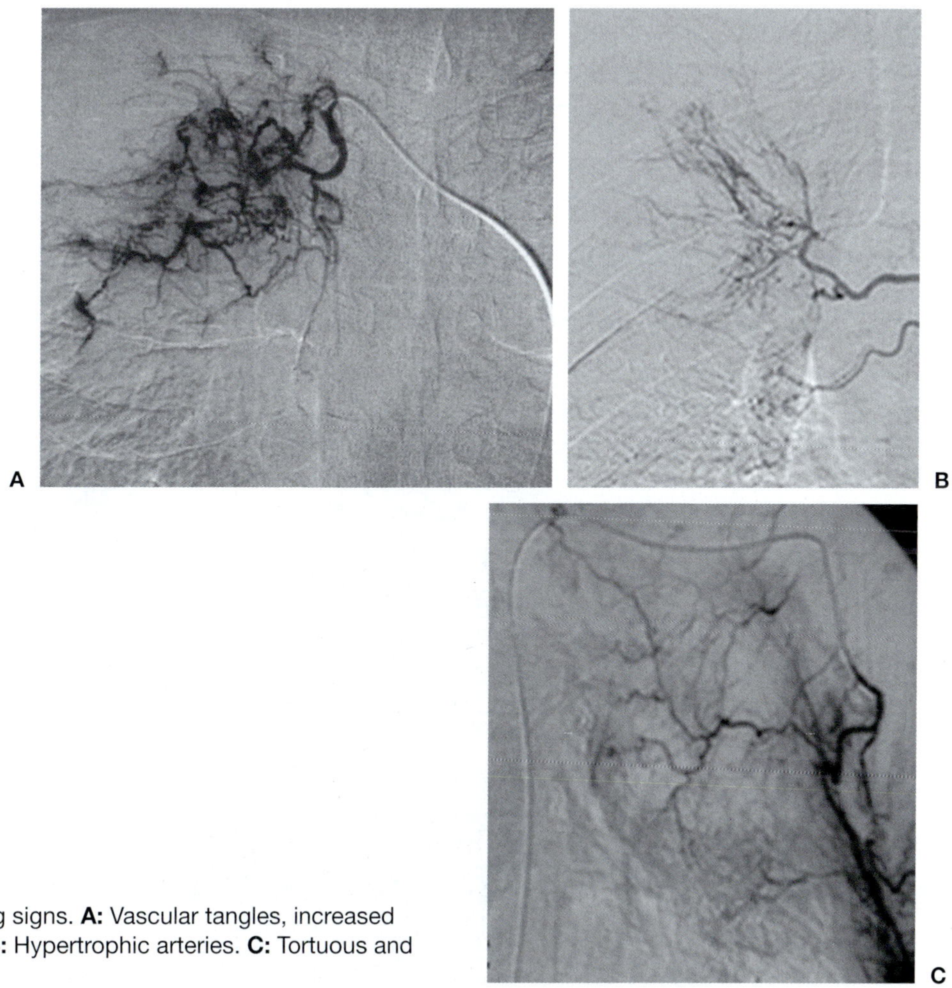

Figure 18.11 Indirect bleeding signs. **A:** Vascular tangles, increased vessel caliber. **B:** Hypertrophic arteries. **C:** Tortuous and irregular blood vessels.

Table 18.3 Direct and Indirect Signs of Bleeding in a Series of 287 Patients

	Direct Signs		Indirect Signs		Total	
Examined Arterial Areas	n	%	n	%	n	%
Bronchial	31	10.6	245	84.1	276	94.8
Mammary	7	2.4	23	7.9	30	10.3
Lateral thoracic	4	1.3	18	6.1	22	7.5
Thoracoacromial	3	4.4	11	3.7	14	4.8
Thoracodorsal	2	2.1	11	3.7	13	4.4
Intercostal	2	2.1	9	3.0	11	3.7
Pulmonary	5	1.7	1	0.3	6	2.0
Right Phrenic	2	2.1	4	1.3	6	2.0
Coronary	0	—	1	0.3	1	0.3
Others	2	2.1	2	2.1	4	1.3

From de Gregorio MA, Medrano J, Mainar A, et al. Endovascular treatment of massive hemoptysis by bronchial artery embolization: short-term and long-term follow-up over a 15-year period. *Arch Bronconeumol*. 2006;42(2):49–56

Of those, 58 (20.2%) presented direct signs of hemorrhage (extravasation and/or aneurysm). The remainder only showed indirect signs that were more or less intense (Table 18.3).

INDICATIONS AND CONTRAINDICATIONS

Not every hemoptysis requires either embolization of bronchial, systemic, or pulmonary arteries. Most small entity hemoptysis require only a correct diagnosis and conservative medical treatment. Massive hemoptysis is the most important indication for invasive treatment by surgery or embolization. There is no agreement in the definition proposed for the term *massive hemoptysis*, being the most commonly used for a blood expectoration greater than 300 to 600 mL in 24 hours. Furthermore, the reliability of patient measurement and reporting of volume of expectorated blood may be limited in real life, therefore a more reasonable practical definition would be any amount of hemoptysis that is life threatening[28,43] (Fig. 18.12).

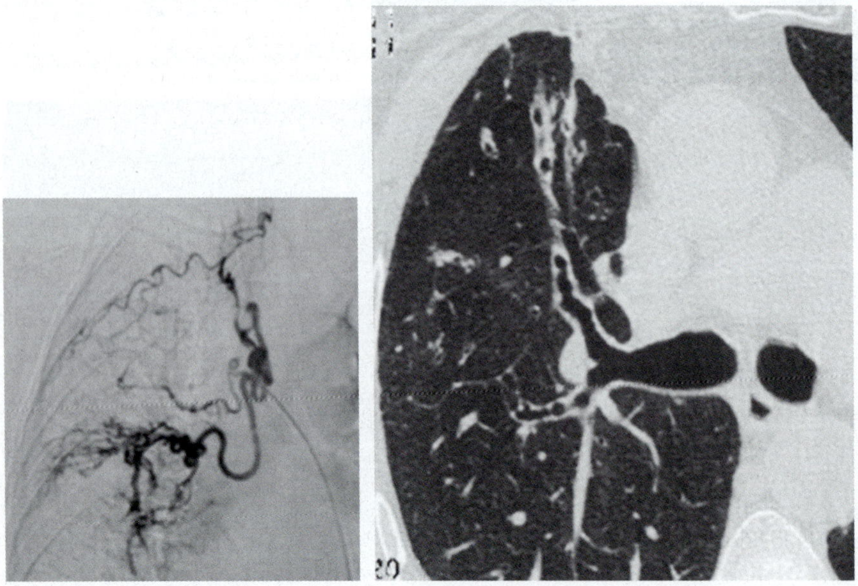

A B

Figure 18.12 A 37-year-old patient with massive hemoptysis (>200 mL in 24 hours). **A:** Irregular and enlarged bronchial arteries in the right superior lobe. **B:** CT image shows bronchiectasias.

Table 18.4 Main Indications for Bronchial and Nonbronchial Hemoptysis Embolization

Massive hemoptysis with curative intent
Life-threatening hemoptysis
Severe hemoptysis previous to surgery
Minor hemoptysis in patients with poor pulmonary reserve
Minor hemoptysis affecting the quality of life of the patient
Relapsing chronic hemoptysis affecting the quality of life of the patient
Hemoptysis of any type in patients with uncontrolled progressive disease

The main indications for embolization treatment are outlined in Table 18.4.

The only real contraindications for bronchial or nonbronchial artery embolization are the usual contraindications for angiography, including intractable coagulopathy, renal dysfunction, and severe contrast allergy. The presence of medullary artery with insurmountable embolization risk, such as a bronchial artery that is too small to be selectivized or a medullary artery that cannot be occluded with a proximal coil, would also contraindicate the technique,. Likewise, inexperience or inability to safely catheterize selectively or embolize the bleeding branches should contraindicate the intervention due to the high risk of embolic agent migration to other territories.[43]

TECHNIQUE

Bronchial and nonbronchial artery embolization requires a thorough detailed examination to discover angiographic pathologic vessels. Both diagnosis and treatment should be performed in a vascular interventional operating room equipped with the best possible imaging technology and the means of constant monitoring and appropriate resuscitation to solve any unexpected issue. The operator must be familiar with the anatomy of thoracic and bronchial arteries as well as the technical considerations and materials of embolization. It can use different arterial access, but perhaps the most used is the right femoral artery. In all cases, an angiogram of thoracic aorta is recommended to demonstrate bronchial artery anatomy and to identify other systemic collateral vessels (Fig. 18.13).

The initial aortogram shows hypertrophied arteries and denotes possible aberrant origins of ectopic arteries that reach the pulmonary parenchyma.[21,53] A methodical selective catheterization of the major bronchial arteries is mandatory even if the aortogram did not show any pathologic bronchial artery.[21] Although 4-Fr to 5-Fr cobra-type curved catheters are the most commonly used for catheterization, several different configurations (e.g., Simmons 1, Headhunter, Michaelson, Yashiro-type, Sos-Omni catheters, etc.) should be available for optimal selection of bronchial arteries.

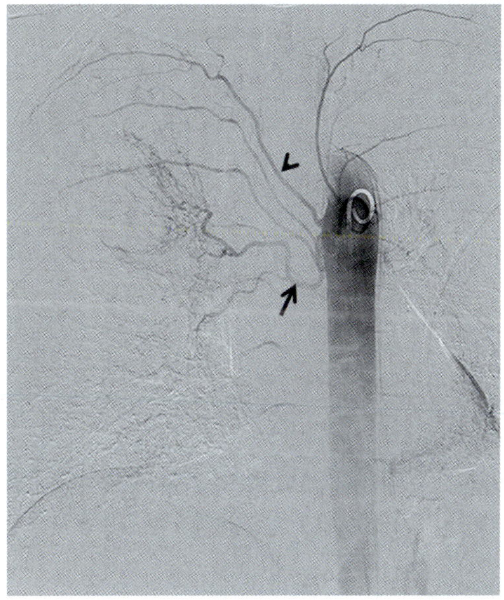

Figure 18.13 Thoracic aortogram. Intercostal branches (*arrowhead*) are observed along with a pathologic intercostobronchial artery (*arrow*).

Most of the authors recommend the routine use of coaxial microcatheters for superselective bronchial artery catheterization. Superselective catheterization allows a safe position and allows the blood flow necessary to achieve distal embolization[1,54,55] (Fig. 18.14).

The use of microcatheters is of particular importance when embolizing the right intercostobronchial trunk to avoid the occlusion of intercostal branches shunting directly to the anterior spinal artery.[56]

To identify the bleeding bronchial artery, it is necessary to selectively catheterize each of the bronchial artery independently and slowly inject small quantities of contrast manually. If all explored bronchial arteries are normal, then the systemic arteries that surround the thorax (internal mammary, lateral thoracic, intercostals, etc.) have to be methodically explored bilaterally; if they are also normal, then we should study the pulmonary arteries. When pleural thickening, peripheral tumors, or peripheral lung scars are detected, it is mandatory to study the systemic vascularization anyway.[21]

It has been established that embolization should always be the most distal possible to prevent recurrences by collateral vessels. The rationale for this approach is that the distal embolization of the bronchopulmonary pathologic anastomosis slows the flow in the smaller vessels, making it easier to occlude them. In fact, several authors contraindicate the use of coils in hemoptysis embolization because they produce a more proximal occlusion and, in case of recurrence, they can complicate the access to the diseased arteries.[52]

In our experience, the proximal occlusion, after distal embolization, reinforces decreasing the bronchial artery flow and ensures its occlusion (Fig. 18.15). In case of recurrence

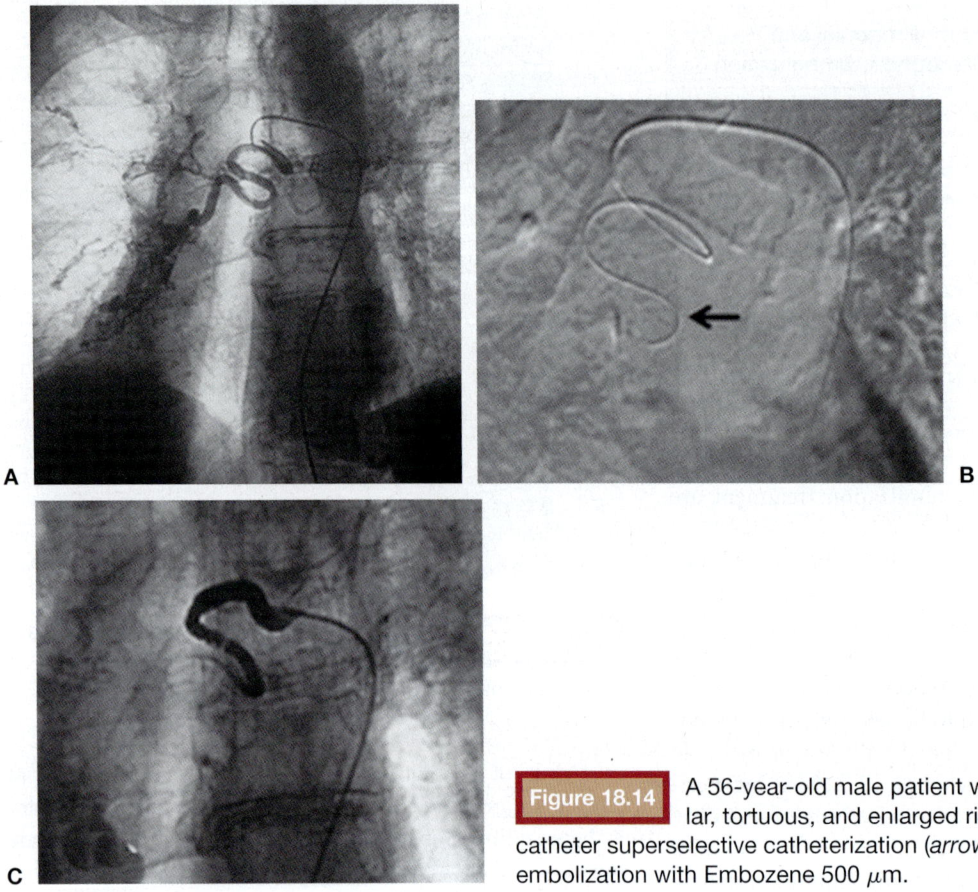

Figure 18.14 A 56-year-old male patient with bronchiectasias. **A:** Irregular, tortuous, and enlarged right bronchial artery. **B:** Microcatheter superselective catheterization (*arrow*). **C:** Angiographic result after embolization with Embozene 500 μm.

by collaterals, that new collaterals are the ones to be closed. With this technique in 15-year follow-up, we observed a lower rate of recurrence (10.4%) than most authors (10% to 55%).[23,57]

Several embolic materials are available for bronchial artery embolization. The use of embolization agents smaller than 300 μm should be avoided. Pump[58] and Bernard et al.[59] have demonstrated that bronchopulmonary anastomoses could allow the flow of particles smaller than this size, so they can produce pulmonary infarction (bronchial artery shunt to pulmonary artery) or systemic embolization (bronchial artery shunt to pulmonary vein).

The main embolic agents used for hemoptysis treatment are absorbable gelatin sponge, polyvinyl alcohol, trisacryl

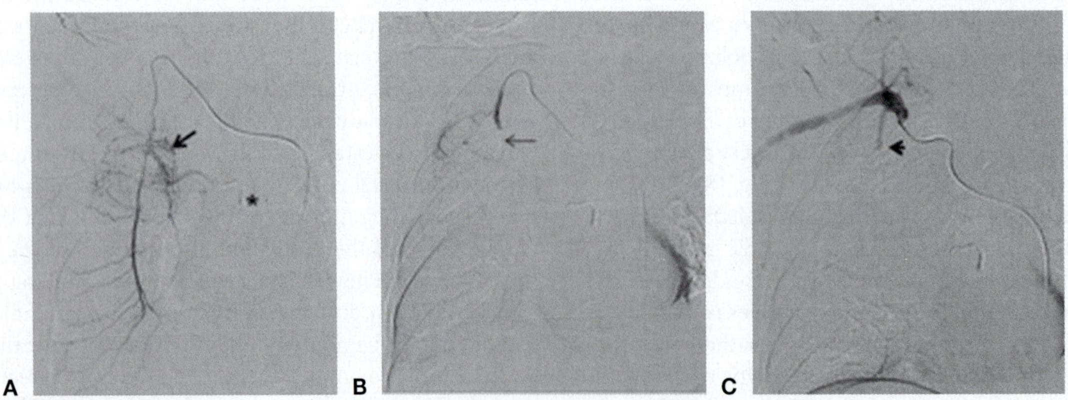

Figure 18.15 Embolization with PVA and microcoils. **A:** Pathologic branches arising from internal mammary artery (*arrow*). Distal embolization with 500-μm microparticles (*asterisk*). **B,C:** Proximal embolization with microcoils (*arrows*).

Table 18.5 Different Types of Embolization Agents

Embolization Agent	Product/Company	Absorbable	Size/Shape	Comments
Gelatin sponge	Gelfoam (Baxter)	Yes	Variable Irregular	High rate of recurrence
Polyvinyl alcohol (PVA)	Contour (Boston Scientific)	None	Variable Nonspherical	Prone to clumping resulting in a proximal occlusion
Trisacryl cross-linked with gelatin	Embosphere Microsphere (Merit Medical)	None	Calibrated/ compressible (33%)	Minimize unwanted proximal embolization and predictable distal embolization
Hydrogel core with lubricious and flexible coating of Polyzene	Embozene Microsphere (CeloNova Biosciences)	None	Calibrated/ spherical	First microspheres with color-coded particle size. Improve visibility and increase procedure safety
Hydrosphere based on a PVA macromere	Bead Block microsphere (Biocompatibles)	None	Calibrated Spherical Compressible	Microspheres synthetic hydrophilic and tinted in blue
N-butyl cyanoacrylate	Histoacryl (B. Braun Medical)	None	Blue liquid polymerizes	Experience required for management
Ethylene vinyl alcohol (EVOH)	Onyx (Covidien)	None	Black liquid EVOH 6% EVOH 8%	Requires solvent dimethyl sulfoxide (DMSO)
Microcoils	Cook Medical, Covidien, Boston Scientific	None	Several sizes and types	Detachable coils are recommended
Hydrocoils	Azur (Terumo Medical)	None	Several sizes	Combines a platinum coil and an expandable hydrogel polymer

microspheres, *N*-butyl cyanoacrylate, ethylene vinyl alcohol, and metal coils[60] (Table 18.5).

Absorbable gelatin sponge (Gelfoam; Baxter, Deerfield, Illinois) is the most economical agent; it is readily available and easy to use. Delivering the material through microcatheters can be difficult. Moreover, it has the disadvantage of producing temporary arterial occlusion with a high rate of recurrence by recanalization when gelatin is reabsorbed in 15 to 30 days.[8,9,54]

Polyvinyl alcohol (PVA) is a nonabsorbable particulate agent available in various particulate sizes. The most common particle size for bronchial artery embolization ranges from 250 to 500 μm. [55,61–63]

Currently used trisacrylic PVA microspheres show a spherical morphology of fairly uniform size, compliant and nonclumping, and easily delivered through microcatheters. There are several companies that sell different types of microspheres with small variations and different characteristics.[64]

Ethylene vinyl alcohol, known as *Onyx* (Covidien, Irvine, California), is a copolymer dissolved in dimethyl sulfoxide and suspended in micronized tantalum powder to provide contrast for visualization under fluoroscopy. The embolic agent Onyx is safer and easier to use than other liquid glues (as Histoacryl; B. Braun Medical, Inc., Bethlehem, Pennsylvania) but has the drawback of its high price.[65]

Histoacryl consists of monomeric *N*-butyl cyanoacrylate, which polymerizes quickly in contact with tissue fluid. Histoacryl is available in two colors: translucent, especially for facial application, and blue, which enables an easy control over the quantity applied. It solidifies in a few seconds upon contact with blood. Its management requires a lot of expertise because the tip of the microcatheter may quickly become trapped in the glue and can be difficult to retrieve.[66,67]

The use of metal coils for bronchial artery embolization in the treatment of hemoptysis is controversial. As it has been already said, many authors advise against its use based on the difficulty of treating a recurrence.[52,60] Other authors defend embolization using microcoils with acceptable rates of recurrence.[68,69]

We use the combination of distal embolization with microspheres and detachable microcoils at the proximal end

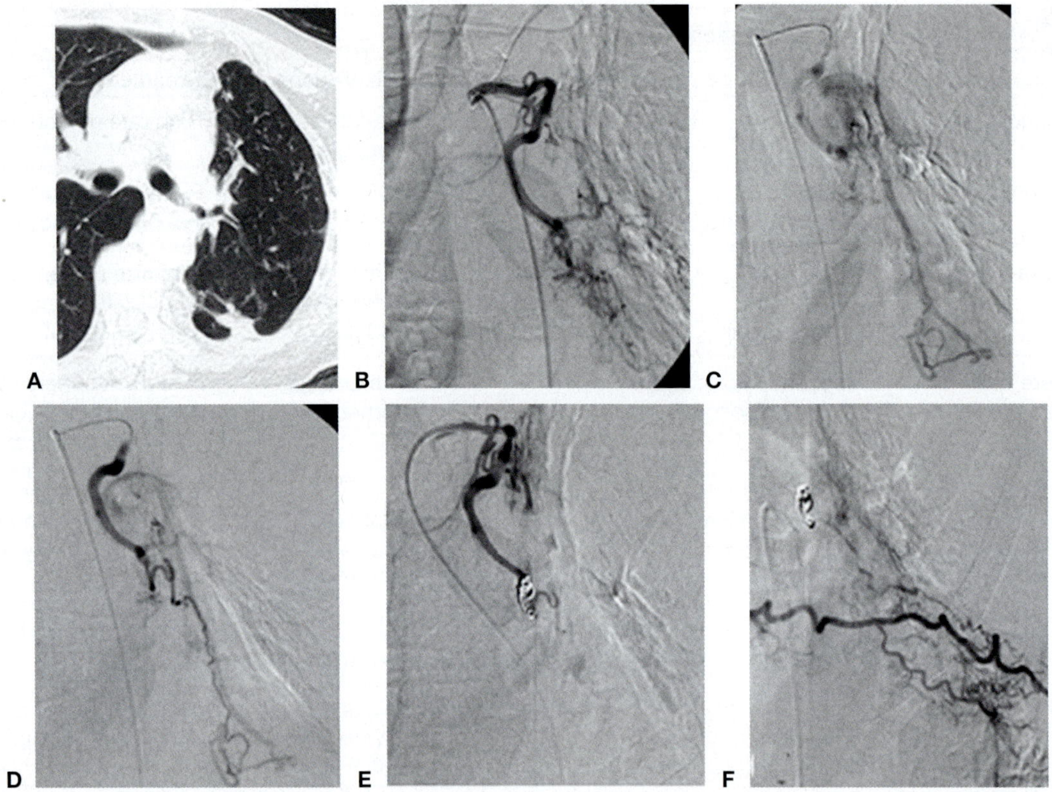

Figure 18.16 A 58-year-old patient with massive hemoptysis. **A:** Chest CT shows scar tissue in left inferior lobe. **B,C:** Left bronchial artery lesions, fistula to the left pulmonary vein branch. **D,E:** Distal embolization with 300-μm PVA and proximal embolization with microcoils. **F:** After a systematic review, a pathologic intercostal artery is also embolized. (Courtesy of Dr. Ignacio Bilbao.)

(Fig. 18.16). Long-term follow-up supports the benefits of this technique.[2,70]

OUTCOMES

Bronchial and nonbronchial systemic artery embolization is the treatment of choice for massive and recurrent hemoptysis. Immediate control of bronchial bleeding is achieved in 73% to 99% of cases[23,57,64,71,72] (Table 18.6).

Technical success achieved with new technologies is very high (>90% of cases), whereas clinical success varies depending on the length of the follow-up. It seems that these new technologies have not improved the clinical long-term outcome, but there are no randomized studies with sufficient clinical evidence to categorically state that. At least, calibrated microparticles and microcatheters seem to have improved the efficacy in arterial occlusion and, especially, the safety.

Immediate control of a massive bleeding rate ranges from 80% to 100% using different embolic agents. The Achilles heel of this procedure is a recurrence up to 50% or even 75%, as stated by some authors. It is difficult to establish the true rate of recurrence if there is no consensus of defining recurrence. If we consider small bloody sputum episodes without clinical significance, our recurrence will be high. Some authors only record episodes of hemoptysis requiring medical management (surgery or embolization).[57,60,73]

Early rebleeding in general is due to incomplete embolization or presence of overlooked collateral vessels. Up to 20% of patients will bleed again in the first month. Late rebleeding (months or years), on the other hand, is due to progression or reactivation of the underlying disease and lesion revascularization by collateral vessels from other bronchial arteries and systemic arteries of the neighborhood.

The main factors for recurrence are improper technique, partial embolization, or embolization of side branches involved in the injury but which are not the origin of the bleeding. Other causes include the use of absorbable embolic agents, acute vascular pathologic processes, or chronic diseases such as tuberculosis, aspergillosis, and cancer.[13,74,75] Also, if the primary disease is not adequately treated, such as in tuberculosis and in aspergillosis lung infections, it is expected to have a higher recurrence rate of bleeding.

Chronic or resistant tuberculosis has high rate of recurrence, whereas acute tuberculosis sensitive to antituberculosis therapy has a favorable outcome with low rate of rebleeding after embolization.[57,75]

Table 18.6 Bronchial Embolization Outcome

Authors	Year	N	Embolic agent	Clinical Success (%)	Recurrence (%)	Follow-up (mo)	Complications (%)
Remy et al.	1977	104	Gelatin sponge	84	28.6	7	11.5
Uflacker et al.	1983	33	Gelatin sponge	100	18.2	24	3
Rabkin et al.	1987	306	PVA Albumin macro aggregates	90.8	33.7	–	0.3
Katoh et al.	1990	33	PVA Gelatin sponge	100	21.1	48	6
Corr	2005	70	Microspheres	87	13	15	8.6
de Gregorio et al.	2006	287	PVA Microcoils	91	10.4	180	28
Poyanli et al.	2007	140	PVA Microcoils	98.5	10	33.6	0
Baltacioğlu et al.	2010	25	NBCA	100	16	63	16
Woo et al.	2013	406	PVA NBCA	92.2 96.5	21.5 1.8	60	34.1 31

PVA, polyvinyl alcohol; NBCA, *N*-butyl cyanoacrylate.

Hemoptysis is the most common symptom in aspergilloma; it occurs in 69% to 83% of all patients, and it ranges from mild to life threatening, with a mortality rate ranging from 2% to 50% and with an early and very high recurrence rate.[57,76]

Patients with lung cancer carry a 10% to 30% risk of developing hemoptysis and are also at risk of recurrence following embolization.[14,77]

It is important to know that hemoptysis is a symptom that can become fatal in patients suffering from a severe pulmonary disease. Embolization is a symptomatic treatment of hemoptysis. It is necessary to medically or surgically resolve the underlying condition, when possible.[52] It is therefore important to identify and embolize all vessels that may be contributing to the abnormal blood supply, including any nonbronchial systemic or pulmonary arteries. The underlying pathology should be treated if possible to achieve long-term hemoptysis control.

POTENTIAL COMPLICATIONS

The most frequent complications of hemoptysis embolization include chest pain (24% to 91%) and dysphagia (1% to 18%). They are temporary symptoms due to ischemic phenomena caused by embolization of intercostal and esophageal branches respectively.[13,21,52]

It is known that the bronchial arteries supply not only the bronchial artery branches but also provide for the vasa vasorum of the aorta, pulmonary artery wall, esophagus, pleura, and spinal cord.[52]

To prevent accidental embolization, we have to work in optimal imaging conditions (adequate equipment, high dose, zoom, and collimation) to identify any leakage to an undesired structure and with the adequate materials for microcatheterization. Every injection should be performed under fluoroscopic control with a slow, careful, and precise infusion of the mixture (iodine contrast and embolic agent, choosing an adequate proportion depending on the contrast concentration and the employed agent).

Subintimal dissection of the aorta or the bronchial artery during hemoptysis embolization is another frequent minor complication, with a reported prevalence of 1% to 6.3%. There are usually no symptoms or problems related to it. This complication can be avoided with the use of soft tip diagnostic catheters, microcatheters coaxially, and gentle hand injections[15,21] (Fig. 18.17).

Probably the most feared and serious complication is the embolization of the anterior spinal artery, which can be caused by transverse myelitis. The prevalence of spinal cord ischemia after hemoptysis embolization is reported to be 1.4% to 6.5%. When the anterior medullary artery (Adamkiewicz artery) is visualized at angiography, embolization should not be performed. Therefore, good imaging and extensive previous diagnostic angiographies or scans are essential.[54,78–80]

As has been already said, sometimes, the medullary artery cannot be visualized at the beginning of the embolization because it is very thin and bronchial flow is dominant. Therefore, embolization should always be performed

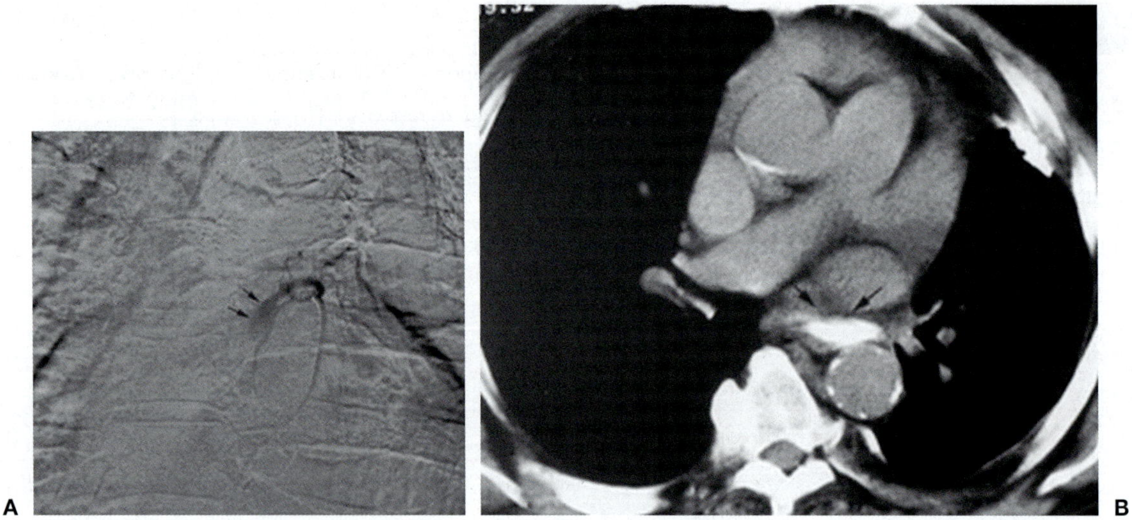

Figure 18.17 Arterial dissection. **A:** Contrast extravazation is observed (*arrows*). **B:** Chest CT confirms the finding (*arrows*).

meticulously, slowly, and under fluoroscopic guidance to stop on time and avoid its accidental embolization.[36]

Another serious but infrequent complication is the posterior cerebral circulation stroke because of embolism to the occipital cortex, either via bronchial artery–pulmonary vein shunt or via collateral vessels between bronchial and vertebral arteries.[81,82]

Other rare complications reported in the literature include aortic and bronchial necrosis, bronchoesophageal fistula, ischemic colitis, and pulmonary infarction.[83,84]

TIPS AND TRICKS

Tips

- Chest CT angiography previous to embolization shortens the procedure length because it helps to locate the bleeding.
- It is useful to include the entire thoracic aorta in the angiography to get the whole picture of bronchial and intercostal arteries and any other anomalous artery arising from the aorta.
- An adequate equipment and radiographic technique that achieve a high image quality is essential to visualize medullary and esophageal arteries.
- Anterior medullary artery can usually be found in the left hemithorax.
- *Always* use a microcatheter coaxial to the diagnostic catheter.
- *Always* use spherical particles greater than 300 μm to avoid leakage to the systemic circulation through shunts.
- Ensure distal embolization.
- *Systematically* check every bronchial and thoracic systemic artery.
- In case of inflammatory or infectious disease such as tuberculosis, do not forget to also check the pulmonary circulation due to the possibility of shunting .

Tricks

- *Do not* introduce the diagnostic catheter (4-Fr to 5-Fr) into the bronchial artery to avoid vasospasm.
- If it is not possible to stabilize the microcatheter, try to use a 5-Fr to 6-Fr guiding catheter in the aorta.
- Try to get as distally as possible with the microcatheter gently using a soft tip 0.014-in microwire.
- Use spherical particles greater than 300 μm, ensure a homogenous mix, and deliver them slowly. *Take your time.*
- Perform control checks gently and slowly to avoid particle lavage to the systemic circulation.
- When a medullary, esophageal, or tracheal artery is visualized, it is possible to close it proximally with a coil to avoid particle embolization.
- Once distal embolization is ensured, some authors recommend proximal coil occlusion. Other authors emphatically advise against it.

SUMMARY

Hemoptysis is a fairly common symptom of a group of respiratory diseases. Fortunately, only a few are massive and/or life threatening. Massive and recurrent hemoptysis are those that require invasive treatment. In the management of hemoptysis, location of the bleeding point is essential. Multidetector CT and bronchoscopy play an important role before angiography. Embolization with nonabsorbable particles is the preferred treatment of massive hemoptysis. Embolization is, in general, a symptomatic treatment: never forget the treatment of the underlying disease, if possible. Surgery is reserved for some difficult cases and embolization failures.

REFERENCES

1. Haponik EF, Fein A, Chin R. Managing life-threatening hemoptysis: has anything really changed? *Chest.* 2000;118:1431–1435.
2. de Gregorio MA, Medrano J, Laborda A, et al. Hemoptysis workup before embolization: single-center experience with a 15-year period follow-up. *Tech Vasc Interv Radiol.* 2007;10: 270–273.
3. Najarian KE, Morris CS. Arterial embolization in the chest. *J Thorac Imaging.* 1998;13:93–104.
4. Marshall TJ, Jackson JE. Vascular intervention in the thorax: bronchial artery embolization for haemoptysis. *Eur Radiol.* 1997;7:1221–1227.
5. Fernando HC, Stein M, Benfield JR, et al. Role of bronchial artery embolization in the management of hemoptysis. *Arch Surg.* 1998;133:862–886.
6. Remy J, Voisin C, Ribet M, et al. Treatment, by embolization, of severe or repeated hemoptysis associated with systemic hypervascularization [in French]. *Nouv Presse Med.* 1973;2:2060–2068.
7. Wholey MH, Chamorro HA, Rao G, et al. Bronchial artery embolization for massive hemoptysis. *JAMA.* 1976;236: 2501–2504.
8. Remy J, Arnaud A, Fardou H, et al. Treatment of hemoptysis by embolization of bronchial arteries. *Radiology.* 1977;122:33–37.
9. Uflacker R, Kaemmerer A, Neves C, et al. Management of massive hemoptysis by bronchial artery embolization. *Radiology.* 1983;146:627–634.
10. Uflacker R, Kaemmerer A, Picon PD, et al. Bronchial artery embolization in the management of hemoptysis: technical aspects and long-term results. *Radiology.* 1985;157:637–644.
11. Keller FS, Rosch J, Loflin TG, et al. Nonbronchial systemic collateral arteries: significance in percutaneous embolotherapy for hemoptysis. *Radiology.* 1987;164:687–692.
12. Hayakawa K, Tanaka F, Torizuka T, et al. Bronchial artery embolization for hemoptysis: immediate and long-term results. *Cardiovasc Intervent Radiol.* 1992;15:154–159.
13. Ramakantan R, Bandekar VG, Gandhi MS, et al. Massive hemoptysis due to pulmonary tuberculosis: control with bronchial artery embolization. *Radiology.* 1996;200:691–694.
14. Mal H, Rullon I, Mellot F, et al. Immediate and long-term results of bronchial artery embolization for life-threatening hemoptysis. *Chest.* 1999;115:996–1001.
15. Kato A, Kudo S, Matsumoto K, et al. Bronchial artery embolization for hemoptysis due to benign diseases: immediate and long-term results. *Cardiovasc Intervent Radiol.* 2000;23:351–357.
16. Jean-Baptiste E. Clinical assessment and management of massive hemoptysis. *Crit Care Med.* 2000;28:1642–1647.
17. Jougon J, Ballester M, Delcambre F, et al. Massive hemoptysis: what place for medical and surgical treatment. *Eur J Cardiothorac Surg.* 2002;22:345–351.
18. de Gracia J, de la Rosa D, Catalán E, et al. Use of endoscopic fibrinogen-thrombin in the treatment of severe hemoptysis. *Respir Med.* 2003;97:790–795.
19. Bidwell JL, Pachner RW. Hemoptysis: diagnosis and management. *Am Fam Physician.* 2005;72:1253–1260.
20. Salajka F. Causes of massive hemoptysis. *Monaldi Arch Chest Dis.* 2001;56:390–393.
21. Yoon W, Kim JK, Kim YH, et al. Bronchial and nonbronchial systemic artery embolization for life-threatening hemoptysis: a comprehensive review. *Radiographics.* 2001;22:1395–1409.
22. Adelman M, Haponik EF, Bleecker ER, et al. Cryptogenic hemoptisis: clinical features, bronchoscopic findings, and natural history in 67 patients. *Ann Intern Med.* 1985;102(6):829–834.
23. de Gregorio MA, Medrano J, Mainar A, et al. Endovascular treatment of massive hemoptysis by bronchial artery embolization: short-term and long-term follow-up over a 15-year period. *Arch Bronconeumol.* 2006;42(2):49–56.
24. Deffenbach ME, Charan NB, Lakshminarayan S, et al. The bronchial circulation: small, but a vital attribute to the lung. *Am Rev Respir Dis.* 1987;135:463–481.
25. Furuse M, Saito K, Kunieda E, et al. Bronchial arteries: CT demonstration with arteriographic correlation. *Radiology.* 1987;162:393–398.
26. Remy J, Remy-Jardin M, Voisin C. Endovascular management of bronchial bleeding. In: Butler J, ed. *The Bronchial Circulation.* New York, NY: Dekker; 1992:667–723.
27. MacIntosh EL, Parrott JC, Unruh HW. Fistulas between the aorta and tracheobronchial tree. *Ann Thorac Surg.* 1991;51: 515–519.
28. Hakanson E, Konstantinov IE, Fransson SG, et al. Management of life-threatening haemoptysis. *Br J Anaesth.* 2002;88:291–295.
29. Pearse EO, Bryan AJ. Massive haemoptysis 27 years after surgery for coarctation of the aorta. *J R Soc Med.* 2001;94:640–641.
30. Bruzzi JF, Rémy-Jardin M, Delhaye D, et al. Multi-detector row CT of hemoptysis. *Radiographics.* 2006;26:3–22.
31. Sancho C, Escalante E, Dominguez J, et al. Embolization of bronchial arteries of anomalous origin. *Cardiovasc Intervent Radiol.* 1998;21:300–304.
32. Morita Y, Takase K, Ichikawa H, et al. Bronchial artery anatomy: preoperative 3D simulation with multidetector CT. *Radiology.* 2010;255:934–943.
33. Remy-Jardin M, Bouaziz N, Dumont P, et al. Bronchial and nonbronchial systemic arteries at multi-detector row CT angiography: comparison with conventional angiography. *Radiology.* 2004;233:741–749.
34. Cauldwell EW, Siekert RG, Lininger RE, et al. The bronchial arteries: an anatomic study of 105 human cadavers. *Surg Gynecol Obstet.* 1948;86:395–412.
35. Rosenthal D. Spinal cord ischemia after abdominal aortic operation: is it preventable? *J Vasc Surg.* 1999;30:391–399.
36. Brown AC, Ray CHE. Anterior spinal cord infarction following bronchial artery embolization. *Semin Intervent Radiol.* 2012; 29:241–244.
37. Ong TH, Eng P. Massive hemoptysis requiring intensive care. *Intensive Care Med.* 2003; 29:317–320.
38. Revel MP, Fournier LS, Hennebicque AS, et al. Replace bronchoscopy in the detection of the site and cause of bleeding in patients with large or massive hemoptysis? *AJR Am J Roentgenol.* 2002;179(5):1217–1224.

39. Cahill BC, Ingbar DH. Massive hemoptysis: assessment and management. *Clin Chest Med.* 1994;15:147–167.
40. Dweik RA, Stoller JK. Role of bronchoscopy in massive hemoptysis. *Clin Chest Med.* 1999;20: 89–105.
41. Hsiao EI, Kirsch CM, Kagawa FT, et al. Utility of fiberoptic bronchoscopy before bronchial artery embolization for massive hemoptysis. *AJR Am J Roentgenol.* 2001;177:861–867.
42. Ponnuswamy I, Sankaravadivelu ST, Maduraimuthu P, et al. 64-detector row CT evaluation of bronchial and non-bronchial systemic arteries in life-threatening haemoptysis. *Br J Radiol.* 2012;85:666–672.
43. Sidhu M, Wieseler K, Burdick TR, et al. Bronchial artery embolization for hemoptysis. *Semin Intervent Radiol.* 2008;25: 310–318.
44. Hayes D Jr, Winkler MA, Kirkby S, et al. Preprocedural planning with prospectively triggered multidetector row CT angiography prior to bronchial artery embolization in cystic fibrosis patients with massive hemoptysis. *Lung.* 2012;190:221–225.
45. Hartmann IJ, Remy-Jardin M, Menchini L, et al. Ectopic origin of bronchial arteries: assessment with multidetector helical CT angiography. *Eur Radiol.* 2007;17:1943–1953.
46. Sbano H, Mitchell AW, Ind PW, et al. Peripheral pulmonary artery pseudoaneurysms and massive hemoptysis. *AJR Am J Roentgenol.* 2005;184:1253–1259.
47. Chun HJ, Byun JY, Yoo SS, et al. Added benefit of thoracic aortography after transarterial embolization in patients with hemoptysis. *AJR Am J Roentgenol.* 2003;180:1577–1581.
48. Vujic I, Pyle R, Parker E, et al. Control of massive hemoptysis by embolization of intercostals arteries. *Radiology.* 1980;137: 617–620.
49. Moore LB, McWey RE, Vujic I. Massive hemoptysis: control by embolization of the thyrocervical trunk. *Radiology.* 1986;161:173–174.
50. Jardin M, Remy J. Control of hemoptysis: systemic angiography and anastomoses of the internal mammary artery. *Radiology.* 1988;168:377–383.
51. Gwon DI, Ko GY, Yoon HK, et al. Inferior phrenic artery: anatomy, variations, pathologic conditions, and interventional management. *Radiographics.* 2007;27:687–705.
52. Chun JY, Morgan R, Belli AM. Radiological management of hemoptysis: a comprehensive review of diagnostic imaging and bronchial arterial embolization. *Cardiovasc Intervent Radiol.* 2010;33:240–250.
53. Phillips S, Ruttley MS. Bronchial artery embolization: the importance of preliminary thoracic angiography. *Clin Radiol.* 2000;55:317–319.
54. Tanaka N, Yamakado K, Murashima S, et al. Superselective bronchial artery embolization for hemoptysis with a coaxial microcatheter system. *J Vasc Interv Radiol.* 1997;8:65–70.
55. White RI Jr. Bronchial artery embolotherapy for control of acute hemoptysis: analysis of outcome. *Chest.* 1999;115: 912–915.
56. McDonald DM. Angiogenesis and remodeling of airway vasculature in chronic inflammation. *Am J Respir Crit Care Med.* 2001;164:S39–S45.
57. Chun JY, Belli AM. Immediate and long-term outcomes of bronchial and non-bronchial systemic artery embolisation for the management of haemoptysis. *Eur Radiol.* 2010;20:558–565.
58. Pump K. Distribution of bronchial arteries in human lung. *Chest.* 1972;62:447–451.
59. Bernard S, Luchtel D, Polissar N, et al. Structure and size of bronchopulmonary anastomoses in sheep lung. *Anat Rec A Discov Mol Cell Evol Biol.* 2005;286:804–813.
60. Sopko DR, Smith TP. Bronchial artery embolization for hemoptysis. *Semin Intervent Radiol.* 2011;28:48–62.
61. Rabkin JE, Astafjev VI, Gothman LN, et al. Transcatheter embolization in the management of pulmonary hemorrhage. *Radiology.* 1987;163:361–365.
62. Katoh O, Kishikawa T, Yamada H, et al. Recurrent bleeding after arterial embolization in patients with hemoptysis. *Chest.* 1990;97:541–546.
63. Poyanli A, Acunas B, Rozanes I, et al. Endovascular therapy in the management of moderate and massive haemoptysis. *Br J Radiol.* 2007;80:331–336.
64. Corr PD. Bronchial artery embolization for life-threatening hemoptysis using tris-acryl microspheres: short-term result. *Cardiovasc Intervent Radiol.* 2005;28:439–441.
65. Loffroy R, Favelier S, Genson PY, et al. Onyx for embolization of life-threatening hemoptysis: a promising but luxury embolic agent. *Cardiovasc Intervent Radiol.* 2012;35(1):221.
66. Pugnale M, Portier F, Lamarre A, et al. Hemomediastinum caused by rupture of a bronchial artery aneurysm: successful treatment by embolization with N-butyl-2 cyanoacrylate. *J Vasc Interv Radiol.* 2001;12:1351–1352.
67. Baltacioğlu F, Cimşit NC, Bostanci K, et al. Transarterial microcatheter glue embolization of the bronchial artery for life-threatening hemoptysis: technical and clinical results. *Eur J Radiol.* 2010;73:380–384.
68. Nistri M, Acquafresca M, Pratesi A, et al. Bronchial artery embolization with detachable coils for the treatment of haemoptysis. Preliminary experience. *Radiol Med.* 2008;113:452–460.
69. Schmidt B, Liebers U, Kröncke T, et al. Bronchial artery embolisation using platinum coils in 52 patients with severe pulmonary hemorrhage [in German]. *Dtsch Med Wochenschr.* 2005;130:440–443.
70. Gimeno MJ, Madariaga B, Alfonso ER, et al. Life-threatening hemoptysis. Treatment with transcatheter embolization. *Arch Bronconeumol.* 1999;35:379–384.
71. Lee S, Chan JW, Chan SC, et al. Bronchial artery embolisation can be equally safe and effective in the management of chronic recurrent haemoptysis. *Hong Kong Med J.* 2008;14:14–20.
72. Woo S, Yoon CJ, Chung JW, et al. Bronchial artery embolization to control hemoptysis: comparison of N-butyl-2-cyanoacrylate and polyvinyl alcohol particles. *Radiology.* 2013;269:594–602.
73. Alexander GR. A retrospective review comparing the treatment outcomes of emergency lung resection for massive haemoptysis with and without preoperative bronchial artery embolization. *Eur J Cardiothorac Surg.* 2014;45:251–255.
74. Hwang HG, Lee HS, Choi JS, et al. Risk factors influencing rebleeding after bronchial artery embolization on the management of hemoptysis associated with pulmonary tuberculosis. *Tuberc Respir Dis (Seoul).* 2013;74:111–119.
75. Yoo DH, Yoon CJ, Kang SG, et al. Bronchial and nonbronchial systemic artery embolization in patients with major hemoptysis: safety and efficacy of N-butyl cyanoacrylate. *AJR Am J Roentgenol.* 2011;196:W199–W204.
76. Kokkonouzis I, Athanasopoulos I, Doulgerakis N, et al. Fatal hemoptysis due to chronic cavitary pulmonary aspergillosis complicated by nontuberculous mycobacterial tuberculosis. *Case Rep Infect Dis.* 2011;2011:837146.

77. Fujita T, Tanabe M, Moritani K, et al. Immediate and late outcomes of bronchial and systemic artery embolization for palliative treatment of patients with nonsmall-cell lung cancer having hemoptysis [published online ahead of print August 5, 2013]. *Am J Hosp Palliat Care.*
78. Wong ML, Szkup P, Hopley MJ. Percutaneous embolotherapy for life-threatening hemoptysis. *Chest.* 2002;121:95–102.
79. Lopez JK, Lee HY. Bronchial embolization for treatment life-threatening hemoptysis. *Semin Intervent Radiol.* 2006;23:223–229.
80. Mesurolle B, Lacombe P, Qanadli S, et al. Angiographic identification of spinal cord arteries before bronchial artery embolization [in French]. *J Radiol.* 1997;78:377–380.
81. Liu SF, Lee TY, Wong SL, et al. Transient cortical blindness: a complication of bronchial artery embolization. *Respir Med.* 1998;92:983–986.
82. Laborda A, Tejero C, Fredes A, et al. Posterior circulation stroke after bronchial artery embolization. A rare but serious complication. *Cardiovasc Intervent Radiol.* 2013;36:1006–1014.
83. Munk PL, Morris C, Nelems B. Left main bronchialesophageal fistula: a complication of bronchial artery embolization. *Cardiovasc Intervent Radiol.* 1990;13:95–97.
84. Remy-Jardin M, Wattinne L, Remy J. Transcatheter occlusion of pulmonary arterial circulation and collateral supply: failures, incidents, and complications. *Radiology.* 1991;180:699–705.

19

Pulmonary Arteriovenous Fistulas

Mary E. Meek • James C. Meek

A pulmonary arteriovenous fistula (PAVF) is a direct connection between a pulmonary artery and pulmonary vein. These high-flow, low pressure, thin-walled fistulae are commonly called *pulmonary arteriovenous malformations* (PAVMs). Complications of untreated PAVFs are related to the right-to-left shunt. Patients may present with hypoxia, exercise intolerance (59%), stroke/transient ischemic attack (TIA) (30%), brain abscess (9%), or hemoptysis (3%).[1] Massive hemoptysis and/or hemothorax occurs in fewer than 8% of patients.[2] Enlargement and rupture of the PAVF occurs more commonly in times of increased cardiac output and hormonal surges such as pregnancy.[3,4] Migraines are present in up to 46% of patients with PAVFs.[1]

Acquired PAVFs occur in hepatopulmonary syndrome and in patients with Glenn or Fontan shunts, malignancy, trauma, amyloidosis, and erosion from Rasmussen aneurysms. Most (>90%) congenital PAVFs are associated with hereditary hemorrhagic telangiectasia (HHT) or an HHT-like disorder.[1] PAVFs are commonly seen in HHT, previously known as *Rendu-Osler-Weber syndrome*. HHT is an autosomal dominant disorder characterized by epistaxis, telangiectasias (commonly on the lips, nose, and fingers), and AVMs (PAVFs, brain, gastrointestinal [GI] tract). A diagnosis of HHT is made based on the Curacao criteria (Table 19.1) or by genetic testing.[5]

Genetic defects associated with HHT and HHT-like syndromes are related to the transforming growth factor beta (TGF-β) pathway. Three mutations have been identified: endoglin (ENG), activin A receptor type II like 1 (ACVRL1 or ALK1), and SMAD4. The ENG mutation is associated with a higher incidence of PAVF and cerebral AVM than the ALK1 mutation.[6] A new genetic mutation in BMP9 has recently been identified in patients with an HHT-like syndrome.[7]

Workup for PAVF is required in all patients with HHT, hypoxia of unknown origin, or evidence of a right-to-left shunt such as a young patient with a brain abscess. Patients may experience orthodeoxia, which is a decrease in oxygen saturation when standing. The workup starts with an Echo–bubble study. Delayed appearance of bubbles in the left heart indicates an extracardiac shunt. If the Echo–bubble study is positive, we proceed with a noncontrast chest computed tomography (CT). Contrast is not necessary for the chest CT. It increases the radiation dose and serves as a risk for intravenous air embolus. The 1-mm axial images should be carefully reviewed to identify any abnormal connection between a pulmonary artery and pulmonary vein. Coronal and sagittal reconstructions can also be helpful.

Due to the need for continuous long-term follow-up, not only of PAVFs but also of the other vascular malformations associated with HHT, we and many other experienced interventionalists believe that these patients should be treated at an HHT Center of Excellence. However, patients will present outside of HHT Centers of Excellence with emergent indications for embolization of their PAVF such as hemoptysis, hemothorax, or brain abscess. It is beyond the scope of this text to discuss the entire workup and management of an HHT patient.[8] Our goal is to provide a basic guide to performing PAVF embolization with the current embolic technology available.

Table 19.1 Curacao Criteria for Hereditary Hemorrhagic Telangiectasia Diagnosis

AVMs	Common: pulmonary, hepatic, cerebral, spinal, GI telangiectasias
Cutaneous telangiectasias	Common: fingertips, nose, lips, tongue
Epistaxis	More than one spontaneous episode, particularly at night
Family history	First-degree relative who meets these criteria

A definite diagnosis is made when three out of the four criteria are present. A probable diagnosis of HHT is made when only two criteria are present. AVMs, arteriovenous malformations; GI, gastrointestinal.

DEVICE/MATERIAL DESCRIPTION

Table 19.2 Commonly Used Embolic Devices

Embolic Device	Pros	Cons
Bentson wire (Cook Medical) (Figs. 19.1–19.3) 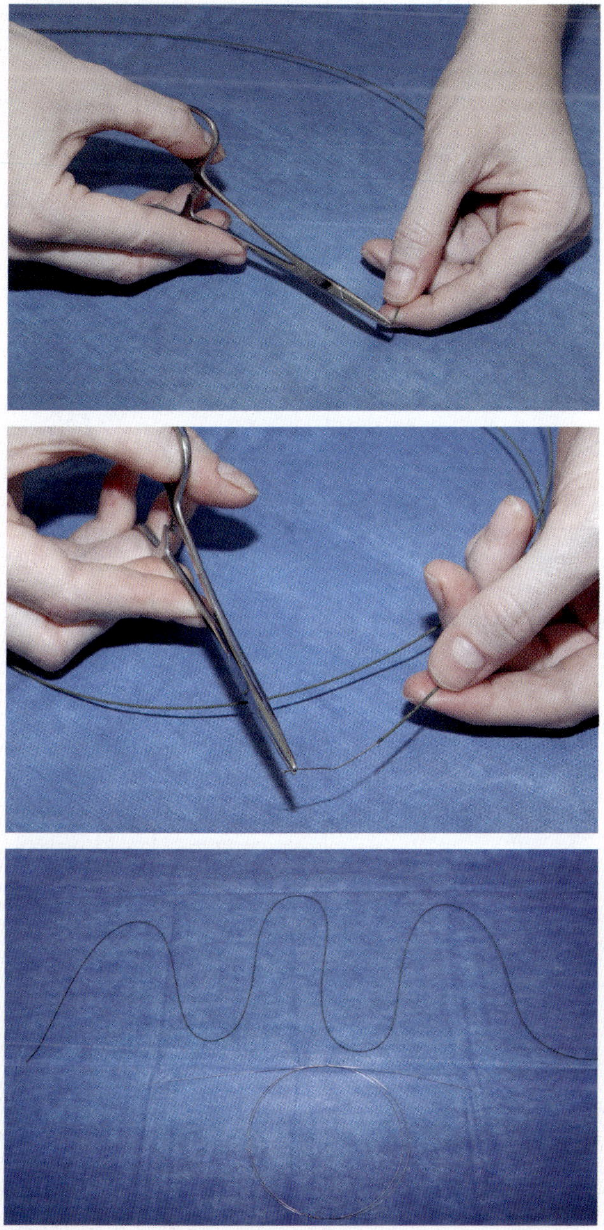 **Figure 19.1–19.3** A Bentson wire can be separated into its two components, the outer portion of which can be used as a coil. Take the back end of the wire and bend it with hemostats until the inner stainless steel core wire is loosened from the outer portion. Strip the soft outer portion away and use a pushable coil. This is off-label and mainly for historical review, but this economical technique can be used when supplies are limited and a large space needs to be filled.	Long lengths, good "filler," low cost	Not a true coil

Continued

Table 19.2 Commonly Used Embolic Devices *(continued)*

Embolic Device	Pros	Cons
Amplatzer Vascular Plug II (St. Jude Medical) (Fig. 19.4) 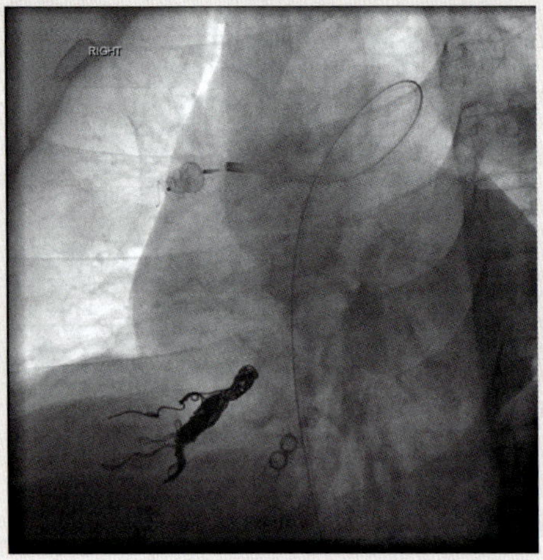 **Figure 19.4** This lesion was reembolized with an AVP II device.	Large diameters (3–22 mm), fast placement, truly detachable	Need large guide catheter (6-Fr to 9-Fr), high cost
Amplatzer Vascular Plug 4 (St. Jude Medical) (Fig. 19.5) 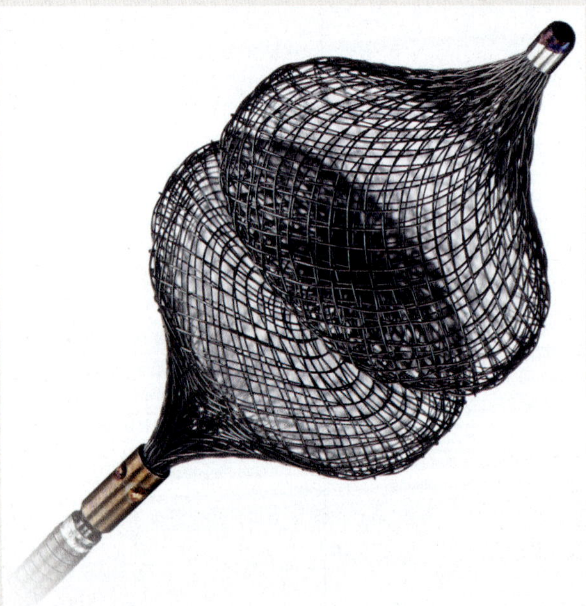 **Figure 19.5** Amplatzer Vascular Plug 4. A device up to 8 mm in diameter will pass through a 0.038-in inner diameter catheter. (Courtesy of St. Jude Medical, Inc., St. Paul, Minnesota.)	Fast placement; truly detachable; can go through a 0.038-in inner diameter catheter, which includes the inner catheter of the White LuMax set	Smaller sizes (4–8 mm), high cost

Continued

Table 19.2 Commonly Used Embolic Devices *(continued)*

Embolic Device	Pros	Cons
Nester coils (Cook Medical) (Figs. 19.6 and 19.7) 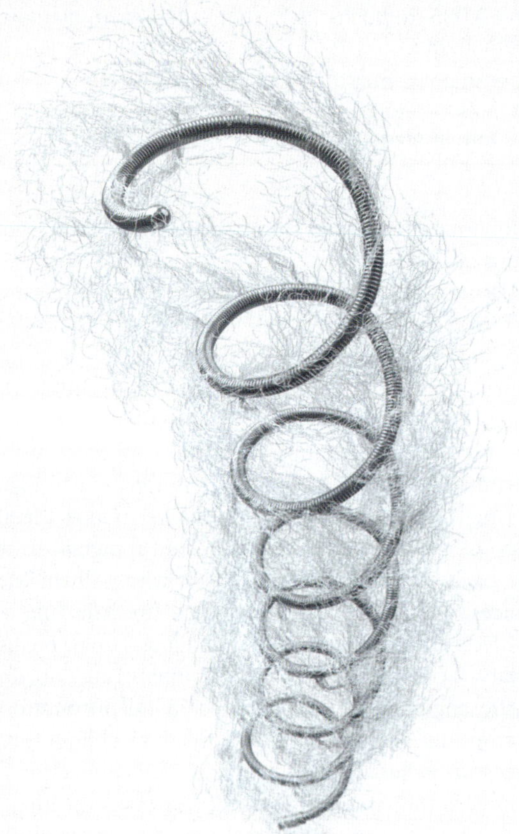 **Figure 19.6** Nester coil. Fibered platinum coil comes in 0.018-in and 0.035-in sizes. This is the "workhorse" of PAVF embolization. A new detachable 0.035-in version is available called the *Retracta*. (Courtesy of Cook Medical, Inc., Bloomington, Indiana.) 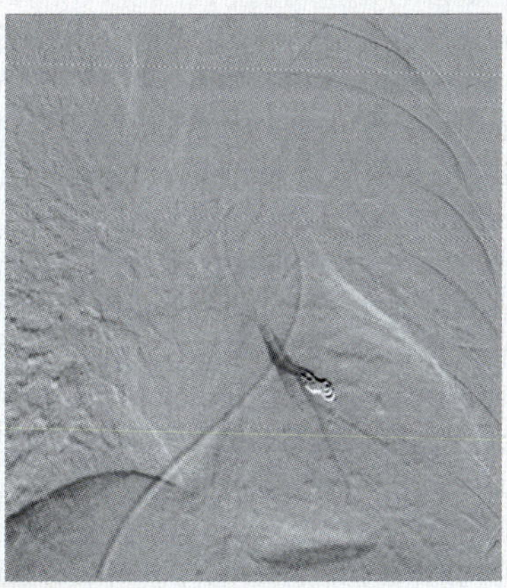 **Figure 19.7** Left PAVF embolized with Nester coils.	0.018-in and 0.035-in sizes, fibered so clot quickly, "go to" coil for PAVF	20 mm is maximum diameter, pushable, requires many coils to get a dense pack

Continued

Table 19.2 Commonly Used Embolic Devices *(continued)*

Embolic Device	Pros	Cons
Ruby Coils (Penumbra)	Very long lengths (up to 60 cm), truly detachable	0.020-in goes through larger microcatheter
Azur hydrogel (Terumo Medical)	0.018-in and 0.035-in, push-able and detachable	15 mm is maximum diameter, more costly than non-gel
Retracta coils (Cook Medical)	0.035-in fibered coils, truly detachable, sizes up to 20 cm long and 20 mm in diameter	Cost similar to AVPs

TECHNIQUE

Embolization for PAVF was first described by Porstmann[9] in 1977 and Taylor et al.[10] in 1978. Dr. White and colleagues[11] further refined the techniques, which led to the development of the White LuMax catheter system (Cook Medical, Inc., Bloomington, Indiana). Early on, coils and detachable balloons were used to close PAVFs. Detachable balloons are no longer available in the United States due to deflation and systemic embolization concerns. The techniques used today are not much different than those described by Dr. White, with the exception of improved embolic devices.[1,11,12] Our goal with adult patients is to embolize as many PAVFs in one outpatient setting as possible within the constraints of contrast load and radiation exposure.[13] In children, we embolize the PAVFs greater than 3 mm in size with the concern that embolization of smaller vessels in the developing lung will result in a "blocked path" to a PAVF that has recruited smaller feeders, making subsequent embolization more difficult.

Right heart and pulmonary artery pressures should be measured to evaluate cardiac physiology. Large right-to-left shunts can cause increased cardiac output and may lead to heart failure. Rarely, pulmonary hypertension (even with PAVFs) may be present. This is felt to be related to the TGF-β family of receptors.[14] If pulmonary hypertension is present, evaluation for a left-to-right shunt, such as in the liver, should be performed.

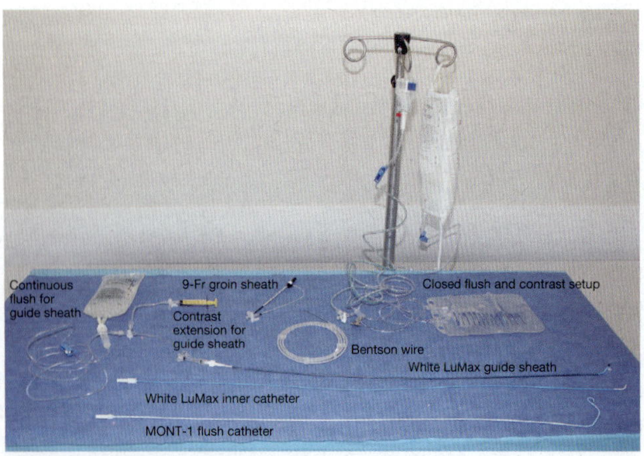

Figure 19.8 Commonly used equipment.

PAVFs represent a right-to-left shunt; therefore, careful attention to technique is critical. Setup should be similar to neuroangiography cases with in-line air filters, continuous flush lines, a closed system for contrast, and double flush technique (Fig. 19.8).

We use a standard right femoral vein approach using a 7-Fr introducer sheath. A diagnostic pulmonary arteriogram is performed with a 7-Fr MONT-1 catheter (Cook Medical, Inc., Bloomington, Indiana). Alternatively, a pigtail catheter over the back end of a shaped Bentson wire (Allwin Medical Devices, Anaheim, California) or a tip-deflecting wire (Cook Medical, Inc., Bloomington, Indiana) may be used. Pulmonary artery pressure measurements are obtained. Diagnostic angiography is performed in full inspiration in the anteroposterior view and the ipsilateral oblique (40 to 60 degrees; we generally use 40 degrees). This projection may seem counterintuitive as it projects the heart over the lung, but this view is best for spreading out the basilar segments where most PAVFs occur. Contrast injection rates range from 20 to 50 mL at 10 to 25 mL per second depending on the size of the pulmonary arteries, size of PAVFs, and presence of pulmonary hypertension. A frame rate of at least six frames per second should be used. It is important to include deep into the lung bases in the field of view as most PAVFs occur in the bases. Each segmental artery should be carefully followed to evaluate for the fistulous connection. A PAVF looks like a long continuation of the pulmonary artery into the pulmonary vein (Fig. 19.9). Frequently, there is an aneurysmal component at the site of the fistula (Fig. 19.10). The feeding vessel is measured. The standard teaching is that anything larger than 3 mm should be embolized. However, typically, the HHT Centers of Excellence use the technique that embolizes as many PAVFs in one setting as possible in the adult patient even sizes smaller than 3 mm as there are reports of embolic events in PAVFs measuring below the 3-mm "standard."[13–15] Over a 260 cm 0.035-in stiff Amplatzer wire, the diagnostic catheter is exchanged for a White LuMax set, which comes in two sizes: 7-Fr or 8-Fr guide catheter with a coaxial angled tip inner catheter. At this point, the patient should receive a bolus of intravenous heparin (~40 IU/kg). The pulmonary artery lower segments are generally easily accessed by "flopping" the Bentson wire down

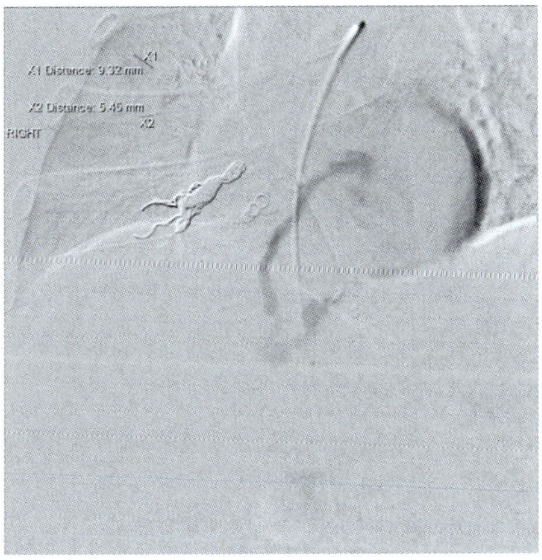

Figure 19.9 Right lower lobe PAVF appears as a long continuation of the pulmonary artery into the pulmonary vein. The irregular and "ragged" appearance of this PAVF is evidence of recent hemorrhage.

into the basilar segment. A hydrophilic angle tip wire such as a Glidewire (Terumo Medical Corporation, Somerset, New Jersey) may facilitate selection of the feeding vessel but should be used with care as dissection can occur. The middle and upper segments are more challenging to cannulate and may require a more sharply angled catheter such as a Judkins right coronary catheter (Cordis) or a left internal mammary catheter.

Detachable Amplatzer Vascular Plugs (AVPs) (St. Jude Medical, Inc., St. Paul, Minnesota) and pushable Nester 0.035-in coils (Cook Medical, Inc., Bloomington, Indiana) are our embolic devices of choice (Figs. 19.5 and 19.6, respectively). Coils and AVPs should be oversized by 20%. The coils should be densely packed and placed as close the fistulous sac as possible, ideally within 1 cm.[16] There are some who believe that packing the aneurysmal fistulous sac has a lower recanalization rate.[17]

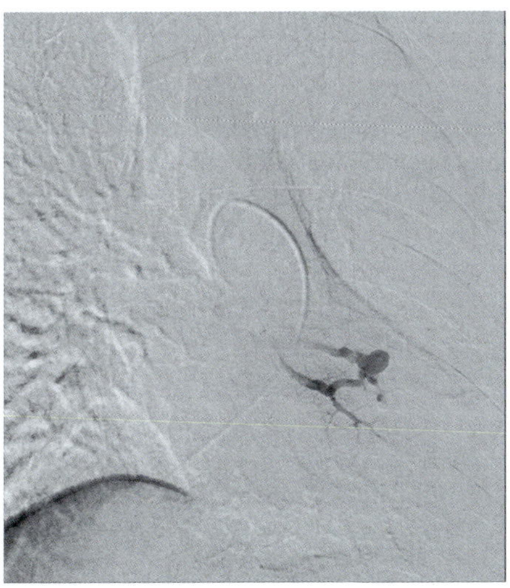

Figure 19.10 Left PAVF with aneurysmal component.

This has yet to be well established in the literature. Occasionally, microcatheters may be needed to deliver 0.018-in coils in a precise location.[18] Many different microcoils are available—both pushable and detachable forms. The anchor technique is used when there is concern about a coil passing through the PAVF and ending up in the systemic circulation. This involves "anchoring" the first loop of the coil into a small side branch of the pulmonary artery that is feeding the PAVF.[1] Alternatively, a large detachable coil may be used as a scaffold to provide stability for placement of more economical pushable coils.

A noncontrast chest CT should be performed 6 months following embolization to evaluate for any residual PAVF patency. The draining vein and aneurysmal sac should disappear or be reduced by 70%. Any reappearance of the draining vein or aneurysmal sac on future follow-up studies performed every 3 to 5 years indicates recanalization. Reperfusion of a previously embolized PAVF is reported about 7% of the time (Fig. 19.11). Causes include not packing the coils densely enough, an accessory vessel that was not embolized, reperfusion from a collateral pulmonary artery vessel, and reperfusion of a collateral bronchial artery vessel. The significance of these recanalized PAVFs is unknown. Some believe that the risk of embolus from these previously treated lesions is less because the coil pack may act as a "filter" and the flow through these lesions is slower. At our institution, we err on the side of caution and reembolize the recanalized PAVFs.

Follow-up chest CT may also reveal the presence of "new" PAVFs, which may or may not be symptomatic. These lesions were likely present on previous studies or were microscopic and have enlarged over time. All accessible lesions greater than 3 mm in diameter should be treated.[11,12]

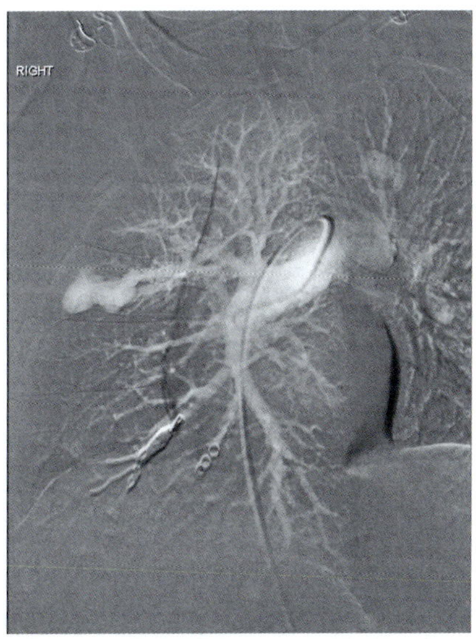

Figure 19.11 Recanalized right middle lobe PAVF 15 years after it was first embolized with only one coil at an outside hospital. The "inverted" contrast image is how we prefer to review the angiographies.

PAVFs are classified as simple or complex.[19] Most (85%) AVFs are classified as simple, meaning that the malformation arises from one or more arteries within a single pulmonary segment. Up to 10% of lesions are considered complex with arterial vessels arising from more than one pulmonary segment, whereas 5% or fewer have involvement of multiple lobes. These are considered diffuse and outcomes in these patients are worse. Pulmonary flow redistribution has been used with some success. This involves the lobar occlusion of pulmonary artery feeding the diffusely involved lobe.[20,21] Lung transplantation, with or without cardiac transplantation depending on presence of high-output heart failure, has been reported for diffuse PAVFs.[22]

POTENTIAL COMPLICATIONS

Patients should be evaluated with a preoperative electrocardiogram (ECG) to look for left bundle branch block (LBBB). Passing the catheters through the heart can induce a right bundle branch block. In a patient with a preexisting LBBB, total heart block can ensue.

Air embolism occurs less than 5% of the time but should always be a concern. Due to its anterior origin, the right coronary artery may be unintentionally embolized with air bubbles or clot causing angina or ECG changes, which can be treated with sublingual nitroglycerin and atropine for bradycardia. Rarely, TIAs may occur. The reported complication rate including angina and TIA is less than 2%. Pleurisy is a common postprocedural complaint (12%). This is treated with anti-inflammatory medication. Rarely, severe, delayed pleurisy occurs.

Coil migration into the systemic arteries has been reported along with successful snare retrieval.[19,23] If this happens, immediately bolus the patient with intravenous heparin for a target activated clotting time near 250 seconds. Proceed with arterial access and retrieval of the embolized coil.

CONCLUSION

Embolization of a PAVF can be technically challenging. Careful attention to preprocedure imaging, high-quality angiography, meticulous technique, and a good knowledge of embolic agents are keys to success.

TIPS AND TRICKS

Angiography

- Use a 2-s injection of 10–25 mL of iodine contrast.
- Use the ipsilateral oblique (40–60 degrees) to spread the basilar pulmonary artery segments.
- The flush catheter typically enters the left pulmonary artery. Curve the back end of a Bentson wire to facilitate steering the MONT-1 catheter to the right side.
- Carefully review your pulmonary angiogram on the workstation. Avoid "search satisfaction" by following each segmental artery out the entire length. Many patients will have multiple PAVFs.
- Invert the contrast image (so it appears white) to better see the PAVFs when reviewing your angiography (Fig. 19.11).
- Do not oversedate the patient as snoring/deep inspiration causes significant motion and may dislodge your carefully placed catheter.

Accessing the Lesion

- Commonly used wires: 0.035-in Rosen (Cook Medical, Inc., Bloomington, Indiana) or 0.035-in stiff Amplatzer for exchanging the MONT-1 for the White LuMax set, Bentson for flopping into basilar segments, semicurved 0.035-in hydrophilic Glidewire (Terumo Medical Corporation, Somerset, New Jersey) for selecting more difficult branches in the upper and middle lobes.
- Use a Judkins right coronary catheter or a left internal mammary catheter to select upper and middle lobe branches.
- If you need to place an AVP II more distally than your Lumax guide will go, you can place a 6-Fr 100-cm Envoy guide catheter (Codman & Shurtleff, Inc., Raynham, Massachusetts), which will allow you to place up to a 12-mm AVP II plug.
- Prowler Plus (Codman & Shurtleff, Inc., Raynham, Massachusetts) is our microcatheter of choice because it has a 0.021-in inner diameter, which allows for placement of pushable 0.018-in Nesters as well as many detachable coils. The Ruby Coils (Penumbra, Inc., Alameda, California) require a larger diameter microcatheter.

Embolization

- Densely pack the coils as close to the fistula as possible (<1 cm).
- We most commonly use AVP II, AVP 4, and Nester coils.
- We do not use the first-generation AVP device due to recanalization concerns.
- A single detachable coil or AVP can be used as a scaffold for the placement of pushable coils to obtain tight packing with reduced cost.
- Anchor technique: place the first portion of a pushable coil into a distal side branch to prevent distal migration of the coil.
- Wait 5 min after placement of device to assess thrombosis.
- Oversize coils and AVPs by at least 20%. Some interventionalists consider using longer coils (with 20%–30% oversize) and oversize the AVP between 30% and 50% in larger and high-flow PAVF.
- Do not use particles or liquids due to the high-flow right-to-left shunt.

REFERENCES

1. Pollack JS, Saluja S, Thabet A, et al. Clinical and anatomic outcomes after embolotherapy of pulmonary arteriovenous malformations. *J Vasc Interv Radiol.* 2006;17:35–45.
2. Ference BA, Shannon TM, White RI, et al. Life-threatening pulmonary hemorrhage with pulmonary arteriovenous malformations and hereditary hemorrhagic telangiectasia. *Chest.* 1994;106(5):1387–1390.
3. Shovlin C, Sodhi V, McCarthy A, et al. Estimates of maternal risks of pregnancy for women with hereditary hemorrhagic telangiectasia (Osler-Weber-Rendu syndrome): suggested approach for obstetric services. *BJOG.* 2008;115:1108–1115.
4. De Gussem EM, Lausman AY, Beder AJ, et al. Outcomes of pregnancy in women with hereditary hemorrhagic telangiectasia. *Obstet Gynecol.* 2014;123:514–520.
5. Shovlin CL, Guttmacher AI, Buscarini E, et al. Diagnostic criteria for hereditary hemorrhagic telangiectasia (Rendu-Osler-Weber syndrome). *Am J Med Genet.* 2000;91(1): 66–67.
6. Sabba C, Pasculli G, Lenato GM, et al. Hereditary hemorrhagic telangiectasia: clinical features in ENG and ALK1 mutation carriers. *J Thromb Haemost.* 2007;5:1149–1157.
7. Wooderchak-Donahue WL, McDonald J, O'Fallon B, et al. BMP9 mutations cause a vascular-anomaly syndrome with phenotypic overlap with hereditary hemorrhagic telangiectasia. *Am J Hum Genet.* 2013;93:530–537.
8. Faughnan ME, Palda VA, Garcia-Tsao G, et al. International guidelines for the diagnosis and management of hereditary hemorrhagic telangiectasia. *J Med Genet.* 2011;48: 73–87.
9. Porstmann W. Therapeutic embolization of arteriovenous pulmonary fistula by catheter technique. In: Kelop O, ed. *Current Concepts in Pediatric Radiology.* Berlin, Germany: Springer; 1977:23–31.
10. Taylor BG, Cockerill EM, Manfredi F, et al. Therapeutic embolization of the pulmonary artery in pulmonary arteriovenous fistula. *Am J Med.* 1978;54:360–365.
11. White RI, Lynch-Nyhan A, Terry P, et al. Pulmonary arteriovenous malformations: techniques and long-term outcome of embolotherapy. *Radiology.* 1988;169:663–669.
12. Trerotola SO, Pyeritz RE. PAVM embolization: an update. *Am J Radiol.* 2010;195:837–845.
13. Trerotola SO, Pyeritz RE, Bernhardt BA. Outpatient single-session pulmonary arteriovenous malformation embolization. *J Vasc Interv Radiol.* 2009;20:1287–1291.
14. Trembath RC, Thomson JR, Machado RD, et al. Clinical and molecular genetic features of pulmonary hypertension in patients with hereditary hemorrhagic telangiectasia. *N Engl J Med.* 2011;345:325–334.
15. Todo K, Moriwaki H, Higashi M, et al. A small pulmonary arteriovenous malformation as a cause of recurrent brain embolism. *Am J Neuroradiol.* 2004;25:428–430.
16. Pollack JS, White RI. Distal cross-sectional occlusion is the "key" to treating pulmonary arteriovenous malformations. *J Vasc Interv Radiol.* 2012;23:1578–1580.
17. Hayashi S, Baba Y, Senokuchi T, et al. Efficacy of venous sac embolization for pulmonary arteriovenous malformations: comparison with feeding artery embolization. *J Vasc Interv Radiol.* 2012;23:1566–1577.
18. Dinkel HP, Triller J. Pulmonary arteriovenous malformations: embolotherapy with superselective coaxial catheter placement and filling of venous sac with Guglielmi detachable coils. *Radiology.* 2002;223(3):709–714.
19. White RI, Pollack JS, Wirth JA. Pulmonary arteriovenous malformations: diagnosis and transcatheter embolotherapy. *J Vasc Interv Radiol.* 1996;7(6):787–804.
20. Faughnan ME, Lui YW, Wirth JA, et al. Diffuse pulmonary arteriovenous malformations: characteristics and prognosis. *Chest.* 2000;11:31–38.
21. Wei CW, Faughnan ME, Menard A, et al. Lobar embolization of diffuse pulmonary arteriovenous malformations in hereditary hemorrhagic telangiectasia: a case report. *J Vasc Interv Radiol.* 2010;21:1105–1108.
22. Fukushima H, Mitsuhashi T, Oto T, et al. Successful lung transplantation in a case with diffuse pulmonary arteriovenous malformations and hereditary hemorrhagic telangiectasia. *Am J Transplant.* 2013;13:3278–3281.
23. Gupta P, Mordin C, Curtis J, et al. Pulmonary arteriovenous malformations: effect of embolization on right-to-left shunt, hypoxemia, and exercise tolerance in 66 patients. *AJR Am J Roentgenol.* 2002;179(2):347–355.

20

Chest Tumors

Shinichi Hori

BACKGROUND

Lung and Mediastinal Malignancy Treatment

Treatment of patients with advanced lung cancer or metastatic lung tumor, usually with serious symptoms such as respiratory distress, pain, or vascular stenosis of the superior vena cava or pulmonary artery, is often attempted. Options commonly taken are palliative radiotherapy or systemic chemotherapy. However, results suggest that these therapies give little benefit. In the case of palliative radiotherapy, the results are indeterminate and any improvement takes a long time to appear. Systemic chemotherapy is often applied despite a history of poor results and serious systemic side effects. Even if these therapies are at first effective, the new lesions created soon cause problems. It is evident that more effective treatment is needed, with fewer ensuing complications.

A new and promising treatment is selective chemoembolization of lung and mediastinal malignancy. Selective catheterization technique of the bronchial artery has shown by Neyazaki et al.[1] in 1969: that blood supply to the primary lung cancer as well as to metastatic pulmonary malignancies has been provided mainly by the bronchial artery. This discovery has been followed up with the following study results. Preoperative induction chemotherapy using bronchial arterial infusion was reported to be effective.[2] Bronchial artery infusion therapy combined with radiotherapy improved the prognosis of locally advanced lung cancer.[3] Bronchial artery infusion for lung cancer was reported to be effective in a study with a small number of patients.[4]

In pathologic situations, the systemic arteries can penetrate into the lung and mediastinum and irrigate neoplastic lesions. Hemoptysis caused by bleeding from the bronchial artery, which shares systemic pressure, is well controlled by the bronchial artery embolization.[5] In another study, the bronchial artery embolization for hemoptysis caused by lung cancer was effective to control bleeding with limited complications.[6,7]

The treatment of specific lesions in the thoracic cage, the mediastinum, and the lung field is now possible due to recent advances in diagnostic apparatus such as the three-dimensional (3-D) computed tomography (CT) scanner to digital angiography and to therapeutic techniques using microcatheters.

In this new approach, selective arterial infusion of antineoplastic agents concentrates the drugs in the target lesion and reduces systemic exposure.[4] Embolization after the infusion helps retention of the drug by inhibiting flushing out by the arterial flow. Selective embolization using new spherical embolic materials does not cause the usual tissue damage because of reduced local irritability. Well-calibrated spherical material will allow controlling the occlusion level, which further avoids usual tissue damage. Arterial blockage may induce necrosis of tumor tissue in some cases. This selective chemoembolization of lung and mediastinal malignancy is a promising treatment procedure for patients who are suffering from various symptoms, such as severe cough or respiratory distress, caused by advanced cancer.

Local Breast Cancer Recurrence and Chest Wall Metastases

Difficult problems for patients are lesions in the chest wall or operated breast after the standard therapy for breast cancer. Patients may see the lesions and or identify them by touch. Usually, they cause intolerable pain, massive bleeding, and infection and seriously restrain the patient's activity. They may invade the mediastinum or form nodular lesions in the lung. Sometimes, surgical resection is necessary to improve symptoms, but it is usually ineffective.[8,9]

A recent advance that has the potential to control tumor growth and active bleeding has been the efficient transarterial administration of drugs (anthracycline, cisplatin, docetaxel) with embolic material. Currently, greater precision is provided during the treatment of individual lesions due to relatively recent advances in angiography, such as superselective microcatheterization and calibrated microspheres.

DEVICES AND MATERIALS

Catheter System

A 4-Fr guiding catheter system is adequate for a transfemoral or transbrachial approach. A Cobra catheter (Terumo, Tokyo) is the first choice for femoral access with less risk of intimal dissection of the aortic wall or occlusion of the bronchial arteries. The Michelson's shape or Shepherd hook type (Terumo, Tokyo) should be the second choice because they provide (higher) risk of intimal damage or temporary occlusion of the orifice of the bronchial artery. A coaxial microcatheter is mandatory for safe and selective catheter insertion. It is extremely important to avoid spasm or temporary occlusion of the bronchial artery. The maintenance of free antegrade flow through the blood vessels is key for effective embolization using flow-directed spherical embolic material.

The use of microcatheters is of particular importance when embolizing the right intercostobronchial trunk. Exclusive superselective catheterization of its bronchial branch will avoid potential occlusion of intercostal branches, which may supply the anterior spinal artery.[10] The embolization of the anterior spinal artery is associated with paraplegia.

Antineoplastic Agent

Different kinds of antineoplastic agents are necessary. Necrotic effects or tumor shrinkage in the mediastinal or pulmonary tumor cannot be expected by embolization alone. The anticancer drugs and their combination are selected according the tumor types or patients' treatment history or allergic reaction. Cisplatin, docetaxel, fluorouracil, anthracycline, or their combination is usually used for primary lung cancer. The total dose of antineoplastic agent can be reduced with selective tumor chemoembolization compared to systemic chemotherapy. We typically perform three sessions on average of chemoembolization.

Embolic Material

The spherical embolic material is the only option among the microparticles. Embolic materials that may cause proximal or permanent occlusion are not recommended. Polyvinyl alcohol (PVA) is not suitable because of the tendency of proximal occlusion. Glue is not suitable due to permanent occlusion. Liquid material such as Lipiodol[11] is potentially dangerous for normal tissue (skin necrosis or damage). Metallic coils will close the arterial access and make it impossible for the sequential procedures, which are always necessary. HepaSphere (QuadraSphere; Merit Medical Systems, Inc., South Jordan, Utah), Embosphere (Merit Medical Systems, Inc., South Jordan, Utah), Embozene (CeloNova BioSciences, Inc., San Antonio, Texas), and Bead Block (Biocompatibles UK Ltd., Farnham, Surrey, United Kingdom) are spherical embolic materials. HepaSphere seems suitable because of its low irritability. The preferable size is 50 to 100 μm in dry state. HepaSphere is an expansible microsphere. The rate of expansion depends on the sodium concentration of the solution. When it contacts with physiologic saline and nonionic contrast material, it becomes four times and six times larger, respectively. The HepaSphere microsphere mixed with the solution with 10% of sodium chloride and nonionic contrast material (1:4) is two times larger. Five milliliters of this solution is put into the 25 mg of vial 10 minutes before use. Further expansion of microsphere up to four times can be expected in the arterial occlusion point. It results in the tight occlusion of the vessel.

Calibrated microspheres seem to improve the efficacy in arterial occlusion at the point of tumor vasculature. Drug-eluting microspheres do not have enough record regarding safety or efficacy. There are no reports to use drug-eluting microspheres for extrahepatic lesions. Our clinical experience is also limited regarding the drug-eluting HepaSphere for mediastinal and chest wall lesions. The role of embolic material is not only for the ischemic effect but also as modulator of chemotherapeutic agents, which can then remain longer in the target lesion than with simple infusion. We are planning to do an animal study to confirm hypothesis. However, it is common to obtain better clinical result from the combination use of antineoplastic agents and microspheres than the solo infusion of drugs.

ANATOMY

Mediastinal Circulation

The main artery for mediastinal circulation is the bronchial artery. There are many variations of bronchial arterial branching from the aorta.[12] The details of the vascular anatomy are well described in the Chapter 18 ("Bronchial Artery Embolization" for hemoptysis management). Hilar lymph nodes and mediastinal tumors are generally supplied by this artery. Lung tumors are also fed by the bronchial artery.[1] The right bronchial artery usually shares a common trunk with the right upper intercostal artery.

The small branches of internal thoracic arteries on both sides may feed the anterior part of the mediastinum. The small branches from the costocervical and thyrocervical arteries may also feed the upper part of the mediastinum. A direct tiny branch from brachiocephalic or subclavian arteries to the mediastinum should also be considered.

The intercostal artery is important if a tumor invades the chest wall. Careful attention to the spinal cord is essential to avoid spinal arterial occlusion, especially when performing embolization of intercostal arteries in the T8–L2 vertebral bodies segment.

The inferior phrenic artery sometimes penetrates the diaphragm and feeds the inferior part of the mediastinum.

Although a thoracic aortogram is recommended to evaluate the branching of the bronchial arteries,[13] a 3-D analysis of dynamic CT with contrast is found to be more useful.

Most lung and mediastinal tumors, regardless of being primary or metastatic tumors, are seen as area of hypervascularity and neovascularity. Sometimes, the neoplastic lesion may show shunting of blood from the bronchial artery branches into pulmonary artery or pulmonary vein.[14]

Chest Wall Circulation

All branches from the subclavian artery, except for the vertebral artery, are involved with recurrent lesions in the chest wall, axillary nodes, and supraclavicular lymph node metastases. The intercostal arteries are potential feeders for chest wall lesions. Almost all chest neoplastic lesions, including lymph node metastases, are identified as hypervascular lesions compared to normal tissue.

TECHNIQUE

There is no specific angiographic technique for embolization of intrathoracic and chest wall malignancies. But compared to other organs, the diameter of their arterial feeders is generally smaller. Infusion and embolization should be done in state of free flow. For this reason, arterial spasm or intimal damage caused by catheterization should be avoided. Operator experience, careful manipulation of the arteries, and catheter insertion with a preshaped microcatheter without microguidewire may help decrease the incidence of complications. Other interventionalists prefer to carefully advance a microcatheter with a microguidewire coaxially through a 4-Fr to 5-Fr diagnostic catheter once the latter is in stable position at the aortic branch ostium (e.g., intercostobronchial or bronchial arteries).

CT examination during selective angiography is reliable for recognizing the anatomy of target arteries. Hybrid angiography suite–CT apparatus provides angiographic and CT examinations in the same room and at the same time, which helps our treatments from cost-effective standpoint. A cone-beam CT function of recent angiography suites may be helpful, but the diagnostic value is not good enough to evaluate tiny arterial supply. Multidirectional digital subtraction angiography (DSA) may also be useful to evaluate the arterial territory, but at the expenses of higher volume of contrast material and radiation dose.

Antineoplastic agents should slowly be infused to the target artery, avoiding backflow. A mixture with contrast material (1:1) is preferable to recognize the flow. Immediately after completion of infusion, embolization should be commenced. Embolic material should be mixed with contrast material to get good opacity to check the free flow state. The end point of embolization is not arterial occlusion but disappearance of tumor vasculature. Flow reduction observed on fluoroscopy during the injection of embolic material is a good sign that the embolization procedure is complete.

Bronchial artery embolization with drug infusion should be repeated (two or three times) to obtain a better local response and to promote a longer survival time.[1]

CLINICAL APPLICATIONS

The main purpose of transarterial treatment for the lung and mediastinal tumors is the reduction of tumor burden. Airway stenosis due to compression or stenosis caused by tumor or direct invasion may cause serious symptoms. The pulmonary hilum lymph node metastases or tumor invasion may result in bronchial stenosis, which may consequently cause insufficiency of sputum expectoration. It may evoke obstructive pneumonia or atelectasis (Fig. 20.1). Irritation of bronchial mucosa causes severe cough or hemosputum. When the tumors compress the trachea, patients complain of respiratory distress or suffocation (Figs. 20.2 and 20.3). Mediastinal invasion or lymph node metastases often cause compression of superior vena cava or pulmonary arteries (see Fig. 20.2). They are always life-limiting factors as bronchial airway stenosis. Reduction of tumor burden by the embolization combined with antineoplastic agents can be obtained as long as superselective administration of drug and embolization can be performed.

Bleeding from the tumor is also serious problem. There are no effective methods to get sufficient hemostasis from the tumor except for selective arterial embolization. The bleeding point can easily be recognized as extravasation or dense tumor vasculature on the DSA images (Fig. 20.4). Immediately after the embolization of bleeding point, complete hemostasis can be obtained.

In cases of local recurrence of breast cancer or chest wall invasion from lung cancer cases, bone destruction including rib, sternum, and spine (Fig. 20.5) is a frequent problem. It usually causes uncontrollable pain. Chemoembolizations can reduce pain probably due to control of excessive blood flow to the hypervascularized lesion.

POTENTIAL COMPLICATIONS

The contraindications for bronchial or nonbronchial artery embolization are the usual contraindications for angiography, including intractable coagulopathy, renal failure, and severe contrast allergy. In addition, the investigation of treatment history and allergic reactions to antineoplastic agents are important to avoid anaphylactic shock during treatment.

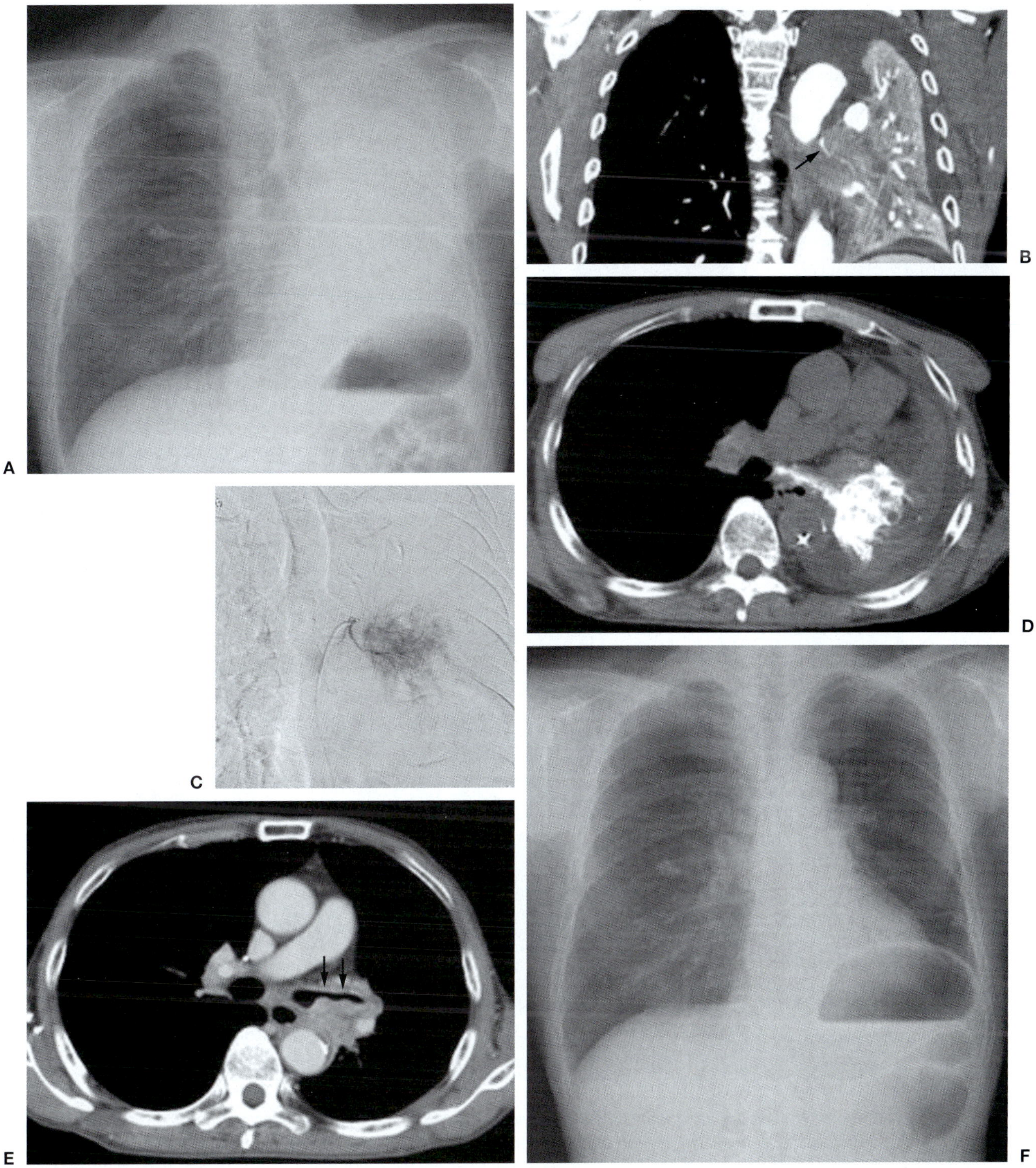

Figure 20.1 A 72-year-old man with non–small cell lung cancer (squamous cell carcinoma, cT4N3M0). **A:** Total collapse of the left lung was found following systemic chemotherapy treatment. He complained of respiratory distress and hemoptysis. **B:** CT coronal view showing a tumor, which was not clearly differentiated from the collapsed lung. The left bronchial artery (*arrow*) was visible at the center of the tumor. Infusion of cisplatin and fluorouracil followed by embolization using HepaSphere was carried out. **C:** Selective bronchial arteriography revealed a similar vascular structure and hypervascularized lesion corresponding to the CT image. **D:** CT scan during selective contrast infusion to the left bronchial artery. The markedly enhanced area corresponds to the tumor in the left hilum. Infusion of cisplatin and fluorouracil followed by embolization using HepaSphere was carried out. **E:** CT scan 1 month after bronchial infusion and embolization. Marked reduction of the hilar tumor and reopening of the left main bronchus (*arrows*) were clearly visible. **F:** Total collapse and mediastinal shift had disappeared in 2 months after treatment.

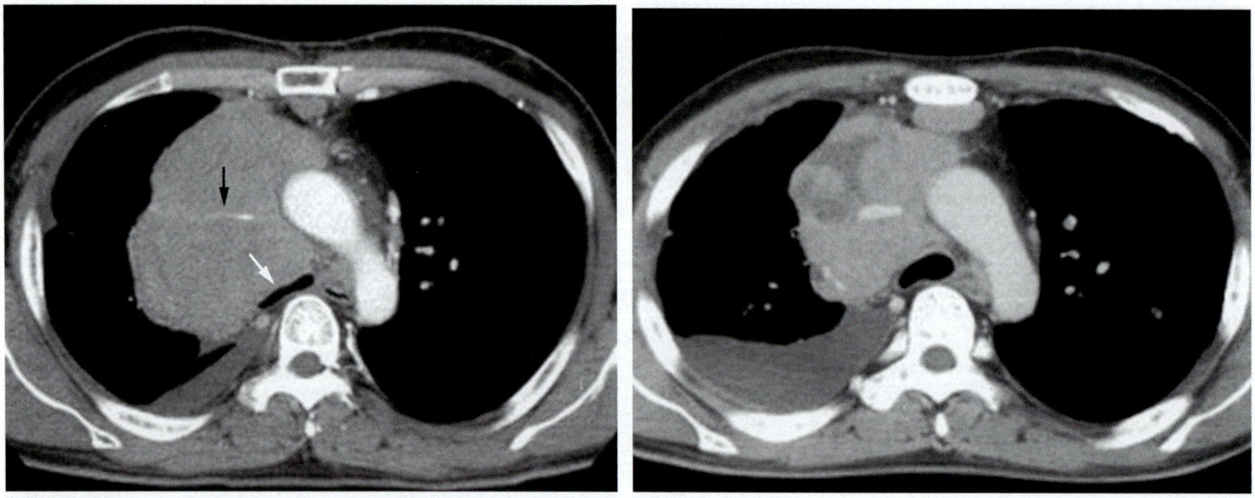

A B

Figure 20.2 A 40-year-old man with atypical carcinoid tumor in the mediastinum. **A:** Tumor compressed trachea (*white arrow*) and superior vena cava (*black arrow*). Both internal thoracic arteries, branches of the right costocervical artery, and two bronchial arteries were embolized with HepaSphere after infusion of cisplatin and fluorouracil. **B:** At 7 months, after four sessions. Marked improvement of vascular and airway compression were obtained due to a considerable reduction of the mediastinal tumor. Respiratory distress and superior vena cava syndrome are improved.

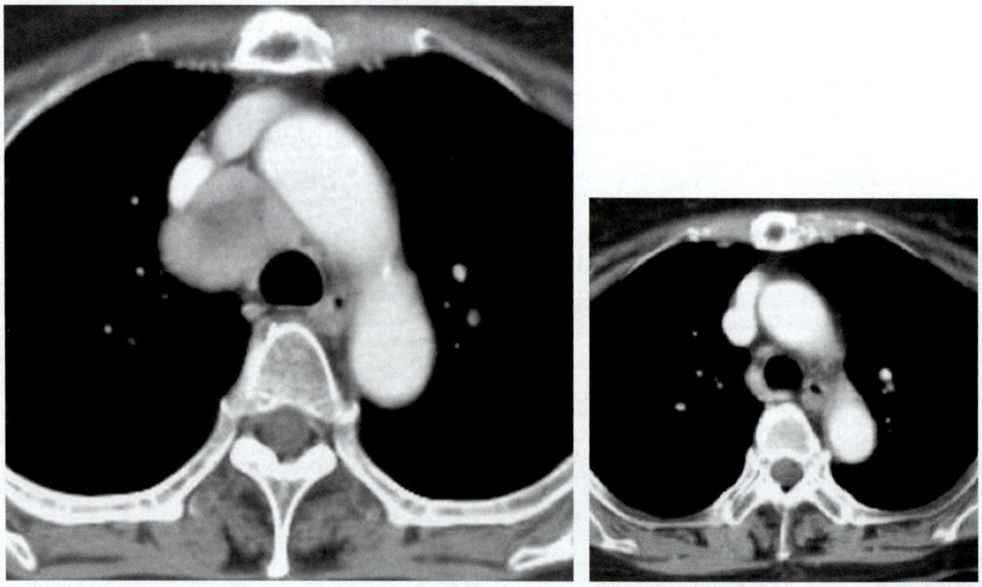

A B

Figure 20.3 A 62-year-old woman with mediastinal lymph node metastases of renal cell carcinoma. **A:** Pretracheal lymph node metastasis caused relocation of the superior vena cava. Patient complained of cough. The right bronchial artery and mediastinal branch of the right internal thoracic artery were embolized with HepaSphere without chemoinfusion. **B:** CT scan 8 years after treatment. Complete remission of the lymph node metastasis was obtained.

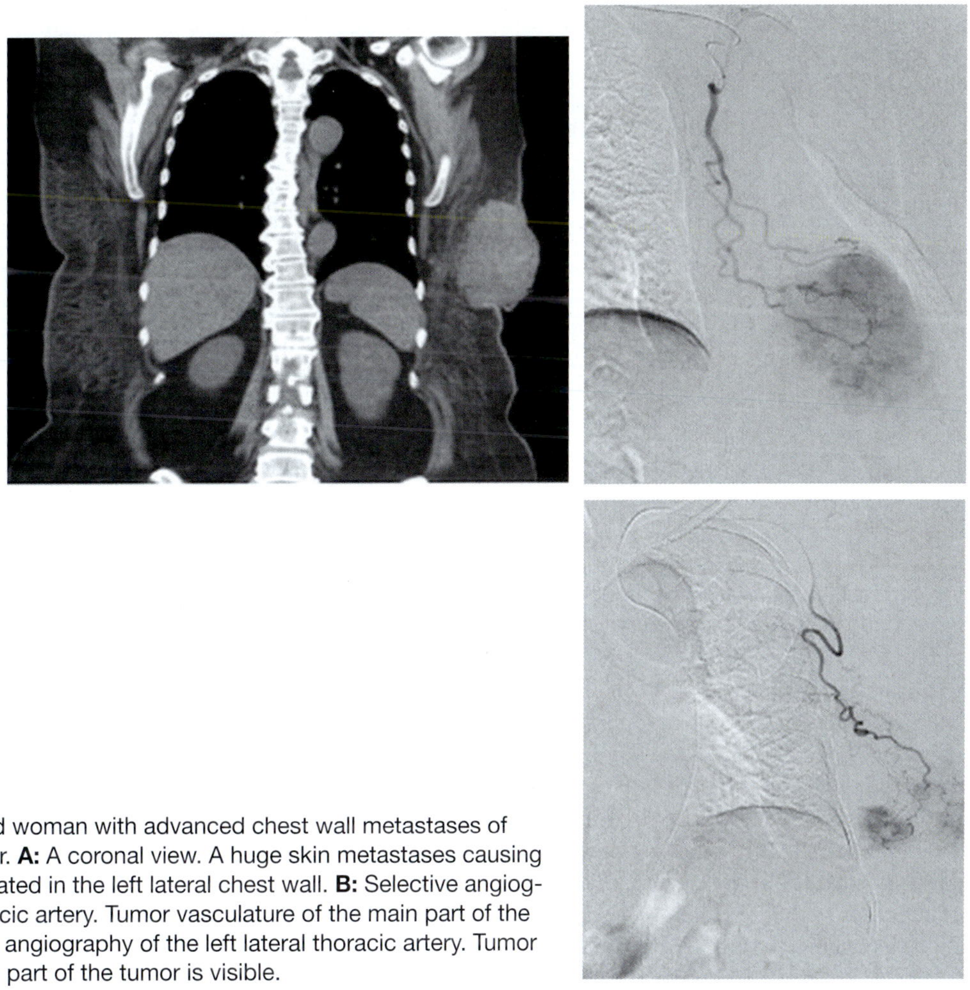

A B C

Figure 20.4 A 61-year-old woman with advanced chest wall metastases of breast cancer. **A:** A coronal view. A huge skin metastases causing bleeding and infection is located in the left lateral chest wall. **B:** Selective angiography of the left dorsal thoracic artery. Tumor vasculature of the main part of the tumor is visible. **C:** Selective angiography of the left lateral thoracic artery. Tumor vasculature of the peripheral part of the tumor is visible.

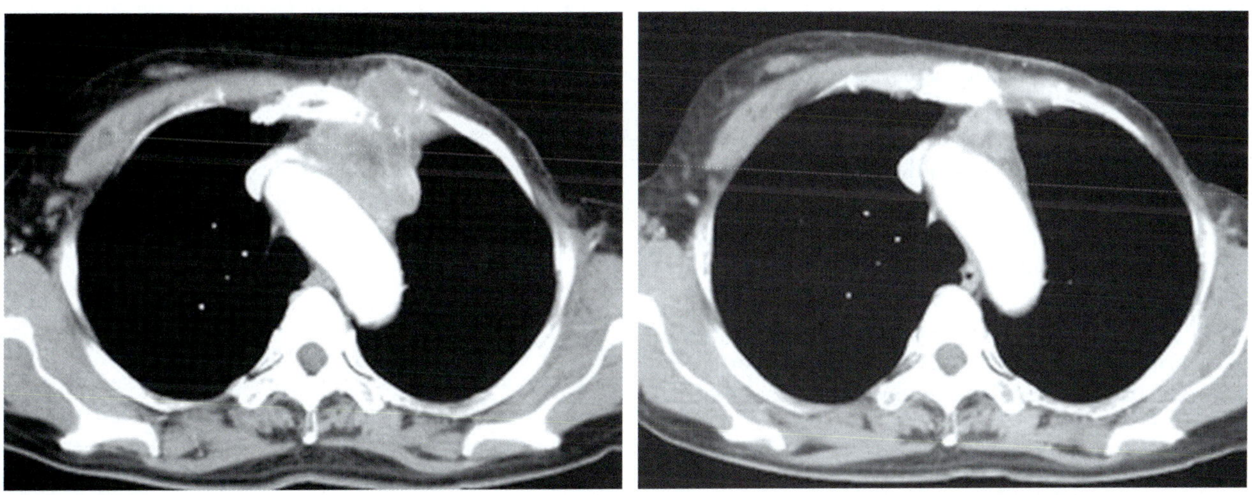

A B

Figure 20.5 A 60-year-old woman with chest wall recurrence of breast cancer. **A:** The tumor in the anterior chest wall invading mediastinum causes severe pain. Infusion of epirubicin and fluorouracil followed by embolization using HepaSphere was repeated three times in 2 months. **B:** CT scan in 3 months after three sessions of treatments. Reduction of tumor effectively relieved pain.

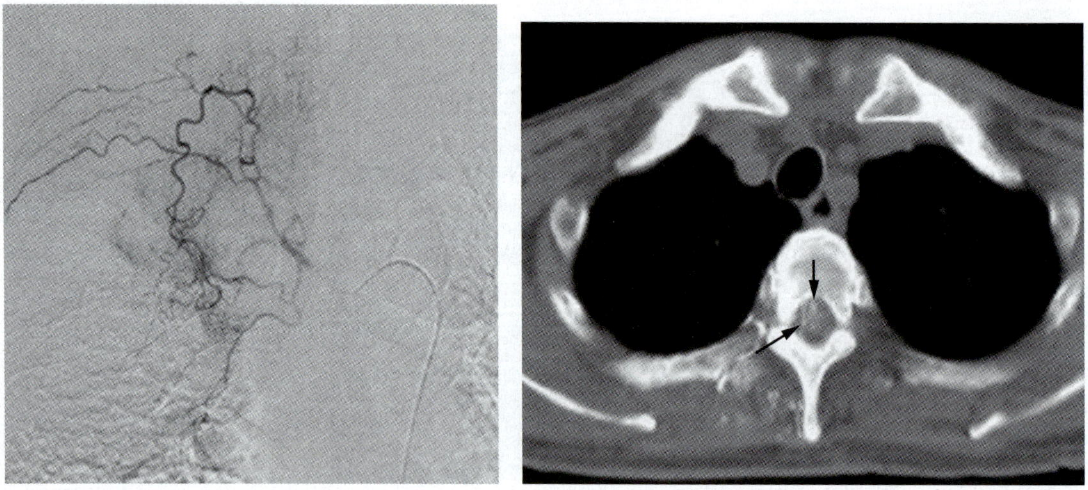

A B

Figure 20.6 A 64-year-old man with lung metastases of colon cancer. **A:** Angiography of common trunk of right intercostal and bronchial arteries. The spinal circulation system was not visible in this examination. **B:** CT scan during contrast infusion of the common trunk of the intercostal and bronchial artery. Both the anterior spinal artery (*short arrow*) and the posterior spinal artery (*long arrow*) were visible. Embolization was carried out in the right bronchial artery.

The spinal cord circulation is an important factor. The branches to the spinal cord from the bronchial artery are seldom found; however, a common trunk with the intercostal artery is common, especially on the right side of the chest (Fig. 20.6). Backflow of embolic material into the intercostal artery should be carefully avoided. The branches from the costocervical artery and thyrocervical artery are also important with regard to communication with the vertebral artery. The mediastinal circulation is changing dynamically during the embolization. The flow velocity and flow direction should carefully be monitored under fluoroscopic observation.[15] Very careful selective injection into these mediastinal branches is critical.

Esophageal enhancement is sometimes visible in bronchial angiography. There are no reported complications caused by arterial infusion or embolization. We have also never experienced esophagitis or dysphagia after these procedures. However, careful observation of esophageal circulation is necessary.

Bronchial to pulmonary artery or pulmonary vein shunting should be considered. Pleural lesions after radiotherapy or inflammation can frequently cause shunting from systemic arteries to pulmonary artery or pulmonary vein. If direct communication is evident, then embolization should be avoided to prevent a systemic embolic showering.

Although rare complications including bronchial necrosis and bronchoesophageal fistula[16] have been reported, we have never had serious complications caused by bronchial wall damage.

TIPS AND TRICKS

- Superselective catheterization with a microcatheter should be always the ultimate goal from the technical standpoint.
- 3-D chest CT and or catheter angiography with rotational CT capabilities should be carefully analyzed to understand the tumor vascularization.
- Review if there are esophageal and anterior spinal branches before starting to embolize any chest blood vessels.
- Antineoplastic agents should slowly be infused to the target artery, avoiding backflow.
- A mixture with contrast material (1:1) is preferable to recognize the flow.
- Immediately after completion of infusion, embolization should be commenced.
- Embolic material should be mixed with contrast material to get good opacity to check the free flow state.
- The end point of embolization is not arterial occlusion but disappearance of tumor vasculature.
- Flow reduction observed on fluoroscopy during the injection of embolic material is a good sign that the embolization procedure is complete.

SUMMARY

Recent advancement of technology including imaging, microcatheter, and embolic material makes it possible to approach transarterially to the lung and mediastinal malignant lesions. Chemoembolization offers considerable improvement of symptoms to patients with less complication compared to the systemic chemotherapy. In the management of advanced chest malignancies, including primary lung cancer, metastatic lung tumors, and chest wall recurrence of breast cancer, transarterial treatment will play an important role to control life-threatening symptoms and increase survival with quality of life.

REFERENCES

1. Neyazaki T, Iked M, Seki Y, et al. Bronchial infusion therapy for lung cancer. *Cancer*. 1969;24:912–922.
2. Osaki T, Oyama T, Takenoyama M, et al. Feasibility of induction chemotherapy using bronchial infusion for locally advanced non-small cell lung cancer: a pilot study. *Surg Today*. 2002;22(9):772–778.
3. Murakami M, Kuroda Y, Sano A, et al. Therapeutic results of non-small cell lung cancer in stage III: combined synchronous irradiation with bronchial artery infusion of CDDP [in Japanese]. *Nihon Igaku Hoshasen Gakkai Zasshi*. 1995;55(1):44–49.
4. Nakanishi M, Umeda Y, Demura Y, et al. Effective use of multi-arterial infusion chemotherapy for advanced non-small cell lung cancer patients: four clinical specified cases. *Lung Cancer*. 2007;55(2):241–247.
5. Park HS, Kim YI, Kim HY, et al. Bronchial artery and systemic artery embolization in the management of primary lung cancer patients with hemoptysis. *Cardiovasc Intervent Radiol*. 2007;30:638–643.
6. Wang GR, Ensor JE, Gupta S, et al. Bronchial artery embolization for the management of hemoptysis in oncology patients: utility and prognostic factors. *J Vasc Intervent Radiol*. 2009;20(6):722–729.
7. De Gregorio MA, Medrano J, Laborda A, et al. Hemoptysis workup before embolization: single-center experience with a 15-year period follow-up. *Tech Vasc Interv Radiol*. 2007;10:270–273.
8. Morimoto K, Takatsuka Y, Sugitachi A, et al. Combined transcatheter arterial embolization and regional chemotherapy for locally advanced carcinoma of the breast. *Acta Radiol Oncol*. 1985;24(3):241–245.
9. Takizawa K, Shimamoto H, Ogawa Y, et al. Development of a new subclavian arterial infusion chemotherapy method for locally or recurrent advanced breast cancer using an implanted catheter-port system after redistribution of arterial tumor supply. *Cardiovasc Intervent Radiol*. 2009;32(5):1059–1066.
10. McDonald DM. Angiogenesis and remodeling of airway vasculature in chronic inflammation. *Am J Respir Crit Care Med*. 2001;164:S39–S45.
11. Fan QS, Huo XK, Wang MQ, et al. Efficacy and safety of transcatheter chemoembolization of the internal thoracic artery in patients with hepatocellular carcinoma. *Chin Med J (Engl)*. 2011;124:1374–1380.
12. Cauldwell EW, Siekert RG, Lininger RE, et al. The bronchial arteries: an anatomic study of 150 human cadavers. *Surg Gynecol Obstet*. 1948;86:395–412.
13. Ghaye B, Dondelinger RF. Imaging guided thoracic interventions. *Eur J Respir J*. 2001;17(8):507–528.
14. Chun JY, Morgan R, Belli AM. Radiological management of hemoptysis: a comprehensive review of diagnostic imaging and bronchial arterial embolization. *Cardiovasc Intervent Radiol*. 2010;33:240–250.
15. Brown AC, Ray CE. Anterior spinal cord infarction following bronchial artery embolization *Semin Intervent Radiol*. 2012;29:241–244.
16. Munk PL, Morris C, Nelems B. Left main bronchial-esophageal fistula: a complication of bronchial artery embolization. *Cardiovasc Intervent Radiol*. 1990;13:95–97.

21

Head and Neck Trauma

Goetz Benndorf

Injuries to the vasculature of the head and neck can be caused by blunt trauma during motor vehicle accidents, falls, assaults, hanging, or sporting injuries[1] and may be associated with significant morbidity and mortality.[2–9] Whereas carotid injuries are associated with 8% to 18 % mortality, injuries to the vertebral arteries can be associated with 17% to 38% mortality.[10] Penetrating vascular trauma is usually caused by sharp objects or instruments, such as knives,[11–17] nail guns,[18] broken glass, arrows,[19] or by bullets from gunshot injuries (GSIs).[20–24] Whereas in Western Europe and Canada, low-velocity stab injuries are the most frequently seen, high-velocity gunshot injuries are by far the dominant cause of penetrating vascular trauma in the United States.[21]

Iatrogenic injuries to the carotid, vertebral, and facial arteries by medical tools or instruments are generally rare but may occur during both diagnostic and therapeutic percutaneous procedures or during open surgical procedures. These include injuries of the carotid during central vein catheter placement,[25,26] inadvertent puncture of the vertebral arteries during cervical epidural steroid injection,[27,28] or injuries to the facial and maxillary arteries during orthognathic surgery.[29–33]

Clustered location of several major arteries, some of which difficult to reach and to control by surgical exposure, is characteristic for the head and neck area. Vascular injuries can result in various lesions with different clinical sequelae ranging from cerebrovascular insults (CVIs) to active extravasation with critical blood loss. Exsanguination and ischemic stroke are the main causal factors of morbidity and mortality for penetrating arterial injury in the head and neck area. Mortality rate is highest in the first 24 hours after presentation, with primary and secondary cerebral ischemic injury accounting for the leading causes of death, followed by exsanguination.[34,35]

Because blunt trauma may result in CVI, and if left untreated can lead to stroke in 30% to 50% of all patients, with severe permanent neurologic deficits in 48% to 58%,[36] early screening and intervention is important to improve clinical outcome.[6]

Nonfatal GSI to the head and neck can be devastating, with mortality in civilian patients ranging from 2% to 29%.[22,37,38] Vascular injury to the carotid or vertebral arteries occurs in 15% to 25% of patients with penetrating injuries to the neck,[39,40] and the stroke rate in patients with arterial injury ranges is reported to be as high as 15%.[9]

Immediate therapeutic measures include hemodynamic control and preventing or decreasing morbidity associated with cerebrovascular insufficiency or embolic phenomena.[20,41]

Iatrogenic vascular trauma can present with local symptoms, stroke, or as acute massive bleeding requiring early therapeutic management.[42] Subacute and chronic lesions such as pseudoaneurysms (PAs) or arteriovenous fistulas (AVFs) can be initially occult and may present with delay from weeks to months.[43] Endovascular treatment (EVT) of vascular lesions following iatrogenic trauma is identical to those caused by penetrating or blunt trauma. Biffl et al.[4] have correlated the degree of blunt injury with clinical outcome (Table 21.1). This grading system may be used to some degree also for penetrating trauma of the carotid and vertebral arteries. However, it is of limited value external carotid artery (ECA) injuries, where luminal narrowing is of no clinical importance, and does not include management of AVFs. The

Table 21.1	Grading for Scale for Blunt Cerebrovascular Injury
Grade I	Irregularity of vessel wall or dissection/intramural hematoma with less than 25% stenosis
Grade II	Intramural thrombus or raised intimal flap or dissection/intramural hematoma with greater than 25% stenosis
Grade III	Pseudoaneurysm
Grade IV	Occlusion
Grade V	Transection

Modified form Biffl WL, Moore EE, Offner PJ, et al. Blunt carotid arterial injuries: implications of a new grading scale. *J Trauma*. 1999;47(5):845–853.

distal internal maxillary artery (IMA) is a relatively frequent location for gunshot-related injuries with massive extravasation that often require emergent endovascular management. Traumatic AVFs in the ECA territory are clinically relatively benign but can cause chronic headaches, bruits, or significant cosmetic problems when involving facial veins.[44] They can usually be electively treated.

TYPES OF INJURIES

Trauma in the head and neck can result in a range of arterial and venous injuries. Although venous injuries can also lead to hematomas and drop in hemoglobin, their clinical presentation is often less dramatic and angiographic detection difficult. They are usually self-limiting and rarely require endovascular or surgical management. Arterial trauma on the other hand can lead to rapid critical blood loss or ischemic deficits due to downstream compromise of the cerebral circulation. The spectrum of vascular injuries is wide and ranges from minor wall irregularities and vasospasm caused by blast effects to the surrounding tissue to partial or complete disruption of arterial blood flow to the central nervous system and rupture or transection with massive extravasation and critical blood loss.

Vessel Injuries without Blood Loss

Minor Wall Irregularities (Grade I)

This most frequently observed injury (~50%) can be seen as simple vasospasm or subtle, minimal luminal irregularities (<25%) that represent minor intimal damages. These small lesions, sometimes only detectable on digital subtraction angiography (DSA), do not notably narrow the arterial lumen or compromise blood flow. Because they can be nevertheless thrombogenic, anticoagulation or antiplatelet therapy becomes necessary when carotid or vertebral arteries are involved. Conservative management with warfarin, heparin, low-molecular-weight heparin (Lovenox), or antiplatelet drugs (acetylsalicylic acid [ASA], clopidogrel) and in some cases follow up imaging is advisable[7,8,45] Because grade I lesion can be associated with strokes in up to 7%,[46] routine screening ideally with four-vessel angiography (DSA) is strongly recommended.

Major Wall Irregularities and Dissections (Grade II)

These injuries can present with angiographic findings identical to spontaneous dissections, including luminal narrowing (>25%) and associated intimal flaps. They may be complicated by rapid intraluminal thrombus formation and thus require a more rigorous anticoagulation regime to prevent thromboembolism.[8] Of note, studies have failed to demonstrate superiority of anticoagulation over antiplatelet therapy in the prevention of stroke,[46,47] which can impact management in trauma patients in whom antiplatelet therapy is generally preferred by surgeons. In select cases, endovascular management such as stent placement may be required.[24,48,49] Routine angiographic follow-up has been recommended, as up to 61% of patients with grade I to II injuries will require change in management. Both, dissections and the formation of PAs are dynamic processes, and thus show morphologic changes over time that influence therapeutic decision making.[46] An early 7 to 10 days FU DSA is helpful to determine the acuteness of a lesion.

Pseudoaneurysms (Grade III)

PAs are small (1 to 3 mm) or large (up to several centimeters) outpouchings of the arterial wall caused by focal arterial damage that can lead to an intramural or extramural hematoma with subsequent recanalization. Depending on the extent of the injury, the wall of the PA may be covered by tunica media, adventitia, or just thrombus material. The latter is considered the "classical pseudoaneurysm," with an angiographic appearance identical to true saccular or fusiform aneurysms. Similar to spontaneous dissections, traumatic PAs, especially with a narrow neck, may heal spontaneously with conservative management including anticoagulation or antiplatelet therapy and follow-up computed tomography angiography (CTA) or DSA.[50,51] Follow-up imaging is important to detect trends of progression or regression that impact therapeutic decision making.[52] A decrease in size usually indicates healing and justifies conservative management. No signs of regression or enlarging PAs may require interventional therapy. Some authors suggest surgical repair,[53] and no clear consensus when to treat asymptomatic dissections or PAs currently exist. However, most operators tend to recommend EVT, and only if there is evidence for worsening on FU imaging.[8,54–57] Treatment options are bare metal or covered stents with or without deployment of coils or liquids into the aneurysmal sac. Covered stents may be used in larger wide-necked lesion but can be associated with parent vessel occlusion.[57] If simple stenting shows no trend of occlusion within 3 to 6 months, coils are usually safe to deploy through the stent meshes,[54] or double stenting is performed.[55] Alternatively, coils can be placed in jailing technique during initial stenting. Recently introduced flow diverter can be used as well but represent a rather expensive solution.[58] Liquids such as *N*-butyl cyanoacrylate ([NBCA] Trufill; DePuy Orthopaedics, Inc., Warsaw, Indiana) and Onyx (Covidien, Irvine, California) can be very efficient to achieve rapid occlusions[43] but have a clearly higher (unnecessary) risk of distal migration into the cerebral circulation.

Depending on availability, both CTA and DSA can be used for screening and follow-up studies. Because detection of minor vascular injuries and visualization of small changes during follow-up can be obscured especially in patients with GSIs and bullet fragments that cause metallic artifacts,[59] the author has a strong preference for DSA. Especially, patients with penetrating trauma are oftentimes of relatively young age without significant underlying vascular diseases, which minimizes the risk of neurologic deficit posed by supra-aortic or cerebral angiography that is less than 1% in experienced hands. In our institution, a protocol with at least one short-term angiogram within 7 to 10 days followed by 4 weeks and 3 months is in place.

Occlusions (Grade IV)

Similar to spontaneous dissections, severe arterial injury may lead to an enlarging hematoma in the vessel wall or in the surrounding tissue and to occlusion the arterial lumen. The consequences of interrupting the carotid blood flow on the cerebral circulation depend to a large degree on the functional status of the circle of Willis, but stroke may occur in up to 50%.[46] Vertebral artery (VA) occlusion can be fully compensated by collateral supply of a contralateral VA or ipsilateral cervical anastomoses. If this collateral circulation is insufficient, cerebellar infarcts or, even worse, a devastating basilar artery occlusion may occur especially in cases with unfavorable anatomy or advanced atherosclerosis.[60] Due to the dual supply to the posterior fossa, complete VA occlusions may be less dangerous than nonocclusive lesions (grades I to III).[46] On the other hand, even a minimal intimal damage is potentially thrombogenic, thus early detection and anticoagulation or antiplatelet therapy can be crucial. Further, it is important to be aware that a completely occluded artery following trauma may recanalize and become a new source of thromboembolic strokes. Therefore, prophylactic anticoagulation may be indicated.

Arteriovenous Fistulas

AVFs are not included in Biffl's grading[4] and rarely caused by blunt trauma. They are more frequently observed following penetrating vascular injuries.[61] Simultaneous injury to arterial and venous vessels creates a channel for arterial blood to reenter the circulation. Traumatic AVFs are usually "single-hole" high-flow lesions that can be small or occult in the beginning, and thus not detectable during initial diagnostic screening, but develop with varying delay.[43,62–64] EVT of traumatic AVFs is more or less identical to the one of congenital lesions and performed using stents, coils, detachable balloons, or embolic liquids depending on location and angioarchitecture of the lesion.[44,65,66] As for all arteriovenous shunting lesions, treatment is effective only when the fistula site itself is permanently occluded (either most distal arterial or most proximal venous segment, or both) and can often be performed as planned procedure (Fig. 21.1).

Injuries with Blood Loss: Rupture, Perforation, Laceration, Transection (Grade V)

Transmural arterial injury causes leakage of blood into either the surrounding structures leading to an expanding hematoma in the soft tissues or into preformed cavities. Both situations can be associated with critical, uncontrollable blood loss and can develop quickly into a life-threatening situation. Open surgery may become necessary in cases with extensive tissue damage and may allow for control of the blood loss in some locations such as common carotid artery (CCA) and proximal internal carotid artery (ICA). Endovascular techniques are more efficient in bleedings arising from the vertebral or internal maxillary arteries and are considered treatment of choice for most of these lesions. If blood leaks into large voluminous spaces, such as the mediastinum, oropharynx, or upper gastrointestinal tract, critical loss can develop very quickly, leading to shock and possible death. Therefore, rapid identification of the bleeding source and immediate occlusion of the bleeding site can become life-saving measure. Especially, injuries of the IMA (Fig. 21.2) are frequently associated with massive bleedings that are difficult to control with packing alone and usually require multiple transfusions.[31–33,52,67–69] In this context, it needs to be clarified that the term *pseudoaneurysm* is sometimes used for ruptures of the IMA or sphenopalatine artery.[29,69] The aneurysm-like appearance is largely caused by a highly unstable hematoma, only supported by nasal or intraoral packing and extremely fragile. Any aggressive manipulation with catheters or guidewires or even the deployment of coils can lead to rerupture. Similarly, transmural injuries of the vertebral or carotid arteries are prone to additional injury or rerupture during intravascular manipulation with tools or occlusive devices if only temporarily occluded by clot.[24] Further, it should be noted that also injuries to small arteries could cause enlarging hematomas of significant size and critical blood loss (Fig. 21.3). For all vessels difficult to reach by surgery, EVT is nowadays the method of choice, employing detachable balloons (currently not available in the United States) or vascular plug devices[70] in larger vessels such as ICA or VA. Embolic liquids such as Onyx or NBCA are preferably used in smaller arteries (e.g., ECA branches). Depending on location and flow conditions, combining liquids with coils as matrix is useful to prevent distal migration (Figs. 21.4 and 21.5).[24] Newer occlusion devices such as the microvascular plug system (MVP) or UNO (Reverse Medical, Irvine, California), resheatable microcatheter-based occlusion systems, may be of use as well.

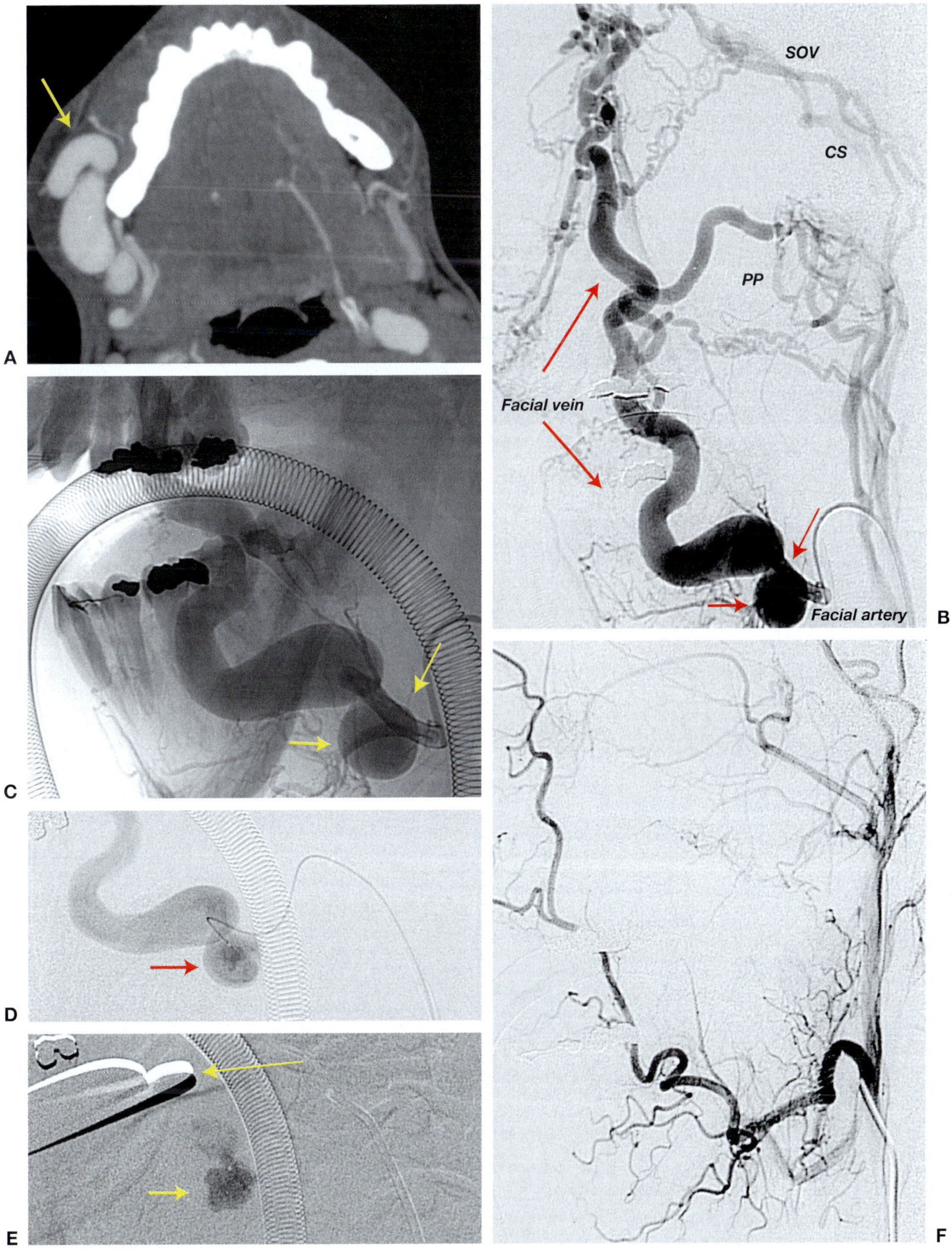

Figure 21.1 Iatrogenic injury. A 33-year-old male presents with a pulsatile mass after bimaxillary surgery 12 months earlier. **A:** Axial CTA shows remarkably enlarged right facial vein coursing over the mandible (*arrow*). **B:** Selective injection into right facial artery reveals a high-flow AVF with only a small stump of the facial artery visualized (*thin arrow*). The draining facial vein (*long arrows*) fills immediately with an initial aneurysmal enlargement (*short arrow*) and flow reversal into the transverse facial and ophthalmic veins (PP, pterygoid plexus; SOV, superior ophthalmic vein; CS, cavernous sinus). **C:** Unsubtracted image shows the stump of the facial artery (*thin arrow*) and the pouch of the facial vein (*short arrow*). **D:** Transarterial microcatheter placement through the fistula into the venous pouch (*arrow*). **E:** Glue cast after injection of glue (60% NBCA–Ethiodol mixture; *short arrow*). Note the hemostatic clamp (*long arrow*) used to compress the draining vein for optimal flow control. **F:** Complete occlusion of the AV shunt with patency of the facial artery.

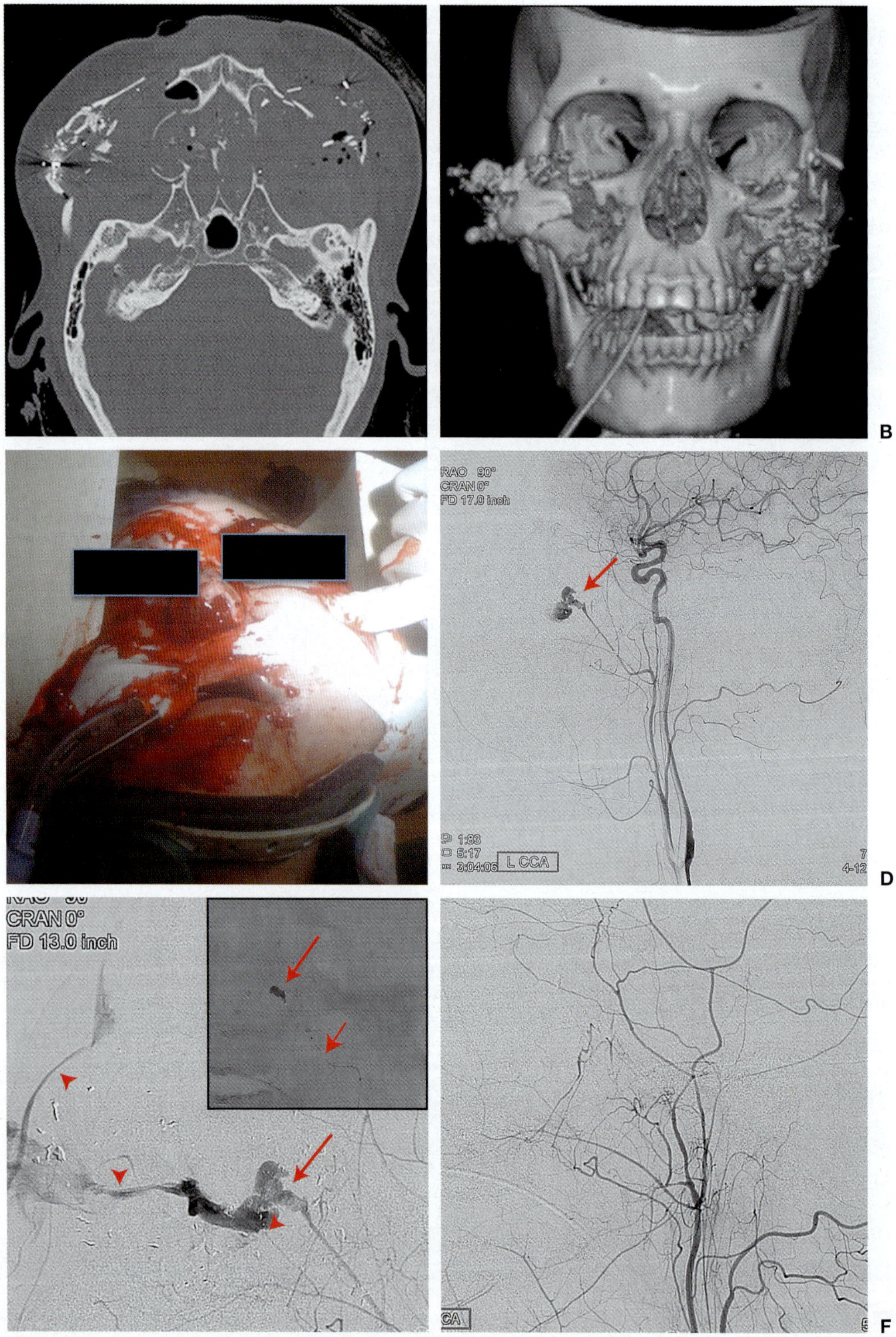

Figure 21.2 Penetrating trauma (GSI). A 39-year-old female after being shot through the face (domestic violence). **A,B:** Axial CT and volume rendering shows extensive destruction of the bilateral facial bones. **C:** Patient presents in the angiography suite with massive bleeding from the nose and through an open wound in her left cheek (compressed manually). **D:** CCA injections reveal significant extravasation from the distal sphenopalatine artery (*arrow*). **E:** Selective ECA injection shows massive extravasation through nasal cavity (*arrowheads*). *Inset:* Glue cast (*long arrow*) after injection of 30% NBCA–Ethiodol mixture and withdrawal of the microcatheter 2 cm more proximal (*short arrow*). **F:** Final ECA run confirms complete occlusion of the ruptured distal IMA. Note the overall extensive vasospasm due to tissue due to tissue swelling from the blast.

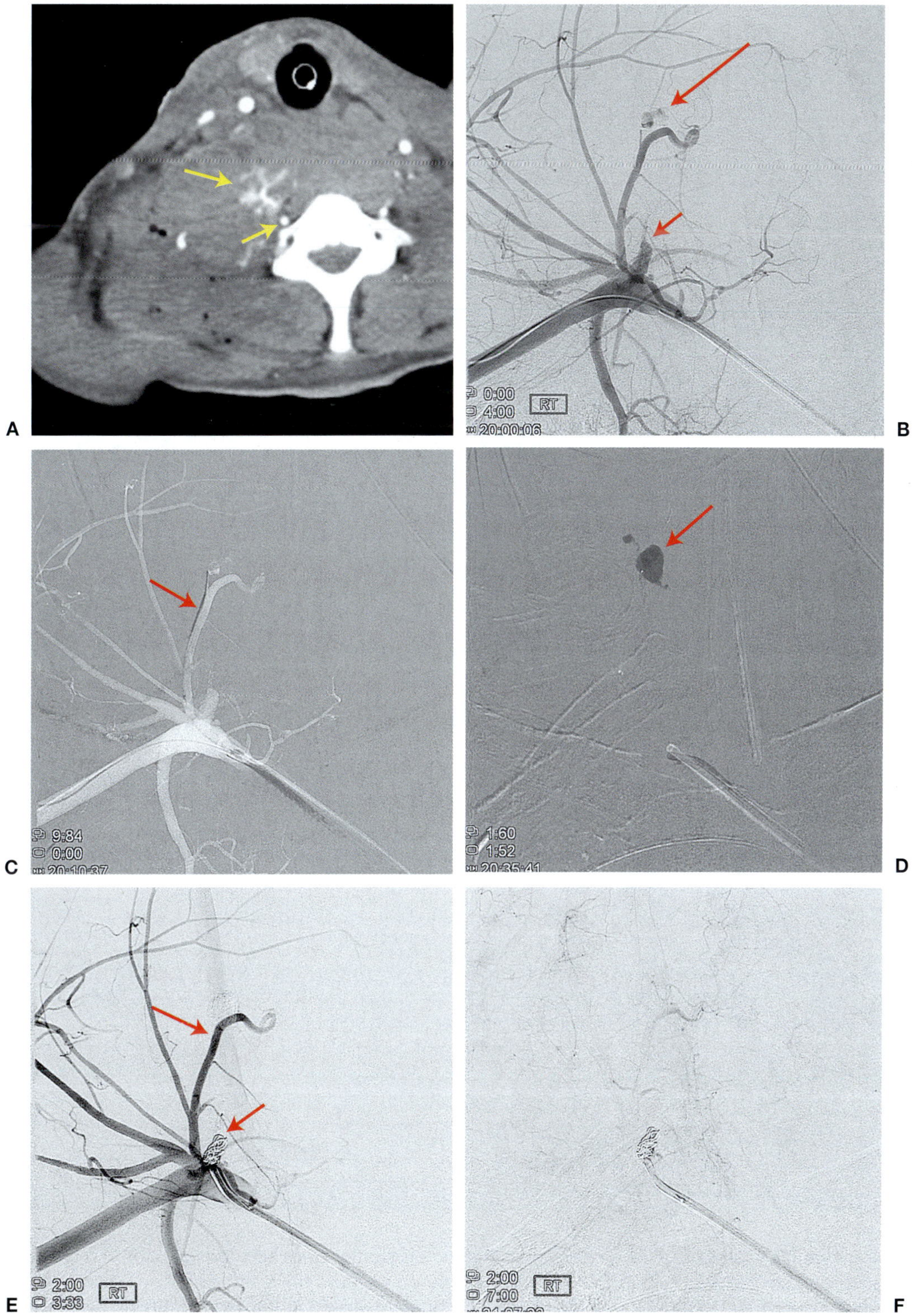

Figure 21.3 Blunt trauma. A 43-year-old male developed massive neck hematoma after motorcycle accident. **A:** Axial CT scan shows contrast leakage into the soft tissue (*long arrow*) next to the right VA (*short arrow*) **B:** Right subclavian artery injection shows a stump of the right VA (*short arrow*) and active extravasation from a small branch of the right inferior thyroid artery (*long arrow*). **C,D:** Road map shows microcatheter navigation into inferior thyroid artery and injection of 30% NBCA–Ethiodol mixture (*arrows*). **E,F:** Control angiogram shows no longer extravasation and complete patency of the inferior thyroid artery (*long arrow*). Note that the VA stump has been also occluded with coils to exclude this injury site as potential additional source for active bleeding (*short arrow*).

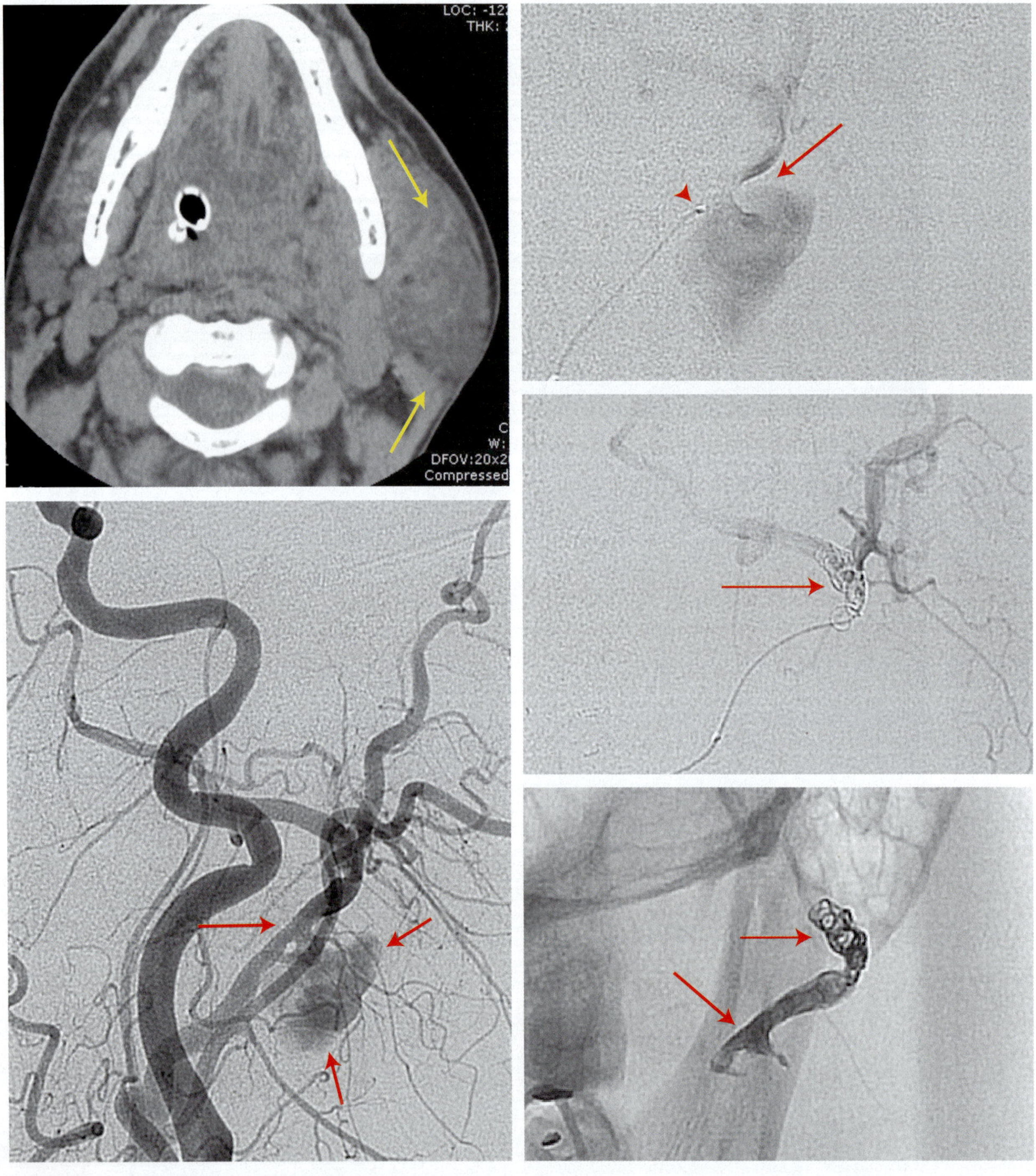

Figure 21.4 Penetrating trauma. **A:** Axial CT shows enlarging hematoma (*arrows*) in the left neck in a 60-year-old male following knife stabbing. **B:** CCA injection, oblique view shows brisk extravasation (*short arrows*) from the main ECA trunk (*long arrow*). **C:** Echelon-10 microcatheter with tip (*arrowhead*) at the level of the injury (*arrow*). **D:** After advancing the microcatheter distal to the bleeding site, coils were packed (*arrow*), followed by an injection of a small amount of Onyx–18 while the catheter was withdrawn proximally 2 cm **(E)**. This allowed occluding the artery proximal and distal to the site of perforation (*thick arrow*). Note that no distal migration of Onyx beyond the coils (*thin arrow*) occurred. *(continued)*

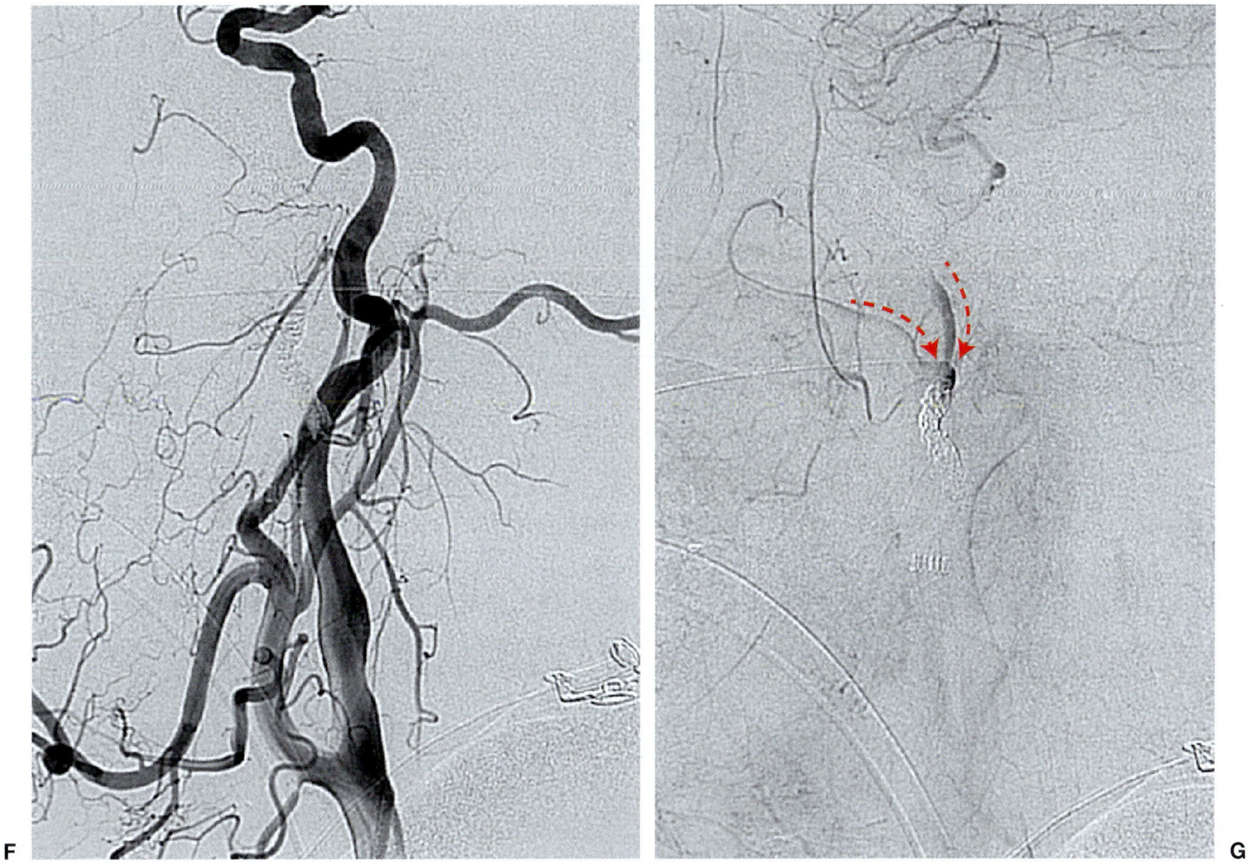

Figure 21.4 *(Continued)* **F:** Final control shows complete occlusion of the ECA at the site of injury. **G:** This late-phase image shows backflow through internal maxillary and superficial temporal arteries, which is blocked by occluding the artery distal to the rupture site (*arrows*).

ENDOVASCULAR TREATMENT

Endovascular management of acute arterial injuries is continuously evolving[49] and employs standard techniques used for treating nontraumatic vascular disorders in the head and neck region. Transfemoral approach with coaxial systems using 5-Fr or 6-Fr guiding catheters and microcatheter–guidewire combination is preferred. In cases with difficult access anatomy, triaxial systems can be used (e.g., 6-Fr Envoy, DePuy Orthopaedics, Inc., Warsaw, Indiana; 0.38 DAC, Concentric Medical, Fremont, California; Excelsior SL-10 microcatheter, Stryker Corporation, Kalamazoo, Michigan). In some cases, ultrasound- or road map–guided direct puncture of the lesion can facilitate access (e.g., scalp lesions).[44] Pressured flushing systems, standard in neurovascular procedures to prevent clot formation and distal thromboembolism, are advisable when embolizing ECA branches. The author regularly uses 1,000 International Units heparin in 1 L saline for flushing of guiding catheters. This can be crucial because additional heparinization is often contraindicated in patients with acute bleedings or suspected additional internal injuries. Although the choice of microcatheters depends mostly on the user's preference, it should be kept in mind that it can become necessary to combine deployment of coils with the injection of liquids (e.g., Echelon; Covidien, Plymouth, Minnesota). Carotid artery or VA stenting is generally a straightforward procedure especially in younger patients. The use of protection devices may not be necessary as the risk of dislodging plaque material from the bifurcation usually does not exist.

TIPS AND TRICKS

- *Selective* injections (ICA, ECA, VA >> CCA, SA) provide more accurate information than global injection when looking for vessel injuries.
- *Check for vessel stumps or abrupt occlusions* in cases with blood loss and negative angiogram (extravasation can be invisible due to packing).
- *Secure* temporary (clot) occluded arteries with additional coils, plugs, liquids, etc.
- *Checking for backflow* through extracranial/intracranial collaterals after proximal/antegrade occlusion is mandatory.

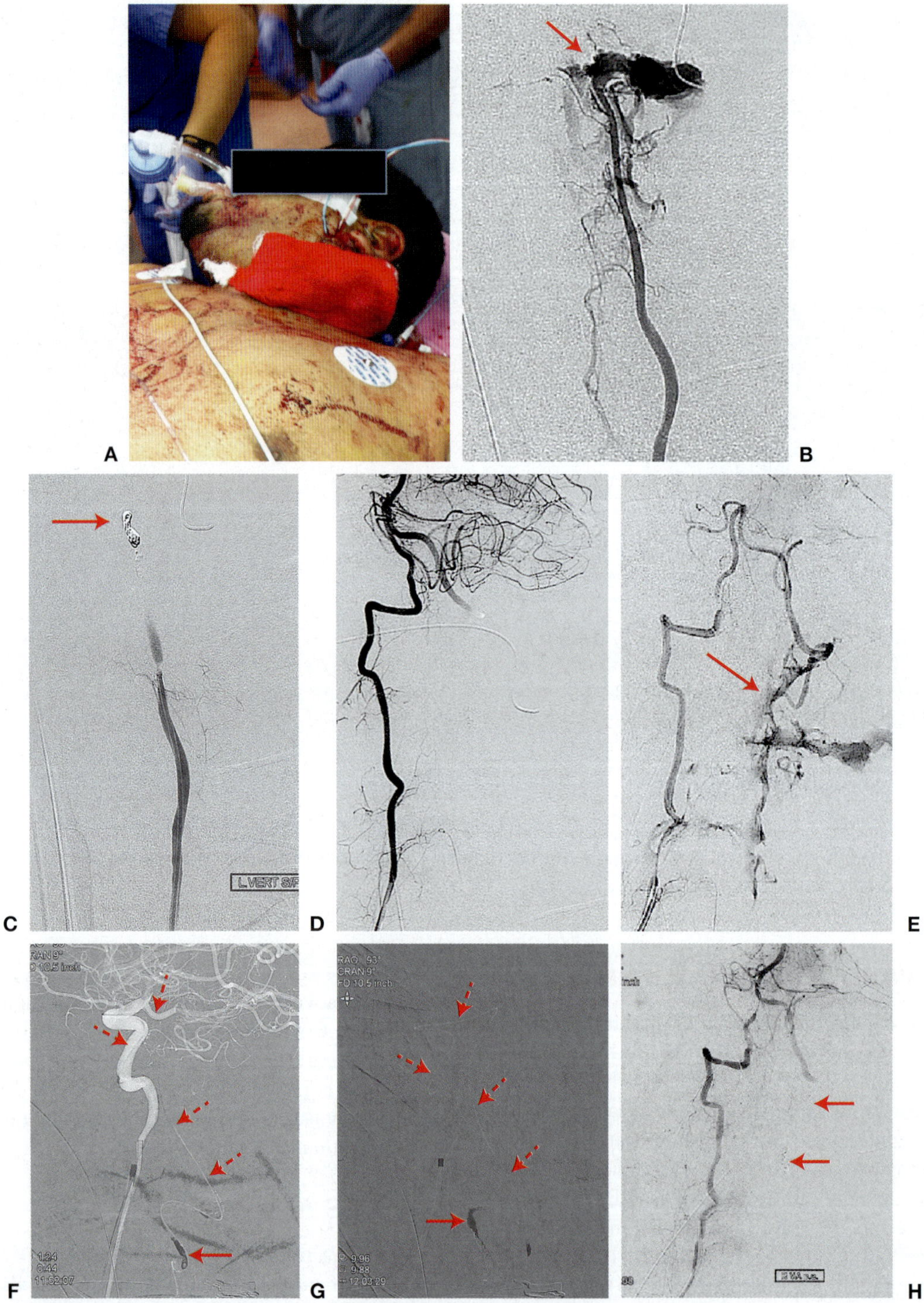

Figure 21.5 A 29-year-old male found on the ground (GCS 3) with a 3-cm stabbing wound in the left neck without palpable pulse. **A:** Patient with open wound in the left neck, actively bleeding. **B:** Left VA injection shows massive extravasation at the level of C3 (*arrow*). **C:** Left VA injection after placement of coils (*arrow*) just proximal to injury site and additional injection of a small amount of glue (30% NBCA–Ethiodol mixture). **D:** Control angiogram of the right VA shows no backflow to the lesion. **E:** Twenty-four hours later, patient starts bleeding again; right VA injection reveals now massive extravasation from retrograde filling (*arrow*). **F:** Acute angle at VA junction prevents cross-catheterization; placement of guiding catheter in ICA and retrograde approach via circle of Willis (*dashed arrows* indicate cavernous ICA–posterior communicating artery–basilar artery–left distal VA) and coil placement (*solid arrow*) is performed. **G:** "Blank road map" after additional glue injection (*solid arrow*) and microcatheter withdrawal (*dashed arrows*). **H:** Control angiogram confirms cessation of the extravasation after "trapping" of the injury site by proximal and distal occlusion (*arrows*).

- *Avoid heparinization* if possible, but flush meticulously guide catheter and microcatheter to avoid thromboembolism.
- Have a large *balloon* occlusion catheter (e.g., Cello; Covidien, Plymouth, Minnesota) ready to prevent massive blood loss while gaining time to prepare microcatheters and embolic agents (coils, liquids).
- *Gentle guidewire manipulation* in injured arteries is mandatory to avoid rerupture (e.g., use double-angle tip Headliner [Terumo Medical Corporation, Somerset, New Jersey] or in general loop techniques).
- Be *cautious with coils* in ruptured arteries or PAs: Most PAs do not have a firm wall and can be easily perforated with guidewires or coils; underpacking may be sufficient and is advised. Consider first the front door–back door technique if possible.
- Glue (NBCA [Trufill])/Onyx: Both agents may be used depending on the operator's comfort level. *Glue occlusion* is *fast* and *permanent* due to immediate tissue reaction (e.g., 30% NBCA–Ethiodol mixture for IMA rupture) and high thrombogenicity. Use concentration greater than 50% for high-flow AVFs; the polymerization would be faster.
- Glue (NBCA [Trufill])/Onyx: *Seal the rupture site* proximally and distally by withdrawing the catheter during injection (trapping). *Avoid proximal occlusion* only.
- Glue (NBCA [Trufill])/Onyx: Advance *guiding catheter into* ECA before removing a microcatheter after injection into IMA.
- Glue (NBCA [Trufill])/Onyx: Be well familiar with so-called *dangerous anastomoses.*
- Glue (NBCA [Trufill])/Onyx: Position the microcatheter *close enough to target* to avoid proximal occlusion or backflow.
- Glue (NBCA [Trufill])/Onyx: If possible and not too time consuming, *block anastomoses* with coils (e.g., occipital artery–VA) before injecting.
- Glue (NBCA [Trufill])/Onyx: Use *flow control* when injecting liquids into AVFs. Superficial veins in face or scalp can be manually compressed using a hemostat clamp.
- *Circle of Willis* approach: Be prepared to perform retrograde approach to a bleeding site through the circle of Willis if antegrade route is blocked, too difficult, or time consuming.
- Consider *removing packings* or *deflating balloons* for repeat angiogram if initial run is negative and there is strong clinical suspicion.
- Consider *removing packings* postembolization in *angiography suite* before sending patient to ICU.
- Use *low-molecular-weight* or antiplatelet (ASA/Plavix) in minor (grade I) injuries to prevent thromboembolism and stroke.

CONCLUSION

The endovascular management of traumatic vascular injuries in the head and neck is technically not more demanding than that of other vascular lesions. However, the scenarios and settings can be fast-paced and dramatic and thus may represent a particular challenge for the inexperienced interventionalist.

REFERENCES

1. Biffl WL, Moore EE, Offner PJ, et al. Blunt carotid and vertebral arterial injuries. *World J Surg.* 2001;25(8):1036–1043.
2. Biffl WL, Moore EE. Identifying the asymptomatic patient with blunt carotid arterial injury. *J Trauma.* 1999;47(6):1163–1164.
3. Biffl WL, Moore EE, Mestek M. Patients with blunt carotid and vertebral artery injuries. *J Trauma.* 1999;47(2):438–439.
4. Biffl WL, Moore EE, Offner PJ, et al. Blunt carotid arterial injuries: implications of a new grading scale. *J Trauma.* 1999;47(5):845–853.
5. DiCocco JM, Fabian TC, Emmett KP, et al. Optimal outcomes for patients with blunt cerebrovascular injury (BCVI): tailoring treatment to the lesion. *J Am Coll Surg.* 2011;212(4):549–557; discussion 557–559.
6. Emmett KP, Fabian TC, DiCocco JM, et al. Improving the screening criteria for blunt cerebrovascular injury: the appropriate role for computed tomography angiography. *J Trauma.* 2011;70(5):1058–1063; discussion 1063–1065.
7. Fabian TC, Patton JH Jr, Croce MA, et al. Blunt carotid injury. Importance of early diagnosis and anticoagulant therapy. *Ann Surg.* 1996;223(5):513–522; discussion 522–525.
8. Harrigan MR, Weinberg JA, Peaks YS, et al. Management of blunt extracranial traumatic cerebrovascular injury: a multidisciplinary survey of current practice. *World J Emerg Surg.* 2011;6:11.
9. Ramadan F, Rutledge R, Oller D, et al. Carotid artery trauma: a review of contemporary trauma center experiences. *J Vasc Surg.* 1995;21(1):46–55; discussion 55–56.
10. Fusco MR, Harrigan MR. Cerebrovascular dissections: a review. Part II: blunt cerebrovascular injury. *Neurosurgery.* 2011;68(2):517–530; discussion 30.
11. Kabanchuk IN, Skorik VT. Knife wound of the neck with injury of the carotid artery [in Russian]. *Klin Khir.* 1989;(4):70.
12. Tu RK, Eskridge JM, Grady MS. Endovascular treatment of a kitchen knife pseudoaneurysm of the cervical internal carotid artery. *AJR Am J Roentgenol.* 1996;166(3):704.
13. Xia X, Zhang F, Lu F, et al. Stab wound with lodged knife tip causing spinal cord and vertebral artery injuries: case report and literature review. *Spine.* 2012;37(15):E931–E934.
14. Mehanna HM, MacGregor FB. The case of the missing carotid artery—a well aimed knife! *J Laryngol Otol.* 1998;112(4):387–388.
15. Sergeev VM. Ligation of the vertebral artery in partial knife wounds [in Russian]. *Zh Vopr Neirokhir Im N N Burdenko.* 1981;(1):53–54.
16. Petrovic P, Nastasic S, Dimkovic D. Knife wounds of the carotid arteries in their cervical segment. Apropos of 3 cases [in French]. *Chirurgie.* 1976;102(10):894–897.

17. Polunin AP, Volkov VG. Knife injury of the common carotid artery [in Russian]. *Vestn Khir Im I I Grek.* 1975;114(3):76.
18. Hiraishi T, Kawaguchi T, Kobayashi T, et al. Unstable stenosis of the internal carotid artery caused by a craniofacial nail-gun injury-case report. *Neurol Med Chir (Tokyo).* 2009;49(12):590–593.
19. Lubarsky M, Helmer R, Knight C, et al. Internal carotid artery dissection following wooden arrow injury to the posterior pharynx. Case report. *J Neurosurg Pediat.* 2008;1(4):334–336.
20. Bell RB, Osborn T, Dierks EJ, et al. Management of penetrating neck injuries: a new paradigm for civilian trauma. *J Oral Maxillofac Surg.* 2007;65(4):691–705.
21. Burgess CA, Dale OT, Almeyda R, et al. An evidence based review of the assessment and management of penetrating neck trauma. *Clin Otolaryngol.* 2012;37(1):44–52.
22. Miller RH, Duplechain JK. Penetrating wounds of the neck. *Otolaryngol Clin North Am.* 1991;24(1):15–29.
23. Sofianos C, Degiannis E, Van den Aardweg MS, et al. Selective surgical management of zone II gunshot injuries of the neck: a prospective study. *Surgery.* 1996;120(5):785–788.
24. Yevich SM, Lee SR, Scott BG, et al. Emergency endovascular management of penetrating gunshot injuries to the arteries in the face and neck: a case series and review of the literature. *J Neurointerv Surg.* 2014;6(1):42–46.
25. Parsons AJ, Alfa J. Carotid dissection: a complication of internal jugular vein cannulation with the use of ultrasound. *Anesth Analg.* 2009;109(1):135–136.
26. Forestner JE. Ipsilateral mydriasis following carotid-artery puncture during attempted cannulation of the internal jugular vein. *Anesthesiology.* 1980;52(5):438–439.
27. Rozin L, Rozin R, Koehler SA, et al. Death during transforaminal epidural steroid nerve root block (C7) due to perforation of the left vertebral artery. *Am J Forensic Med Pathol.* 2003;24(4):351–355.
28. Ziai WC, Ardelt AA, Llinas RH. Brainstem stroke following uncomplicated cervical epidural steroid injection. *Arch Neurol.* 2006;63(11):1643–1646.
29. Avelar RL, Goelzer JG, Becker OE, et al. Embolization of pseudoaneurysm of the internal maxillary artery after orthognathic surgery. *J Craniofac Surg.* 2010;21(6):1764–1768.
30. Hacein-Bey L, Blazun JM, Jackson RF. Carotid artery pseudoaneurysm after orthognathic surgery causing lower cranial nerve palsies: endovascular repair. *J Oral Maxillofac Surg.* 2013;71(11):1948–1955.
31. Jo HW, Kim YS, Kang DH, et al. Pseudoaneurysm of the facial artery occurred after mandibular sagittal split ramus osteotomy. *J Oral Maxillofac Surg.* 2013;17(2):151–154.
32. Kim YW, Baek MJ, Kim HD, et al. Massive epistaxis due to pseudoaneurysm of the sphenopalatine artery: a rare postoperative complication of orthognathic surgery. *J Laryngol Otol.* 2013;127(6):610–613.
33. Lanigan DT, Hey JH, West RA. Major vascular complications of orthognathic surgery: false aneurysms and arteriovenous fistulas following orthognathic surgery. *J Oral Maxillofac Surg.* 1991;49(6):571–577.
34. Acosta JA, Yang JC, Winchell RJ, et al. Lethal injuries and time to death in a level I trauma center. *J Am Coll Surg.* 1998;186(5):528–533.
35. Sauaia A, Moore FA, Moore EE, et al. Epidemiology of trauma deaths: a reassessment. *J trauma.* 1995;38(2):185–193.
36. Biffl WL, Moore EE, Ryu RK, et al. The unrecognized epidemic of blunt carotid arterial injuries: early diagnosis improves neurologic outcome. *Ann Surg.* 1998;228(4):462–470.
37. Pereira C, Boyd JB, Dickenson B, et al. Gunshot wounds to the face: level I urban trauma center: a 10-year level I urban trauma center experience. *Ann Plast Surg.* 2012;68(4):378–381.
38. Biffl WL, Moore EE, Rehse DH, et al. Selective management of penetrating neck trauma based on cervical level of injury. *Am J Surg.* 1997;174(6):678–682.
39. Asensio JA, Valenziano CP, Falcone RE, et al. Management of penetrating neck injuries. The controversy surrounding zone II injuries. *Surg Clin North Am.* 1991;71(2):267–296.
40. Munera F, Soto JA, Palacio DM, et al. Penetrating neck injuries: helical CT angiography for initial evaluation. *Radiology.* 2002;224(2):366–372.
41. Wang AC, Charters MA, Thawani JP, et al. Evaluating the use and utility of noninvasive angiography in diagnosing traumatic blunt cerebrovascular injury. *J Trauma Acute Care Surg.* 2012;72(6):1601–1610.
42. Benndorf G. Endovascular management of a major vascular complication after orthognatic surgery. *Interv Neuroradiol.* 1998;4(4):307–310.
43. Lee SR, Metwalli ZA, Yevich SM, et al. Variability in evolution and course of gunshot injuries to the neck and impact on management. A case report. *Interv Neuroradiol.* 2013;19(4):489–495.
44. Benndorf G, Lehmann TN, Lanksch WR. Treatment of external carotid artery fistula by percutaneous venous approach. *Interv Neuroradiol.* 1999;5(3):251–256.
45. Cothren CC, Biffl WL, Moore EE, et al. Treatment for blunt cerebrovascular injuries: equivalence of anticoagulation and antiplatelet agents. *Arch Surg.* 2009;144(7):685–690.
46. Biffl WL, Ray CE Jr, Moore EE, et al. Treatment-related outcomes from blunt cerebrovascular injuries: importance of routine follow-up arteriography. *Ann Surg.* 2002;235(5):699–706; discussion 706–707.
47. Kennedy F, Lanfranconi S, Hicks C, et al. Antiplatelets vs anticoagulation for dissection: CADISS nonrandomized arm and meta-analysis. *Neurology.* 2012;79(7):686–689.
48. Biffl WL, Moore EE, Ray C, et al. Emergent stenting of acute blunt carotid artery injuries: a cautionary note. *J Trauma.* 2001;50(5):969–971.
49. DuBose J, Recinos G, Teixeira PG, et al. Endovascular stenting for the treatment of traumatic internal caroid injuries: expanding experience. *J Trauma.* 2008;65(6):1561–1566.
50. Guillon B, Brunereau L, Biousse V, et al. Long-term follow-up of aneurysms developed during extracranial internal carotid artery dissection. *Neurology.* 1999;53(1):117–122.
51. Tekiner A, Gokcek C, Bayar MA, et al. Spontaneus resolution of a traumatic vertebral artery pseudoaneurysm. *Turk Neurosurg.* 2011;21(1):90–93.
52. Lee CY, Yim MB, Benndorf G. Traumatic pseudoaneurysm of the pharyngeal artery: an unusual cause of hematemesis and hematochezia after craniofacial trauma. *Surg Neurol.* 2006;66(4):444–446; discussion 446.
53. Garg K, Rockman CB, Lee V, et al. Presentation and management of carotid artery aneurysms and pseudoaneurysms. *J Vasc Surg.* 2012;55(6):1618–1622.

54. Phatouros CC, Sasaki TY, Higashida RT, et al. Stent-supported coil embolization: the treatment of fusiform and wide-neck aneurysms and pseudoaneurysms. *Neurosurgery*. 2000;47(1): 107–113; discussion 113–115.
55. Benndorf G, Wellnhofer E, Schneider GH. Doubled stenting for effective occlusion of a dissecting carotid artery aneurysm. *Interv Neuroradiol*. 2000;6(4):343–348.
56. Berne JD, Reuland KR, Villarreal DH, et al. Internal carotid artery stenting for blunt carotid artery injuries with an associated pseudoaneurysm. *J Trauma*. 2008;64(2):398–405.
57. Cox MW, Whittaker DR, Martinez C, et al. Traumatic pseudoaneurysms of the head and neck: early endovascular intervention. *J Vasc Surg*. 2007;46(6):1227–1233.
58. Rahal JP, Dandamudi VS, Heller RS, et al. Use of concentric Solitaire stent to anchor Pipeline flow diverter constructs in treatment of shallow cervical carotid dissecting pseudoaneurysms. *J Clin Neurosci*. 2014;21:1024–1028.
59. DiCocco JM, Emmett KP, Fabian TC, et al. Blunt cerebrovascular injury screening with 32-channel multidetector computed tomography: more slices still don't cut it. *Ann Surg*. 2011;253(3):444–450.
60. Desouza RM, Crocker MJ, Haliasos N, et al. Blunt traumatic vertebral artery injury: a clinical review. *Eur Spine J*. 2011;20(9):1405–1416.
61. Amirjamshidi A, Rahmat H, Abbassioun K. Traumatic aneurysms and arteriovenous fistulas of intracranial vessels associated with penetrating head injuries occurring during war: principles and pitfalls in diagnosis and management. A survey of 31 cases and review of the literature. *J Neurosurg*. 1996;84(5): 769–780.
62. Perry MO. Complications of missed arterial injuries. *J Vasc Surg*. 1993;17(2):399–407.
63. Fox CJ, Gillespie DL, Weber MA, et al. Delayed evaluation of combat-related penetrating neck trauma. *J Vasc Surg*. 2006;44(1):86–93.
64. Johnson ON, Fox CJ, O'Donnell S, et al. Arteriography in the delayed evaluation of wartime extremity injuries. *Vasc Endovascular Surg*. 2007;41(3):217–224.
65. Redekop G, Marotta T, Weill A. Treatment of traumatic aneurysms and arteriovenous fistulas of the skull base by using endovascular stents. *J Neurosurg*. 2001;95(3):412–419.
66. Herrera DA, Vargas SA, Dublin AB. Endovascular treatment of traumatic injuries of the vertebral artery. *AJNR Am J Neuroradiol*. 2008;29(8):1585–1589.
67. Manafi A, Ghenaati H, Dezham F, et al. Massive repeated nose bleeding after bimaxillary osteotomy. *J Craniofac Surg*. 2007;18(6):1491–1493.
68. Pappa H, Richardson D, Niven S. False aneurysm of the facial artery as complication of sagittal split osteotomy. *J Craniomaxillofac Surg*. 2008;36(3):180–182.
69. Silva AC, O'Ryan F, Beckley ML, et al. Pseudoaneurysm of a branch of the maxillary artery following mandibular sagittal split ramus osteotomy: case report and review of the literature. *J Oral Maxillofac Surg*. 2007;65(9):1807–1816.
70. Ross IB, Buciuc R. The vascular plug: a new device for parent artery occlusion. *AJNR Am J Neuroradiol*. 2007;28(2):385–386.

22

Thoracoabdominal Trauma

Lawrence J. Keating • Ashley Adamovich

ABDOMINAL TRAUMA

BACKGROUND

During the past three decades, management of traumatic abdominal organ injury has evolved from a predominantly surgical approach to a strategy of nonoperative therapy in most cases. There is now broad consensus that most patients with injuries to solid abdominal viscera who are hemodynamically stable are candidates for nonoperative management (NOM), although debate persists about the specifics including when to use angiography and which patients should proceed directly to surgery. The change in philosophy has been in large part a result of rapid advances in imaging capabilities, specifically computed tomography (CT), and the increasing capability of interventional radiology to treat vascular injuries using minimally invasive endovascular techniques. During the 1980s, diagnostic peritoneal lavage (DPL) was obviated by the development and availability of CT. With concurrent expansion in the capabilities of interventional radiology, the risks of surgery began to outweigh the risks of conservative management, defined as observation with or without angiography and embolization, in many cases.

The Organ Injury Scale (OIS)—created by a committee of the American Association for the Surgery of Trauma (AAST) in 1987 and since updated and validated for the liver, kidney, and spleen using National Trauma Data Bank (NTDB)—is the most commonly used grading system for evaluation of abdominal trauma (Table 22.1).[1] The current scale was revised in 1994 for the spleen and liver, partly to reflect the increasing reliance on CT for diagnosis and grading. It provides a common nomenclature for studies and outcomes research that is used almost exclusively in the trauma literature, although it is imperfect, particularly when used to assign prognostic value, which is not its fundamental objective.[1,2] It is designed primarily to allow comparison of equivalent injuries managed differently.[3] In a study designed to evaluate and compare injury grading scales, Barquist et al.[4] found significant inter-reader variability among radiologists in higher grade injuries as well as a tendency to underestimate injury grades based on CT compared to operative findings. Contrast extravasation indicating continuing hemorrhage and vascular injuries such as pseudoaneurysm or arteriovenous fistula are prognostic factors and may be indications for nonoperative interventions such as angioembolization but are not specifically described in the scale. Modifications addressing these concerns including a new CT grading system for splenic injuries and substratification of the renal OIS grade IV into IVa (high risk) and IVb (low risk) have been proposed but not yet widely adopted.[5,6]

The OIS enables accurate outcomes comparisons among institutions with differing protocols, but urgent decisions in the trauma setting are typically made based on clinical status combined with imaging findings. Current surgical guidelines support emergency surgery for hemodynamically unstable patients (hypotension and tachycardia unresponsive to ongoing fluid and packed red blood cell resuscitation) and a trial of NOM for stable patients in settings where monitored beds and surgical teams are readily available.[6–10]

The new standard of conservative management has been supported and improved by the increasing availability and effectiveness of angiography with embolization. By 2005, up to 85% of traumatic injuries involving liver, spleen, and kidney were managed nonsurgically.[10] Shafi et al.[11] studied operative intervention and mortality rates at 152 level I and level II trauma centers and demonstrated that hospitals with higher risk-adjusted mortality rates tend to also have the highest rates of surgical intervention for abdominal trauma. Various conclusions can be drawn from this, but the lowest

Table 22.1 American Association for the Surgery of Trauma Organ Injury Scale I

Organ	Grade[a]	Injury Type	Description of Injury
Spleen	I	Hematoma	Subcapsular, <10% surface area
		Laceration	Capsular tear, <1 cm parenchymal depth
	II	Hematoma	Subcapsular, 10%–50% surface area; intraparenchymal, <5 cm diameter
		Laceration	Capsular tear, 1–3 cm depth; does not involve trabecular vessel
	III	Hematoma	Subcapsular, >50% surface area or expanding; ruptured subcapsular or parenchymal hematoma; intraparenchymal hematoma, >5 cm or expanding
		Laceration	>3 cm parenchymal depth or involving trabecular vessels
	IV	Laceration	Laceration involving segmental or hilar vessels producing major devascularization (>25% of spleen)
	V	Hematoma	Completely shattered spleen
		Laceration	Hilar vascular injury devascularizes spleen
Liver	I	Hematoma	Subcapsular, <10% surface area
		Laceration	Capsular tear, <1 cm parenchymal depth
	II	Hematoma	Subcapsular, 10%–50% surface area; intraparenchymal, <10 cm in diameter
		Laceration	Capsular tear, 1–3 cm; parenchymal depth, <10 cm in length
	III	Hematoma	Subcapsular, >50% surface area of ruptured subcapsular or parenchymal hematoma; intraparenchymal hematoma, >10 cm or expanding
		Laceration	>3 cm parenchymal depth
	IV	Laceration	Parenchymal disruption involving 25%–75% hepatic lobe or 1–3 Couinaud segments
	V	Laceration	Parenchymal disruption involving >75% of hepatic lobe or >3 Couinaud segments within a single lobe
		Vascular	Juxtahepatic venous injuries (i.e., retrohepatic vena cava/central major hepatic veins)
	VI	Vascular	Hepatic avulsion
Kidney	I	Contusion	Microscopic or gross hematuria, urologic studies normal
		Hematoma	Subcapsular, nonexpanding without parenchymal laceration
	II	Hematoma	Nonexpanding perirenal hematoma confined to renal retroperitoneum
		Laceration	<1 cm parenchymal depth of renal cortex without urinary extravasation
	III	Laceration	>1 cm parenchymal depth of renal cortex without collecting system rupture or urinary extravasation
	IV	Laceration	Parenchymal laceration extending through renal cortex, medulla, and collecting system
		Vascular	Main renal artery or vein injury with contained hemorrhage
	V	Laceration	Completely shattered kidney
		Vascular	Avulsion of renal hilum that devascularizes the kidney

[a]Advance one grade for bilateral injuries up to grade III.
From Tinkoff G, Esposito TJ, Reed J, et al. American Association for the Surgery of Trauma Organ Injury Scale I: spleen, liver, and kidney, validation based on the National Trauma Data Bank. *J Am Coll Surg*. 2008;207:646–655.

mortality rates will occur when we have the best understanding of which patients need operative versus conservative management. Because randomized trials are impractical in this setting, collective experience in the form of retrospective studies is our principal guide.

SPLEEN

The spleen may be the most commonly injured organ in blunt abdominal trauma.[12] Aristotle considered the spleen an unnecessary organ and this was the prevailing view until recently.[13] From the first splenectomy for trauma by Nicholaus Matthias in 1678 until the 1970s, removal of the injured spleen was accepted, if not standard, practice. The notion that without splenectomy most patients with splenic injury would bleed to death because the spleen cannot heal nor be easily repaired was rarely questioned.[13] Interest in splenic preservation increased after the description in 1952 by King and Schumacker[14] of overwhelming postsplenectomy infection (OPSI) in infants. Upadhyaya and Simpson performed the first case-control study of operative versus nonoperative management for pediatric splenic injury and demonstrated the safety of the latter approach in 1968.[13] Children were found to recover from these injuries surprisingly well, and by the late 1980s, the conservative management of pediatric splenic trauma was universally accepted, a change largely predating the radiologic advances that were crucial to the broad adoption of this strategy in adults.[14,15]

New understanding about the spleen's role in immunocompetence encouraged early efforts at salvage in adult trauma patients. OPSI, although rare, with a lifetime risk of less than 0.05%, carries a mortality rate of 50%.[12,16] Less severe infectious complications are more common, including abscess, wound infection, and pneumonia, all of which are increased after splenectomy, compared to splenic preservation after trauma.[17] The reasons for this remain incompletely understood. The spleen represents one-quarter to one-half of the lymphoid tissue in the body; is a reservoir of macrophages, which remove bacteria and red blood cells infected with parasites; and produces vital immunomodulators such as opsonins, which are needed to clear encapsulated organisms. Asplenic patients are probably more susceptible to gram-negative bacteria and fungi as well.[12] Splenectomized patients should be immunized against *Streptococcus pneumoniae*, meningococcus, *and Haemophilus influenzae* type B, the encapsulated organisms for which vaccines are currently available.[12,16,17]

The trend toward conservative management of splenic injury coincided with the development of endovascular techniques to achieve hemostasis and support organ preservation. Although balloon occlusion and gelatin foam embolization had been previously reported,[18,19] in 1981, Sclafani[20] described endovascular occlusion of the proximal main splenic artery with coils, and he predicted that this would improve the outcomes of NOM. In 1991, Sclafani and his colleagues[21] reported a striking 97% splenic salvage rate with routine angiography and selective proximal splenic artery occlusion in patients with splenic lacerations diagnosed with CT.

The specific indications and most appropriate candidates for NOM and adjunctive angioembolization have been a topic of debate and many retrospective studies in the intervening period; the object has been to elucidate the vital factors which contribute to the success or failure of conservative management. Failure is indicated by continued or recurrent splenic bleeding, often referred to as *delayed splenic rupture*. Peitzman et al.[22] found that the success of NOM is directly correlated with increasing hematocrit and blood pressure and inversely correlated with OIS grade and quantity of hemoperitoneum. Advanced age has been shown to be a risk factor; Renzulli et al.[23] found age older than 55 years to be the only independent risk factor for failure of NOM. The direct relationship between increasing OIS grade and failure rate of conservative therapy has been demonstrated in multiple retrospective analyses.[22,24–27]

Patient Selection

Most large trauma centers include splenic artery embolization (SAE) as a variable component of NOM. Much of the current literature supports angiography for hemodynamically stable patients with CT findings suggesting contrast extravasation and/or grade IV or V injuries. Several studies have demonstrated that in low-grade injuries (OIS I to III), angioembolization does not result in an improvement in outcomes, whereas in higher grade injuries, a marked improvement is seen.[25–27] For example, Requarth et al.[27] showed that although failure of nonoperative management (FNOM) was less than 5% in OIS grades I and II injuries with or without SAE, it rose with each OIS grade to 83.1% in grade V observation-only patients but only to 25% in patients who underwent SAE.

Although most trauma centers include angiography and embolization as an adjunct to NOM of splenic trauma in hemodynamically stable patients, there are no randomized trials. Thus, the Eastern Association for the Surgery of Trauma (EAST) assigns a level 2 recommendation to use SAE in grades IV and V injuries or whenever contrast extravasation is noted on CT.[8] Bhullar et al.[28] supported this recommendation in a 2013 study, pointing out that significantly higher failure rate of NOM in grades IV and V injuries may be affected by the fact that many centers do not perform angiography in cases where extravasation is not noted on CT. Although evidence of active bleeding is more common in higher grade injuries, it may be seen in lower grade (OIS I to III) injuries as well.

Technique

If the splenic artery is clearly identified on the admission CT, a flush aortogram may not be necessary before splenic artery selection. Typically, a Cobra (Angiodynamics, Latham, New York) or reverse curve catheter such as an Sos or Mikaelsson (Angiodynamics, Latham, New York) is used to select the celiac axis. Splenic angiography should be performed with automated injection. If angiography reveals active extravasation, then selective distal coil embolization may be performed using a microcatheter with microcoils and/or gelfoam, followed by proximal main splenic artery coil embolization (Fig. 22.1). If there is no evidence of active hemorrhage, then only proximal main SAE is performed using coils, either via the main catheter or a microcatheter.

The rationale for proximal main SAE is reduction of splenic blood pressure, facilitating hemostasis without causing infarction. The abundant arterial supply to the spleen makes this possible. Perfusion is maintained by pancreatic, omental, and short gastric arteries at relatively lower pressure, which gives splenic vascular injuries an opportunity to heal; as the collateral arteries enlarge, pressure is believed to eventually return to preembolization levels, although when this happens is unknown.[29,30] Requarth and colleagues[30] conducted a study demonstrating significant variability in the distal splenic arterial pressure during proximal balloon occlusion of the splenic artery. They concluded that some patients, such as those with celiac stenosis, might already have well-developed splanchnic collaterals, which would negate the impact of proximal splenic artery occlusion on parenchymal pressure. Interestingly, their results suggest that it may be reasonable to perform splenic

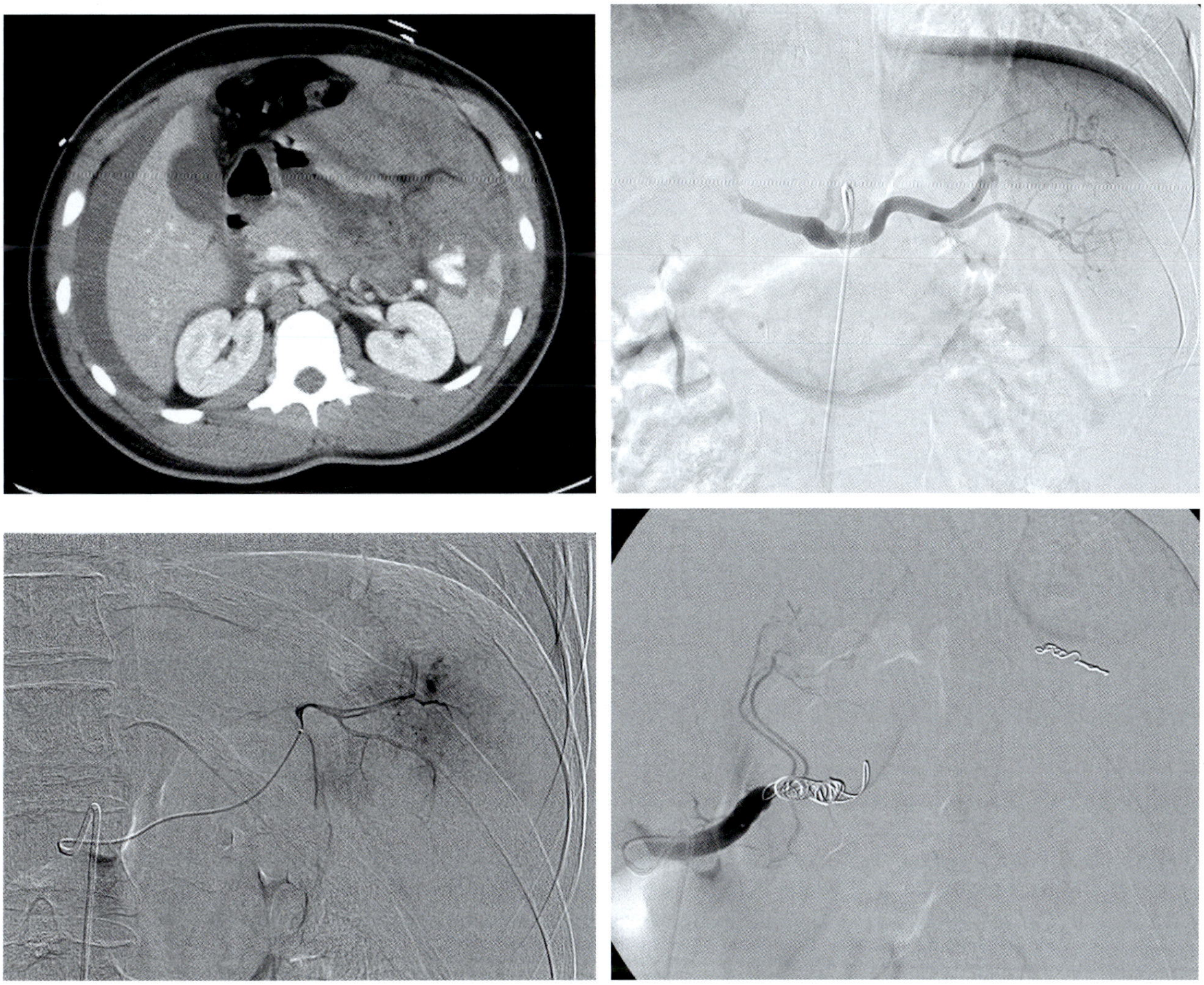

A B C D

Figure 22.1 A 20-year-old male, involved in snowboarding accident. **A:** CT demonstrates a grade III splenic laceration, active extravasation, and hemoperitoneum. **B:** Splenic angiography did not demonstrate active extravasation. **C:** Selective microcatheter injection demonstrates pseudoaneurysm. **D:** Pseudoaneurysm was excluded with detachable coils proximal and distal to the injury and proximal SAE was performed with 6- to 12-mm detachable coils.

artery balloon occlusion with pressure measurements in all splenic trauma patients before deciding whether to embolize; patients who do not demonstrate a significant decrease in splenic artery pressure during balloon occlusion may be better served with either surgery or observation.

The diameter of the splenic artery should be measured and coils oversized by at least 2 mm to avoid coil migration and increased risk of splenic infarction. Appropriate sizing is difficult. Detachable coils allow the operator to retract a partially deployed coil if it appears that migration is likely. For proximal main SAE, coils should be placed distal to the dorsal pancreatic artery and proximal to the greater pancreatic artery (often called by its Latin name *arteria pancreatica magna*), although the ideal location is not known (Fig. 22.2). The dorsal pancreatic artery is usually the largest splenic artery branch to the pancreas and there is at least a small risk that occluding this vessel could lead to pancreatic ischemia.[29] It also gives rise to distal branches that become a collateral source of splenic perfusion after occlusion of the splenic artery. However, there is variability in the anatomic origins of these pancreatic branches, and they cannot always be identified with certainty. The omental and short gastric arteries, left gastroepiploic artery, and other branches from the inferior and caudal pancreatic artery will also serve as collateral blood sources for the spleen after proximal embolization.[29,30] Postembolization angiography should demonstrate occlusion of the main splenic artery with delayed splenic parenchymal perfusion via collateral flow.

Results

In a comprehensive retrospective analysis of 33 blunt splenic injury outcomes articles from 1994 to 2009 by

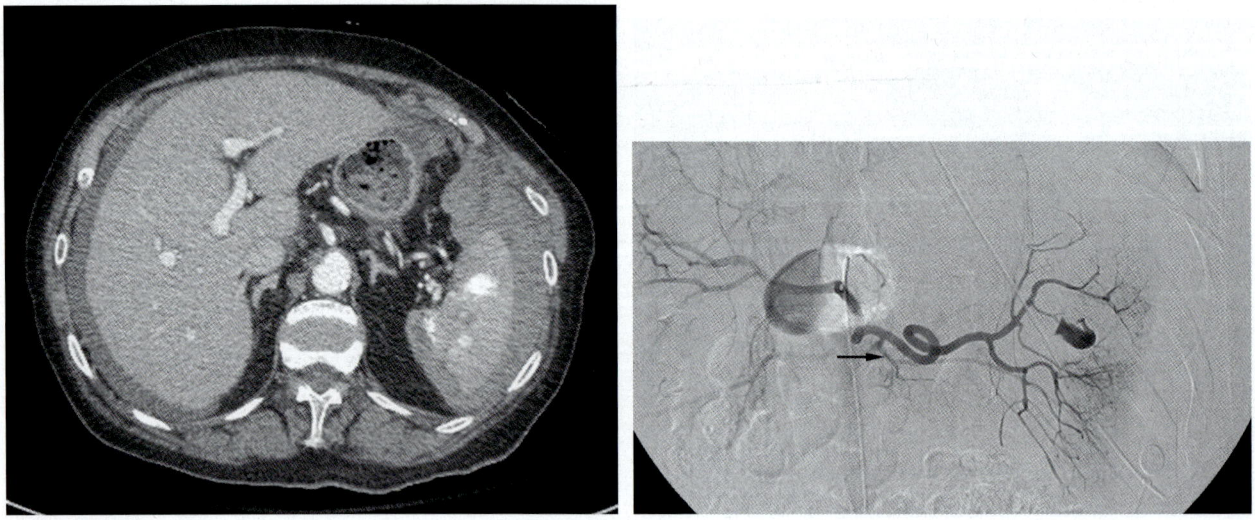

Figure 22.2 A 16-year-old male, tackled in football practice. **A:** CT shows a grade IV splenic laceration with active extravasation and hemoperitoneum. **B:** Celiac arteriography shows the splenic artery and dorsal pancreatic artery (*arrow*). There is active extravasation of contrast from a segmental artery, which was subsequently occluded with helical 2- to 4-mm microcoils.

Requarth et al.,[27] patients were stratified based on type of NOM (with or without SAE) as well as splenic injury grade. They found the overall failure rate of observational management to be 17%, with much worse rates of 44% and 83% in grades IV and V injuries, respectively.[27] However, SAE significantly decreased the failure rates in grades IV and V to 17% and 25%, respectively.[27] Bhullar et al.[28] found a 4% failure rate in patients with high-grade splenic injuries who underwent SAE, including those with contrast blush on CT, only 9% of whom ultimately required laparotomy (splenectomy or splenorrhaphy). In one of the largest single-center studies using a protocol of selective embolization in patients with CT evidence of vascular injury or active bleeding, Sabe et al.[31] reported an NOM success rate of 97%. Banerjee et al.[32] compared outcomes across four level I trauma centers with varying rates of embolization and found that SAE is an independent predictor of spleen salvage; centers in which it was used more had higher NOM success rates. Haan et al.[33] published another large single-center study which demonstrated 90% success overall with NOM and over 80% success in grades IV and V splenic injuries. Many of the successful cases had CT scans demonstrating pseudoaneurysm or active extravasation and were treated with SAE. However, in patients with traumatic arteriovenous fistula (AVF), failure rates were high (40%) even after SAE. They concluded that AVF requires direct embolization and that proximal SAE is insufficient in these cases.[33]

In cases of late rebleeding after observation or SAE, it appears that many, if not most, centers favor splenectomy even though conservative management has become standard therapy for acute splenic injury. The reasons for this are unclear but likely reflect a reluctance to continue with a "failed" strategy. In a paper by Liu et al.,[34] 15 cases of "delayed splenic rupture" were reviewed. Twelve were treated nonoperatively with 83% success rate, and 5 of these underwent SAE with 80% success rate. These results are comparable to those of primary NOM with or without SAE and they conclude that embolization is a reasonable strategy for late rebleeding.[34]

The most common complication directly related to SAE is splenic infarction, of which there is a higher risk when distal embolization is performed.[35,36] The clinical significance of these typically small or segmental splenic infarcts is unclear, as most ultimately resolve without further intervention.[35] In a meta-analysis by Schnuringer et al.,[35] no difference in the rate of major complications such as large infarct or abscess requiring splenectomy was found when comparing proximal and distal embolization techniques. Other complications are predominantly technical and rare, including arterial dissection, coil migration into the aorta, and femoral artery pseudoaneurysm.[36]

Protocols regarding observation, discharge, and follow-up imaging vary but typically include inpatient stay of 3 to 5 days, as recommended by Peitzman et al.[22] Rebleeding, the most common cause of failure, most often occurs within 3 days of injury.[37,38] Smith et al.[38] demonstrated that 95% of failures would be detected within 3 days. Significantly improving this risk is unlikely because statistically, to detect 99% of failures, 30-day observation would be required.[38] Most surgeons do not perform routine postdischarge imaging.[9] This is supported by a study by Haan and colleagues[37] examining splenic pseudoaneurysms after NOM. In their series, distal splenic embolization was only performed if free extravasation of contrast was seen at angiography. Pseudoaneurysm, AVF, and extravasation confined to the spleen were treated with proximal SAE. Patients found to have persistent or new pseudoaneurysms on follow-up CT after NOM had similar splenic salvage rates (94%) without additional therapies. Most pseudoaneurysms had resolved on follow-up imaging.[37]

Finally, the question of immunocompetence after splenic angioembolization has been addressed in several papers. Although our understanding of immunomodulating functions of the spleen is incomplete, authors of several studies have concluded that there is no evidence that immune function is significantly affected by SAE.[17,39] Therefore, immunization is not recommended for these patients.

TIPS AND TRICKS

- When performing a proximal SAE, ideal coil deployment is between the dorsal pancreatic and great pancreatic artery (also known as *arteria pancreatica magna*). Given the anatomic variability and often poor visualization of these branches, a good rule of thumb is to deposit coils at the junction of the proximal and middle third of the splenic artery.
- Sizing coils for a proximal SAE can be difficult. Detachable coils or Amplatzer Vascular Plugs (St. Jude Medical, Inc., St. Paul, Minnesota) may be partially deployed and retrieved if they do not "hold," which helps to avoid distal coil migration.
- Selective distal coil occlusion should only be performed if there is active extravasation, pseudoaneurysm, or AVF. Given the likelihood in high-grade injuries of other vascular lesions that may not be evident on angiography due to thrombus or vasospasm, this should be followed by proximal SAE.

LIVER

Hepatic arterial embolization, similar to splenic embolization, is an important adjunct in the NOM of liver trauma, although technique, rationale, and complications are different. Owing to the greater inherent difficulty of controlling hemorrhage from hepatic compared to splenic injury, angiography and embolization may play a larger role during and after surgery.[40] This is because high-OIS-grade liver injuries often produce arterial bleeding, which is well controlled by transarterial embolization, as well as venous bleeding, which is not.[41] Juxtahepatic venous hemorrhage often requires laparotomy, sometimes with perihepatic packing and temporary closure ("damage control") for the most critical patients.[40–42] In many modern operating rooms which are equipped with adequate fluoroscopy, embolization of deep, surgically inaccessible arterial bleeding can be accomplished immediately after laparotomy.

Identifying the patients with injuries to the retrohepatic inferior vena cava and hepatic veins therefore is vital. In a 2003 paper by Mohr et al.,[43] patients with juxtahepatic venous injuries had the highest mortality rates among liver injuries. However, according to Hagiwara and colleagues,[41] CT has low specificity and positive predictive value for venous injury. In their 2002 prospective study of liver trauma patients, the highest sensitivity, specificity, and positive predictive value of juxtahepatic venous injury was resuscitative requirement of greater than 2 L of fluids per hour.[41] Although most would agree that these patients are not stable and should be brought to the operating room, in a 2009 paper by Misselbeck and colleagues,[44] 52% of patients who underwent laparotomy for hepatic injury demonstrated continued postoperative arterial bleeding requiring embolization. In the same study, patients with CT evidence of active extravasation were 20 times more likely to have positive angiograms compared to those with no evidence of active hemorrhage on CT.[44] The 2012 EAST guidelines assign a level 2 recommendation to angiography with embolization in patients who are transient responders to resuscitation as an "adjunct to potential operative intervention."[7]

Technique

Hepatic angiography should generally begin with flush aortography due to the high incidence of variable anatomy. A 5-Fr catheter is used to select the celiac axis and angiography is performed from the common hepatic artery. Even if there is no evidence of hemorrhage, selective angiography should be performed with a microcatheter targeting areas of extravasation identified on CT. In contrast to proximal splenic artery occlusion in which decreasing blood pressure to the spleen is the primary goal, the goal in hepatic injury is to embolize distally where there is evidence of hemorrhage (Fig. 22.3). The dual arterial and portal venous blood supply to the liver likely confers some protection from ischemic complications, but proximal hepatic artery occlusion is typically unnecessary and may be detrimental, particularly in patients with preexisting liver disease or compromised portal venous blood flow.

The choice of embolic material depends on the extent of the injury and how distal the microcatheter can be placed. If there is a wide area of arterial extravasation or the patient is decompensating, relatively proximal embolization with particles or gelfoam slurry may be necessary to achieve rapid hemostasis. However, it must be understood that this will increase the risk of hepatic failure or necrosis requiring operative debridement. If the hemorrhage is focal, superselective catheterization is preferable. Microcoils, particles, and gelfoam have all been used successfully. However, the presence of bile is a unique and possibly complicating feature of liver lacerations because it inhibits granulation and scar formation, thereby arresting the normal reparative process.[45] Biloma formation is a known complication of hepatic trauma,

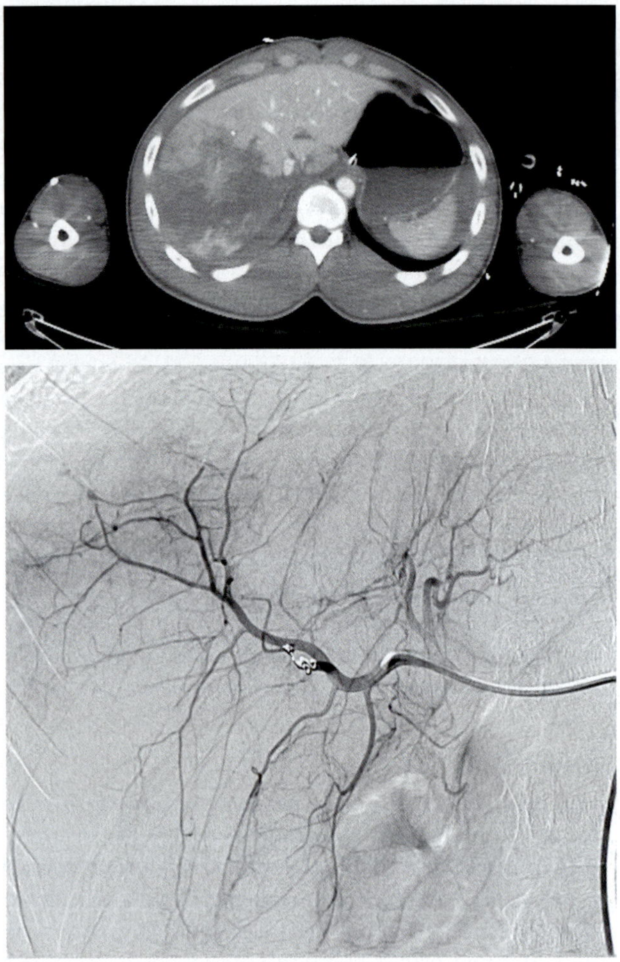

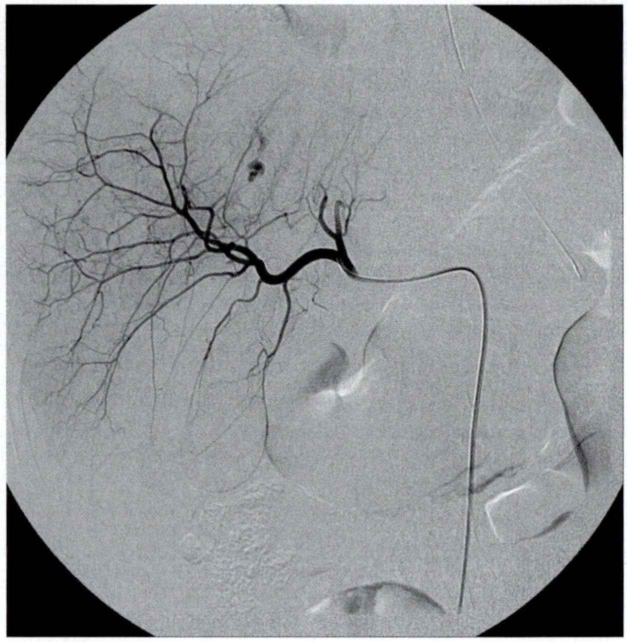

A B C

Figure 22.3 A 20-year-old male, fell from three stories. **A:** CT demonstrates a grade IV hepatic laceration in the posterior right hepatic lobe with active extravasation. **B:** Right hepatic angiogram demonstrates extravasation. **C:** Selective coil embolization using 2-mm pushable coils.

occurring after 2% to 8% of cases.[46] Theoretically, therefore, use of gelfoam, which causes temporary vascular occlusion, may increase the risk of pseudoaneurysm formation because in the presence of bile, there may not be sufficient time for healing of vascular injuries before recanalization occurs. Hagiwara et al.[46] presented evidence supporting this theory in a small review of 11 patients with posttraumatic biloma; pseudoaneurysm formation was significantly more likely in patients initially treated with gelfoam embolization compared to those embolized with metallic coils. Although this was a small retrospective study, their conclusion that in the liver, permanent coil embolization is preferable to gelfoam when technically feasible is worth considering.[46]

Results

The safety and efficacy of hepatic arterial embolization for hemodynamically stable trauma patients has been established.[40,41,43,44,47] Clinical success rates of greater than 90% have been reported by several investigators.[48–50] Complications of severe hepatic injury, such as biloma, necrosis, and abscess, have been reported to occur in up to 50% of cases and are similar to those which could be attributed to embolization. Mohr et al.[43] reported the occurrence of such complications in 58% of hepatic trauma patients in her series and concluded that liver-related morbidity is not increased or decreased by angioembolization. Gallbladder ischemia and necrosis, however, can often be attributed directly to embolization; Mohr et al.[43] and Misselbeck et al.[44] both describe gallbladder-related complications, all of which occurred in patients who underwent selective right hepatic artery embolization. This can be avoided with judicious use of particles and superselective embolization distal to the cystic artery origin when treating injuries to branches of the right hepatic artery.

Hepatic necrosis after trauma often requires open debridement, but bilomas and abscesses can be effectively managed using interventional radiology techniques.[51] In the patients who undergo hepatic artery embolization, the risk of these complications can be mitigated with more selective technique. Bile leaks complicated 23% of cases in the series by Mohr et al.[43] and were managed by interventional radiologists with percutaneous drainage for a median of 1 month. Carrillo and colleagues[51] brought attention to the importance of interventional radiologic techniques for management of these more common complications.

TIPS AND TRICKS

- Microcoils should be used for superselective embolization to limit necrosis.
- If there is a large territory with multifocal arterial injuries, realize that particles or gelfoam may be necessary for hemostasis but will increase the risk of liver failure and may lead to necrosis requiring operative debridement.
- When embolizing the right hepatic artery, the catheter should be positioned distal to the cystic artery to avoid gallbladder necrosis.

KIDNEY

In comparison with hepatic and splenic injuries, renal injuries are less common, occurring in 1% to 5% of all traumas.[52] Hemorrhagic renal injuries requiring intervention are more commonly iatrogenic, that is, related to percutaneous nephrostomy, biopsy, nephrostolithotomy, etc., than traumatic.[53] As in all solid organ injuries, conservative management with selective angioembolization is now the standard in patients with grades I to IV injuries who are hemodynamically stable. A common theme throughout this chapter is organ preservation; patients with renal injuries who undergo laparotomy are more likely to have a nephrectomy, the implications of which may ultimately be severe, particularly in the event of future trauma, nephrolithiasis, malignancy, or other renal insult.[54] In one series of patients with renal trauma, 28% of patients undergoing nephrectomy developed renal failure.[55] Grades I and II injuries are managed conservatively (observation-only), with near 100% success rate.[54] In grades III and IV injuries, management depends on imaging findings and clinical status.

The optimal management of grade V lesions is uncertain, and published results are variable. Many surgeons advocate nephrectomy in grade V, particularly renovascular lesions. Breyer et al.[56] reported a failure rate of 100% (5/5) for angioembolization of grade V injuries. Brewer et al.[57] reported 100% success rate of angioembolization for grade V injuries in unstable patients. These differences in outcomes may be due to inhomogeneity of grade V injuries, with renal pedicle avulsion, for example, likely requiring surgery.[58] Hagiwara et al.[59] reported on his success with angioembolization in all grade III through grade V renal injuries in which it was attempted. Eight of the patients in this series were grade IV or grade V, and each of these was successfully embolized.[59] In the study by Brewer et al.,[57] nine hemodynamically unstable patients with grade V parenchymal and renovascular injuries were successfully embolized with no further interventions required. Most of these patients, however, underwent main renal artery occlusion with coils. Follow-up after a mean of 2.7 years revealed no adverse effects of the embolizations.[60]

Complete renal embolization is an alternative to nephrectomy in patients who may be poor surgical candidates, with low complication rates and few long-term sequelae. In a 1999 paper by Hom et al.,[61] eight patients underwent complete renal embolization for various reasons including recurrent bleeding from tumor or angiomyolipoma, none of which related to trauma. Most of the patients required narcotics for pain control for up to 48 hours, but in mean follow-up of 30 months, no abscess, hypertension, or renal failure developed.[61] Main renal artery embolization for trauma, however, is essentially a nonoperative nephrectomy with the benefits limited to avoidance of exploratory laparotomy. Optimal management of grade V vascular renal injury remains uncertain and for now depends on individual trauma center expertise and availability of interventional radiologists.

OIS grade and clinical status are important but imperfect indicators for the need for intervention, particularly with regard to OIS grades III and IV injuries. Several retrospective studies have helped to clarify this issue by identifying specific CT findings indicative of the need for intervention, either angiographic or surgical.[6,62,63] Contrast extravasation and perirenal hematoma rim distance (PRD) were found to be significant predictors of intervention in the studies by Dugi et al.[6] and Nuss et al.[62] In the study by Dugi et al.,[6] medial as opposed to lateral laceration site was also found to be a significant predictor of the need for intervention. Most recently, Lin et al.[63] found that the combination of contrast extravasation and extent of hematoma "remarkably increased the predictive value of the need for intervention." Dugi et al.[6] recommended substratifying the OIS grade IV into grades IVa (low risk) and IVb (high risk: PRD >3.5 cm, contrast extravasation, and medial renal laceration), with IVb indicating the need for angioembolization or surgery. These CT findings could also be used to upgrade grade III injuries with two or more risk factors to IVb injuries.[6]

Technique

Arterial lacerations and pseudoaneurysms in the kidney, like those in the liver or spleen, are preferably treated with coil embolization of the artery as close as possible to the site of injury (Fig. 22.4). Given the variability in arterial supply to the kidney, flush aortography is typically necessary. A Cobra or reverse curve (Sos or Mikaelsson, for example) catheter is most commonly used to select the renal artery. If extravasation, pseudoaneurysm, or AVF is present, the injured artery is selected using a microcatheter, and embolization with microcoils is performed as close to the injury as possible. In cases of extravasation from the main renal artery, a covered stent may be deployed. If this is suspected based on CT findings or clinical status, starting with a longer 6-Fr or 7-Fr sheath or shaped guiding catheter, which can be advanced to the renal artery ostium for stent delivery, will save time. As described earlier, main renal artery embolization may be required in renal hilar injuries; close communication

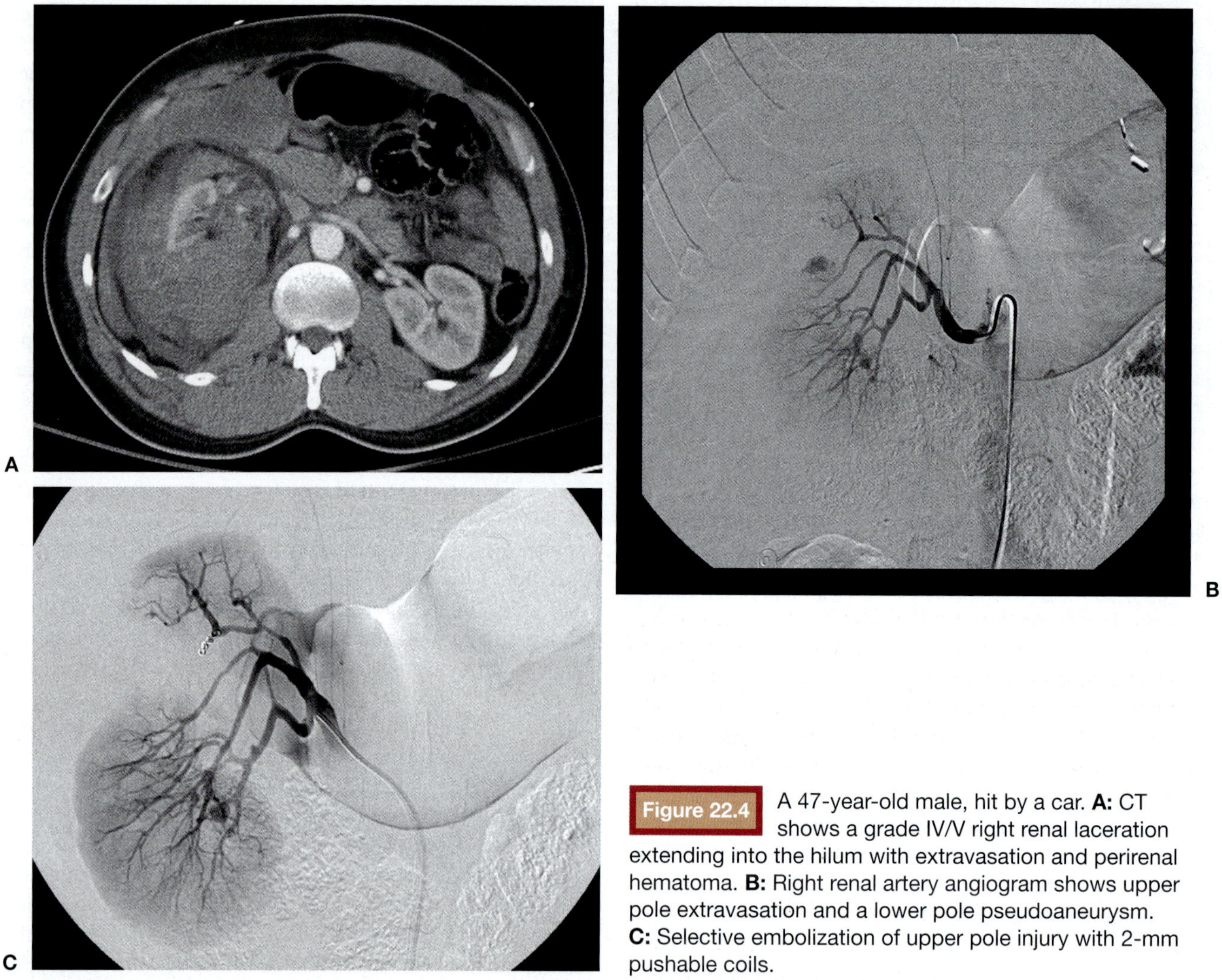

Figure 22.4 A 47-year-old male, hit by a car. **A:** CT shows a grade IV/V right renal laceration extending into the hilum with extravasation and perirenal hematoma. **B:** Right renal artery angiogram shows upper pole extravasation and a lower pole pseudoaneurysm. **C:** Selective embolization of upper pole injury with 2-mm pushable coils.

between the interventional radiologist and trauma surgeon is particularly important in these cases to determine the optimal course of action.

Results

Reported outcomes of transarterial embolization for renal vascular injury are excellent and demonstrate the effectiveness of this therapy in fulfilling the dual goals of hemostasis and preservation of renal function. In a series of five patients with nontraumatic arterial injury and pseudoaneurysm who underwent transarterial coil embolization, Poulakis et al.[53] demonstrated 100% success rate in cessation of bleeding and return to preinjury creatinine values. Average estimated area of renal infarct in follow-up CT was 5%.[53] Segmental renal arteries are considered end arteries, so infarcts typically occur after renal angioembolization, but they tend to be subclinical and are reported to decrease in size over time.[64,65] This process may represent collateral blood flow restoring perfusion to initially ischemic parenchyma (i.e., these may not actually be true end arteries) or contraction of scar tissue.[65] There is a significant association between OIS grade based on initial CT and decrease in renal function in patients managed expectantly with or without embolization, with overall poor functional outcome in grade V as well as certain grade IV injuries.[66,67] One may therefore conclude that embolization in grade V injuries is unlikely to significantly affect the degree of renal function preservation. Several studies have demonstrated that superselective angioembolization of renal arterial injuries does not result in a clinically significant long-term decrease in renal function.[53,64,65]

Huber et al.[68] analyzed 26 studies of renal embolization for traumatic and nontraumatic hemorrhage and found 89% primary success rate and 82% success rate in repeat angioembolization for those who failed the initial therapy. In patients who failed angioembolization and did not undergo repeat attempt, 100% underwent nephrectomy. Based on this data, they concluded that patients who fail angioembolization should undergo a repeat session instead of laparotomy.[68]

In the largest such study of renal trauma patients to date, Hotaling et al.[69] analyzed NTDB data of renal injuries from 2002 to 2007 and also found high success rates for repeat angioembolization.

Finally, the type of renal vascular injury, penetrating versus blunt, may play a role in outcomes of expectant management and influence the decision to intervene. Specifically, penetrating renal trauma may require a more aggressive approach due to the higher likelihood of arterial laceration. This was the conclusion of Muir et al.[70] who reported a 20% failure of observation in penetrating renal trauma and support the use of early angiography in this setting. In a study by Bjurlin et al.[71] reviewing 98 penetrating renal injuries, selective NOM resulted in lower mortality rate, shorter mean intensive care unit and hospital stays, and fewer blood transfusions compared with nephrectomy; angioembolization was not a part of the protocol at their institution. Most of the cited studies of renal trauma did not substratify patients based on mechanism of injury.

TIPS AND TRICKS

- Microcatheters should be used for superselective coil occlusion to preserve renal function.

THORACIC TRAUMA

BACKGROUND AND PATIENT SELECTION

Blunt and penetrating thoracic trauma often results in persistent intrathoracic hemorrhage and hemothorax, for which exploratory thoracotomy has historically been the "gold standard" treatment.[72] However, many patients are poor candidates for surgery due to associated injuries or comorbidities. In patients with slow or intermittent arterial bleeding, thoracotomy may fail to identify and control the source.[72,73] Excluding injuries to the aorta and great vessels, which are also often treated endovascularly with stent grafts, a common cause of hemothorax is intercostal arterial injury, which is well suited to transcatheter embolization. Compared with the literature regarding solid organ injury, embolization for thoracic trauma has received little attention. Several case reports and small retrospective series have demonstrated its safety and effectiveness.[72–75]

Up to 85% of patients who survive blunt or penetrating thoracic trauma require only conservative measures, including tube thoracostomy, adequate volume resuscitation, and serial chest radiographs.[72] Chest tube output of between 500 and 1,000 mL over a defined period is considered a threshold for thoracotomy.[74] In keeping with the theme of this chapter, transarterial embolization is an effective alternative in the hemodynamically stable patient and can obviate the need for thoracotomy.

According to Hagiwara et al.,[74] common causes of hemothorax after thoracic trauma are intercostal arterial lacerations and pulmonary lacerations. Differentiating between the two is important in the patient with significant chest tube output (>200 mL per hour) because embolization would not be helpful if the bleeding is secondary to pulmonary laceration. In their study of 154 patients who underwent contrast-enhanced CT, contrast extravasation and large displacement of a fractured rib were associated with intercostal arterial injury, and 5 out of 5 of these patients were successfully embolized.[74] Their findings support CT in patients with chest tube output of greater than 200 mL per hour and embolization if there is contrast extravasation on CT.[74] Other authors rely on chest tube output or hemoglobin and less on CT findings.[72,73]

TECHNIQUE

Intercostal arteries as well as bronchial arteries are not typically well seen with aortography given their small size. Reverse curve catheters such as Mikaelsson are often used. The intercostal arteries are small, and at times, 5-Fr may be too large to actually select the artery; in these cases, a microwire and microcatheter may be advanced coaxially into the artery. If extravasation or pseudoaneurysm is identified, superselective catheterization with microcoil embolization and/or particles is performed. Achieving hemostasis may be difficult because of collateral flow via internal mammary, musculophrenic, inferior phrenic, and adjacent intercostal arteries that can cause rebleeding.[73] Thus, if there is injury to the intercostal artery with extravasation or pseudoaneurysm, coils should be placed distal (Fig. 22.5) and proximal to the injury and consideration should be given to occluding the adjacent intercostal artery as well.[73] If the source of bleeding is ventral, then the internal mammary artery should be interrogated; this will also allow imaging of the musculophrenic artery, which is a branch of the internal mammary. The inferior phrenic artery may also anastomose with lower anterior intercostal arteries. The use of particles should be reserved for cases in which superselective catheterization is unsuccessful. This also requires particular caution because anterior segmental medullary arteries arise from various posterior intercostal arteries and supply portions of the anterior spinal cord. If these arteries are occluded, paralysis will likely result, the extent of which depends on the level of the spinal cord affected. The largest, or major, anterior segmental medullary artery (artery of Adamkiewicz) is typically present at the level of T10 on the left, but it may arise anywhere from T8 to T12, and embolization of this artery will cause anterior spinal cord ischemia and bilateral lower extremity paralysis.[76]

Catheterization of the internal mammary artery and other small branches of the subclavian artery such as the pectoral or lateral thoracic arteries may be difficult, often requiring placement of a 90-cm sheath or ipsilateral access via the

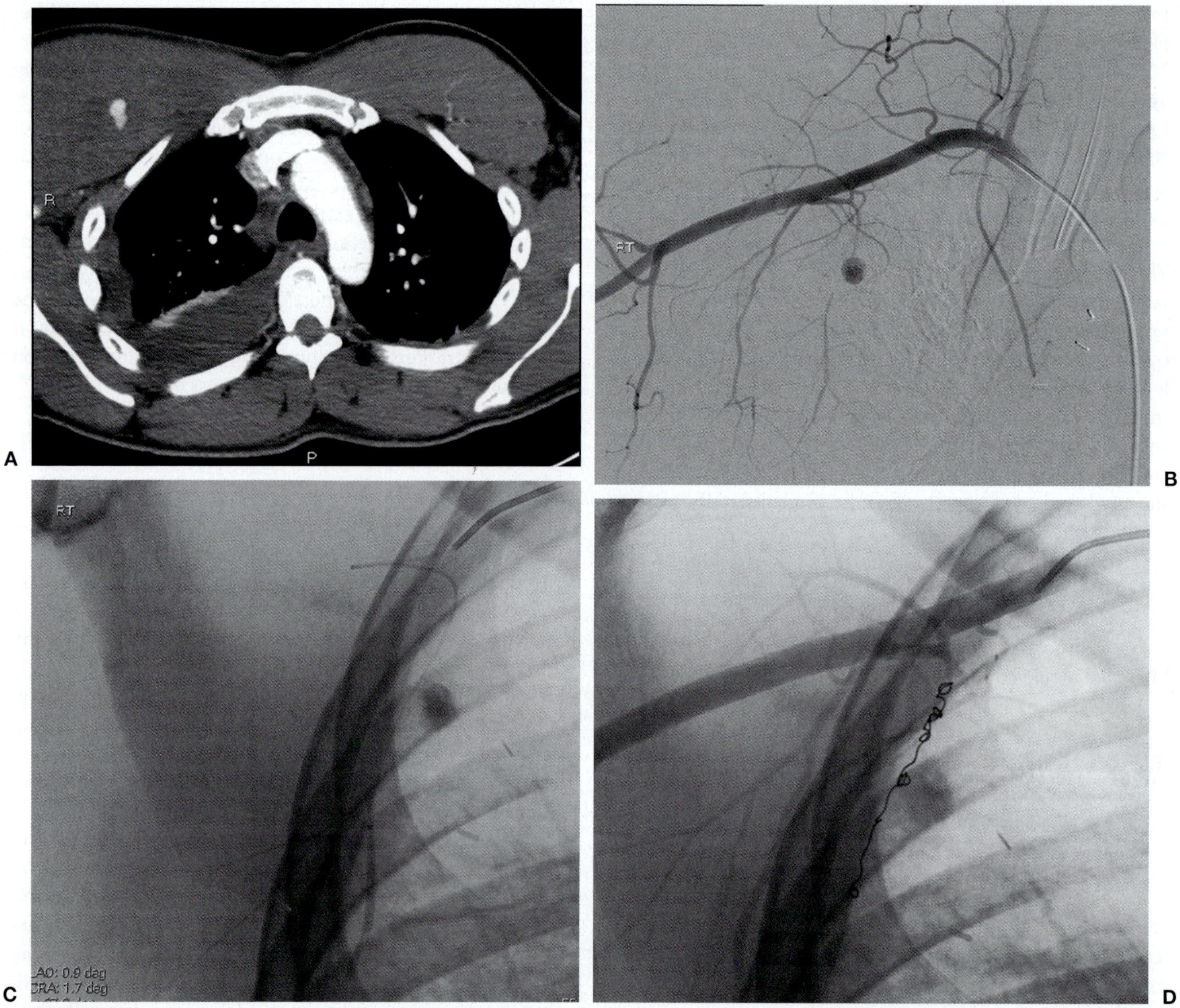

Figure 22.5 A 38-year-old male, with penetrating right chest injury. **A:** CT with extravasation in right pectoralis muscle. **B:** Subclavian angiogram demonstrates pseudoaneurysm arising from right pectoral artery, a branch of the thoracoacromial artery. **C:** Microcatheter placed distal to the pseudoaneurysm. **D:** Exclusion of the pseudoaneurysm with microcoils. (Courtesy of Kevin Daly, MD, Tufts Medical Center.)

radial or brachial artery. If access is via the femoral artery, an arch aortogram may be useful, particularly in older patients who may have difficult arch anatomy.

RESULTS

There is a paucity of series examining arterial embolization after thoracic trauma. Retrospective studies by Carrillo et al.[72] and Chemelli et al.,[73] cited earlier, demonstrate feasibility and efficacy of embolization in blunt and penetrating chest injuries, predominantly involving intercostal and internal mammary arterial injuries. Injuries to other anterior thoracic arteries originating from the subclavian artery, such as pectoral and lateral thoracic arteries, may be considered in the same category. The larger study by Chemelli et al.[73] demonstrated 87.5% primary technical success rate of arterial embolization in a combination of traumatic and iatrogenic thoracic injuries. Other literature is largely limited to case reports involving, for example, pulmonary artery pseudoaneurysms[77] (which most commonly result from iatrogenic injury), esophageal hematoma,[78] and a report by Hagiwara and Iwamoto[75] of successful embolization of bleeding from thoracic vertebral fractures via intercostal arteries.

These cases, relatively rare compared to solid organ injuries of the abdomen, do not lend themselves well to large retrospective studies. However, the basic principles and techniques of embolization are the same. The most significant variables in thoracic cases are the location of injury and presence of collateral vessels, which may cause rebleeding. When superselective catheterization is possible, every attempt should be made to exclude the injury by deploying coils across (distal and proximal to) the injury.

TIPS AND TRICKS

Thorax

- For bronchial or intercostal artery embolization, look for branches with the "hairpin turn" of the anterior segmental medullary arteries; embolization proximal to these arteries must be avoided as it may cause anterior spinal cord ischemia, which can lead to paralysis.

General

- When embolizing traumatic pseudoaneurysms, the injured artery should be embolized from a point just distal to the pseudoaneurysm to a point just proximal to the pseudoaneurysm to completely exclude the area of injury.

REFERENCES

1. Tinkoff G, Esposito TJ, Reed J, et al. American Association for the Surgery of Trauma Organ Injury Scale I: spleen, liver, and kidney, validation based on the National Trauma Data Bank. *J Am Coll Surg*. 2008;207:646–655.
2. Esposito TJ, Tinkoff G, Reed J, et al. American Association for the Surgery of Trauma Organ Injury Scale (OIS): past, present, and future. *J Trauma Acute Care Surg*. 2013;74:1163–1174.
3. Moore EE, Cogbill TH, Jurkovich GJ, et al. Organ injury scale: spleen and liver (1994 revision). *J Trauma*. 1995;38:323–324.
4. Barquist ES, Pizano LR, Feuer W, et al. Inter- and intra-rater reliability in computed axial tomographic grading of splenic injury: why so many grading scales? *J Trauma*. 2004;56:334–338.
5. Marmery H, Shanmuganathan K, Alexander MT, et al. Optimization of selection for nonoperative management of blunt splenic injury: comparison of MDCT grading systems. *AJR Am J Roentgenol*. 2007;189:1421–1427.
6. Dugi DD, Morey AF, Gupta A, et al. American Association for the Surgery of Trauma grade 4 renal injury substratification into grades 4a (low risk) and 4b (high risk). *J Urol*. 2010;183:592–597.
7. Stassen NA, Bhullar I, Cheng JD, et al. Selective nonoperative management of blunt hepatic injury: an Eastern Association for the Surgery of Trauma practice management guideline. *J Trauma Acute Care Surg*. 2012;73:S288–S293.
8. Stassen NA, Bhullar I, Cheng J, et al. Selective nonoperative management of blunt splenic injury: an Eastern Association for the Surgery of Trauma practice management guideline. *J Trauma Acute Care Surg*. 2012;73:S294–S300.
9. Olthof DC, van der Vlies CH, Joosse P, et al. Consensus strategies for the nonoperative management of patients with blunt splenic injury: a Delphi study. *J Trauma Acute Care Surg*. 2013;74:1567–1574.
10. Moore FA, Davis JW, Moore EE, et al. Western Trauma Association (WTA) critical decisions in trauma: management of adult blunt splenic trauma. *J Trauma*. 2008;65:1007–1011.
11. Shafi S, Parks J, Ahn C, et al. More operations more deaths? Relationship between operative intervention rates and risk-adjusted mortality at trauma centers. *J Trauma*. 2010;69:70–77.
12. Skattum J, Naess PA, Gaarder C. Nonoperative management and immune function after splenic injury. *Br J Surg*. 2012;99:59–65.
13. Upadhyaya P. Conservative management of splenic trauma: history and current trends. *Pediatr Surg Int*. 2003;19:617–627.
14. King H, Shumacker HB Jr. Splenic Studies 1. Susceptibility to infection after splenectomy performed in infancy. *Ann Surg*. 1952;136:239–242.
15. Pearl RH, Wesson DE, Spence LJ, et al. Splenic injury: a 5-year update with improved results and changing criteria for conservative management. *J Pediatr Surg*. 1989;24:121–125.
16. Malhotra AK, Carter RF, Lebman DA, et al. Preservation of splenic immunocompetence after splenic artery angioembolization for blunt splenic injury. *J Trauma*. 2010;69:1126–1131.
17. Demetriades D, Scalea TM, Degiannis E, et al. Blunt splenic trauma: splenectomy increases early infectious complications: a prospective multicenter study. *J Trauma*. 2012;72:229–234.
18. Wholey MH. The technology of balloon catheters in interventional angiography. *Radiology*. 1977;125:671–676.
19. Katzen BT, Rossi P, Passariello R, et al. Transcatheter therapeutic arterial embolization. *Radiology*. 1976;120:523–531.
20. Sclafani SJA. The role of angiographic hemostasis in salvage of the injured spleen. *Radiology*. 1981;141:645–650.
21. Sclafani SJA, Weisberg A, Scalea TM, et al. Blunt splenic injuries: nonsurgical treatment with CT, arteriography, and transcatheter arterial embolization of the splenic artery. *Radiology*. 1991;181:189–196.
22. Peitzman AB, Heil B, Rivera L, et al. Blunt splenic injury in adults: multi-institutional study of the Eastern Association for the Surgery of Trauma. *J Trauma*. 2000;49:177–189.
23. Renzulli P, Gross T, Schnuringer B, et al. Management of blunt injuries to the spleen. *Br J Surg*. 2010;97:1696–1703.
24. Olthof DC, Joose P, van der Vlies CH, et al. Prognostic factors for failure of nonoperative management in adults with blunt splenic injury: a systematic review. *J Trauma Acute Care Surg*. 2013;74:546–557.
25. Jeremitsky E, Kao A, Carlton C, et al. Does splenic embolization and grade of splenic injury impact nonoperative management in patients sustaining blunt splenic trauma? *Am Surg*. 2011;77:215–220.
26. Bhullar IS, Frykberg ER, Siragusa D, et al. Selective angiographic embolization of blunt splenic traumatic injuries in adults decreases failure rate of nonoperative management. *J Trauma*. 2012;72:1127–1134.
27. Requarth JA, D'Agostino RB, Miller PR. Nonoperative management of adult blunt splenic injury with and without splenic artery embolotherapy: a meta-analysis. *J Trauma*. 2011:71: 898–903.
28. Bhullar IS, Frykberg ER, Tepas III JJ, et al. At first blush: absence of computed tomography contrast extravasation in grade IV or V adult blunt splenic trauma should not preclude angioembolization. *J Trauma Acute Care Surg*. 2013;74:105–112.
29. Hamers RL, Van DenBerg FG, Groeneveld ABJ. Acute necrotizing pancreatitis following inadvertent extensive splenic artery embolization for trauma. *Br J Radiol*. 2009;82:e11–e14.

30. Requarth JA. Distal splenic artery hemodynamic changes during transient proximal splenic artery occlusion in blunt splenic injury patients: a mechanism of delayed splenic hemorrhage. *J Trauma*. 2010;69:1423–1426.
31. Sabe AA, Cloridge JA, Rosenblum DI, et al. The effects of splenic artery embolization on nonoperative management of blunt splenic injury: a 16-year experience. *J Trauma*. 2009;67:565–572.
32. Banerjee A, Duane TM, Wilson SP, et al. Trauma center variation in splenic artery embolization and spleen salvage: a multicenter analysis. *J Trauma Acute Care Surg*. 2013;75:69–75.
33. Haan JM, Bochicchio GV, Kramer N, et al. Nonoperative management of blunt splenic injury: a five-year experience. *J Trauma*. 2005;58:492–498.
34. Liu P, Liu H, Hsieu T, et al. Nonsurgical management of delayed splenic rupture after blunt trauma. *J Trauma*. 2012;72: 1019–1023.
35. Schnuringer B, Inaba K, Konstantinidis A, et al. Outcomes of proximal versus distal splenic artery embolization after trauma: a systematic review and meta-analysis. *J Trauma*. 2011;70: 252–260.
36. Ekeh AP, Khalaf S, Ilyas S, et al. Complications arising from splenic artery embolization: a review of an 11-year experience. *Am J Surg*. 2013;205:250–254.
37. Haan JM, Marmery H, Shanmuganathan K, et al. Experience with splenic main coil embolization and significance of new or persistent pseudoaneurysm: reembolize, operate, or observe. *J Trauma*. 2007;63:615–619.
38. Smith J, Armen S, Cook C, et al. Blunt splenic injuries: have we watched long enough? *J Trauma*. 2008;64:656–665.
39. Tominaga GT, Simon FJ, Dandan IS, et al. Immunologic function after splenic embolization, is there a difference? *J Trauma*. 2009;67:289–293.
40. Johnson JW, Graciac VH, Gupta R, et al. Hepatic angiography in patients undergoing damage control laparotomy. *J Trauma*. 2002;52:1102–1106.
41. Hagiwara A, Murata A, Matsuda T, et al. The efficacy and limitations of transarterial embolization for severe hepatic injury. *J Trauma*. 2002;52:1091–1096.
42. Higa G, Friese R, O'Keefe T, et al. Damage control laparotomy: a vital tool once overused. *J Trauma*. 2010;69:53–59.
43. Mohr AM, Lavery RF, Barone A, et al. Angiographic embolization for liver injuries: low mortality, high morbidity. *J Trauma*. 2003;55:1077–1082.
44. Misselbeck TS, Teicher EJ, Cipolle MD, et al. Hepatic angioembolization in trauma patients: indications and complications. *J Trauma*. 2009;67:769–773.
45. Sandblum P, Mirkovitch V, Gardiol D. The healing of liver wounds. *Ann Surg*. 1976;183:679–684.
46. Hagiwara A, Tarui T, Murata A, et al. Relationship between pseudoaneurysm formation and biloma after successful transarterial embolization for severe hepatic injury: permanent embolization using stainless steel coils prevents pseudoaneurysm formation. *J Trauma*. 2005;59:49–55.
47. Ciraulo DL, Luk S, Palter M, et al. Selective hepatic arterial embolization of grade IV and V blunt hepatic injuries: an extension of resuscitation in the nonoperative management of traumatic hepatic injuries. *J Trauma*. 1998;45:353–359.
48. Malhotra AK, Fabian TC, Croce MA, et al. Blunt hepatic injury: a paradigm shift from operative to nonoperative management in the 1990s. *Ann Surg*. 2000;231:804–813.
49. Velmahos GC, Toutouzas K, Radin R, et al. High success with nonoperative management of blunt hepatic trauma. *Arch Surg*. 2003;138:475–481.
50. Van der Wilden GM, Velmahos GC, Emhoff T, et al. Successful nonoperative management of the most severe blunt liver injuries. *Arch Surg*. 2012;147:423–428.
51. Carrillo EH, Spain DA, Wohltmann CD, et al. Interventional techniques are useful adjuncts in nonoperative management of hepatic injuries. *J Trauma*. 1999;46:619–624.
52. Shoobridge JJ, Corcoran NM, Martin KA, et al. Contemporary management of renal trauma. *Rev Urol*. 2011;13(2):65–72.
53. Poulakis V, Ferakis N, Becht E, et al. Treatment of renal-vascular injury by transcatheter embolization: immediate and long-term effects on renal function. *J Endourol*. 2006;20(6):405–409.
54. Santucci RA, Fisher MB. The literature increasingly supports expectant (conservative) management of renal trauma—a systematic review. *J Trauma*. 2005;59:491–501.
55. Narrod JA, Moore EE, Posner M, et al. Nephrectomy following trauma—impact on patient outcome. *J Trauma*. 1985;25: 842–844.
56. Breyer BN, McAninch JW, Elliott SP, et al. Minimally invasive endovascular techniques to treat acute renal hemorrhage. *J Urol*. 2008;179:2248–2252.
57. Brewer ME Jr, Strnad BT, Daley BJ, et al. Percutaneous embolization for management of grade 5 renal trauma in hemodynamically unstable patients: initial experience. *J Urol*. 2009;181:1737–1741.
58. Altman AL, Haas C, Dinchman KH, et al. Selective nonoperative management of blunt grade 5 renal injury. *J Urol*. 2000;164:27–31.
59. Hagiwara A, Sakaki S, Goto G, et al. The role of interventional radiology in the management of blunt renal injury: a practical protocol. *J Trauma*. 2001;51:526–531.
60. Stewart AF, Brewer ME Jr, Daley BJ, et al. Intermediate-term follow-up of patients treated with percutaneous embolization for grade 5 blunt renal trauma. *J Trauma*. 2010;69:468–470.
61. Hom D, Eiley D, Lumerman JH, et al. Complete renal embolization as an alternative to nephrectomy. *J Urol*. 1999;161: 24–27.
62. Nuss GR, Morey AF, Jenkins AC, et al. Radiographic predictors of the need for angiographic embolization after traumatic renal injury. *J Trauma*. 2009;67:578–582.
63. Lin WC, Lin CH, Chen JH, et al. Computed tomographic imaging in determining the need of embolization for high-grade blunt renal injury. J *Trauma Acute Care Surg*. 2012;74:230–235.
64. Sofocleous CT, Hinrics C, Hubbi B, et al. Angiographic findings and embolotherapy in renal arterial trauma. *Cardiovasc Intervent Radiol*. 2005;28:39–47.
65. Chatziliannou A, Brountzos E, Primetis E, et al. Effects of superselective embolization for renal vascular injuries on renal parenchyma and function. *Eur J Vasc Endovasc Surg*. 2004;28:201–206.
66. Fiard G, Rambeaud JJ, Descotes JL, et al. Long-term renal function assessment with dimercapto-succinic acid scintigraphy after conservative treatment of major renal trauma. *J Urol*. 2012;187:1306–1309.
67. Tasian GE, Aaronson DS, McAninch JW. Evaluation of renal function after major renal injury: correlation with the American Association for the Surgery of Trauma injury scale. *J Urol*. 2010;183:196.

68. Huber J, Paternik S, Hallscheidt P, et al. Selective transarterial embolization for post traumatic renal hemorrhage: a second try is worthwhile. *J Urol.* 2011;185:1751–1755.
69. Hotaling JM, Sorensen MD, Smith TG, et al. Analysis of diagnostic angiography and angioembolization in acute management of renal trauma using a national data set. *J Urol.* 2011;185:1316–1320.
70. Muir MT, Inaba K, Ong A, et al. The need for early angiography in patients with penetrating renal injuries. *Eur J Trauma Emerg Surg.* 2012;38:275–280.
71. Bjurlin MA, Jeng EI, Goble SM, et al. Comparison of nonoperative management with renorrhaphy and nephrectomy in penetrating renal injuries. *J Trauma.* 2011;71:554–558.
72. Carrillo E, Heniford T, Senler S, et al. Embolization therapy as an alternative to thoracotomy in vascular injuries of the chest wall. *Am Surg.* 1998;64:1142–1148.
73. Chemelli AP, Thaurer M, Wiedermann F, et al. Transcatheter arterial embolization for the management of iatrogenic and blunt traumatic injuries. *J Vasc Surg.* 2009;49:1505–1513.
74. Hagiwara A, Yanagawa Y, Kaneko N, et al. Indications for transcatheter arterial embolization in persistent hemothorax caused by blunt trauma. *J Trauma.* 2008;65:589–594.
75. Hagiwara A, Iwamoto S. Usefulness of transcatheter arterial embolization for intercostal arterial bleeding in a patient with burst fractures of the thoracic vertebrae. *Emerg Radiol.* 2009;16:489–491.
76. Ozoilo K, Stein M. Paraplegia complicating embolization for bleeding intercostal artery in penetrating trauma. *Inj Ex.* 2013;44:70–73.
77. Block M, Lefkowitz T, Ravenel J, et al. Endovascular coil embolization for acute management of traumatic pulmonary artery pseudoaneurysm. *J Thorac Cardiovasc Surg.* 2004;128:784–785.
78. Shim J, Jang JY, Hwangbo Y, et al. Recurrent massive bleeding due to dissecting intramural hematoma of the esophagus: treatment with therapeutic angiography. *World J Gastroenterol.* 2009;15:5232–5235.

23

Pelvic Trauma

Pierre E. Bize • Yann Lachenal • Alban Denys

Pelvic hemorrhage is usually related to unstable pelvic fractures, which are observed in up to 25% of all polytrauma patients.[1] Because pelvic fractures are usually caused by high-energy trauma and often associated with injuries in other parts of the body, their management requires a multidisciplinary approach and triage decision between all bleeding sites. Despite the advances made in all disciplines of resuscitative medicine and surgery, the mortality rate following pelvic ring injuries ranges from 20% to 40%.[2–5]

Pelvic trauma represents a particular physiologic condition in the trauma spectrum. Usually, the pelvic compartment represents a closed space in which tamponade occurs rapidly, limiting the extension of bleeding. But in case of pelvic ring disruption, this tamponade effect does not occur, and it has been demonstrated that a gap of only 3 cm in the pelvic symphysis increases the volume of the pelvic compartment of as much as 1.5 L.[6]

Then, in case of pelvic fracture, patients can bleed up to 4 L of blood in a closed, difficult-to-reach compartment. According to the Advanced Trauma Life Support (ATLS) recommendation, the external stabilization of the pelvis should be performed in any case where there is suspicion or clinical evidence of pelvic fracture.[7] This can be achieved at the patient's arrival in the hospital or before using dedicated pelvic belts. A chest and pelvic x-ray should be obtained in the emergency room in all trauma patients to rule out hemothorax or pneumothorax and assess the presence or absence of evident pelvic fractures. Hemodynamically stable patient should then undergo computed tomography (CT) scan for a throughout workup. Hemodynamically unstable patients should benefit from a focused assessment by sonography for trauma (FAST) to look for free peritoneal fluid. Unstable patients with free abdominal fluid should be rushed to the operating room for exploratory laparotomy. However, note that if the peritoneum is not breached, the bleeding can be completely occult at FAST. In case of hemodynamically unstable patients without any other seriously bleeding injury and with no, or not enough, free intraperitoneal fluid to explain instability, retroperitoneal bleeding from the pelvis should be suspected.[5]

Bleeding in the pelvis can occur from arteries, veins, or directly from the broken bones. The immobilization of the pelvic ring with a strap or an external fixator helps restore the tamponade effect and has been shown to restore hemodynamic stability in polytrauma patients suffering from pelvic fractures.[8] However, tamponade is efficient only in case of bleeding from broken bones or lacerated veins. In patients with persistent hemodynamic instability despite pelvic ring immobilization, an arterial bleeding should be suspected. In this case, four treatment options are usually described: immediate external surgical fixation, direct surgical vessel ligation, retroperitoneal packing, and transcatheter arterial embolization (TAE).[9] There is no consensus on which of these treatment options is the most efficient in restoring hemodynamic stability, but there is a growing evidence in the literature suggesting that external fixation should be performed first and does not preclude any other subsequent adjuvant treatment.[9] However, this can be ponderated when arterial lesions are evidenced on the CT scanner and when surgical procedure is complex and would delay arterial bleeding control by TAE.

Figure 23.1 describes the decision-making algorithm proposed by Geeraerts et al.[5]

There are many classifications of pelvic fractures based on the underlying traumatic mechanism or on the presence or absence of posterior ring elements instability.[10] The classification of Pennal et al.[11] describes three types of underlying mechanism: type 1 (anteroposterior compression), resulting in transverse opening of the pelvic ring (open book fracture) and risk of lesion of the internal iliac artery (IIA); type 2

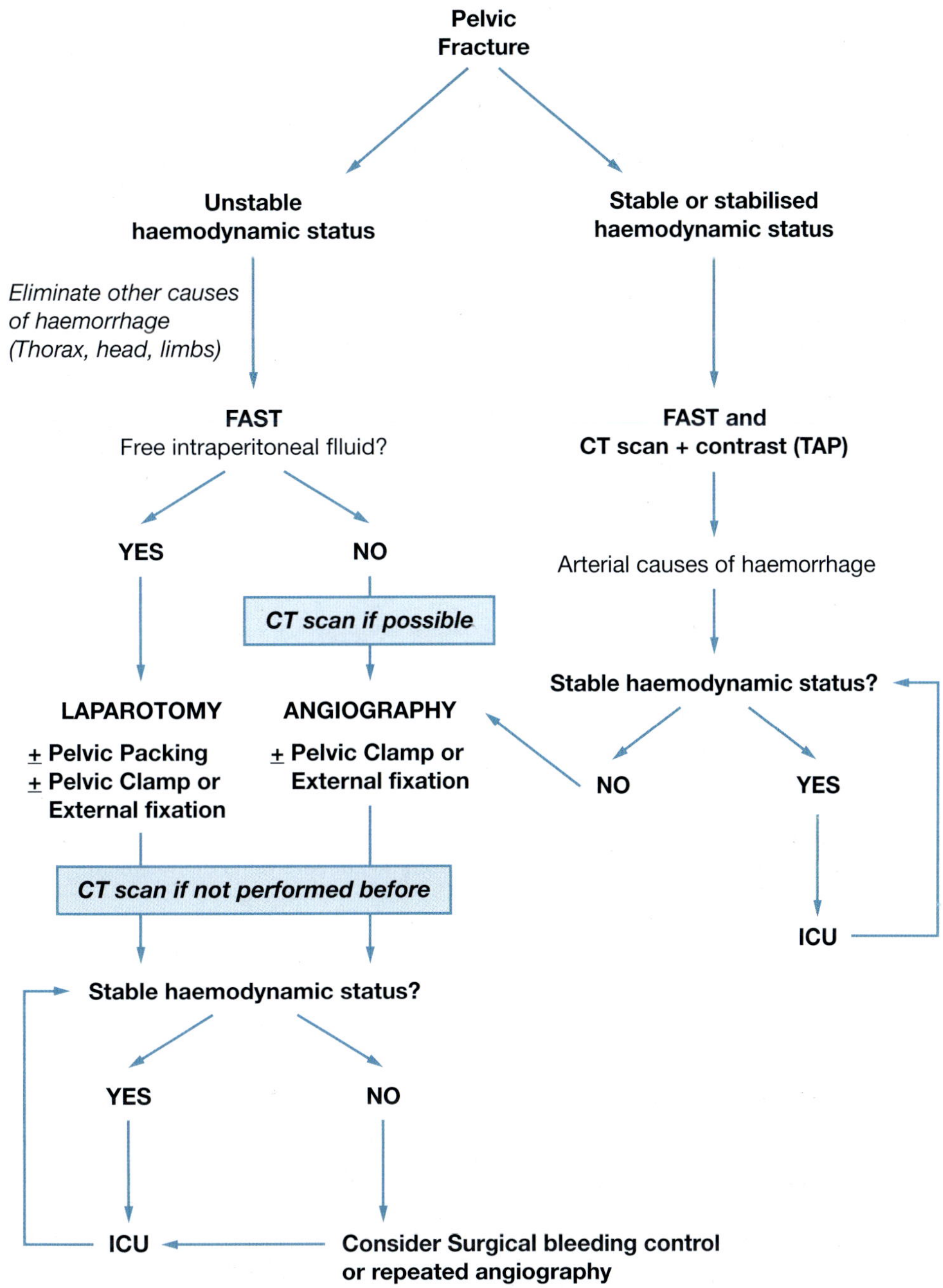

Figure 23.1 Decision-making algorithm for initial management of blunt pelvic trauma patients as proposed by Geeraerts et al.[5] FAST, focused assessment with sonography for trauma; CT, computed tomography; ICU, intensive care unit; TAP, thoracoabdominal–pelvic. (From Geeraerts T, Chhor V, Cheisson G, et al. Clinical review: initial management of blunt pelvic trauma patients with haemodynamic instability. *Crit Care*. 2007;11[1]:204.)

(lateral compression), with risk of lesion of the iliac vessels and retropubic venous plexus; and type 3 (vertical shearing), with structural instability of the posterior ring elements. The classification of Burgess et al.[12] adds a fourth category for mixed fractures with high risk of vascular lesions. The anteroposterior compression type and the vertical shear type of pelvic fracture are more often associated with vascular lesions.[13] However, there seems to be no correlation between the type of fracture and vascular injury. The probability of vascular injury rather seems to be related to the amount of energy that caused the trauma.[4] The anatomy of the IIA and its branching pattern is highly variable and needs to be well known. Figure 23.2 displays the classical anatomy of the IIA and its branches. The most commonly affected vessels are, in descending order of frequency, the superior gluteal, the lateral sacral, the iliolumbar, the obturator, and the vesical and inferior gluteal arteries.[5]

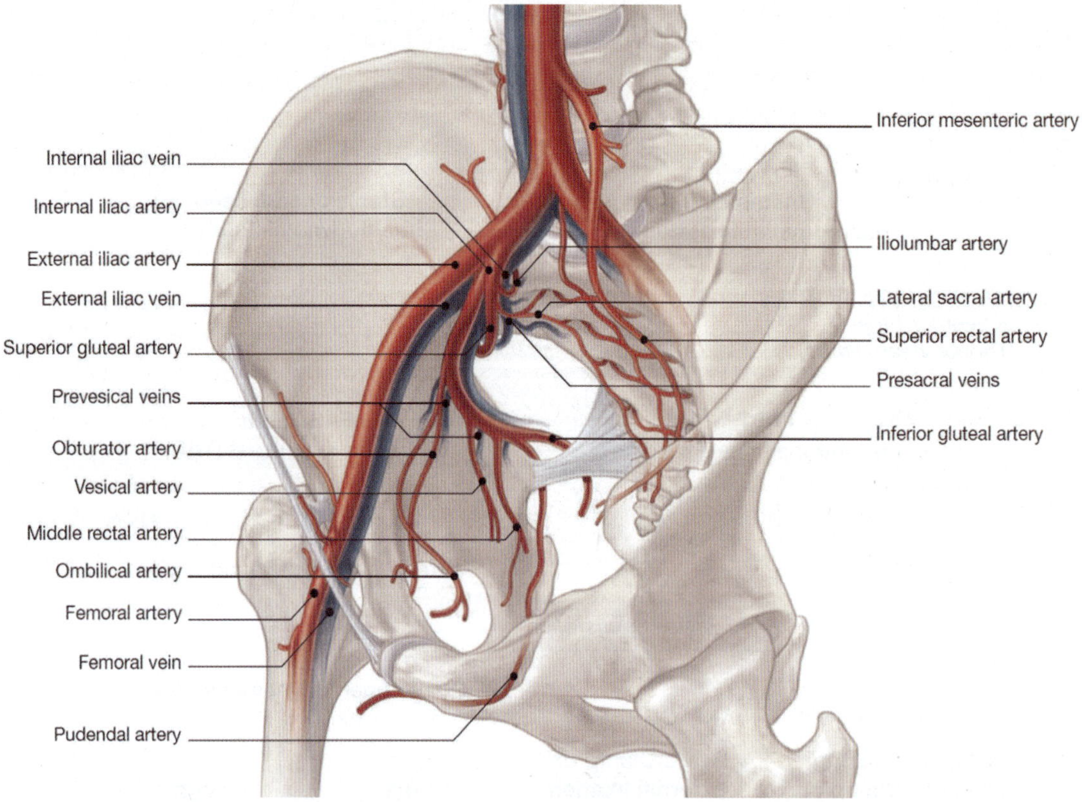

Figure 23.2 Anatomical description of the main pelvic arteries and veins. (From Geeraerts T, Chhor V, Cheisson G, et al. Clinical review: initial management of blunt pelvic trauma patients with haemodynamic instability. *Crit Care*. 2007;11[1]:204.)

The aberrant obturator artery from the external iliac artery is a frequently overlooked source of bleeding in patients with pelvic fracture. This anatomical variant is thought to be present in 14% to 36% of cases.[14] Figure 23.3 displays the angiographic aspect of the aberrant obturator artery.

The success rate of transcatheter embolization ranges from 59% to 100% and is best assessed by the rapid improvement of the hemodynamic status in the angiography suite.[15] Care should be taken to recontrol the efficacy of the embolization once the hemodynamic stability has been restored as arterial spasm might mask adequate management of vascular injury or bleeding and the embolized vessels might reopen when the vasoconstriction diminishes.

DEVICE AND MATERIAL DESCRIPTION

Gelatin sponge pledgets is used as the preferred embolic agent, but *N*-butyl cyanoacrylate (NBCA) glue can be an efficient alternative in extremely unstable patients. Particulate agents should not be used in this setting because of the potential important ischemia that they may induce. Ischemia of the large muscular territories of the buttocks and thighs have been described. Coils should be used only in case of superselective occlusion of a single peripheral vessel. In case of a disrupted vessel, the "front door/back door" technique should be used to avoid continuous bleeding from collateral reperfusion. Coils should not be used in the proximal IIA as they will not be efficient because of the important collateralization in this anatomical region.

TECHNIQUE

Vascular access in patients with pelvic fracture can be challenging in the presence of soft tissue lesions at or near the usual site of puncture and because of compression or external fixation devices. Choice of the side of arterial puncture is usually the opposite of the bone lesions. In case of nonpalpable femoral pulse, ultrasound guidance should be used promptly. In these cases, vascular access can also be obtained from the brachial or radial arteries. The Seldinger technique is used to gain vascular access with a 5-Fr or 6-Fr introducer sheath. In case of selecting radial or brachial arterial access, use of introducer sheaths larger than 5-Fr should be avoided. The contralateral side is embolized first as the contralateral catheterization of the IIA is usually easier and the rapid control of bleeding will help stabilize the hemodynamic status of the patient. The contralateral IIA can be easily catheterized with a Cobra 2 catheter Terumo Europe, Leuven Belgium. Digital subtraction angiography (DSA) images will allow appreciation of the vascular anatomy of the IIA. Vascular lesions and active bleeding may be identified at this point.

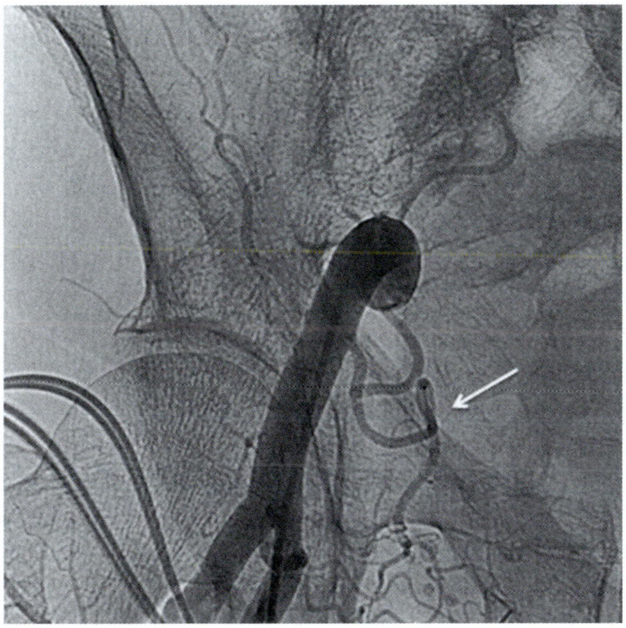

Figure 23.3 Angiography of the external iliac artery demonstrating an aberrant obturator artery arising from the inferior epigastric artery. The aberrant obturator artery can be recognized as it travels above the iliopubic bone to give branches to the inner aspect of the obturator foramen (*arrow*). This artery can be the source of persistent bleeding after embolization of the IIA.

If the patient's hemodynamic status allows, superselective catheterization of the main target vessel should always be attempted with a microcatheter. It will allow selective embolization with 0.018-in coils. Once the contralateral side is embolized, a Waltman loop may be formed in the aorta and the catheterization of the ipsilateral IIA is performed. When the patient is hemodynamically stable, multiple DSAs from different angles can be obtained to identify the site of active bleeding or vascular injury (e.g., pseudoaneurysm/sudden cutoff of any branch close to the bone fracture), which will be then catheterized and embolized superselectively. But when the patient is hemodynamically unstable, we recommend to perform just a single DSA in the posteroanterior view to confirm proper localization of the catheter in the IIA before proximal embolization is performed. In this setting, both IIAs should be occluded as rapidly as possible with Gelfoam pledgets (Ethicon, Somerville, New Jersey).

In case of hemodynamically unstable patients with multiple bleeding sites, the use of an aortic occlusion balloon catheter (e.g., Equalizer; Boston Scientific Corporation, Natick, Massachusetts) can be a lifesaver. This type of balloon can be placed even without any kind of imaging guidance in the aorta after obtaining common femoral access using Seldinger technique in the emergency department (ED). The balloon catheter is advanced 30 cm upward using the umbilicus of the patient as the target level then inflated and pulled backward until resistance is felt when the balloon reaches the aortic bifurcation. This will immediately control most bleeding in the lower body while other procedures can take place.

TAE of upper abdominal organs can be performed while an occlusion balloon is inflated by inserting a 5-Fr catheter between the balloon and the aortic wall (Fig. 23.4). Once the other bleeding sources are controlled, the balloon can be deflated and the IIA embolized.

Particular attention should be paid to "missing arteries." One example is the truncated superior gluteal artery in case of anteroposterior compression type fracture. This artery must be embolized using the front door and back door technique with coils.

One must know that some arteries are at more risk of complications: the inferior gluteal artery feeds the sciatic nerve roots and the inferior and median rectal arteries are the feeding vessels of the rectal lower third and anal canal.

CLINICAL APPLICATIONS

Scenario 1

Hemodynamically stable patient with localized source of bleeding on CT scan. This patient should benefit from selective TAE of the injured vessel first. TAE is a quick procedure that will prevent occurrence of secondary hemodynamic instability and allow the patient to undergo surgical internal stabilization of the pelvis, which can be a long and complex procedure.

Scenario 2

Patient with marginal hemodynamic stability (transiently responding to fluid resuscitation) with localized source of bleeding on CT scan. This patient should benefit from both external pelvic fixation and nonselective embolization of both IIAs. Which should be performed first remains debated, but external fixation is a quick procedure that can be performed in the ED and in our opinion, should be performed first.[9] Because external fixation only takes care of venous and osseous bleeding and arterial bleeding is the main cause of hemodynamic instability, TAE should be performed as soon as possible after external fixation.

Scenario 3

Polytrauma patient with marginal hemodynamic stability with multiple pelvic and extrapelvic sources of bleeding on CT scan and no indication for emergent laparotomy. This patient should benefit from external fixation and TAE or laparotomy for bleeding control. It has been demonstrated that in this particular setting, TAE can be efficient in controlling multiple bleeding sources and has the advantage of avoiding the physiologic insult of laparotomy in fragile patients.[16] Figure 23.5 displays the case of a patient with hemodynamic instability and clinically evident pelvic fracture that was treated by TAE of both IIAs with Gelfoam pledgets before being scanned.

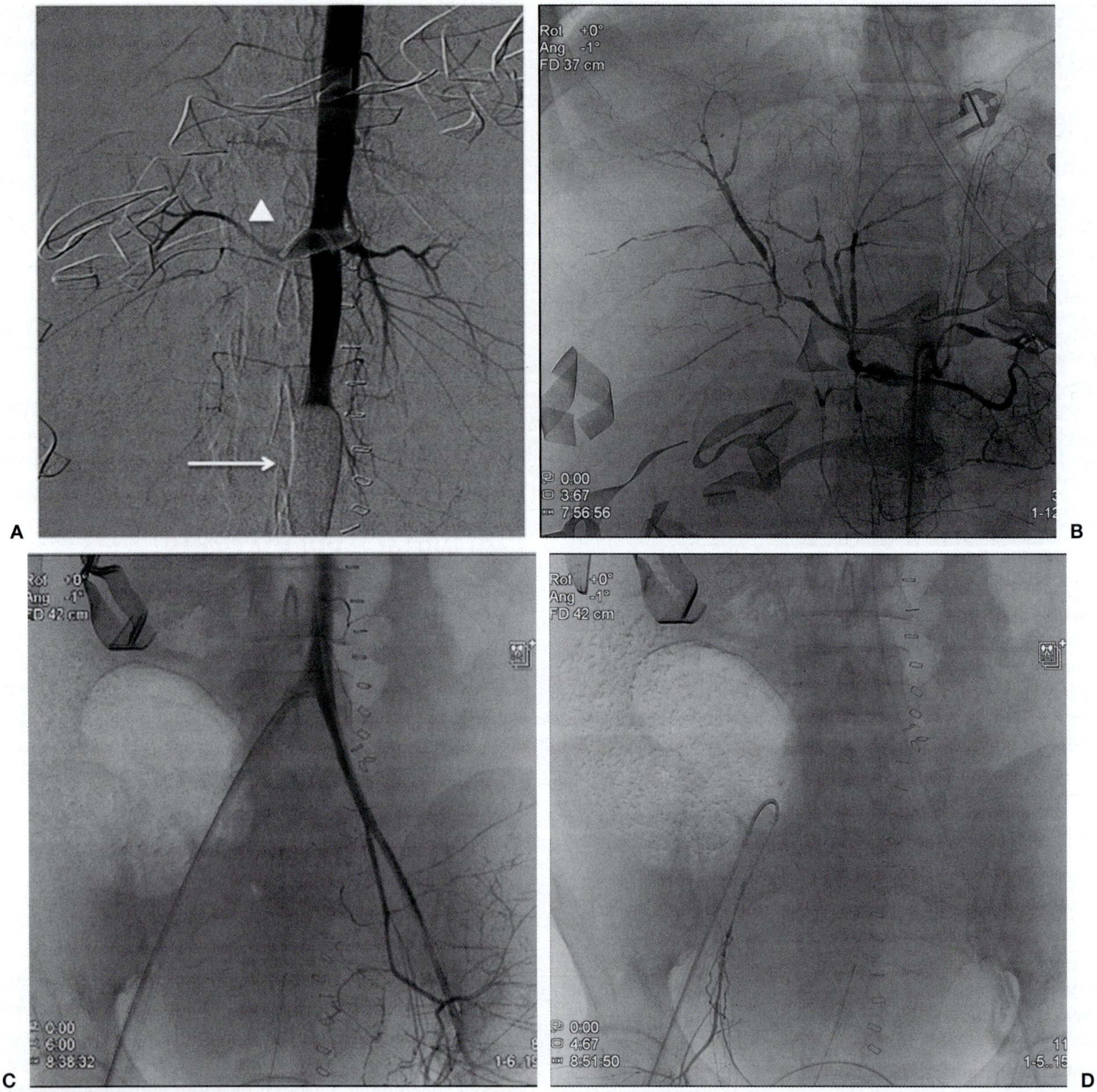

Figure 23.4 Angiographic images of a severely hypotensive 37-year-old female patient with liver laceration and pelvic bleeding. Initially, the patient underwent damage control laparotomy with liver packing. **A:** Due to persistent hemodynamic instability, an aortic occlusion balloon was placed in the aorta (*arrow*) to control the pelvic bleeding. A Cobra catheter (*arrowhead*) was advanced between the occlusion balloon and the aortic wall to perform selective angiograms of both renal arteries, the celiac trunk, and hepatic and splenic arteries. **B:** The hepatic artery was embolized with NBCA. **C,D:** The occlusion balloon was deflated and both IIAs were embolized with NBCA.

POTENTIAL COMPLICATIONS

In the setting of polytraumatized patients with complex pelvic ring fractures, it is difficult to establish with certainty if the observed complication was caused by the trauma itself or by the embolization. Major complications related to TAE in the pelvic territory are observed in less than 5%.[5] These complications mostly consist of puncture-related hematomas, skin necrosis, rhabdomyolysis, pelvic or perineal infections, and nerve injuries. Travis et al.[17] found no significant differences in the complication rates between embolized and nonembolized patients within 30 days from injury as well as during the 18.4-month follow-up. Nevertheless, a significantly higher rate of moderate complications such as buttock, thigh, and perineal paresthesia in the embolized patients group was observed. There was

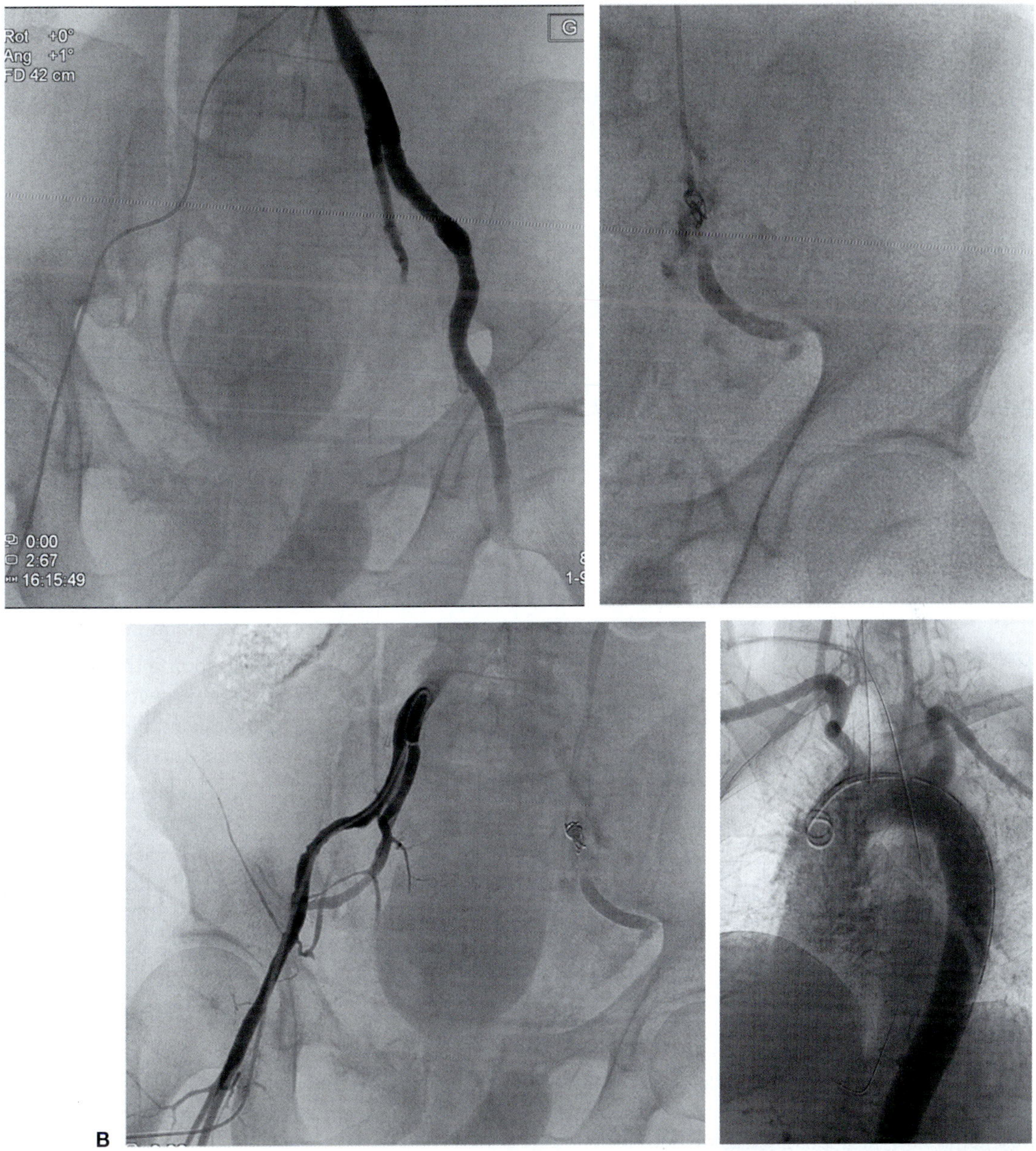

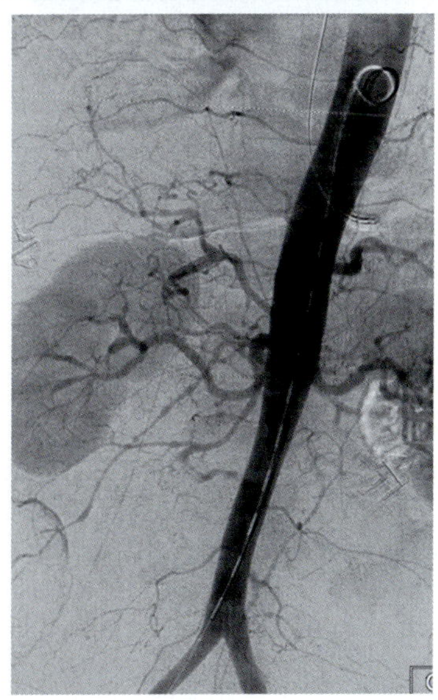

Figure 23.5 A 58-year-old male who had a paragliding accident. Pelvic fracture was evident on clinical examination at the site of the accident. A pelvic compression strap was applied suppress "IN THE PELVIS" and the patient was transferred to the hospital. Initial assessment revealed a marginally stable patient who required heavy fluid resuscitation. There was no evidence of other injuries; the patient underwent TAE of the left IIA with Gelfoam pledgets **(A)** and coils **(B)**. The right IIA was catheterized after a Waltman maneuver **(C)** and embolized with Gelfoam pledgets. Because the patient did not have a CT scan at admission because of hemodynamic instability, we performed a thoracoabdominal aortogram and selective visceral angiograms to rule out additional vascular injuries **(D,E)**. At the completion of the procedure, the patient was hemodynamically stable.

TIPS AND TRICKS

Hemodynamically stable patient	Perform CT scan to identify bleeding vessels	• Embolize selectively the identified bleeding vessels with Gelfoam or coils. • Consider the front door and back door technique. • Look for missing vessels and treat them. • Beware of the inferior gluteal artery and the inferior and median rectal arteries.
Patient with marginal hemodynamic stability	Perform CT scan to identify bleeding vessels	• External pelvic fixation • Nonselective embolization of both IIAs with Gelfoam pledgets or slurry • Use ultrasound guidance whenever needed. • Both IIAs can be catheterized from the same access point using the Waltman maneuver.
Hemodynamically unstable patient (CT might not be available)	Suspected isolated pelvic trauma	• Embolize the IIA ipsilateral to the suspected bleeding site with Gelfoam pledgets ipsilateral to the suspected bleeding site or slurry.
	Suspected multiple bleeding sites	• Use an aortic occlusion balloon catheter. • Upper abdominal organs can be embolized while the occlusion balloon is inflated by inserting a 5-Fr catheter between the balloon and the aortic wall.

no significant difference between patients who underwent superselective embolization or nonselective embolization of the IIA. Ischemic complications such as rhabdomyolysis and skin necrosis are probably more frequent in patients with poor collateral supply, such as patient with extensive atherosclerosis. Rare complications reported in the literature include bladder necrosis,[18] necrosis of the femoral head,[19] paresis in the territory of the sciatic nerve,[20] and nontarget embolization. Inadvertent embolization of a persistent sciatic artery has also been described.[21] A few cases of paraplegia have been reported.[15,22]

CONCLUSION

TAE should be integrated in the multidisciplinary management of patients with pelvic trauma. The indication for TAE should be based on the hemodynamic status of the patient above all. TAE has many advantages in this particular setting: it can quickly control hemorrhage in a difficult-to-reach anatomical compartment and it can be associated with embolization of other bleeding sites without exposing the patient to the risk of an emergency surgical procedure.

REFERENCES

1. Inaba K, Sharkey PW, Stephen DJ, et al. The increasing incidence of severe pelvic injury in motor vehicle collisions. *Injury*. 2004; 35(8)759–765.
2. Velmahos GC, Toutouzas KG, Vassliu P, et al. A prospective study on the safety and efficacy of angiographic embolization for pelvic and visceral injuries. *J Trauma*. 2002;53(2):303–308.
3. Demetriades D, Karaiskakis M, Toutouzas K, et al. Pelvic fractures: epidemiology and predictors of associated abdominal injuries and outcomes. *J Am Coll Surg*. 2002;195(1):1–10.
4. Cook RE, Keating JF, Gillespie I. The role of angiography in the management of haemorrhage from major fractures of the pelvis. *J Bone Joint Surg Br*. 2002;84(2):178–182.
5. Geeraerts T, Chhor V, Cheisson G, et al. Clinical review: initial management of blunt pelvic trauma patients with haemodynamic instability. *Crit Care*. 2007;11(1):204.

6. Burk DL Jr, Meats DC, Herbert DL, et al. Pelvic and acetabular fractures: examination by angled CT scanning. *Radiology*. 1984; 153(2):548.
7. Bell RM, Krantz BE, Weigelt JA. ATLS: a foundation for trauma training. *Ann Emerg Med*. 1999;34(2):233–237.
8. Vermeulen B, Peter R, Hoffmeyer P, et al. Prehospital stabilization of pelvic dislocations: a new strap belt to provide temporary hemodynamic stabilization. *Swiss Surg*. 1999;5(2):43–46.
9. Abrassart S, Stern R, Peter R. Unstable pelvic ring injury with hemodynamic instability: what seems the best procedure choice and sequence in the initial management? *Orthop Traumatol Surg Res*. 2013;99(2):175–182.
10. Young JW, Resnik CS. Fracture of the pelvis: current concepts of classification. *AJR Am J Roentgenol*. 1990;155(6):1169–1175.
11. Pennal GF, Tile M, Waddell JP, et al. Pelvic disruption: assessment and classification. *Clin Orthop Relat Res*. 1980;(151):12–21.
12. Burgess AR, Eastridge BJ, Young JW, et al. Pelvic ring disruptions: effective classification system and treatment protocols. *J Trauma*. 1990;30(7):848–856.
13. Broadwell SR, Ray CE. Transcatheter embolization in pelvic trauma. *Semin Intervent Radiol*. 2004;21(1):23–35.
14. Requarth JA, Miller PR. Aberrant obturator artery is a common arterial variant that may be a source of unidentified hemorrhage in pelvic fracture patients. *J Trauma*. 2011;70(2):366–372.
15. Karadimas EJ, Nicolson T, Kakagia DD, et al. Angiographic embolisation of pelvic ring injuries. Treatment algorithm and review of the literature. *Int Orthop*. 2011;35(9):1381–1390.
16. Bize PE, Duran R, Madoff DC, et al. Embolization for multicompartmental bleeding in patients in hemodynamically unstable condition: prognostic factors and outcome. *J Vasc Interv Radiol*. 2012;23(6):751–760.e4.
17. Travis T, Monsky WL, London J, et al. Evaluation of short-term and long-term complications after emergent internal iliac artery embolization in patients with pelvic trauma. *J Vasc Interv Radiol*. 2008;19(6):840–847.
18. Sieber PR. Bladder necrosis secondary to pelvic artery embolization: case report and literature review. *J Urol*. 1994;151(2):422.
19. Obaro RO, Sniderman KW. Case report: avascular necrosis of the femoral head as a complication of complex embolization for severe pelvic haemorrhage. *Br J Radiol*. 1995;68(812):920–922.
20. Hare WS, Holland CJ. Paresis following internal iliac artery embolization. *Radiology*. 1983;146(1):47–51.
21. Hsu WC, Lim KE, Hsu YY. Inadvertent embolization of a persistent sciatic artery in pelvis trauma. *Cardiovasc Intervent Radiol*. 2005;28(4):518–520.
22. Palacios-Jaraquemada JM. Buttock necrosis and paraplegia after bilateral internal iliac artery embolization for postpartum hemorrhage. *Obstet Gynecol*. 2012;120(5):1210; author reply 1210.

24

Extremity Trauma

Jaime All • John F. Angle

Embolotherapy for extremity trauma is a well-established and essential tool for the management of hemorrhage and vascular injury with potential for hemorrhage. Familiarity with clinical presentation, pretreatment imaging, and angiographic findings are all essential components to interventionalists providing these services. Embolization technique and the similarities and important differences between pelvic and extremity injury will be discussed.

PELVIC TRAUMA

Within the context of a multispecialty approach to the care of the trauma patient, the transcatheter arterial embolization (TAE) is an essential tool in the treatment of traumatic pelvic arterial injury.[1] Many trauma centers have developed algorithms based on the nature of the injury, computed tomography (CT) findings, and other injuries.[2–5] Some trauma scenarios are best treated with TAE first, others are supplemented with TAE, and many will not benefit from early pelvic angiography.[2–7] Blunt or penetrating pelvic trauma may lead to vascular injury, with blunt injuries being much more common in most geographic areas. Blunt trauma resulting in pelvic fracture is associated with vascular injury in up to 40% of patients, and hemorrhage is still the highest cause of mortality (50% to 74% of patients).[8–10] With blunt pelvic injury, the source of hemorrhage may be venous, arterial, or from cancellous bone.[7,11] TAE is only indicated for the treatment of arterial hemorrhage and is indicated in approximately 3% to 10% of cases.[2,8,12,13] In the correct clinical setting, angiography with TAE is effective in controlling pelvic hemorrhage in 85% to 97% of cases.[6] Patients embolized within 3 hours of arrival have a statistically improved survival rate as compared to those receiving intervention outside of the initial 3-hour window.[14]

Indications for TAE in the setting of pelvic trauma include pelvic fractures and hemodynamic instability after exclusion of other sources of hemorrhage outside of the pelvis, active extravasation of contrast on computed tomography angiography (CTA) in the presence of pelvic fracture regardless of hemodynamic status, prior TAE for pelvic trauma with ongoing hemodynamic instability after other sources of hemorrhage have been excluded, and patients older than 60 years of age with a high-risk pelvic fracture pattern.[6,12,15,16]

Motor vehicle collisions and pedestrians hit by motor vehicles account for most blunt arterial injury.[12] Domestic falls are a less common cause, but the need for pelvic vascular injury evaluation in this population is well documented.[7,12,16] This is particularly true for the elderly because age is an independent predictor of active bleeding and indication for TAE, regardless of hemodynamic stability.[12,16] Additionally, osteoporosis in elderly women may result in increased rate of pelvic fracture, even when the mechanism of injury is less dramatic.[17] The prevalence of chronic anticoagulation for cerebrovascular and cardiovascular disease in this patient population may also necessitate early intervention.

Types of vascular injury seen with blunt pelvic trauma include complete or partial transection, arteriovenous fistula, pseudoaneurysm, dissection, and traumatic thrombosis. The different angiographic appearances of traumatic vascular injury are listed in Table 24.1.[1,18–20] Vascular injury typically occurs in relationship to adjacent osseous fractures or shearing forces against the ligamentous structures of the pelvis.[19] It is important to note that disruption of the osseous pelvis significantly enlarges what is normally a confined space. This allows for a larger volume of hemorrhage to accumulate rapidly, and thus early intervention is necessary to prevent exsanguination.[7] It is worth repeating that pelvic hemorrhage is usually from venous or fractured cancellous bone, and this type of low-pressure hemorrhage is best controlled

Table 24.1 Angiographic Appearance of Traumatic Vascular Injury

Type of Injury	Appearance on Angiography
Transection	Brisk extravasation of contrast. Partial or complete transection may result in vasospasm. The appearance cannot be distinguished from traumatic thrombosis or vasospasm without transection.
Dissection	Luminal irregularity with an intimal flap.
Pseudoaneurysm	Contrast filling an irregular outpouching in communication with the vessel lumen.
Arteriovenous fistula	Early filling of a vein adjacent to the contrast opacified artery. This may have an associated pseudoaneurysm.
Thrombosis	Abrupt cutoff of the vessel. This cannot be distinguished from vasospasm.
Hemorrhage originating from cancellous bone	Group of small round collections of contrast, clustered together. This is seen within the region of osseous or ligamentous injury.
Vasospasm	May have several appearances, including contour irregularity of the vessel lumen, abrupt narrowing of the vessel, or abrupt cutoff.

with external fixation or compression with pelvic binding. The goal of these methods is to reestablish the normal tamponading effect of the retroperitoneum, although some recent studies call into question the overall efficacy with this approach.[6,19,21] Peritoneal pelvic packing has been introduced as an additional method of treating pelvic hemorrhage. Some centers have questioned; whether pelvic packing should replace TAE, most use TAE as an adjunctive treatment, and others suggest TAE first with fixation secondarily.[2–7,21] From a practical standpoint, we push for angiography first if active extravasation is seen on CT and suggest deferring the fixation, which can make angiography very difficult to perform. Regardless of the algorithm or combinations of treatment employed, early control of pelvic arterial hemorrhage has a strong association with improved outcome, and TAE continues to occupy a central role in the treatment of traumatic pelvic hemorrhage.[1–6,14]

As many as 50% of patients with pelvic fracture have additional injuries, so pelvic fracture should be treated as an indicator of polytrauma (Fig. 24.1).[21] An algorithm approach to the care of the trauma patient, although institution-dependent, must weigh the severity of multiple injuries and therefore mandates a multidisciplinary approach. Most would prioritize an intra-abdominal source of hemorrhage over intrapelvic bleeding, although a few have argued to the contrary.[4,6,22] However, it is accepted that exploratory laparotomy in the setting of unaddressed pelvic hemorrhage can lead to rapid expansion of the pelvic hematoma.[9] Additionally, some solid organ injury within the abdomen may be treated at the time of pelvic embolization, such as a splenic or renal laceration. Regardless of when TAE is performed, consideration must be given to the possibility of additional organ injury, and this should guide the goal of the procedure in terms of the degree of vessel selectivity. Failure of hemodynamic status to correct following embolization should prompt search for additional sources of bleeding.

Historically, fracture patterns were felt to be important diagnostic indicators in pelvic trauma.[9,19] More recent studies have shown that arterial hemorrhage can occur with any of the fracture patterns, as well as in the less severe subtypes, and may occur in the absence of fracture.[22] Those most worrisome (and those which are considered high-grade at our institution) are vertical shear and types II and III lateral compressions and anterior posterior compressions.[9,19,23] It is still important for the interventionalist to recognize these patterns because they may suggest which vessel is the culprit, even in the absence of active extravasation at angiography. At the most basic level, anterior fracture patterns are associated with injury to the anterior division of the internal iliac artery, and posterior fractures are associated with injuries to the posterior division.[1,23] The importance of fracture pattern recognition has been largely supplanted by CT, which has superior diagnostic sensitivity, and adds a wealth of additional data over conventional radiography.[24,25] Advances in technology have allowed for rapid image acquisition and processing, thereby allowing for the imaging of patients whose status may be tenuous and, in some centers, even those who are unstable.

Examples of penetrating pelvic injuries include gunshot wounds, stab wounds, or iatrogenic injury (such as with percutaneous drainage tube placement and placement of orthopedic hardware).[26] Penetrating injuries are more likely to result in transection or pseudoaneurysm formation, with or without arteriovenous fistula.[27] Traumatic pseudoaneurysms are at high risk for rupture and should all be treated, preferably with endovascular methods when possible.[18]

EXTREMITY INJURY

Traumatic vascular injury to the extremity may also cause life-threatening hemorrhage, but, more commonly than in the pelvis, it may result in vessel occlusion with signs of acute limb ischemia. Iatrogenic injury accounts for 74% of embolization procedures performed in the extremity.[28] Many of these are associated with orthopedic procedures, which

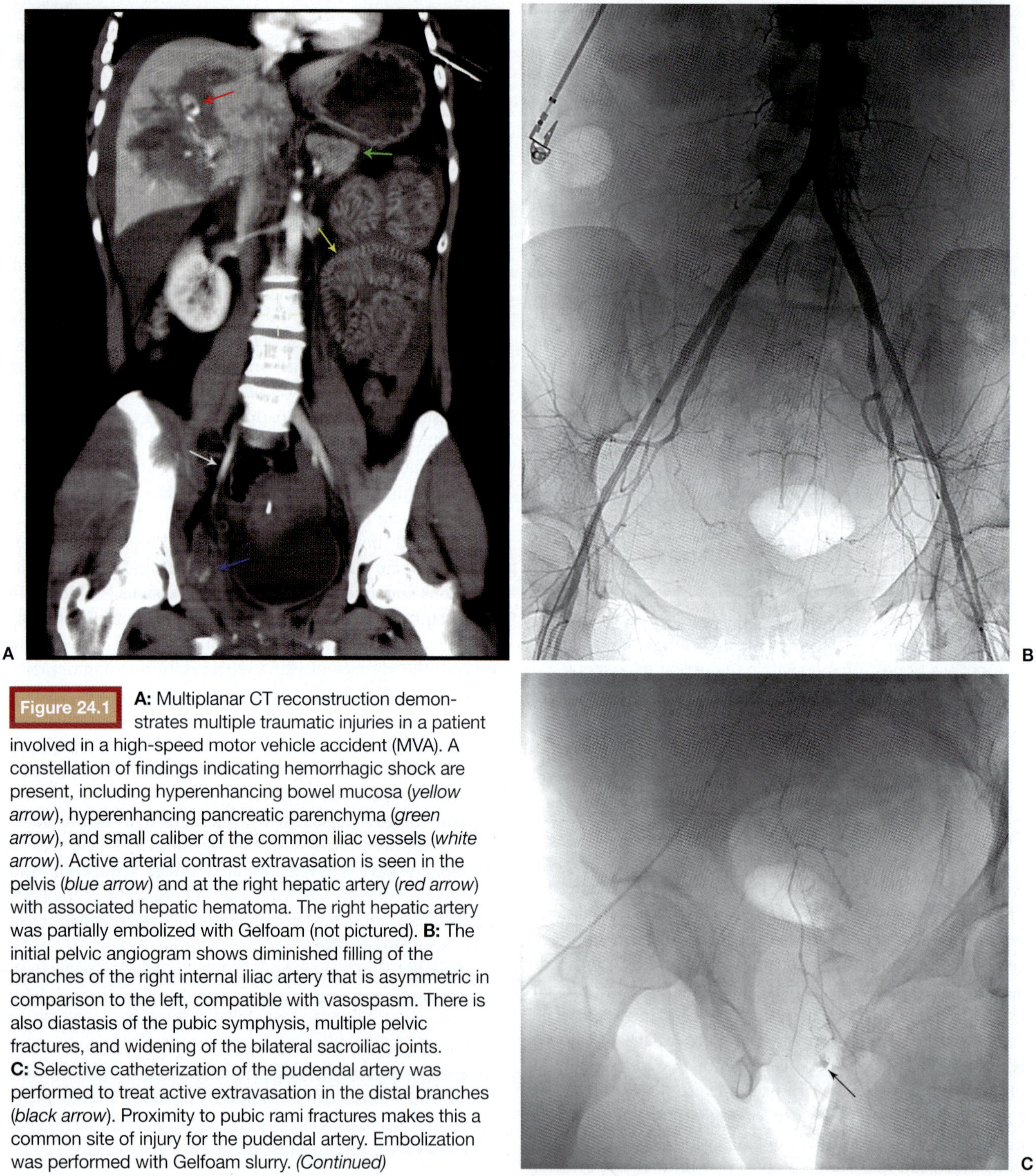

Figure 24.1 **A:** Multiplanar CT reconstruction demonstrates multiple traumatic injuries in a patient involved in a high-speed motor vehicle accident (MVA). A constellation of findings indicating hemorrhagic shock are present, including hyperenhancing bowel mucosa (*yellow arrow*), hyperenhancing pancreatic parenchyma (*green arrow*), and small caliber of the common iliac vessels (*white arrow*). Active arterial contrast extravasation is seen in the pelvis (*blue arrow*) and at the right hepatic artery (*red arrow*) with associated hepatic hematoma. The right hepatic artery was partially embolized with Gelfoam (not pictured). **B:** The initial pelvic angiogram shows diminished filling of the branches of the right internal iliac artery that is asymmetric in comparison to the left, compatible with vasospasm. There is also diastasis of the pubic symphysis, multiple pelvic fractures, and widening of the bilateral sacroiliac joints. **C:** Selective catheterization of the pudendal artery was performed to treat active extravasation in the distal branches (*black arrow*). Proximity to pubic rami fractures makes this a common site of injury for the pudendal artery. Embolization was performed with Gelfoam slurry. *(Continued)*

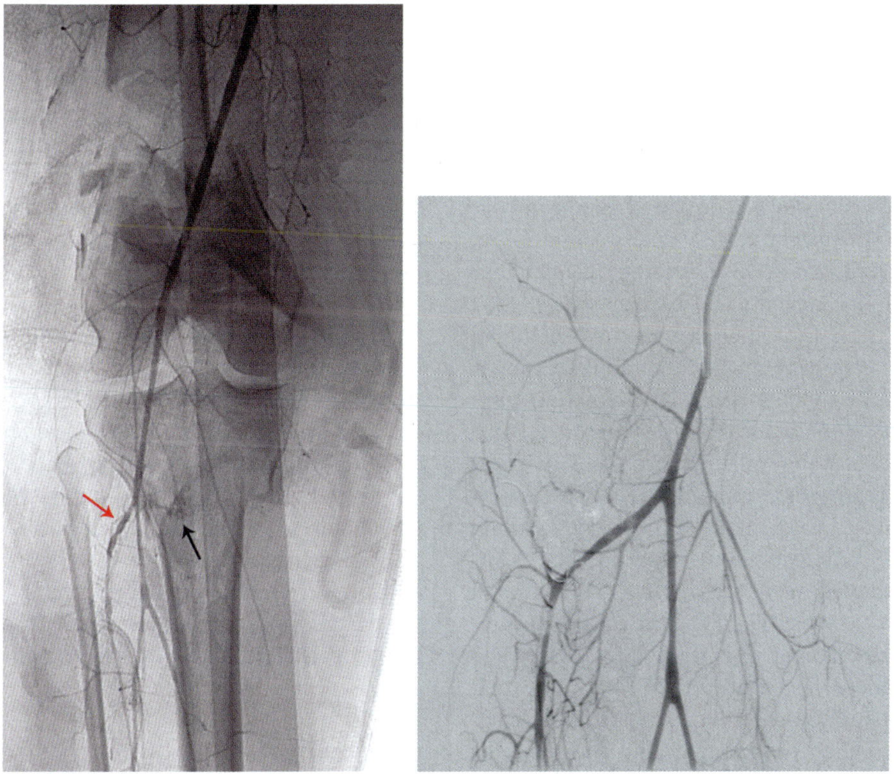

D E

Figure 24.1 *(Continued)* **D:** A right lower extremity angiogram of the same patient demonstrates comminuted fractures. Vasospasm is indicated by the irregular contour of the anterior tibial artery (*red arrow*). Active extravasation from a small branch of the anterior tibial artery is also present (*black arrow*). The small caliber of the popliteal artery can be an indicator of compartment syndrome; however, in this patient, it is more likely secondary to hypovolemia given the concurrent abdominal and pelvic findings. **E:** No contrast extravasation is evident following superselective embolization with microcoils.

are likely to increase as our aging population requires an increasing number of major joint procedures. Arterial injury associated with orthopedic procedures typically involves a branch vessel in the pelvis or lower extremities, rather than a major artery, and is thus ideally suited to treatment via endovascular methods.[28]

Traumatic arterial injury of the extremity is divided into penetrating or blunt trauma. The distinction between the two has important clinical implications. Penetrating injury (more common) results in pseudoaneurysm, arteriovenous fistula, and partial or complete transection.[29] Outside of iatrogenic causes, glass is the most common source of penetrating injury followed by gunshot wounds and stab wounds.[30] Blunt injury is often seen with associated orthopedic trauma such as fracture and dislocation. The vascular injury seen with blunt trauma is typically dissection, pseudoaneurysm, or occlusion secondary to intramural hematoma or traumatic thrombosis.[31] Diagnosis of arterial injury in the setting of a penetrating mechanism is usually more straightforward as there is obvious external evidence of injury. Hard signs of injury are more likely to be present, such as active external hemorrhage, enlarging hematoma, or obvious indicators of limb ischemia.[27] Signs of limb ischemia include pallor, abnormal peripheral pulses, unequivocal neurologic defects, and a thrill or bruit.[32]

Blunt peripheral arterial injury is more likely to be occult with delayed diagnosis and concomitant traumatic injuries to the head and body, which may take precedence over the extremity.[31] Diagnosis of blunt arterial injury requires a higher index of suspicion and recognition of soft signs of vascular injury. These include (1) discrepancies in the ankle–brachial index performed with Doppler ultrasound and (2) adjacent injury, including fracture, nerve injury, or stable hematoma.[18] Duplex ultrasonography may be beneficial for characterization of some specific vascular injuries, but CTA provides clinically important additional information about extremity osseous and soft tissue structures.[27,33] Additionally, newer CT scanners can acquire arterial phase imaging of the extremities during the concomitant CTA evaluation of the chest, abdomen, and pelvis. Conventional angiography for diagnostic evaluation of acute arterial injury has largely been replaced by CTA, given the excellent sensitivity of CTA.[33]

Vascular injury is more common in the lower extremity than the upper extremity, and the femoral and popliteal arteries are the most common sites of vascular traumatic injury.[34] Knee dislocation is a common cause of occult lower extremity arterial injury.[32] In the upper extremity, the brachial artery is the most commonly injured vessel followed by the radial and ulnar arteries.[30] The arteries of the forearm typically do not require intervention for occlusive traumatic injury secondary to collateral flow at the palmar arch.[30] Blunt brachial artery injury is most commonly seen in children in the setting of elbow dislocation or displaced supracondylar fractures.[35] Injury to the axillary artery is less common but can be seen with severe anterior dislocation of the glenohumeral joint.[31] Additional damage to the branch vessels of the axillary artery can also be seen with this mechanism of injury.

With respect to extremity treatment, embolotherapy is predominantly indicated for hemorrhage originating from branch vessels that do not provide distal perfusion.[18,29] Pseudoaneurysms and arteriovenous fistulas, even those without active extravasation, are often appropriate indications for embolization as well.[18,29] Acute injury of the larger vessels is more often treated surgically, although endovascular treatment with stent graft placement is increasing.[36] Branches of the profunda femoral artery are an ideal site for endovascular treatment of acute traumatic hemorrhage because these do not provide direct perfusion to the distal extremity and are traditionally difficult to access via a surgical approach.[19] The branches surrounding the shoulder and the profunda brachial artery are similarly potential candidates for TAE in the upper extremity.[28,37]

TECHNIQUE

Preprocedural Planning

Familiarity with the trauma history and all available medical information including prior imaging is essential to assisting the trauma team in assessing the appropriateness and timing of angiography. The local algorithm for the treatment of the trauma patient should also be clearly understood. The interventionalist should be familiar with Advanced Trauma Life Support (ATLS) protocol and have an appropriate level of critical care support in the angiography suite.

Embolic materials used in trauma are almost always coils, microcoils, or Gelfoam (Pfizer Inc., New York, New York). Alternative large vessel occlusion devices such as the Amplatzer 4 Vascular Plug (St. Jude Medical, Inc., St. Paul, Minnesota) have seen increasing usage. Some authors have described the use of liquid embolic agents such as Onyx (Covidien, Irvine, California) and *N*-butyl cyanoacrylate (Trufill; Codman & Shurtleff, Inc., Raynham, Massachusetts), with the potential advantages of achieving vessel occlusion in the setting of coagulopathy and providing distal control when distal catheterization is not possible.[38,39] Cost, a steep learning curve, and a potentially narrow safety profile are noteworthy considerations in the use of liquid embolic agents. Catheter-directed thrombin has also been described for the treatment of traumatic pseudoaneurysms of branches of the internal iliac artery.[40] We feel that the efficacy and safety profile of autologous clot, Onyx, or glue are better choices when distal control cannot be achieved. Small particles, including Gelfoam particles, have little or no role in the treatment of acute trauma, and the use of alcohol in the trauma patient is contraindicated.[18,19] Additional embolic agents that are mostly of historical interest include clipped pieces of silk suture and segments of the outer winding of a 0.035-in Bentson guidewire (Cook Medical, Inc., Bloomington, Indiana).

Periprocedural considerations should include anticipating the impact of CTA contrast within the urinary bladder. If there is suspicion for urethral injury, pelvic angiography should not be delayed and consideration should be given to delaying cystography until after the embolization procedure to avoid extravasation of contrast.[19]

Examination of the extremity color, temperature, and pedal pulses (radial and ulnar pulses if upper extremity access is planned) should be assessed by the interventionalist performing the procedure. Any postprocedure change should prompt query into a potential complication, such as reflux of embolic agents into the extremity vessels or access site vascular injury.

SITE OF ACCESS AND DIAGNOSTIC IMAGING

Pelvic binders vary among institutions. Some are made of fabric, and a hole can be cut through them for femoral access. Others are leather binders, which may have to be undone before obtaining access. Most pelvic embolizations can be performed via a single common femoral artery access site. If there is known unilateral pelvic or lower extremity injury, contralateral femoral access is preferred. If injuries or external devices preclude the preferred femoral access, the procedure can be performed via a brachial or even popliteal or radial artery access. More recently, dual access has been advocated to allow placement of a temporary occlusion balloon within the infrarenal abdominal aorta while pelvic or lower extremity hemorrhage is treated.[7,11] We advocate the use of ultrasound guidance for all arterial punctures. When used routinely, it adds little time to the procedure and avoids the complications encountered with suboptimal access (e.g., retroperitoneal hematoma or arteriovenous fistula). This is especially important when dealing with hemorrhagic shock, as these patients already have little cardiovascular reserve and may not tolerate iatrogenic injury superimposed on traumatic injury. Ultrasound guidance also increases the likelihood that a closure device can be successfully used at the end of the procedure.

Often in the acute setting, renal function has not yet been assessed, and the risk of contrast nephropathy becomes a secondary concern. In a patient with known renal insufficiency, nonselective and selective pelvic and lower extremity angiography may be performed with carbon dioxide (CO_2).

The procedure should start with nonselective angiography to quickly localize sites of hemorrhage and serves as a road map for vessel selection. Additionally, the initial imaging is useful in differentiating traumatic injury from guidewire-induced vasospasm. Fractures should prompt selective angiography at potential sites of vascular injury. For instance, the superior gluteal artery is the most commonly injured vessel with a posterior fracture pattern, and this is typically injured as it passes under the sciatic notch. It is commonly injured with open book fractures.[19]

Appropriate angiographic imaging of the internal iliac artery requires orthogonal selective views. The anterior division is best imaged with a contralateral oblique view of approximately 45 degrees. This can be thought of as looking at the iliac wing en face. An ipsilateral anterior oblique view is important to identify the superior gluteal artery and the internal pudendal artery. It should be stressed that, although initial nonselective pelvic angiogram is an important part of pelvic or extremity evaluation, selective angiography is crucial to achieving appropriate angiographic sensitivity.

Hemorrhage from pelvic trauma is most often associated with the internal iliac artery, but some have advocated that a selective angiogram of the external iliac artery should also be obtained.[41] Although the external iliac artery is not usually a source of pelvic hemorrhage, the external pudendal, deep iliac circumflex, inferior epigastric, and the circumflex femoral arteries may be injured.[1,3,42] The more inferior lumbar arteries as well as the inferior mesenteric or even the gonadal arteries are other rare sources of pelvic bleeding.

Following completion of contralateral pelvic vessel evaluation, selection of the ipsilateral common iliac artery should be obtained with a reverse curve catheter or a tightly curved catheter such as the Rim catheter (AngioDynamics, Latham, New York). Imaging of the bilateral iliac vessels should always be obtained. This avoids continued hemorrhage resulting from reperfusion of the injured vessel via anastomoses with the contralateral pelvic arteries. It also rules out additional injury, which may have been occult on initial CT imaging.

Pelvic Embolotherapy

The decision to embolize should be based on angiographic findings of vessel injury but not limited to active extravasation. This aggressive approach may even include embolization of potential sources of hemorrhage identified on CT. Less selective or nonselective internal iliac embolization is recommended by some if the patient is hemodynamically unstable or if multiple sites of active extravasation are identified. Nonselective embolization of the internal iliac arteries is performed with the injection of Gelfoam, often followed by coils with the tip positioned in the internal iliac artery. Nonselective embolization is probably not appropriate for most pelvic trauma and is not appropriate for the profunda artery given the risk of ischemia. At the very least, CT will usually direct the operator to nonselectively embolize either the anterior or posterior division of the internal iliac artery.

Gelfoam, widely considered the workhorse of trauma embolotherapy, is a temporary agent that allows for potential recanalization within a few weeks. This may allow for reclaimed tissue perfusion once the acute injury has had time to heal. It is also inexpensive and readily available. Gelfoam is typically delivered as slurry. This is mixed in a three-way stopcock with a half-strength mixture of contrast and normal saline. More agitation will create a Gelfoam mixture that is less coarse. If the target of embolization with Gelfoam is distal, the Gelfoam mixture should be kept coarse. This achieves hemostasis through occlusion proximal to the end capillary bed, thereby mitigating against the complication of tissue necrosis.[6,43] Gelfoam can also be delivered in the form of 2- to 3-mm pledgets termed *torpedoes*. This is achieved by front-loading a 2- to 3-mm piece of Gelfoam into the tip of a 1-mL syringe of half-strength contrast. The torpedoes may be soaked in contrast before injection. This can be used to achieve occlusion of larger caliber vessels and may reduce the risk of ischemia. The delivery of Gelfoam should be followed with a contrast injection after every few 0.1- to 0.3-mL injections of slurry or every few torpedoes, with the goal of sluggish flow and not complete stasis of contrast.[19,29] This technique helps limit reflux of embolic agents into other branches.

The administration of Gelfoam into internal iliac artery branches is typically followed by selective branch occlusion with coils (Fig. 24.2). The theory is that the coils prevent very early recanalization of the vessel but are proximal enough to not cause ischemia. The problem with coils is that they may block access to bleeding vessels if repeat embolization is needed. If a 4-Fr or 5-Fr catheter has been advanced to the target vessel, then 0.035-in coils such as a Nester or Tornado (Cook Medical, Inc., Bloomington, Indiana) can be used. These 0.035-in coils have Dacron fibers to promote thrombogenesis. The 0.035-in coils should be pushed and not injected. Superselective catheterization of the target vessel is typically accomplished with a 0.021-in lumen 3-Fr microcatheter (e.g., Cantata; Cook Medical, Inc., Bloomington, Indiana). A high-flow microcatheter, which typically has a 0.025-in lumen, such as the Progreat Omega (Terumo Medical Corporation, Somerset, New Jersey), provides the ability to perform rapid power injection. The slightly larger inner lumen introduces concerns with compatibility of 0.018-in microcoils (e.g., Nester or Tornado) with high-flow microcatheters because coils can fold over and become wedged within larger lumen microcatheters. This will potentially make arterial branch access difficult for the operator to obtain.

Microcoils can be deployed conventionally by using a pushing wire such as the TruPush (Cordis Corporation, Bridgewater, New Jersey). Microcoils can also be injected, which may expedite the procedure, but the safety of this

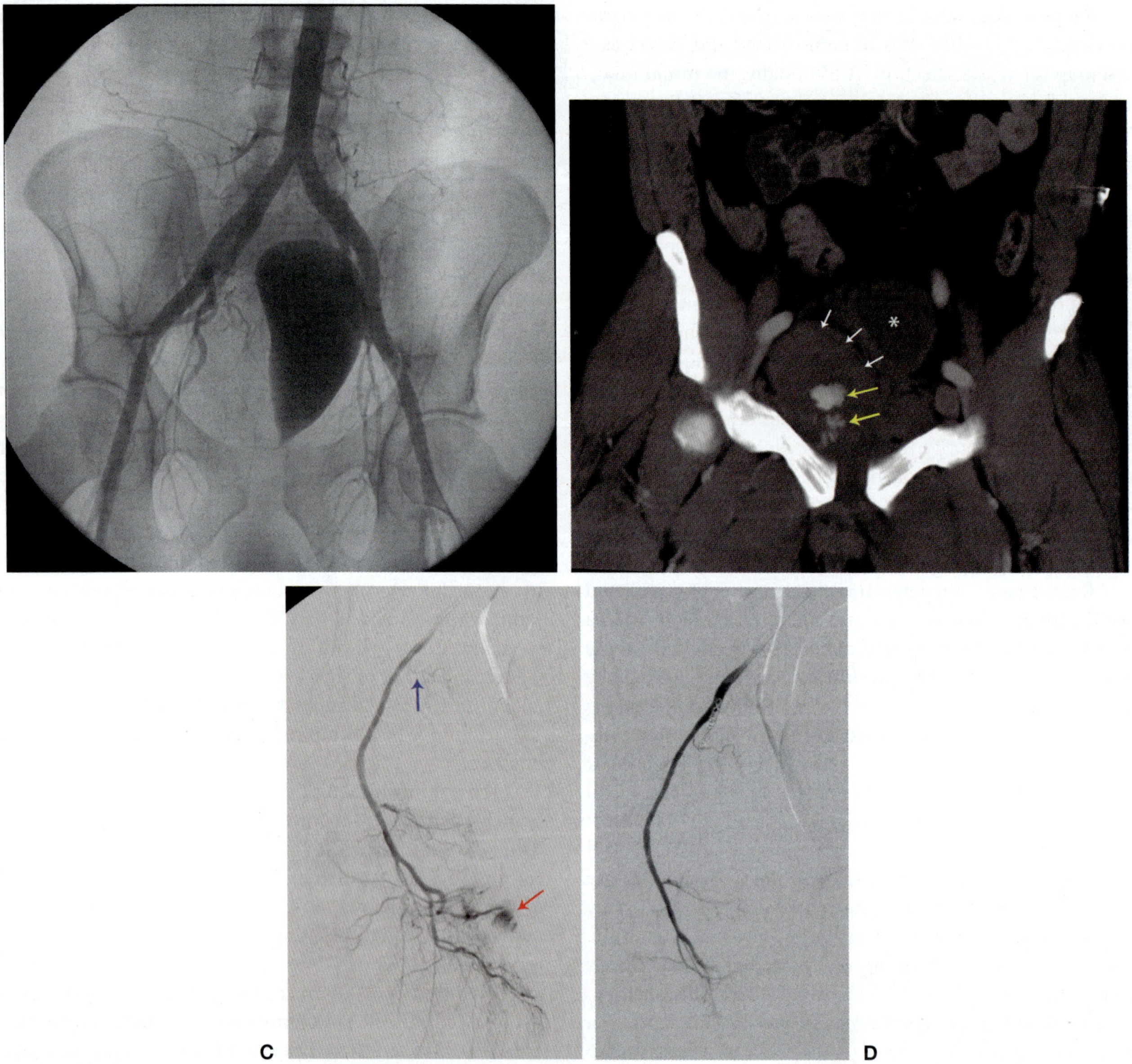

Figure 24.2 **A:** Pelvic angiography for a patient with an open book pelvic fracture sustained after an MVA shows an elevated and elongated appearance of the bladder secondary to mass effect from pelvic sidewall hematoma. **B:** A coronal image from the same patient's CT scan shows the sidewall hematoma (*white arrows*) with mass effect on the bladder (indicated by an *asterisk*) as well as active arterial extravasation (*yellow arrows*). **C:** A selective angiogram of the obturator artery shows active extravasation distally (*red arrow*). Notice that this is not appreciated on the nonselective pelvic angiogram, demonstrating the value of selective interrogation. Extravasation from the vesical branches (*blue arrow*) arising from the obturator artery was also present (not shown on this image). **D:** No persistent extravasation is seen following administration of Gelfoam and coils within the proximal obturator artery. Coil placement is proximal to the origin of the vesical branches. The pudendal artery remains patent following the superselective embolization.

technique requires a stable delivery location (i.e., not close to the origin of the vessel) and low risk of refluxing Gelfoam.

The proximity of the microcatheter to the vessel origin during embolization influences the choice of embolization materials. If the catheter is near the origin of the accessed vessel, detachable coils (e.g., the Axiom Concerto coil; Covidien, Irvine, California), although often more expensive, may be considered to help prevent herniation of the coil into the parent vessel.

Attempts should always be made to advance the microcatheter distal to the site of injury. This allows for coils first to be deployed distal to the injury, followed by Gelfoam, and then additional coils proximally (the so-called Gelfoam

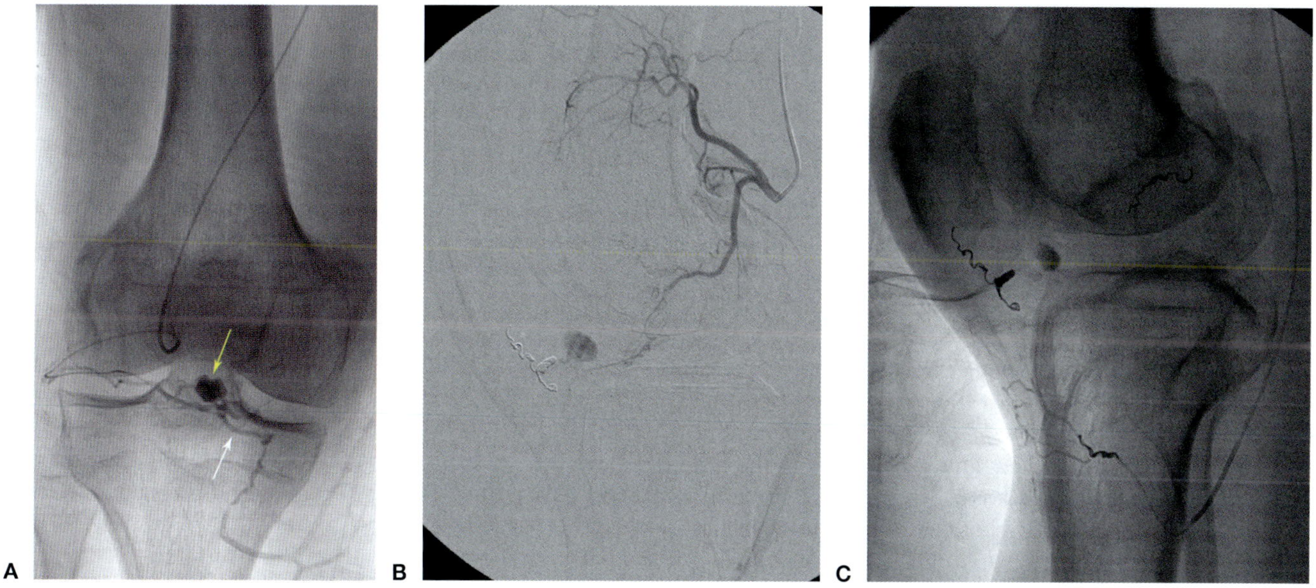

Figure 24.3 The patient developed progressive painful swelling following arthroscopy for a meniscal tear. **A:**. Contrast injection through a microcatheter positioned within the lateral inferior genicular artery demonstrates a pseudoaneurysm (*yellow arrow*) with an arteriovenous fistula, as evidenced by an early draining vein (*white arrow*). **B:** This was treated with the Gelfoam sandwich technique, with microcoils placed distal to the pseudoaneurysm, then Gelfoam followed by additional microcoils across the neck of the pseudoaneurysm into the proximal vessel. Coil embolization of collateral vessels supplying the pseudoaneurysm was also required. **C:** Postembolization angiography demonstrates stagnant contrast within the pseudoaneurysm sac without continued filling.

sandwich technique) (Fig. 24.3). Gelfoam, or in very select circumstances glue or Onyx, and proximal coils without distal coiling can be used if the lesion cannot be crossed. If a traumatic pseudoaneurysm begins expanding subsequent to proximal coiling, endovascular treatment options are limited to percutaneous embolization of the additional branches that are backfilling the pseudoaneurysm. Coils should not be used directly within a traumatic pseudoaneurysm sac due to the potential for rupture as well as reexpansion.[18] However, if the anatomy of the pseudoaneurysm allows, coiling can be performed across the neck of a pseudoaneurysm.

Traumatic arteriovenous fistula may occur when a vein and artery are injured simultaneously, either in the pelvis or extremities. Angiographically, this is appreciated as abnormal early venous return concurrent with the opacification of the arteries. Treatment is similar to pseudoaneurysms, with distal and proximal coil embolization of the artery, but rarely, treatment may require access through both the arterial and venous systems. Although coils can be used in this situation, there is a risk of coil migration in the venous system and subsequent migration centrally. Other options include exclusion of the fistulous connection with an arterial stent graft or use of an Amplatzer Vascular Plug.[44] The Amplatzer Vascular Plug can be particularly useful for the treatment of AVF because of its low risk of migration. The Amplatzer 4 device has a 5-Fr delivery profile. It is the authors' opinion that the use of detachable coils with simultaneous balloon occlusion of venous outflow carries a risk of massive coil migration when the balloon is deflated.

Extremity Embolotherapy

Preprocedural assessment with CT may be obtained but is not necessarily commonplace. CTA of the extremity and runoff vessels is reliably sensitive for evaluation of traumatic vascular injury and can be obtained with a single contrast bolus used for concurrent CT imaging of the chest, abdomen, and pelvis.

Although the upper and lower extremities do not differ significantly in terms of the specific methods of treatment, a few differences bear mentioning. First, a double flush technique should be used whenever the catheter is proximal to the cerebral circulation, including the vertebral and thyrocervical trunk. This is accomplished by first aspirating the catheter with a 20-mL syringe hooked up to a stopcock and then using a second 20-mL syringe to make an additional aspiration of a few milliliters. The catheter is then flushed with the second 20-mL syringe, with the stopcock turned off while actively injecting to prevent any blood accumulation in the catheter tip. Second, CO_2 should not be used during evaluation of the upper extremity due to the risk of reflux in the cerebral vasculature.

The distal anastomoses of the radial and ulnar arteries via the deep and superficial palmar arches can allow embolization of an upper extremity runoff vessel. Although this is a rare clinical situation where surgical options are usually preferred, perfusion of the hand can be maintained if either the radial artery or ulnar artery is sacrificed so long as the palmar arches are sufficient. Patency of the palmar arches and collateral circulation (with Allen test) should be confirmed on physical exam as well as with angiography before intervention. If the distal anastomoses are satisfactory, embolotherapy, such as with the Gelfoam sandwich technique, can be undertaken within the radial or ulnar artery for the purpose of treating traumatic injury. Coil occlusion distal to site of hemorrhage is critical to prevent Gelfoam embolization to the digits. A single runoff vessel to the lower extremity may be sacrificed in a similar fashion so long as the other two runoff vessels are patent and there are no confounding factors such as multifocal flow-limiting stenoses in the setting of peripheral vascular disease.

Angiographic evaluation should begin with nonselective angiography through a sidehole catheter positioned within the aortic arch for the upper extremity or within the infrarenal abdominal aorta for the lower extremity. Subsequent angiographic evaluation should then be obtained in the proximal vessel, either the axillary artery or external iliac artery. As with the pelvis, initial diagnostic angiographic imaging should be carefully scrutinized for the presence of variant anatomy, vascular injury in areas predicted by preprocedure imaging, and also for potential additional sites of injury, which may have been occult on initial imaging or physical examination. Selective angiography is typically obtained with the use of a glidewire and an angle-tipped catheter such as a Kumpe catheter (AngioDynamics, Latham, New York). A Headhunter catheter (AngioDynamics, Latham, New York) is often used in the selection of the upper extremity.

Trauma is complicated by decreased cardiac output, hypovolemia, and vasospasm, but paradoxically, the injection rate and volume of contrast within the extremity may need to be increased over what is normally used. Slow flow may indicate vascular injury and vasospasm or, in the lower leg, raise suspicion for compartment syndrome.

Large vessel injury, such as the brachial artery, even if diagnosed angiographically, may be preferentially treated surgically depending on the institution. Endovascular treatment within the larger vessels is typically limited to stent graft placement. The use of stent grafts for the purpose of excluding the focal site of traumatic injury is being used more frequently.[36] Embolotherapy of side branches near or in the site of injury may be required to prevent endoleak.

The branches of the profunda femoral arteries, muscular branches, and geniculate arteries are an ideal application of embolotherapy for trauma within the extremity.[18] Treatment here can often be accomplished without compromising perfusion of the treated extremity. The endovascular treatment of traumatic injury within the extremity is approached in much the same way as treatment within the pelvis, but with careful attention to primary or accidental embolization of the runoff vessels.

Following embolization, the success of the procedure should be assessed with both postembolization angiography and examination of the extremities. Any change in the peripheral vascular exam should be further interrogated, with possible angiography of the involved limb. Routine postprocedure care includes keeping the accessed extremity steady, which can sometimes be challenging in a patient going to the operating room or suffering disorientation.

DEVICE AND MATERIALS

- Nonselective multi-sidehole catheters: Pigtail (AngioDynamics, Latham, New York) or Sos-Omni (AngioDynamics, Latham, New York)
- Selective catheters: Cobra (AngioDynamics, Latham, New York), multipurpose (AngioDynamics, Latham, New York), Bernestein (AngioDynamics, Latham, New York), JB1 (AngioDynamics, Latham, New York), or Headhunter for the upper extremity; Cobra, multipurpose, Bernestein, Rim, Kumpe, or Sos-Omni for the lower extremity
- Microcatheters: Cantata, Renegade (Boston Scientific Corporation, Natick, Massachusetts), high-flow Renegade, Direxion (Boston Scientific Corporation, Natick, Massachusetts), Progreat, Progreat Omega, Prowler (Cordis Corporation, Bridgewater, New Jersey)
- Embolization materials: Gelfoam in slurry or torpedo form (Gelfoam particles are not used), Nester coils and microcoils, Tornado coils and microcoils, Amplatzer occlusion devices

POTENTIAL COMPLICATIONS

Rebleeding after pelvic TAE should be considered the most important adverse event because it occurs in 15% to 20% of patients and is associated with mortality increasing from 15% to 30%.[2] Predictors of recurrent pelvic arterial hemorrhage include hemoglobin less than 7.5 g/dL before the procedure, more than 6 units of packed red blood cells (PRBCs) after the procedure, or a superselective embolization.[2] This last predictor of rebleeding is contrary to the authors' opinion on the advantages of superselective embolization.[2] Injured vessels may be in vasospasm or otherwise go undetected during angiography. These missed arterial injuries can manifest as delayed hemorrhage after resuscitation restores intravascular volume. Vasospasm or delayed migration/packing of Gelfoam may also contribute to rebleeding. We continue to advocate superselective embolization but also recommend aggressive embolization of occluded vessels, which may be due to traumatic thrombosis or vasospasm. Leaving the vascular sheath in place should also be considered when there is concern the embolization is incomplete or the patient still needs resuscitation.

Complication directly related to embolization is tissue ischemia within the treatment vascular bed or other territories secondary to nontarget embolization. This uncommon complication is manifested in pelvic embolizations as gluteal muscle necrosis, sacral skin breakdown, ischemic necrosis of the bladder wall and rectum, or necrosis of the femoral head.[42,43,45–47] Nerve injury following TAE for trauma has been reported, but shear injury from the trauma itself rather than procedure-related ischemic changes may account for many of these reported pelvic TAE complications.[42] Impotence in the male patient is likewise usually considered a consequence of the initial traumatic injury rather than nerve injury caused by pelvic TAE.[48,49]

Because of the possibility of inducing tissue necrosis, selective embolization should be performed if the patient's hemodynamic status permits, and the patient should be adequately observed for signs of ischemic changes in the days that follow. Long-term follow-up is also required as buttock claudication may be associated with pelvic TAE but not be observed until patient is well into rehabilitation exercises.[50]

The most important step in reducing the risk of tissue ischemia is the appropriate choice of embolic agent. This should be small enough to effectively occlude the site of bleeding but large enough to avoid the terminal capillary bed. The use of nonpermanent embolic agents (Gelfoam) may potentially aid in reducing the risk of tissue necrosis by allowing for recanalization of the vessel over the course of a few weeks.

Nontarget embolization most often occurs when the rate of embolization is too fast and embolic material refluxes proximal to the catheter tip. Anastomotic vessels not appreciated on angiography can also contribute to nontarget embolization. Nontarget embolization of unintended pelvic vessels is typically well tolerated secondary to pelvic collateral vessels. In contrast, embolic material introduced into the outflow vessels of the extremity, or used during an intervention for the extremity, can jeopardize the perfusion of the limb. Endovascular coils, if placed within a proximal segment of vessel, can herniate into the parent vessel, thereby resulting in unintended occlusion distal to the point of herniation. Coils can also embolize through arteriovenous fistulae. The operator must have familiarity with coil retrieval if providing arterial embolization services.

Knowledge of variant anatomy is easy to forget in the high-stress setting of trauma embolization, but failure to recognize variants can lead to profound ischemia. In the pelvis, the two most important variants are (1) the persistent sciatic artery and (2) the corona mortis.

The persistent sciatic artery (PSA) is a rare congenital variant branch of the internal iliac artery that exits the pelvis through the obturator foramen.[51,52] When this is present, the ipsilateral external iliac and common femoral arteries are hypoplastic. The PSA may give rise to the popliteal artery and provide most of the blood flow to the lower extremity or it may supplement the dominant femoral arterial system. In either case, it should be recognized angiographically. This can also be detected on physical exam if normal posterior tibial and dorsalis pedis pulses are present with an absent or diminished ipsilateral femoral pulse.

The corona mortis (or, more ominously translated, "the crown of death") is an anatomic variant consisting of an obturator artery originating from the external iliac artery or an anastomotic connection between the obturator artery and either the inferior epigastric artery or external iliac artery.[53,54] (It takes its name not from its reputation with interventionalists but rather from the propensity for disastrous injury it used to have during orthopedic procedures.) This can also refer to a connection between the veins of the pelvis, which is more common than the arterial variant. Close proximity to the superior pubic ramus predispose this vessel to acute traumatic injury. This vessel is a potential source of hemorrhage fed by the external iliac artery as well as a source for back bleeding subsequent to embolization targeting the internal iliac branches.

Variant anatomy within the extremity is also important to keep in mind. Important variants include a high takeoff of the radial or ulnar arteries in the upper extremity and a takeoff of the anterior or posterior tibial artery in the lower extremity.[55]

Attention to diagnostic images must also include the recognition of acquired variant anatomy, which is actually far more common. A patient with peripheral vascular disease may have runoff vessels supplied entirely through collateral flow from the profunda femoral artery. Although the branches of the profunda can normally be sacrificed without great consequence, in this setting, their occlusion would be a disaster.

Upper extremity angiography alone introduces a small risk of stroke. Embolization of proximal upper extremity branches raises this risk of stroke. Extreme caution must be taken to know the runoff of any proximal subclavian arteries being considered for embolization and to avoid particles and liquids when working near the vertebral arteries or spinal arteries.

TIPS AND TRICKS

Pelvic Trauma

- In pelvic trauma, both internal iliac arteries should be imaged even if the prior CT indicates unilateral injury.
- A compliant occlusion balloon may be placed in the infrarenal aorta at the start of the procedure to limit ongoing hemorrhage during portions of the pelvic embolization procedure.

Extremity Trauma

- Extremity arterial embolization can be safely performed in profunda, muscular, or genicular branches.
- Trauma to the vessels of the lower leg or forearm, although uncommon, can be treated with endovascular occlusion so long as appropriate collateralization at the palmar or plantar arches is confirmed.
- Superselective embolization is almost always preferred, so long as the patient status will allow it, to prevent early rebleeding and reduce risk of ischemia.
- If the microcatheter is in stable position, microcoils can be injected to expedite the procedure.

- The use of high-flow microcatheters allows for power injections to be performed.
- Microcoil compatibility with high-flow microcatheter must be confirmed.
- Detachable coils are particularly helpful as the first coil (to confirm stability and appropriate packing) and as the last coil (to avoid herniation into the parent vessel).
- Renal protection may be aided by the use of CO_2 during certain portions of the exam.
- A Gelfoam slurry should be kept coarse, particularly if the target is relatively less selective.
- Gelfoam torpedoes provide a more proximal particle embolization.
- Consider leaving the arterial access if hypothermia or rapid PRBC administration has caused a coagulopathy or if repeat angiography in the next 12–24 h is likely.
- Closure devices can be used in the trauma setting to avoid the time constraint of manual pressure. The use of a closure device does not preclude the use of repeat short interval access at the same site.

REFERENCES

1. Hoffer EK. Transcatheter embolization in the treatment of hemorrhage in pelvic trauma. *Semin Intervent Radiol.* 2008;25(3):281–292.
2. Fang JF, Shih LY, Wong YC, et al. Repeat transcatheter arterial embolization for the management of pelvic arterial hemorrhage. *J Trauma.* 2009;66(2):429–435.
3. Hagiwara A, Minakawa K, Fukushima H, et al. Predictors of death in patients with life-threatening pelvic hemorrhage after successful transcatheter arterial embolization. *J Trauma.* 2003;55(4):696–703.
4. Jeske HC, Larndorfer R, Krappinger D, et al. Management of hemorrhage in severe pelvic injuries. *J Trauma.* 2010;68(2):415–420.
5. Karadimas EJ, Nicolson T, Kakagia DD, et al. Angiographic embolisation of pelvic ring injuries. Treatment algorithm and review of the literature. *Int Orthop.* 2011;35(9):1381–1390.
6. Cullinane DC, Schiller HJ, Zielinski MD, et al. Eastern association for the surgery of trauma practice management guidelines for hemorrhage in pelvic fracture—update and systematic review. *J Trauma.* 2011;71(6):1850–1868.
7. Kos S, Gutzeit A, Hoppe H, et al. Diagnosis and therapy of acute hemorrhage in patients with pelvic fractures. *Semin Musculoskelet Radiol.* 2013;17(4):396–406.
8. Cook RE, Keating JF, Gillespie I. The role of angiography in the management of haemorrhage from major fractures of the pelvis. *J Bone Joint Surg Br.* 2002;84(2):178–182.
9. Eastridge BJ, Starr A, Minei JP, et al. The importance of fracture pattern in guiding therapeutic decision-making in patients with hemorrhagic shock and pelvic ring disruptions. *J Trauma.* 2002;53(3):446–450.
10. Smith W, Williams A, Agudelo J, et al. Early predictors of mortality in hemodynamically unstable pelvis fractures. *J Orthop Trauma.* 2007;21(1):31–37.
11. Frevert S, Dahl B, Lonn L. Update on the roles of angiography and embolisation in pelvic fracture. *Injury.* 2008;39(11):1290–1294.
12. Starr AJ, Griffin DR, Reinert CM, et al. Pelvic ring disruptions: prediction of associated injuries, transfusion requirement, pelvic arteriography, complications, and mortality. *J Orthop Trauma.* 2002;16(8):553–561.
13. Miller PR, Moore PS, Mansell E, et al. External fixation or arteriogram in bleeding pelvic fracture: initial therapy guided by markers of arterial hemorrhage. *J Trauma.* 2003;54(3):437–443.
14. Agolini SF, Shah K, Jaffe J, et al. Arterial embolization is a rapid and effective technique for controlling pelvic fracture hemorrhage. *J Trauma.* 1997;43(3):395–399.
15. Biffl WL, Smith WR, Moore EE, et al. Evolution of a multidisciplinary clinical pathway for the management of unstable patients with pelvic fractures. *Ann Surg.* 2001;233(6):843–850.
16. Kimbrell BJ, Velmahos GC, Chan LS, et al. Angiographic embolization for pelvic fractures in older patients. *Arch Surg.* 2004;139(7):728–732; discussion 732–733.
17. Sarin EL, Moore JB, Moore EE, et al. Pelvic fracture pattern does not always predict the need for urgent embolization. *J Trauma.* 2005;58(5):973–977.
18. Bauer JR, Ray CE. Transcatheter arterial embolization in the trauma patient: a review. *Semin Intervent Radiol.* 2004;21(1):11–22.
19. Ben-Menachem Y, Coldwell DM, Young JW, et al. Hemorrhage associated with pelvic fractures: causes, diagnosis, and emergent management. *AJR Am J Roentgenol.* 1991;157(5):1005–1014.
20. Niola R, Pinto A, Sparano A, et al. Arterial bleeding in pelvic trauma: priorities in angiographic embolization. *Curr Probl Diagn Radiol.* 2012;41(3):93–101.
21. Suzuki T, Smith WR, Moore EE. Pelvic packing or angiography: competitive or complementary? *Injury.* 2009;40(4):343–353.
22. Blackmore CC, Cummings P, Jurkovich GJ, et al. Predicting major hemorrhage in patients with pelvic fracture. *J Trauma.* 2006;61(2):346–352.
23. Metz CM, Hak DJ, Goulet JA, et al. Pelvic fracture patterns and their corresponding angiographic sources of hemorrhage. *Orthop Clin North Am.* 2004;35(4):431–437, v.
24. Pinto A, Niola R, Tortora G, et al. Role of multidetector-row CT in assessing the source of arterial haemorrhage in patients with pelvic vascular trauma. comparison with angiography. *Radiol Med.* 2010;115(4):648–667.
25. Roy-Choudhury SH, Gallacher DJ, Pilmer J, et al. Relative threshold of detection of active arterial bleeding: in vitro comparison of MDCT and digital subtraction angiography. *AJR Am J Roentgenol.* 2007;189(5):W238–W246.
26. Katsanos K, Sabharwal T, Carrell T, et al. Peripheral endografts for the treatment of traumatic arterial injuries. *Emerg Radiol.* 2009;16(3):175–184.
27. Doody O, Given MF, Lyon SM. Extremities—indications and techniques for treatment of extremity vascular injuries. *Injury.* 2008;39(11):1295–1303.

28. Maleux G, Herten PJ, Vaninbroukx J, et al. Value of percutaneous embolotherapy for the management of traumatic vascular limb injury. *Acta Radiol.* 2012;53(2):147–152.
29. Aksoy M, Taviloglu K, Yanar H, et al. Percutaneous transcatheter embolization in arterial injuries of the lower limbs. *Acta Radiol.* 2005;46(5):471–475.
30. Franz RW, Skytta CK, Shah KJ, et al. A five-year review of management of upper-extremity arterial injuries at an urban level I trauma center. *Ann Vasc Surg.* 2012;26(5):655–664.
31. Peck MA, Rasmussen TE. Management of blunt peripheral arterial injury. *Perspect Vasc Surg Endovasc Ther.* 2006;18(2):159–173.
32. Levy BA, Zlowodzki MP, Graves M, et al. Screening for extermity arterial injury with the arterial pressure index. *Am J Emerg Med.* 2005;23(5):689–695.
33. Pieroni S, Foster BR, Anderson SW, et al. Use of 64-row multidetector CT angiography in blunt and penetrating trauma of the upper and lower extremities. *Radiographics.* 2009;29(3):863–876.
34. Fox N, Rajani RR, Bokhari F, et al. Evaluation and management of penetrating lower extremity arterial trauma: an eastern association for the surgery of trauma practice management guideline. *J Trauma Acute Care Surg.* 2012;73(5)(suppl 4):S315–S320.
35. Sidhu MK, Hogan MJ, Shaw DW, et al. Interventional radiology for paediatric trauma. *Pediatr Radiol.* 2009;39(5):506–515.
36. Piffaretti G, Benedetto F, Menegolo M, et al. Outcomes of endovascular repair for blunt thoracic aortic injury. *J Vasc Surg.* 2013;58(6):1483–1489.
37. Carrafiello G, Lagana D, Mangini M, et al. Percutaneous treatment of traumatic upper-extremity arterial injuries: a single-center experience. *J Vasc Interv Radiol.* 2011;22(1):34–39.
38. Mavili E, Donmez H, Ozcan N, et al. Endovascular treatment of lower limb penetrating arterial traumas. *Cardiovasc Intervent Radiol.* 2007;30(6):1124–1129.
39. Yoo DH, Jae HJ, Kim HC, et al. Transcatheter arterial embolization of intramuscular active hemorrhage with N-butyl cyanoacrylate. *Cardiovasc Intervent Radiol.* 2012;35(2):292–298.
40. Juszkat R, Zielinski M, Wykretowicz M, et al. Traumatic inferior gluteal artery aneurysm managed with emergency transcatheter thrombin injection. *Cardiovasc Intervent Radiol.* 2010;33(3):607–609.
41. Johnson GE, Sandstrom CK, Kogut MJ, et al. Frequency of external iliac artery branch injury in blunt trauma: improved detection with selective external iliac angiography. *J Vasc Interv Radiol.* 2013;24(3):363–369.
42. Auerbach AD, Rehman S, Kleiner MT. Selective transcatheter arterial embolization of the internal iliac artery does not cause gluteal necrosis in pelvic trauma patients. *J Orthop Trauma.* 2012;26(5):290–295.
43. Yasumura K, Ikegami K, Kamohara T, et al. High incidence of ischemic necrosis of the gluteal muscle after transcatheter angiographic embolization for severe pelvic fracture. *J Trauma.* 2005;58(5):985–990.
44. Shetty R, Lotun K. Treatment of an iatrogenic femoral artery pseudoaneurysm with concomitant arteriovenous fistula with percutaneous implantation of an Amplatzer Vascular Plug. *Catheter Cardiovasc Interv.* 2013;81(1):E53–E57.
45. Travis T, Monsky WL, London J, et al. Evaluation of short-term and long-term complications after emergent internal iliac artery embolization in patients with pelvic trauma. *J Vasc Interv Radiol.* 2008;19(6):840–847.
46. Takahira N, Shindo M, Tanaka K, et al. Gluteal muscle necrosis following transcatheter angiographic embolisation for retroperitoneal haemorrhage associated with pelvic fracture. *Injury.* 2001;32(1):27–32.
47. Suzuki T, Kataoka Y, Minehara H, et al. Transcatheter arterial embolization for pelvic fractures may potentially cause a triad of sequela: gluteal necrosis, rectal necrosis, and lower limb paresis. *J Trauma.* 2008;65(6):1547–1550.
48. Ramirez JI, Velmahos GC, Best CR, et al. Male sexual function after bilateral internal iliac artery embolization for pelvic fracture. *J Trauma.* 2004;56(4):734–739; discussion 739–741.
49. Ellison M, Timberlake GA, Kerstein MD. Impotence following pelvic fracture. *J Trauma.* 1988;28(5):695–696.
50. Rayt HS, Bown MJ, Lambert KV, et al. Buttock claudication and erectile dysfunction after internal iliac artery embolization in patients prior to endovascular aortic aneurysm repair. *Cardiovasc Intervent Radiol.* 2008;31(4):728–734.
51. Brantley SK, Rigdon EE, Raju S. Persistent sciatic artery: embryology, pathology, and treatment. *J Vasc Surg.* 1993;18(2):242–248.
52. Hsu WC, Lim KE, Hsu YY. Inadvertent embolization of a persistent sciatic artery in pelvis trauma. *Cardiovasc Intervent Radiol.* 2005;28(4):518–520.
53. Smith JC, Gregorius JC, Breazeale BH, et al. The corona mortis, a frequent vascular variant susceptible to blunt pelvic trauma: identification at routine multidetector CT. *J Vasc Interv Radiol.* 2009;20(4):455–460.
54. Requarth JA, Miller PR. Aberrant obturator artery is a common arterial variant that may be a source of unidentified hemorrhage in pelvic fracture patients. *J Trauma.* 2011;70(2):366–372.
55. Uflacker R, ed. *Atlas of Vascular Anatomy: An Angiographic Approach.* 2nd ed. Philadelphia, PA: Lippincott Williams & Wilkins; 2006.

25

Spine and Bone Trauma

Pierre E. Bize • Yann Lachenal • Alban Denys

Transcatheter arterial embolization (TAE) has proven to be useful in the treatment of hemodynamically stable polytrauma patients.[1,2] It has also proven to be useful in selected hemodynamically unstable patients who responded at least transiently to fluid resuscitation.[3,4] However, the place of TAE in the treatment algorithm of polytrauma patients remains to be defined.[5–12] TAE has several advantages in selected trauma patients. It can control several sources of bleeding from one single vascular puncture, avoiding unnecessary surgical exposure in those fragile patients, thus avoiding hypothermia, which is often a problem in this setting. It can be performed in the angiography suite while other resuscitation maneuvers are carried on. It can be performed without major risks in patients with impaired coagulation, which is also quite frequent in polytranfused patients. As opposed to solid organ or pelvic bone fractures, there is little information on the role of TAE in the treatment of paraspinal bleeding associated with spine trauma or with fractures of other bones such as in the limbs.[13–21]

DEVICE AND MATERIALS

Bleeding associated with spine or bone fractures is usually of osseous or venous origin and is self-limited. However, some cases of bleeding from an arterial injury can be associated with significant blood loss. Arterial bleeding in the paraspinal space and in the limbs may have originated from muscular branches and thus can be embolized with gelatin sponge or even glue. Particulate agents such as Bead Blocks (Biocompatible, Farnham UK) are not usually recommended because they might cause ischemia and rhabdomyolysis. Coils are convenient when there is a single well-identified vessel that can be selectively catheterized, such as the intercostal or the lumbar arteries. However, when using coils, one should use the "front door/back door" embolization technique to prevent further bleeding from retrograde flow. This technique consists of placing the coil beyond and before the vascular lesion. However, glue and gelatin sponge are perfectly suitable in this particular situation, with the advantage of being able to control the bleeding from both the antegrade and retrograde flow more quickly and at a lower cost.

TECHNIQUE

The target vessel should be identified from the computed tomography (CT) with contrast as it might be difficult to identify bleeding vessels by digital subtraction angiography (DSA) in hypotensive patients. Arterial access is gained usually from one of the common femoral arteries. When bleeding from a lower limb is present and other vessels need to be embolized, it is best to choose the contralateral common femoral artery and to catheterize the bleeding side by crossover. Antegrade puncture of the common femoral artery on the bleeding side is not convenient as it will render catheterization of other bleeding vessels uneasy if not impossible. In case of nonpalpable pulse, ultrasound guidance should be used promptly. The Seldinger technique is used to gain vascular access, and a 5-Fr or 6-Fr introducer sheath is inserted in the common femoral artery. The choice of catheter curvature will depend on the vessel to be embolized. A Cobra C2 (Glidecath, Terumo Europe, Leuven Belgium) catheter usually allows catheterization of the lumbar arteries and also allows crossover to the contralateral iliac and femoral arteries. Vascular anomalies such as irregular vessel walls, dissection, pseudoaneurysm, or active bleeding should be looked for by selective catheterization using a 4-Fr or 5-Fr catheter. If no abnormality and no active bleeding is seen in the suspected vascular territory, a forceful hand injection can reveal the bleeding from an injured vessel, which was occluded by spasm, dissection, or clot. In case of

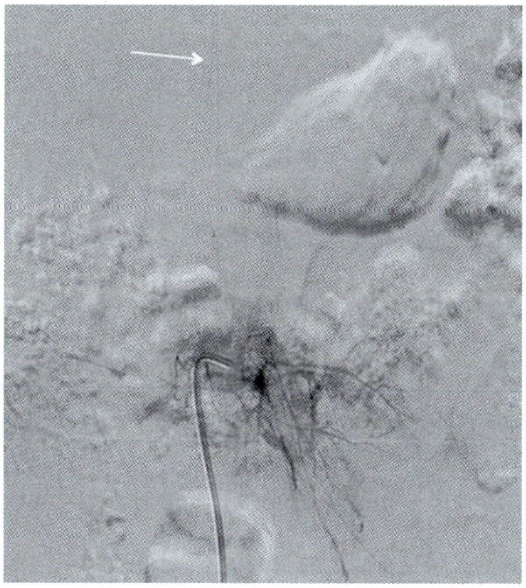

Figure 25.1 Typical hairpin appearance of an anterior spinal artery upon injection of contrast media in a lumbar artery (*arrow*).

superselective catheterization, a microcatheter allowing the use of 0.018-in coils should be used. In case of embolization of a lumbar artery with coils, care should be taken to embolize the lumbar arteries above and below the bleeding level to avoid retrograde filling of the embolized artery by collateral flow from the upper and lower levels.

In the paraspinal space, always look for spinal arteries, especially in the dorsolumbar region. The anterior and posterior spinal arteries supply the spinal cord. The anterior spinal artery receives blood from a large segmental vessel originating from one of the last intercostal arteries known as the *Adamkiewicz artery* (typically located between the vertebral bodies T8–L2 segment). The posterior spinal artery receives many segmental feeders known as the *radiculospinal arteries*, which can be recognized by their "hairpin" shape on angiography (Fig. 25.1). When present, embolization should take place from beyond the origin of the radiculospinal artery. Coils or large gelatin sponge torpedoes are best used in this situation. If particulate agents are to be used, they should be greater than 350 μm in size.[22]

CLINICAL APPLICATIONS

TAE of arterial bleeding associated with spine or peripheral bone fracture can be convenient in patients with other bleeding sites that also need to be treated by embolization or in patients with altered coagulation status. One typical scenario is a patient with a ruptured spleen associated with rib and lumbar transverse apophysis fractures. Another scenario would be a patient with a fractured bone and an impaired coagulation status. TAE could resolve the hemorrhage quickly while the coagulation status is restored before reparative surgery.

Bleeding in the Paraspinal Space

In trauma patients, bleeding in the paraspinal space is usually associated with vertebral fractures. Paraspinal bleeding originates mostly from the broken bone itself or from the azygos and hemiazygos veins and perispinal venous plexuses. These bleeding sources are not amenable to embolization, but they are usually self-limiting.[19] However, bleeding in the paraspinal space when associated with bleeding in other territories can lead to significant blood loss.[21,23] Care should be taken to look for an arterial bleeding source when interpreting a CT scan in a polytrauma patient with a significant hematoma in the paraspinal space. In the absence of other sources of bleeding such as the renal or the internal iliac arteries and their branches, the most frequently involved arteries in this setting are the intercostal and lumbar arteries.[21,23,24] If the bleeding vessel can be identified from multislice CT imaging, TAE can be used to control bleeding in the paraspinal space. TAE is particularly useful in patients with other bleeding sites. As it is the case for abdominal organ lesions, a good CT with arterial enhancement and multiplanar reconstruction will guide the embolization procedure and make it quicker and easier, avoiding the time-consuming catheterization of all lumbar and pelvic arteries. Figure 25.2 displays the case of a woman on anticoagulants with a vertebral fracture and paraspinal hematoma with active bleeding treated by TAE. Another interesting use of TAE is the treatment of bleeding from penetrating wounds such as stab wounds or gunshot wounds.[1,18,25] When surgery is not absolutely mandatory, such as in case of hollow viscus perforation, TAE can avoid surgery and quickly control bleeding from the injured vessels. Figure 25.3 displays the case of a patient who sustained a stab wound in the paraspinal region and was treated by TAE only.

Bleeding Associated with Trauma of the Limbs

Most bleeding associated with bone fracture are from osseous or venous origin and is self-limited. However, in case of a penetrating injury, fractures, and joint dislocation, arterial lesions can occur and should be searched for. Angiography is considered to be excellent in revealing vascular lesions in the extremities. These lesions consist of occlusion, extravasation, pseudoaneurysm, and arteriovenous fistula. Intraluminal filling defects such as thrombi and intimal flaps can also be visualized.[1]

The bleeding in limb trauma can fall in two categories: (1) major vessel injuries, such as the superficial femoral artery or the brachial artery, with immediate threat for the involved limb; and (2) bleeding from secondary muscular branches. The first category is definitely not to be treated by any kind of endovascular procedure but necessitates immediate surgical vascular repair. If surgery is not immediately available or feasible, a tourniquet should be used to control

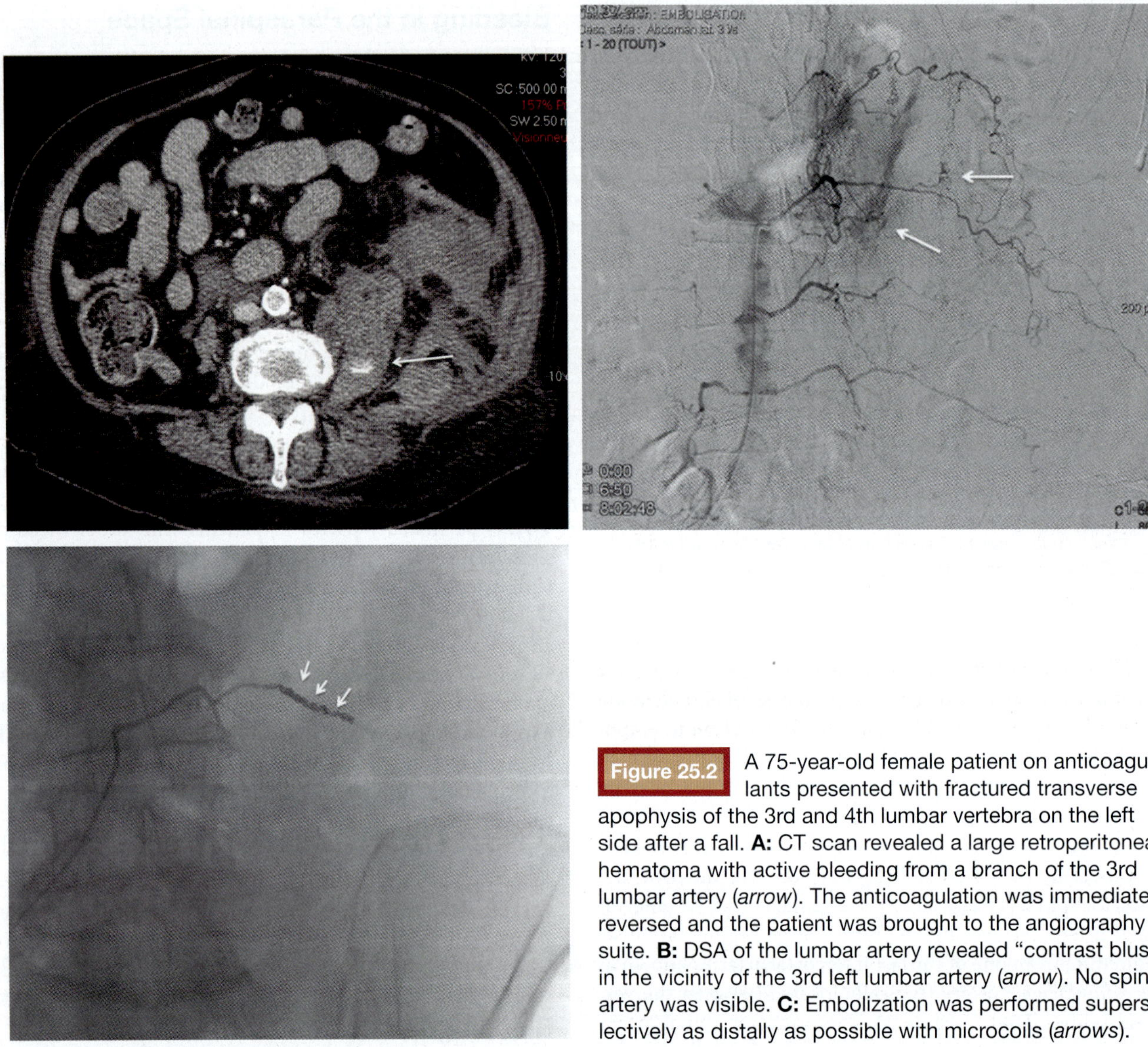

Figure 25.2 A 75-year-old female patient on anticoagulants presented with fractured transverse apophysis of the 3rd and 4th lumbar vertebra on the left side after a fall. **A:** CT scan revealed a large retroperitoneal hematoma with active bleeding from a branch of the 3rd lumbar artery (*arrow*). The anticoagulation was immediately reversed and the patient was brought to the angiography suite. **B:** DSA of the lumbar artery revealed "contrast blush" in the vicinity of the 3rd left lumbar artery (*arrow*). No spinal artery was visible. **C:** Embolization was performed superselectively as distally as possible with microcoils (*arrows*).

the bleeding. In the second category, muscular bleeding is usually self-limited by tamponade effect from the muscular fascia and might not necessitate TAE. TAE might become necessary if there is evidence of growing hematoma, compartment syndrome, or impaired coagulation status. However, even in these cases, surgery has the advantage of addressing the compartment syndrome that often results from accumulation of large quantities of blood in the fascia by performing fasciotomies. When the fascia is ruptured, such as in an open trauma, TAE can be an option if direct surgical control of the bleeding cannot be performed immediately.

Upper Extremity

The brachial artery should not be embolized as it supplies blood to the hand and the collateral supply at this level is usually not sufficient to preserve viability of the hand territory. Segments of the ulnar and radial arteries can be embolized with coils after angiographic confirmation that the palmar arch is patent. Glue, gelatin sponge, and particulate agents should definitely not be used in the upper limbs because they will cause irreversible ischemia in the hands.[22] Muscular branches in the upper extremity can be embolized without risk due to extensive collateralization.

Lower Extremity

The common and superficial femoral arteries should not be embolized as they supply the lower extremity and their occlusion could result in irreversible ischemic damage. The deep femoral artery should be preserved whenever possible as it also contributes in an important way to the perfusion of the lower extremity. Superselective embolization of muscular branches, leaving the main trunk patent, is the

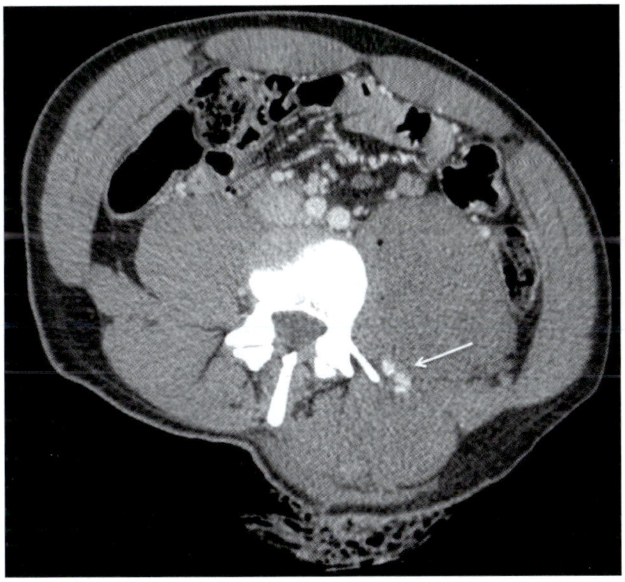

A

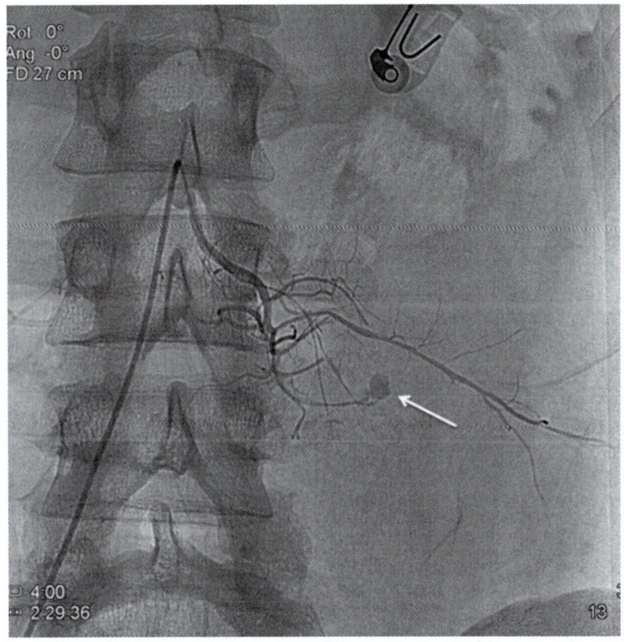

B

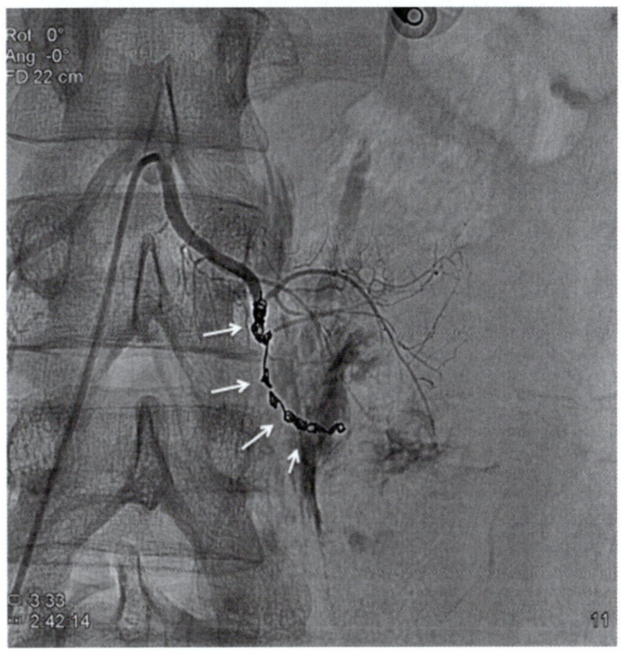

C

Figure 25.3 A 20-year-old male with a stab wound in the left paraspinal region was brought to the emergency department. The patient was hemodynamically stable but there was clinical evidence of ongoing arterial bleeding from the wound. **A:** CT scan revealed active bleeding from the 3rd left lumbar artery (*arrow*). **B:** Angiography confirmed contrast extravasation from this vessel (*arrows*). There was no visible spinal artery. **C:** The bleeding vessel was embolized with microcoils as close as possible to the vascular injury.

preferred way to perform TAE in this territory. In case of cataclysmic bleeding from the deep femoral artery, a transient embolic agent such as gelatin foam should be used. Below the knee, one vessel of the trifurcation is considered sufficient to maintain sufficient perfusion in the foot. Surgical repair of these vessels is considered difficult and surgical treatment often consists of ligation of the injured vessel. Hence, embolization is an alternative as long as one vessel is patent. In case of disruption, the front door/back door technique should be used to prevent continuous bleeding from retrograde flow.

POTENTIAL COMPLICATIONS

The most common complication after embolization of a muscular arterial territory is ischemia and rhabdomyolysis, often accompanied by pain and inflammatory syndrome. Paresis or even paralysis of the treated limb can occur due to nerve ischemia from TAE.[26]

In the paraspinal space, the most dreadful complication is paraplegia from inadvertent embolization of a spinal artery.[19] To avoid the risk of spinal cord ischemia, spinal branches from the segmental arteries should be sought for and embolization should be performed as distally as possible.

TIPS AND TRICKS

Paraspinal Space

- Bleeding in the paraspinal space originates mostly from broken bone and veins. These bleeding sources are not amenable to embolization but usually self-limited. Embolize only when there's a good reason.
  - Anticoagulation therapy
  - Multiple bleeding sites
  - Bleeding vessel clearly identified on CT
- Use coaxial microcatheter technique to navigate through potentially small and tortuous arteries.
- Special attention should be paid to the T8–L2 level where the Adamkiewicz artery may be. Embolization of this artery may lead to paraplegia due to ischemia of the spinal cord.
- Perform superselective and precise embolization as close as possible to the target lesion.
- The posterior spinal artery feeders can have a hairpin shape on DSA (Fig. 25.3).
- Preferably use coils for precise embolization, which should take place from beyond the origin of the radiculospinal artery.

Limbs

- Bleeding associated with bone fracture are from osseous or venous origin and self-limited.
- In case of a penetrating injury, fractures, and joint dislocation, look for arterial lesions.
- Major vessel injuries with immediate threat for the involved limb
  - Immediate surgical vascular repair
  - If surgery is not an option, a tourniquet should be used to control the bleeding.
- Bleeding from secondary muscular branches is usually self-limited; embolize when with the following:
  - Growing hematoma
  - Altered coagulation status
  - Multiple bleeding sites
- Surgery is the best choice in case of compartment syndrome.
- Do not occlude the brachial and common and superficial femoral arteries.
- Always check collaterals and assess blood supply to the extremity of the limb.

CONCLUSION

The use of TAE in trauma patients with bleeding in the paraspinal space or in the limbs is marginal. However, in certain situations such as in those patients with multiple bleeding sites or those under anticoagulation treatment, TAE could be an efficient way to limit blood loss. Special care should be taken in the paraspinal space to not embolize any spinal artery and in the limbs to not cause ischemia distally.

REFERENCES

1. Bauer JR, Ray CE. Transcatheter arterial embolization in the trauma patient: a review. *Semin Intervent Radiol.* 2004;21(1):11–22.
2. Ben-Menachem Y, Handel SF, Thaggard A III, et al. Therapeutic arterial embolization in trauma. *J Trauma.* 1979;19(12):944–952.
3. Bize PE, Duran R, Madoff DC, et al. Embolization for multicompartmental bleeding in patients in hemodynamically unstable condition: prognostic factors and outcome. *J Vasc Interv Radiol.* 2012;23(6):751–760.e4.
4. Hagiwara A, Murata A, Matsuda T, et al. The usefulness of transcatheter arterial embolization for patients with blunt polytrauma showing transient response to fluid resuscitation. *J Trauma.* 2004;57(2):271–276; discussion 276–277.
5. Karadimas EJ, Nicolson T, Kakagia DD, et al. Angiographic embolisation of pelvic ring injuries. Treatment algorithm and review of the literature. *Int Orthop.* 2011;35(9):1381–1390.
6. Letoublon C, Morra I, Chen Y, et al. Hepatic arterial embolization in the management of blunt hepatic trauma: indications and complications. *J Trauma.* 2011;70(5):1032–1036; discussion 1036–1037.
7. Niola R, Pinto A, Sparano A, et al. Arterial bleeding in pelvic trauma: priorities in angiographic embolization. *Curr Probl Diagn Radiol.* 2012;41(3):93–101.

8. Lui B, Schlicht S, Vrazas J. Role of embolization in the management of splenic trauma. *Australas Radiol.* 2004;48(3):401–403.
9. Broadwell SR, Ray CE. Transcatheter embolization in pelvic trauma. *Semin Intervent Radiol.* 2004;21(1):23–35.
10. Greco L, Francioso G, Pratichizzo A, et al. Arterial embolization in the treatment of severe blunt hepatic trauma. *Hepatogastroenterology.* 2003;50(51):746–749.
11. Totterman A, Dormagen JB, Madsen JE, et al. A protocol for angiographic embolization in exsanguinating pelvic trauma: a report on 31 patients. *Acta Orthop.* 2006;77(3):462–468.
12. Monnin V, Sengel C, Thony F, et al. Place of arterial embolization in severe blunt hepatic trauma: a multidisciplinary approach. *Cardiovasc Intervent Radiol.* 2008;31(5):875–882.
13. Armstrong NN, Zarvon NP, Sproat IA, et al. Lumbar artery hemorrhage: unusual cause of shock treated by angiographic embolization. *J Trauma.* 1997;42(3):544–545.
14. Haydu P, Chang J, Knox G, et al. Transcatheter arterial embolization of a traumatic lumbar artery false aneurysm. *Surgery.* 1978;84(2):288–291.
15. Panetta T, Sclafani SJ, Goldstein AS, et al. Percutaneous transcatheter embolization for arterial trauma. *J Vasc Surg.* 1985;2(1):54–64.
16. Siablis D, Panagopoulos C, Karamessini M, et al. Delayed diagnosis of a false aneurysm after lumbar arterial injury: treatment with endovascular embolization: a case report. *Spine (Phila Pa 1976).* 2003;28(4):E71–E73.
17. Sofocleous CT, Hinrichs CR, Hubbi B, et al. Embolization of isolated lumbar artery injuries in trauma patients. *Cardiovasc Intervent Radiol.* 2005;28(6):730–735.
18. Zamora CA, Sugimoto K, Mori T, et al. Lumbar artery injury after self-stabbing in a hara-kiri suicide attempt: treatment by selective microcatheter embolization. *J Trauma.* 2005;58(2):384–387.
19. Morita S, Tsuji T, Fukushima T, et al. Arterial embolization of an extrapleural hematoma from a dislocated fracture of the lumbar spine: a case report. *Scand J Trauma Resusc Emerg Med.* 2009;17:27.
20. Hamid RS, ul HT, Chishti I, et al. Post traumatic avulsion of lumbar artery: a rare cause of retroperitoneal haemorrhage treated by glue embolization. *J Pak Med Assoc.* 2010;60(6):487–489.
21. Holting T, Buhr HJ, Richter GM, et al. Diagnosis and treatment of retroperitoneal hematoma in multiple trauma patients. *Arch Orthop Trauma Surg.* 1992;111(6):323–326.
22. Burdick TR, Hoffer EK, Kooy T, et al. Which arteries are expendable? The practice and pitfalls of embolization throughout the body. *Semin Intervent Radiol.* 2008;25(3):191–203.
23. Grieco JG, Perry JF Jr. Retroperitoneal hematoma following trauma: its clinical importance. *J Trauma.* 1980;20(9):733–736.
24. Goins WA, Rodriguez A, Lewis J, et al. Retroperitoneal hematoma after blunt trauma. *Surg Gynecol Obstet.* 1992;174(4):281–290.
25. Velmahos GC, Demetriades D, Chahwan S, et al. Angiographic embolization for arrest of bleeding after penetrating trauma to the abdomen. *Am J Surg.* 1999;178(5):367–373.
26. Hare WS, Holland CJ. Paresis following internal iliac artery embolization. *Radiology.* 1983;146(1):47–51.

26

Iatrogenic Lesions

Yann Lachenal • Alban Denys • Pierre E. Bize

BACKGROUND

With the increasing number of minimally invasive diagnostic and therapeutic procedures, iatrogenic complications have become more frequent.[1–6] These complications can have no clinical impact and remain silent but can also have dramatic outcomes. Transarterial embolization (TAE) is in first line for treatment of vascular lesions such as active hemorrhage, pseudoaneurysm (PA), arteriovenous fistula (AVF), and arteriocavitary fistula. It is then of the highest importance for the interventional radiologist to know them, recognize them and be able to manage them.[2,5–12]

Iatrogenic Vascular Access Lesions

The common femoral artery is the most frequent arterial access of vascular procedures, with an overall complication rate around 6%.[13] Other vascular access locations are less used and have a complication rate estimated from 2% to 36% for brachial access,[14–16] 7.7% to 15.7% for popliteal access,[17–19] and less than 3% for transradial access.[13] The most frequent vascular complications are hematoma, AVF, PA, distal embolization, dissection, and thrombosis.[2] There are different ways to manage common femoral artery access–related injuries, but the discussion will focus on iatrogenic lesions that require embolization.

Iatrogenic Renal Lesions

Iatrogenic traumas are the main cause of transplanted and native kidney vascular injuries.[20–23] Hemorrhagic complications are frequent, with perirenal hematoma larger than 2 cm seen in 12.5% and macroscopic hematuria seen in 3.8% of patients after percutaneous biopsy.[24,25] Because of their prevalence, percutaneous biopsies are the leading cause of iatrogenic vascular injury in kidney, despite reported rate of transfusion and embolization in recent studies of 0.9% and 0.2% to 0.6%, respectively.[25,26] Major hemorrhagic complications requiring transfusions and/or embolization are seen in 12.5% of transjugular kidney biopsy,[27,28] 1% to 4% of percutaneous nephrostomy,[29] 12% to 14% of percutaneous lithotripsy,[29] 6% of partial nephrectomy,[30] 5% of radiofrequency ablation,[31] and 0.7% to 2.6% of cryoablation.[32,33]

Iatrogenic Liver Lesions

Iatrogenic traumas are currently the main etiology of hemorrhagic complications seen in the liver. This situation finds its origin in the increasing number of percutaneous procedures over the last few decades.[1,6] Major hemorrhagic complications have been described after percutaneous (biopsy, percutaneous transhepatic cholangiography [PTC], percutaneous transhepatic biliary drainage [PTBD], radiofrequency ablation [RFA]), endovascular (transjugular hepatic biopsy, transjugular intrahepatic portosystemic shunts [TIPS]), endoscopic (retrograde cholangiography, endoscopic retrograde cholangiopancreatography [ERCP]), and laparoscopic (cholecystectomy) interventions as well as open surgery (pancreatobiliary surgery, liver transplantation) with an incidence of 0.3% to 6%.[1,8,34–43]

Arterioportal fistula (APF) is the most frequent arterial injury type. Iatrogenic injuries are mostly intrahepatic.[43,44] The rate of APF is 4.2% in the first week following liver biopsy.[45] Most seem to close spontaneously, whereas only a minority progresses.[45–47] Clinically, only 17% of APF are symptomatic,[44] with findings related to hemobilia and portal hypertension, such as gastrointestinal bleeding, ascites, abdominal pain, and diarrhea.[48,49] Diagnosis and management are decided after Doppler ultrasound (US) examination (see the section "Clinical Applications").

Arteriohepatic vein fistulas (AHFs) are rare and not well studied. Their finding is often incidental on computed tomography (CT) in patients who had a liver biopsy in the past. AHFs may lead to high-output cardiac failure by increasing cardiac load, but they usually stay clinically silent as vascular shunt is insignificant.[43,45]

PA of hepatic artery is usually of iatrogenic origin. Percutaneous procedures are the leading cause of intrahepatic lesions, whereas endoscopic procedures, laparoscopy, hepatobiliary surgery, and liver transplantations are the cause of extrahepatic lesions.[43,50] The right hepatic artery is the most common artery involved.[50]

Iatrogenic Splenic Lesions

Most splenic injuries are caused by trauma or pancreatitis. Iatrogenic lesions contribute only to a minority of cases and are caused by splenic biopsy and abdominal surgery.[51] Incidence of major complications after splenic biopsy is 2.2%, most of which are hemorrhagic.[52] The rate of splenic injuries during abdominal surgery is 0.5%.[53] These lesions are usually recognized and treated surgically immediately. Therefore, the incidence of splenic injuries not recognized during surgery that would require TAE is not known.[54] The spectrum of arterial injuries is the same as for blunt trauma: active bleeding, PA, and AVF. Clinical presentation is variable and extends from absence of symptoms to hemodynamic collapse. AVF can additionally show symptoms of portal hypertension such as abdominal pain, gastroesophageal varices, and intestinal bleeding.[55]

Iatrogenic Pulmonary Lesions

Hemorrhagic complications are seen in up to 23% of lung biopsies,[56] but massive hemorrhages are encountered in less than 0.5% of patients after biopsy[35,57] and less than 1% after RFA.[58,59] Hemoptysis is the main clinical manifestation. Mortality after biopsy is low (0.07%)[57] and is due rather to asphyxia than to exsanguination when caused by lung hemorrhage. Hemorrhagic lung complications are often self-limiting and usually do not require endovascular treatment. Lesions to the pulmonary artery with formation of a PA after Swan-Ganz catheter placement and RFA have been described and treated successfully with embolization, but these lesions remain rare.[58–60]

DEVICE/MATERIAL DESCRIPTION

The choice of embolic agent that will be used depend mostly on the type of lesion that will be treated and on operator preference. Gelatin sponge is effective and inexpensive. Vascular occlusion is transitory and lasts a few days with progressive recanalization of occluded artery. This property is its main drawback, because if healing of the arterial injury is not complete, bleeding can reappear. *N*-butyl cyanoacylate (NBCA) is effective and permanent. Occlusion is immediate. Because of its liquid nature, it flows through vessels with blood and occludes vessels more distally than coils. In liver and other organs, this property is useful if catheter access is limited. Drawbacks are the long learning curve to use glue and the risk of nontarget embolization. Coils are very effective and provide a permanent occlusion. However, they can't be positioned as far as liquid agents. Covered stents are used to treat arterial parietal injuries without occluding the feeding artery. Often, materials are mixed to increase embolization efficacy. Situations in which these various embolic agents should be used will be discussed in more detail in the "Clinical Applications" section.

TECHNIQUE

Iatrogenic Vascular Access Lesions

PAs are not usually treated by TAE but rather by US-guided compression, direct thrombin injection (see "Tips and Tricks"), stent graft insertion, or surgical repair. AVFs are not usually treated by embolization but by US-guided compression, direct thrombin injection, or stent graft placement over the neck of the fistula. In this case, stent diameter should be oversized 1 mm larger in normal artery and 2 mm in calcified artery.[2] Retroperitoneal hemorrhage can usually be treated with a stent graft when it is caused by a leak from a major vessel such as the common femoral or the external iliac artery. The stent graft diameter should be oversized as stated earlier. When the bleeding occurs from a secondary branch (as the circumflex iliac artery) usually perforated by an inappropriate guidewire manipulation, this secondary branch can usually be embolized with coils, Gelfoam (Ethicon, Johnson & Johnson, Somerville, New Jersey) or a mix of them.

Iatrogenic Renal Lesions

Catheterization of the renal artery is performed with a Cobra, Renal Double Curve (RDC), H-Stick, or Simmons 5-Fr support catheters (Cordis, Johnson & Johnson Medical, Waterloo, Belgium). Catheter choice depends on the orientation of the renal artery. Glide catheters should be avoided as they do not provide strong support. Images can show active retroperitoneal or calyceal hemorrhage, arterial transection, PA, AVF, or deformation of renal parenchyma by subcapsular or perirenal hematoma. Iatrogenic lesions are usually unifocal, so superselective catheterization with 3-Fr or less coaxial microcatheter is the rule. PA should ideally be embolized with microcoils filling the PA and extending proximally in the afferent artery. When selective catheterization is not feasible, embolization of afferent artery is enough. The classical technique of PA embolization using sandwich technique is not necessary as kidney vascularization is terminal with few collaterals. NBCA can be used to fill PA and extend in the feeding artery. It should be used if lesions are multiple or too distal in location to be reachable with a microcatheter.[10] Gelfoam alone should be avoided as it resorbs over a few days, but it can be mixed with coils to improve efficacy of embolization. AVF embolization is most often performed with microcoils (Fig. 26.1). Care must be taken in the choice of type and size of coils as there is a risk of coil migration and nontarget embolization. They must be oversized 1.5 times the diameter of the target vessel. For high-flow fistulas, the first coil should

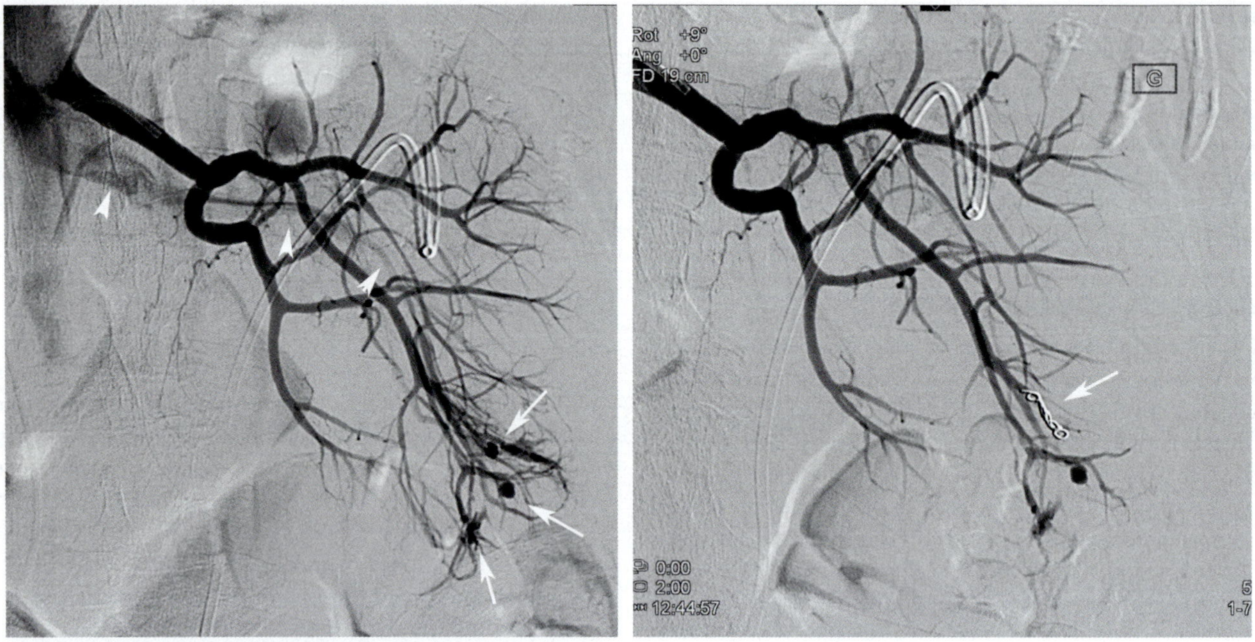

A B

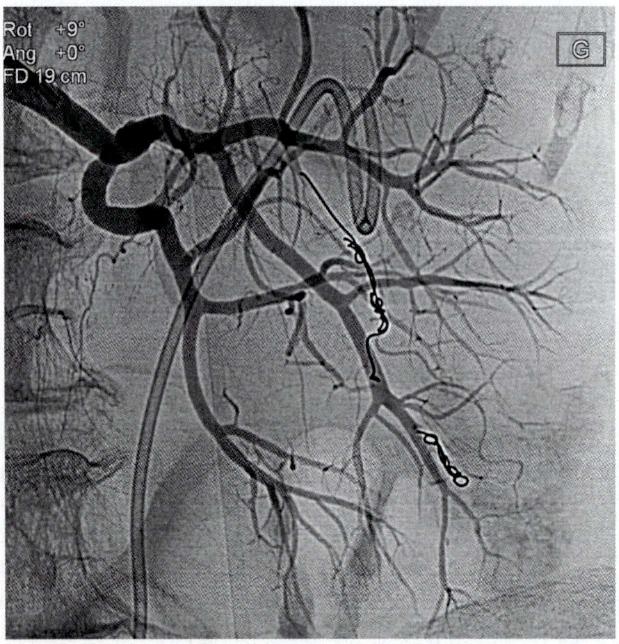

C

Figure 26.1 Persisting macrohematuria in a 65 years old male after kidney biopsy. A double J catheter has been positioned in the urinary tract earlier to treat urinary obstruction by blood. **A:** DSA with contrast injection through 5-Fr Cobra C2 support catheter positioned in left renal artery demonstrates three pseudoaneurysmal lesions (*thin arrows*) in lower part of the left kidney associated with an early venous return (*arrowheads*) related to the presence of an AVF. **B:** Renal DSA through support catheter after embolization of one of the injured arteries with microcoils (*arrow*). Two pseudoaneurysmal lesions are still visible. **C:** After placement of additional microcoils, total exclusion of vascular anomalies is achieved.

be detachable and have enough length for a good control of its stability before its release and to build a frame. Afterward, pushable coils of smaller size are used to fill the frame. NBCA can be used, with usual caution. Gelfoam or particles should be avoided. Vascular plugs are sometimes used, but their delivery may be impossible in tortuous vessels. In case of arteriocalyceal fistula with active hemorrhage, embolization of feeding artery with microcoils or NBCA is usually efficient.

Iatrogenic Liver Lesions

Single curve, Cobra, Sidewinder, or Simmons 5-Fr support catheters (Cordis, Johnson & Johnson Medical, Waterloo, Belgium) are used to access celiac trunk. Catheterization should be delicate to avoid dissection. After a digital subtraction angiographic (DSA) serie by support catheter with patient in apnea, navigation to the target lesion is performed with a 3-Fr or less coaxially inserted microcatheter. DSA may show PA, APF, arteriobiliary fistula, artery transection, and active bleeding.

Hepatic PA embolization approach depends on location of vascular injury.

If the PA is extrahepatic (common hepatic artery, proper hepatic artery and its right and left branches), exclusion can be performed with a covered stent 4 to 6 mm diameter depending on artery size (Coronary Graftmaster covered stent [Abbott Vascular, Diegem, Belgium] or Advanta V12 covered stent [Atrium, Rastatt, Germany]) or by filling the lesion with coils or NBCA to preserve permeability of the injured artery. This approach is mandatory in transplanted livers as they are very sensitive to ischemia. However, sacrifice of the left or right branch of the hepatic artery can be considered in native liver, because intrahepatic collaterals from one side to the other open immediately after vascular occlusion and oxygenation by portal vein is usually sufficient if this vein is patent and that portal venous flow is not hepatofugal.

If the vascular injury is intrahepatic, treatment depends on selectivity of microcatheterization. If possible, microcoils or NBCA should extend across the PA's neck in distal and proximal artery to avoid backflow vascularization of the PA by collaterals. Catheterization of the PA itself should be avoided because of the risk of rupture by microcatheter tip. To facilitate stasis and thrombosis, Gelfoam can be used between coils ("sandwich technique") or to fill the PA feeding vessel. As the PA does not have walls, a basic principle is to avoid treating the PA sac like a true aneurysm would be treated. Attention should be paid to embolize the feeder(s) vessel(s) if possible. If only the PA sac is embolized (the exception is embolization of common femoral artery with direct thrombin percutaneous injection), there is a tendency to recanalization and reexpansion of the PA sac around the embolic agent as the feeder vessel can transmit pressure to the soft tissues surrounding the PA. If microcatheter positioning close to the lesion is not possible, Gelfoam or NBCA should be used in association or not with coils. Finally, direct percutaneous puncture of the PA with injection of thrombin or coils has been described for unreachable lesions.[43,61]

Embolization of APF should be performed with microcatheter closely positioned to the fistulous site. Embolization is usually made with coils, but other embolic agents have been used (detachable balloon, NBCA, Onyx [EV3 Europe SAS/International, Paris, France], microspheres [Bead-Block, Biocompatibles, Farnham, UK] and Gelfoam).[62] The fistulous tract is sometimes very short and it becomes unavoidable to embolize the feeding artery, so great caution should be taken before embolization of a lesion in an operated or transplanted liver because of the risk of ischemia. Decrease of flow through fistula rather than complete occlusion is sometimes enough to prevent the progression of APF.[43] Deployment of coils must be done carefully because of risk of migration.

The approach to arteriobiliary fistula or artery transection with active bleeding is the same as for PA (Fig. 26.2).

Iatrogenic Spleen Lesions

Access to celiac trunk is performed with 4-Fr or 5-Fr support catheter, usually a Cobra C2 or a Simmons 1 or 2. If possible, direct catheterization and DSA of splenic artery should be performed first to save time and contrast. A vascular lesion might appear as a PA, AVF, contrast extravasation, artery transection, or splenic parenchymal deformation by hematoma. Number, topography, and accessibility of lesions are assessed to determine indication for proximal and/or distal splenic artery embolization (see the section "Clinical Applications"). A 3-Fr or smaller microcatheter is coaxially inserted to access embolization chosen site selectively. Splenic artery diameter usually measures 7 to 8 mm, so proximal embolization of the main splenic artery should be performed with 10- to 12-mm diameter coils. Attention should be paid that hypovolemic patients have spastic arteries, which can lead to underestimation of true lumen diameter. The superior polar splenic artery can have a proximal origin and should be checked for hemorrhage. Coils should be deployed between dorsal and magna pancreatic arteries to keep collateral flow to spleen. Anchoring of the first coil in a small branch is useful to avoid coil migration. The first coil must be long enough (usually 10 to 14 cm long) to build a solid frame before packing with smaller coils. The end point is stagnation of contrast upstream in splenic artery. For distal embolization of the splenic artery, a 3-Fr or smaller microcatheter is positioned as close as possible to the target lesion. PA should ideally be embolized "front door and back door" with embolic material (coils or NBCA) covering its neck. As intrasplenic collaterals are not numerous, if catheterization of the "back door" is not possible, embolization of the "front door" artery is often efficient and enough, especially if liquid embolic agent such as glue is selected. Catheterization of the PA itself should be avoided to minimize rupture risk. AVF are usually embolized with coils positioned in the fistula or just proximal to it. Care should be taken to avoid coil migration in venous flow. Active hemorrhage should embolized with coils, NBCA, or Gelfoam. For multiple lesions in the same splenic segment, segmental artery embolization with NBCA, gelfoam slurry, or coils is indicated. For lesions that are in different segments, superselective embolization can be performed if time and access are granted; otherwise, proximal embolization is efficient (Fig. 26.3). PVA particles should usually be avoided as they may cause profound parenchymal ischemia.

Iatrogenic Pulmonary Lesions

Because they are usually self-limiting, hemorrhagic complication of lung biopsies are often treated conservatively. To avoid filling of the airways with blood, patients presenting with hemoptysis after lung biopsy should be laid on the punctured side. Close monitoring of blood oxygen level should be performed as the main risk for these patients is suffocation. If blood oxygen level drops, cleaning of the airways with rigid fibroscopy should be performed promptly. Pulmonary artery PA from Swan-Ganz insertion or RFA can be treated by coil embolization from a venous peripheral puncture.

CLINICAL APPLICATIONS

Iatrogenic Vascular Access Lesions

Patient-related risk factors for vascular complications are hypertension, female gender, emergency procedures, high bifurcation of femoral artery, and anticoagulation. Technical risk factors are left groin puncture, method of puncture, arterial entry site, size of sheath, anticoagulation, and use of

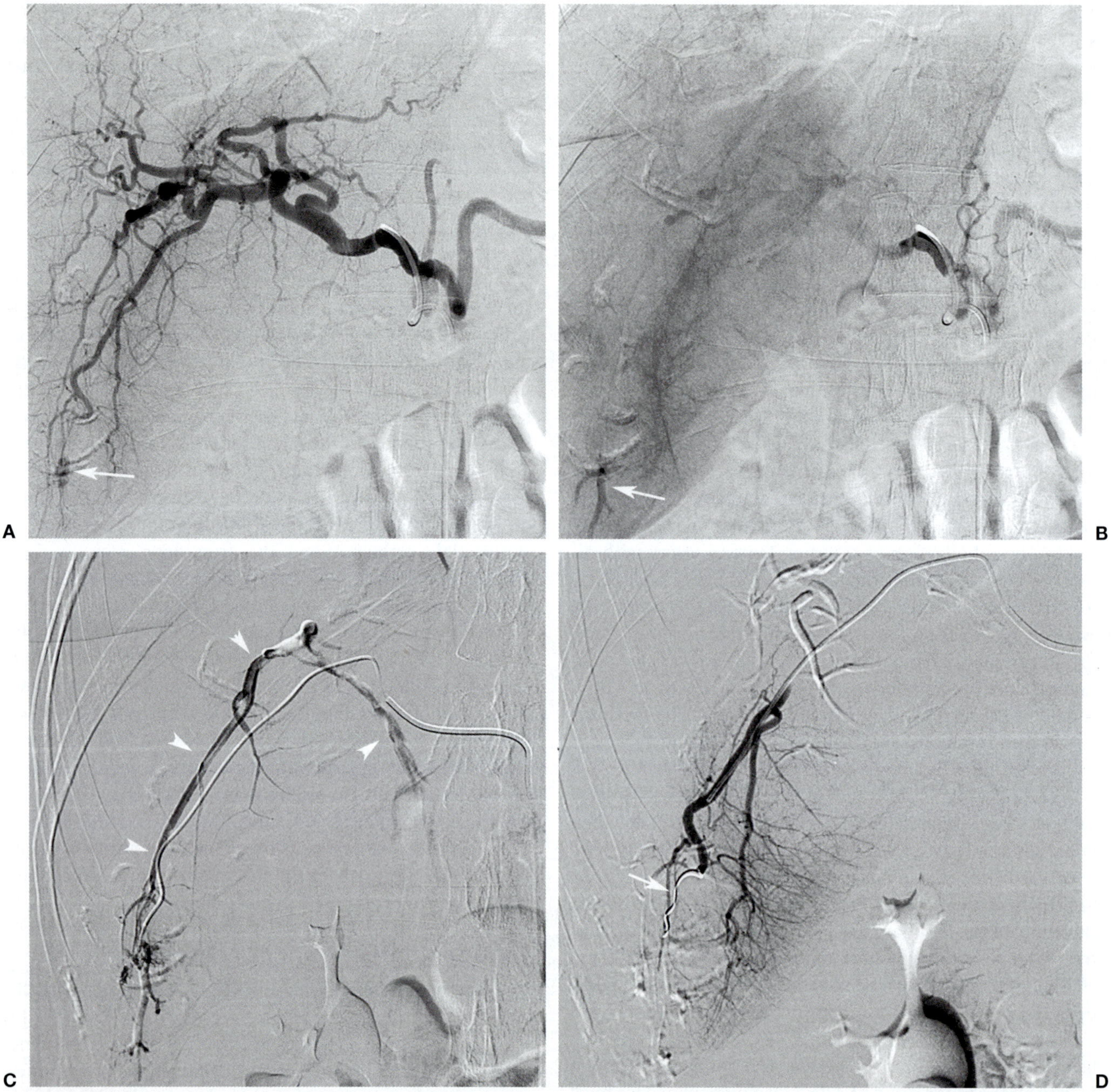

Figure 26.2 Hemobilia in a 55 years old male patient after liver biopsy. **A:** Hepatic artery DSA shows a PA lesion in periphery of segment 6 (*arrow*). **B:** During parenchymal phase, contrast is noted flowing in a bile duct (*arrow*). **C:** Catheterization of the injured artery with a 2.7-Fr microcatheter inserted coaxially in the 5-Fr support catheter. The microcatheter is positioned as close as possible to the vascular lesion. Contrast injection shows opacification of the bile duct up to the main bile duct (*arrowheads*). **D:** Contrast injection in the injured artery after placement of a microcoil (*arrow*) across arterial injury's neck. Vascular lesions have disappeared.

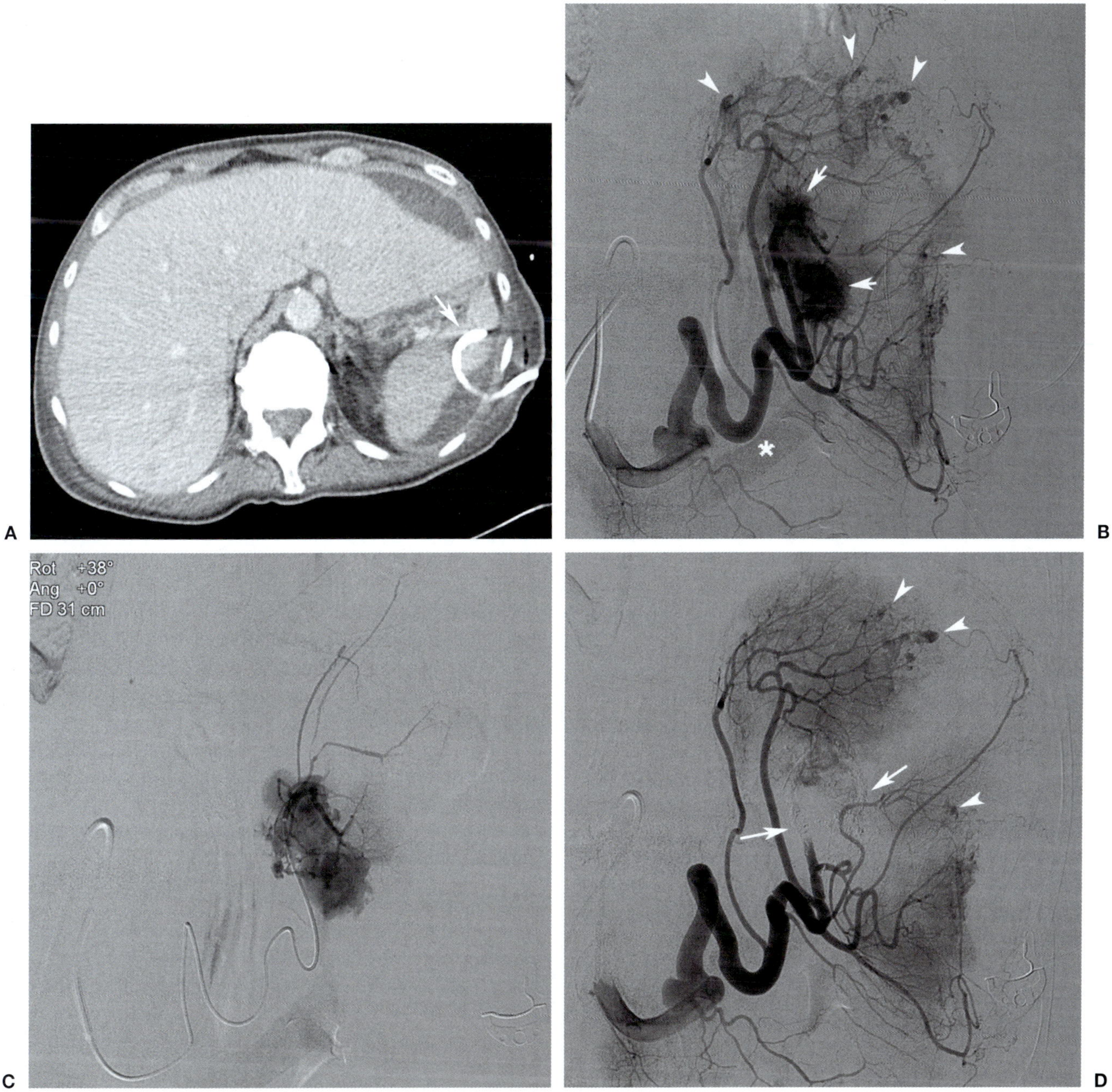

Figure 26.3 72 years old female patient with perisplenic fluid collection that needed percutaneous drainage. **A:** Contrast CT shows a malpositioned drain (*arrow*) with extremity located in the spleen. Notice peritoneal enhancement in a context of peritonitis. **B:** Splenic DSA through a 5-Fr support Simmons 2 catheter shows pooling of contrast at the center of image in relation to a large PA (*arrows*). In the upper pole of the spleen, multiple small PAs are seen (*arrowheads*). Arterial phase shows early enhancement of splenic veins compatible with AVFs (*asterisk*). **C:** Superselective microcatheterization of the feeding artery of the large PAs. **D:** DSA after embolization and exclusion with NBCA of the splenic segmental branch feeding the large PA (*arrows*). Multiple small PAs remain in the cranial pole of spleen (*arrowheads*). Superselective catheterization was not possible. (*Continued*)

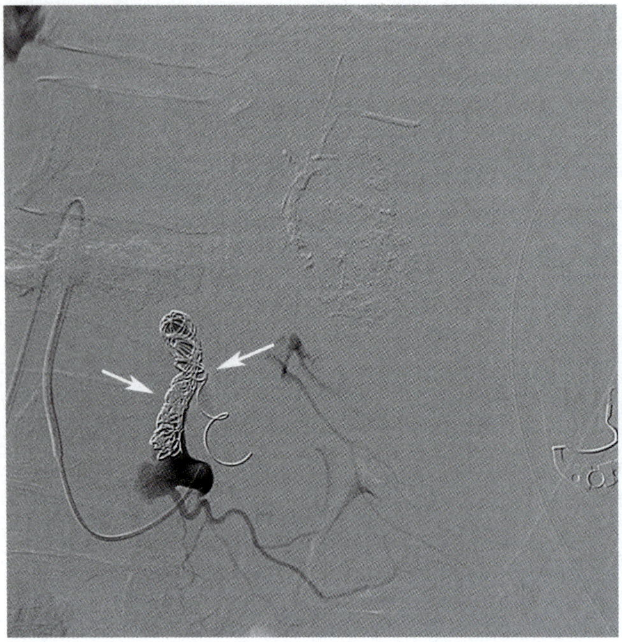

E

Figure 26.3 (*Continued*) **E:** Proximal embolization of the splenic artery with coils was performed successfully (*arrows*). Distally, arterial pressure is dropped by a factor of 2, which usually allows natural coagulation to take place and repair the vascular lesions.

closure device.[11,63–65] Hematoma of the groin is usually self-limiting. Small hematomas are frequent, but in up to 2.8% of patients, blood transfusion or invasive treatment is required.[65] Clinically, immediate or delayed tumefaction appears around the arterial puncture site and increases the diameter of the thigh. Rarely, hematoma is hard to control even with manual compression. US or angio-CT is needed to exclude PA.

Pseudoaneurysm

PAs are seen in 1.2% to 8% of femoral punctures.[63,66] Clinical manifestation is a palpable, painful, pulsatile, or thrilling mass, which can grow over time. Complications related to PA are rupture, distal embolization of thrombus, infection, skin necrosis, and nerve and vessel compression.[67] Diagnosis is confirmed with Doppler US.[11] In symptomatic patients, PA must be treated quickly. But in asymptomatic patients, it has been shown that most PAs less than 1.8 cm diameter spontaneously thrombose in less than 2 months.[68,69] PA bigger than 1.8 cm and PA in anticoagulated patients, regardless of the size, must be treated.[68,69] Due to its noninvasiveness, US-guided compression is considered as the first-line treatment. US-guided thrombin injection can be a valuable adjunct to US-guided compression (see "Tips and Tricks") and has a success rate of 90% to 100%.[2] However, surgery remains indicated in case of failure of other techniques.

Arteriovenous Fistulas

AVF between the femoral artery and vein is seen in less than 1% of inguinal punctures.[63,64] The risk increases with low femoral artery puncture. AVFs are rarely symptomatic, but they can present with high-output cardiac failure, limb edema, claudication, or aneurysmal dilatation of femoral and iliac artery and veins. Diagnosis is confirmed by Doppler US.[11] AVF should be treated because they tend to increase with time and can cause complications such as venous hypertension in the affected limb or high-output cardiac failure.[2] They are usually treated by US-guided compression as first-line treatment. Covered stent placement and surgical repair are options in case of failure. There is concern about long-term patency of those stents and their resistance in a flexure point such as the groin, so this option might be interesting in older patients and in patients with contraindication to surgery, but surgical repair is preferred for younger patients.

Retroperitoneal Hemorrhage

Retroperitoneal hemorrhage occurs generally when arterial puncture is performed above the inguinal ligament. This complication can be life-threatening as there is no exteriorization of blood. Clinical signs (tachycardia, hypotension, abdominal pain, confusion, agitation) might appear only late after intervention. Incidence is low, less than 1% of femoral punctures. Noncontrast CT must be performed to make diagnosis and guide treatment.[11]

Retroperitoneal bleeding is usually self-limited, but in some cases, such as in patients with toubled coagulation status, it should be treated if size of hematoma is increasing.

Iatrogenic Renal Lesions

Clinical manifestations are related to hemodynamic consequences of blood loss and urinary obstruction: hematuria, flank pain, and hypovolemia. AVF can also lead to progressive renal failure or to new or uncontrollable hypertension as a consequence of blood steal and relative ischemia of renal parenchyma. Cardiac failure caused by high-flow shunting is also possible.[70,71] These symptoms may be delayed for years after an intervention.[72,73] Lesion types are artery transection with active bleeding, PA, arteriocalyceal fistula, AVF, or an association of these.[23] Superselective embolization is the treatment of choice. The procedure is safe and effective, with a technical success rate of over 90% and clinical success rate over 80%.[20,22,23,74–79] Surgery remains indicated in case of failure of endovascular treatment. The right timing for embolization is unclear. Hemorrhage is usually self-limiting. For mildly symptomatic, stable, and well-responding transfused patients, it is acceptable to wait 72 hours after intervention before going to embolization. For persisting or uncontrollable hematuria, retroperitoneal hemorrhage, deteriorating renal function, and unstable patients, emergency embolization is required.[74,76,80] CT with contrast and US can categorize lesion types and help to plan embolization but are not mandatory before angiography. The approach is different in asymptomatic patients. Some older series with a limited number of patients have reported a spontaneous closure of AVF up to 75% and of PA up to 100% a few weeks postintervention.[81–84] The risk of spontaneous enlargement and rupture of AVF and PA, and the fact that TAE is a safe procedure, should make this technique the first-line treatment in the management of these types of lesions.[74]

Iatrogenic Liver Lesions

Clinical manifestations include hemobilia, systemic hypotension, gastrointestinal bleeding, and perihepatic hematoma.[1,8] Hemobilia has 94% positive predictive value for arterial injury[1] and is the most frequent clinical sign, but its classic triad of abdominal pain, jaundice, and gastrointestinal bleeding is present in only 22% of patients.[6] Clinical presentation may be delayed from days to months after intervention, but approximately 80% of vascular complications are discovered within 2 weeks after an intervention.[8] At laboratory, arterial injuries should be suspected particularly if there is a 5% decrease of hematocrit level or abnormality/worsening of the hepatic tests after the intervention.[1,48] It should also be noted that a large proportion of vascular injuries may remain clinically silent.[6,45] TAE is currently the treatment of choice for these lesions, with a technical and clinical success rate of 75% to 100%.[8,10,42,48,85–87] Surgery remains available in cases of failure of TAE, but has a higher morbidity and mortality. Embolization in transplanted liver and after pancreatico-biliary operation should be evaluated very carefully as liver are and particularly bile ducts become very sensitive to ischemia, as they are primarily vascularized by hepatic arteries.[48]

Angiographic findings are active bleeding, PA, APF, AHF (rare), arteriobiliary fistula, and nonspecific lesions.[45] Complex injuries are defined by a mix of more than one lesion type.[88] Symptomatic APF requires embolization. Estimation of the hemodynamic consequences of the fistula with Doppler US should be made.[43,48] A significant shunt is defined by a low arterial resistive index (RI) or a drop of RI ≥ 0.10 compared to previous examinations and by reversal of flow in portal vein or first-order branch, with or without arterialization of spectral flow.[43,48] Angiography confirms presence and estimates shunt during intervention. APF is considered significant if contrast flows back to portal vein or first-order branch.[44,49] In conclusion, in asymptomatic patients with large and hemodynamically significant APF, embolization is required, whereas in others, surveillance is probably enough.[43,44,48,49] Hepatic artery PAs have a reported rupture rate[50] as high as 76% and a mortality rate of 16% to 43%.[50,89] In consequence, treatment is required regardless of symptomatology. However, in transplanted liver and after pancreatico-biliary surgery if PA is small, asymptomatic, and nonevoluting, a conservative attitude may be indicated.[43] Arteriobiliary fistulas are managed as PA.

Iatrogenic Spleen Lesions

Splenic TAE has a high technical success rate close to 100% and a high clinical success rate of around 91.1%.[12] The natural evolution of splenic PA is unclear. It appears that an unknown proportion of PA spontaneously thromboses.[51,90,91] As PAs have a high rupture and mortality risk, recommendation is embolization of all PA independently of symptomatology.[51] The spontaneous evolution of AVFs is also unclear. It seems logical to embolize them, unless they are present for a long time and are asymptomatic.

Regardless the lesion types, proximal embolization of the splenic artery is indicated when the splenic artery is too tortuous to allow microcatheterization of the spleen, when bleeding is diffuse or multifocal, or when hemodynamic instability is severe and time is lacking. Distal embolization is indicated when bleeding is unifocal or paucifocal.[92] After proximal TAE of the splenic artery, the spleen remains vascularized through short gastric, gastroepiploic, and pancreatic collaterals, but pressure in the splenic artery is reduced by a factor of 2, allowing coagulation to occur naturally.[93–95]

COMPLICATIONS

Iatrogenic Vascular Access Lesions

Thrombus leakage during thrombin percutaneous injection through PA neck with distal nontarget embolization is a known complication. So, in lesions with wide neck, a balloon can be used to cover the PA neck during thrombin injection (see the section "Clinical Applications"). In case of AVF, embolization material may flow directly to the right atrium and lungs or even the left atrium in case of patent foramen ovale. This is why US-guided compression, surgical repair, and, in selected patients, covered-stent placement is preferred when neck is wide. Stent graft deformation and fracture can occur if deployed in flexure points. Care should also be taken before stent graft deployment because of risk of occlusion of unwanted vessels (typically deep femoral artery).[2]

Iatrogenic Renal Lesions

Ischemic parenchymal territory after embolization is estimated from less than 50% in older series[23] to less than 10% in recent ones.[76] Moreover, there is a partial reperfusion of the ischemic territory after some time due to collateral vascular supply.[20,76] Studies have failed to demonstrate any effect of embolization on worsening of renal function and blood pressure.[20,21,74,75,77–79,96,97] Other complications are nontarget embolization, coil migration, artery dissection, thrombosis, postembolization syndrome, abdominal compartment syndrome, and renal abscess.[98]

Iatrogenic Liver Lesions

Usually, the complication rate after TAE in the liver is low because of the dual vascularization of liver by portal vein and hepatic artery. Moreover, intraparenchymal arterial collaterals are opening immediately after embolization.[99] So, in the native liver, parenchymal necrosis is rare, occurring only in 4.2% of patients after TAE.[8] Transitory ischemia of liver parenchyma is reflected by transient increase of liver enzymes and explains part of the postembolization syndrome, which is seen in 20% of patients.[3,8,42] Patients who have undergone pancreatic, biliary, or hepatic surgery or liver transplantation, as well as those with underlying liver disease, have a higher risk of liver necrosis and failure.[100] Embolization is contraindicated in patients with portal vein thrombosis because of the risk of ischemia.[44] As the bile ducts are vascularized by the hepatic artery, ischemia after TAE may lead to wall necrosis with stenosis or fistulas. As consequence, there is an increased risk of biloma, cholangitis, hepatic abscess, or peritonitis.[5] A small series shows 6.7% hepatic abscess formation after TAE for hepatic arterial injuries.[87] Nontarget embolization may lead to gallbladder, pancreas, or spleen ischemia or inflammation.

Celiac trunk and hepatic artery dissection with or without occlusion may occur, especially in patients with arcuate ligament syndrome and fibromuscular dysplasia, both infrequent entities.

Iatrogenic Spleen Lesions

Postembolization syndrome occurs in 30% of patients with fever, abdominal pain, slowed transit, and sometimes pancreatitis.[101] Other complications such as abscess formation, spleen infarction, and abnormal fluid collections are seen in 3.8% to 7%, 10% to 43%, and 43% of patients, respectively.[12,102–104]

TIPS AND TRICKS

Minimally Invasive Treatment of Vascular Access Complications

- *US-guided compression of PA*: The probe is positioned over the neck of the PA and a pressure is applied until flow disappearance inside the PA. Pressure is maintained until complete thrombosis. This method is not invasive and has few complications but also has drawbacks. It takes time as the compression should be applied during at least 20–30 min and can be very painful; the failure rate is between 30% and 40% in anticoagulated patients.[105] Strong analgesia with intravenous opioids should be considered.
- *Direct percutaneous thrombin injection:* Under US guidance, a small-diameter needle (19–21 gauge) is inserted in the PA and positioned at its center. Color Doppler US should show the needle tip in the part of the PA with blood flowing away from the neck to minimize thromboembolic risks. 500–1,000 International Units of thrombin should be injected in small pushes. This dose is usually enough to completely embolize the PA. If the PA is multiloculated, embolization should begin with the farthest loculus from PA neck. The coagulation status of the patient does not seem to affect thrombin injection efficacy. The risk of thrombin leakage in the femoral artery and distal embolization is low.[106] To protect the limb from distal thromboembolic event, in PAs with large and short neck or complex PA, an occlusion balloon can be inserted from a contralateral arterial access. It should be inflated to occlude the neck of the PA during thrombin injection.[107] The balloon should stay inflated for 10–15 min afterward. US Doppler should be used to confirm disappearance of flow in the aneurysm before and after thrombin injection. Neck width larger than 3 mm in diameter has been proposed as the minimal diameter for this technique (Fig. 26.4).[108]

Renal and Splenic Pseudoaneurysms

- PA in the renal and splenic vasculature can usually be treated with proximal embolization only because parenchymal vascularization is almost terminal with few collaterals.

Arterial Embolization in the Liver

- Before performing embolization in the native liver, care should be taken to verify permeability of the portal vein and direction of the portal vein flow because of the risk of ischemia. It is particularly important in liver to embolize front door and back door vessels because liver has many intraparenchymal collaterals and there is a risk of recanalization of lesion.[87] Embolization with coils or thrombin of a PA through a direct percutaneous transhepatic approach has been described in cases where TAE was not feasible.[109]

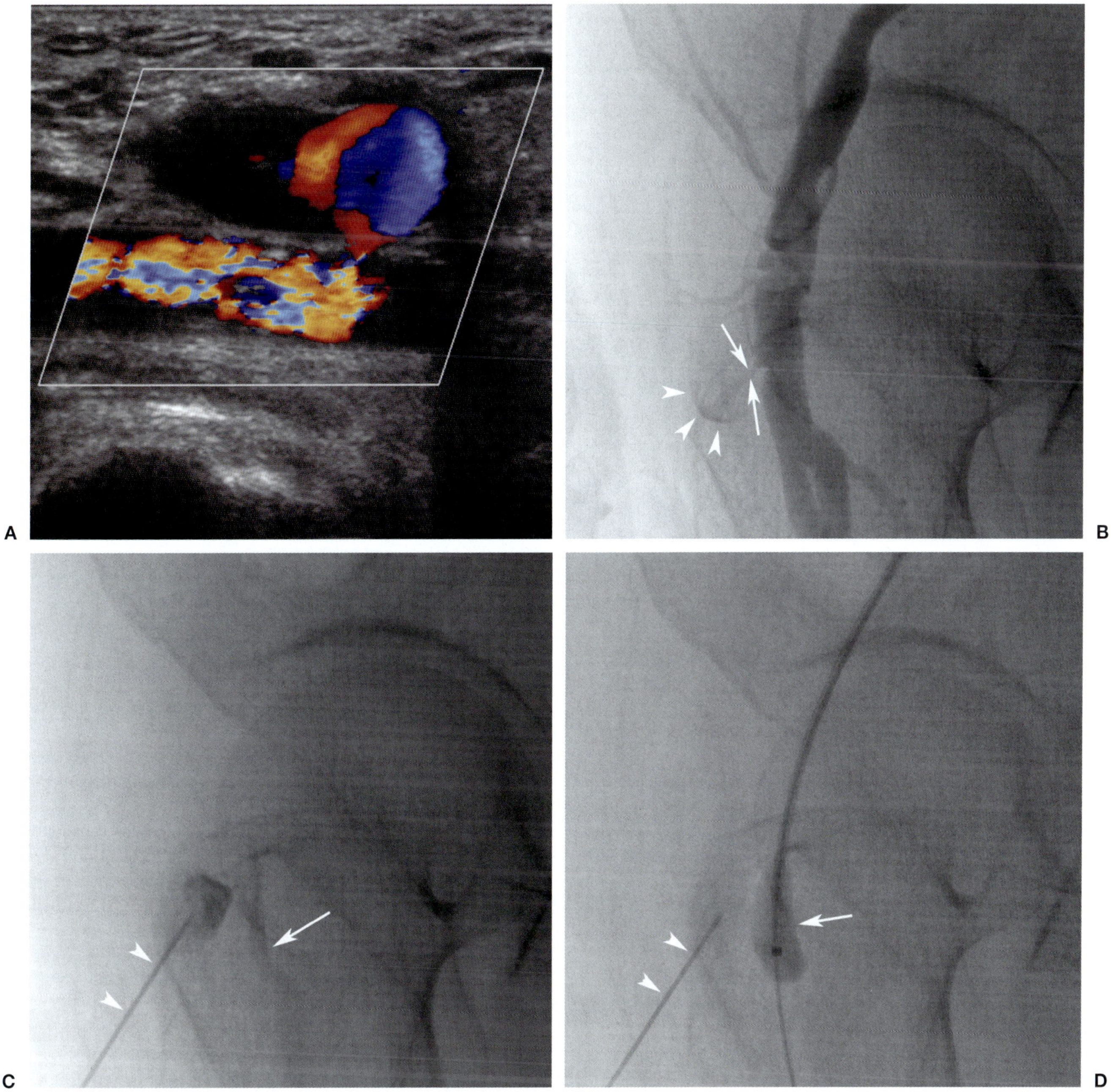

Figure 26.4 65 years old woman stented in left superficial femoral artery with right retrograde femoral access and crossover a few weeks ago. She has now a pulsatile thrilling mass near the previous puncture site. **A:** Doppler US shows the characteristic "yin-yang" image of a PA with a neck width measured in its largest part of 3 to 5 mm. **B:** Angiography was performed through contralateral inguinal access. Image shows high-flow jet of contrast through PA neck (*arrows*). PA is opacified by contrast (*arrowheads*). **C:** A needle (*arrowheads*) is positioned in the PA under US guidance. A small volume of contrast injected through the needle demonstrates flow going back in the superficial femoral artery (*arrow*). **D:** A compliant balloon (*arrow*) is positioned against the PA neck and is inflated. The needle (*arrowheads*) remains located in the PA and can be used as a marker for accurate balloon positioning. *(Continued)*

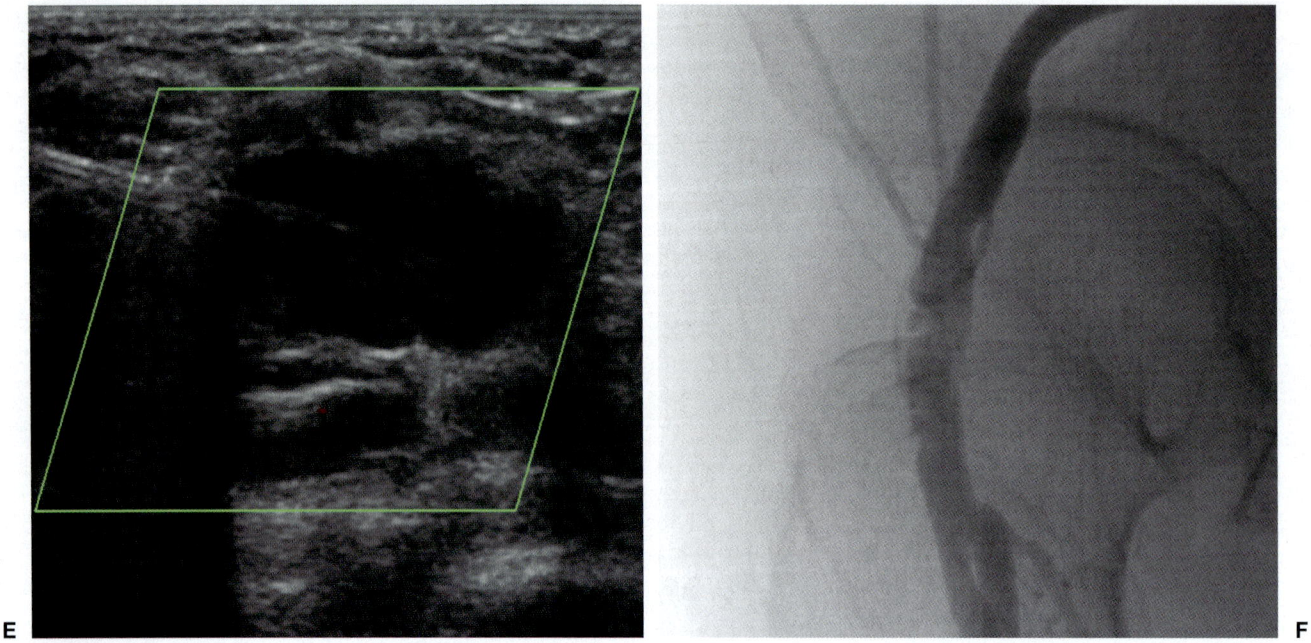

Figure 26.4 (Continued) **E:** 500 to 1,000 units of human thrombin are injected under US control. Control image shows absence of Doppler signal after thrombin injection. **F:** Final DSA shows complete exclusion of PA.

REFERENCES

1. Fidelman N, Bloom AI, Kerlan RK Jr, et al. Hepatic arterial injuries after percutaneous biliary interventions in the era of laparoscopic surgery and liver transplantation: experience with 930 patients. *Radiology*. 2008;247(3):880–886.
2. Tsetis D. Endovascular treatment of complications of femoral arterial access. *Cardiovasc Intervent Radiol*. 2010;33(3):457–468.
3. Srivastava DN, Sharma S, Pal S, et al. Transcatheter arterial embolization in the management of hemobilia. *Abdom Imaging*. 2006;31(4):439–448.
4. Hidalgo F, Narvaez JA, Rene M, et al. Treatment of hemobilia with selective hepatic artery embolization. *J Vasc Interv Radiol*. 1995;6(5):793–798.
5. Petroianu A. Arterial embolization for hemorrhage caused by hepatic arterial injury. *Dig Dis Sci*. 2007;52(10):2478–2481.
6. Green MH, Duell RM, Johnson CD, et al. Haemobilia. *Br J Surg*. 2001;88(6):773–786.
7. Saad NE, Saad WE, Davies MG, et al. Pseudoaneurysms and the role of minimally invasive techniques in their management. *Radiographics*. 2005;25(suppl 1):S173–S189.
8. Choi SH, Gwon DI, Ko GY, et al. Hepatic arterial injuries in 3110 patients following percutaneous transhepatic biliary drainage. *Radiology*. 2011;261(3):969–975.
9. Song HH, Won YD, Kim YJ. Transcatheter N-butyl cyanoacrylate embolization of pseudoaneurysms. *J Vasc Interv Radiol*. 2010;21(10):1508–1511.
10. Kish JW, Katz MD, Marx MV, et al. N-butyl cyanoacrylate embolization for control of acute arterial hemorrhage. *J Vasc Interv Radiol*. 2004;15(7):689–695.
11. Stone PA, Campbell JE. Complications related to femoral artery access for transcatheter procedures. *Vasc Endovascular Surg*. 2012;46(8):617–623.
12. Dasgupta N, Matsumoto AH, Arslan B, et al. Embolization therapy for traumatic splenic lacerations. *Cardiovasc Intervent Radiol*. 2012;35(4):795–806.
13. Feldman DN, Swaminathan RV, Kaltenbach LA, et al. Adoption of radial access and comparison of outcomes to femoral access in percutaneous coronary intervention: an updated report from the national cardiovascular data registry (2007-2012). *Circulation*. 2013;127(23):2295–2306.
14. Hildick-Smith DJ, Khan ZI, Shapiro LM, et al. Occasional-operator percutaneous brachial coronary angiography: first, do no arm. *Catheter Cardiovasc Interv*. 2002;57(2):161–165; discussion 166.
15. Ernst S, Fischbach R, Brochhagen HG, et al. Transbrachial thrombolysis, PTA and stenting in the lower extremities. *Cardiovasc Intervent Radiol*. 2003;26(6):516–521.
16. Alvarez-Tostado JA, Moise MA, Bena JF, et al. The brachial artery: a critical access for endovascular procedures. *J Vasc Surg*. 2009;49(2):378–385; discussion 385.
17. Ye M, Zhang H, Huang X, et al. Retrograde popliteal approach for challenging occlusions of the femoral-popliteal arteries. *J Vasc Surg*. 2013;58(1):84–89.
18. Fanelli F, Lucatelli P, Allegritti M, et al. Retrograde popliteal access in the supine patient for recanalization of the superficial femoral artery: initial results. *J Endovasc Ther*. 2011;18(4):503–509.
19. Noory E, Rastan A, Schwarzwalder U, et al. Retrograde transpopliteal recanalization of chronic superficial femoral artery occlusion after failed re-entry during antegrade subintimal angioplasty. *J Endovasc Ther*. 2009;16(5):619–623.

20. Sam K, Gahide G, Soulez G, et al. Percutaneous embolization of iatrogenic arterial kidney injuries: safety, efficacy, and impact on blood pressure and renal function. *J Vasc Interv Radiol.* 2011;22(11):1563–1568.
21. Mavili E, Donmez H, Ozcan N, et al. Transarterial embolization for renal arterial bleeding. *Diagn Interv Radiol.* 2009; 15(2):143–147.
22. Pappas P, Leonardou P, Papadoukakis S, et al. Urgent superselective segmental renal artery embolization in the treatment of life-threatening renal hemorrhage. *Urol Int.* 2006;77(1):34–41.
23. Fisher RG, Ben-Menachem Y, Whigham C. Stab wounds of the renal artery branches: angiographic diagnosis and treatment by embolization. *AJR Am J Roentgenol.* 1989;152(6):1231–1235.
24. Ishikawa E, Nomura S, Hamaguchi T, et al. Ultrasonography as a predictor of overt bleeding after renal biopsy. *Clin Exp Nephrol.* 2009;13(4):325–331.
25. Corapi KM, Chen JL, Balk EM, et al. Bleeding complications of native kidney biopsy: a systematic review and meta-analysis. *Am J Kidney Dis.* 2012;60(1):62–73.
26. Tondel C, Vikse BE, Bostad L, et al. Safety and complications of percutaneous kidney biopsies in 715 children and 8573 adults in Norway 1988-2010. *Clin J Am Soc Nephrol.* 2012;7(10): 1591–1597.
27. Thompson BC, Kingdon E, Johnston M, et al. Transjugular kidney biopsy. *Am J Kidney Dis.* 2004;43(4):651–662.
28. See TC, Thompson BC, Howie AJ, et al. Transjugular renal biopsy: our experience and technical considerations. *Cardiovasc Intervent Radiol.* 2008;31(5):906–918.
29. Saad WE, Moorthy M, Ginat D. Percutaneous nephrostomy: native and transplanted kidneys. *Tech Vasc Interv Radiol.* 2009; 12(3):172–192.
30. Richstone L, Montag S, Ost MC, et al. Predictors of hemorrhage after laparoscopic partial nephrectomy. *Urology.* 2011; 77(1):88–91.
31. Gervais DA, McGovern FJ, Arellano RS, et al. Radiofrequency ablation of renal cell carcinoma: part 1, indications, results, and role in patient management over a 6-year period and ablation of 100 tumors. *AJR Am J Roentgenol.* 2005;185(1):64–71.
32. Atwell TD, Farrell MA, Leibovich BC, et al. Percutaneous renal cryoablation: experience treating 115 tumors. *J Urol.* 2008; 179(6):2136–2140; discussion 2140–2131.
33. Rosenberg MD, Kim CY, Tsivian M, et al. Percutaneous cryoablation of renal lesions with radiographic ice ball involvement of the renal sinus: analysis of hemorrhagic and collecting system complications. *AJR Am J Roentgenol.* 2011; 196(4):935–939.
34. Burke DR, Lewis CA, Cardella JF, et al. Quality improvement guidelines for percutaneous transhepatic cholangiography and biliary drainage. *J Vasc Interv Radiol.* 2003;14(9, pt 2): S243–S246.
35. Gupta S, Wallace MJ, Cardella JF, et al. Quality improvement guidelines for percutaneous needle biopsy. *J Vasc Interv Radiol.* 2010;21(7):969–975.
36. Kalambokis G, Manousou P, Vibhakorn S, et al. Transjugular liver biopsy—indications, adequacy, quality of specimens, and complications—a systematic review. *J Hepatol.* 2007;47(2): 284–294.
37. Gaba RC, Khiatani VL, Knuttinen MG, et al. Comprehensive review of TIPS technical complications and how to avoid them. *AJR Am J Roentgenol.* 2011;196(3):675–685.
38. Watanabe M, Usui S, Kajiwara H, et al. Current pancreatogastrointestinal anastomotic methods: results of a Japanese survey of 3109 patients. *J Hepatobiliary Pancreat Surg.* 2004;11(1): 25–33.
39. Saad WE, Wallace MJ, Wojak JC, et al. Quality improvement guidelines for percutaneous transhepatic cholangiography, biliary drainage, and percutaneous cholecystostomy. *J Vasc Interv Radiol.* 2010;21(6):789 795.
40. Takaki H, Yamakado K, Nakatsuka A, et al. Frequency of and risk factors for complications after liver radiofrequency ablation under CT fluoroscopic guidance in 1500 sessions: single-center experience. *AJR Am J Roentgenol.* 2013;200(3): 658–664.
41. Kodama Y, Shimizu T, Endo H, et al. Complications of percutaneous transhepatic portal vein embolization. *J Vasc Interv Radiol.* 2002;13(12):1233–1237.
42. Nicholson T, Travis S, Ettles D, et al. Hepatic artery angiography and embolization for hemobilia following laparoscopic cholecystectomy. *Cardiovasc Intervent Radiol.* 1999;22(1):20–24.
43. Saad WE. Management of nonocclusive hepatic artery complications after liver transplantation. *Tech Vasc Interv Radiol.* 2007; 10(3):221–232.
44. Saad WE, Davies MG, Rubens DJ, et al. Endoluminal management of arterioportal fistulae in liver transplant recipients: a single-center experience. *Vasc Endovascular Surg.* 2007; 40(6):451–459.
45. Saad WE, Davies MG, Ryan CK, et al. Incidence of arterial injuries detected by arteriography following percutaneous right-lobe ultrasound-guided core liver biopsies in human subjects. *Am J Gastroenterol.* 2006;101(11):2641–2645.
46. Hellekant C, Olin T. Vascular complications following needle puncture of the liver. An angiographic investigation in the rabbit. *Acta Radiol Diagn (Stockh).* 1973;14(5):577–582.
47. Okuda K, Musha H, Nakajima Y, et al. Frequency of intrahepatic arteriovenous fistula as a sequela to percutaneous needle puncture of the liver. *Gastroenterology.* 1978;74(6): 1204–1207.
48. Saad W, Lippert A, Davies M, et al. Prevalence, presentation, and endovascular management of hemodynamically or clinically significant arterio-portal fistulae in living and cadaveric donor liver transplant recipients. *Clin Transplant.* 2012; 26(4):532–538.
49. Vauthey JN, Tomczak RJ, Helmberger T, et al. The arterioportal fistula syndrome: clinicopathologic features, diagnosis, and therapy. *Gastroenterology.* 1997;113(4):1390–1401.
50. Tessier DJ, Fowl RJ, Stone WM, et al. Iatrogenic hepatic artery pseudoaneurysms: an uncommon complication after hepatic, biliary, and pancreatic procedures. *Ann Vasc Surg.* 2003; 17(6):663–669.
51. Tessier DJ, Stone WM, Fowl RJ, et al. Clinical features and management of splenic artery pseudoaneurysm: case series and cumulative review of literature. *J Vasc Surg.* 2003;38(5):969–974.
52. McInnes MD, Kielar AZ, Macdonald DB. Percutaneous image-guided biopsy of the spleen: systematic review and meta-analysis of the complication rate and diagnostic accuracy. *Radiology.* 2011;260(3):699–708.
53. Eaton MA, Valentine J, Jackson MR, et al. Incidental splenic injury during abdominal vascular surgery: a case-controlled analysis. *J Am Coll Surg.* 2000;190(1):58–64.

54. Gayer G, Galperin-Aizenberg M. Iatrogenic splenic injury in postoperative patients: a series of case reports. *Emerg Radiol.* 2008; 15(2):109–113.
55. Chen B, Tang CW, Zhang CL, et al. Melena-associated regional portal hypertension caused by splenic arteriovenous fistula. *World J Gastroenterol.* 2012;18(16):1996–1998.
56. Heck SL, Blom P, Berstad A. Accuracy and complications in computed tomography fluoroscopy-guided needle biopsies of lung masses. *Eur Radiol.* 2006;16(6):1387–1392.
57. Tomiyama N, Yasuhara Y, Nakajima Y, et al. CT-guided needle biopsy of lung lesions: a survey of severe complication based on 9783 biopsies in Japan. *Eur J Radiol.* 2006;59(1):60–64.
58. Yamakado K, Takaki H, Takao M, et al. Massive hemoptysis from pulmonary artery pseudoaneurysm caused by lung radiofrequency ablation: successful treatment by coil embolization. *Cardiovasc Intervent Radiol.* 2010;33(2):410–412.
59. Sakurai J, Mimura H, Gobara H, et al. Pulmonary artery pseudoaneurysm related to radiofrequency ablation of lung tumor. *Cardiovasc Intervent Radiol.* 2010;33(2):413–416.
60. Abreu AR, Campos MA, Krieger BP. Pulmonary artery rupture induced by a pulmonary artery catheter: a case report and review of the literature. *J Intensive Care Med.* 2004;19(5):291–296.
61. Merhav H, Zajko AB, Dodd GD, et al. Percutaneous transhepatic embolization of an intrahepatic pseudoaneurysm following liver biopsy in a liver transplant patient. *Transpl Int.* 1993; 6(4):239–241.
62. Kumar A, Ahuja CK, Vyas S, et al. Hepatic arteriovenous fistulae: role of interventional radiology. *Dig Dis Sci.* 2012; 57(10):2703–2712.
63. Ohlow MA, Secknus MA, von Korn H, et al. Incidence and outcome of femoral vascular complications among 18,165 patients undergoing cardiac catheterisation. *Int J Cardiol.* 2009; 135(1):66–71.
64. Kelm M, Perings SM, Jax T, et al. Incidence and clinical outcome of iatrogenic femoral arteriovenous fistulas: implications for risk stratification and treatment. *J Am Coll Cardiol.* 2002; 40(2):291–297.
65. Doyle BJ, Ting HH, Bell MR, et al. Major femoral bleeding complications after percutaneous coronary intervention: incidence, predictors, and impact on long-term survival among 17,901 patients treated at the Mayo Clinic from 1994 to 2005. *JACC Cardiovasc Interv.* 2008;1(2):202–209.
66. Mlekusch W, Haumer M, Mlekusch I, et al. Prediction of iatrogenic pseudoaneurysm after percutaneous endovascular procedures. *Radiology.* 2006; 240(2):597–602.
67. Morgan R, Belli AM. Current treatment methods for postcatheterization pseudoaneurysms. *J Vasc Interv Radiol.* 2003; 14(6):697–710.
68. Kent KC, McArdle CR, Kennedy B, et al. A prospective study of the clinical outcome of femoral pseudoaneurysms and arteriovenous fistulas induced by arterial puncture. *J Vasc Surg.* 1993; 17(1):125–131; discussion 131–123.
69. Toursarkissian B, Allen BT, Petrinec D, et al. Spontaneous closure of selected iatrogenic pseudoaneurysms and arteriovenous fistulae. *J Vasc Surg.* 1997;25(5):803–808; discussion 808–809.
70. McAlhany JC Jr, Black HC Jr, Hanback LD Jr, et al. Renal arteriovenous fistula as a cause of hypertension. *Am J Surg.* 1971; 122(1):117–120.
71. Maldonado JE, Sheps SG, Bernatz PE, et al. Renal arteriovenous fistula. A reversible cause of hypertension and heart failure. *Am J Med.* 1964;37:499–513.
72. Chazen MD, Miller KS. Intrarenal pseudoaneurysm presenting 15 years after penetrating renal injury. *Urology.* 1997; 49(5):774–776.
73. Alcazar R, de la Torre M, Peces R. Symptomatic intrarenal arteriovenous fistula detected 25 years after percutaneous renal biopsy. *Nephrol Dial Transplant.* 1996;11(7):1346–1348.
74. Perini S, Gordon RL, LaBerge JM, et al. Transcatheter embolization of biopsy-related vascular injury in the transplant kidney: immediate and long-term outcome. *J Vasc Interv Radiol.* 1998;9(6):1011–1019.
75. Loffroy R, Guiu B, Lambert A, et al. Management of post-biopsy renal allograft arteriovenous fistulas with selective arterial embolization: immediate and long-term outcomes. *Clin Radiol.* 2008;63(6):657–665.
76. Chatziioannou A, Brountzos E, Primetis E, et al. Effects of superselective embolization for renal vascular injuries on renal parenchyma and function. *Eur J Vasc Endovasc Surg.* 2004; 28(2):201–206.
77. Poulakis V, Ferakis N, Becht E, et al. Treatment of renal-vascular injury by transcatheter embolization: immediate and long-term effects on renal function. *J Endourol.* 2006;20(6):405–409.
78. Beaujeux R, Saussine C, al-Fakir A, et al. Superselective endo-vascular treatment of renal vascular lesions. *J Urol.* 1995; 153(1):14–17.
79. Maleux G, Messiaen T, Stockx L, et al. Transcatheter embolization of biopsy-related vascular injuries in renal allografts. Long-term technical, clinical and biochemical results. *Acta Radiol.* 2003;44(1):13–17.
80. Dorffner R, Thurnher S, Prokesch R, et al. Embolization of iatrogenic vascular injuries of renal transplants: immediate and follow-up results. *Cardiovasc Intervent Radiol.* 1998;21(2):129–134.
81. Ekelund L. Spontaneous closure of arteriovenous fistulae following percutaneous renal biopsy. An experimental investigation in the rabbit. *Acta Radiol Diagn (Stockh).* 1971;11(3):289–294.
82. Ekelund L. Arteriovenous fistulae secondary to renal biopsy. An experimental study in the rabbit. *Acta Radiol Diagn (Stockh).* 1970;10(3):218–224.
83. Ekelund L, Lindholm T. Arteriovenous fistulae following percutaneous renal biopsy. *Acta Radiol Diagn (Stockh).* 1971;11(1):38–48.
84. Bennett AR, Wiener SN. Intrarenal arteriovenous fistula and aneurysm. A complication of percutaneous renal biopsy. *Am J Roentgenol Radium Ther Nucl Med.* 1965;95(2):372–382.
85. Monsignore LM, Scarpelini S, Santos JS, et al. Urgent percutaneous transcatheter embolization of hemorrhagic hepatic lesions with N-butyl cyanoacrylate. *Diagn Interv Radiol.* 2012; 18(4):403–409.
86. Finley DS, Hinojosa MW, Paya M, et al. Hepatic artery pseudoaneurysm: a report of seven cases and a review of the literature. *Surg Today.* 2005;35(7):543–547.
87. Tzeng WS, Wu RH, Chang JM, et al. Transcatheter arterial embolization for hemorrhage caused by injury of the hepatic artery. *J Gastroenterol Hepatol.* 2005;20(7):1062–1068.
88. Saad WE, Davies MG, Darcy MD. Management of bleeding after percutaneous transhepatic cholangiography or transhepatic biliary drain placement. *Tech Vasc Interv Radiol.* 2008; 11(1):60–71.

89. Messina LM, Shanley CJ. Visceral artery aneurysms. *Surg Clin North Am.* 1997;77(2):425–442.
90. Raghavan A, Wong CK, Lam A, et al. Spontaneous occlusion of post-traumatic splenic pseudoaneurysm: report of two cases in children. *Pediatr Radiol.* 2004;34(4):355–357.
91. Dror S, Dani BZ, Ur M, et al. Spontaneous thrombosis of a splenic pseudoaneurysm after blunt abdominal trauma. *J Trauma.* 2002;53(2):383–385.
92. van der Vlies CH, Hoekstra J, Ponsen KJ, et al. Impact of splenic artery embolization on the success rate of nonoperative management for blunt splenic injury. *Cardiovasc Intervent Radiol.* 2012;35(1):76–81.
93. Bessoud B, Denys A. Main splenic artery embolization using coils in blunt splenic injuries: effects on the intrasplenic blood pressure. *Eur Radiol.* 2004;14(9):1718–1719.
94. Bessoud B, Duchosal MA, Siegrist CA, et al. Proximal splenic artery embolization for blunt splenic injury: clinical, immunologic, and ultrasound-Doppler follow-up. *J Trauma.* 2007; 62(6):1481–1486.
95. Madoff DC, Denys A, Wallace MJ, et al. Splenic arterial interventions: anatomy, indications, technical considerations, and potential complications. *Radiographics.* 2005;25(suppl 1): S191–S211.
96. Kessaris DN, Bellman GC, Pardalidis NP, et al. Management of hemorrhage after percutaneous renal surgery. *J Urol.* 1995; 153(3, pt 1):604–608.
97. Phadke RV, Sawlani V, Rastogi H, et al. Iatrogenic renal vascular injuries and their radiological management. *Clin Radiol.* 1997;52(2):119–123.
98. Breyer BN, McAninch JW, Elliott SP, et al. Minimally invasive endovascular techniques to treat acute renal hemorrhage. *J Urol.* 2008;179(6):2248–2252; discussion 2253.
99. Mays ET, Wheeler CS. Demonstration of collateral arterial flow after interruption of hepatic arteries in man. *N Engl J Med.* 1974; 290(18):993–996.
100. Cho SK, Kim SS, Do YS, et al. Ischemic liver injuries after hepatic artery embolization in patients with delayed postoperative hemorrhage following hepatobiliary pancreatic surgery. *Acta Radiol.* 2011;52(4):393–400.
101. Guillon R, Garcier JM, Abergel A, et al. Management of splenic artery aneurysms and false aneurysms with endovascular treatment in 12 patients. *Cardiovasc Intervent Radiol.* 2003; 26(3):256 260.
102. Ekeh AP, Khalaf S, Ilyas S, et al. Complications arising from splenic artery embolization: a review of an 11-year experience. *Am J Surg.* 2013; 205(3):250–254; discussion 254.
103. Ekeh AP, McCarthy MC, Woods RJ, et al. Complications arising from splenic embolization after blunt splenic trauma. *Am J Surg.* 2005;189(3):335–339.
104. Haan JM, Biffl W, Knudson MM, et al. Splenic embolization revisited: a multicenter review. *J Trauma.* 2004;56(3): 542–547.
105. Eisenberg L, Paulson EK, Kliewer MA, et al. Sonographically guided compression repair of pseudoaneurysms: further experience from a single institution. *AJR Am J Roentgenol.* 1999; 173(6):1567–1573.
106. Sadiq S, Ibrahim W. Thromboembolism complicating thrombin injection of femoral artery pseudoaneurysm: management with intraarterial thrombolysis. *J Vasc Interv Radiol.* 2001; 12(5):633–636.
107. Loose HW, Haslam PJ. The management of peripheral arterial aneurysms using percutaneous injection of fibrin adhesive. *Br J Radiol.* 1998;71(852):1255–1259.
108. Elford J, Burrell C, Freeman S, et al. Human thrombin injection for the percutaneous treatment of iatrogenic pseudoaneurysms. *Cardiovasc Intervent Radiol.* 2002;25(2):115–118.
109. Souftas VD, Prassopoulos P. Computed-tomography-guided direct percutaneous transhepatic embolization of a bleeding hepatic artery branch aneurysm. *Acta Radiol.* 2006; 47(5): 461–464.

27

Peripheral Vascular Malformations

Jose Luiz Orlando • Francisco Ramos • Bruno C. Odisio

Peripheral vascular malformations arise as a result of a focal vascular differentiation embryologic failure leading to an abnormal development of the vascular system. They are responsible for important functional and aesthetic changes that often impact on the individual's daily routine. Diagnosis and treatment of this condition is still considered challenging in view of the various presentations and complexity levels of lesions.

CLASSIFICATION AND DESCRIPTION

Mulliken and Glowacki[1,2] described in 1982 a useful classification system, which gained acceptance by the scientific community based on the histologic findings, the flow characteristics, and the clinical aspects of the vascular anomalies. According to this classification, vascular anomalies fall into two major categories: hemangiomas and vascular malformations.[1,2] Hemangiomas are not included in the scope of the this chapter and therefore will not be discussed.

Vascular malformations arise from dysplastic vascular channels. These channels, generally presented at birth, will grow in proportion to the development of the individual and will never suffer involution.[1,3] Although congenital, in approximately 10% of patients, the lesions cannot be identified at birth, appearing later triggered by hormonal stimuli during adolescence and gestation or exacerbating their symptoms after infection, thrombosis, or local trauma.[4] The vascular malformations were initially classified according to the prevalence of the vascular channels in five different forms: venous, lymphatic, capillary, arterial, or combined. In 1993, Jackson et al.,[5] based on the classification system by Mulliken and Glowacki,[1,2] reclassified vascular malformations considering its hemodynamic characteristics, dividing them into low- and high-flow lesions. The low-flow lesions are classified as venous malformation, lymphatic capillaries, or venolymphatic forms (capillary venous and the lymphatic–venous capillary lesions); the high-flow lesions are divided in arteriovenous malformations (AVMs) and arteriovenous fistulas.[6] In 1996, this classification system was adopted and expanded by the International Society for the Study of Vascular Anomalies and is currently widely used.[7]

PATHOPHYSIOLOGY

The most accepted theory for the origin of vascular malformations is that they are caused by a total or partial agenesis of the capillary bed of a given territory. This agenesis would be associated with primitive persistent arteriovenous communications that constitute the AVM nidus.[8] The AVMs are basically characterized by presenting abnormal communications between the arterial and venous system, without the interposition of the capillary network. These shunts are, in most cases, multiple and configured as a conglomerate of vessels known as *vascular nidus*.[9] The advent of digital subtraction selective angiography along with the development of microcatheterization techniques allowed the angioarchitecture of these lesions to be identified with greater precision. The

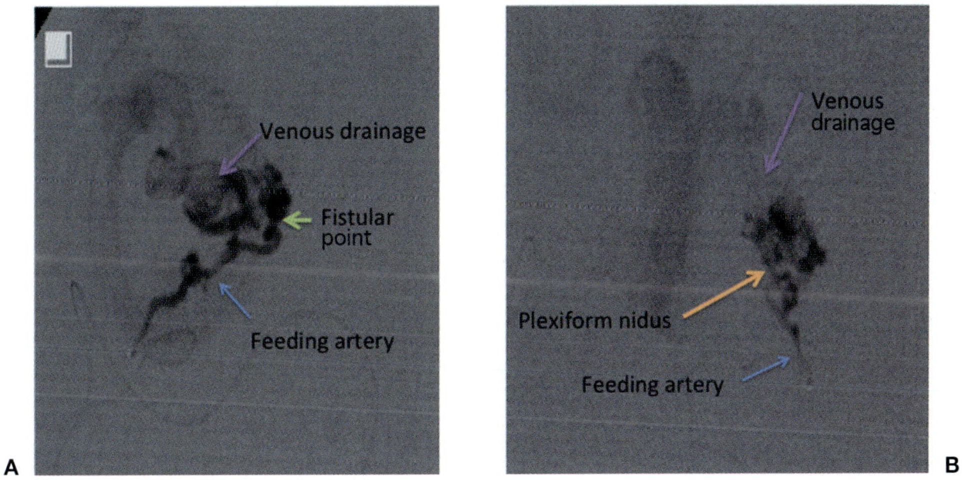

Figure 27.1 Selective digital subtraction angiography using an AVM using a 1.5-Fr microcatheter demonstrating a direct fistula **(A)** and plexiform nidus **(B)**.

angioarchitecture is divided into three distinct segments: nourishing artery(ies), a nidus, and the draining vein(s).[10]

The nourishing arteries can be classified as direct or indirect branches and can present as single or multiple branches. The direct branches directly supply the region of the vascular nidus and, in general, have a large diameter. The indirect branches supply the nidus and the surrounding tissues and may have blood flow opposite to its natural direction through anastomoses with neighboring arteries, where other arterial segments participate in the nutrition of the tissue. In this case, the preexisting arterioarterial anastomosis increases their caliber and promotes the passage of blood flow in a reversed direction. This compensatory phenomenon, characterized by the recruitment of collateral vessels to reconstruct the arterial supply distal to the AVM, is usually present in high-flow AVMs.[11]

The vascular nidus represents the core of the AVM and is interposed between the distal segment of the feeding artery(ies) and the proximal segment of the draining vein(s).[12] These arteriovenous communications are called *shunts* and are responsible for the secondary angiopathy induced by the increased blood flow. The nidus is a complex vascular structure and can be presented in three distinct patterns (Fig. 27.1):

- Plexiform: composed of a tangle of arteriolar and venular structures with a coiled and wrapped aspect. In this pattern, the supplying arteries ends in a cluster of multiple vessels with arteriovenous communications in which one or multiple channels emerge as the venous drainage.
- Fistulas: characterized by the presence of communication between artery and vein called arteriovenous fistulas. In this case, one or multiple arteries of anomalous path starting from a truncal artery empties into the venous system directly or in a venous lake located, for example, in the compartment muscle or subcutaneous tissue.
- Mixed pattern: a combination of both patterns mentioned earlier, with a predominance of one over the other. The nidus may also be constituted by one or more compartments.

The AVM draining veins corresponds mostly to the topography of the lesion and can be classified as deep or shallow. Drainage can occur from multiple compartments to a single main draining vein or smaller caliber accessory veins. Additionally, a single drainage vein from the AVM may branch into other veins, which can be confused with multiple draining veins (Fig. 27.2).

CLINICAL EVALUATION

Vascular malformations can occur anywhere in the body and can have either a localized or extensive distribution pattern. Commonly, its diagnosis is the result of a clinical history and detailed physical examination. The clinical presentation of peripheral AVMs is diverse and can range from asymptomatic to disabling pain cases. The presence of pain may be related to the presence of mass effect, varicose veins, thrombophlebitis, bone erosion, and mixed-origin ulcers caused by venous hypertension due to ischemia caused by preferential blood flow to the vascular malformation in detriment of the normal tissues.[1,13]

The lesions on the extremities are characterized by the presence of pulsatile tumor of firm consistency and slightly compressible, with thrill or murmur that result from turbulent blood flow.[14] Other characteristic findings of these injuries are a wide arterial pulse and the presence of a prominent proximal venous drainage, generally elongated and tortuous. Additionally, changes may occur secondary to the ischemia and the venous hypertension such as edema, skin pigmentation, stasis eczema, ulcers, and gangrene[13,15] (Fig. 27.3). The hypertrophy of the involved extremity is a frequent finding

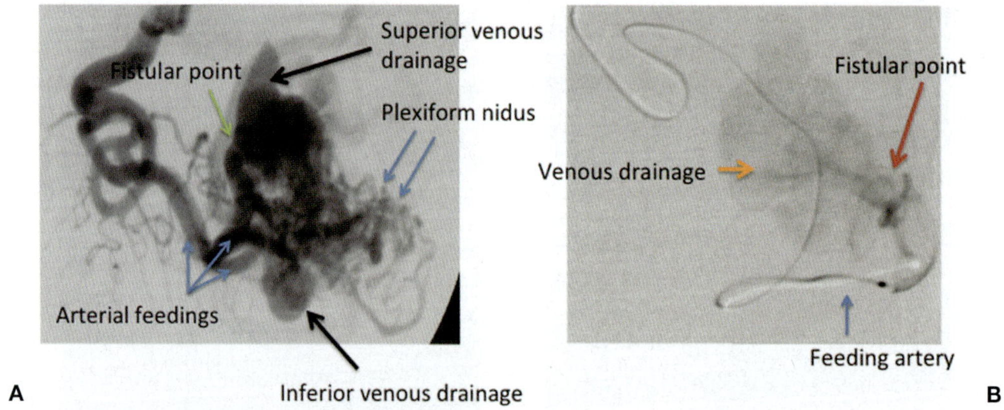

Figure 27.2 Selective digital subtraction angiography using an AVM using a 1.5-Fr microcatheter. **A:** AVM with multiple compartment—fistular and plexiform nidus. **B:** High-flow fistula.

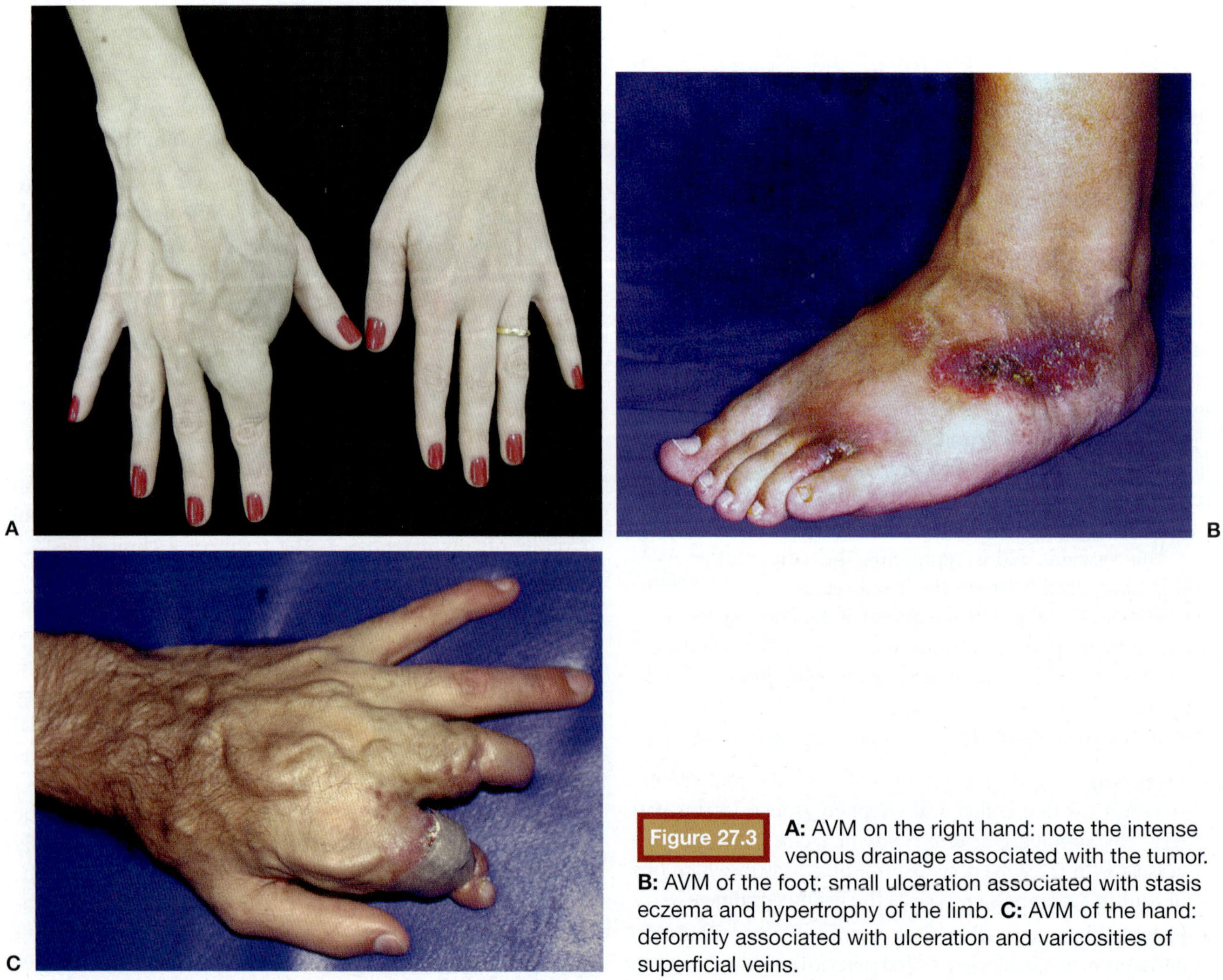

Figure 27.3 **A:** AVM on the right hand: note the intense venous drainage associated with the tumor. **B:** AVM of the foot: small ulceration associated with stasis eczema and hypertrophy of the limb. **C:** AVM of the hand: deformity associated with ulceration and varicosities of superficial veins.

and may be evident only in late childhood.[16,17] Pelvic AVMs are characterized by an increased soft tissue mass and can cause severe pain, pelvic congestion, sexual dysfunction, and hemorrhage.[18–20] In the presence of a large number of high-flow fistulae, congestive heart failure can occur in varying degrees as a result of cardiac overload.[21]

IMAGING EVALUATION

The use of different imaging modalities is an essential tool for differentiating between the different types of vascular malformations and between these and soft tissue tumors, assessing the exact extension of the lesions, and correlating the findings with other anatomical structures involved. The most common imaging modalities used in the diagnosis of vascular abnormalities are the ultrasonography (US), magnetic resonance imaging (MRI), computed tomography (CT), and angiography.

US is considered the imaging modality of choice for the initial evaluation of patients with soft tissue lesions of possible vascular origin.[22,23] The US Doppler allows characterizing the morphologic and hemodynamic aspects of the vascular malformations. The color mapping allows distinguishing the afferent arteries constituted of elongated and tortuous vessels, the nidus that is characterized by a conglomerate of vessels in the core of the lesion, and the draining veins. The hemodynamic changes in high-flow vascular malformations are characterized by the presence of a biphasic pattern with high systolic and diastolic velocities, indicating low resistance due to the presence of shunts. The nidus is recognized by the presence of high-velocity turbulent flow with a mosaic of colors. The venous segment of the malformation presents with a high-flow monophasic pattern that might be associated with some pulsatile pattern (Fig. 27.4). The MRI allows for assessment of the extent of the injury and its relationship to adjacent anatomical structures. It is also useful in differentiating between lesions of high and low flow.[3,24] AVMs are characterized as areas of absence of signal (flow-void) on T1 and T2 weighted sequences corresponding to the nurturing arteries and the nidus[15,25] (Fig. 27.5). MRI can also help in the differential diagnosis of tumors. Noteworthy are the proliferative hemangiomas that, despite showing hyperintense signal on T2 sequences and intermediate signal on T1 and areas of flow voids, has a well-defined and lobulated contours.[3,23,26] Other tumors such as sarcomas, neuroblastomas, hemangiopericytomas, fibrosarcomas, and rhabdomyosarcomas exhibit features of tissue invasion that can be associated with perilesional edema.[23,27–29] CT provides limited information regarding the extent of the lesion, generally underestimating its size and its flow characteristics when compared to MRI. The use of ionizing radiation is also another disadvantage associated with this method. CT can be useful in the differential diagnosis with soft tissue tumors to evaluate its mass effect and provide more detailed evaluation of changes in the adjacent structures such as bone erosions, periosteal

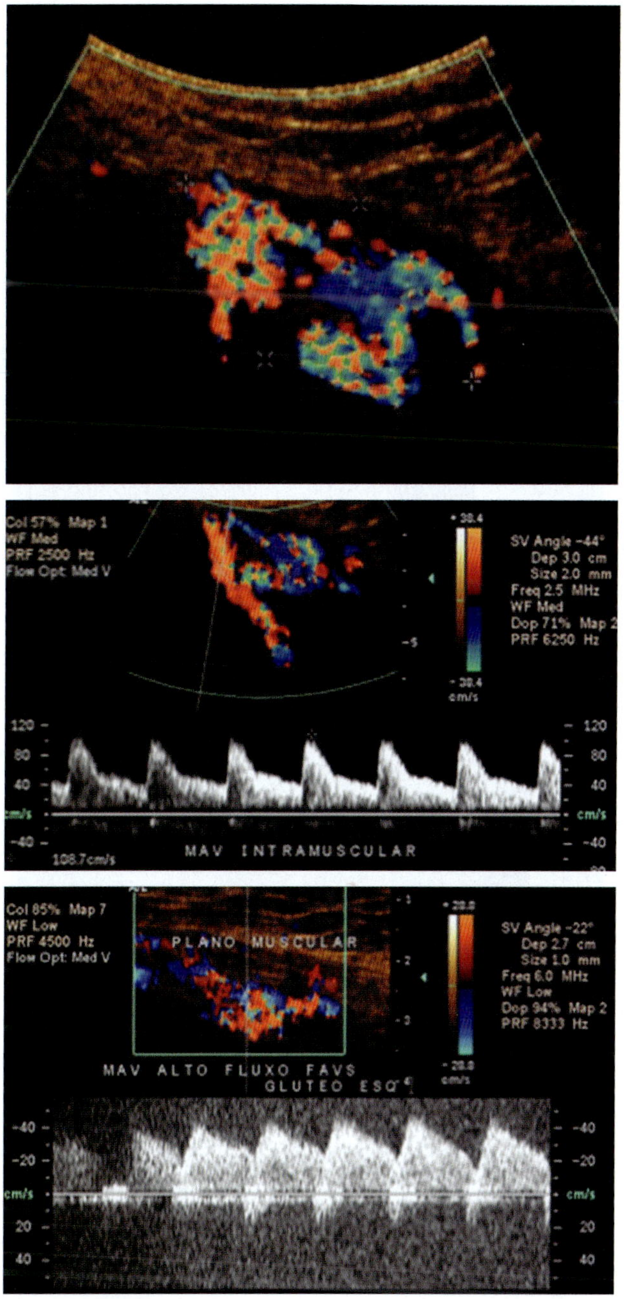

Figure 27.4 **A:** Doppler US: high-flow AVM within the gluteal muscle. Vascular plexiform nidus with multiple arteriovenous fistulas, characterized by a color mosaic pattern. **B:** Gluteal muscle artery nourishing the nidus with anomalous arterial pattern of low resistance (biphasic). **C:** Spectral analysis showing swirled stream. Fistular pattern within the nidus.

reaction, pathologic fractures, and presence of phleboliths. The phlebolith lesions are characteristic of venous malformations.[30] The use of angiography involves the selective catheterization of all pedicles involved for a complete study of the extension of the lesion and its flow characteristics. The

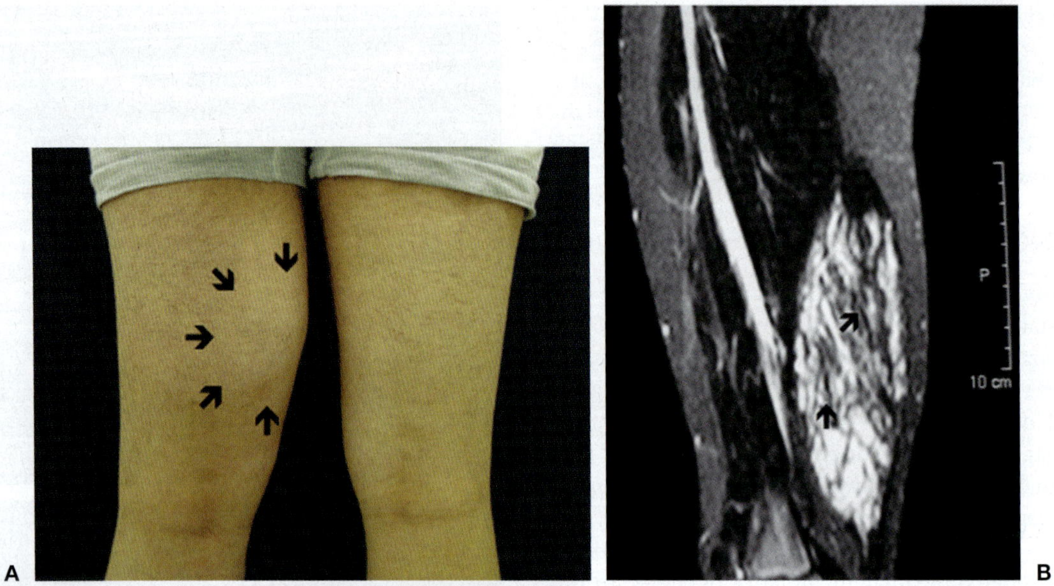

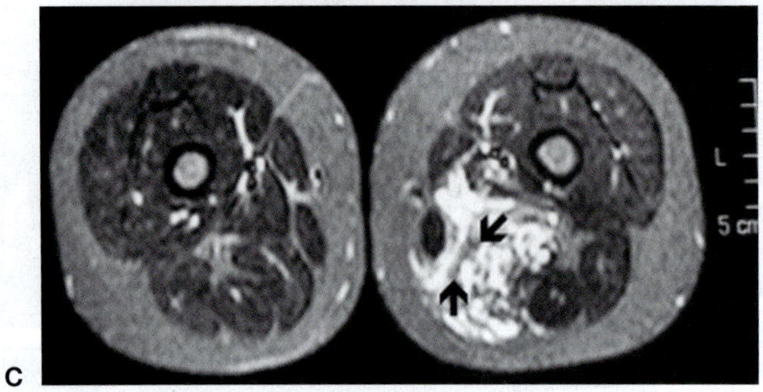

Figure 27.5 **A:** A 19-year-old male patient with an AVM located in the medial aspect of the left thigh (*black arrows*). **B:** Sagittal MRI of the right thigh: lesion with hypersignal T2 within the semimembranous muscle plane (*black arrows*). **C:** T2 axial MRI of the thighs: flow-void areas (*black arrows*) within lesion.

angiographic findings of AVMs include feeding artery(ies) with increased caliber and tortuous path, a conglomerate of arteries and veins (nidus), and an early venous filling segment characterized by elongated and large-caliber veins[12,31] (Fig. 27.6). An alternative access by direct puncture of the nidus transcutaneously allows for evaluation of extension and flow characteristics[31,32] (Fig. 27.7).

TREATMENT

The treatment of AVMs is still a challenge for surgeons and interventional radiologists.[33,34] Surgical treatment is usually associated with some technical difficulties due to the absence of a cleavage plane between the lesion and surrounding tissue, bleeding, and inaccessible location. Surgical ligation of the nourishing arteries is ineffective and often results in recurrence of the lesion by the recruitment of numerous arterial and venous branches.[17,18,20,35–38] The introduction of selective catheterization techniques created the possibility of implementing the treatment of vascular malformations through embolization. The evolution and development of new products and the introduction of microcatheters with smaller diameters allows greater selectivity of feeding vessels, making embolization the treatment of choice for vascular AVMs.[15,19,39] For a proper treatment planning, it is essential to perform a diagnostic angiography for the study of the vascular anatomy of the lesion and its hemodynamic pattern.[21,40] The goal of AVM embolization is the occlusion of the feeding vessels of the vascular nidus, avoiding areas of nontarget embolization (Fig. 27.8). The choice of the embolic material should be based on the lesion's angioarchitecture, size, length, number of involved vessels, flow characteristics, and pattern of venous drainage.[12,41] The limitations to a satisfactory embolization include the presence of elongated and tortuous branches and aneurysms that hinder the progression of the catheter (Figs. 27.9 and 27.10) and the presence of indirect branches or anastomoses nourishing the malformation that prevent the placement of the microcatheter within the nidus (Fig. 27.11). Additionally, these indirect branches may also supply adjacent normal tissues, increasing the risk of nontarget embolization. Most AVMs present both types of nurturing branches, and success of treatment depends on the ability to select the vascular nidus with the microcatheter.[12]

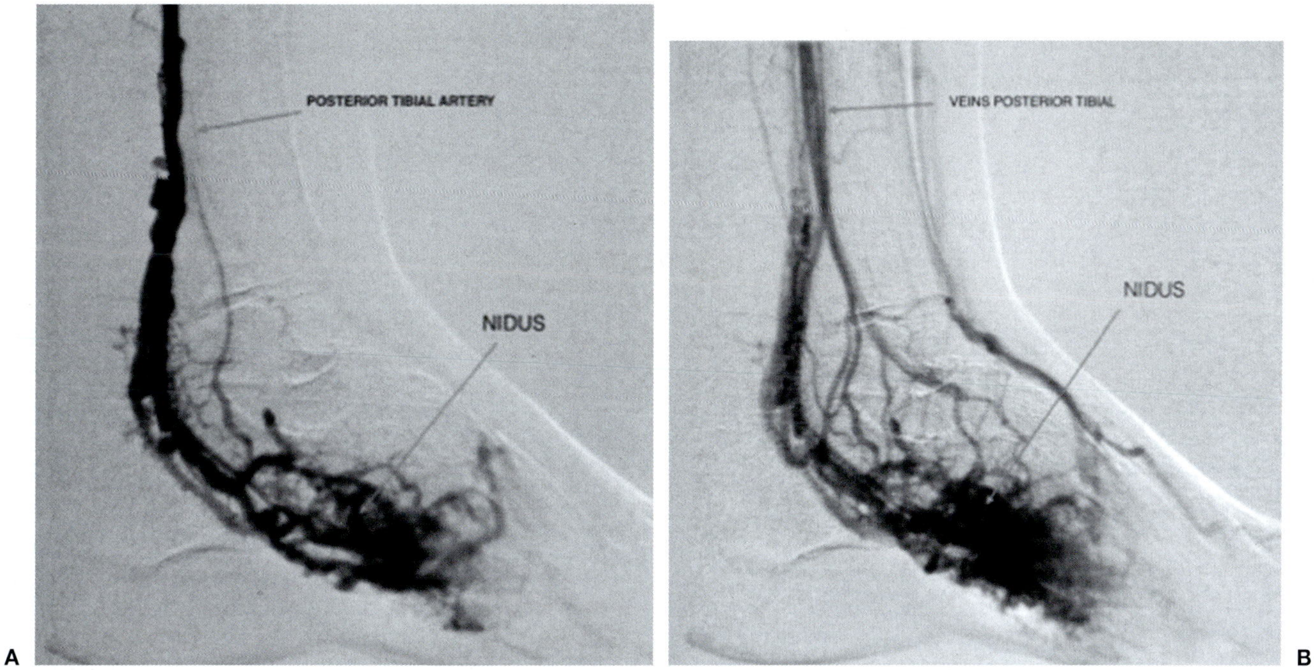

Figure 27.6 Selective angiography of the left posterior tibial artery. **A:** Enlarged arterial caliber with opacification of the vascular nidus. **B:** There is early venous filling.

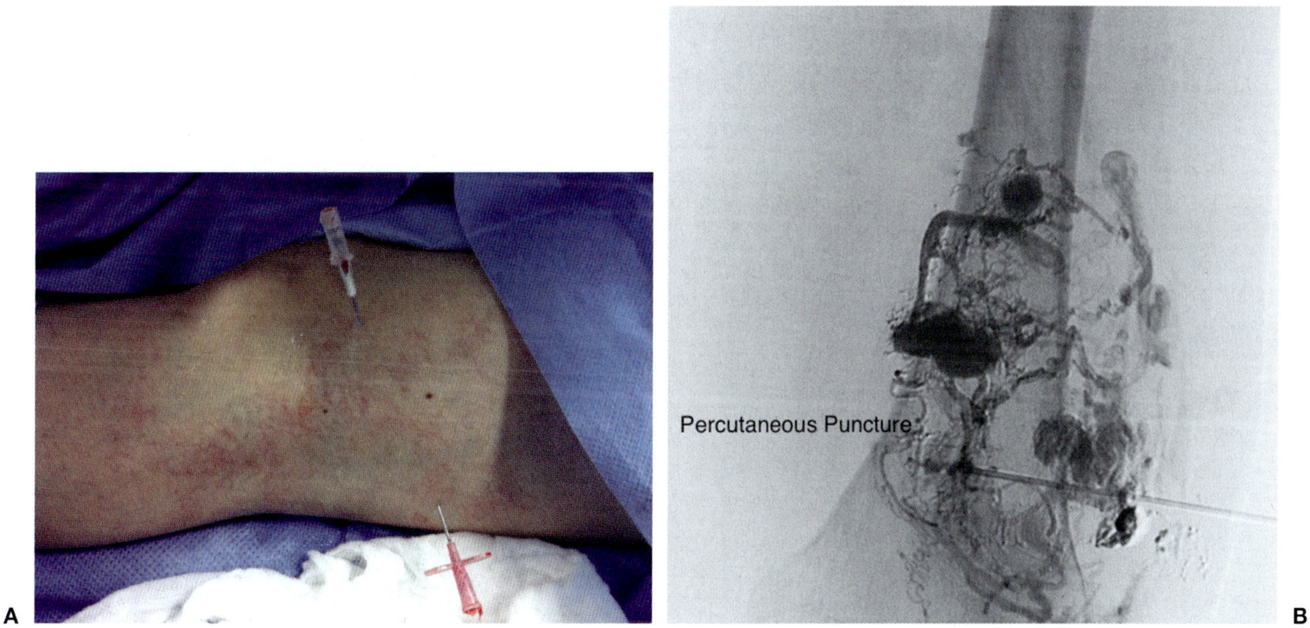

Figure 27.7 AVM of the left thigh. **A:** Direct puncture of the lesion **B:** Transcutaneous angiography shows opacification of the vascular nidus.

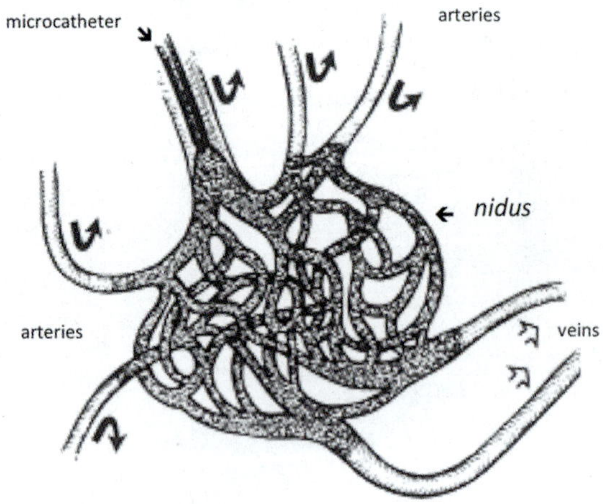

Figure 27.8 Schematic representation of the vascular nidus.

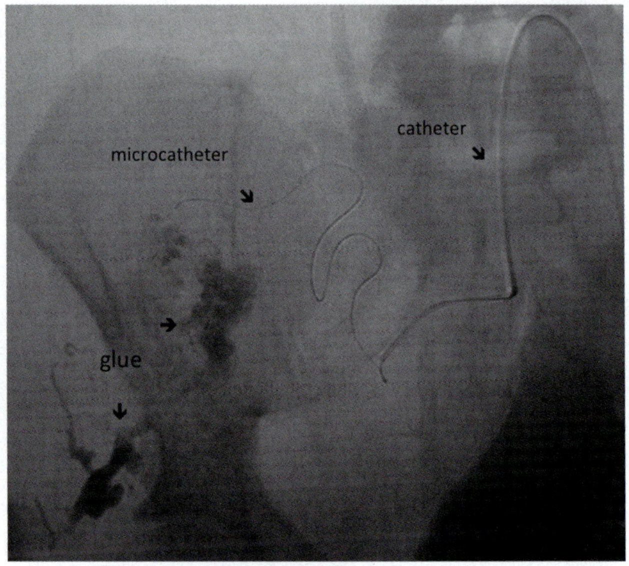

Figure 27.9 Iliac arteriography of a pelvic AVM: Observe the elongated and tortuous branches of the right hypogastric artery that demonstrate the importance of microcatheters and coaxial technique.

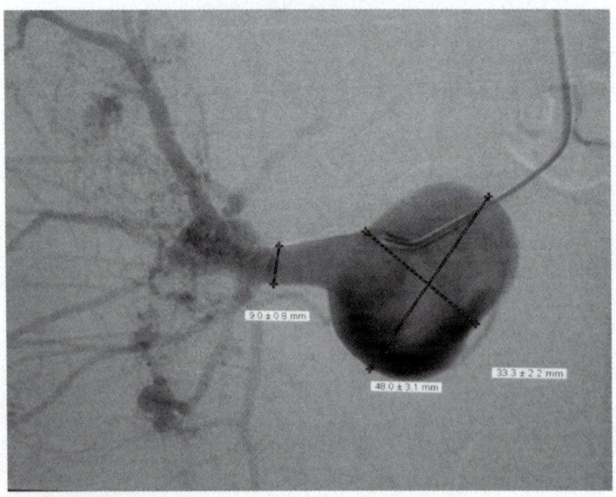

Figure 27.10 Right internal iliac artery aneurysm associated to arteriovenous fistulas.

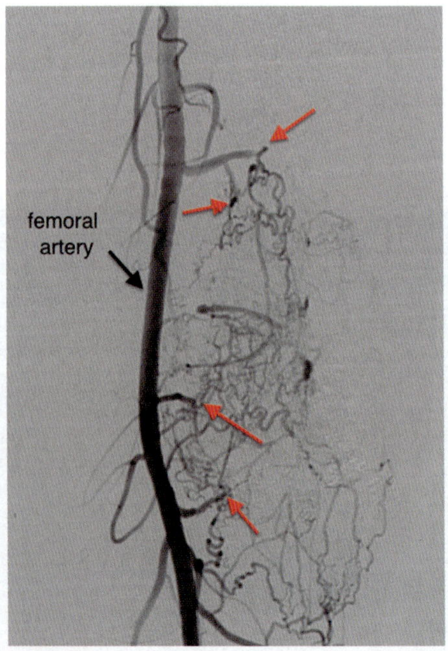

Figure 27.11 Superficial femoral artery angiography: indirect branches for arterio-arterial anastomoses (*red arrows*).

DEVICE/MATERIAL DESCRIPTION

Guiding Catheters and Introducer Sheaths

Guiding catheters or long introducer sheaths are frequently used to secure access. It also provides stability during catheter exchanges, which is especially useful in situations when the embolic agents occlude the catheter. A guiding catheter or a long introducer sheath is typically tracked over a 0.035-in guidewire and secured close to or at the orifice of the feeding branches, such as a branch of hypogastric artery for a pelvic AVM and a branch of profunda femoral artery for a thigh AVM.

Coaxial Catheter System

Successful embolization of the nidus of an AVM often requires selective catheterization of numerous arterial feeding branches. This is facilitated by using coaxial microcatheter systems. The microcatheter is coaxially introduced through 4-Fr or 5-Fr diagnostic catheter and can be manipulated into the terminal feeding artery. Embolic agents are then delivered via a variety of end-hole microcatheters ranging from 1.5-Fr to 3.0-Fr (most commonly 2-Fr to 2.4-Fr).

Embolic Agents

Glue or tissue adhesive, such as *N*-butyl cyanoacrylate (NBCA) (Histoacryl; B. Braun Melsungen AG, Melsungen, Germany) and Glubran 2 (GEM Srl, Viareggio, Italy),[42] is classified as a liquid, adhesive, nonabsorbable, permanent embolic agent. Tissue adhesives offer great versatility due to the ability to use different dilutions (i.e., proportion of Ethiodol and glue in the solution) in various types of AVM. The tissue adhesive consists of an N-Butil-2 monomer linked with ciano group and connected to carbon radicals that, when in contact with ionic substances such as normal saline or blood, activates the glue polymerization process through the union of molecules of ethylene.[43] The liquid nature of this agent allows its passage through microcatheters which, when released very near or within the region of the nidus, initiates a polymerization process that forms a framework around it, occluding blood circulation. Its association with iodized poppy seed oil (Lipiodol UF; Guerbet USA, Bloomington, Indiana) gives radiopacity to the solution and retards the polymerization time, facilitating its handling.[44] In the mixture of glue and Lipiodol, the higher the proportion of Lipiodol (for example 3:1 of Lipiodol/glue, respectively), the longer it will take for the glue to get polymerized (solid). The reverse is also true. The higher the concentration of glue (for example 1:3 of Lipiodol/glue, respectively), the faster will be the polymerization time (see Chapter 9).

Onyx (Covidien, Irvine, California) is a liquid, nonadhesive, nonabsorbable, permanent embolic agent.[45] Onyx is composed of a certain percentage of ethylene vinyl alcohol (EVOH) copolymer dissolved in dimethyl sulfoxide (DMSO) and suspended micronized tantalum powder to provide contrast for visualization under fluoroscopy. It was approved in 2005 for the treatment of AVMs by the U.S. Food and Drug Administration. Its use has been progressively extended to other pathologies.[46] It is recommended using specific delivery microcatheters compatible with DMSO: Marathon, Rebar, or UltraFlow HPC (Covidien, Irvine, California).

Its composition consists of 48 mol/L of ethylene and 52 mol/L of vinyl alcohol dissolved in DMSO and associated with the tantalum powder at a concentration of 35% weight per volume to make the product radiopaque.

This product is commercially available in different concentrations The density of Onyx is defined by the concentration of the EVOH varying from 6% to 8%. Onyx is available in three formulations: Onyx 18 (EVOH concentration of 6%), Onyx 34 (8% EVOH), and Onyx HD500 (20% EVOH). Peripheral AVMs are usually treated with Onyx 18. Use of this product requires preparation for a period of 20 minutes in a mixer provided by the manufacturer so that the copolymer is mixed homogeneously with the tantalum powder. The active principle of Onyx precipitates upon contact with saline, water, or blood. The solvent DMSO prevents precipitation of Onyx (see Chapter 10).

TECHNIQUE

The access route for embolization is initially established by puncture and catheterization of the artery ipsilateral or contralateral depending on the location of the lesion. The microcatheters are introduced through larger caliber catheters (coaxial system) and kept under continuous infusion in saline. Heparin is used at a dose of 100 units per kilogram of weight with a maintenance bolus dose of 1,000 units per hour. The anticoagulation is used routinely in our practice, but currently, there is no consensus about using it in all AVM embolization cases. The guiding catheter is positioned selectively in the feeding vessel proximal to the lesion, from which are introduced microcatheters ranging from 1.5-Fr to 3.0-Fr depending on the vessel to be treated. Road mapping technique can be used for superselective nidus microcatheterization.

Tissue Adhesive Embolization Technique

The cyanoacrylate is diluted in Lipiodol in proportions ranging from 1:1 to 1:8 depending on the lesion flow characteristics.[44,47] The microcatheter is filled with dextrose 5% until immediately before embolization. This maneuver is intended to prevent early polymerization of the glue on the catheter upon contact with blood (dextrose has similar role as the DMSO has in Onyx embolization). The injection of glue through the microcatheter is performed in a slow fashion and under fluoroscopic control until it reaches the end of the microcatheter. The progression of glue inside the nidus is influenced by the dilution and injection pressure applied in the plunger of the syringe. One of the risks associated with cyanoacrylate embolization is the possibility of the catheter adhering to the vessel, preventing its withdrawal. Maneuvers used to minimize this risk include the use of solutions with a lower concentration of cyanoacrylate and heating to reduce its viscosity. Under microcatheter aspiration (negative pressure applied in the syringe connected to the hub of the microcatheter), it also should be quickly pulled out as soon as a satisfactory embolization is achieved.

Onyx Embolization Technique

The first step is to purge the catheter with saline to clear any contrast residue and then prime with solvent solution DMSO. The amount of DMSO required for this will be determined by prior knowledge of the internal lumen of the catheter to be used (microcatheter dead space information is available in the package label). After filling the microcatheter with DMSO, Onyx is aspirated into a syringe provided by the manufacturer and connected to the microcatheter, forming an interface between the DMSO present within the microcatheter and the syringe with Onyx. This is done with the intent of preventing early polymerization and catheter occlusion by the contact of Onyx with blood or saline in the microcatheter. It is recommended that the injection of Onyx is to be performed at a rate of 0.1 to 0.2 mL per minute to promote a slow release and contact of the DMSO with arterial endothelium. The contact of DMSO with the endothelium of the vessel may cause vasospasm, angionecrosis, and/or pain, which is more likely to happen if the injection of the solvent occurs quickly.[48] The injection pressure should be sufficient enough to promote progression of the Onyx within the artery and prevent reflux toward the catheter. Reflux is acceptable but should not involve more than 1.0 to 1.5 cm of the distal aspect of the microcatheter. Despite the fact that Onyx is not being considered an adhesive agent, its prolonged injection time followed by reflux around the microcatheter can create difficulties in removing the catheter. The removal of the catheter after the end of the embolization should occur smoothly and progressively. Abrupt maneuvers to remove it increase the risk of rupture of the artery or catheter, increasing the morbidity related to treatment.

Direct Puncture Using Tissue Adhesive Embolization Technique

Catheter embolization can be contraindicated due to lack of an arterial access. It can be related to previous surgical bandages, inadequate embolization proximal to the nidus, presence of marked tortuosity of the vessels supplying the vascular nidus, and the presence of arteriovenous anastomoses that may preclude selective catheterization. For direct puncture of the lesion, various needle lengths can be used according to the depth of the lesion. Superficial lesions can be addressed under direct vision. Deep lesions generally require ultrasound or angiography guidance. The choice of embolic agents relies on the same criteria already established in the intra-arterial embolization and experience of the operator.

CLINICAL APPLICATIONS

The treatment of AVMs is indicated in symptomatic cases or in those with deformities that interfere with daily activities. For a successful embolization, it is necessary to know the angioarchitecture of the lesion, selective catheterization of the supplying vessel(s), and injection of the embolic agent within the nidus. In our experience, the use of systemic heparin and perfusion catheter with saline solution helps to prevent thromboembolic complications. General anesthesia, spinal block, or conscious sedation is mandatory to keep the patient comfortable and steady during the procedure. The angiography is the standard test to characterize the vascular nidus and define treatment. The presence of early opacification of the draining vein(s) during the arterial phase is compatible with arteriovenous fistula. In the presence of a plexiform nidus, a cluster of anomalous and tortuous vessels is generally identified preceding the opacification of the draining veins. In low-flow lesions, it is necessary to perform selective microcatheterization of the branches of small caliber directly related to nutrition of the AVM to define its angioarchitecture.

Embolization may be performed with liquid or solid embolic agents. Liquid agents are the most suitable for the permanent occlusion of AVMs. The embolization success depends on the proper use of the technique and selective occlusion of the malformation without compromising the perfusion of surrounding normal tissues. Onyx has a particularly good applicability in the treatment of AVMs with massive plexiform nidus or nourished by multiple branches. Contrarily, it is not used in the presence of high-flow arteriovenous fistulas, where cyanoacrylate typically is a better embolic agent, with or without flow control techniques assistance.

Cyanoacrylate acts differently from Onyx and promotes vascular occlusion through the process of polymerization, which varies according to the concentration used in dilution with Lipiodol. The technique of injection of cyanoacrylate can vary from slow to fast depending on the dilution chosen and the pattern of intralesional flow. For plexiform AVM lesions, bulky lesions, or low-flow lesions, we recommend using the cyanoacrylate, which can be diluted to low concentrations (15% to 20%). On the other hand, cyanoacrylate can be used in higher concentration solution, ranging from 50% to 70%, in the embolization of high-flow fistulas. In slow-flow lesions nourished by arteries of small caliber in which it is not always possible to position the microcatheter in the nidus, the injection of diluted cyanoacrylate (20% to 30% concentration) is usually effective, allowing satisfactory penetration within the distal aspect of the lesion. Flow reduction techniques may help obtain better control of the injection of the embolic agent. Blood pressure cuffs, tourniquets, or local external compression performed proximal to the lesion can also be used and can contribute to the prevention of nontarget embolization. It favors the agent penetration within the nidus as it delays the progression of the embolic agent into the draining veins. Postembolization angiography is necessary to check the effectiveness of the procedure and at the same time assess the need for reintervention.

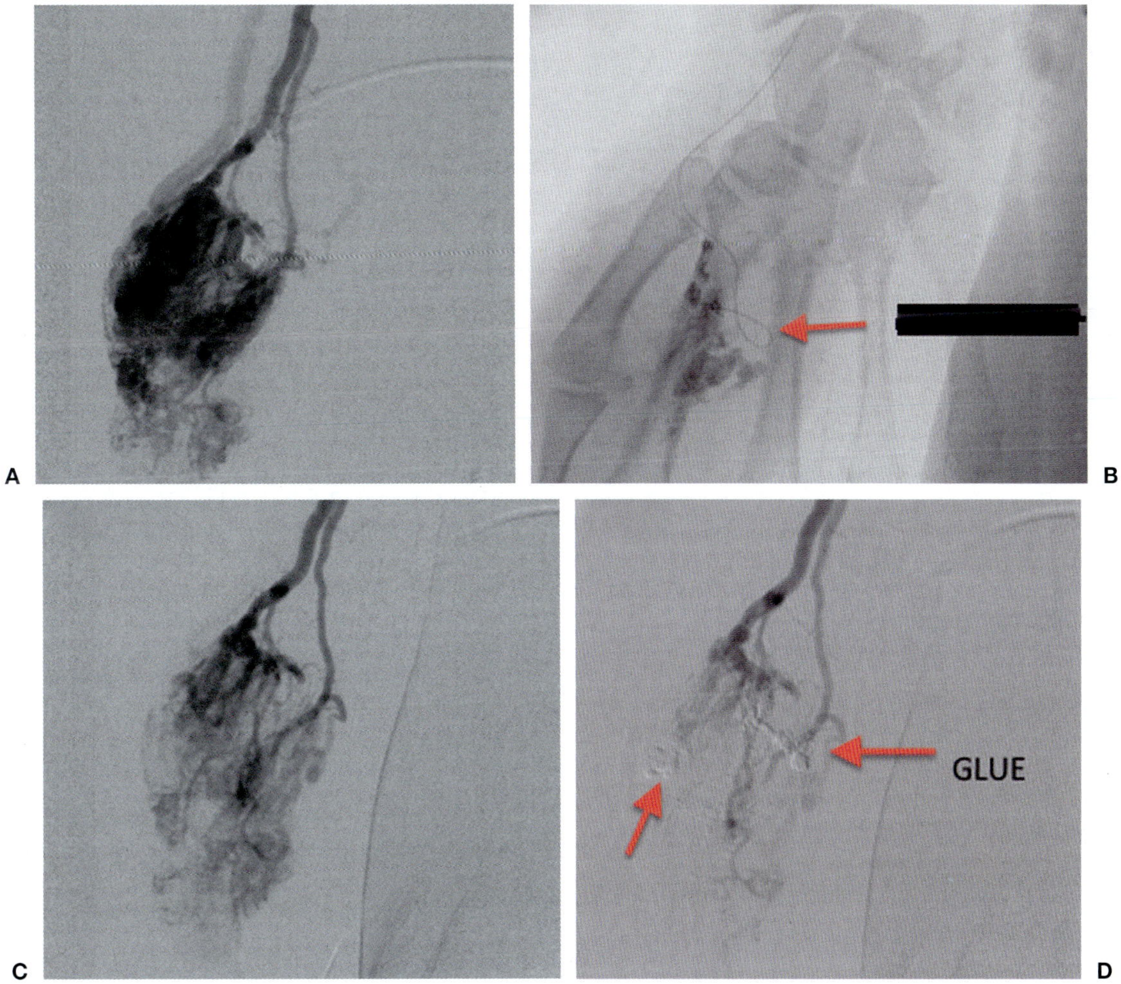

Figure 27.12 Angiography of the right hand with catheter placed within the radial artery. **A:** Enlarged and elongated supplying arteries; vascular nidus associated with early venous filling. **B:** Microcatheter 1.5-Fr positioned selectively within the nidus (*arrow*). **C:** Control arteriography after embolization with partial devascularization of the lesion. **D:** Postembolization cast of glue (*arrows*).

There is no consensus in the literature about the ideal way to perform AVM embolization. The treatment may be carried out in a single session to obtain occlusion of the entire lesion or in multiple sessions. Multiple sessions are generally indicated in lesions of great extension to reduce the side effects related to hemodynamic alterations that are responsible for the appearance of edema or hemorrhage.[49] The use of particulate agents, such as microparticles, has a temporary effect in promoting vessel occlusion, lasting only a few days, and is not sufficient to promote complete thrombosis, causing recurrence. In addition, high-flow AVMs with large fistulas can promote migration of the particulate agents into the venous system, pulmonary circulation, and potentially to the systemic circulation in case of right-to-left heart shunt, without occluding the fistula. Coils also have limited use because of technical difficulties in obtaining suitable deployment within the fistula, often leading to a proximal occlusion of the artery. In fact, in addition to not occluding the fistula, it also creates a proximal mechanical barrier that potentially precludes proper selective catheterization of the fistula to perform future embolizations of the lesion. For these reasons, the use of particles and coils are not indicated for the treatment of AVMs. The results of embolization may vary from the complete disappearance of symptoms and control of the lesion until partial improvement, meaning a palliative measurement in the treatment of complex lesions, providing comfort and improved quality of life for the patient[50–52] (Fig. 27.12).

POTENTIAL COMPLICATIONS

Although infrequent, complications occurring after AVM embolization are still present in the daily practice. Patients should be informed of the potential risks of treatment. Skin necrosis is one of the potential complications and can be aggravated by infection and bleeding. Other potentially more

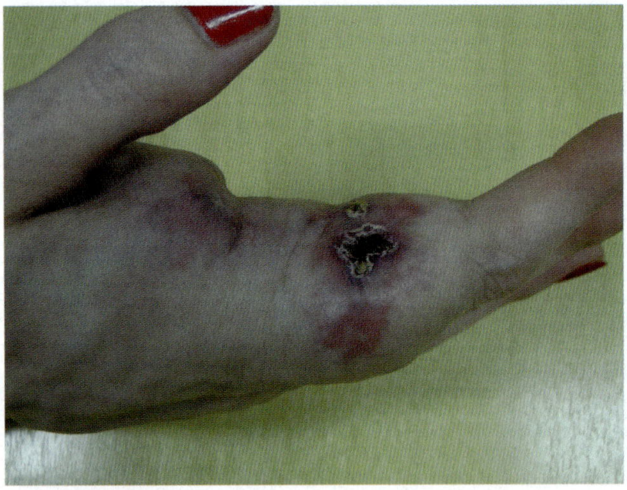

Figure 27.13 Trophic lesion in the healing phase after one session of percutaneous embolization with glue mixed with Lipiodol (1:4) of an anomalous ramus arising from the ulnar artery.

serious complications include ischemia of organs and tissues as a result of nontarget embolization[12,53] (Fig. 27.13). Although less frequent in the treatment of AVMs than in embolization or visceral tumors, the postembolization syndrome can occur after AVM embolization. Symptoms and signs such as pain, fever, leukocytosis, and nausea occur shortly after the procedure and usually resolve within a few days; however, they may persist for more than a week.[13]

TIPS AND TRICKS

Tips

Angiographic Findings	Characteristics
Arteriovenous fistula	Immediate opacification of artery and vein
Nidus	Conglomerate of arteries and veins
Arterioarterial anastomosis	Large artery that supplies the nidus via a smaller caliber artery
Indirect branches	Arterial branch that supplies normal surrounding tissues and the nidus

Tricks

Angioarchitecture	Flow	Embolic Agent
Plexiform	High	Onyx 18; Glue 33%–50%
	Low	Glue 15%–20%
Fistula	High	Glue 33%–50%
Mixed	High	Onyx 18
	Low	Onyx 18; Glue 15%–20%

CONCLUSION

Despite the advances of percutaneous embolization in the treatment of vascular malformations and the low incidence of complications associated with it, only symptomatic patients should be considered for treatment,[51] avoiding the treatment of AVM for cosmetic reasons.

REFERENCES

1. Mulliken JB, Glowacki J. Hemangiomas and vascular malformations in infants and children: a classification based on endothelial characteristics. *Plast Reconstr Surg*. 1982;69(3):412–422.
2. Mulliken JB, Glowacki J. Classification of pediatric vascular lesions. *Plast Reconstr Surg*. 1982;70(1):120–121.
3. Moukaddam H, Pollak J, Haims AH. MRI characteristics and classification of peripheral vascular malformations and tumors. *Skeletal Radiol*. 2009;38(6):535–547.
4. Gloviczki P, Duncan A, Kalra M, et al. Vascular malformations: an update. *Perspect Vasc Surg Endovasc Ther*. 2009;21(2):133–148.
5. Jackson IT, Carreno R, Potparic Z, et al. Hemangiomas, vascular malformations, and lymphovenous malformations: classification and methods of treatment. *Plast Reconstr Surg*. 1993;91(7):1216–1230.
6. Belov S. Anatomopathological classification of congenital vascular defects. *Semin Vasc Surg*. 1993;6(4):219–224.
7. Enjolras O. Classification and management of the various superficial vascular anomalies: hemangiomas and vascular malformations. *J Dermatol*. 1997;24(11):701–710.
8. Van den Bergh R, van der Eecken H. Anatomy and embryology of cerebral circulation. *Prog Brain Res*. 1968;30(20):1–25.
9. Houdart E, Gobin YP, Casasco A, et al. A Proposed angiographic classification of intracranial arteriovenous-fistulas and malformations. *Neuroradiology*. 1993;35(5):381–385.
10. Alvarez H, Valavanis A. *Interventional Neuroradiology*. Berlin, Germany: Springer-Verlag; 1993.
11. Berenstein A, Lasjaunias P. *Surgical Neuroangiography 4 Endovascular Treatment of Cerebral Lesions*. Berlin, Germany: Springer-Verlag; 1992. http://dx.doi.org/10.1007/978-3-642-71864-9.
12. Valavanis A, Müller-Forrell W. Diagnostic and interventional neuroradiology of brain arteriovenous malformations: implications of angioarchitecture for embolization. In: Bock WJ, Lumenta C, Brock M, et al, eds. *Advances in Neurosurgery*. Berlin, Germany: Springer-Verlag; 1991:35–40.
13. Rosen RR, Riles TS, Berenstein A. Congenital vascular malformations. In: Rutherford RB, ed. *Vascular Surgery*. Philadelphia, PA: W. B. Saunders; 1995:1218–1232.
14. Upton J, Coombs CJ, Mulliken JB, et al. Vascular malformations of the upper limb: a review of 270 patients. *J Hand Surg Am*. 1999;24(5):1019–1035.
15. Ernemann U, Kramer U, Miller S, et al. Current concepts in the classification, diagnosis and treatment of vascular anomalies. *Eur J Radiol*. 2010;75(1):2–11.
16. Belov S. Haemodynamic pathogenesis of vascular-bone syndromes in congenital vascular defects. *Int Angiol*.1990;9(3):155–161.
17. Abdool-Carrim AT, Cuschieri RJ, Vohra R, et al. Management of congenital arteriovenous malformations. *J R Coll Surg Edinb*. 1990;35(1):39–41.

18. Morgan RF, Horowitz JH, Wanebo HJ, et al. Surgical management of vascular malformations of the head and neck. *Am J Surg.* 1986;152(4):424–429.
19. Jacobowitz GR, Rosen RJ, Rockman CB, et al. Transcatheter embolization of complex pelvic vascular malformations: results and long-term follow-up. *J Vasc Surg.* 2001;33(1):51–55.
20. Malan E. Surgical problems in the treatment of congenital arterio-venous fistulae. *J Cardiovasc Surg (Torino).* 1965;5(6)(suppl):251–255.
21. Yakes WF, Rossi P, Odink H. How I do it. Arteriovenous malformation management. *Cardiovasc Intervent Radiol.* 1996;19(2):65–71.
22. Dubois J, Patriquin HB, Garel L, et al. Soft-tissue hemangiomas in infants and children: diagnosis using Doppler sonography. *AJR Am J Roentgenol.* 1998;171(1):247–252.
23. Dubois J, Alison M. Vascular anomalies: what a radiologist needs to know. *Pediatr Radiol.* 2010;40(6):895–905.
24. Dobson MJ, Hartley RW, Ashleigh R, et al. MR angiography and MR imaging of symptomatic vascular malformations. *Clin Radiol.* 1997;52(8):595–602.
25. Ohgiya Y, Hashimoto T, Gokan T, et al. Dynamic MRI for distinguishing high-flow from low-flow peripheral vascular malformations. *AJR Am J Roentgenol.* 2005;185(5):1131–1137.
26. Dubois J, Garel L. Imaging and therapeutic approach of hemangiomas and vascular malformations in the pediatric age group. *Pediatr Radiol.* 1999;29(12):879–893.
27. Kransdorf MJ, Jelinek JS, Moser RP Jr, et al. Soft-tissue masses: diagnosis using MR imaging. *AJR Am J Roentgenol.* 1989;153(3):541–547.
28. Navarro OM, Laffan EE, Ngan BY. Pediatric soft-tissue tumors and pseudo-tumors: MR imaging features with pathologic correlation: part 1. Imaging approach, pseudotumors, vascular lesions, and adipocytic tumors. *Radiographics.* 2009;29(3):887–906.
29. Siegel MJ. Magnetic resonance imaging of musculoskeletal soft tissue masses. *Radiol Clin North Am.* 2001;39(4):701–720.
30. Flors L, Leiva-Salinas C, Maged IM, et al. MR imaging of soft-tissue vascular malformations: diagnosis, classification, and therapy follow-up. *Radiographics.* 2011;31(5):1321–1340; discussion 1340–1341.
31. Rosen. Abnormal arteriovenous communications. In: Baum S, Pentecost M, eds. *Abrams' Angiography: Vascular and Interventional Radiology.* Boston, MA: Little Brown; 1997:998–1030.
32. Boxt LM, Levin DC, Fellows KE. Direct puncture angiography in congenital venous malformations. *AJR Am J Roentgenol.* 1983;140(1):135–136.
33. Hyodoh H, Hori M, Akiba H, et al. Peripheral vascular malformations: imaging, treatment approaches, and therapeutic issues. *Radiographics.* 2005;25(suppl 1):S159–S171.
34. Legiehn GM, Heran MK. Classification, diagnosis, and interventional radiologic management of vascular malformations. *Orthop Clin North Am.* 2006;37(3):435–474, vii–viii.
35. Szilagyi DE, Smith RF, Elliott JP, et al. Congenital arteriovenous anomalies of the limbs. *Arch Surg.* 1976;111(4):423–429.
36. Lee BB, Bergan JJ. Advanced management of congenital vascular malformations: a multidisciplinary approach. *Cardiovasc Surg.* 2002;10(6):523–533.
37. Yamada S, Brauer FS, Colohan AR, et al. Concept of arteriovenous malformation compartments and surgical management. *Neurol Res.* 2004;26(3):288–300.
38. Loose DA. Surgical correction of vascular malformations of the lower extremity [in German]. *Kongressbd Dtsch Ges Chir Kongr.* 2001;118:507–515.
39. Donnelly LF, Adams DM, Bisset GS III. Vascular malformations and hemangiomas: a practical approach in a multidisciplinary clinic. *AJR Am J Roentgenol.* 2000;174(3):597–608.
40. Uflacker, R. Embolização de malformação arteriovenosa, hemangiomas e fistulas arteriovenosas. In: *Radiologia Intervencionista.* São Paulo, Brasil: Savier; 1987:270–288.
41. Coldwell DM, Stokes KR, Yakes WF. Embolotherapy: agents, clinical applications, and techniques. *Radiographics.* 1994;14(3):623–643; quiz 645–646.
42. Raffi L, Simonetti L, Cenni P, et al. Use of Glubran 2 acrylic glue in interventional neuroradiology. *Neuroradiology.* 2007;49(10):829–836.
43. Pollak JS, White RI Jr. The use of cyanoacrylate adhesives in peripheral embolization. *J Vasc Interv Radiol.* 2001;12(8):907–913.
44. Widlus DM, Lammert GK, Brant A, et al. In vivo evaluation of iophendylate-cyanoacrylate mixtures. *Radiology.* 1992;185(1):269–273.
45. Yamashita K, Taki W, Iwata H, et al. Characteristics of ethylene vinyl alcohol copolymer (EVAL) mixtures. *AJNR Am J Neuroradiol.* 1994;15(6):1103–1105.
46. Guimaraes M, Wooster M. Onyx (ethylene-vinyl alcohol copolymer) in peripheral applications. *Semin Intervent Radiol.* 2011;28(3):350–356.
47. Brothers MF, Kaufmann JC, Fox AJ, et al. n-Butyl 2-cyanoacrylate—substitute for IBCA in interventional neuroradiology: histopathologic and polymerization time studies. *AJNR Am J Neuroradiol.* 1989;10(4):777–786.
48. Siekmann R. Basics and principles in the application of Onyx LD Liquid Embolic System in the endovascular treatment of cerebral arteriovenous malformations. *Interv Neuroradiol.* 2005;11(suppl 1):131–140.
49. Picard L. Brain AVMs endovascular treatment. *Interv Neuroradiol.* 2003;9(suppl 2):205–207.
50. Tan KT, Simons ME, Rajan DK, et al. Peripheral high-flow arteriovenous vascular malformations: a single-center experience. *J Vasc Interv Radiol.* 2004;15(10):1071–1080.
51. Rockman CB, Rosen RJ, Jacobowitz GR, et al. Transcatheter embolization of extremity vascular malformations: the long-term success of multiple interventions. *Ann Vasc Surg.* 2003;17(4):417–423.
52. White RI Jr, Pollak J, Persing J, et al. Long-term outcome of embolotherapy and surgery for high-flow extremity arteriovenous malformations. *J Vasc Interv Radiol.* 2000;11(10):1285–1295.
53. Yakes WF. Endovascular management of high-flow arteriovenous malformations. *Semin Intervent Radiol.* 2004;21(1):49–58.

28

Dysfunctional Hemodialysis Accesses

Dheeraj K. Rajan • Ricardo Yamada

In 2006, the last update of the Kidney Disease Outcomes Quality Initiative along with the Fistula First program reinforced the concept of arteriovenous fistula (AVF) as the preferred hemodialysis (HD) access, given its longer durability, less risk of infection, and less overall cost compared with arteriovenous grafts (AVGs).[1,2] Unfortunately, AVF primary failure can reach up to 53% according to one series.[3] Therefore, multiple strategies have been implanted to improve outcome, including better patient selection, refined surgical techniques, and access surveillance. Recently, endovascular techniques have been successfully used to improve AVF development, including collateral veins embolization. In addition, primary failure is not the only obstacle encountered among HD accesses, and percutaneous embolization has also been applied to solve other access-related problems such as arterial "steal syndrome" and traumatic fistula formation adjacent to main AVG.

NONMATURED FISTULA

Anatomic Considerations

The ideal AVF is the one that can be easily cannulated, providing sufficient blood flow with satisfactory long-term patency. Objective parameters have been established to evaluate those characteristics, and they include minimal flow of 600 mL per minute, diameter bigger than 6 mm, and location approximately 6 mm from the skin surface.[4] To achieve these goals, quality of the vessels being used is a key factor. The minimum diameter before AVF creation for arteries should be 2.0 mm and for veins 2.5 mm, as shown by Wong et al.[5] who demonstrated that fistulas created with vessels smaller than 1.6 mm were associated with early failure. Also, too calcified arteries and/or preexisting focal venous/arterial stenoses can prevent fistula maturation.

The most common and preferred AVF is the radiocephalic fistula, which is created just above the wrist. The cephalic vein is cut and the portion going up to the forearm is anastomosed to the side of the radial artery in an end-to-side anastomosis. The distal end directed to the hand is then ligated. The second most used AVF is the brachiocephalic fistula, created just above the elbow. Again, this is an end-to-side anastomosis, in which the proximal end of the cephalic vein is anastomosed to the side of the brachial artery. The distal cephalic vein is ligated. Finally, the least common AVF is the brachiobasilic fistula, in which the end of the basilic vein is anastomosed to the side of the brachial artery. Because the basilic vein has a deep course, it needs to be mobilized to the subcutaneous tissue where it can be easily accessed.

Pathophysiology

Basically, fistula creation bypasses a high-resistance vascular bed, diverting blood flow toward a low-resistance venous circuit, which is now receiving "arterialized" inflow. In response to this new environment, progressive arterial and vein dilation are expected over time to accommodate this high blood volume in this new low-resistance system. Initially, vein dilation results from the increased blood pressure within it. In addition, a second component plays an important role and that is called *beneficial vascular remodeling*.[6,7]

In this process, the increased blood flow induces an increased longitudinal shear stress against the vein wall, and this promotes endothelial cell quiescence and secretion of anti-inflammatory and anticoagulant agents. This will, ultimately, result in vein dilation and reduction in neointimal hyperplasia.

On the other hand, reduction in both blood flow and longitudinal shear stress leads to endothelial cell activation and release of inflammatory and procoagulant factors, which will result in neointimal hyperplasia and vasoconstriction, an opposite process called *negative vascular remodeling*. Another important part of this process is the degree of medial hypertrophy, which is determined mainly by the transmural pressure. It has been demonstrated that increased intraluminal pressure activates smooth muscle cells, cytokine expression, and production of extracellular matrix components.[8] The final result is thickening of the muscular layer of the vessel wall. Therefore, fistula final lumen diameter is determined by the combination of three components: vein dilation, neointimal hyperplasia, and medial hypertrophy. Most of the times, lumen loss due to intimal hyperplasia and medial hypertrophy is compensated by vein dilation, and the final diameter is large enough to promote the necessary blood flow for an efficient dialysis.

Blood flow through the fistula is the major determinant of beneficial vascular remodeling and, in consequence, fistula maturation. Some anatomic problems can prevent adequate flow within the fistula, halting fistula development, and the most common are stenotic lesions and presence of accessory veins.[9] According to Beathard et al.,[9] outflow venous stenosis is found in 78% of the patients with a failed-to-mature fistula, and presence of accessory veins is found in 46% of patients. In these scenarios, percutaneous balloon angioplasty has been proven to be a useful tool in facilitating fistula maturation and, more recently, accessory vein embolization has become a valuable option.

CLINICAL APPLICATIONS

Nonmatured Arteriovenous Fistula Embolization

It has been confirmed that presence of accessory veins is the second most anatomic factor that prevents fistula maturation.[9,10] In the setting of an AVF, accessory veins divert flow from the main venous channel, which in turn reduces the resistance and blood flow within the venous segment above the branch(es). Flow reduction leads to decreased longitudinal shear stress, which triggers negative vascular remodeling, causing exacerbated neointimal hyperplasia and vasoconstriction. Ultimately, AVF maturation may be compromised. According to Turmel-Rodrigues et al.,[11] filling of an accessory vein would not be a cause of poor fistula maturation but only a consequence of an underlying outflow venous stenosis, therefore vein obliteration would not be necessary as long as the stenotic lesion is fixed. Nonetheless, Beathard et al.[10] in their series of 100 patients described 12 failed fistulas in which isolated accessory veins without outflow stenoses were the only anatomic culprit factors. All of them were obliterated with 100% success rate. Accordingly, other series have shown that accessory vein obliteration was effective in promoting fistula maturation.[12,13]

Thus, obliteration of those accessory veins has been applied when AVF fails to mature despite venous stenosis correction or when those accessory channels are the only anatomic abnormality. Initially, vein ligation was the only option. For that, after fistulography, accessory vein location is identified and marked on the skin surface. A small incision is made and after fluoroscopic vein visualization, ligation is performed with 4-0 silk and the skin incision is closed with 4-0 sutures. A less invasive technique has been described without skin incision using two 2-0 polypropylene sutures and inserting the needles into the skin adjacent to the vein and advancing them under the accessory vein until they reach the skin on the opposite side. The notches are then set on the skin surface and ligation is confirmed with a fistulogram. With these techniques, successful fistula maturation has been described as high as 100% with the first technique[9] and 88 % with the last one.[12]

Vein ligation is an excellent option for superficial veins as they can be easily reached with a small surgical incision or even transcutaneously. For deeper veins, ligation is not well suited as damage to muscles, nerves, or tendons can occur. For that location, embolization is a better option because these veins can be selectively catheterized and then occluded. On the other hand, coil embolization of very superficial veins can lead to skin irritation/erosion given the close proximity between the embolic agent and cutaneous tissue (Fig. 28.1).

Embolization has been found to be a valid option by Nikam et al.,[13] who treated dysfunctional fistulas with coil embolization alone or in combination with angioplasty when necessary, achieving fistula maturation in 10 out of 14 patients. The technique for fistula embolization has been previously described, with the use of pushable fibered coils as the preferred embolic device.[14] To prevent distal coil migration,

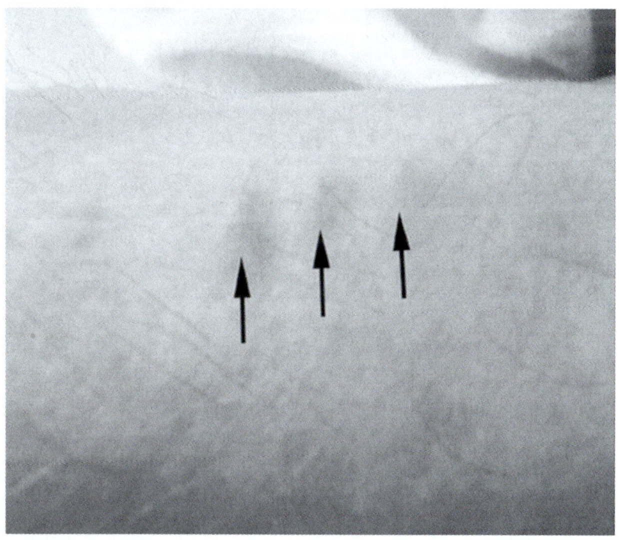

Figure 28.1 Cutaneous deformity (*black arrows*) from recent coil embolization of a superficial vein, which can lead to skin irritation/erosion.

at least 2-mm upsizing should be applied and, ideally, compact packing should be obtained to occlude flow efficiently (Fig. 28.2). Another important technical point is to maintain a safe distance from the point of embolization and the main outflow vein. There should be at least 5-mm distance to avoid outflow vein stenosis due to postembolization inflammatory reaction and also to prevent misplacement of the embolic agent within the main outflow vein (Fig. 28.3).

Other options of embolic devices, taking into consideration a more controlled deployment, are detachable coils and

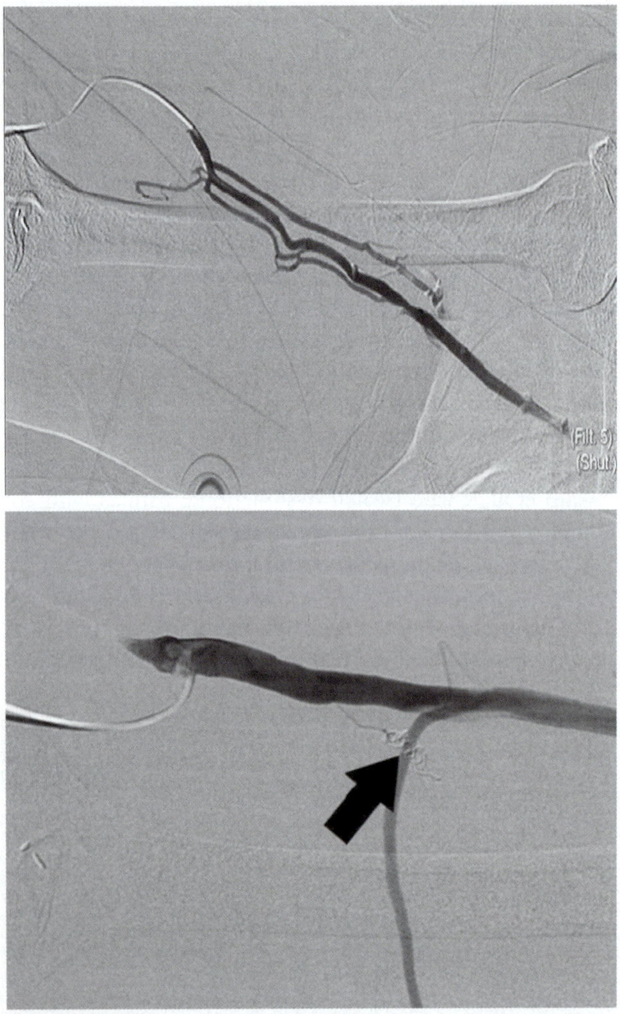

A

B

Figure 28.2 **A:** Nonmaturing fistula characterized by reduced caliber of the main outflow vein and multiple collateral pathways in the upper arm. **B:** Venogram post coil embolization of one of the collateral veins (*black arrow*). Note the point of embolization at a safe distance from the main outflow vessel, avoiding compromise. Also, note absence of flow within the embolized vessel and prevention of distal migration, giving correct coil oversizing. (From Rajan DK, ed. *Essentials in Percutaneous Dialysis Interventions*. Dordrecht, The Netherlands: Springer; 2011:323–339.)

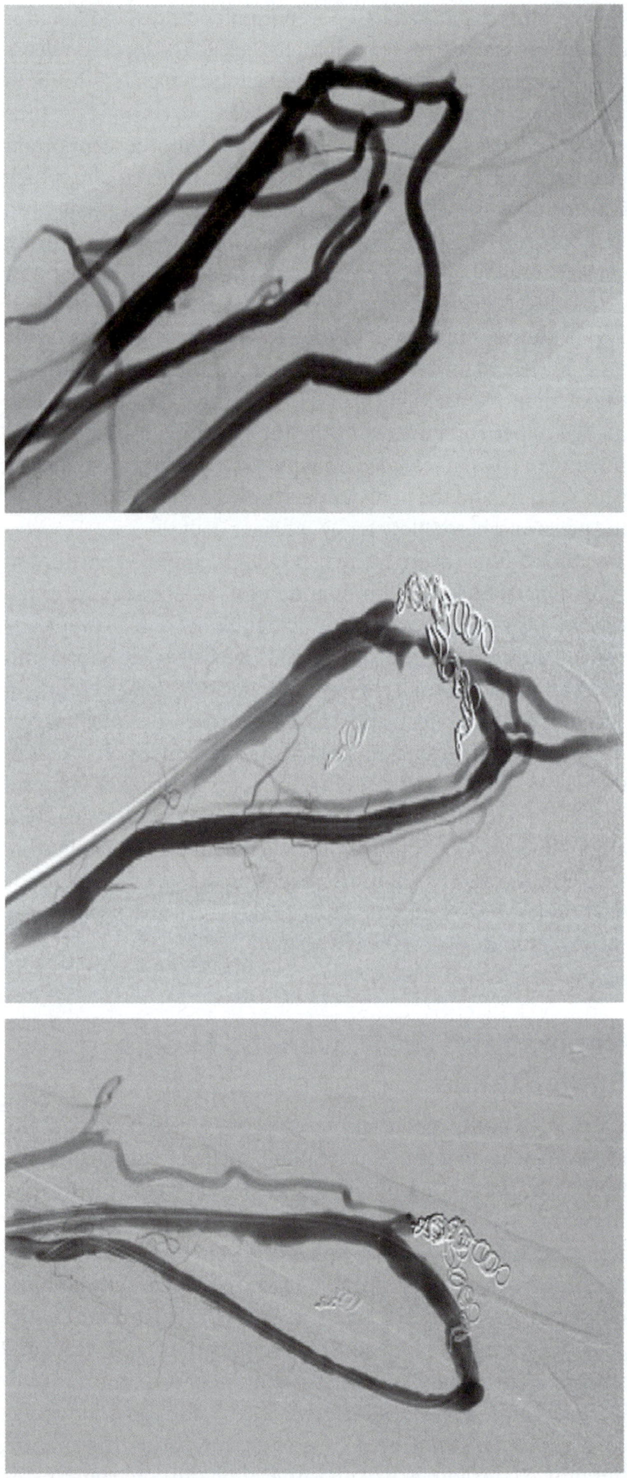

A

B

C

Figure 28.3 **A:** Nonmaturing fistula with multiple collateral veins. **B:** Follow-up venogram a few weeks after coil embolization of two collateral veins showing narrowing of the main outflow vessel due to peri-inflammatory reaction associated with coil deployment in its proximity. **C:** Venogram post balloon angioplasty demonstrating caliber and flow improvement of the previous narrowed segment. Note persistent occlusion of both embolized collateral vessels.

the Amplatzer Vascular Plug (St. Jude Medical, Inc., St. Paul, Minnesota). Powell et al.[15] reported using the Amplatzer Vascular Plug to occlude a tributary vein that was diverting flow from the cephalic vein and preventing fistula maturation. This device is made of a self-expandable nitinol mesh that expands within the vessel, achieving the necessary wall apposition. This helps secure the device in place, avoiding distal embolization. For that, the manufacturer advises 30% to 50% upsizing to achieve ideal wall apposition and safe deployment. In addition, the delivery mechanism permits deployment, retrieval/reposition, and redeployment of the plug, if necessary. The second generation of the device, the Amplatzer Vascular Plug II, is believed to promote faster vessel occlusion compared with the first generation[15] due to increased surface area and thrombogenicity. The device size varies from 3 to 22 mm, which requires up to a 7-Fr sheath or 9-Fr guiding catheter. The latest generation, the Amplatzer Vascular Plug 4, has a low-profile system, allowing delivery of up to a 8-mm plug through a 5-Fr diagnostic catheter.

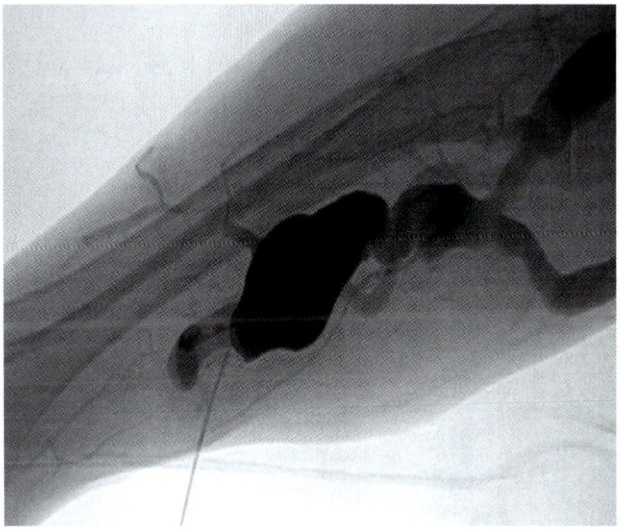

Figure 28.4 Radiocephalic fistula with total blood flow diversion from the radial artery into the fistula and complete absence of antegrade flow distally. This patient was completely asymptomatic regarding hand perfusion, given adequate blood supply through the ulnar artery.

Embolization for Steal Syndrome

Steal syndrome occurs when the AVF prevents adequate blood supply to the hand. It is a rare complication and its incidence ranges from 1.7% to 8%, depending on multiple factors, with fistula location being a major factor.[16] AVFs at the level of the elbow have higher incidence of steal syndrome compared with the ones located on the wrist. Symptoms and signs include numbing, tingling, pain, and weakness; decreased temperature; and diminished pulses. In severe cases, ulceration can occur. A high index of suspicion should be maintained as those signs and symptoms may be nonspecific and misinterpreted as diabetic neuropathy.

Initially after fistula creation, there is reduction of the distal tissue perfusion, which in turn induces collateral circulation development and peripheral vasodilation. These compensatory mechanisms in combination with a competent ulnar artery and palmar arch permit adequate tissue perfusion in most cases. Unfortunately, in a minority of patients, the hemodynamic changes after AVF creation are not adequately compensated by those mechanisms, leading to insufficient distal blood perfusion to meet the metabolic requirements.

This new hemodynamic environment is part of the complex pathophysiology of steal syndrome, in which the major determinant is the difference between fistula's resistance and the resistance of the hand's capillary circulation. Because fistula resistance is lower than the resistance of the distal capillary bed, most or even all blood from the donor artery will be diverted into the AVF, but that should not be an issue, as the ulnar artery and the palmar arch can guarantee adequate hand perfusion (Figs. 28.4 and 28.5A).

However, lack of blood supply can result from either insufficient antegrade blood flow or complete retrograde flow in the artery distal to the fistula.[17] The first uncompensated scenario occurs when decreased or absent antegrade flow in the donor artery distal to the fistula is not compensated by a diseased ulnar artery and/or incompetent palmar arch (Fig. 28.5B). A second scenario takes place when fistula's resistance is so low that not only the whole blood flow from the donor artery is diverted into the outflow vein but also the flow from the ulnar artery, which is directed into the fistula through the palmar arch and distal donor artery in a retrograde fashion (Fig. 28.5C). The last scenario occurs when a proximal stenosis in the donor artery is present, preventing adequate distal flow to the extremity, which is more common in upper arm fistulas (Figs. 28.5D and 28.6A).

Depending on the underlying cause, different treatment strategies should be applied, and arteriography plays an important role in understanding flow dynamics in each particular patient. For example, proximal stenosis in the donor artery can be managed with balloon angioplasty alone (Fig. 28.6). When distal retrograde flow (as shown in Fig. 28.5C) is the underlying problem, surgical or endovascular approaches can be performed.

Initially, surgical strategies aimed to increase fistula resistance by banding, plicating, or lengthening were attempted. Unfortunately, those techniques have been shown to be of little help and were associated with increased risk of fistula thrombosis.[18] In 1988, Schanzer et al.[19] described a new surgical technique consisting of ligation of the artery distal to the fistula and creation of a distal bypass, the so-called distal revascularization and interval ligation (DRIL) procedure. In consequence, resistance ratio between the fistula and peripheral circulation is decreased.[19] This technique has been validated by other authors with series of cases demonstrating symptom resolution and preserved fistula patency.[20]

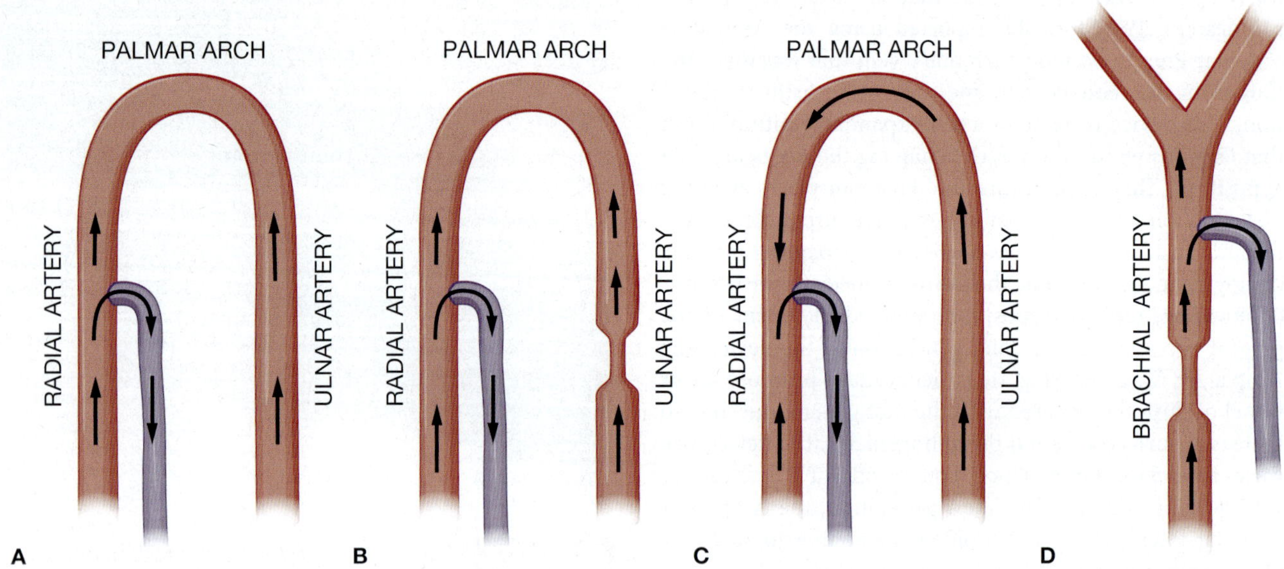

Figure 28.5 **A:** Normal fistula flow pattern with sufficient antegrade distal blood flow from the radial and ulnar arteries. **B:** Stenotic lesion in the ulnar artery and insufficient antegrade flow from the radial artery, preventing adequate tissue perfusion distally. **C:** Very low-resistance fistula. In this situation, total blood flow from the radial artery and ulnar artery are diverted into the fistula through the palmar arch and distal radial artery in a retrograde fashion. **D:** Brachiocephalic fistula. Stenotic lesion in the brachial artery proximal to the fistula leading to insufficient blood flow distally.

Recently, Plumb et al.[21] described a less invasive approach using coil embolization to prevent retrograde flow from the distal arterial into the AVF. In their report, a 46-year-old patient with a radiocephalic fistula presented with steal syndrome, and arteriography showed retrograde flow within the distal radial artery as well as in some collateral arterial vessels. The radial artery distal to the fistula and those collateral vessels were embolized with fibered coils during three different sessions, and the patient remained asymptomatic after 6 months follow-up. According to them, the advantage of the endovascular approach was the possibility of collateral circulation embolization, which was contributing to the steal syndrome and would not be suited for surgical ligation. Since then, other case reports have demonstrated use of coil embolization in treating these patients,[22,23] accomplishing 100% symptom relief. In addition, Miller et

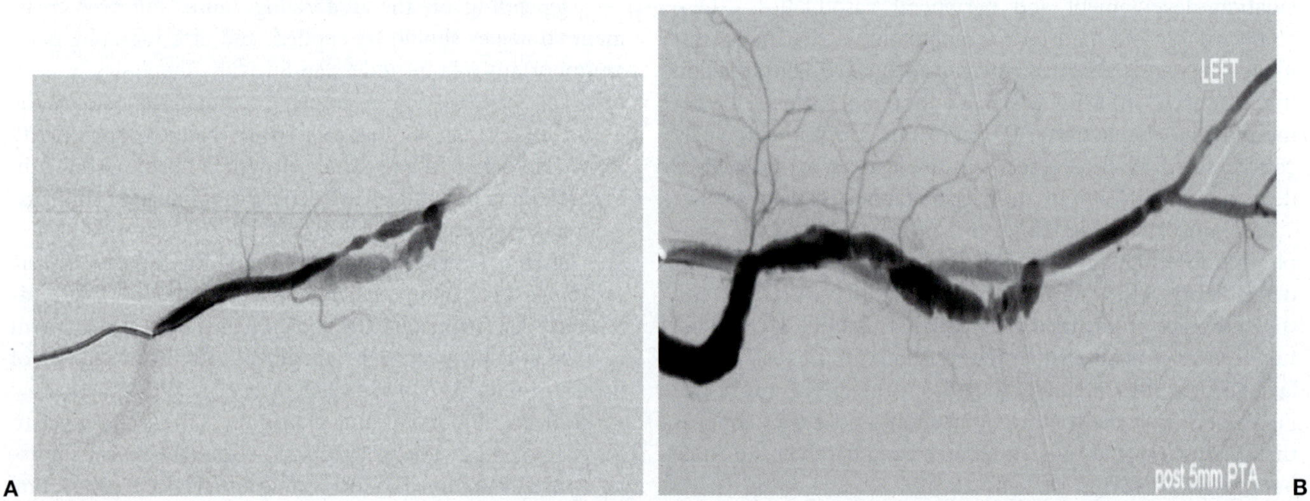

Figure 28.6 **A:** Upper extremity arteriogram showing significant stenosis in the brachial artery proximal to the fistula and lack of sufficient arterial flow distally. Patient was complaining of left hand pain and numbness exacerbated during dialysis. **B:** Arteriogram post angioplasty with a 5-mm balloon demonstrated caliber improvement and satisfactory distal arterial blood supply.

al.[22] suggested that coil embolization was preferred over arterial ligation as first-line therapy as it is safe, effective, and a quicker alternative.

Another endovascular technique that has been described to treat steal syndrome is coil embolization of deep collateral drainage veins.[24] This is based on the concept that collateral veins impose lower fistula resistance and occluding these collateral channels would increase system resistance, which in turn decreases blood shunt. Kariya et al.[24] have successfully demonstrated effectiveness of this approach when dealing with deep accessory veins not suitable for future dialysis access. In their series of five patients, pushable coils were used in four patients and detachable coils were used in one patient based on location and flow velocity, adding more safety to the procedure.[24] Especially in this high flow velocity environment, one should always consider the use of detachable coils.

In more unusual and extreme situations associated with severe symptoms, based on case-by-case analysis, complete access occlusion is required due to failure of more conservative options or when dialysis is not required anymore.[15,25,26] Traditionally, surgical ligation is the preferable option, but in some circumstances, such as presence of extensive ischemic changes and/or arm swelling, surgery is not always possible. In these cases, the fistula can be closed by endovascular methods.

Coils and *N*-butyl cyanoacrylate (NBCA) have been used for this purpose, and more recently, the Amplatzer Vascular Plug device became another option. Combined use of these embolic devices has also been reported.[26,27] Regardless of the chosen embolic agent, precise deployment should be done as close as possible to the arterial anastomotic site without extending into the artery to avoid both aneurysm formation in the remnant venous stump and thrombosis of the arterial side. To achieve this goal, some important maneuvers and/or tools can be applied, such as external compression of the outflow vein until complete flow stasis, inflation of an occlusion balloon, and use of embolic agents with controlled delivery system, such as detachable coils and the Amplatzer Vascular Plug. In fact, the vascular plug allows for very precise deployment, which can be performed under road mapping and/or ultrasound guidance,[26] with the possibility of retrieval and redeployment in case of inappropriate position.

Traumatic Fistula Embolization

Fistulous connections between the AVG and nearby native veins do not have a well-known incidence, with limited literature reporting an incidence ranging from 0.027% to 9% (Fig. 28.7).[28,29] Their formation is related to repeated needle punctures and/or pseudoaneurysm rupture in a setting of high intragraft pressure due to an outflow venous stenosis.[30]

Most of the time, a graft-to-vein fistula (GVF) is an asymptomatic condition without clinical significance. Nonetheless, in some circumstances, these abnormal communications can result in decreased access flow,

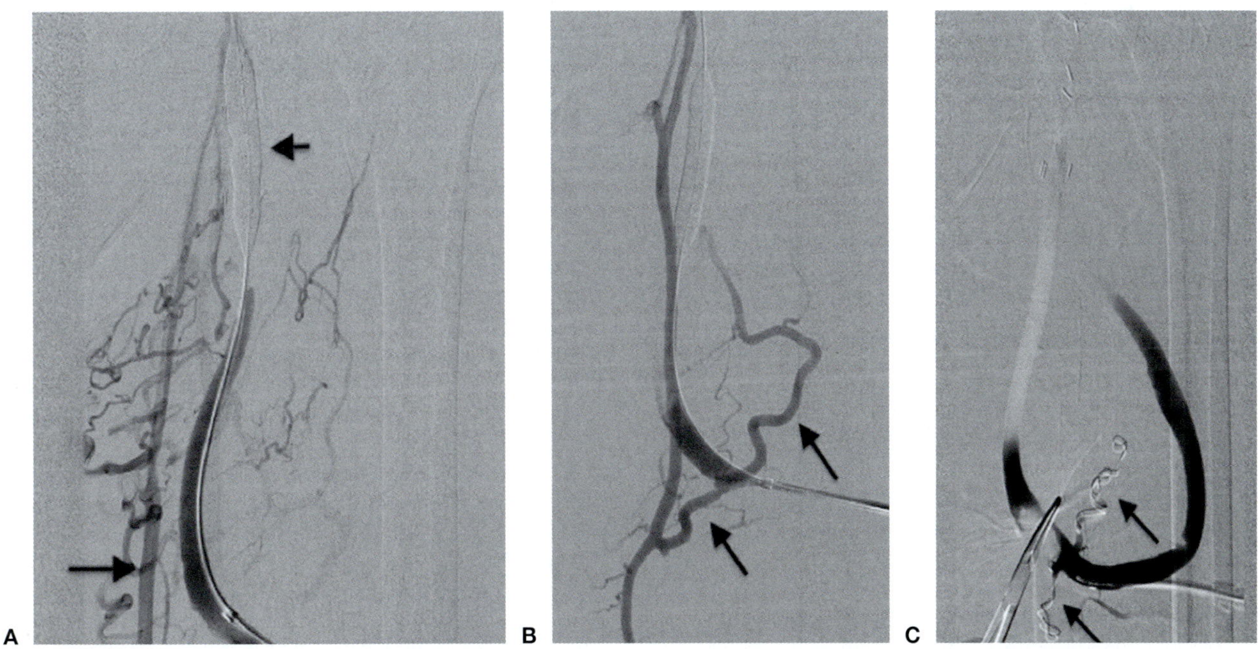

A B C

Figure 28.7 **A:** Patient with a left thigh graft presenting with painful lower extremity swelling for the past 6 months. Contrast injection through a vascular sheath with an inflated angioplasty balloon within the distal portion of the graft (*short arrow*) demonstrates multiple small GVFs and retrograde opacification of the great saphenous vein (*long arrow*). **B:** Contrast injection showing two important GVFs coming off the graft (*black arrows*). **C:** Postembolization image confirming successful occlusion of the two GVFs and mash of deployed coils (*black arrows*).

decreased HD adequacy, and increased risk of graft thrombosis.[30] Clinically, some patients can present with palpable thrill on the arterial limb only and dilated superficial veins on the forearm (or the thigh in patients with groin loop grafts), indicating that the venous limb is likely thrombosed and the flow is maintained through the fistulous connections.[28] This situation can be associated with difficult graft cannulation during dialysis, poor clearance, and upper/lower extremity edema.

In such cases, intervention is required, and treatment of the outflow venous stenosis/occlusion, which is almost always present, is mandatory. In fact, balloon angioplasty and/or stent placement might be the only necessary treatment modalities, as normalization of intragraft pressure can result in closure of fistulous communication.[31] In situations when angioplasty is not sufficient or presence of the abnormal communication is the only problem, closure of the fistula is required. That can be achieved by surgical ligation as described by Min et al.[32] or percutaneous coil embolization as described by Harris.[33]

Given the rarity of this entity and yet unclear clinical significance, necessity of GVF closure is still not well established. Recently, Margoles et al.[34] described a case series of 12 patients with GVF in whom coil embolization was performed in 5 of them. Together with the previous experience in the literature, the authors proposed an algorithm to clarify the need for GVF closure based on presence of stenosis, arm swelling/partial thrombosis, and flow measurements. Basically, patients with symptoms and/or inadequate access flow, who did not respond to angioplasty or who did not present with outflow stenosis, should have their GVF closed.[34]

TIPS AND TRICKS

Tips

- Do not extend the coil to the collateral/vein interface. The inflammatory reaction may cause stenosis of the AVF.
- Consider embolization of venous collaterals only when areas of stenosis have been excluded, including the inflow artery within nonmaturing AVFs.
- Err on the side of shorter coil length used rather than longer coils to prevent extension into the vascular access.
- Amplatzer Vascular Plug use should be reserved for deep vein and prosthetic graft embolization.

Tricks

- To prevent forward migration of a coil, anchoring the leading edge within a branch vein helps secure the location.
- When using embolization coils, to pack the coil properly, rotate the catheter and gently pull back slowly as you pack the coil.

CONCLUSION

Percutaneous interventions to dialysis accesses such a balloon angioplasty and mechanical thrombectomy are very well-established and widely used tools to increase access functionality and durability. Embolization has become another important tool in the armamentarium of percutaneous techniques in treating different problems related to dialysis access, as shown in this chapter. Proper knowledge of malfunctioning access pathophysiology and hemodynamics as well as familiarity with embolization technique and different available devices are crucial for successful outcomes.

REFERENCES

1. National Kidney and Urologic Diseases Information Clearinghouse. Kidney disease statistics for the United States. National Institute of Diabetes and Digestive and Kidney Diseases, National Institutes of Health Web site. http://kidney.niddk.nih.gov/kudiseases/pubs/kustats/#7. Published 2012. Updated November 15, 2012. Accessed May 13, 2013.
2. Navuluri R, Regalado S. The KDOQI 2006 Vascular Access update and Fistula First program synopsis. *Semin Intervent Radiol.* 2009;26(2):122–124.
3. Allon M, Robbin ML. Increasing arterio-venous fistulas in hemodialysis patients: problems and solutions. *Kidney Int.* 2002; 62(4):1109–1124.
4. Vascular Access 2006 Work Group. Clinical practice guidelines for vascular access. *Am J Kidney Dis.* 2006;48(suppl 1): S176–S247.
5. Wong V, Ward R, Taylor J, et al. Factors associated with early failure of arterio-venous fistulae for haemodialysis access. *Eur J Vasc Endovasc Surg.* 1996;12(2):207–213.
6. Dixon BS. Why don't fistulas mature? *Kidney Int.* 2006;70(8): 1413–1422.
7. Roy-Chaudhury P, Spergel LM, Besarab A, et al. Biology of arterio-venous fistula failure. *J Nephrol.* 2007;20(2):150–163.
8. Lehoux S, Castier Y, Tedgui A. Molecular mechanisms of the vascular responses to haemodynamic forces. *J Intern Med.* 2006;259(4):381–392.
9. Beathard GA, Arnold P, Jackson J, et al; for the Physician Operators Forum of RMS Lifeline. Aggressive treatment of early fistula failure. *Kidney Int.* 2003;64(4):1487–1494.
10. Beathard GA, Settle SM, Shields MW. Salvage of the nonfunctioning arterio-venous fistula. *Am J Kidney Dis.* 1999;33(5): 910–916.
11. Turmel-Rodrigues L, Mouton A, Birmelé B, et al. Salvage of immature forearm fistulas for haemodialysis by interventional radiology. *Nephrol Dial Transplant.* 2001;16(12): 2365–2371.
12. Faiyaz R, Abreo K, Zaman F, et al. Salvage of poorly developed arterio-venous fistulae with percutaneous ligation of accessory veins. *Am J Kidney Dis.* 2002;39(4):824–827.
13. Nikam M, Popuri RK, Inaba A, et al. Arterio-venous fistula failure: is there a role for accessory draining vein embolization? *J Vasc Access.* 2012;13(4):498–503.
14. Rajan DK, ed. *Essentials in Percutaneous Dialysis Interventions.* Dordrecht, The Netherlands: Springer; 2011:323–339.

15. Powell S, Narlawar R, Odetoyinbo T, et al. Early experience with the Amplatzer Vascular Plug II for occlusive purposes in arterio-venous hemodialysis access. *Cardiovasc Intervent Radiol.* 2010;33(1):150–156.
16. Zibari GB, Rohr MS, Landreneau MD, et al. Complications from permanent hemodialysis vascular access. *Surgery.* 1988; 104(4):681–686.
17. Wixon CL, Hughes JD, Mills JL. Understanding strategies for the treatment of ischemic steal syndrome after hemodialysis access. *J Am Coll Surg.* 2000;191(3):301–310.
18. De Caprio JD, Valentine RJ, Kakish HB, et al. Steal syndrome complicating hemodialysis access. *Cardiovasc Surg.* 1997;5(6): 648–653.
19. Schanzer H, Schwartz M, Harrington E, et al. Treatment of ischemia due to "steal" by arterio-venous fistula with distal artery ligation and revascularization. *J Vasc Surg.* 1988;7(6):770–773.
20. Wixon CL, Mills JL Sr, Berman SS. Distal revascularization-interval ligation for maintenance of dialysis access and restoration of distal perfusion in ischemic steal syndrome. *Semin Vasc Surg.* 2000;13(1):77–82.
21. Plumb TJ, Lynch TG, Adelson AB. Treatment of steal syndrome in a distal radiocephalic arterio-venous fistula using intravascular coil embolization. *J Vasc Surg.* 2008;47(2):457–459.
22. Miller GA, Khariton K, Kardos SV, et al. Flow interruption of the distal radial artery: treatment for finger ischemia in a matured radio-cephalic AVF. *J Vasc Access.* 2008;9(1):58–63.
23. Shukla PA, Contractor S, Huang JT, et al. Coil embolization as a treatment alternative for dialysis-associated steal syndrome. *Vasc Endovascular Surg.* 2012;46(7):546–549.
24. Kariya S, Tanigawa N, Kojima H, et al. Transcatheter coil embolization for steal syndrome in patients with hemodialysis access. *Acta Radiol.* 2009;50(1):28–33.
25. Bui JT, Gaba RC, Knuttinen MG, et al. Amplatzer vascular plug for arterio-venous hemodialysis access occlusion: initial experience. *J Vasc Access.* 2009;10(1):5–10.
26. Ozyer U, Harman A, Aytekin C, et al. Application of the AMPLATZER vascular plug in endovascular occlusion of dialysis accesses. *Cardiovasc Intervent Radiol.* 2009;32(5):967–973.
27. Owens CA, Bui JT, West DL, et al. Use of the Amplatzer Vascular Plug as a coil constrainer during endovascular occlusion of a dialysis shunt. *Cardiovasc Intervent Radiol.* 2007;30(4):754–756.
28. Standage BA, Schuman ES, Quinn SF, et al. Single limb patency of polytetrafluoroethylene dialysis loop grafts maintained by traumatic fistulization. *Ann Vasc Surg.* 1998;12(4):364–369.
29. Dousset V, Grenier N, Douws C, et al. Hemodialysis grafts: color Doppler flow imaging correlated with digital subtraction angiography and functional status. *Radiology.* 1991;181(1):89–94.
30. Haddad NJ, Vachharajani TJ, Van Cleef S, et al. Iatrogenic graft to vein fistula (GVF) formation associated with synthetic arterio-venous grafts. *Semin Dial.* 2010;23(6):643–647.
31. Kanterman RY, Vesely TM. Graft-to-vein fistulas associated with polytetrafluoroethylene dialysis grafts: diagnosis and clinical significance. *J Vasc Interv Radiol.* 1995;6(2):267–271.
32. Min SK, Park YH, Lee HH, et al. Iatrogenic fistula between prosthetic haemodialysis access graft and autogenous vein: unusual cause of graft thrombosis. *Nephrol Dial Transplant.* 2004;19(10):2647–2649.
33. Harris V. Percutaneous coil embolization of an iatrogenic fistula from a polytetrafluoroethylene dialysis shunt to the superficial venous system. *J Vasc Interv Radiol.* 1993;8:138–141.
34. Margoles HR, Shlansky-Goldberg RD, Soulen MC, et al. A proposed management algorithm for fistulae between hemodialysis access circuits and adjacent veins. *J Vasc Access.* 2012;13(3): 374–380.

Section F Gastrointestinal Arterial Embolization

29

Upper Gastrointestinal Bleeding

Rakesh C. Navuluri • Brian Funaki

Approximately 100,000 cases of upper gastrointestinal bleeding require inpatient admission annually in the United States. When medical management and endoscopic therapy are inadequate, endovascular intervention can be lifesaving. This chapter begins with a brief review of the preangiographic workup of patients with upper gastrointestinal bleeding. This will be followed by a detailed discussion of the angiographic technique, including a closer look at the use of various embolic agents. The primary focus will be on nonvariceal (arterial) hemorrhage with brief consideration given to variceal (venous) hemorrhage.

BACKGROUND

Upper gastrointestinal bleeding (UGIB) is defined by a bleeding source proximal to the ligament of Treitz. UGIB accounts for 76% of gastrointestinal (GI) bleeding events.[1] The incidence of UGIB in the United States is estimated at 102 per 100,000 per year, with a mortality rate of 5% based on data from 1991.[2] UGIB can be divided into arterial (nonvariceal) and venous (variceal) etiologies. This is an important point of differentiation and a major branch in the management decision tree. Causes of arterial UGIB include peptic ulcer disease (up to 40%), Mallory-Weiss tear (15%), hemorrhagic gastritis, pancreatitis-related pseudoaneurysms, neoplasm, aortoduodenal fistula, and trauma. Other rare causes of arterial UGIB include hemobilia from iatrogenic injury and hemosuccus pancreaticus related to chronic pancreatitis. Venous causes include variceal bleeding secondary to portal venous hypertension (e.g., due to cirrhosis or Budd-Chiari syndrome) or splenic vein thrombosis (Table 29.1).

Symptoms

Typical UGIB symptoms include hematemesis or melena. Hematochezia, although commonly attributed to lower GI sources, can also occur depending on the bleeding rate and transit time of blood through the bowel. Patients with nonvariceal bleeding commonly present with coffee-ground emesis and history of nonsteroidal anti-inflammatory drug use. Variceal bleeding is likely to present with clinical signs of cirrhosis, painless hematemesis, and a greater degree of hemodynamic instability.

Algorithm

Current treatment algorithms call for immediate medical stabilization followed by endoscopic diagnosis and intervention. Refractory cases should be referred for either transvenous or transarterial endovascular intervention, depending on the source of bleeding identified at endoscopy. Although surgery is generally considered the last option, endovascular intervention may be reattempted following failed surgery.

Medical

Stabilization of blood pressure is the immediate objective in managing patients with UGIB. Fluid resuscitation should be instituted without delay. Patients with hemodynamically significant bleeding should also be immediately typed and crossed to allow for transfusion of blood products as necessary. The goal of transfusion in this setting is to raise the hemoglobin level above 7 g/dL. Any existing coagulopathy (international normalized ratio [INR] >1.5 or platelet count <50,000/μL) should also be corrected.[3] It is important to

Table 29.1 Etiology of Upper Gastrointestinal Bleeding

Arterial (Nonvariceal)	Venous (Variceal)
Peptic ulcer disease	Cirrhosis
Mallory-Weiss tear	Budd-Chiari syndrome
Hemorrhagic gastritis	Splenic vein thrombosis
Neoplasm	
Inflammatory pseudoaneurysms	
Aortoduodenal fistula	
Iatrogenic injury	
Trauma	
Hemobilia	
Hemosuccus pancreaticus	

note that units of packed red blood cells (pRBCs) do not contain the factors and platelets needed for thrombogenesis. If these are not replaced during large-volume blood transfusions, a dilutional coagulopathy will result, which may affect the success of subsequent embolization procedures.

Insertion of a nasogastric tube can help to confirm an upper GI source of bleeding. If variceal bleeding is suspected, a Minnesota tube (or Sengstaken-Blakemore tube) can be placed to tamponade esophageal varices. It has been reported to have variable success in achieving hemostasis but is a good option in stabilizing patients in the emergent setting before interventional procedures.

An estimated 10% to 15% of cases require intervention beyond medical management to control bleeding.[4] To help sustain the success of subsequent interventional procedures, various medication regimens may be instituted. Administration of proton pump inhibitors (PPIs) have been shown to reduce the rate of rebleeding and surgery in high-risk patients with nonvariceal UGIB.[5] This is because hemostasis within the stomach and duodenum is impeded by low intragastric pH. Low pH has been shown to inhibit platelet function and activate pepsin, which disaggregates platelet plugs.[6] The use of portal pressure–reducing medications such as somatostatin, octreotide, or vasopressin can improve outcomes in patients with variceal UGIB.[7]

Endoscopy

Endoscopy should be the initial intervention as it allows for localization of bleeding and determination of etiology via visual inspection and biopsy. It can be particularly helpful in differentiating arterial and venous sources of hemorrhage. Endoscopy can also identify upper and midesophageal sources of bleeding that are not amenable to embolization such as esophagitis. Beyond its diagnostic use, endoscopy also offers several therapeutic options. Hemostasis can be achieved endoscopically via thermocoagulation, sclerosant injection, or clips (banding). Endoscopic clip placement, even if ineffectual, can aid subsequent endovascular intervention by directing the interventional radiologist to the area of concern.

Endoscopy performed within 24 hours of presentation is associated with improved patient outcome and decreased hospital stay. However, the source of bleeding may not be seen in up to 24% of patients at the first endoscopic exam.[8] Although endoscopic treatment is reported to be effective in 85% to 90% of patients,[9] repeat bleeding occurs in 15% to 20%, most commonly in the first 72 hours after treatment.[10] Endoscopic predictors of rebleeding include visualized active bleeding, nonbleeding visible vessel, adherent clot, ulcer size greater than 2 cm, and ulcer location in the posterior midgastric body or posterior duodenal bulb[11–13] (Table 29.2). Recurrent bleeding should be followed with a second endoscopic treatment before endovascular intervention is undertaken.[14] Further bleeding after a second endoscopic treatment should be referred to interventional radiology. Alternatively, the inability to visualize the bleeding source at endoscopy due to the severity of bleeding warrants urgent endovascular intervention.

Localization

Localization of bleeding before angiography is important for several reasons. First, it decreases procedure time by allowing for a more targeted approach. This consequently reduces radiation exposure as well as contrast load used during angiography. Minimizing contrast dose is critical in patients with borderline azotemia. Second, it has also been shown to directly impact the success rate of endovascular therapy.[15] Last, it permits empiric embolization to be undertaken even if active bleeding is not seen at angiography.

If the source of bleeding cannot be identified, angiography may be deferred. However, in the setting of hemodynamic instability or in patients requiring more than 5 units of pRBCs, angiography should be performed immediately. In these circumstances, angiography is the most practical diagnostic tool because it offers the option of concomitant therapy.[16] If the clinical situation permits, localization with computed tomography angiography may be considered before proceeding to conventional angiography.

Computed Tomography Angiography

Compared with conventional angiography, computed tomography angiography (CTA) has the advantage of greater availability, speed, and noninvasiveness. It also does not suffer from bowel or respiratory motion artifact. In an animal

Table 29.2 Endoscopic Predictors of Rebleeding

Visible active bleeding
Nonbleeding visible vessel
Adherent clot
Ulcer size greater than 2 cm
Ulcer location in posterior midgastric body or posterior duodenal bulb

model, CTA has been shown to detect bleeding rates as low as 0.3 mL per minute—better than conventional angiography.[17] No studies specific to UGIB have been performed to date, but a study by Yoon et al.[18] found CTA to have a sensitivity of 90.9%, a specificity of 99%, and an accuracy of 97.6% in localizing hemorrhage when considering both upper and lower GI sources. CTA, unlike conventional angiography, may also detect lesions, such as ulcers, masses and aneurysms, that are not bleeding at the time of the study. The ability to characterize the inciting lesion can have a significant impact on treatment planning. If, for example, a mass lesion is seen, particle embolization may be performed where it might otherwise be avoided in the treatment of GI hemorrhage to avoid bowel necrosis. CTA also has the benefit of providing information on the vascular anatomy for preinterventional planning. For example, a steep takeoff of the celiac artery may necessitate the use of a Waltman loop or even brachial artery access. Stenotic or tortuous mesenteric arteries indicate that a guiding catheter will be helpful. Similarly, occlusion of the celiac axis may require embolization of the pancreaticoduodenal arcade via the superior mesenteric artery (SMA) (Fig. 29.1).

CTA protocols are similar to those for endoleak evaluation. A noncontrast series is followed by intravenous contrast-enhanced series in arterial and delayed phases. A positive CTA study will show hyperdense contrast material (>90 HU) within the bowel lumen on the arterial

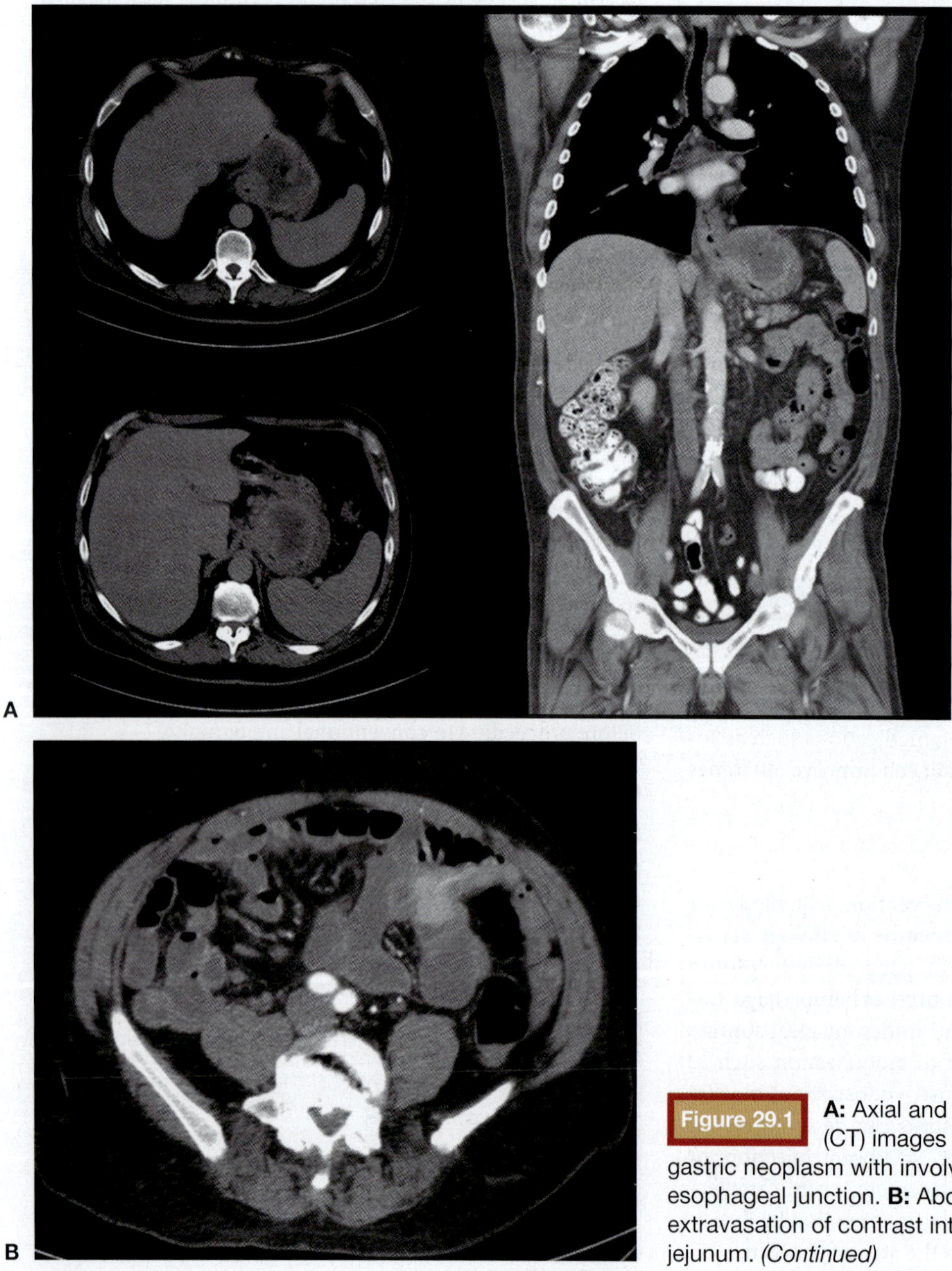

Figure 29.1 **A:** Axial and coronal computed tomography (CT) images of the abdomen demonstrate a gastric neoplasm with involvement of the fundus and gastroesophageal junction. **B:** Abdominal CTA demonstrating active extravasation of contrast into the lumen of the proximal jejunum. *(Continued)*

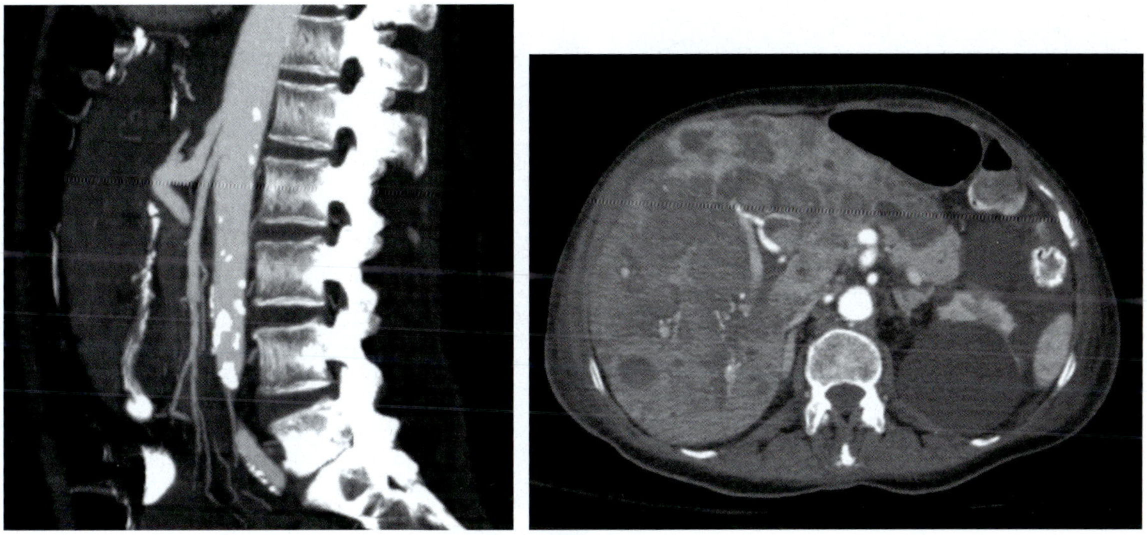

Figure 29.1 *(Continued)* **C:** Sagittal CT image of the abdomen demonstrating acute angulation of the celiac artery from the abdominal aorta. **D:** CT abdomen demonstrating an arteriobiliary fistula within the liver.

phase that increases on the delayed phase.[19] This provides up to a 90-second window of time to evaluate for contrast extravasation—depending on the timing of the delayed series—compared with a 10-second window of evaluation for conventional angiography. Oral contrast should *not* be given during the exam because it will obscure intravenous contrast extravasation into the bowel lumen.

The primary drawback of CTA is the necessity of intravenous iodinated contrast, which may elicit a hypersensitivity reaction or cause renal injury.[20] Typically, 1.5 mL/kg (up to 150 mL) is administered. This can be prohibitive in patients with poor renal function, particularly when considering the additional contrast required in a subsequent endovascular procedure. Radiation dose is another drawback to consider.

Nuclear Medicine

Radionuclide scintigraphy may be helpful in identifying sources of chronic GI bleeding, which are otherwise not detectable by endoscopy or conventional angiography. Technetium 99m (Tc-99m)–labeled red blood cell scans can detect bleeding rates as low as 0.2 mL per minute, compared with 0.5 mL per minute for angiography, and can be particularly useful in the setting of intermittent GI bleeding. Unlike angiography and CTA, bleeding scans allows for interrogation over a multiple-hour window, which increases sensitivity for detection of GI bleeding. In patients with hemodynamic instability, studies with an immediate tracer blush are more likely to have a positive angiogram than studies with a delayed blush.[21] It is worth noting that positive scintigrams can also occur in cases of variceal bleeding (Fig. 29.2).

In terms of localizing bleeding within the upper GI tract, nuclear medicine is limited by the low resolution of imaging as well as confounding factors such as uptake of free technetium by the gastric mucosa. Consequently, at our institution, we do not routinely recommend radionuclide scintigraphy for localizing the site of bleeding in the upper GI tract.

Once active hemorrhage is documented and localized with a diagnostic radiology study, patients should be transferred immediately to the angiography suite. At our institution, we strive to perform angiography within 1 hour of radiologic diagnosis of active GI bleeding.

Angiography Indications

The primary indication for conventional angiography is the inability to control the source of bleeding endoscopically. Angiography is favored over surgery as the treatment of choice after failed endoscopic therapy, particularly in high-risk surgical patients.[16] It is minimally invasive, associated with lower mortality,[22] and there has been shown to be no difference in outcome between patients managed with surgery versus arterial embolization.[23,24]

Angiography is also warranted in instances where the bleeding site cannot be identified by endoscopy or CTA and the patient is hemodynamically unstable as it may be lifesaving. Endovascular embolization is also the primary treatment for hepatobiliary bleeding.

Preangiography

Before angiography, the patient's renal and coagulation statuses should be assessed. Elevated partial thromboplastin time and prothrombin time/INR as well as thrombocytopenia should be corrected. Embolization is less likely to succeed in the setting of coagulopathy because the most common embolic agent used—coils—causes vessel obstruction by providing a scaffold for thrombus formation rather than by pure mechanical occlusion.[16] Furthermore, several studies

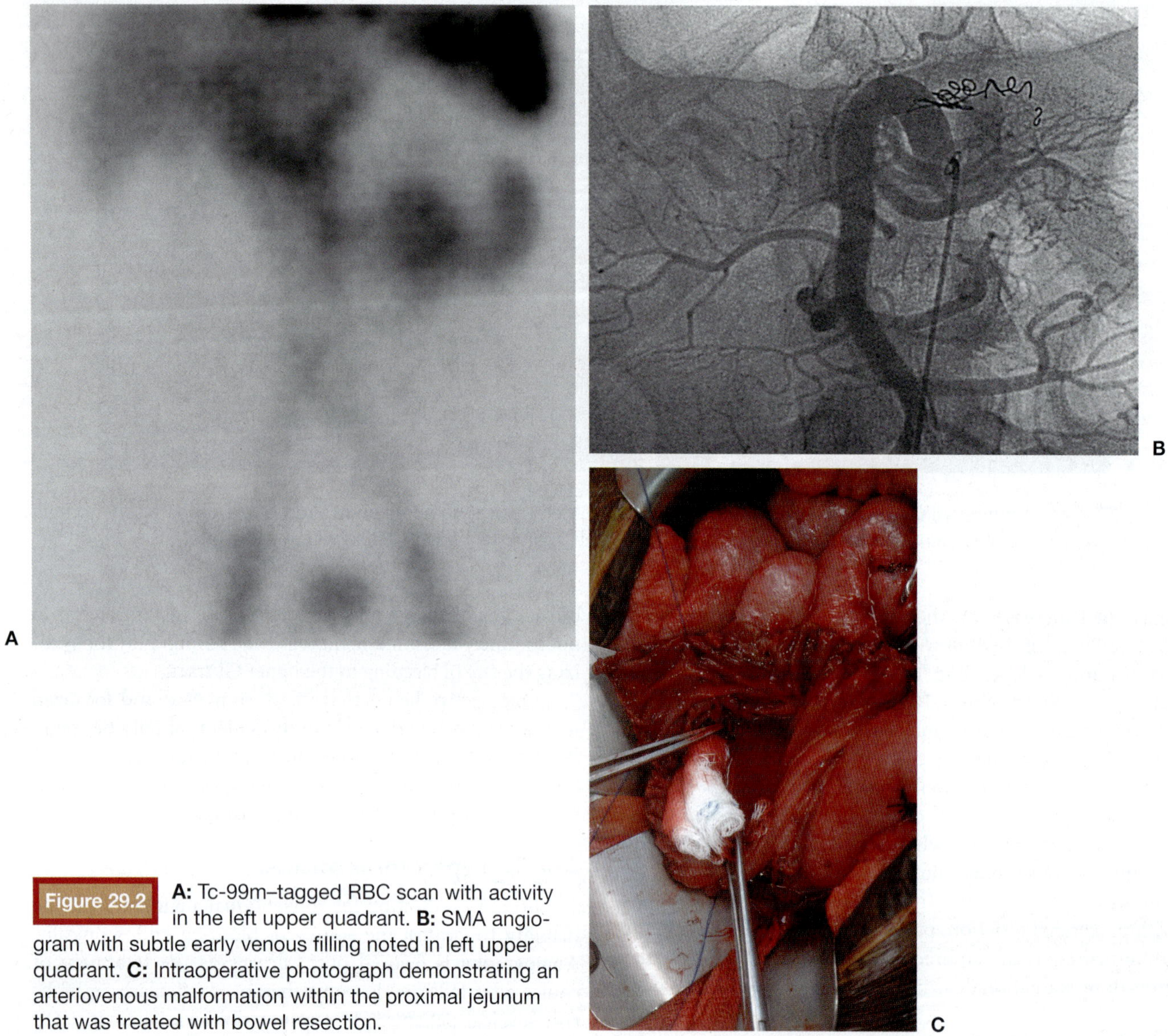

Figure 29.2 **A:** Tc-99m–tagged RBC scan with activity in the left upper quadrant. **B:** SMA angiogram with subtle early venous filling noted in left upper quadrant. **C:** Intraoperative photograph demonstrating an arteriovenous malformation within the proximal jejunum that was treated with bowel resection.

have demonstrated preinterventional coagulopathy to have a negative effect on clinical success.[25,26] Embolotherapy has been reported to be nearly three times more likely to fail in patients with coagulopathy.[27] If necessary, blood products may be given intraprocedurally to expedite the procedure.

Even in the setting of uncorrectable coagulopathy, embolization often remains the best option for treatment. In these scenarios, alternative embolic agents including placement of a Gelfoam sandwich or the application of glue or Onyx (Micro Therapeutics Inc., Irvine, California) may prove effective.

ANGIOGRAPHY AND EMBOLOTHERAPY

Review of imaging, such as CTA, before intervention can profoundly expedite cases by demonstrating vascular occlusions or variant anatomy. One should also consider the angle at which the mesenteric vessels arise from the aorta.

The right common femoral artery is the default access site for mesenteric angiography. We begin with a mapping aortogram to obtain a survey of the vascular anatomy. This is helpful in identifying the ostia of the mesenteric vessels and in guiding subsequent catheter selection. This step takes only a few minutes to accomplish and can save valuable time later on in the procedure. If recent imaging of the vascular anatomy is available, either as a CTA or conventional angiogram, an initial aortogram can be skipped in favor of a selective mesenteric angiogram to decrease contrast load in patients with poor renal function or to expedite the procedure. Contrast extravasation is rarely visible on the mapping aortogram. We use a 5-Fr nonmarking pigtail catheter (Cook Medical Inc., Bloomington, Indiana) placed through a 5-Fr

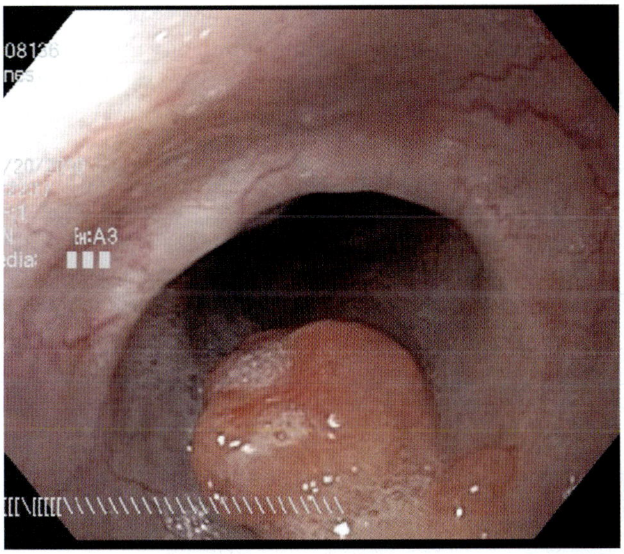

A

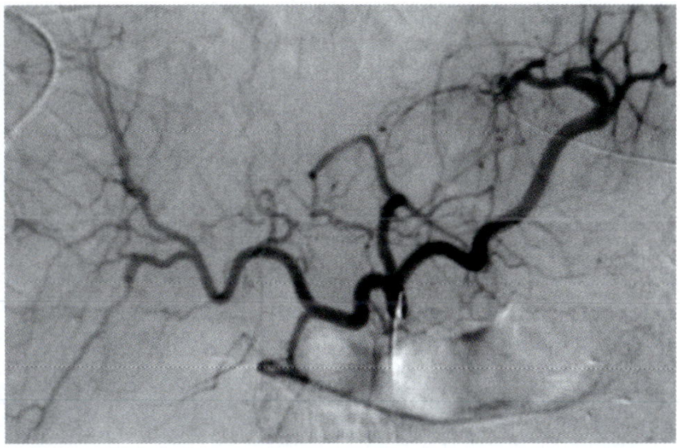

B

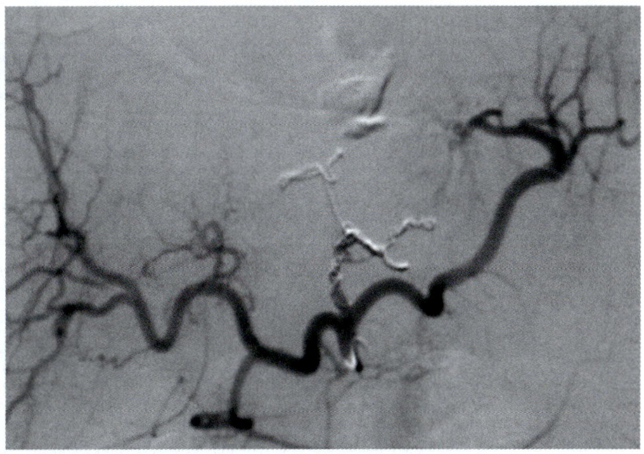

C

Figure 29.3 **A:** Esophagogastroduodenoscopy (EGD) photograph of a distal esophageal diverticular mass lesion. **B:** Celiac arteriogram demonstrates a replaced left hepatic artery arising from the left gastric artery. **C:** Postembolization celiac arteriogram: Neovascularity corresponding to the mass lesion was embolized with 500- to 700-μm particles as well as microcoils. Additional active extravasation arising from branch of replaced left hepatic artery necessitated microcoil embolization of the replaced left hepatic artery.

vascular sheath. The pigtail should be positioned just below the level of the diaphragm. Power injection is performed at a rate of 20 mL per second, for a total volume of 30 mL.

Although not required, 1 mg glucagon can be administered before angiography to limit peristalsis motion artifacts on digital subtraction angiography (DSA). For similar reasons, breath hold during DSA is ideal to limit respiratory motion. However, this is not always feasible depending on the patient's condition and level of sedation.

We favor the use of Rosch celiac (RC-1) or visceral selective (VS1) catheters (Cook Medical Inc., Bloomington, Indiana) to select the celiac artery and SMA. It is important to seat the catheter just beyond the ostium of the mesenteric vessel. If advanced too far, early branching vessels may not be imaged on the angiogram. Power injection of contrast is used for all angiograms to optimize detection of active bleeding. Celiac artery and SMA angiogram injection rates are typically 5 mL per second, for a total volume of 20 to 25 mL. DSA is carried out until the portal venous phase to document patency of the portal vein. This can be important to document in cases that potentially require hepatic artery embolization (Fig. 29.3). Delayed angiograms may also reveal varices that were not readily apparent by endoscopy. If there is hemobilia related to recent percutaneous biliary drain placement, removal of the tube over a guidewire may be necessary before angiography as the relative tamponade effect of the tube may obscure visualization of the bleeding vessel.

If no evidence of bleeding is found at celiac angiography, superselective catheterization of the suspected second-order branch (gastroduodenal artery [GDA] or left gastric) is undertaken. A microcatheter is preferred in these circumstances to avoid inducing vasospasm before the culprit vessel is identified. If these studies are also negative, an SMA arteriogram is performed before terminating the exam.

Angiography can detect bleeding rates as low as 0.5 mL per minute. The primary angiographic findings of bleeding are visualization of active contrast extravasation and contrast pooling in the venous phase. A review of studies by Loffroy et al.[28] found that angiographic evidence of active extravasation was seen in 54% of cases. Other indirect signs of bleeding on angiography include pseudoaneurysm, vessel spasm or cutoff, early venous filling, and hypervascularity (Table 29.3).

The presence of an abnormal blush may indicate an inflammatory process. This can represent a bleeding source if such an entity was suspected on prior endoscopy.[28] In cases of hemorrhagic neoplasm, tumoral blush and neovascularity may be identified. Not uncommonly, trial subselection of vessels is necessary to demonstrate bleeding.

In theory, carbon dioxide (CO_2) angiography is more sensitive than conventional angiography with iodinated contrast

Table 29.3 Angiographic Signs of Hemorrhage
Active extravasation
Contrast pooling
Pseudoaneurysm
Vasospasm, abrupt vessel cutoff
Hypervascularity

because the lower viscosity of CO_2 should predispose it to extravasating through endothelial injuries (Fig. 29.4). However, in practice, CO_2 imaging is degraded by fragmentation of the CO_2 bolus and patient motion related to discomfort caused by the CO_2 injection. It also has poorer spatial resolution, which may impair subsequent endovascular treatment.[29]

In one study, a negative bleeding focus was noted in 52% of cases, with a lower incidence in UGIB (46%) compared with lower GI bleeding (66%).[30] Failure to localize a bleeding source may be attributed to slow or intermittent nature of the hemorrhage. In such cases, provocative angiography can aid in detection. Several techniques have been reported, including the administration of anticoagulants, vasodilators, and fibrinolytics, to temporarily augment bleeding and increase diagnostic sensitivity. However, this is rarely, if ever, used for UGIB because, unlike lower GI bleeding, angiography for UGIB is nearly always preceded by endoscopy, which

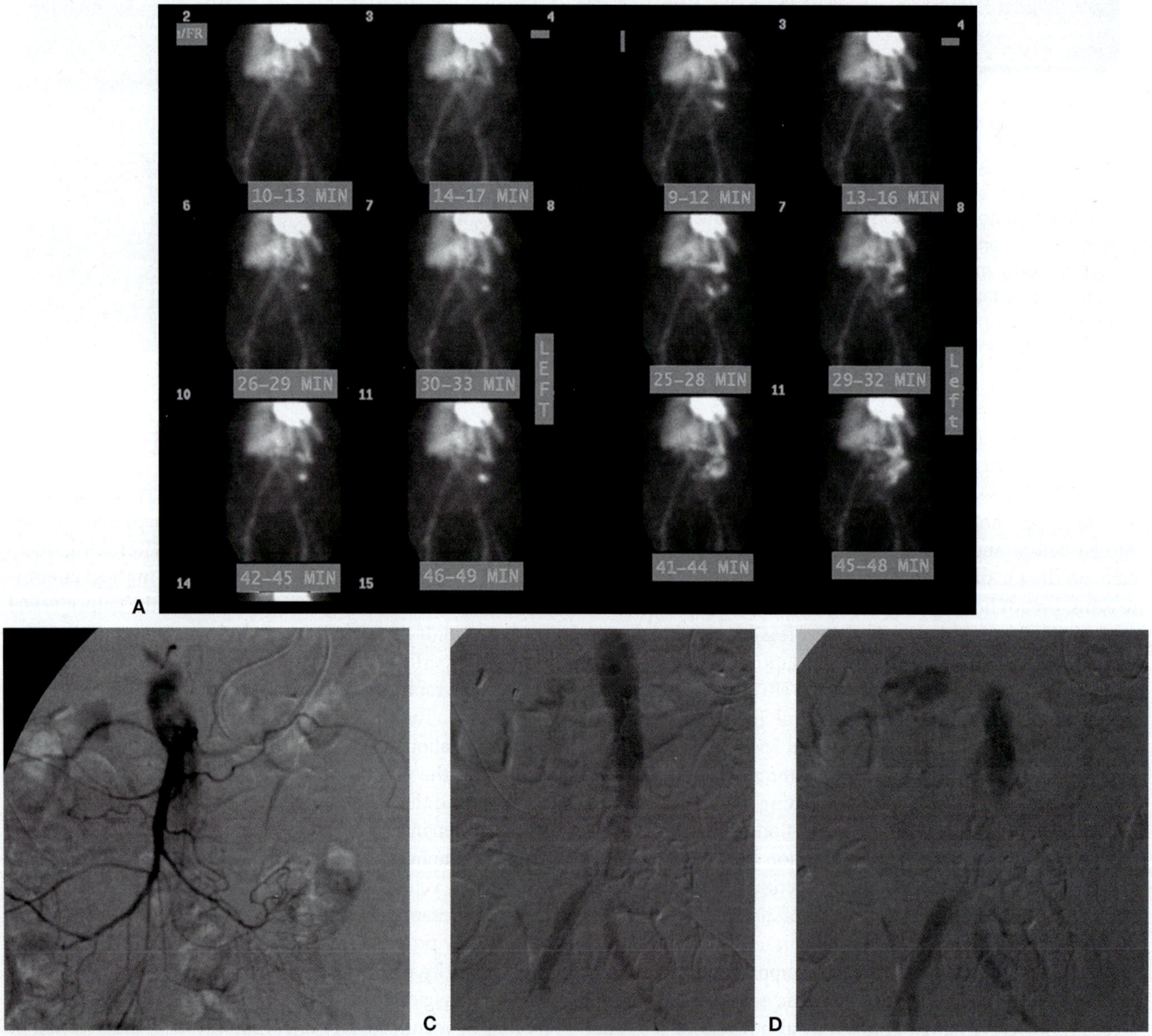

Figure 29.4 **A:** Tc-99M–tagged RBC scan with activity in left upper quadrant. **B:** Initial arteriograms of celiac artery (not shown) and SMA show no evidence of hemorrhage. **C,D:** CO_2 arteriogram of SMA reveals extravasation in the right upper quadrant. *(Continued)*

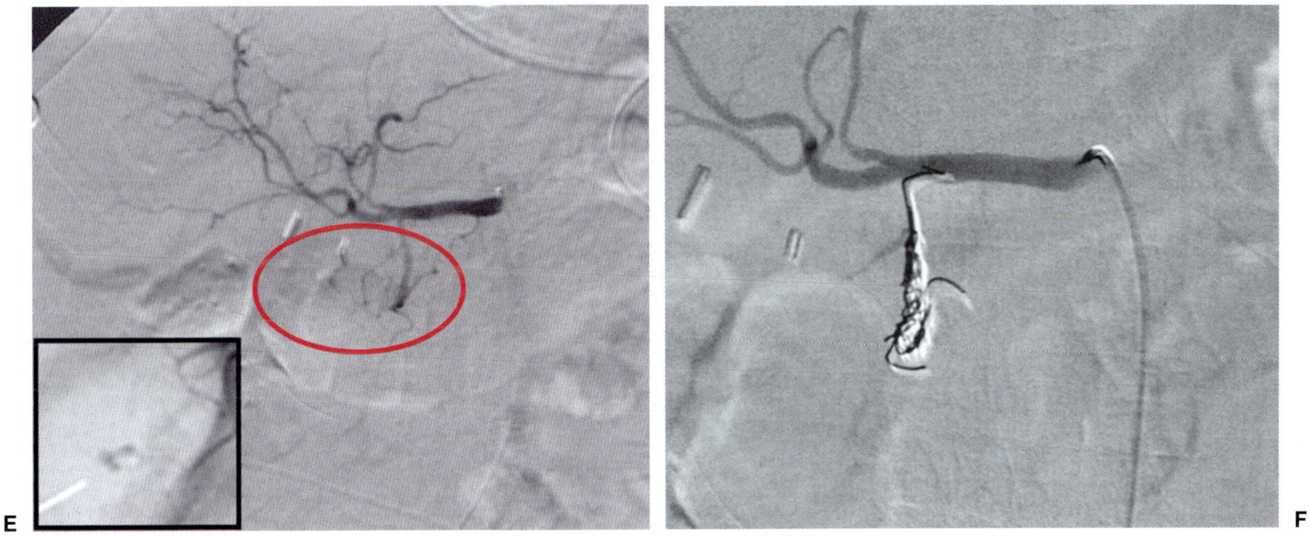

Figure 29.4 *(Continued)* **E:** Repeat celiac arteriogram revealed active extravasation of iodinated contrast from the superior pancreaticoduodenal artery. **F:** Coil embolization of the gastroduodenal artery.

commonly elucidates the source of bleeding. Moreover, the feasibility of empiric embolization in the upper GI tract does not justify the risks of provocative angiography.

If no arterial abnormality is seen, empiric embolization of the vessels supplying the area of concern can be performed. Empiric embolization is performed in 46% of endovascular cases of UGIB.[28] This technique is low risk due to the rich collateral circulation of the upper GI tract. The two arteries targeted for empiric embolization are the left gastric artery and the GDA. The left gastric artery, which runs along the lesser curve of the stomach, supplies the distal esophagus, cardia, fundus, and incisura. There is collateralization with branches of the short gastric and right gastric arteries, which typically arise from the splenic and hepatic arteries respectively. The GDA supplies the remainder of the stomach and duodenum through the right gastroepiploic artery and branches of the pancreaticoduodenal arcade. There is collateralization with the left gastroepiploic artery, which arises from the distal splenic artery, and branches from the SMA. The SMA provides duodenal supply via the pancreaticoduodenal arcades[28] (Table 29.4). There has been shown to be no statistical difference in outcomes between patients treated with empiric embolization versus embolization after angiographically demonstrated contrast extravasation.[26,31,32] An alternative to empiric embolization in cases of negative angiography is to target branches supplying the area of endoscopically placed clips.

Although the number of arteries embolized may not impact clinical success of embolotherapy,[25] it may affect subsequent surgical therapy. For example, embolization of both the left gastric and gastroduodenal arteries for treatment of a large gastric ulcer may impair attempts at subsequent partial gastrectomy in favor of total gastrectomy (Fig. 29.5).

Superselection of vessels may be necessary to identify bleeding. This typically requires coaxial placement of a 3-Fr microcatheter through a 5-Fr catheter. At our institution, we commonly employ a Renegade (Boston Scientific Corporation, Natick, Massachusetts) or a Progreat (Terumo, Tokyo, Japan) microcatheter. The Renegade microcatheter is available in two types: HI-FLO and STC. The Renegade HI-FLO has a larger diameter (0.027 in) and is best suited for cases where particulate agents are used. The slightly smaller diameter (0.021 in) of the Renegade STC is preferred for the deployment of microcoils as the narrower lumen helps guard against intracatheter coil "formation," particularly when using detachable coils. Particles can be administered through the Renegade STC with the caveat that the smaller diameter can lead to aggregation of particles and occlusion of the catheter. In such cases, the catheter can be carefully flushed with a 1-mL

Table 29.4 Blood Supply[a] of Upper Gastrointestinal Tract

Artery	Segment of Upper Gastrointestinal Tract
Inferior thyroid arteries	Cervical esophagus
Bronchial arteries, intercostals arteries, direct aortic branches	Midesophagus
Left gastric artery and inferior phrenic arteries	Distal esophagus
Left gastric artery	Stomach (cardia, fundus, incisura)
Gastroduodenal artery	Stomach (body, antrum, pylorus) and duodenum

[a]Vessels targeted during embolization

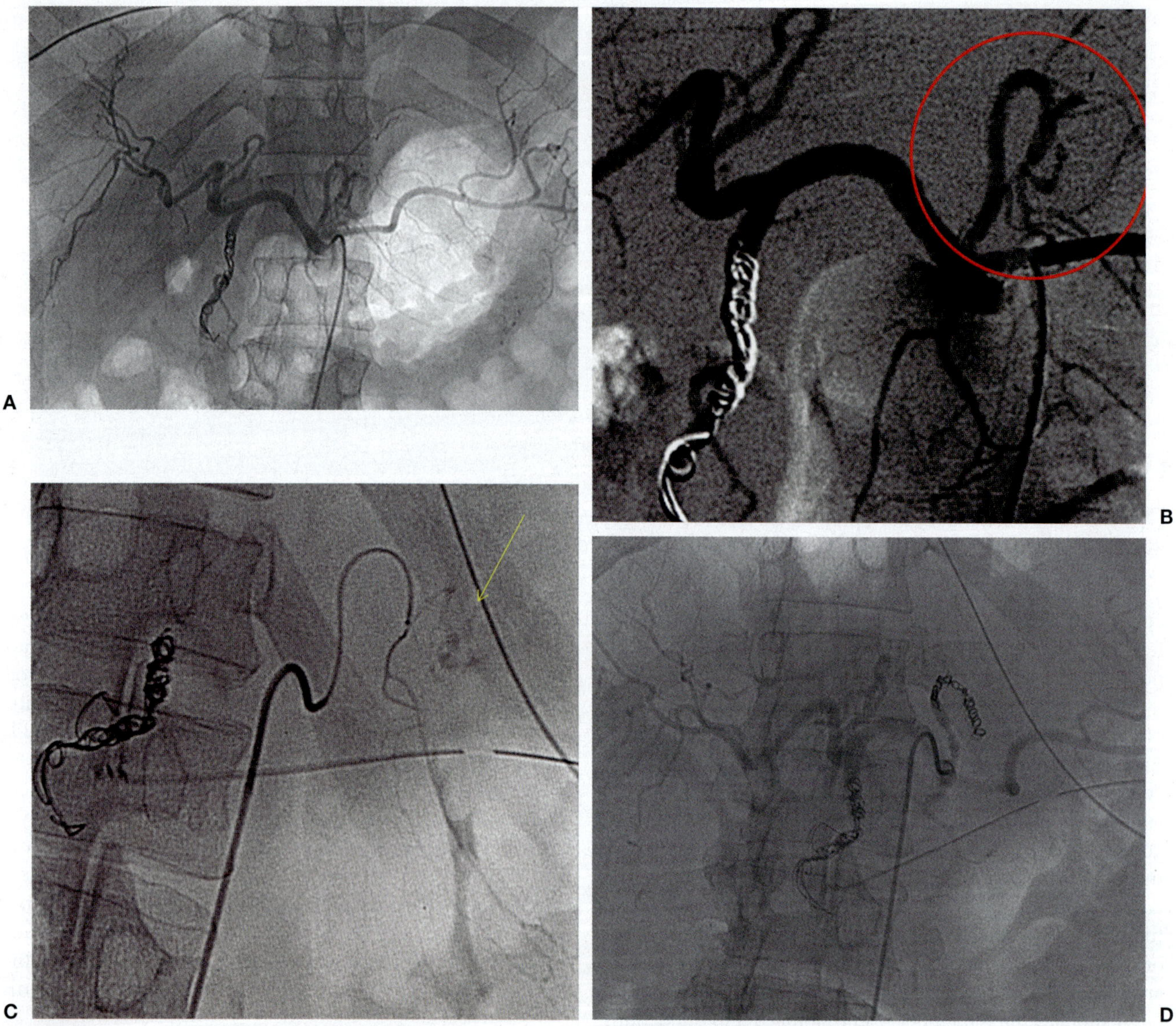

Figure 29.5 Endoscopy found an ulcer along the lesser curve at the incisura with active bleeding from a visible vessel. **A:** Celiac arteriogram shows previous coil embolization of the GDA but no active extravasation. **B:** Closer inspection of left gastric artery reveals vasospasm and pseudoaneurysm of left gastric artery branches. **C:** Superselection of the branch in question with a microcatheter uncovers active extravasation (*arrow*). **D:** Coil embolization of the left gastric artery. The patient continued to bleed despite technically successful embolization. This necessitated surgical intervention. Due to embolization of both the GDA and left gastric artery, total gastrectomy was favored over partial gastrectomy.

saline-filled syringe. The Progreat microcatheter is also available in various sizes, including 2.8-Fr (0.027 in) and 2.4-Fr (0.022 in). The former is available to order as a coaxial system that comes preloaded with a hydrophilic microwire.

Selecting the Gastroduodenal Artery

The GDA most commonly arises from the common hepatic artery. Less common variants include branches off the right hepatic artery or directly off the celiac axis.[33] In many cases, the GDA is accessible with a 5-Fr catheter. The catheter is advanced from the celiac artery ostium into the proper hepatic artery over a Glidewire (Terumo, Tokyo, Japan). Care should be taken to avoid arterial dissection when using a Glidewire; this is especially true for patients with surgically altered anatomy (e.g., liver transplantation). Rotating the reverse curve catheter counterclockwise as it is being advanced can help when negotiating a tortuous common hepatic artery. Once in the proper hepatic artery, the catheter is carefully withdrawn until the tip engages the GDA.

Selecting the Left Gastric Artery

Normal celiac anatomy, with the left gastric artery being the smallest of the three primary branches of the hepatogastrosplenic trunk, is seen in 89% of patients. Less common variants include direct aortic origin (4.4%) and separate gastrosplenic and hepaticomesenteric trunks (2.6%).[34] The left gastric artery courses cranially in a direction counter to the orientation of the celiac trunk. This feature can make it particularly challenging to catheterize. We favor accessing the celiac trunk with a VS1 catheter. The catheter is then carefully withdrawn until the tip is directed cranially and engages the origin of the left gastric artery. A microwire and microcatheter are then advanced into the vessel (Fig. 29.6).

Embolization

Embolization should be carried out both distal and proximal to the site of injury to prevent continued bleeding through a "back door." For example, GDA embolization performed for management of a duodenal ulcer calls for coil embolization distally into the right gastroepiploic artery with extension proximally into the GDA. Adequate embolization is confirmed by superior mesenteric arteriogram to exclude back door bleeding through the pancreaticoduodenal arcade.

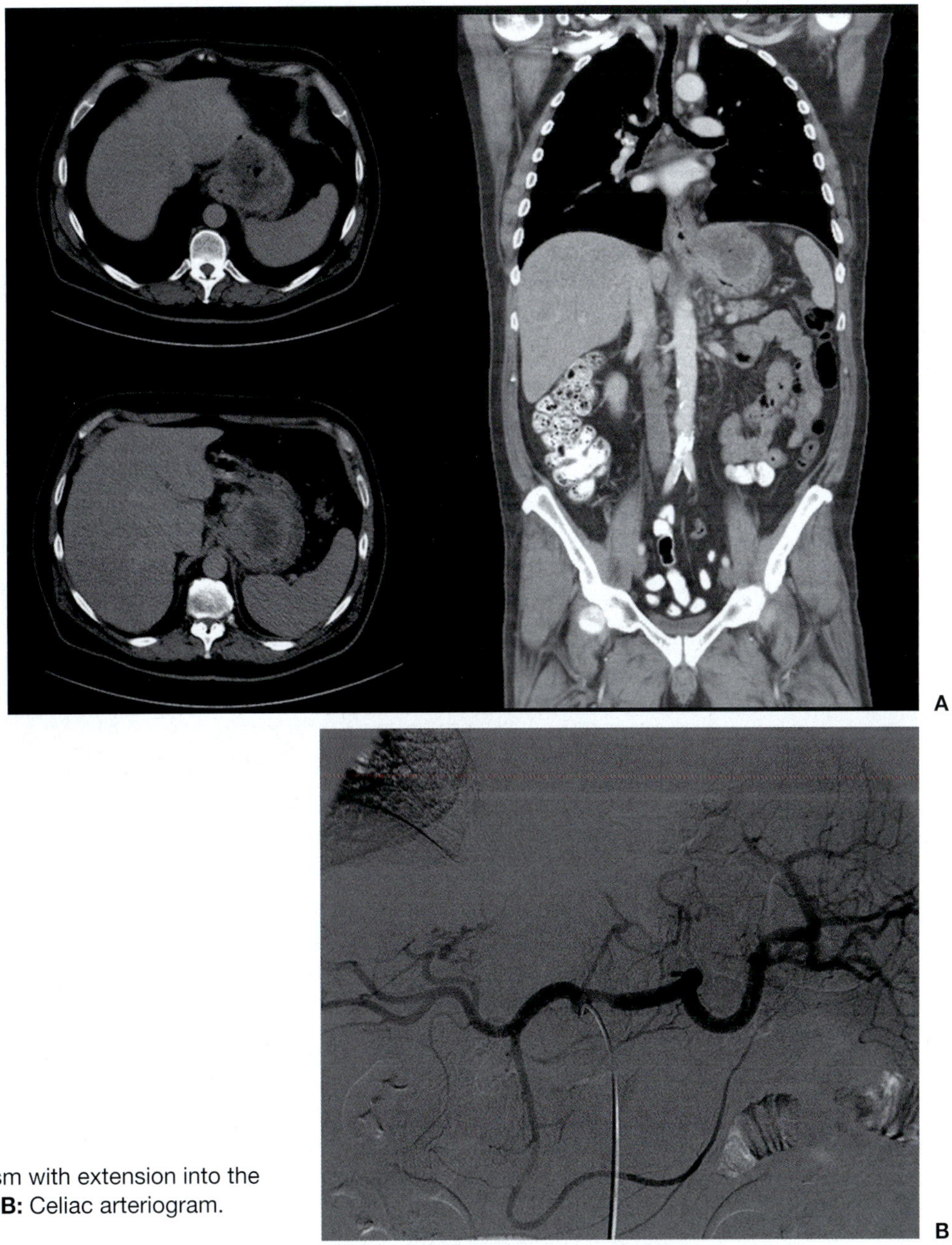

Figure 29.6 **A:** Gastric neoplasm with extension into the distal esophagus. **B:** Celiac arteriogram.

(Continued)

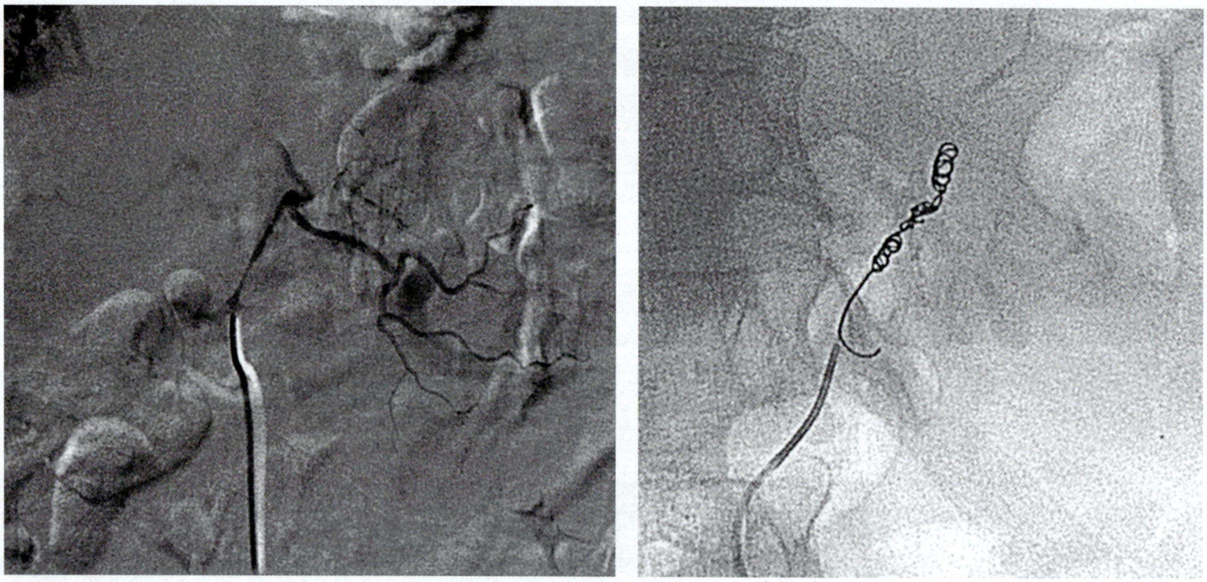

C B

Figure 29.6 *(Continued)* **C:** Left gastric arteriogram demonstrates hypervascularity consistent with neoplasm. **D:** Successful particle and coil embolization of the left gastric artery.

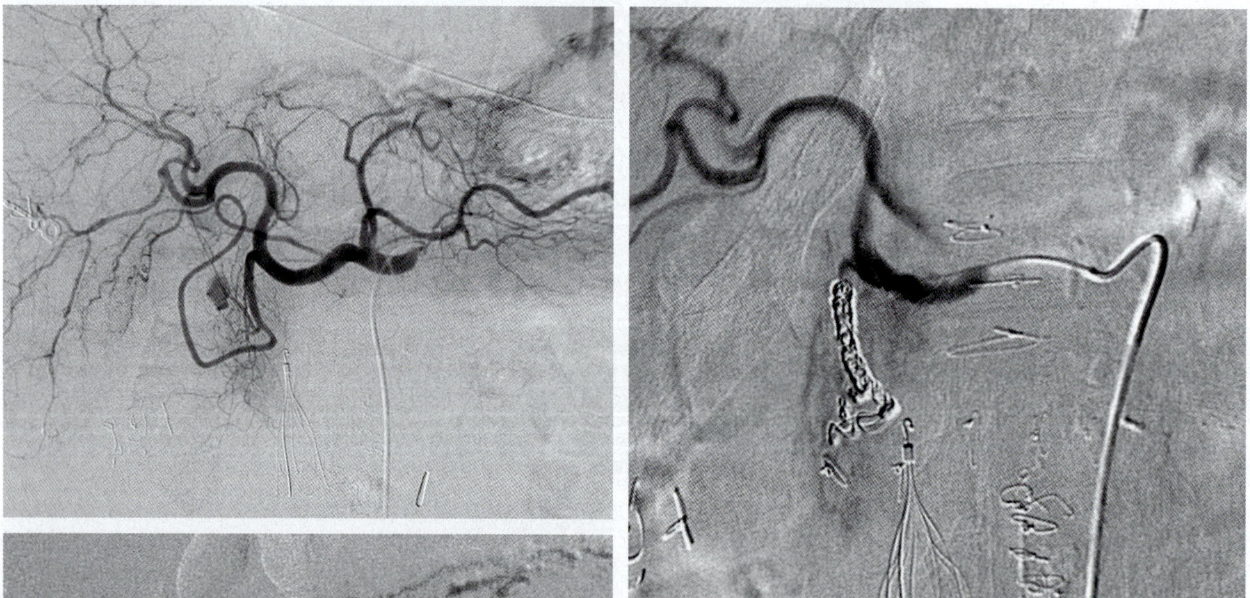

A B

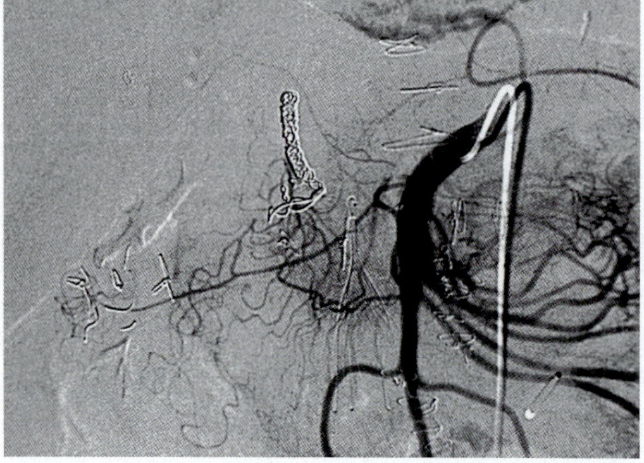

C

Figure 29.7 **A:** Celiac arteriogram with active contrast extravasation and pooling from a pancreaticoduodenal branch off the GDA. **B:** Common hepatic arteriogram after coil embolization of the GDA demonstrates resolution of the hemorrhage. **C:** SMA angiogram confirms no retrograde filling of the duodenal lesion.

If bleeding persists, the inferior pancreaticoduodenal arcade should be superselected via an SMA approach and embolization should be performed as distally as possible. Likewise, embolization performed via the SMA should be checked with a celiac angiogram before concluding the case (Fig. 29.7).

Distal catheterization can be limited by vasospasm and vessel tortuosity. The latter can be overcome by the use of soft-tipped microwires—the 0.014-in Hi-Torque Balance Middle Weight (BMW) guidewire (Abbott Vascular, Santa Clara, California) is a favorite of the authors. The use of road mapping technique when attempting to subselect vessels can also be helpful. Vasospasm can be managed by infusion of 200 μg nitroglycerin into the affected artery. Although vasospasm may temporarily mask bleeding in the targeted vessel, it can occasionally be a blessing in disguise by revealing bleeding from an adjacent artery.

HEMOBILIA

Hemobilia is a sign of an arteriobiliary fistula and most commonly results from iatrogenic injury or trauma. Hemosuccus pancreaticus, or bleeding via the pancreatic duct, is rare and usually associated with pancreatitis or splenic artery aneurysm. Embolotherapy is the first-line treatment for hemobilia and hemosuccus pancreaticus as endoscopy is limited by its inability to reach the injured vessel.[16]

Embolization of the hepatic artery for hemobilia is generally well tolerated due to the dual blood supply of the liver

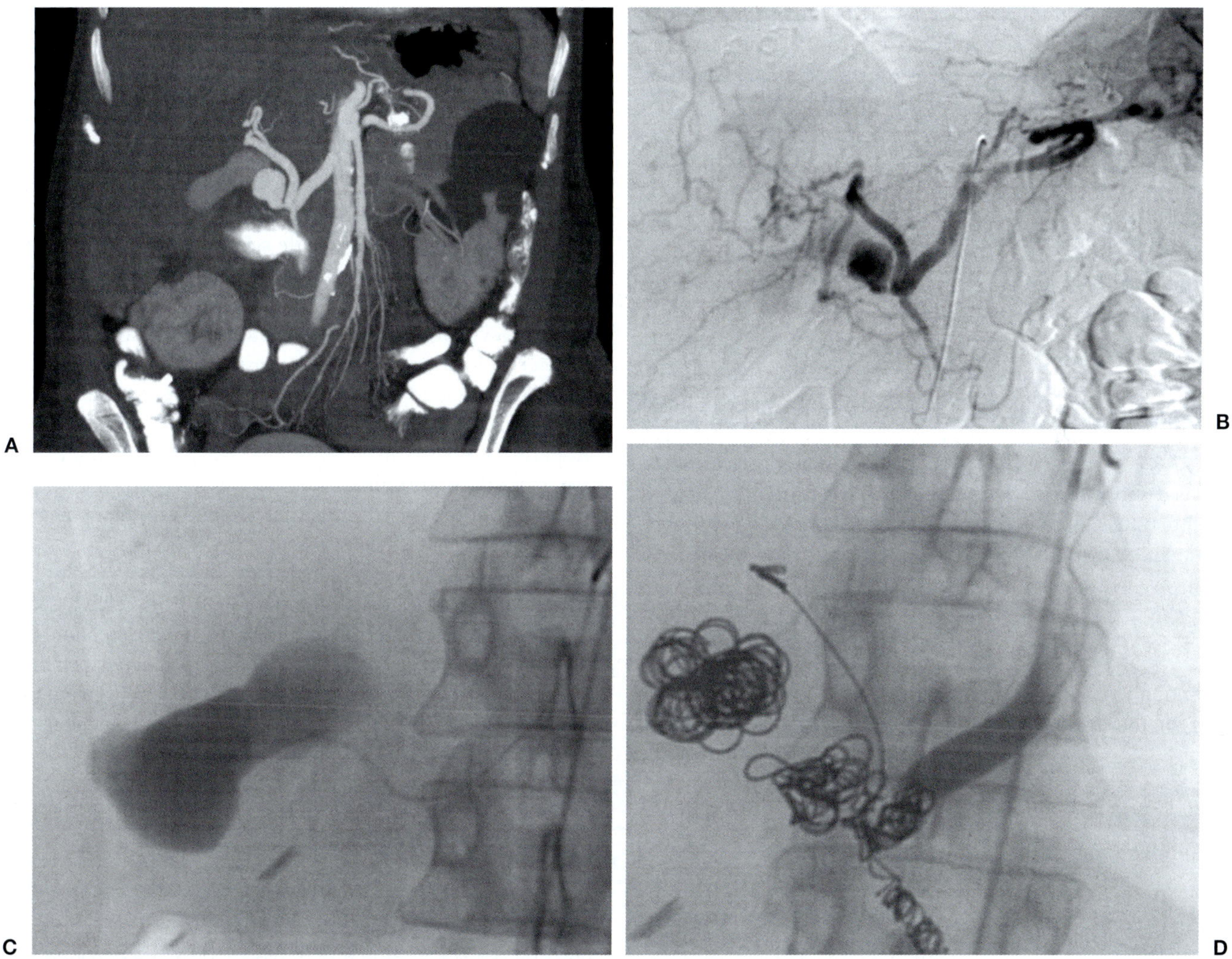

Figure 29.8 A 71-year-old female with a history of laparoscopic cholecystectomy complicated by hepatic artery pseudoaneurysm and treated with a covered stent. The patient was transferred from an outside hospital where active hemobilia was confirmed by EGD. **A:** CT of the abdomen demonstrates arteriobiliary fistula. **B:** Celiac arteriogram with pooling of contrast within the pseudoaneurysm. Subtle opacification of the dilated biliary duct can also be noted. **C:** Microcatheter is advanced across the pseudoaneurysm and into the bile duct, confirming location of arteriobiliary fistula. **D:** Coil embolization of pseudoaneurysm proved unsuccessful. Covered stent placement across the pseudoaneurysm could not be achieved to do the hairpin curve of common and proper hepatic arteries. Emergent coil embolization of proper hepatic artery was performed. Embolization was extended into GDA to prevent retrograde flow into the pseudoaneurysm.

(75% via the portal vein and 25% via the hepatic artery) (Fig. 29.8). However, in the absence of a patent portal vein with centripetal flow, hepatic artery embolization risks hepatocyte ischemia. For this reason, it is imperative that delayed arteriography of the celiac axis is performed before embolization of any hepatic branches is undertaken. Nontarget embolization of the cystic artery via reflux of embolic material (e.g., Gelfoam slurry) can be associated with cholecystitis. When possible, superselection of the targeted hepatic artery branches should be done to reduce the risk of cystic artery embolization. Hepatic abscess formation following hepatic artery embolization has also been reported.[35]

Even with normal portal hepatic perfusion, arterial embolization can be complicated by biliary ischemia in rare instances. Unlike hepatocytes, the intrahepatic bile ducts do not have a dual blood supply. They are perfused via a peribiliary capillary plexus, which arises from hepatic arterial branches.[36] Consequently, there is a risk of biliary necrosis, stenosis, or cholangitis when embolizing the hepatic artery. The risk is theoretically greater with smaller embolic agents (e.g., particles), which cause very distal occlusion. Thus, we recommend embolization with coils when possible.

Evaluation of hemosuccus pancreaticus should involve interrogation of both the celiac artery and SMA. Angiographic findings include opacification of the main pancreatic duct or the presence of aneurysm or pseudoaneurysm.[37] Pseudoaneurysms are commonly a result of chronic pancreatitis and typically occur in the splenic, gastroduodenal, or pancreaticoduodenal arteries. In one series, embolotherapy was successful in providing immediate hemostasis in 77.8% of cases.[37] The risk of splenic infarction should be considered when embolization of a splenic artery aneurysm is attempted. Embolotherapy of an aneurysm or pseudoaneurysm may also be undertaken as a presurgical measure to improve hemodynamic control.

ESOPHAGEAL BLEEDING

Although very uncommon, embolization for arterial bleeding of the cervical and midesophagus has been reported. Cases typically involve bleeding ulcers.[38–40] However, studies are limited by lack of long-term data and small patient populations. The risk of ischemia is thought to be low due to the extensive collateral capillary network created by the complex arterial supply of the esophagus[41] (Table 29.4).

EMBOLIC AGENTS

There is no conclusive evidence to indicate that one embolic agent is superior to the others. In practice, operator familiarity with each agent and institutional availability determine what is used. The goal of embolotherapy is to reduce blood flow to the site of bleeding without causing bowel ischemia. This is an important principle to keep in mind when deciding on an embolic agent (Table 29.5).

Coils

Coils are the most commonly used embolic agent as well as the agent of choice at our institution. They can be precisely positioned and are associated with minimal risk of infarction because they do not affect the microvasculature. They are, however, permanent and may prevent reaccessing the target vessel should bleeding recur.

Coils are available in a wide selection of sizes, allowing one to correctly match the targeted vessel diameter. It is advisable to err on the side of slightly oversizing the coils as there is inevitably some degree of vasospasm associated with catheterization. Once the vasospasm resolves, blood flow can resume around an inadvertently undersized coil and GI hemorrhage will recur. Grossly oversized coils will not form properly within the vessel lumen and will provide a less effective scaffold for thrombus.

We favor the use of standard 0.035-in coils when possible. These larger diameter coils expedite vessel occlusion by their inherent size, and the additional steps involved in positioning the microcatheter are avoided. Moreover, 0.035-in coils are less costly than their microcoil counterparts, not to mention the added cost of the microcatheter equipment through which they are deployed. The obvious limitation to using 0.035-in coils is the inability to access the target vessel using a 5-Fr catheter alone.

Table 29.5 Embolic Agents

Embolic Agent	Benefit	Drawback
Coils	– Precise positioning – Minimal risk of ischemia	– Less effective in coagulopathic patients – Less effective when used alone
Gelatin sponge	– Temporary; useful for surgically altered anatomy or hepatic arteries – Expedites coil embolization (Gelfoam sandwich)	– High rate of bleeding recurrence when used alone
Particles	– Bleeding GI tumors	– Bowel ischemia – Nontarget embolization
Liquid embolics	– Patients with uncorrected coagulopathy	– Requires experienced operator

GI, gastrointestinal.

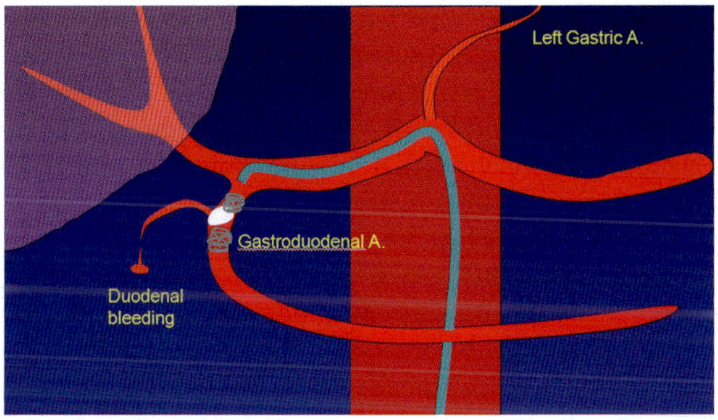

Figure 29.9 Illustration of a Gelfoam sandwich.

Coil placement can be alternated with infusion of a slurry of gelatin sponge (Gelfoam; Pfizer, New York, New York) to create a "Gelfoam sandwich." This technique helps expedite embolization and is especially useful in patients with underlying coagulopathy in whom thrombus is slow to develop on the fibered coil scaffolding. The Gelfoam sandwich technique also helps limit the number of coils needed to embolize larger and longer vessels such as the GDA (Fig. 29.9).

When the diameter of the target vessel is in doubt or there is a dubious landing zone for coil placement, detachable coils are a useful tool. We prefer the Interlock Fibered IDC Occlusion System (Boston Scientific Corporation, Natick, Massachusetts). These allow the operator to retract and reposition coils or even completely retrieve the coil before final placement. They have the additional advantage of not requiring a separate pusher wire. This can be useful when working with limited support staff.

If inappropriately positioned, coils can preclude subsequent endovascular access to the targeted lesion or vessel. In such instances, surgical intervention may be the only remaining treatment option should bleeding recur. Fortunately, if bleeding continues after coil embolization, it is usually much less severe and the patient is more hemodynamically stable, thus allowing for surgical or endoscopic therapy to be undertaken in more optimal conditions.

Gelatin Sponge

Use of Gelfoam alone provides a variable degree of short-term hemostasis as embolized vessels will recanalize over 2 to 6 weeks.[27,42] In theory, this should cause a lesser degree of bowel ischemia compared with other embolic agents. However, because of the rich collateralization of upper GI arterial system, there is less concern for bowel ischemia when treating UGIB. Thus, permanent agents, such as coils, are used without hesitation. Patients with prior bowel surgery (e.g., Whipple procedure) are an exception to this rule. This population has altered vascular anatomy and collateral circulation may be diminished or absent. In such cases, coil embolization may be relegated to the second option after Gelfoam pledgets because of the heightened concern for bowel ischemia. Keep in mind, however, that bowel necrosis can occur within 8 to 12 hours in the setting of acute mesenteric ischemia. Thus, any decision to perform embolization in patients with surgically altered anatomy should be made after consultation with surgical colleagues.

As previously noted, gelatin sponge is used most commonly as a component of a Gelfoam sandwich in conjunction with coils. Gelfoam may also be useful when embolizing hepatic arteries in the setting of compromised portal vein patency. In these cases, Gelfoam may be a better option to address acute hemorrhage while allowing for future blood flow to hepatocytes and bile ducts after recanalization of the vessel.

Gelfoam pledgets can be administered using a microcatheter. We recommend using one of a larger caliber (≥0.27 in) to avoid catheter occlusion. A 1-mL syringe of saline can be helpful to clear catheter occlusions when administering Gelfoam. Note that nontarget embolization is a potential negative repercussion to using Gelfoam in this manner.

Particles

Neoplasm-induced hemorrhage is the lone setting in which the use of particles is generally agreed to be safe and possibly advantageous. Although surgery is the only definitive treatment for neoplasm, particle embolization can be used as temporizing measure in cases of emergent GI hemorrhage from primary or metastatic GI tumors.[43] Particle embolization has also been successful in shrinking and devascularizing tumors before surgical resection.[44]

Unlike with benign lesions of the GI tract, ischemia at the arteriole or capillary level is sought when treating bleeding tumors. Use of particle sizes as small as 200 μm has been reported to be technically successful in the embolization of primary GI tumors and is not associated with bowel ischemia or postembolization syndrome.[44] Care must be taken to ensure no arteriovenous shunting is present on preembolization selective angiography. This is especially true when using smaller particle sizes. The authors recommend using particles no smaller than 500 μm to avoid the risk of bowel ischemia from nontarget embolization. Reflux into nontarget arteries should also be strictly avoided.

Because of their small size and potential to reach the level of the intramural vasculature, particulate agents, such as polyvinyl chloride or trisacryl gelatin microspheres, are theoretically associated with an increased risk of bowel infarction and organ necrosis. For this reason, we advise against the use of particulate agents in the treatment of nontumoral UGIB.

Liquid Embolics

The primary advantage of *N*-butyl cyanoacrylate, or glue, (TruFill NBCA; Cordis Neurovascular, Miami Lakes, Florida) and ethylene vinyl alcohol copolymer (Onyx) is that they cause mechanical occlusion of vessels and do not rely on the patient's ability to form thrombus. They work by polymerizing upon exposure to an ionic environment (blood) and immediately forming a cast of the vessel, causing permanent occlusion. Thus, they are ideal agents when the patient has an uncorrected coagulopathy. Their potential use is affirmed when considering that coagulopathy is associated with a 2.9-fold greater risk of embolization failure and a 9.6-fold greater risk of death from bleeding after embolization.[27]

Glue and Onyx are also suitable in cases complicated by small and tortuous vasculature where precise delivery of coils is not possible. They can also be delivered through smaller (0.010 in) catheters than microcoils, which may be beneficial in small, tortuous, or spastic vessels.[45] These agents are also useful when embolizing pseudoaneurysms with multiple branch vessels that cannot be completely excluded with coils. Embolization of all collateral vessels is necessary in these cases to prevent continued bleeding through retrograde pathways.

The microcatheter should be positioned as close as possible to the site of bleeding. When using NBCA, the degree of dilution with iodized oil should be determined based on the distance of embolization target from the catheter as well as the rate of injection by the operator. A greater ratio of Ethiodol to NBCA increases the polymerization time, allowing it to travel more distally. Polymerization of NBCA occurs within seconds.[46] Alternatively, coil embolization before NBCA infusion can be done to help control the flow of glue or to prevent nontarget embolization.[47] The end point of infusion is extravasation from the bleeding site or complete filling of the target vessel. Only a small amount of the NBCA–iodized oil mixture, on the order of 1 mL, is typically needed. Once injection is complete, the microcatheter should be removed immediately to prevent adherence to the catheter wall.

The primary concern in using glue or NBCA is that the extent of vascular penetration can be difficult to control, resulting in increased risk of ischemia and nontarget embolization. Conversely, if adequate embolization distal to the target is not achieved, recurrent bleeding may result from collateral flow. Consequently, these agents require more operator experience and diligence. In a study by Lang et al.,[42] a high prevalence of duodenal stricture as a late complication of embolization using 6-cyanoacrylate was postulated to be secondary to the embolization technique used by the operators, in which terminal muscular branches were embolized. Yata et al.[47] found evidence of ulcers in 3 of 10 patients who underwent postembolization endoscopic evaluation within the first week after treatment. However, all cases showed improvement on follow-up endoscopy and none required surgical intervention. Interestingly, the same study also reported hepatic abscesses in 2 of 2 patients who underwent hepatic artery embolization. Both were successfully treated by percutaneous drainage.

NBCA has been reported to successfully achieve immediate hemostasis in 88% to 94% of cases of UGIB, with recurrent bleeding seen in only 6% to 7%.[47,48] Jae et al.[49] reported an 83% clinical success rate in patients with underlying coagulopathy and acute UGIB. It is this subset of patients in whom we recommend liquid embolic agents.

Onyx is a much more forgiving liquid embolic agent compared with NBCA. It is less likely to result in catheter adhesion and its lavalike consistency allows for more controlled infusion by the operator.[50] The extent of distal diffusion within the vasculature depends on the rate of injection. Onyx may be impractical from a cost perspective as it is itself more expensive and also requires the use of dimethyl sulfoxide–compatible catheters (Fig. 29.10).

VASOPRESSIN

Vasopressin causes vasoconstriction of the smooth muscle of the splanchnic blood vessels and the bowel wall which, in turn, decreases perfusion to the site of vascular injury to allow for clot formation. Thus, as with embolotherapy, procedural success depends on a normal coagulation cascade. Historically, vasopressin infusion was considered in cases where embolization was not technically achievable. However, unlike for lower GI bleeding, vasopressin has not been shown to be effective for UGIB. The relatively larger vessels from which UGIB usually arises may not constrict to the same degree as smaller branches associated with lower GI bleeding.[51]

POSTANGIOGRAPHY

If a patient is on aspirin, it should be resumed when the cardiovascular risks outweigh the risk of rebleeding. This determination should be made after consultation with all those involved in the care of the patient. A PPI should be considered in patients who developed acute GI bleeding while taking aspirin or clopidogrel (in spite of the potential clopidogrel–PPI interaction).

OUTCOMES

A review of studies by Loffroy et al.[28] found that the overall technical and clinical success of embolization in UGIB were 93% and 67% respectively, with a 33% rebleeding rate. Repeat embolization was successful in approximately half of these patients with rebleeding.[28] Technical failure can be attributed to difficult anatomy such as vessel tortuosity or stenosis. Schenker et al.[25] demonstrated that patients who underwent clinically successful embolotherapy were 13.3 times more likely to survive than those with unsuccessful procedures. The same study found sixfold greater success rate of embolotherapy when done for trauma or iatrogenic injury.[25] This suggests that focal vascular injuries respond better to embolotherapy than inflammatory or neoplastic processes. Schenker et al.[25] also found that patients with successful embolization had one-sixth the mortality rate of those with failed embolization.

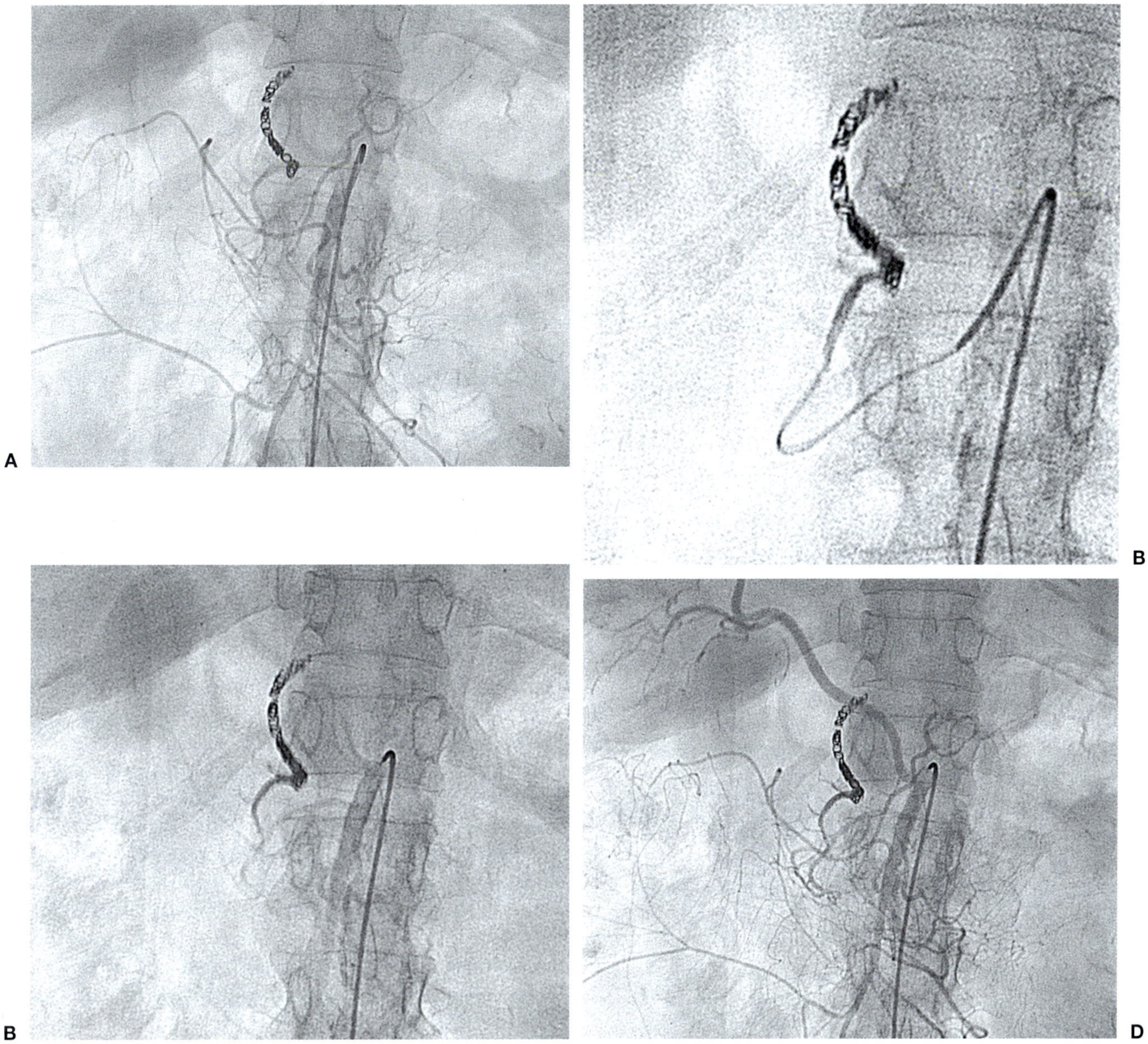

Figure 29.10 **A:** Superior mesenteric arteriogram with evidence of continued bleeding via branches of the pancreaticoduodenal arcade despite coil embolization of the GDA. **B:** Microcatheter advanced into the pancreaticoduodenal arcade with infusion of Onyx. **C:** Spot fluoroscopic image obtained after completion of Onyx infusion. **D:** Postembolization SMA arteriogram confirms technically successful embolization.

The incidence of surgical intervention for patients with clinically unsuccessful arterial embolization is 9% to 20%.[28,52,53]

One study found UGIB to be more resistant to hemostasis, with a higher rate of early rebleeding, than lower GI hemorrhage.[25] This was hypothesized to be secondary to refilling of injured vessels through collateral circulation distal to the point of embolization. It is also important to remember that embolization does not treat the underlying pathology of UGIB such as peptic ulcer disease. In these patients, gastric acid suppression and treatment of *Helicobacter pylori* are important adjuncts to prevent recurrence of bleeding. UGIB also tends to be more profuse than lower GI bleeding and is associated with greater risk factors (i.e., sicker patients), leading to treatment failure. Factors associated with clinical failure of arterial embolization include bleeding secondary to trauma or invasive procedures, multiorgan failure, use of anticoagulants, underlying coagulopathy, longer time interval between onset of bleed and embolization, increased number of pRBC transfusions, postinterventional administration of fresh frozen plasma (FFP), hypovolemic shock and/or vasopressor use, corticosteroids, and the use of coils as the lone embolic agent[24,25,28,52,54,55] (Table 29.6).

Table 29.6 Factors Associated with Clinical Failure of Embolization
Bleeding due to trauma or invasive procedures
Multiorgan failure
Use of anticoagulants
Underlying coagulopathy
Longer time interval between bleeding onset and embolization
Increased number of pRBC transfusions
Postintervention administration of FFP
Hypovolemic shock and/or vasopressor use
Using coils alone as embolic agent

pRBC, packed red blood cells; FFP, fresh frozen plasma.

No prospective comparison of embolic agents has been performed to date. There is, however, some evidence that coils, when combined with polyvinyl alcohol particles or Gelfoam, are associated with lower bleeding recurrence compared with the use of coils alone.[26] The authors recommend using a Gelfoam sandwich technique, in part, for this reason. These agents are widely available and most interventionalists are well versed in how to deploy them. Moreover, option of retractable coils can make up for inexperience.

The overall postembolization complication rate is 6% to 9%.[52,56] Complications include access site hematoma, arterial dissection, contrast nephropathy, and nontarget embolization. Bowel ischemia or infarction can be caused by embolization too far distal in the vascular bed. This is of concern primarily when using particles or liquid embolic agents. Additionally, one must be cognizant that the normally rich collateral blood supply of the upper GI tract that protects against ischemia is compromised in patients who have had prior surgery or radiation therapy. A review of studies by Mirsadraee et al.[56] found mortality rate secondary to technical failure or procedural complication ranged from 0% to 33%.

EMBOLIZATION VERSUS SURGERY

Endovascular embolization has become the de facto second-line treatment after endoscopy because it is minimally invasive and avoids laparotomy in critically ill patients, although it is interesting to note that no significant survival benefit over surgery has been demonstrated in the literature. Although transarterial embolization is associated with fewer complications, it has a higher rebleeding rate when compared with surgery.[57,58] The available data is only retrospective in nature and nearly always confounded by older patient populations with more comorbidities in the embolization groups.

VARICEAL BLEEDING

Acute variceal bleeding is associated with a high early mortality rate of up to 30%.[59,60] Variceal sources of GI bleeding are distinct from arterial bleeding both in etiology and endovascular treatment. For these reasons, it is important to distinguish between nonvariceal and variceal sources of hemorrhage at the outset. Sources of variceal UGIB include gastroesophageal varices from portal venous hypertension and gastric varices from splenic vein thrombosis. Thirty percent of patients with portal hypertension who present with UGIB actually have an arterial source of bleeding.[61]

Active variceal hemorrhage accounts for about one-third of all deaths related to cirrhosis.[62] Variceal bleeding stops spontaneously only in approximately 50% of patients, which is considerably less than in arterial UGIB.[63–65] Following cessation of active hemorrhage, there is a high risk of recurrent hemorrhage. The greatest risk is within the first 48 to 72 hours, and over 50% of all early rebleeding episodes occur within the first 10 days.[66] Each episode of bleeding carries a 30% mortality, with mortality rates approaching 70% to 80% in patients with continued bleeding.[67,68] The risk of rebleeding is high (60% to 70%) until the gastroesophageal varices are treated.[69] Risk factors for early rebleeding include age older than 60 years, renal failure, large varices, and severe initial bleeding as defined by a hemoglobin level below 8 g/dL at admission.[66] The goals of management during an active bleeding episode are hemodynamic resuscitation, prevention and treatment of complications, and treatment of bleeding.

Endoscopic therapy is currently the definitive treatment of choice for active variceal hemorrhage and can be performed at the time of diagnostic endoscopy. Two forms of endoscopic treatment are commonly used: sclerotherapy and variceal band ligation. Urgent endoscopic and/or pharmacologic treatments nevertheless fail to control bleeding in approximately 10% to 20% of patients, and more definitive therapy such as portosystemic shunt creation must be immediately instituted.[7] Although balloon tamponade is an effective way to achieve short-term hemostasis, due to complications of rebleeding upon balloon deflation, its use is generally reserved for temporary stabilization until more definitive treatment can be instituted.

Transjugular Intrahepatic Portosystemic Shunt

Portal venous hypertension is most commonly attributable to cirrhosis and Budd-Chiari syndromes. Reduction of the portal–venous gradient usually necessitates a transjugular intrahepatic portosystemic shunt (TIPS) creation with or without concomitant variceal embolization. A portosystemic gradient less than 12 mm Hg is associated with a lower risk of bleeding recurrence. Embolization of varices is not routinely performed at the time of TIPS at our institution unless it is in the setting of acute ongoing variceal bleeding. A retrospective study by Tesdal et al.[70] demonstrated that the incidence of rebleeding is lower in cases of TIPS with variceal embolization compared with TIPS alone. However, this study did not reveal a statistically significant difference in survival between the two cohorts. We routinely place 10-mm diameter Viatorr stents (W. L. Gore & Associates, Inc., Newark, Delaware) and dilated them as needed to achieve the desired portosystemic gradient. This is typically achieved at 8 mm. If bleeding recurs in the short-term, the stent is fully dilated to 10 mm and additional attempts at variceal embolization are made.

Balloon-Occluded Retrograde Transvenous Obliteration

Gastric varices represent a slightly different pathology and hemodynamic issue than esophageal varices. Most gastric varices are due to portal hypertension, whereas others are secondary to splenic vein thrombosis. Balloon-occluded retrograde transvenous obliteration (BRTO) is a highly effective and minimally invasive treatment for gastric varices, particularly in patients who are not suitable candidates for TIPS due to poor hepatic reserve. BRTO is widely accepted in Japan, with growing use worldwide. This technique uses an occlusion balloon to control the blood flow through prominent draining veins of portosystemic shunts (most commonly a gastrorenal shunt) contributing to the gastric varices. With the shunt outflow occluded, the goal is to sufficiently fill the variceal complex with a sclerosing agent and obliterate the gastric varices without refluxing into the systemic or portal circulation. Successful treatment relies on an understanding of the anatomy and hemodynamic patterns of the gastric varices. For a detailed discussion of BRTO, please refer to Chapter 31.

TIPS AND TRICKS

Gastroduodenal Artery Embolization

- Embolize distally into the GDA at its junction with the right gastroepiploic artery; this is commonly demarcated by a right angle turn of the vessel.
- Gelfoam sandwich—alternating deposition of coils and Gelfoam slurry—can expedite embolization of a lengthy vessel such as the GDA.
- Embolize as close to the GDA–hepatic artery junction as possible to ensure occlusion of all pancreaticoduodenal branches.
- Use retractable coils near GDA–hepatic artery junction to guard against coil placement into the hepatic artery.
- Check the SMA for back door bleeding.

Accessing the Left Gastric Artery

- Select the celiac artery using a reverse curve catheter (e.g., VS1).
- Carefully pull back the catheter so that the tip of the reverse curve catheter is directed cranially and engages the left gastric artery.
- Advance a microwire and microcatheter coaxially through the reverse curve catheter and into the left gastric artery.

REFERENCES

1. Peura DA, Lanza FL, Gostout CJ, et al. The American College of Gastroenterology Bleeding Registry: preliminary findings. *Am J Gastroenterol.* 1997;92:924–928.
2. Longstreth GF. Epidemiology of hospitalization for acute upper gastrointestinal hemorrhage: a population-based study. *Am J Gastroenterol.* 1995;90:206–210.
3. Barnert J, Messmann H. Diagnosis and management of lower gastrointestinal bleeding. *Nat Rev Gastroenterol Hepatol.* 2009;6(11):637–646.
4. Billingham RP. The conundrum of lower gastrointestinal bleeding. *Surg Clin North Am.* 1997;77:241–252.
5. Leontiadis GI, Sharma VK, Howden CW. Proton pump inhibitor treatment for acute peptic ulcer bleeding. *Cochrane Database Syst Rev.* 2006;(1):CD002094.
6. Green FW, Kaplan MM, Curtis LE, et al. Effect of acid and pepsin on blood coagulation and platelet aggregation. A possible contributor prolonged gastroduodenal mucosal hemorrhage. *Gastroenterology.* 1978;74(1):38–43.
7. Garcia-Tsao G, Sanyal AJ, Grace ND, et al; Practice Guidelines Committee of American Association for Study of Liver Diseases; Practice Parameters Committee of American College of Gastroenterology. Prevention and management of gastroesophageal varices and variceal hemorrhage in cirrhosis. *Am J Gastroenterol.* 2007;102(9):2086–2102.
8. Vreeburg RM, Snel P, de Bruijne JW, et al. Acute upper gastrointestinal bleeding in the Amsterdam area: incidence, diagnosis, and clinical outcome. *Am J Gastroenterol.* 1997;92:236–243.
9. Bjorkman DJ, Zaman A, Fennerty MB, et al. Urgent vs. elective endoscopy for acute non-variceal upper-GI bleeding: an effectiveness study. *Gastrointest Endosc.* 2004;60:1–8.
10. Lim J, Ahmed A. Endoscopic approach to the treatment of gastrointestinal bleeding. *Tech Vasc Interv Radiol.* 2005;7:123–129.
11. Greenspoon J, Barkun A. A summary of recent recommendations on the management of patients with nonvariceal upper gastrointestinal bleeding. *Pol Arch Med Wewn.* 2010;120(9):341–346.
12. Lau JY, Sung JJ, Lam YH, et al. Endoscopic treatment compared with surgery in patients with recurrent bleeding after initial endoscopic control of bleeding ulcers. *N Engl J Med.* 1999;11(340):751–756.
13. Laine L, Peterson WL. Bleeding peptic ulcer. *N Engl J Med.* 1994;331:717–727.
14. Laine L, Jensen DM. Management of patients with ulcer bleeding. *Am J Gastroenterol.* 2012;107(3):345–360.
15. Gunderman R, Leef J, Ong K, et al. Scintigraphic screening prior to visceral arteriography in acute lower gastrointestinal bleeding. *J Nucl Med.* 1998;39:1081–1083.
16. Millward SF. ACR appropriateness criteria on treatment of acute nonvariceal gastrointestinal tract bleeding. *J Am Coll Radiol.* 2008;5:550–554.
17. Kuhle W, Sheiman R. Detection of active colonic hemorrhage with use of helical CT: findings in a swine model. *Radiology.* 2003;228:743–752.
18. Yoon W, Jeong YY, Shin SS, et al. Acute massive gastrointestinal bleeding: detection and localization with arterial phase multidetector row helical CT. *Radiology.* 2006;239:160–167.

19. Yann G, Rodallec MH, Boulay-Coletta I, et al. Multidetector CT angiography in acute gastrointestinal bleeding: why, when and how. *Radiographics.* 2011;31:E35–E47.
20. ACR Committee on Drugs and Contrast Media. *Manual on Contrast Media: Version 7.* Reston, VA: American College of Radiology; 2010.
21. Ng DA, Opelka FG, Beck DE, et al. Predictive value of technetium Tc 99m-labeled red blood cell scintigraphy for positive angiogram in massive lower gastrointestinal haemorrhage. *Dis Colon Rectum.* 1997;40:471–477.
22. Eriksson L, Ljungdahl M, Sundbom M, et al. Transcatheter arterial embolization versus surgery in the treatment of upper gastrointestinal bleeding after therapeutic endoscopy failure. *J Vasc Interv Radiol.* 2008;19:1413–1418.
23. Ripoll C, Banares R, Beceiro I, et al. Comparison of transcatheter arterial embolization and surgery for treatment of bleeding peptic ulcer after endoscopic treatment failure. *J Vasc Interv Radiol.* 2004;15:447–450.
24. Defreyne L, Vanlangenhove P, De Vos M, et al. Embolization as a first approach with endoscopically unmanageable acute nonvariceal gastrointestinal hemorrhage. *Radiology.* 2001;218(3): 739–748.
25. Schenker MP, Duszak R Jr, Soulen MC, et al. Upper gastrointestinal hemorrhage and transcatheter embolotherapy: clinical and technical factors impacting success and survival. *J Vasc Interv Radiol.* 2001;12:1263–1271.
26. Aina R, Oliva VL, Therasse E, et al. Arterial embolotherapy for upper gastrointestinal hemorrhage: outcome assessment. *J Vasc Interv Radiol.* 2001;12:195–200.
27. Encarnacion CE, Kadir S, Beam CA, et al. Gastrointestinal bleeding: treatment with gastrointestinal arterial embolization. *Radiology.* 1992;183:505–508.
28. Loffroy R, Rao P, Ota S, et al. Embolization of acute nonvariceal upper gastrointestinal hemorrhage resistant to endoscopic treatment: results and predictors of recurrent bleeding. *Cardiovasc Intervent Radiol.* 2010;33:1088–1100.
29. Sandhu C, Buckenham TM, Belli AM. Using CO2-enhanced arteriography to investigate acute gastrointestinal hemorrhage. *AJR Am J Roentgenol.* 1999;173(5):1399–1401.
30. Kim JH, Shin JH, Yoon H, et al. Angiographically negative acute arterial upper and lower gastrointestinal bleeding: incidence, predictive factors, and clinical outcomes. *Korean J Radiol.* 2009;10:384–390.
31. Padia SA, Geisinger MA, Newman JS, et al. Effectiveness of coil embolization in angiographically detectable versus nondetectable sources of upper gastrointestinal hemorrhage. *J Vasc Interv Radiol.* 2009;20:461–466.
32. Dixon S, Chan V, Shrivastava V, et al. Is there a role for empiric gastroduodenal artery embolization in the management of patients with active upper GI hemorrhage? *Cardiovasc Intervent Radiol.* 2013;36:970–977.
33. Loffroy RF, Abualsaud BA, Lin MD, et al. Recent advances in endovascular techniques for management of acute nonvariceal upper gastrointestinal bleeding. *World J Gastrointest Surg.* 2011;3(7):89–100.
34. Song SY, Chung JW, Yin YH, et al. Celiac axis and common hepatic artery variations in 5002 patients: systematic analysis with spiral CT and DSA. *Radiology.* 2010;255:278–288.
35. Tzeng WS, Wu RH, Chang JM, et al. Transcatheter arterial embolization for hemorrhage caused by injury of the hepatic artery. *J Gastroenterol Hepatol.* 2005;20:1062–1068.
36. Sakamoto I, Iwanaga S, Nagaoki K, et al. Intrahepatic biloma formation (bile duct necrosis) after transcatheter arterial chemoembolization. *Am J Roentgenol.* 2003;181:79–87.
37. Lermite E, Regenet N, Tuech J, et al. Diagnosis and treatment of hemosuccus pancreaticus: development of endovascular management. *Pancreas.* 2007;34(2):229–232.
38. Park JH, Kim HC, Chung JW, et al. Transcatheter arterial embolization of arterial esophageal bleeding with the use of *N*-butyl cyanoacrylate. *Korean J Radiol.* 2009;10:361–365.
39. Kos X, Trotteur G, Dondelinger RF. Delayed esophageal hemorrhage caused by a metal stent: treatment with embolization. *Cardiovasc Intervent Radiol.* 1998;21(5):428–430.
40. Michal JA, Brody WR, Walter J, et al. Transcatheter embolization of an esophageal artery for treatment of a bleeding esophageal ulcer. *Radiology.* 1980;134:246.
41. Vogten JM, Overtoom TT, Lely RJ, et al. Superselective coil embolization of arterial esophageal hemorrhage. *J Vasc Interv Radiol.* 2007;18(6):771–773.
42. Lang EK. Transcatheter embolization in management of hemorrhage from duodenal ulcer: long-term results and complications. *Radiology.* 1992;182:703–707.
43. Fidelman N, Freed RC, Nakakura EK, et al. Arterial embolization for the management of gastrointestinal hemorrhage from metastatic renal cell carcinoma. *J Vasc Interv Radiol.* 2010;21: 741–744.
44. Kurihara N, Kikuchi K, Tanabe M, et al. Partial resection of the second portion of the duodenum for gastrointestinal stromal tumor after effective transarterial embolization. *Int J Clin Oncol.* 2005;10:433–437.
45. Frodsham A, Berkmen T, Ananian C, et al. Initial experience using *N*-butyl cyanoacrylate for embolization of lower gastrointestinal hemorrhage. *J Vasc Interv Radiol.* 2009;20: 1312–1319.
46. Pollack JS, White RI. The use of cyanoacrylate adhesives in peripheral embolization. *J Vasc Interv Radiol.* 2001;12(8):907–913.
47. Yata S, Ihaya T, Kaminou T, et al. Transcatheter arterial embolization of acute arterial bleeding in the upper and lower gastrointestinal tract with *N*-butyl-2-cyanoacrylate. *J Vasc Interv Radiol.* 2013;24:422–431.
48. Lee CW, Liu KL, Wang HP, et al. Transcatheter arterial embolization of acute upper gastrointestinal tract bleeding with *N*-butyl-2-cyanoacrylate. *J Vasc Interv Radiol.* 2007;18:209–216.
49. Jae HJ, Chung JW, Jung AY, et al. Transcatheter arterial embolization of nonvariceal upper gastrointestinal bleeding with *N*-butyl cyanoacrylate. *Korean J Radiol.* 2007; 8:48–56.
50. Lenhart M, Paetzel C, Sackmann M, et al. Superselective arterial embolization with a liquid polyvinyl alcohol copolymer in patients with acute gastrointestinal hemorrhage. *Eur Radiol.* 2010;20(8):1994–1999.
51. Darcy M. Treatment of lower gastrointestinal bleeding: vasopressin infusion versus embolization. *J Vasc Interv Radiol.* 2003;14:535–543.
52. Lundgren JA, Matsushima K, Lynch FC, et al. Angiographic embolization of nonvariceal upper gastrointestinal bleeding: predictors of clinical failure. *J Trauma.* 2011;70:1208–1212.

53. Jairath V, Kahan BC, Logan RFA, et al. National audit of the use of surgery and radiological embolization after failed endoscopic haemostasis for non-variceal upper gastrointestinal bleeding. *Br J Surg*. 2012;99(12):1672–1680.
54. Poultsides GA, Kim CJ, Orlando R III, et al. Angiographic embolization for gastroduodenal hemorrhage: safety, efficacy, and predictors of outcome. *Arch Surg*. 2008;143:457–461.
55. Mensel B, Kuhn J, Kraft M, et al. Selective microcoil embolization of arterial gastrointestinal bleeding in the acute situation: outcome, complications, and factors affecting treatment success. *Eur J Gastroenterol Hepatol*. 2012;24(2):155–163.
56. Mirsadraee S, Tirukonda P, Nicholson A, et al. Embolization for non-variceal upper gastrointestinal tract haemorrhage: a systematic review. *Clin Radiol*. 2011;66(6):500–509.
57. Ang D, Teo EK, Tan A, et al. A comparison of surgery versus transcatheter angiographic embolization in the treatment of nonvariceal upper gastrointestinal bleeding uncontrolled by endoscopy. *Gastroenterol Hepatol*. 2012;24:929–938.
58. Wong TC, Wong KT, Chiu PW, et al. A comparison of angiographic embolization with surgery after failed endoscopic hemostasis to bleeding peptic ulcers. *Gastrointest Endosc*. 2011;73:900–908.
59. de Franchis R. Evolving consensus in portal hypertension. Report of the Baveno IV consensus workshop on methodology of diagnosis and therapy in portal hypertension. *J Hepatol*. 2005;43:167–176.
60. Garcia-Tsao G, Sanyal AJ, Grace ND, et al. Prevention and management of gastroesophageal varices and variceal hemorrhage in cirrhosis. *Hepatology*. 2007;46:922–938.
61. Lee E, Laberge J. Differential diagnosis of gastrointestinal bleeding. *Tech Vasc Interv Radiol*. 2004;7(3):112–122.
62. Avgerinos A, Armonis A. Balloon tamponade technique and efficiency in variceal hemorrhage. *Scand J Gastroenterol Suppl*. 1994;207:11.
63. Brett BT, Hayes PC, Jalan R. Primary prophylaxis of variceal bleeding in cirrhosis. *Eur J Gastroenterol Hepatol*. 2001;13:349.
64. Gines P, Cardenas A, Arroyo V, et al. Management of cirrhosis and ascites. *N Engl J Med*. 2004;350:1646.
65. Infante-Rivard C, Esucola S, Villeneuve JP. Role of endoscopic variceal sclerotherapy in the long term management of variceal bleeding: a metaanalysis. *Gastroenterology*. 1989;96:1087.
66. de Franchis R, Primignani M. Why do varices bleed? *Gastroenterol Clin North Am*. 1992;21(1):85.
67. Smith JL, Graham DY. Variceal hemorrhage: a critical evaluation of survival analysis. *Gastroenterology*. 1982;82:968.
68. DeDombal FT, Clarke JR, Clamp SE, et al. Prognostic factors in upper GI bleeding. *Endoscopy*. 1986;18:6s.
69. Graham DY, Smith JL. The course of patients after variceal hemorrhage. *Gastroenterology*. 1981;80:800.
70. Tesdal IK, Filser T, Weiss C, et al. Transjugular intrahepatic portosystemic shunts: adjunctive embolization of collateral vessels in the prevention of variceal rebleeding. *Radiology*. 2005;236(1):360–367.

30

Lower Gastrointestinal Bleeding

Michael Bret Anderson

Lower gastrointestinal (GI) bleeding is defined by intraluminal bleeding distal to the ligament of Treitz (the suspensory ligament of the duodenum composed of a band of smooth muscle extending from the junction of the duodenum and jejunum to the left crus of the diaphragm). The severity of lower GI bleeding can range from clinically insignificant to massive and life threatening. Although *upper* GI bleeding is four times as common as *lower* GI bleeding, lower tract bleeding still accounts for 21 adult hospital admissions per 100,000 persons per year. Primarily affecting older adults, the mean age of presentation is 63 to 77 years. Approximately 80% to 90% of cases will resolve with conservative medical therapy; however, up to 25% of patients will rebleed during or after the hospital admission. The mortality of lower GI bleeding is reported from 2% to 4%.[1]

Common etiologies of lower GI hemorrhage in the adult population include diverticular disease, hemorrhoids, arteriovenous malformation (AVM) and angiodysplasia, postpolypectomy bleeding, inflammatory bowel disease, neoplasm, infection, ulcers, and aortoenteric fistula.[2] Meckel diverticulum is encountered in the pediatric and young adult population (Table 30.1).

Lower tract varices are an uncommon source of lower GI bleeding and are generally treated with a similar approach to the more typical upper tract varices of portal hypertension.[3]

The colon is the source of bleeding in 80% of lower GI tract hemorrhages. When the source of bleeding is the large bowel, the distribution is rather evenly distributed, with one-third originating in the ascending colon, one-third in the transverse colon, and one-third in the rectosigmoid.[4]

Endoscopy is generally considered first-line treatment for both upper and lower GI bleeding.[5] Although colonoscopy is useful and recommended for the evaluation and possibly the treatment of "slow" or chronic recurrent bleeding, its usefulness can be limited in the setting of acute lower GI arterial bleeding. Intraluminal blood and retained stool can impair visibility and make it difficult to reach the ascending colon, which is a common site of lower GI hemorrhage. Additionally, the lower GI tract to include all the small bowel distal to the ligament of Treitz cannot be fully evaluated with conventional endoscopy.[1]

Surgery, alternatively, does not carry the same limitations as endoscopy. However, emergent surgery for active arterial bleeding in the lower tract is associated with significant morbidity and mortality (20% to 30%), with mortality reported greater than 40% in some studies.[6,7] In the event the site of bleeding cannot be localized intraoperatively, empiric resection might be required with selection of a partial or subtotal colectomy. If in fact the site of bleeding is not resected, hemorrhage is most likely to recur.[8]

The use of catheter angiography to diagnose GI bleeding was first described in 1963.[9] The infusion of vasoconstrictive drugs followed soon thereafter. Then in 1970, autologous clot was first used as an embolic agent in the treatment of upper GI bleeding.[10]

For maximum benefit and optimal outcomes, a multidisciplinary approach should be considered. A team including gastroenterology, interventional radiology, and surgery is recommended to provide the best care to the patient with lower GI bleeding (Fig. 30.1).

IMAGING (FIGS. 30.2 TO 30.8)

Given its sensitivity to detect GI bleeding at rates as low as 0.04 mL per minute, nuclear medicine radionuclide scintigraphy ("bleeding scan") with technetium 99m (Tc 99m)–labeled red blood cells (RBCs) is often used to detect and localize GI hemorrhage. Tc 99m RBC scintigraphy has a reported 93% sensitivity and 95% specificity for detecting the site of GI bleeding.[11] Scintigraphy is also of benefit in the

Table 30.1 Most Common Causes of Lower Gastrointestinal Bleeding

Most Common Causes of Lower Gastrointestinal Bleeding
Diverticulosis
Hemorrhoids
AVM/angiodysplasia
Postpolypectomy bleeding
Inflammatory bowel disease
Neoplasm
Infection
Ulceration
Aortoenteric/graft-enteric fistula
Meckel diverticulum

AVM, arteriovenous malformation.

patient demonstrating a pattern of recurrent hemorrhage who intermittently ceases to bleed. Because imaging is performed over the course of at least 1 to 2 hours, Tc 99m RBC studies increase the chances of "catching" active bleeding and therefore localizing the site before intervention.

However, in recent years, with the evolution of multidetector-row helical computed tomography (MDCT), contrast-enhanced computed tomography angiography (CTA) has become a rapid, noninvasive, and accurate tool to diagnose and localize GI bleeding. CT mesenteric angiography has been shown, in the setting of hemodynamically significant GI bleeding, to provide an overall location-based sensitivity, specificity, and accuracy in the detection and localization of GI bleeding of 91%, 99%, and 97%, respectively.[12] In addition, CT provides the anatomic detail and diagnostic information of cross-sectional imaging that is not obtained with scintigraphy or catheter angiography alone. When the underlying etiology of bleeding is unknown, CT is very helpful in diagnosis. Given the multiple possible etiologies of lower GI hemorrhage, CTA can potentially limit the time and contrast volume that will be required in the angiography suite to localize and treat the source of bleeding. Knowing the etiology of the hemorrhage also allows preprocedure planning for the technique and embolic materials that will most likely be used to achieve embolization.

TECHNIQUE

In contrast to the vascular supply of the upper GI tract that is well-collateralized by a rich network of branch vessels of the celiac axis and the superior mesenteric artery (SMA), the lower GI tract is at greater risk of iatrogenic ischemic insult secondary to embolization and surgical procedures. The extensive arcades of the SMA and the inferior mesenteric artery (IMA) provide some protection via collateralized supply in the lower GI tract.[13]

Historical use of embolotherapy for the control of lower GI bleeding was complicated by the risk of ischemic colitis or frank bowel infarction, and embolization gave way for a time to the preferred method of catheter-directed vasopressin infusion. However, with the development of microcatheter technology, superselective embolization has emerged as the first-line therapy in the treatment of patients with severe lower GI bleeding refractory to conservative management.

There are essentially no absolute contraindications to superselective embolization. Relative contraindications include significant coagulopathy (in that embolotherapy is to a degree reliant on the native clotting of the patient) and severe contrast allergy (although rapid steroid pretreatment can be performed).[14]

Appropriate resuscitation efforts should be carried out before and throughout the course of the angiographic procedure to include large-bore intravenous (IV) access, correction of

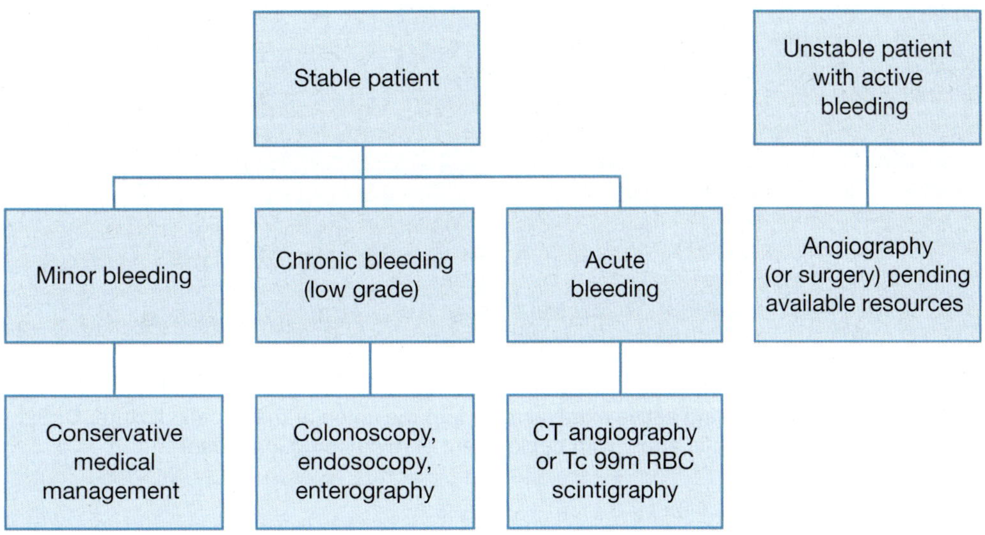

Figure 30.1 Team approach to management of patients with lower GI bleeding. CT, computed tomography; Tc 99m, technetium 99m; RBC, red blood cell.

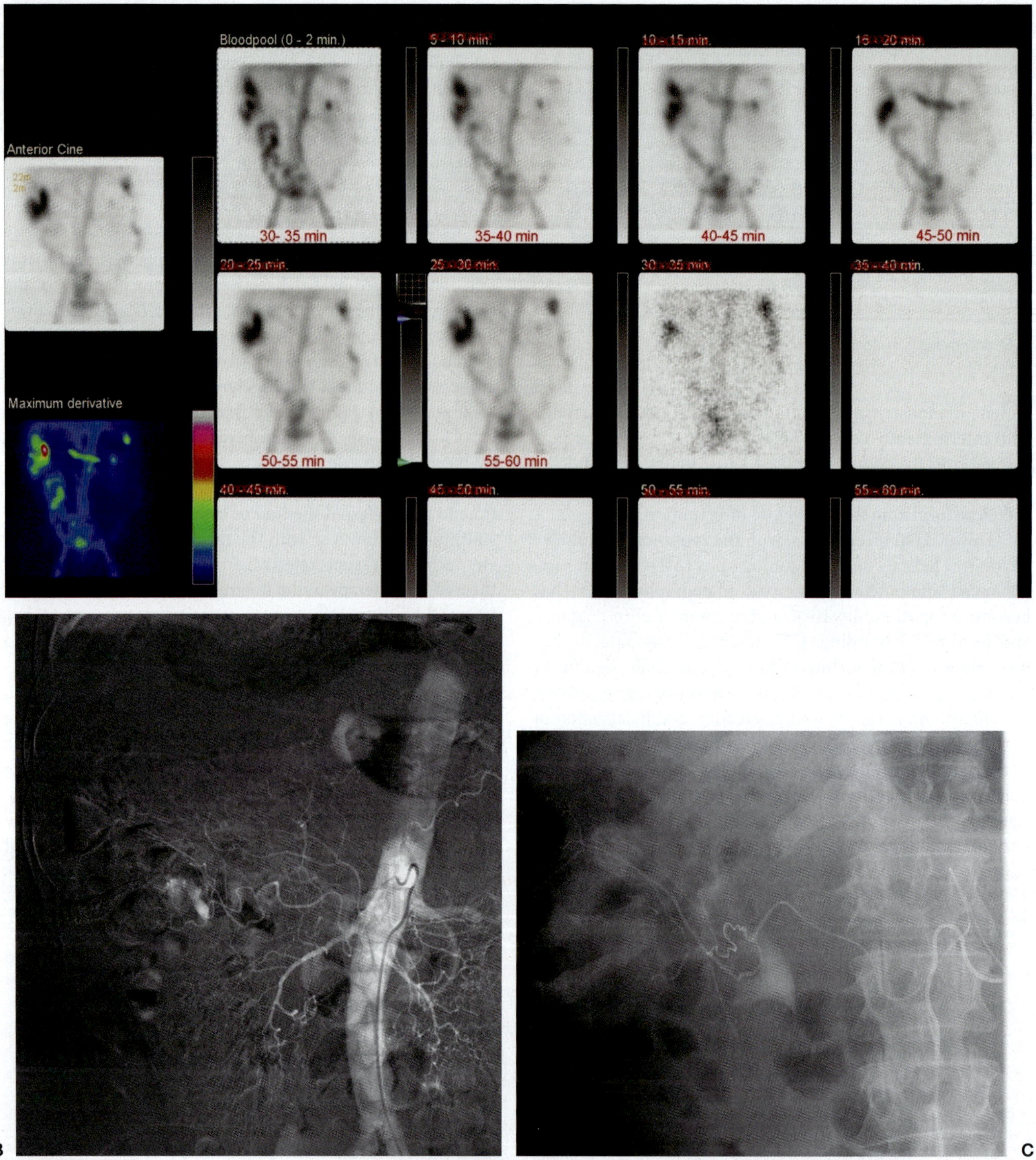

A

B

C

Figure 30.2 **A:** Nuclear medicine Tc 99m RBC scintigraphy demonstrating GI bleeding localized to the hepatic flexure. **B:** SMA angiogram revealing active extravasation into the colon at the hepatic flexure. **C:** Superselective catheterization of a branch of the right colic artery with deployment of microcoil. *(Continued)*

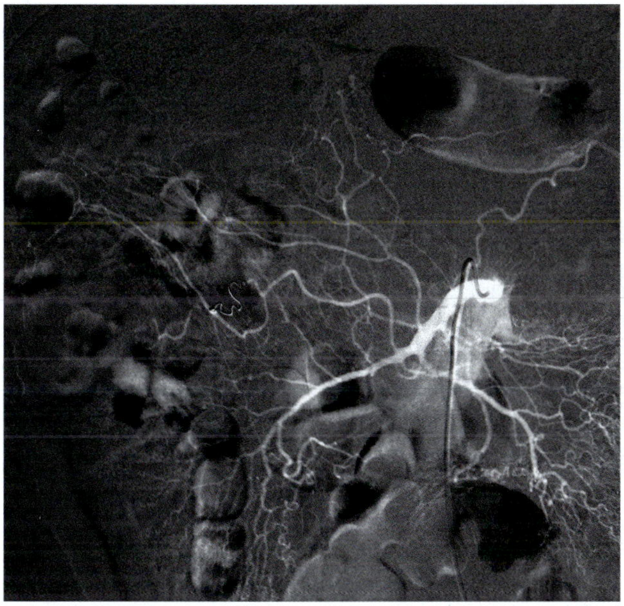

D

Figure 30.2 *(Continued)* **D:** After coiling, SMA angiogram demonstrates no further extravasation with preserved flow to the adjacent colon.

coagulopathy, and transfusions as needed. Continuous cardiorespiratory monitoring throughout the procedure is required. Blood loss must be recorded throughout the exam, and blood products should be transfused as warranted.[15] General anesthesia may be required and can prove helpful in visualization by limiting respiratory and GI motion artifact. Foley catheter placement should also be considered to monitor urine output as well as improve visualization of the pelvis.

Initially, a 5-Fr catheter (a Mickelson [Boston Scientific, Marlborough, Massachusetts] or Cobra 2 [Angiodynamics, Latham, New York] catheter are most commonly chosen at the author's institution) should be used to select the SMA or IMA and arteriography is performed. Selecting the IMA first to interrogate its distribution in the pelvis before the urinary bladder filling with contrast material may be helpful. Preprocedure imaging is of course valuable in directing the operator to where the search should begin for the source of bleeding. Glucagon in a dose of 0.25 to 2 mg IV may be administered to limit peristalsis of the bowel if motion interferes with detection of extravasation.[16] Acquisition of images in digital subtraction mode with images reviewed in native display is often helpful to differentiate motion artifact from true extravasation.

When a source of active bleeding is identified, a 3-Fr or smaller diameter microcatheter should be positioned coaxially via the 5-Fr catheter and directed to the site of extravasation. The most feared complication of lower GI embolization is bowel ischemia; therefore, embolization should only be attempted when adequate selective catheterization can be achieved. If the microcatheter cannot be advanced distally to the level of the marginal artery or vasa rectae ("border of the colon"), then there is an increased risk of ischemia. Performing an arteriogram at this point—before embolization—is advised to ensure adjacent vascular arcades provide adequate perfusion to the bowel proximal and distal to the site of embolization.[13] Embolization is considered technically successful when conducted to the point of cessation of arterial extravasation. Embolization can be performed with microcoils, Gelfoam (Pharmacia & Upjohn, Kalamazoo, Michigan), and polyvinyl alcohol particles. Of note, particles smaller than 250 μm should not be used to avoid end-organ embolization.[1,13,17]

A

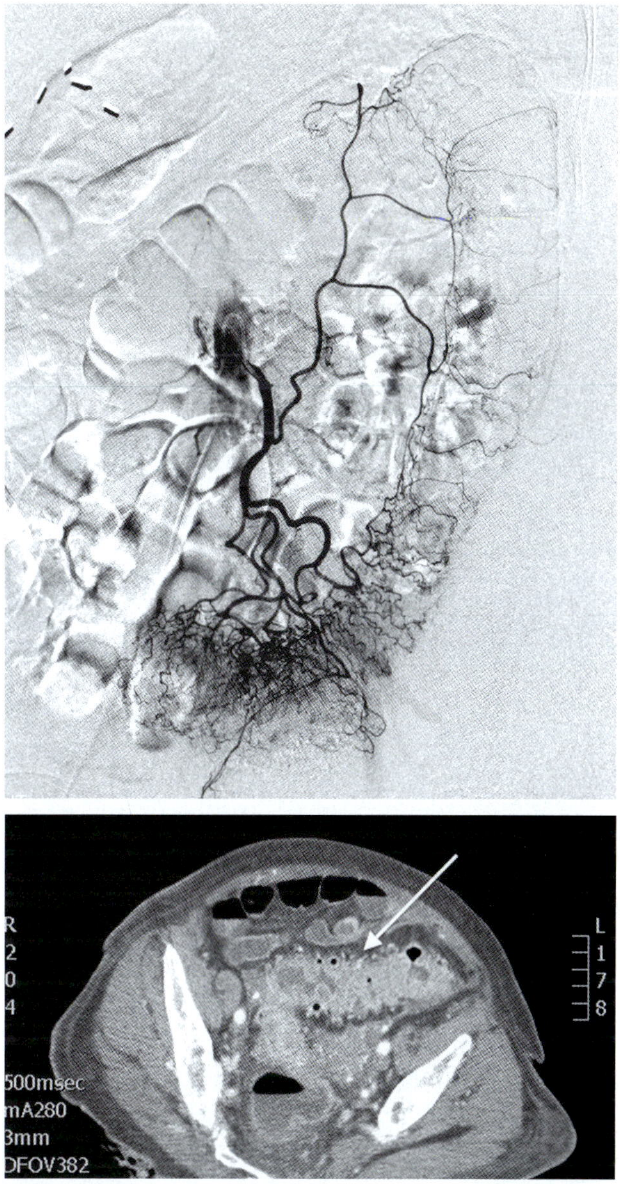

B

Figure 30.3 **A:** Selective IMA angiogram demonstrating characteristic appearance of inflammation/hyperemia of sigmoid diverticulitis without active extravasation. **B:** CT imaging in same patient correlating findings of diverticulitis (*white arrow*) without active bleeding.

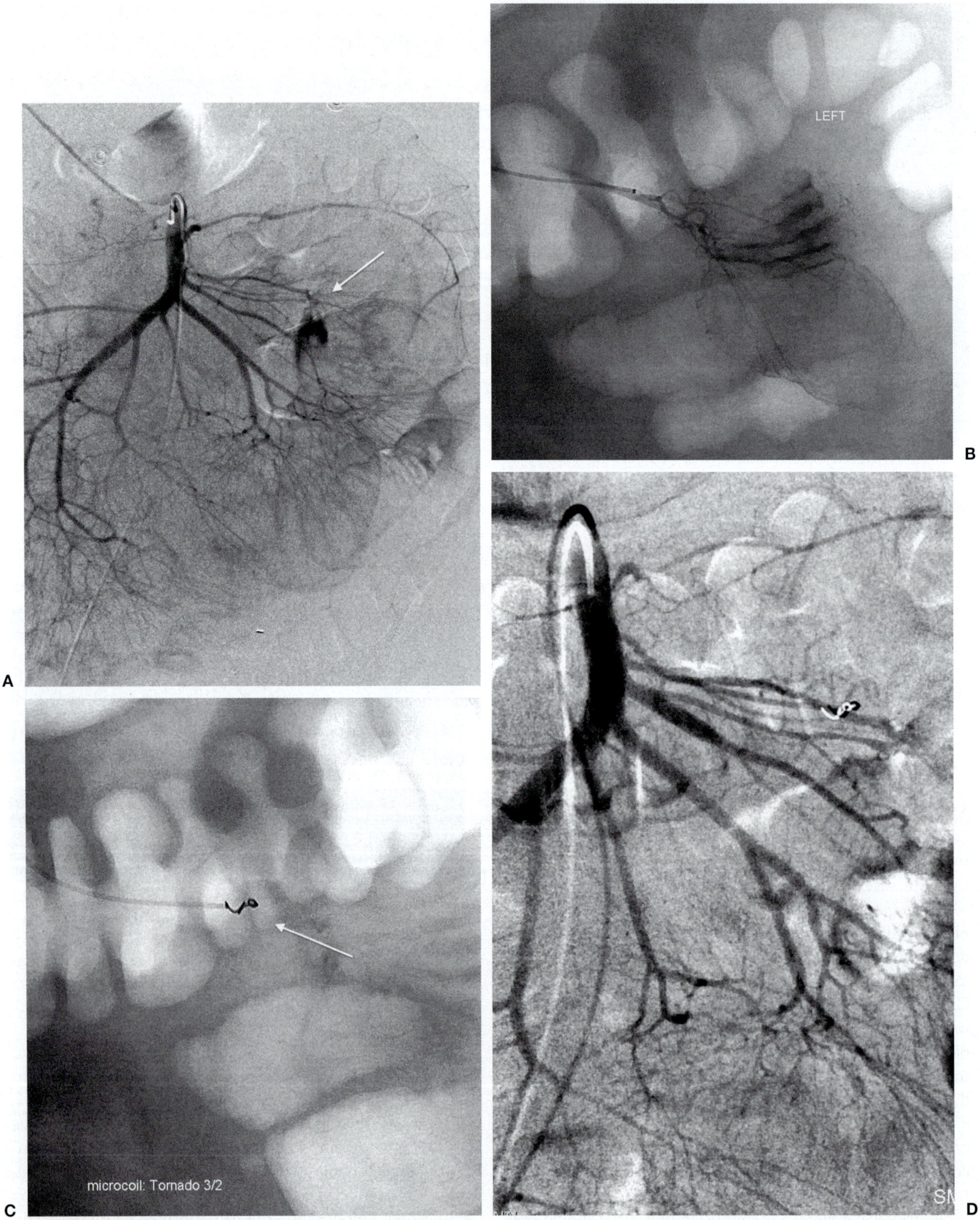

Figure 30.4 **A:** SMA angiogram, with use of glucagon IV, in a patient with known graft-versus-host disease (GVHD) demonstrating active bleeding from a jejunal branch (*white arrow*) in the left midabdomen. **B:** Superselective microcatheter angiogram showing intraluminal extravasation of contrast. **C:** Microcoil and Gelfoam embolization (*arrow*). **D:** SMA angiogram post coiling shows cessation of bleeding.

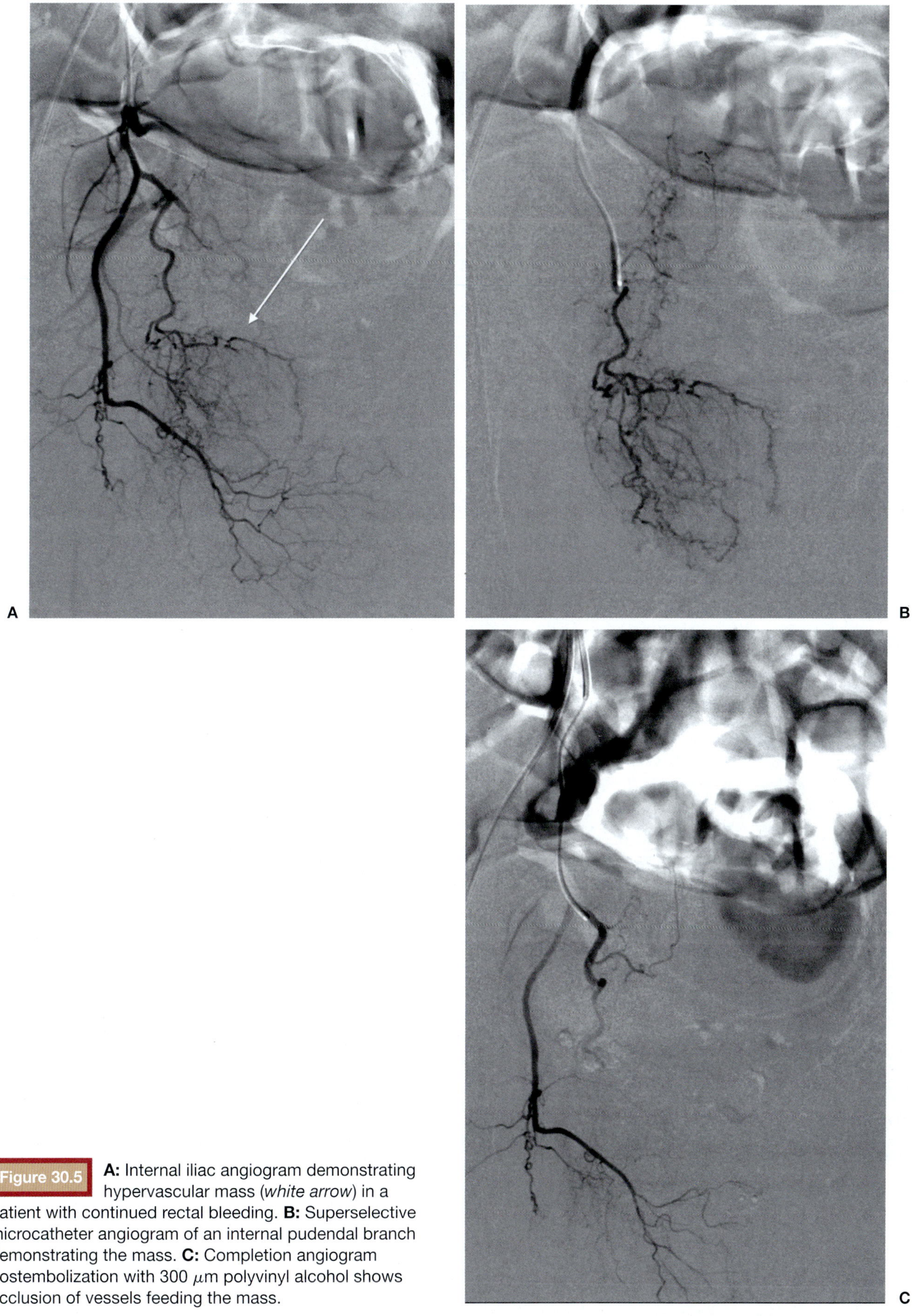

Figure 30.5 **A:** Internal iliac angiogram demonstrating hypervascular mass (*white arrow*) in a patient with continued rectal bleeding. **B:** Superselective microcatheter angiogram of an internal pudendal branch demonstrating the mass. **C:** Completion angiogram postembolization with 300 μm polyvinyl alcohol shows occlusion of vessels feeding the mass.

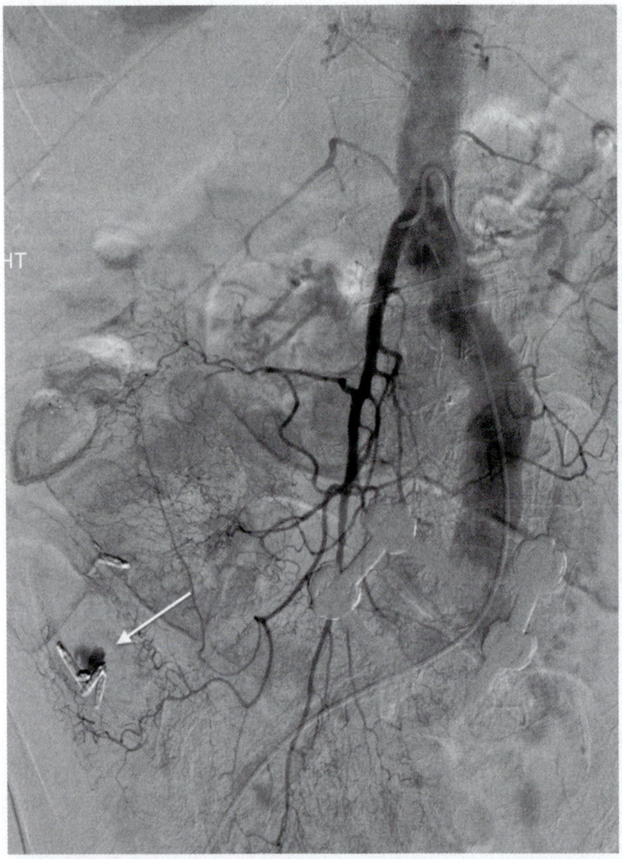

A

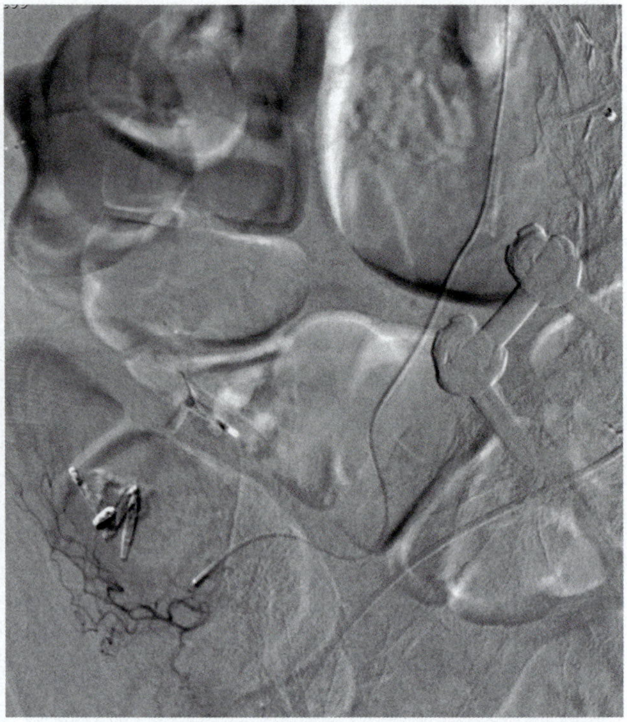

B

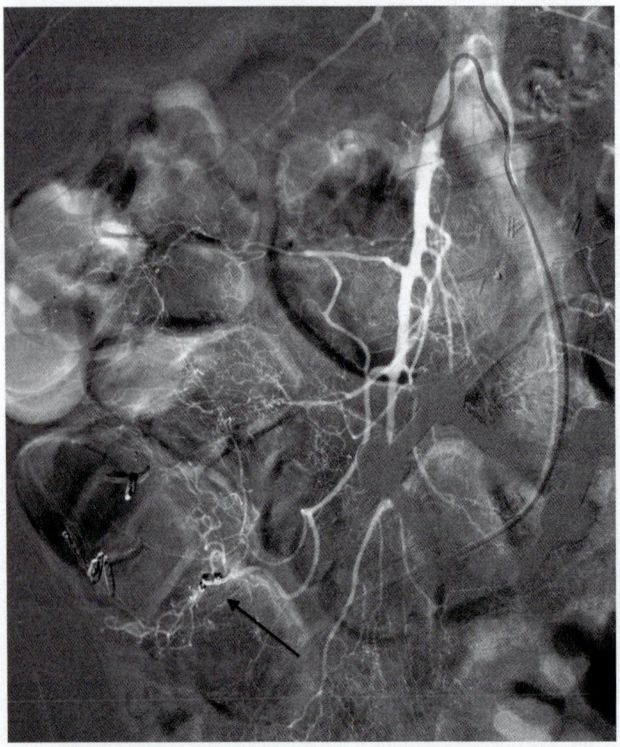

C

Figure 30.6 **A:** SMA angiogram in a patient with postpolypectomy lower GI bleeding demonstrating active bleeding (*white arrow*) from a branch of the ileocolic artery at the site of polypectomy. **B:** Superselective angiogram of the ileocolic branch to the site of bleeding. **C:** Post microcoil (*black arrow*) embolization, there is no further active bleeding seen.

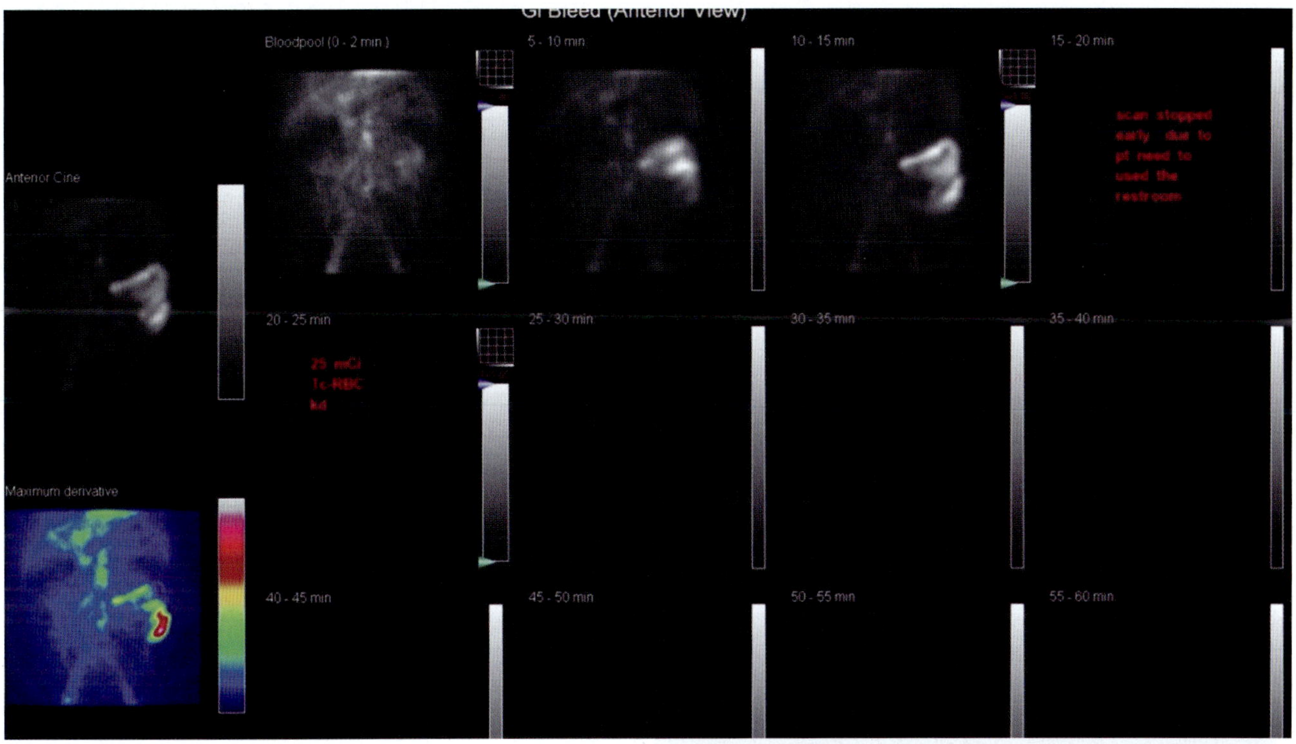

A

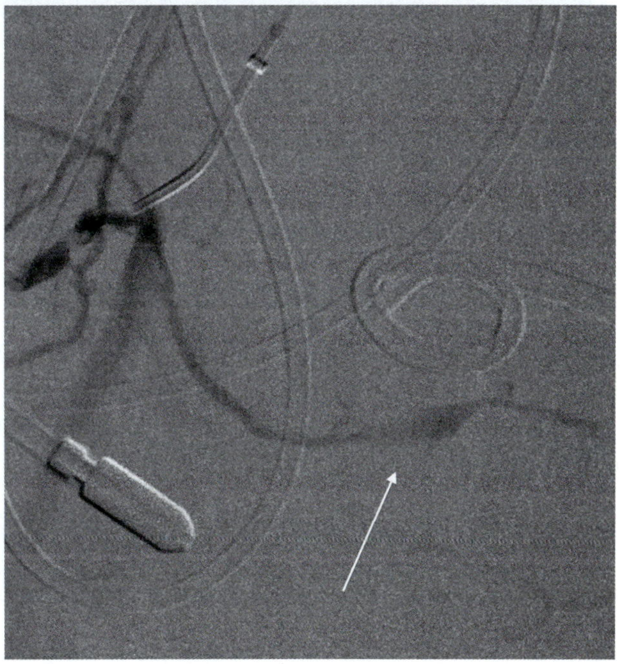

B

Figure 30.7 **A:** Tc 99m RBC scan shows active bleeding in the jejunum of the left midabdomen. **B:** SMA angiogram reveals a jejunal branch pseudoaneurysm (*white arrow*). *(Continued)*

Although the use of *N*-butyl cyanoacrylate (NBCA), commonly referred to as *glue*, has been shown to be safe and effective in other applications including bleeding in the *upper* GI tract,[18] in the *lower* GI tract, its use remains controversial based on the risk of nonselective, or too extensive, embolization. The use of NBCA, however, as an alternative agent in the lower tract when standard embolic agents are not feasible in the coagulopathic, unstable patient has been reported.[19]

In the event that superselective catheterization cannot be achieved, vasopressin infusion may be used as an alternative therapy. Vasopressin (Pitressin), an anterior pituitary hormone that causes smooth muscle contraction and water retention, can be infused to induce vasoconstriction and control bleeding in the colon or small intestine. Its use, however, is labor and time intensive. Positioning the catheter in either the proximal SMA or IMA, infusion is initiated at 0.2 unit

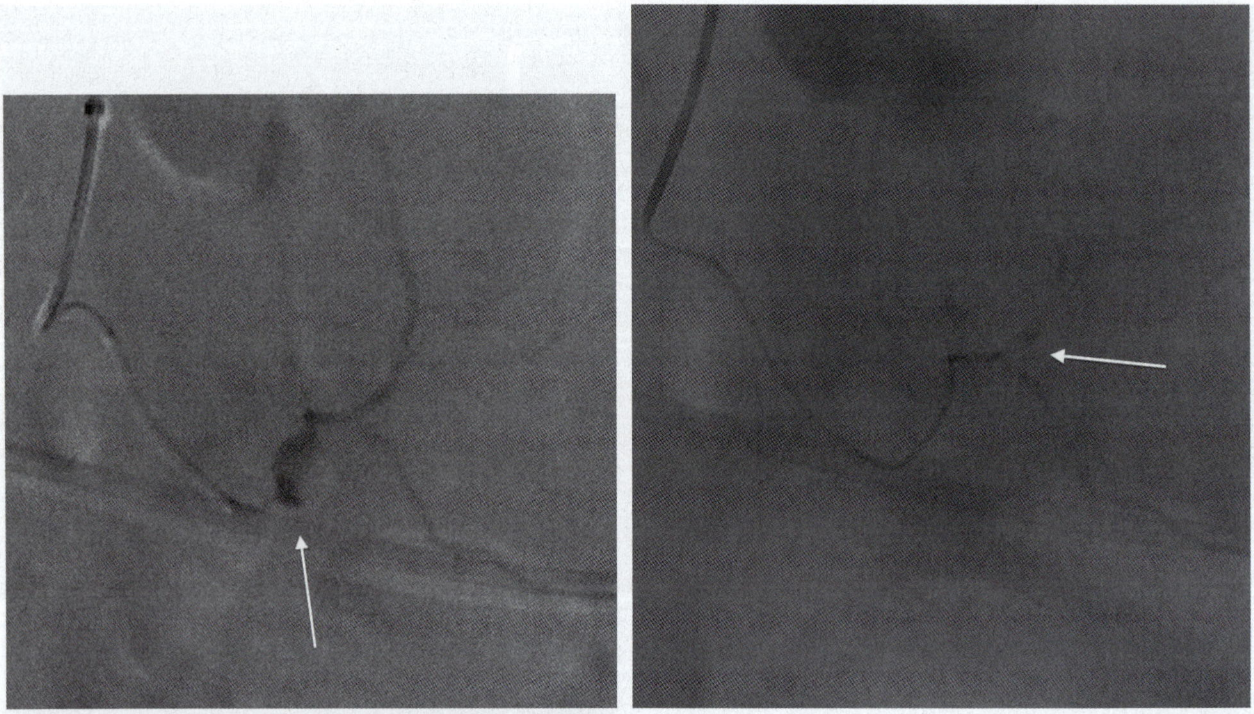

C D

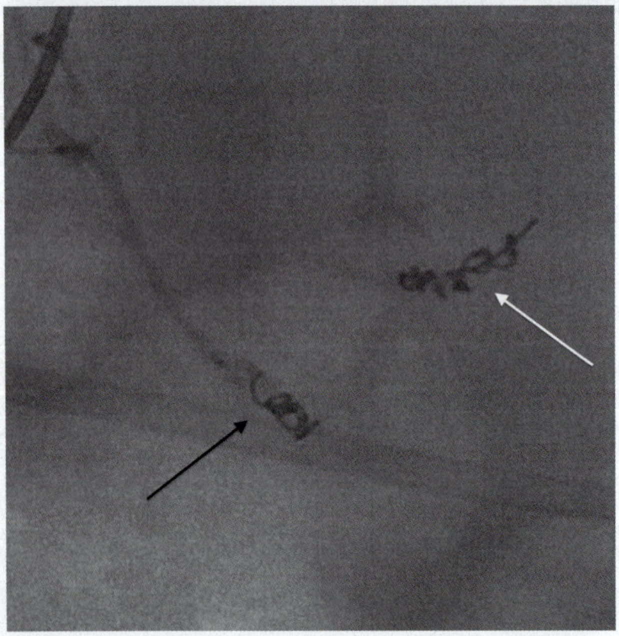

E

Figure 30.7 *(Continued)* **C,D:** A microcatheter is selectively advanced to positions proximal and then distal to the pseudoaneurysm (*white arrows*). **E:** Microcoils deployed distal (*white arrow*) then proximal (*black arrow*) to exclude the pseudoaneurysm.

per minute, repeating angiography every 20 to 30 minutes to evaluate for continued bleeding. The vasopressin infusion is increased by 0.1 unit per minute until the bleeding ceases or the maximum dose of 0.4 unit per minute is reached. Once bleeding is controlled, the vasopressin should be administered at the effective dose and then gradually tapered over time. As an example, if 0.4 unit per minute controls the hemorrhage, then infuse at 0.4 unit per minute × 12 hours, taper to 0.3 unit per minute × 12 hours, then 0.2 unit per minute × 12 hours, then 0.1 unit per minute × 12 hours, and then discontinued if there is no evidence of further GI bleeding. The catheter should remain secured in place and saline should be infused an additional 6 to 12 hours.[5,14]

Contraindications to vasopressin infusion include active myocardial ischemia, bowel ischemia, and limb ischemia. Patients must be monitored in the intensive care unit (ICU) and might experience significant abdominal cramping secondary to the smooth muscle constriction.[19] Vasopressin should not be used to treat AVMs or pseudoaneurysms but can be up to 90% effective in treating diverticular bleeding

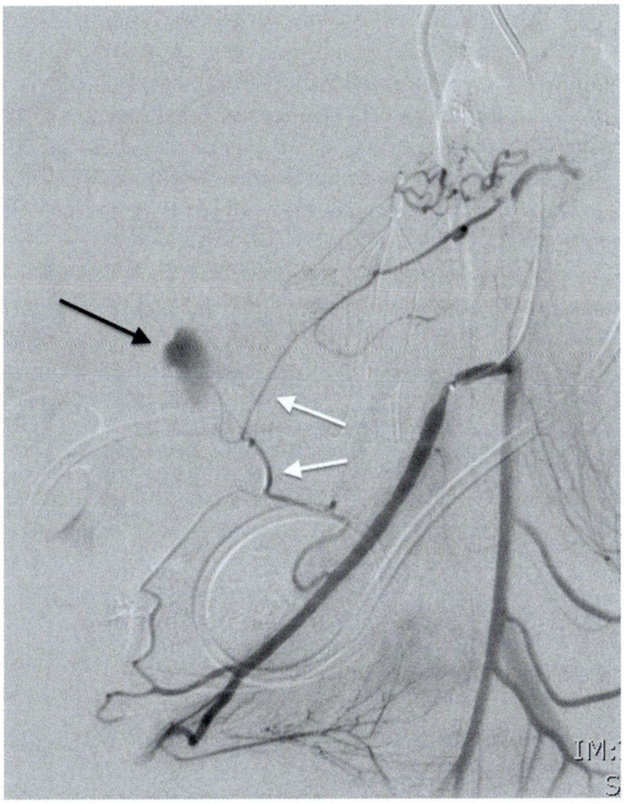

A

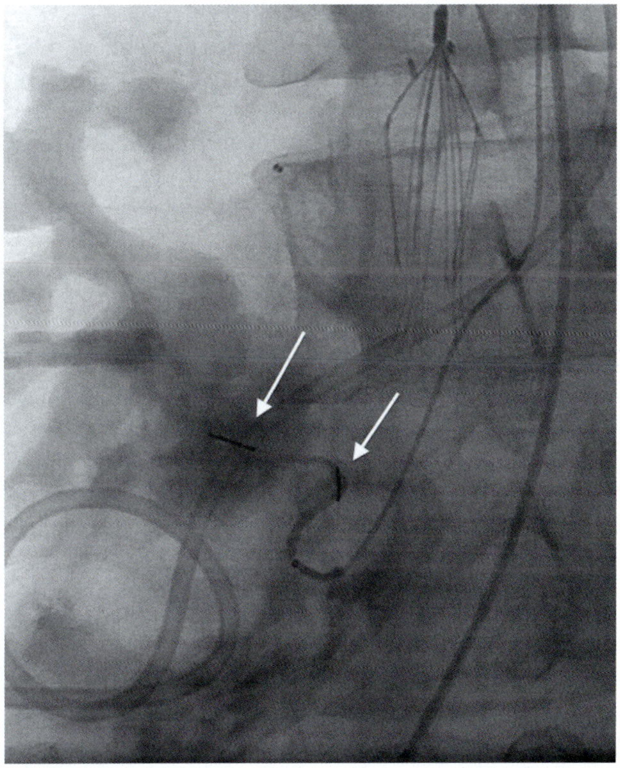

B

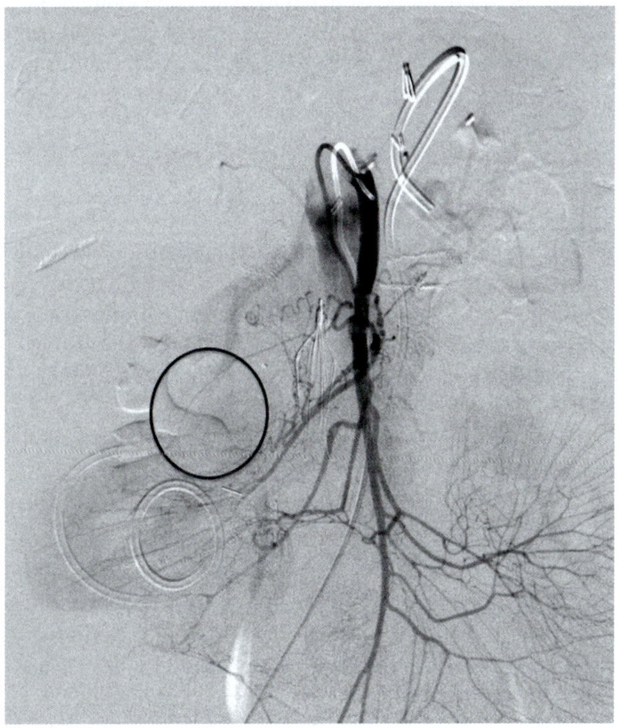

C

Figure 30.8 **A:** SMA angiogram reveals active extravasation (*black arrow*). Note two separate feeding vessels (*white arrows*) and spasm about the tip of the microcatheter. **B:** Superselective embolization with two Hilal (Cook Medical Inc., Bloomington, Indiana) microcoils (*white arrows*). **C:** Completion angiogram shows no further extravasation.

and postpolypectomy bleeding.[20,21] Unfortunately, half of these patients may rebleed at a later time.[21–23]

It is not uncommon for mesenteric angiography to be negative for active bleeding at the time the exam is performed. When active bleeding is not demonstrated at the time of angiography, provocative maneuvers to induce a prohemorrhagic state can be employed; if bleeding is induced, then the site can be localized and potentially treated. The technique consists of adding anticoagulants, vasodilators, and fibrinolytics during angiography to provoke bleeding. Provocative angiography is likely to be most useful in the small percentage of lower GI hemorrhage patients who require multiple admissions and repeat transfusions but remain undiagnosed by standard endoscopic and radiologic examination.[24] The use of provocative angiography, initially described in 1982,[25] has been shown to be safe and effective.[26,27] However, the protocols employed and reported rates of success vary significantly, and therefore it is suggested that provocative maneuvers should be reserved for those operators experienced with this technique. It is also recommended that surgical "back up" be available in the rare event that uncontrollable bleeding is encountered.

In the event neither embolization nor vasopressin infusion can be safely performed, but the source of bleeding is identified, then the site can be localized for the surgeon. A catheter can be positioned and left in place to facilitate intraoperative methylene blue injection. Alternatively, a coil can be deployed to later be identified by palpation or transillumination of the mesentery at the time of surgery.[28,29]

POTENTIAL COMPLICATIONS AND RESULTS

The most worrisome and serious complication of lower GI tract embolization is bowel infarction. An overly aggressive embolization, vasopressin combined with embolization, arterial dissection, and surgically altered collateral flow about anastomotic bleeding sites have all been implicated in cases of bowel infarction. Postprocedure abdominal pain, passage of bloody stools, and occasionally fever and leukocytosis can be encountered after lower GI tract embolization. Although these signs and symptoms are not uncommonly secondary to the underlying pathology or mild ischemia, the abdominal exam and laboratory values must be closely monitored to detect early signs of ischemia or infarction. Strict bowel rest is recommended until clinically cleared.[2] Other potential complications include nontarget embolization, arterial dissection, hematoma/vascular access complications, and contrast-induced nephropathy.[30]

Development of bowel stricture postembolization (identified at endoscopy) has also been reported.[31] These strictures are not necessarily symptomatic but if required can potentially be treated with endoscopic dilation. Since 1990, with the use of microcatheters and superselective technique, a minor complication rate of 15.3% and major complication rate of 1.3% have been reported.[21]

Technical success as defined by the cessation of active extravasation at angiography has been reported from 73% to 100%. In recent years, with the use of microcatheters, the reported technical success rate has reached an average of 88%. The *clinical* success rate, defined as prolonged cessation of bleeding postembolization, is reported slightly lower with an average of 83%. Clinical success is superior in the colon (86% to 100%) to the overall success rate (60% to 100%).[21]

In 1974, embolization therapy for lower GI hemorrhage was reported for the first time[32] and since has been reported in greater than 50 publications. Superselective mesenteric embolization for lower GI bleeding, although at times technically challenging, can be safely performed in the appropriately selected patient with a favorable technical and clinical rate of success. The risk of bowel infarction exists, but the rate of intestinal injury is low. The procedure allows for rapid control of bleeding and can be repeated if continued or recurrent bleeding occurs. Superselective embolization should be considered the transcatheter treatment of choice in active lower GI bleeding.

TIPS AND TRICKS

- Be superselective to avoid bowel ischemia/infarction.
- Use a team management approach with collaboration among gastroenterology, surgery, and interventional radiology.
- When able, obtain CT angiogram or Tc 99m scintigraphy to localize bleeding before angiography.
- Acquire images in digital subtraction; review images in native display.
- Glucagon 1 mg IV can be used to limit motion artifact of bowel peristalsis.
- Image the IMA first before contrast collects in the urinary bladder.
- If the source of bleeding is not identified, check the celiac axis. Brisk upper GI bleeding can mimic lower GI bleeding.
- Papaverine 25 mg intra-arterial can be used to treat catheter-induced vasospasm.
- In the setting of intermittent bleeding and a previously negative arteriogram, a return trip to angiography when the patient is clinically actively bleeding can be successful. Provocative bleeding maneuvers can be employed based on the operator's expertise.
- In the severely coagulopathic patient, Gelfoam pledgets deployed between coils can potentially provide occlusion of the selected vessel and increase the chances of hemostasis. Early results show that NBCA (glue) can also be useful in the setting of severe coagulopathy.
- In the appropriate patient when selective embolization cannot be achieved, vasopressin infusion can be considered. In some situations, vasopressin can be

used to temporarily diminish bleeding and possibly increase the patient's chance of receiving definitive surgery/intervention.

- If selective embolization cannot be safely performed, but the site of bleeding is identified, a catheter can be placed for intraoperative methylene blue injection. Alternatively, a coil can be placed to be identified later by palpation or transillumination of the mesentery at time of surgery.

REFERENCES

1. Rockey D. Lower gastrointestinal bleeding. *Gastroenterology*. 2006;130:165–171.
2. Gould J. Angiography and embolization in lower gastrointestinal bleeding. *Appl Radiol*. 2004;33(12).
3. Yuki N, Kubo M, Noro Y, et al. Jejunal varices as a cause of massive gastrointestinal bleeding. *Am J Gastroenterol*. 1992; 87(4):514–517.
4. Walker T, Salazar G, Waltman A. Angiographic evaluation and management of acute gastrointestinal hemorrhage. *World J Gastroenterol*. 2012;18(11):1191–1201.
5. Cherian M, Mehta P, Kalyanpur T, et al. Arterial interventions in gastrointestinal bleeding. *Semin Intervent Radiol*. 2009;26(3): 184–196.
6. Taylor F, Epstein L. Treatment of massive diverticular hemorrhage. *Arch Surg*. 1969;98:505–508.
7. Rozycki G, Tremblay L, Feliciano D, et al. Three hundred consecutive emergent celiotomies in general surgery patients. *Ann Surg*. 2002;235:681–688.
8. Klein R, Gallagher D. Massive colonic bleeding from diverticular disease. *Am J Surg*. 1969;118:553–557.
9. Nusbaum M, Baum S. Radiographic demonstration of unknown sites of gastrointestinal bleeding. *Surg Forum*. 1963;14:374–375.
10. Rosch J, Keller F, Kaufman J. The birth, early years, and future of interventional radiology. *J Vasc Interv Radiol*. 2003;14: 841–853.
11. Bunker S, Lull R, Tanasescu D, et al. Scintigraphy of gastrointestinal hemorrhage. *AJR Am J Roentgenol*. 1984;143(3):543–548.
12. Yoon W, Jeong Y, Shin S. Acute massive gastrointestinal bleeding: detection and localization with arterial phase multidetector row helical CT. *Radiology*. 2006;239(1):160–167.
13. Funaki B. Microcatheter embolization of lower gastrointestinal hemorrhage. *Cardiovasc Intervent Radiol*. 2004;27:591–599.
14. Uflacker R. *Visceral and Non-Vascular Percutaneous Therapy*. Philadelphia, PA: Lippincott Williams & Wilkins; 2002.
15. Funaki B. On-call treatment of acute gastrointestinal hemorrhage. *Semin Intervent Radiol*. 2006; 23(3):215–222.
16. Oppenheimer J, Ray C Jr, Kondo K. Miscellaneous pharmaceutical agents in interventional radiology. *Semin Intervent Radiol*. 2010;27(4):422–430.
17. Uflacker R. Transcatheter embolization for treatment of acute lower gastrointestinal bleeding. *Acta Radiol*. 1987;28:425–430.
18. Jae HJ, Chung JW, Jung AY, et al. Transcatheter arterial embolization of nonvariceal upper gastrointestinal bleeding with n-butyl cyanoacrylate. *Korean J Radiol*. 2007;8(1):46–56.
19. Frodsham A, Berkmen T, Ananian C, et al. Initial experience using N-butyl cyanoacrylate for embolization of lower gastrointestinal hemorrhage. *J Vasc Interv Radiol*. 2009;20(10): 1312–1319.
20. Kaufman J. Visceral arteries. In: Kaufman J, Lee M, eds. *Vascular and Interventional Radiology: The Requisites*. Philadelphia, PA: Mosby; 2004:286–322.
21. Darcy M. Treatment of lower gastrointestinal bleeding: vasopressin infusion versus embolization. *J Vasc Interv Radiol*. 2003; 14:535–543.
22. Baum S, Nusbaum M. The control of gastrointestinal hemorrhage by selective mesenteric arterial infusion of vasopressin. *Radiology*. 1971;98:497–505.
23. Athanasoulis C, Baum, S, Rösch J, et al. Mesenteric arterial infusions of vasopressin for hemorrhage from colonic diverticulosis. *Am J Surg*. 1975;129:212–216.
24. Johnston C, Tuite D, Pritchard R, et al. Use of provocative angiography to localize site in recurrent GI bleeding. *Cardiovasc Intervent Radiol*. 2007;30:1042–1046.
25. Rösch J, Keller FS, Wawrukiewicz A, et al. Pharmacoangiography in the diagnosis of recurrent massive lower gastrointestinal bleeding. *Radiology*. 1982;145:615–619
26. Bloomfield R, Smith T, Schneider A, et al. Provocative angiography in patients with gastrointestinal hemorrhage of obscure origin. *Am J Gastroenterol*. 2000;95(10):2807–2812.
27. Kim C, Suhocki P, Miller M Jr, et al. Provocative mesenteric angiography for lower gastrointestinal hemorrhage. *J Vasc Interv Radiol*. 2010;21(4):477–483.
28. Athanasoulis C, Moncure A, Greenfield A, et al. Intraoperative localization of small bowel bleeding sites with combined use of angiographic methods and methylene blue injection. *Surgery*. 1980;87:77–84.
29. Schmidt S, Boskind J, Smith D, et al. Angiographic localization of small bowel angiodysplasia with use of platinum coils. *J Vasc Interv Radiol*. 1993;4:737–739.
30. Tan K, Strong D, Shore T, et al. The safety and efficacy of mesenteric embolization in the management of acute lower gastrointestinal hemorrhage. *Ann Coloproctol*. 2013;29(5):205–208.
31. Mitty H, Efremidis S, Keller R. Colonic stricture after transcatheter embolization for diverticular bleeding. *AJR Am J Roentgenol*. 1979;133:519–521.
32. Bookstein J, Chlosta E, Foley D, et al. Transcatheter hemostasis of gastrointestinal bleeding using modified autogenous clot. *Radiology*. 1974;113:277–285.

Section G Gastrointestinal Venous Embolization

31

Portal Vein Embolization

David Li • Richard H. Marshall • David C. Madoff

The hepatitis C epidemic in the United States has contributed to a dramatic rise of hepatocellular carcinoma (HCC), with HCC increasing in incidence at a rate of 4.5% per year from 1980 to 2005.[1,2] HCC has a poor prognosis and is the third leading cause of cancer-related mortality despite being the sixth most common cancer worldwide.[3] Given both its increased incidence and poor prognosis, the mortality rate from primary liver cancer has increased more than any other major cancer in the United States over the past several decades.[1] In addition, the liver remains a common site of metastases from colorectal carcinoma and other primary tumors.[4] Surgical resection of primary tumors and metastases confined to the liver remains the mainstay of curative therapy.[5,6]

In recent years, advances in hepatobiliary surgical techniques have led to improved morbidity and mortality in patients after hepatic resection.[7,8] Despite these advances, major hepatic resection (i.e., greater than three Couinaud segments) places patients at risk for developing complications related to liver insufficiency in the perioperative period. The anticipated volume of liver which remains after surgery, termed the *future liver remnant* (FLR), has been shown to be a strong, independent predictor of postoperative complications.[9,10]

Portal vein embolization (PVE) is a well-established procedure to redirect portal blood flow to the intended FLR for patients who are candidates for extensive liver resection to promote hypertrophy of nonembolized segments that will remain after resection.[11–13] When needed, this increased FLR volume is associated with improved biliary excretion, albumin uptake, and postoperative liver function in patients undergoing major hepatectomy.[14–16] PVE has also been shown to improve the functional reserve of the FLR before surgery; reduce perioperative morbidity; and allow for safe, potentially curative hepatectomy in patients previously considered ineligible for resection based on anticipated small remnant liver volumes.[17–20] This chapter summarizes the mechanism of action, current indications, outcomes, techniques, and complications related to PVE.

MECHANISM OF ACTION

The liver is unique for its enormous capacity for regeneration: even a loss of as much as two-thirds of the liver parenchyma can be compensated with complete recovery of liver function within 2 weeks.[21] Regeneration of the liver depends on portal blood flow delivering multiple mitogenic factors, the most potent hepatotrophic agents being hepatocyte growth factor (HGF) and tumor growth factor alpha (TGF-α).[22,23] Comitogenic factors, such as insulin and glucagon, are transported via the portal system and act in concert with hepatotrophic agents to stimulate cytokine release and ultimately hepatocyte proliferation. The synergistic action of insulin with HGF accounts for the observation that hepatic regeneration rates are slower in diabetic as compared to nondiabetic patients.[24,25]

Regeneration of the liver depends on both the stimulus of injury and the condition of the liver parenchyma. Hepatocyte proliferation is directly proportional to the degree of severity of the insult to the liver: minor injuries (i.e., $<10\%$ parenchymal involvement) induce only localized mitotic reactions, whereas major injuries (i.e., $>50\%$ parenchymal involvement) induce multiple mitotic waves throughout the entire liver.[21] Liver regeneration rates depend on the time

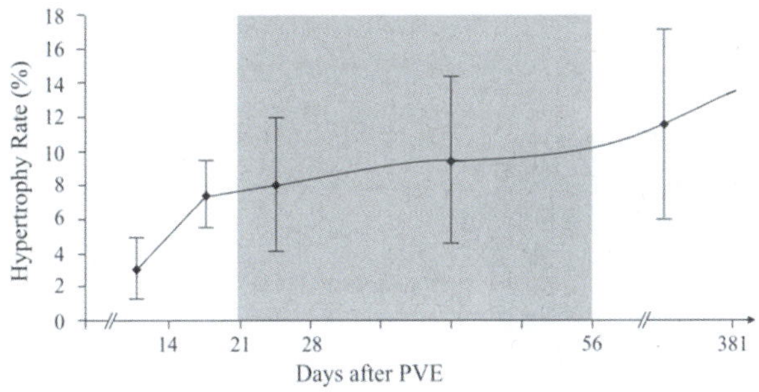

Figure 31.1 Degree of hypertrophy of the sFLR over time after PVE with kinetics of FLR growth, plotted as median degree of hypertrophy after PVE (with interquartile ranges). The *shaded zone*, days 22 to 56 after PVE, represents the "plateau" period during which the degree of hypertrophy did not change significantly between measurement points. (Used with permission from Ribero D, Abdalla EK, Madoff DC, et al. Portal vein embolization before major hepatectomy and its effects on regeneration, resectability and outcome. *Br J Surg*. 2007;94[11]:1386–1394.)

from injury, with the greatest rate of regeneration after PVE occurring within the first 2 weeks (Fig. 31.1).[10] Hepatocyte removal or necrosis is a stronger stimulus for liver regeneration as compared to cell-mediated apoptosis.[26,27] Apoptosis is the predominant mechanism of cell death in PVE, thus regeneration after PVE occurs at a slower rate compared with hepatectomy.[10] In addition, PVE is known to cause minimal pain and fever as compared to the postembolization syndrome associated with transarterial embolization where necrosis is the primary mechanism of cell death.[28] Cirrhotic livers are known to have both a reduced rate and capacity for liver regeneration.[29] Both a suboptimal hepatocyte microenvironment with fibrosis reducing delivery of portal flow and a blunted response of the diseased hepatocytes to hepatotrophic factors are thought to contribute to the reduced regeneration ability of cirrhotics.[30] One novel approach to augmentation of liver regeneration rates in the setting of PVE has been the use of stem cells. Esch et al.[31] reported greater absolute and relative FLR volumes after adjuvant stem cell infusion in conjunction with PVE in a small cohort of patients.

FUTURE LIVER REMNANT DETERMINATION

PVE is indicated when the anticipated FLR is insufficient to support hepatic function, particularly in the perioperative period, before the liver has had time to regenerate. Accurate calculation of the FLR is essential in triaging the potential hepatectomy candidates for whom PVE is indicated. Liver volume is directly correlated with a patient's size; hence, normalizing the anticipated liver volume to a patient's size results in a more accurate assessment of the FLR.[32,33] This principle led to the proposal and clinical validation of a standardized FLR (sFLR) by Vauthey et al.,[33] expressed as a ratio of the FLR over the total *estimated* functioning liver volume (TELV): sFLR = FLR/TELV.

Computed tomography (CT) volumetry serves as the standard for FLR measurement as it is accurate within ±5% of estimating normal liver parenchymal volumes (Fig. 31.2).[33,34] Several methods have been used to measure TELV, including those based on CT volumetry, body surface area (BSA), or body weight. Vauthey et al. derived the following formula for estimating TELV by analyzing liver size and BSA in 292 Western adults: $TELV = -794.41 + 1{,}267.28 \times BSA$, which has been demonstrated to be the least biased and most accurate in adult patients by meta-analysis as compared to similar formulas.[35,36] Other formulas for determining TELV from CT volumetry are both tedious and imprecise because measurements of the tumor volume must be performed and excluded from the overall liver volume using this method. Ribero et al.[37] verified that CT volumetry was less accurate than BSA for calculating sFLR by identifying a subset of patients for whom CT volumetry underestimated the risk of hepatic insufficiency. Chun et al.[38] found the body weight method to be equally as predictive as BSA; however, a more recent study comparing direct volumetric liver measurement and estimated liver volume based on BSA found the TELV method to be superior ($P < .005$).[39]

INDICATIONS

Outcomes in Healthy Livers

Multiple studies have demonstrated that hepatectomy in a setting of sFLR less than 20% is associated with increased postoperative complications.[10,13,40] As a result, the National Comprehensive Cancer Network treatment guidelines from 2013 (category IIA) endorse an sFLR of greater than 20% as a minimum threshold for patients without underlying liver disease to safely undergo hepatectomy, with consideration for PVE to be performed on patients below that threshold.[5] Ribero et al.[10] found that both sFLR less than 20% and degree of sFLR hypertrophy after PVE less than 5% predicted outcome after resection in a series of 112 patients (Fig. 31.3). Kishi et al.[40] published a series of 301 consecutive patients who underwent extended right hepatectomy and found that patients with a preoperative sFLR less than 20% had significantly higher rates of postoperative liver insufficiency and death from liver failure compared with patients with sFLR greater than 20% ($P < .05$). In addition, patients who underwent PVE before surgery to increase their sFLR from less than 20% to greater than 20% had statistically equivalent rates of liver insufficiency as patients with greater than 20% at baseline (Fig. 31.4). This study confirmed both the sFLR threshold of less than 20% being associated with increased perioperative complications and the beneficial role of PVE in reducing perioperative complication rates in those patients who hypertrophy their liver to an sFLR greater than 20%.

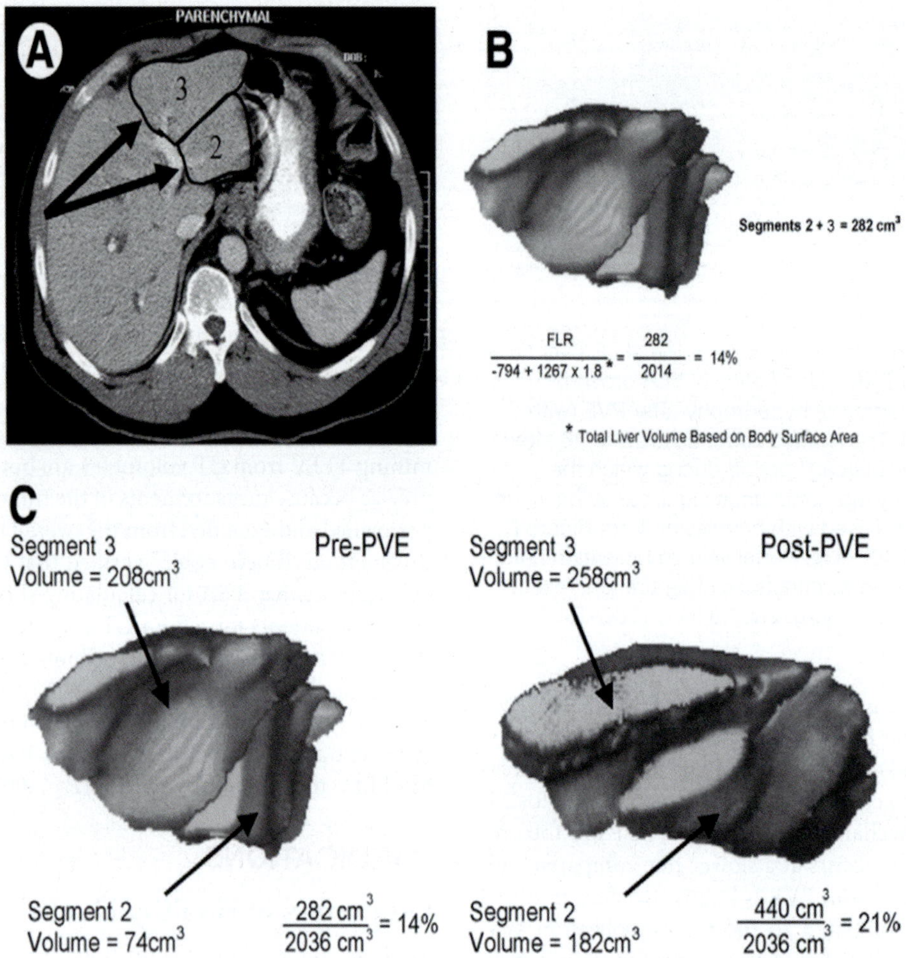

Figure 31.2 Hyperytrophy of the future liver remnant after PVE as determined by three-dimensional (3-D) reconstruction of CT images. **A:** 3-D volumetric measurements determined by outlining hepatic segmental contours and then calculating the volumes as determined from the surface measurements of each slice. *Arrows* point to outlining of borders of segments 2 and 3 of the liver. **B:** Formula for calculating total liver volume based on patient's BSA. **C:** Before embolization (*left*), the volume of segments 2 and 3 was 282 cm^3 (14% of total liver volume [2,036 cm^3]). After embolization (*right*), the volume of segments 2 and 3 was 440 cm^3 (21% of total liver volume [2,036 cm^3]). (Modified with permission Vauthey JN, Chaoui A, Bilimoria MM, et al. Standardized measurement of the future liver remnant prior to extended liver resection: methodology and clinical associations. *Surgery*. 2000;127[5]:512–519.)

Recently, Shindoh et al.[41] have proposed the kinetic growth rate (defined as degree of hypertrophy at initial volume assessment divided by number of weeks elapsed after PVE) as a predictor of postoperative complications after hepatectomy as compared to the sFLR. They analyzed a series of 107 patients who underwent right PVE and subsequent right hemihepatectomy or extended right hepatectomy and found the kinetic growth rate to be the most accurate predictor of postoperative hepatic insufficiency and mortality when compared to sFLR or degree of hypertrophy measurements using receiver operating characteristic analysis (Fig. 31.5). Of the three measures, a kinetic growth rate cutoff value of less than 2.0% per week demonstrated the highest accuracy (81%), with sensitivity of 100% and specificity of 71% in predicting postoperative hepatic insufficiency.

Outcomes in Diseased Livers

Liver regeneration occurs at a reduced rate and capacity in diseased livers.[21,29,30,42] This observation has directly correlated to clinical outcomes. De Meijer et al.[43] performed a meta-analysis of four studies involving 1,000 patients and found that patients with greater than 30% steatosis of the liver had significantly higher risk of postoperative complications and postoperative death compared with patients without steatosis (relative risk and 95% confidence interval 2.01 and 1.66 to 2.44 vs. 2.79 and 1.19 to 6.51). Similarly, several series evaluating outcomes after extensive hepatic resection demonstrated higher rates of both postoperative hepatic insufficiency and mortality in cirrhotic patients.[44,45] Hence, higher sFLR cutoffs are considered for patients with additional risk

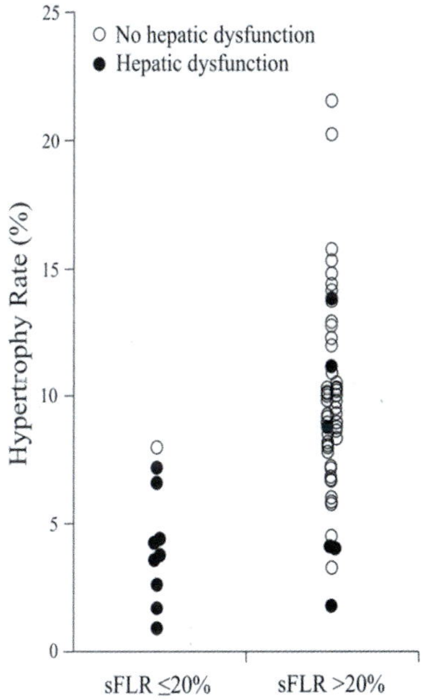

Figure 31.3 Presence of hepatic dysfunction by sFLR volume and degree of hypertrophy. (Used with permission from Ribero D, Abdalla EK, Madoff DC, et al. Portal vein embolization before major hepatectomy and its effects on regeneration, resectability and outcome. *Br J Surg*. 2007;94[11]:1386–1394.)

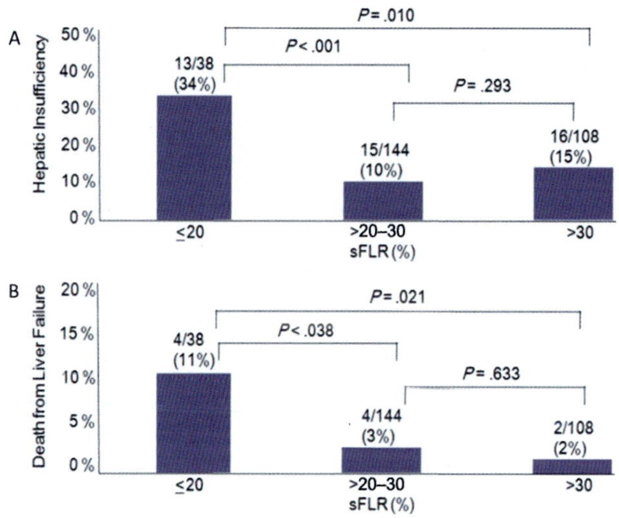

Figure 31.4 Rates of hepatic insufficiency **(A)** and death **(B)** by preoperative sFLR volume. (Modified with permission from Kishi Y, Abdalla EK, Chun YS, et al. Three hundred and one consecutive extended right hepatectomies: evaluation of outcome based on systematic liver volumetry. *Ann Surg*. 2009;250[4]:540–548.)

factors such as hepatic steatosis, hepatotoxic chemotherapy exposure, and compensated cirrhosis.

Cirrhosis

For patients with well-compensated cirrhosis (i.e., Child-Pugh class A) who are considered for resection, an sFLR greater than 40% is recommended. In support of this recommendation, Shirabe et al.[46] demonstrated that all cases (n = 7) of postoperative hepatic insufficiency occurred when the FLR was calculated to be less than 250 mL/m^2 (which corresponds to a calculated sFLR of <40%) in a series of 80 cirrhotic patients who underwent major hepatic resection. A prospective alternative allocation trial in which 28 patients with chronic liver disease were allocated to PVE or no PVE before resection further validated the higher minimum sFLR cutoff of less than 40%; the PVE group had a mean sFLR size of 35% and

Figure 31.5 Receiver operating characteristic curves for measured volume parameters in the prediction of postoperative hepatic insufficiency. Area under the curve (*AUC*) calculated for kinetic growth rate (*KGR*), degree of hypertrophy (*DH*), and standardized future liver remnant (*sFLR*). *P* values represent asymptotic significance (null hypothesis, AUC = 0.500). SE, standard error. (Modified with permission from Shindoh J, Truty MJ, Aloia TA, et al. Kinetic growth rate after portal vein embolization predicts posthepatectomy outcomes: toward zero liver-related mortality in patients with colorectal liver metastases and small future liver remnant. *J Am Coll Surg*. 2013;216[2]:201–209.)

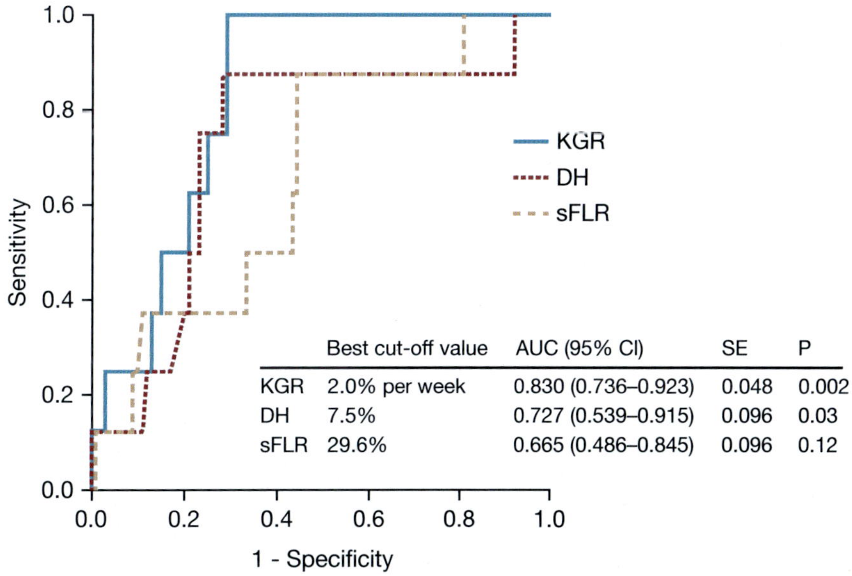

	Best cut-off value	AUC (95% CI)	SE	P
KGR	2.0% per week	0.830 (0.736–0.923)	0.048	0.002
DH	7.5%	0.727 (0.539–0.915)	0.096	0.03
sFLR	29.6%	0.665 (0.486–0.845)	0.096	0.12

demonstrated significantly lower incidence of complications including liver failure.[47]

Chemotherapy

Accelerated tumor growth after PVE has been reported for both primary and metastatic liver tumors.[48–51] Progression of disease after PVE may preclude curative intent surgery; a 20% dropout rate after first-stage resection due to progression of disease has already been reported in two-stage hepatectomy series.[52,53] Neoadjuvant chemotherapy can be administered in an attempt to provide tumor control in the interim between PVE and resection; however, concerns have been raised about its potential deleterious effect on liver function, liver hypertrophy, and lack of efficacy in preventing progression of disease.

Two separate series, one by Pawlik et al.[54] and another by Vauthey et al.,[55] have demonstrated an association of oxaliplatin with sinusoidal dilation and irinotecan with steatohepatitis. In the series by Vauthey et al.,[55] the presence of steatohepatitis in patients who had undergone resection was correlated to increased 90-day mortality (14.7% vs. 1.6%; $P = .001$; odds ratio [OR] = 10.5; 95% CI, 2.0 to 36.4). Given these findings, Shindoh et al.[56] performed a retrospective analysis on a series of 194 patients with colorectal liver metastasis to determine the optimal FLR for patients treated with neoadjuvant chemotherapy. The authors found that both long duration of chemotherapy (defined as >12 weeks) and sFLR less than or equal to 30% were predictors of hepatic insufficiency (OR = 5.4, $P = .004$; OR 6.3, $P = .019$, respectively) (Fig. 31.6). No cases of postoperative mortality and only two cases of postoperative hepatic insufficiency were reported if the sFLR is greater than 30%, indicating that an sFLR greater than 30% may be a more appropriate cutoff value in patients who have received neoadjuvant chemotherapy, particularly if the duration of treatment is more than 12 weeks.

In addition, the effect of systemic neoadjuvant chemotherapy on liver hypertrophy after PVE has been addressed by several studies. Zorzi et al.[57] reviewed FLR hypertrophy after PVE in patients with colorectal liver metastases who underwent PVE either with concomitant neoadjuvant chemotherapy (n = 43) or without chemotherapy (n = 22) before resection. The chemotherapy group, which included 26 patients treated in part with the vascular endothelial growth factor (VEGF) receptor blocker bevacizumab, demonstrated similar rates of hypertrophy when compared to the no chemotherapy group at 4 weeks after PVE. Similarly, Covey et al.[58] also reported on patients with colorectal liver metastases who underwent PVE either with (n = 47) or without (n = 53) neoadjuvant chemotherapy. Both groups showed no significant difference in median contralateral liver growth after PVE. However, in a small series of 15 consecutive patients by Beal et al.,[59] the volume increase of the anticipated FLR was reduced in the setting of chemotherapy (median of 89 vs. 135 mL, range of 7 to 149 vs. 110 to 254 mL; $P = .016$).

Chemotherapy has not been proven to prevent progression of disease between PVE and resection. A recent study examined the effect of chemotherapy on disease progression between the first and second stages of a two-stage hepatectomy.[60] Of the initial 47 patients who underwent first-stage resection, 25 patients (53.2%) were treated with subsequent chemotherapy compared to 22 (46.8%) patients who did not receive interval chemotherapy. Eleven patients (23.4%) failed to complete second-stage hepatectomy due to progression of disease. There was no statistically significant difference in the number of patients with progression of disease between the groups treated or not treated with interval chemotherapy (n = 12 vs. n = 13; $P = .561$). The authors concluded that chemotherapy after stage 1 resection does not guarantee lower progression of disease rates, within the limitation that the study groups were not randomized.

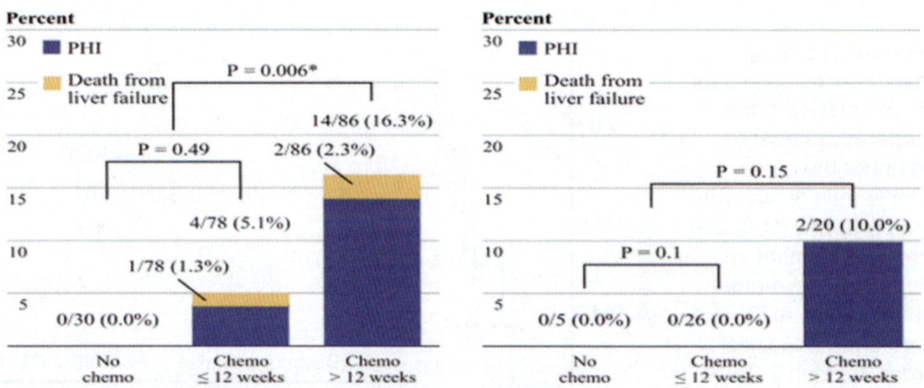

Figure 31.6 Postoperative liver insufficiency and mortality from liver failure in patients who underwent extended right hepatectomy in the setting of colorectal metastases, stratified to those undergoing no chemotherapy, chemotherapy, or long duration (>12 weeks) chemotherapy. Cutoffs for resection eligibility: (1) sFLR greater than 20% cutoff and (2) sFLR greater than 30% cutoff. PHI, post-operative hepatic insufficiency. (Used with permission from Shindoh J, Tzeng CW, Aloia TA, et al. Optimal future liver remnant in patients treated with extensive preoperative chemotherapy for colorectal liver metastases. *Ann Surg Oncol*. 2013;20[8]:2493–2500.)

TWO-STAGE HEPATECTOMY AND OUTCOMES OF EMBOLIZATION VERSUS LIGATION OF THE PORTAL VEIN

Two-stage hepatectomy has been developed to increase the number of patients with bilobar colorectal liver metastasis amenable for resection.[61] During the first-stage treatment, tumor within the projected FLR is resected or, in some cases, ablated. Once the FLR is cleared of tumor, portal blood flow is directed toward the FLR either by portal vein ligation (PVL) or PVE of the ipsilateral tumor-bearing liver. Once adequate FLR hypertrophy is achieved, the second stage hepatectomy targets the remainder of liver metastases, typically requiring a right or extended right hepatectomy. Brouquet et al.[52] studied the outcomes of 65 patients with colorectal metastases who underwent first-stage hepatectomy, 47 of whom completed the second-stage resection in comparison to nonsurgical patients. Both study groups had disease confined to the liver and demonstrated an objective response to systemic chemotherapy. The overall 5-year survival rate of the surgical group was 51% compared to 15% for the medical group ($P = .005$). For the 47 patients who completed the second-stage resection, 5-year survival was improved to 64%. Hence, resection conferred a clear additional survival benefit.

As an alternative to PVE, intraoperative right PVL has been performed during the initial stage of two-stage hepatectomy or as a separate surgical intervention as a means of inducing FLR hypertrophy.[62–64] Results from comparative studies between PVE and PVL are mixed, with some studies demonstrating comparable liver hypertrophy, while others showing a liver hypertrophy benefit from PVE.

Both Aussilhou et al.[65] (PVE: n = 18; PVL: n = 17) and Capussotti et al.[66] (PVE: n = 31; PVL: n = 17) retrospectively compared patients who underwent PVE with patients who underwent PVL during the first stage of a two-stage hepatectomy and found comparable increases in left liver volume in the two groups. Other studies have found inferior FLR hypertrophy after PVL compared to PVE. Broering et al.[67] found that increase in left lateral liver volume was significantly higher for the PVE (n = 17) group compared to PVL (n = 17) (188 ± 81 mL vs. 123 ± 58 mL; $P = .012$) before extended right hepatectomy. In addition, hospital stay was significantly shorter for PVE compared to PVL (4 ± 2.9 days vs. 8.1 ± 5.1 days; $P < .01$). Robles et al.[68] also compared left lobe hypertrophy in two-stage hepatectomy patients who underwent PVL (n = 23) versus PVE (n = 18). This group found that PVE resulted in improved median percentage increase of the FLR compared to PVL (40% vs. 30%, $P < .05$).[68] The inferior hypertrophy after PVL may be explained by portal–portal shunts, which can lead to recanalization of the ligated right portal vein.[69]

CONTRAINDICATIONS

PVE is as an adjunctive procedure to major hepatectomy. Hence, contraindications to PVE mirror those of hepatectomy. Severe portal hypertension precluding surgery is the only absolute contraindication to PVE. Also, in cases where tumor obstructs the portal system in the liver to be resected, PVE is not necessary as portal flow is already redirected to the FLR.[70,71] Relative contraindications include uncorrectable coagulopathy, renal failure, and extrahepatic metastasis. Two-stage hepatectomy has expanded the patients with bilobar hepatic disease burden eligible for PVE and potential curative resection as will be further detailed in the following discussion; however, diffuse hepatic disease burden remains a contraindication to PVE.

TECHNICAL CONSIDERATIONS

Portal Venous Anatomy and Access Routes

Knowledge of standard portal vein anatomy and common variations is essential for both PVE and surgical planning.[71] In standard anatomy, the splenic and superior mesenteric veins join to form the main portal vein, which divides into the left and right branches at the hepatic hilum. The right portal branch subdivides into anterior and posterior divisions, which supply Couinaud segments 5/8 and 6/7, respectively. The left portal branch subdivides into branches, which supply segments 4, 3, and 2. In one series of 200 patients studied with CT portography, standard anatomy (type I) was identified 65% of the time (Fig. 31.7).[71,72] In the most common variation (type III), the right posterior portal vein is the first branch of the main portal vein, followed by bifurcation of the right anterior and left portal branches.

PVE has traditionally been performed via one of three approaches, termed *transileocolic*, *contralateral*, and *ipsilateral* techniques. The original approach, the transileocolic approach, is a surgical procedure where a right lower quadrant incision is used to access a major venous ileocolic branch via direct puncture, allowing for catheter manipulation to the portal vein. This approach has the advantage of avoiding puncture through the liver. However, the surgery has generally been replaced by the less invasive percutaneous contralateral and ipsilateral techniques, which are performed using ultrasound-guided transhepatic puncture.

The contralateral approach accesses the portal system via the FLR (Fig. 31.8A), preferably a peripheral branch of segment. The major advantage of the contralateral approach is easier catheter manipulation to the tumor-bearing liver because of fewer acute angles between access and target portal branches.[12,73] In addition, embolization is performed with the catheter pointed toward the direction of flow. The major disadvantage of the contralateral approach is risk of damage to the FLR during access and catheter manipulation, which could potentially make a patient unresectable.

The ipsilateral approach accesses the portal system through the tumor-bearing liver, thus avoiding potential damage to the FLR during instrumentation (Fig. 31.8B).

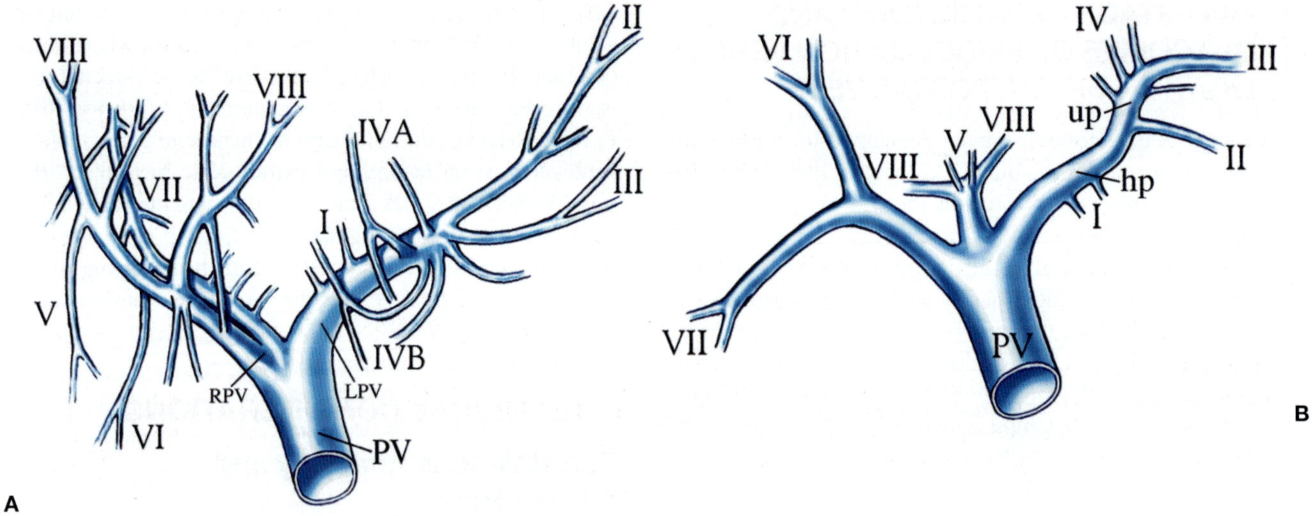

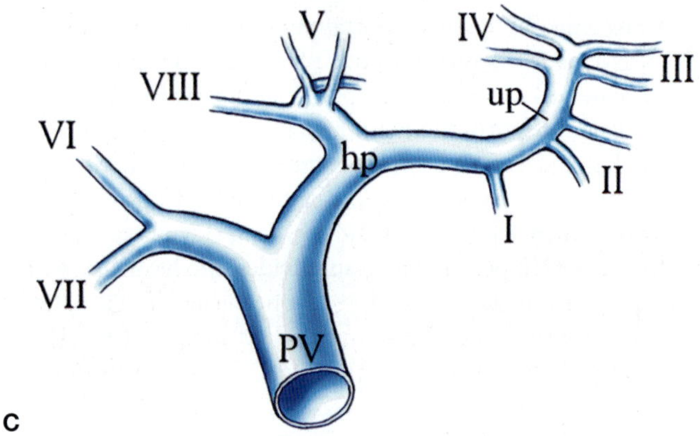

Figure 31.7 Portal venous anatomy variations, left portal vein (*LPV*), right anterior portal vein (RAPV), right posterior portal vein (RPPV). **A:** Conventional anatomy (type I). **B:** Trifurcation (type II) **C:** RPPV as first branch of main portal vein (type III). RPV, right portal vein; PV, portal vein; up, umbilical (vertical) part; hp, horizontal part. (Used with permission from Madoff DC, Hicks ME, Vauthey JN, et al. Transhepatic portal vein embolization: anatomy, indications, and technical considerations. *Radiographics*. 2002;22[5]:1063–1076.)

As demonstrated by Madoff et al.,[74,75] the acute angles encountered between access and target portal branches during ipsilateral access can be overcome with the use of commercially available reverse curve catheters and microcatheters. In addition, catheterization of segment 4 is more straightforward via the ipsilateral approach should embolization of segment 4 be required (further detailed in the following text).

For the ipsilateral approach, access through the anterior segment of the right portal vein is associated with a lower complication rate and thus preferred.[76] Care must be taken to

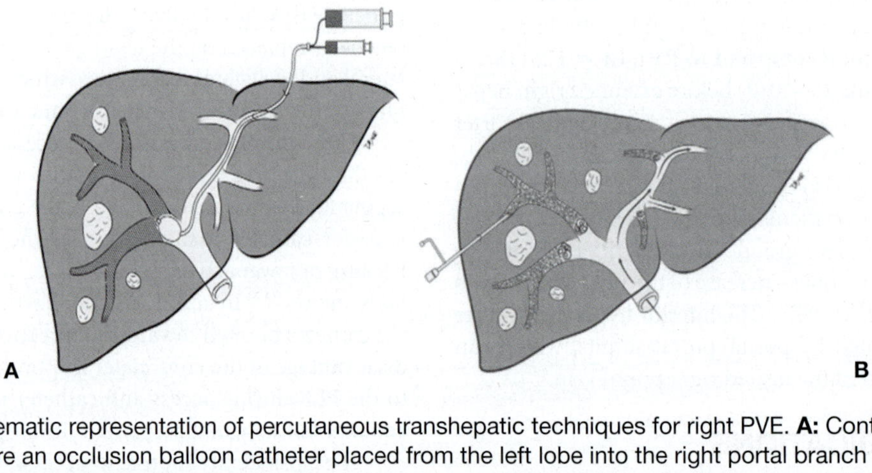

Figure 31.8 Schematic representation of percutaneous transhepatic techniques for right PVE. **A:** Contralateral technique where an occlusion balloon catheter placed from the left lobe into the right portal branch allows anterograde delivery of embolic agents. **B:** Modified ipsilateral technique where a 6-Fr vascular sheath is placed into a right portal branch through which an angled 5-Fr catheter can be navigated into the left portal system and a reverse curve 5-Fr catheter can be used for embolization of right portal vein branches. Microcatheters can be used whenever needed.

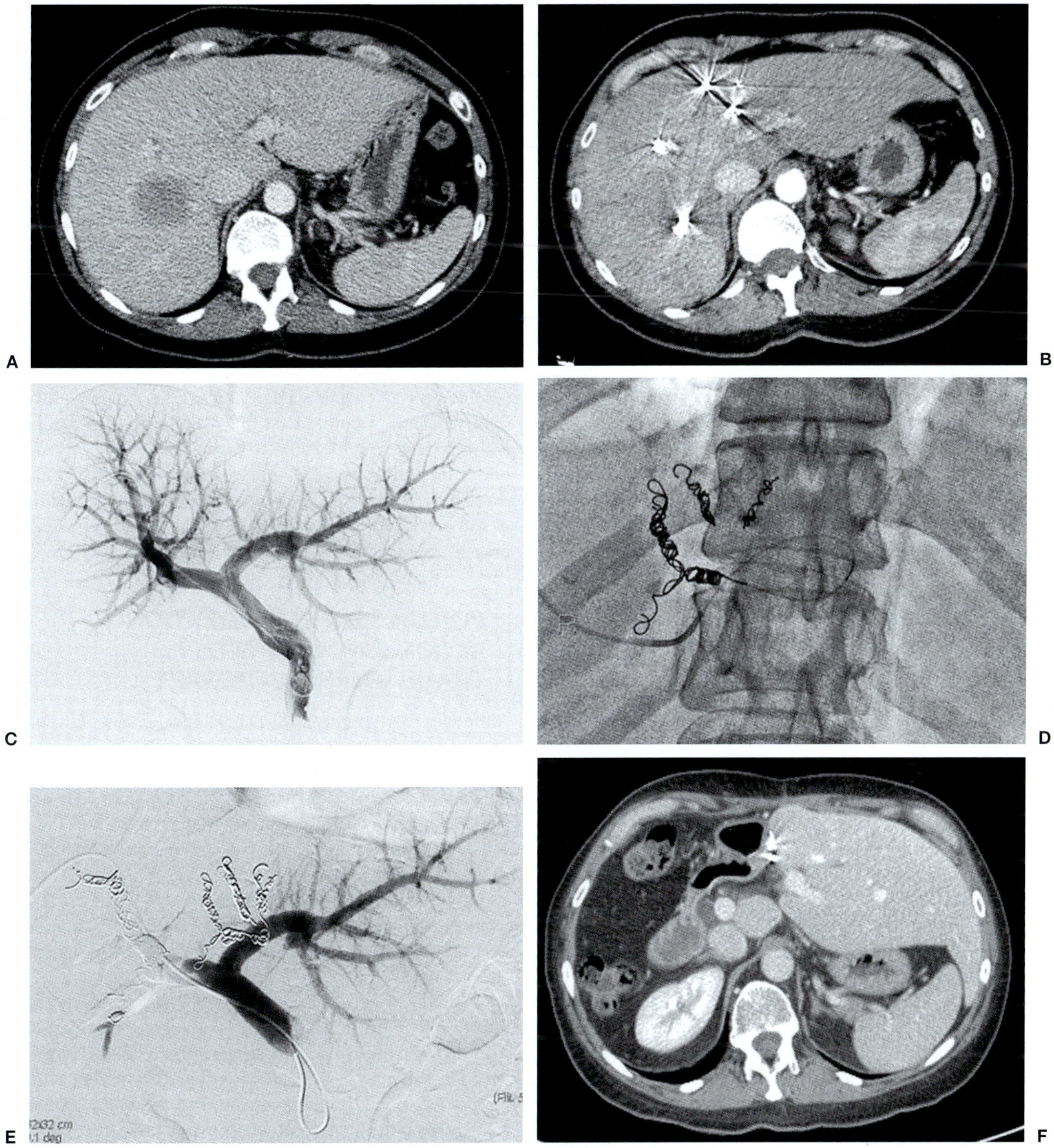

Figure 31.9 Transhepatic ipsilateral right PVE extended to segment 4 using trisacryl particles and coils performed in a 48-year-old female with cholangiocarcinoma involving segments 4, 5, and 7. **A:** Contrast-enhanced CT image of the liver with a lesion centered in segment 7 and the normal-appearing left lateral liver before PVE. **B:** CT obtained after PVE demonstrates hypertrophy of the FLR (sFLR growth from 27% to 35%, KGR 4%). **C:** Anteroposterior flush portogram obtained through a 5-Fr flush catheter within the main portal vein via ipsilateral approach demonstrates patent conventional portal anatomy. **D:** Intraprocedural fluoroscopic image from PVE depicts coil placement into segment 4 branches via a microcatheter. **E:** Final portogram shows occlusion of the portal vein branches to segments 4 to 8 with continued patency of the veins supplying the left lateral liver. **F:** CT image obtained after uncomplicated extended right hepatectomy shows massive hypertrophy of the remnant liver.

avoid access through tumor to prevent peritoneal seeding. Figure 31.9 depicts a PVE performed via a transhepatic ipsilateral approach extending to segment 4 using trisacryl microspheres and coils in a patient with cholangiocarcinoma. Ultrasound-guided puncture of a distal branch of the right portal system is performed and the needle exchanged over a wire for a 5-Fr or 6-Fr vascular sheath. A flush catheter can then be advanced into the main portal vein and flush portography and pressure measurements performed. A 5-Fr reverse curve catheter such as an SOS-2 (Angiodynamics) or a Simmons 1 (Terumo) is subsequently inserted via the sheath and used to catheterize the right portal vein branches for embolization.

Embolization Extended to Include Segment 4

Before extended right hepatectomy, some authors have argued for extending right PVE to include segment 4 (RPVE + 4) as a means of improving hypertrophy of segments 2 and 3.[77] The drawback is that catheter manipulation into branches feeding segment 4 is more technically demanding and inadvertent reflux of embolic material to the FLR has been reported.[78,79] Capussotti et al.[78] evaluated 26 patients who underwent RPVE (n = 13) or RPVE + 4 (n = 13) and found no difference in the volume increase ($P = .20$) or rate of increase ($P = .40$) of segments 2 and 3 in the two groups. However, recent studies comparing RPVE and RPVE + 4 have reported improved hypertrophy of segments 2 and 3 when segment 4 is also embolized, without increased incidence of complications.[10,80,81] Kishi et al.[80] compared patients who underwent RPVE (n = 15) versus those who underwent RPVE + 4 (n = 58). Compared to RPVE alone, the RPVE + 4 group demonstrated a greater absolute increase in segments 2 and 3 volume (median, 106 mL vs. 141 mL; $P = .044$) as well as a higher hypertrophy rate for segments 2 and 3 (median, 26% vs. 54%; $P = .021$). The complication rates were similar for RPVE and RPVE + 4 groups (7% vs. 10%; $P > .99$) and no PVE complication precluded resection.

EMBOLIZATION MATERIALS

Various materials and devices exist for embolization, and some of these have been adapted for the portal system. Commonly reported agents include polyvinyl alcohol, gelfoam, fibrin glue, *N*-butyl cyanoacrylate (NBCA), polidocanol foam, microspheres, Ethiodol, coils, and Amplatzer Vascular Plugs (St. Jude Medical, Inc., St. Paul Minnesota) among others.[82,83] An ideal material will provide permanent portal venous embolization that is safe and well tolerated by the patient.[74] The two agents most commonly discussed currently are NBCA and microspheres in combination with coils. To date, there has been no prospective randomized trial comparing the two.

Multiple studies have demonstrated the safety and effectiveness of small particle embolization of the liver with both PVA and microspheres.[20,84] After catheterization of the portal system, embolization of distal small veins is performed with 100- to 300-μm particles. More proximal veins are embolized with larger particles with a goal of near stasis of flow or stasis. Coils are placed behind particles to prevent later particle dislodgement and recanalization.

NBCA has been shown to produce portal venous occlusion for more than 4 weeks[85] and has been shown to induce a larger FLR when compared coils and gelatin sponge.[73] NBCA induces an inflammatory reaction resulting in peribiliary fibrosis,[73] and rates of liver regeneration are believed to be as good as or better than other embolic agents. However, preparation and administration require advanced knowledge and experience, and the inflammatory reaction sometimes renders surgical resection more difficult.[73] Nontarget embolization has been reported and a technique has been developed to prevent backflow by placing a nitinol plug.[86] NBCA is mixed with ethiodized oil and is delivered through an end-hole angiographic catheter from second- or third-order portal branch to prevent nontarget embolization. Straight catheters are preferred by some operators to prevent gluing of catheters into the liver, and great care must be taken to prevent embolization of NBCA to nontarget areas.

PORTAL VEIN EMBOLIZATION IN CONJUNCTION WITH TRANSARTERIAL THERAPY

Although PVE typically leads to reliable rates of hypertrophy, liver regeneration can be variable, especially when comorbidities such as underlying hepatic dysfunction or diabetes are present. When FLR hypertrophy is inadequate after PVE, adjunct therapies such as transarterial embolization (TAE) can be performed. The mechanism of TAE is complementary as a component of inflammation and necrosis is added to the apoptosis-mediated cell death induced by PVE to stimulate liver hypertrophy. In fact, arterial embolization alone has been shown to induce hypertrophy of the FLR, although to a lesser degree compared to PVE.[87]

Nagino et al.[77] first described the use of TAE to improve FLR volume in two patients with cholangiocarcinoma who demonstrated inadequate hypertrophy following PVE. In both patients, PVE in the setting of underlying liver disease led to negligible hypertrophy of the FLR at 58 days (patient 1) and 14 days (patient 2). After TAE, the FLR volume increased from 470 to 685 mL (46%) 2 weeks after TAE (patient 1) and from 649 to 789 mL (22%) 3 weeks after TAE (patient 2) and both patients underwent successful curative resection. In this study, only half of the target segments were treated due to the potential risk of hepatic infarction given that both portal and arterial systems were disrupted. Similarly, Gruttadauria et al.[88] reported inadequate hypertrophy after PVE in two patients with colorectal metastasis who demonstrated improved hypertrophy after TAE, allowing for subsequent successful hepatectomy.

TAE can also be performed as a staged procedure before PVE, with an interval of 2 to 3 weeks between the procedures to help prevent hepatic infarction.[89,90] Aoki et al.[89] reported the use of sequential transcatheter arterial chemoembolization (TACE) followed within 2 weeks by PVE in 17 patients with HCC. Sixteen of the 17 patients were able to undergo staged hepatectomy with no episodes of postoperative hepatic insufficiency. Analysis of the explanted livers demonstrated profound tumor necrosis without substantial injury to the noncancerous liver, and the authors therefore encourage the aggressive use of this strategy in patients with large HCC and chronically injured livers. In this patient population, the rationale for performing TACE before PVE includes prevention of tumor progression after PVE, reduction of arterioportal shunts that may limit the effectiveness of the subsequent PVE, and boosting the regenerative stimulus in chronically diseased livers. Ogata et al.[90] performed sequential TACE and PVE versus PVE alone in a series of 36 patients with HCC and chronic liver disease before right hepatectomy. Patients in the combined chemoembolization (TACE) and PVE group (n = 18) demonstrated a higher mean increase in percentage of FLR volume (12% vs. 8%; $P = .022$) than those who underwent PVE alone (n = 18). The incidence of complete tumor necrosis (83% vs. 6%; $P < .001$) and 5-year disease-free survival rate (37% vs. 19%; $P = .041$) were also significantly higher in patients who underwent TACE and PVE.

POTENTIAL COMPLICATIONS

In 2010, the Society of Interventional Radiology established quality improvement guidelines for transcatheter embolization, including a suggested threshold for PVE-related major complications of 6% and morbidity of 11%.[91] Most published complication rates fall well below this range.[92] A meta-analysis by Abulkhir et al.[17] pooled data from 37 studies from 1990 to 2005 for a total of 1,088 subjects who underwent PVE and found the pooled procedure-related morbidity and mortality to be 2.2% and 0%, respectively. In this analysis, percutaneous PVE was performed in most cases (72%); the remainder was performed via the transileocolic technique. Complications of PVE are similar to other image-guided transhepatic procedures and include subscapular hematoma, hemoperitoneum, hemobilia, abscess formation, cholangitis and sepsis, arterioportal shunts, arterioportal fistula, and pneumothorax. In addition, PVE-specific complications include nontarget embolization, recanalization of embolized segments, and extension of portal vein thrombosis to involve the left or main branches. Kodama et al.[76] compared complication rates between contralateral (n = 11) and ipsilateral approaches (n = 36) in a series of 47 patients who underwent PVE. Contralateral approach PVE was associated with an 18.1% complication rate as compared to 13.9% for ipsilateral PVE. Although the difference did not reach statistical significance, the authors recommended ipsilateral approach due to the potential for injury to the FLR during contralateral approach. Di Stefano et al.[93] reported on 188 patients who underwent contralateral approach PVE and found a 12.8% adverse event rate and only one major complication (complete portal vein thrombosis) directly related to the contralateral approach that precluded surgery.[93] Ribero et al.[10] reported on 112 patients who underwent ipsilateral approach PVE and found an 8.9% adverse event rate. Accounting for the fact that Di Stefano et al.[93] included clinically occult CT findings in their complications, the rates are comparable between the two studies.

TIPS AND TRICKS

- Not all livers are created equal.
  - There is significant variation in segmental and portal venous anatomy (see Fig. 31.7)
  - Volumetry cutoffs need to be adjusted depending on the underlying baseline liver function: For normal livers, PVE should be considered for sFLR less than 20%; for cirrhotics, PVE should be considered for sFLR less than 40%.
  - Chemotherapy affects baseline liver function, and PVE should be considered for sFLR less than 30%, especially if chemotherapy duration is more than 3 mo (see Fig. 31.6).
- PVE is an adjunctive technique to surgery.
  - Contraindications to surgery serve as contraindications to PVE.
  - Two-stage hepatectomy has increased the number of surgically resectable candidates, thus expanding the number of patients eligible for PVE.
- There are multiple ways to measure liver regeneration; choose one that is accurate and clinically relevant.
  - Liver volumes must be normalized to a patient's size.
  - sFLR as calculated with CT volumetry has been clinically validated as an accurate and reproducible measure of postoperative hepatic insufficiency (see Fig. 31.2).
  - Kinetic growth rate may serve as a more accurate predictor of postoperative hepatic insufficiency (see Fig. 31.5).
- Choose your percutaneous approach wisely (contralateral vs. ipsilateral).
  - Ipsilateral approach avoids FLR injury and allows easy access to segment 4 (see Fig. 31.8).
  - Contralateral approach allows direct access to right portal vein branches.
- Choose your embolic agent at your discretion.
  - No clear evidence to suggest improved efficacy of a particular embolic agent.
  - Choice should depend on operator experience/comfort level and anatomic considerations including variant anatomy and extent of embolization.

- Embolize the entire tumor-bearing liver.
  - Right PVE in addition to segment 4 embolization (RPVE + 4) results in increased liver hypertrophy as compared to RPVE.
  - When performing RPVE + 4, start with segment 4; if RPVE is performed first and there is thrombosis in the left portal vein, it is potentially catastrophic.
  - There are no reports of increased complications with RPVE + 4 as compared to RPVE alone.
- PVE does not preclude TAE; in fact, they may be complementary.
  - Transarterial embolotherapy can be done in a staged fashion before PVE to prevent tumor progression and boost the regenerative stimulus of chronically diseased livers.
  - In select cases, transarterial embolotherapy can be performed after PVE to further promote liver hypertrophy.

SUMMARY

PVE is well established worldwide as an adjunctive procedure before hepatectomy to induce FLR hypertrophy. PVE has been shown to reduce perioperative morbidity and allows for safe, potentially curative hepatectomy in patients previously considered ineligible for resection based on anticipated small remnant livers. PVE continues to demonstrate an essential adjunctive role to major hepatectomy, even as advances in hepatobiliary surgical techniques evolve and indications for curative hepatectomy expand, given its high safety profile and proven efficacy at promoting liver remnant hypertrophy.

REFERENCES

1. Altekruse SF, McGlynn KA, Reichman ME. Hepatocellular carcinoma incidence, mortality, and survival trends in the United States from 1975 to 2005. *J Clin Oncol*. 2009;27(9):1485–1491.
2. Nathan H, Segev DL, Mayo SC, et al. National trends in surgical procedures for hepatocellular carcinoma: 1998-2008. *Cancer*. 2012;118(7):1838–1844.
3. Parkin DM, Bray F, Ferlay J, et al. Global cancer statistics, 2002. *CA Cancer J Clin*. 2005;55(2):74–108.
4. Simard EP, Ward EM, Siegel R, et al. Cancers with increasing incidence trends in the United States: 1999 through 2008 [published online ahead of print January 4, 2012]. *CA Cancer J Clin*.
5. Benson AB III, Abrams TA, Ben-Josef E, et al. NCCN clinical practice guidelines in oncology: hepatobiliary cancers. *J Natl Compr Canc Netw*. 2009;7(4):350–391.
6. Benson AB III, Bekaii-Saab T, Chan E, et al. Metastatic colon cancer, version 3.2013: featured updates to the NCCN Guidelines. *J Natl Compr Canc Netw*. 2013;11(2):141–152; quiz 152.
7. Tsao JI, Loftus JP, Nagorney DM, et al. Trends in morbidity and mortality of hepatic resection for malignancy. A matched comparative analysis. *Ann Surg*. 1994;220(2):199–205.
8. Vauthey JN, Pawlik TM, Abdalla EK, et al. Is extended hepatectomy for hepatobiliary malignancy justified? *Ann Surg*. 2004; 239(5):722–730.
9. Shoup M, Gonen M, D'Angelica M, et al. Volumetric analysis predicts hepatic dysfunction in patients undergoing major liver resection. *J Gastrointest Surg*. 2003;7(3):325–330.
10. Ribero D, Abdalla EK, Madoff DC, et al. Portal vein embolization before major hepatectomy and its effects on regeneration, resectability and outcome. *Br J Surg*. 2007;94(11):1386–1394.
11. Makuuchi M, Thai BL, Takayasu K, et al. Preoperative portal embolization to increase safety of major hepatectomy for hilar bile duct carcinoma: a preliminary report. *Surgery*. 1990;107(5):521–527.
12. de Baere T, Roche A, Vavasseur D, et al. Portal vein embolization: utility for inducing left hepatic lobe hypertrophy before surgery. *Radiology*. 1993;188(1):73–77.
13. Abdalla EK, Barnett CC, Doherty D, et al. Extended hepatectomy in patients with hepatobiliary malignancies with and without preoperative portal vein embolization. *Arch Surg*. 2002; 137(6):675–680.
14. Hirai I, Kimura W, Fuse A, et al. Evaluation of preoperative portal embolization for safe hepatectomy, with special reference to assessment of nonembolized lobe function with 99mTc-GSA SPECT scintigraphy. *Surgery*. 2003;133(5):495–506.
15. Ijichi M, Makuuchi M, Imamura H, et al. Portal embolization relieves persistent jaundice after complete biliary drainage. *Surgery*. 2001;130(1):116–118.
16. Uesaka K, Nimura Y, Nagino M. Changes in hepatic lobar function after right portal vein embolization. An appraisal by biliary indocyanine green excretion. *Ann Surg*. 1996;223(1):77–83.
17. Abulkhir A, Limongelli P, Healey AJ, et al. Preoperative portal vein embolization for major liver resection: a meta-analysis. *Ann Surg*. 2008;247(1):49–57.
18. Azoulay D, Castaing D, Krissat J, et al. Percutaneous portal vein embolization increases the feasibility and safety of major liver resection for hepatocellular carcinoma in injured liver. *Ann Surg*. 2000;232(5):665–672.
19. Azoulay D, Castaing D, Smail A, et al. Resection of nonresectable liver metastases from colorectal cancer after percutaneous portal vein embolization. *Ann Surg*. 2000;231(4):480–486.
20. Madoff DC, Abdalla EK, Gupta S, et al. Transhepatic ipsilateral right portal vein embolization extended to segment IV: improving hypertrophy and resection outcomes with spherical particles and coils. *J Vasc Interv Radiol*. 2005;16(2, pt 1):215–225.
21. Koniaris LG, McKillop IH, Schwartz SI, et al. Liver regeneration. *J Am Coll Surg*. 2003;197(4):634–659.
22. Michalopoulos GK, DeFrances MC. Liver regeneration. *Science*. 1997;276(5309):60–66.
23. Huh CG, Factor VM, Sánchez A, et al. Hepatocyte growth factor/c-met signaling pathway is required for efficient liver regeneration and repair. *Proc Natl Acad Sci U S A*. 2004;101(13):4477–4482.
24. Nagino M, Nimura Y, Kamiya J, et al. Changes in hepatic lobe volume in biliary tract cancer patients after right portal vein embolization. *Hepatology*. 1995;21(2):434–439.
25. Imamura H, Shimada R, Kubota M, et al. Preoperative portal vein embolization: an audit of 84 patients. *Hepatology*. 1999; 29(4):1099–1105.
26. Lee KC, Kinoshita H, Hirohashi K, et al. Extension of surgical indications for hepatocellular carcinoma by portal vein embolization. *World J Surg*. 1993;17(1):109–115.

27. Tashiro S. Mechanism of liver regeneration after liver resection and portal vein embolization (ligation) is different? *J Hepatobiliary Pancreat Surg.* 2009;16(3):292–299.
28. Ikeda K, Kinoshita H, Hirohashi K, et al. The ultrastructure, kinetics and intralobular distribution of apoptotic hepatocytes after portal branch ligation with special reference to their relationship to necrotic hepatocytes. *Arch Histol Cytol.* 1995;58(2):171–184.
29. Yamanaka N, Okamoto E, Kawamura E, et al. Dynamics of normal and injured human liver regeneration after hepatectomy as assessed on the basis of computed tomography and liver function. *Hepatology.* 1993;18(1):79–85.
30. Duncan AW, Soto-Gutierrez A. Liver repopulation and regeneration: new approaches to old questions. *Curr Opin Organ Transplant.* 2013;18(2):197–202.
31. Esch JS, Schmelzle M, Fürst G, et al. Infusion of CD133+ Bone marrow-derived stem cells after selective portal vein embolization enhances functional hepatic reserves after extended right hepatectomy: a retrospective single-center study. *Ann Surg.* 2012;255(1):79–85.
32. Johnson TN, Tucker GT, Tanner MS, et al. Changes in liver volume from birth to adulthood: a meta-analysis. *Liver Transpl.* 2005;11(12):1481–1493.
33. Vauthey JN, Chaoui A, Bilimoria MM, et al. Standardized measurement of the future liver remnant prior to extended liver resection: methodology and clinical associations. *Surgery.* 2000;127(5):512–519.
34. Soyer P, Roche A, Elias D, et al. Hepatic metastases from colorectal cancer: influence of hepatic volumetric analysis on surgical decision making. *Radiology.* 1992;184(3):695–697.
35. Vauthey JN, Abdalla EK, Doherty DA, et al. Body surface area and body weight predict total liver volume in Western adults. *Liver Transpl.* 2002;8(3):233–240.
36. Ribero D, Chun YS, Vauthey JN. Standardized liver volumetry for portal vein embolization. *Semin Intervent Radiol.* 2008; 25(2):104–109.
37. Ribero D, Amisano M, Bertuzzo F, et al. Measured versus estimated total liver volume to preoperatively assess the adequacy of the future liver remnant: which method should we use? *Ann Surg.* 2013;258:801–806.
38. Chun YS, Ribero D, Abdalla EK, et al. Comparison of two methods of future liver remnant volume measurement. *J Gastrointest Surg.* 2008;12(1):123–128.
39. Shah A, Goffette P, Hubert C, et al. Comparison of different methods to quantify future liver remnants after preoperative portal vein embolization to predict postoperative liver failure. *Hepatogastroenterology.* 2011;58(105):109–114.
40. Kishi Y, Abdalla EK, Chun YS, et al. Three hundred and one consecutive extended right hepatectomies: evaluation of outcome based on systematic liver volumetry. *Ann Surg.* 2009;250(4):540–548.
41. Shindoh J, Truty MJ, Aloia TA, et al. Kinetic growth rate after portal vein embolization predicts posthepatectomy outcomes: toward zero liver-related mortality in patients with colorectal liver metastases and small future liver remnant. *J Am Coll Surg.* 2013;216(2):201–209.
42. Fausto N, Campbell JS, Riehle KJ. Liver regeneration. *Hepatology.* 2006;43(2)(suppl 1):S45–S53.
43. de Meijer VE, Kalish BT, Puder M, et al. Systematic review and meta-analysis of steatosis as a risk factor in major hepatic resection. *Br J Surg.* 2010;97(9):1331–1339.
44. Tanabe G, Sakamoto M, Akazawa K, et al. Intraoperative risk factors associated with hepatic resection. *Br J Surg.* 1995;82(9): 1262–1265.
45. Tjandra JJ, Fan ST, Wong J. Peri-operative mortality in hepatic resection. *Aust N Z J Surg.* 1991;61(3):201–206.
46. Shirabe K, Shimada M, Gion T, et al. Postoperative liver failure after major hepatic resection for hepatocellular carcinoma in the modern era with special reference to remnant liver volume. *J Am Coll Surg.* 1999;188(3):304–309.
47. Farges O, Belghiti J, Kianmanesh R, et al. Portal vein embolization before right hepatectomy: prospective clinical trial. *Ann Surg.* 2003;237(2):208–217.
48. Elias D, De Baere T, Roche A, et al. During liver regeneration following right portal embolization the growth rate of liver metastases is more rapid than that of the liver parenchyma. *Br J Surg.* 1999;86(6):784–788.
49. Kokudo N, Tada K, Seki M, et al. Proliferative activity of intrahepatic colorectal metastases after preoperative hemihepatic portal vein embolization. *Hepatology.* 2001;34(2):267–272.
50. Hayashi S, Baba Y, Ueno K, et al. Acceleration of primary liver tumor growth rate in embolized hepatic lobe after portal vein embolization. *Acta Radiol.* 2007;48(7):721–727.
51. Simoneau E, Aljiffry M, Salman A, et al. Portal vein embolization stimulates tumour growth in patients with colorectal cancer liver metastases. *HPB (Oxford).* 2012;14(7):461–468.
52. Brouquet A, Abdalla EK, Kopetz S, et al. High survival rate after two-stage resection of advanced colorectal liver metastases: response-based selection and complete resection define outcome. *J Clin Oncol.* 2011;29(8):1083–1090.
53. Narita M, Oussoultzoglou E, Jaeck D, et al. Two-stage hepatectomy for multiple bilobar colorectal liver metastases. *Br J Surg.* 2011;98(10):1463–1475.
54. Pawlik TM, Olino K, Gleisner AL, et al. Preoperative chemotherapy for colorectal liver metastases: impact on hepatic histology and postoperative outcome. *J Gastrointest Surg.* 2007;11(7):860–868.
55. Vauthey JN, Pawlik TM, Ribero D, et al. Chemotherapy regimen predicts steatohepatitis and an increase in 90-day mortality after surgery for hepatic colorectal metastases. *J Clin Oncol.* 2006;24(13):2065–2072.
56. Shindoh J, Tzeng CW, Aloia TA, et al. Optimal future liver remnant in patients treated with extensive preoperative chemotherapy for colorectal liver metastases. *Ann Surg Oncol.* 2013; 20(8):2493–2500.
57. Zorzi D, Chun YS, Madoff DC, et al. Chemotherapy with bevacizumab does not affect liver regeneration after portal vein embolization in the treatment of colorectal liver metastases. *Ann Surg Oncol.* 2008;15(10):2765–2772.
58. Covey AM, Brown KT, Jarnagin WR, et al. Combined portal vein embolization and neoadjuvant chemotherapy as a treatment strategy for resectable hepatic colorectal metastases. *Ann Surg.* 2008;247(3):451–455.
59. Beal IK, Anthony S, Papadopoulou A, et al. Portal vein embolisation prior to hepatic resection for colorectal liver metastases and the effects of periprocedure chemotherapy. *Br J Radiol.* 2006;79(942):473–478.
60. Muratore A, Zimmitti G, Ribero D, et al. Chemotherapy between the first and second stages of a two-stage hepatectomy for colorectal liver metastases: should we routinely recommend it? *Ann Surg Oncol.* 2012;19(4):1310–1315.

61. Jaeck D, Oussoultzoglou E, Rosso E, et al. A two-stage hepatectomy procedure combined with portal vein embolization to achieve curative resection for initially unresectable multiple and bilobar colorectal liver metastases. *Ann Surg*. 2004;240(6):1037–1049.
62. Kianmanesh R, Farges O, Abdalla EK, et al. Right portal vein ligation: a new planned two-step all-surgical approach for complete resection of primary gastrointestinal tumors with multiple bilateral liver metastases. *J Am Coll Surg*. 2003;197(1):164–170.
63. Schnitzbauer AA, Lang SA, Goessmann H, et al. Right portal vein ligation combined with in situ splitting induces rapid left lateral liver lobe hypertrophy enabling 2-staged extended right hepatic resection in small-for-size settings. *Ann Surg*. 2012;255(3):405–414.
64. Homayounfar K, Liersch T, Schuetze G, et al. Two-stage hepatectomy (R0) with portal vein ligation—towards curing patients with extended bilobular colorectal liver metastases. *Int J Colorectal Dis*. 2009;24(4):409–418.
65. Aussilhou B, Lesurtel M, Sauvanet A, et al. Right portal vein ligation is as efficient as portal vein embolization to induce hypertrophy of the left liver remnant. *J Gastrointest Surg*. 2008; 12(2):297–303.
66. Capussotti L, Muratore A, Baracchi F, et al. Portal vein ligation as an efficient method of increasing the future liver remnant volume in the surgical treatment of colorectal metastases. *Arch Surg*. 2008;143(10):978–982.
67. Broering DC, Hillert C, Krupski G, et al. Portal vein embolization vs. portal vein ligation for induction of hypertrophy of the future liver remnant. *J Gastrointest Surg*. 2002;6(6):905–913.
68. Robles R, Marín C, Lopez-Conesa A, et al. Comparative study of right portal vein ligation versus embolisation for induction of hypertrophy in two-stage hepatectomy for multiple bilateral colorectal liver metastases. *Eur J Surg Oncol*. 2012;38:586–593.
69. Denys AL, Abehsera M, Sauvanet A, et al. Failure of right portal vein ligation to induce left lobe hypertrophy due to intrahepatic portoportal collaterals: successful treatment with portal vein embolization. *AJR Am J Roentgenol*. 1999;173(3):633–635.
70. Thakrar PD, Madoff DC. Preoperative portal vein embolization: an approach to improve the safety of major hepatic resection. *Semin Roentgenol*. 2011;46(2):142–153.
71. Madoff DC, Hicks ME, Vauthey JN, et al. Transhepatic portal vein embolization: anatomy, indications, and technical considerations. *Radiographics*. 2002;22(5):1063–1076.
72. Covey AM, Brody LA, Getrajdman GI, et al. Incidence, patterns, and clinical relevance of variant portal vein anatomy. *AJR Am J Roentgenol*. 2004;183(4):1055–1064.
73. de Baere T, Roche A, Elias D, et al. Preoperative portal vein embolization for extension of hepatectomy indications. *Hepatology*. 1996;24(6):1386–1391.
74. Madoff DC, Abdalla EK, Vauthey JN. Portal vein embolization in preparation for major hepatic resection: evolution of a new standard of care. *J Vasc Interv Radiol*. 2005;16(6):779–790.
75. Madoff DC, Hicks ME, Abdalla EK, et al. Portal vein embolization with polyvinyl alcohol particles and coils in preparation for major liver resection for hepatobiliary malignancy: safety and effectiveness—study in 26 patients. *Radiology*. 2003; 227(1):251–260.
76. Kodama Y, Shimizu T, Endo H, et al. Complications of percutaneous transhepatic portal vein embolization. *J Vasc Interv Radiol*. 2002;13(12):1233–1237.
77. Nagino M, Kanai M, Morioka A, et al. Portal and arterial embolization before extensive liver resection in patients with markedly poor functional reserve. *J Vasc Interv Radiol*. 2000;11(8):1063–1068.
78. Capussotti L, Muratore A, Ferrero A, et al. Extension of right portal vein embolization to segment IV portal branches. *Arch Surg*. 2005;140(11):1100–1103.
79. van Gulik TM, van den Esschert JW, de Graaf W, et al. Controversies in the use of portal vein embolization. *Dig Surg*. 2008;25(6):436–444.
80. Kishi Y, Madoff DC, Abdalla EK, et al. Is embolization of segment 4 portal veins before extended right hepatectomy justified? *Surgery*. 2008;144(5):744–751.
81. Mueller L, Hillert C, Möller L, et al. Major hepatectomy for colorectal metastases: is preoperative portal occlusion an oncological risk factor? *Ann Surg Oncol*. 2008;15(7):1908–1917.
82. van Lienden KP, van den Esschert JW, de Graaf w, et al. Portal vein embolization before liver resection: a systematic review. *Cardiovasc Intervent Radiol*. 2013;36(1):25–34.
83. Guiu B, Bize P, Gunthem D, et al. Portal vein embolization before right hepatectomy: improved results using n-butyl-cyanoacrylate compared to microparticles plus coils. *Cardiovasc Intervent Radiol*. 2013;36(5):1306–1312.
84. Cazejust J, Bessoud B, Le Bail M, et al. Preoperative portal vein embolization with a combination of trisacryl microspheres, gelfoam and coils [published online ahead of print September 2, 2013]. *Diagn Interv Imaging*.
85. Matsuoka T, Nakatsuka H, Nakamura K, et al. Long-term embolization of the portal vein with isobutyl-2-cyanoacrylate in hepatoma [in Japanese]. *Nihon Igaku Hoshasen Gakkai Zasshi*. 1986;46(1):72–74.
86. Bent CL, Low D, Matson MB, et al. Portal vein embolization using a nitinol plug (Amplatzer vascular plug) in combination with histoacryl glue and iodinized oil: adequate hypertrophy with a reduced risk of nontarget embolization. *Cardiovasc Intervent Radiol*. 2009;32(3):471–477.
87. Denecke T, Seehofer D, Steffen IG, et al. Arterial versus portal venous embolization for induction of hepatic hypertrophy before extended right hemihepatectomy in hilar cholangiocarcinomas: a prospective randomized study. *J Vasc Interv Radiol*. 2011;22(9):1254–1262.
88. Gruttadauria S, Luca A, Mandala L, et al. Sequential preoperative ipsilateral portal and arterial embolization in patients with colorectal liver metastases. *World J Surg*. 2006;30(4):576–578.
89. Aoki T, Imamura H, Hasegawa K, et al. Sequential preoperative arterial and portal venous embolizations in patients with hepatocellular carcinoma. *Arch Surg*. 2004;139(7):766–774.
90. Ogata S, Belghiti J, Farges O, et al. Sequential arterial and portal vein embolizations before right hepatectomy in patients with cirrhosis and hepatocellular carcinoma. *Br J Surg*. 2006;93(9):1091–1098.
91. Angle JF, Siddigi NH, Wallace MJ, et al. Quality improvement guidelines for percutaneous transcatheter embolization: Society of Interventional Radiology Standards of Practice Committee. *J Vasc Interv Radiol*. 2010;21(10):1479–1486.
92. Denys A, Bize P, Demartines N, et al. Quality improvement for portal vein embolization. *Cardiovasc Intervent Radiol*. 2010; 33(3):452–456.
93. Di Stefano DR, de Baere T, Denus A, et al. Preoperative percutaneous portal vein embolization: evaluation of adverse events in 188 patients. *Radiology*. 2005;234(2):625–630.

32

Balloon-Occluded Retrograde Transvenous Obliteration

Luke R. Wilkins • Wael E. Saad

Gastric and esophageal varices can have multiple etiologies. Most (90%) patients have underlying cirrhosis and portal hypertension. This patient population has a 30% risk of developing varices, with gastric varices representing 10% to 20%. Although the bleeding risk associated with gastric varices is less than that associated with esophageal varices, gastric varices are accompanied with higher rates of morbidity and mortality.[1] Treating patients with gastric variceal bleeding necessitates a multidisciplinary team approach, including hepatologists, endoscopists, diagnostic radiologists, and interventional radiologists.[1,2]

Although upper gastrointestinal (GI) endoscopy is the first-line diagnostic and management tool for upper GI bleeding secondary to varices, endovascular treatment is playing an ever-increasing role in definitive treatment.[1,2] From the perspective of interventional radiology, there has been a significant amount of controversy regarding the optimal therapeutic management of patients with gastric variceal bleeding.[3–7] Whereas the West (United States and Europe) typically prefers decompression of the portal circulation as the primary treatment approach (i.e., transjugular intrahepatic portosystemic shunt [TIPS]), the East (Japan and South Korea) focuses on the gastric varices themselves, sclerosing them via the balloon-occluded retrograde transvenous obliteration (BRTO) procedure.[3,8]

Although this chapter will focus on the obliteration (sclerotherapy and/or embolotherapy) of gastric varices, given the complexity and variability of gastric varices, the preprocedural clinical management, endoscopic management, and the preprocedural imaging will also be discussed.

DEVICE/MATERIAL DESCRIPTION

Embolization Agents/Sclerosants

Many agents are available for use in variceal obliteration. Examples include ethanolamine oleate (EO, Oldamin; Grelan Pharmaceutical Co., Ltd., Tokyo, Japan), sodium tetradecyl sulfate (Sotradecol; AngioDynamics, Queensbury, New York), polidocanol foam (Polidocasklerol; ZERIA Pharmaceutical Co., Ltd., Tokyo, Japan), and *N*-butyl cyanoacrylate. EO is the original agent used for BRTO and remains the agent of choice in Asia.[9–11] Five percent EO is the most common concentration used and is made with 10% EO and the same dose of contrast medium.[9,11] EO causes hemolysis with the release of free hemoglobin which may result in renal tubular disturbances and acute renal failure. The administration of 4,000 units of haptoglobin (Green Cross, Osaka, Japan) intravenously will prevent renal insufficiency by binding circulating free hemoglobin. Additional reported complications include pulmonary edema, disseminated intravascular coagulation, and cardiogenic shock.[10,12,13] Consequently, some authors recommend limiting EO to a volume of 40 mL per procedure. Routine use of this agent in the United States is markedly limited as haptoglobin is not approved by the U.S. Food and Drug Administration (FDA).

Sodium tetradecyl sulfate (STS) has been extensively used for sclerotherapy of superficial lower extremity varicose veins in both liquid and foam forms.[14,15] Additional uses include treatment of venous malformations, male varicoceles, and pelvic congestion syndrome.[16–19] There are many potential advantages of STS foam, including minimal administered doses, contact with variceal wall, density of material, and efficiency of endothelial damage. A recent study demonstrated a marked decrease in amount of STS given when comparing the liquid mixture (34.1 mL, range 10 to 65 mL) to the foam mixture (10 mL, range 1 to 20 mL). This lower dose may correspond to decreased systemic effects of hemolysis and renal failure without significantly affecting technical success. Further, STS foam is thought to provide improved contact with the variceal wall in comparison to liquid sclerosing agents. This has been demonstrated in the treatment of lower extremity varicose veins where foam sclerotherapy was found to be far more effective than liquid sclerotherapy by improved displacement of the blood volume along with providing a larger surface area of the sclerosant to contact the venous endothelium.[15] In vivo studies have demonstrated pathologic damage to the endothelium to be rapid and occur within the first 2 minutes of contact, followed by intimal edema, progressive intimal separation from the tunica media, and microthrombi formation in the following 30 minutes.[20] In addition, the foam sclerosants have a tendency to ascend immediately into nondependent gastric varices when compared with more dense liquid sclerosants.

Sotradecol is available in 1% and 3% concentrations. Although a recent study suggested that there is no added benefit in using 3% versus 1% concentration, 3% Sotradecol is often favored as it provides the highest dose possible to the varix.[15] Although there is no standard method of foam preparation, it is recommended that 3% Sotradecol be mixed with gas (air or carbon dioxide [CO_2]) along with Lipiodol for added visualization in the following ratio: 2 mL STS : 1 mL Lipiodol : 3 mL air/CO_2.[13] Although many observe that room air remains in foam solution longer than CO_2, there remains concern that room air may potentially embolize to the lungs or the systemic circulation via a patent foramen ovale as it comes out of solution.[21,22] Alternative sclerosant mixtures include foam EO (10 mL of 10% EO : 10 mL iodinated contrast medium : 20 mL of air) and foam polidocanol (2 mL of 3% polidocanol : 8 mL of air).

With regard to occlusion balloons, there are several options available in the United States and include the Coda (Cook Medical, Inc., Bloomington, Indiana), Python occlusion balloon (Applied Medical, Rancho Santa Margarita, California), Equalizer (Boston Scientific Corporation, Natick, Massachusetts), and flow-directed occlusion balloon catheters (Cook Medical, Inc., Bloomington, Indiana).

Complete details on inventory (sclerosants and catheters) are beyond the scope of this chapter; however, they are discussed in detail by Saad et al.,[23] including specifications for balloon occlusion catheters.

TECHNIQUE

Procedural Steps

Access is usually achieved via the right femoral or internal jugular vein using standard angiographic technique and placement of a 6-Fr to 12-Fr sheath. More commonly, access is through a right femoral vein approach. However, some institutions use the jugular vein approach exclusively. Preprocedure imaging may aid in deciding which approach provides the best angle for selecting the shunt.

During a conventional BRTO, the gastrorenal shunt (GRS) is catheterized via the left renal vein using a balloon occlusion catheter (a compliant balloon mounted on a catheter). Balloon occlusion catheters with a reverse curve are available in Asia and provide easier and more stable access into the shunt. These catheters are not readily available in the United States, and it is suggested that stable access into the inferior vena cava (IVC) or distal renal vein be secured with an appropriately sized sheath (6-Fr to 12-Fr). The renal vein may be selected with a 5-Fr diagnostic catheter (Cobra; AngioDynamics, Queensbury, New York). The diagnostic catheter can then be exchanged for an angled-tip catheter, which may be used to select the shunt. Alternatively, a 5-Fr Simmons 2 catheter (AngioDynamics, Queensbury, New York) may be used to select the renal vein and withdrawn until the tip engages the shunt. A 0.035-in stiff guidewire (TAD II [Mallinckrodt Inc., St. Louis, Missouri] or Rosen [AngioDynamics, Queensbury, New York]) is advanced into the shunt as far as possible and the angled-tip catheter is exchanged for an occlusion balloon that is sized to occlude the communicating GRS of interest. The diameter of occlusion balloons ranges from 8.5 to 32 mm. Selection of the proper occlusion balloon would optimally occur at the time of preprocedure imaging (as detailed earlier). A new technique for selection of the shunt from the left renal vein via a femoral approach using a straight reinforced sheath is called the *PRESS technique* (Pullback RE-inforced Straight Sheath).[24,25] The left renal vein is selected with a catheter (usually Cobra-shaped) and a 0.035-in Rosen wire is advanced into the left renal vein into the left renal hilum. The Cobra catheter is exchanged for a reinforced sheath. Pullback venography through the sheath as it is withdrawn over the anchoring Rosen wire is performed. The anchoring wire and the shape of the reinforced sheath allows the sheath to "scrape" the superior aspect of the left renal vein. The sheath will then "pop" into the shunt.[24,25]

Balloon occlusion venography may then be performed to define the type of varix/varices and the anatomy of the venous drainage. As will be discussed in greater detail in the section entitled "Preprocedure Imaging," venous drainage patterns may be classified into type A, B, or C (Fig. 32.1). Type D drainage patterns lack a definable shunt and are unable to be treated via the BRTO procedure.[5,26]

Following balloon occlusion venography, the sclerosant may be infused. The goal of sclerosant infusion is filling of the extent of the varix with the embolization end point of minimal filling of the afferent portal vein branch(s). Although the injection of the sclerosing agent can be performed with or without the use of a microcatheter, it is recommended

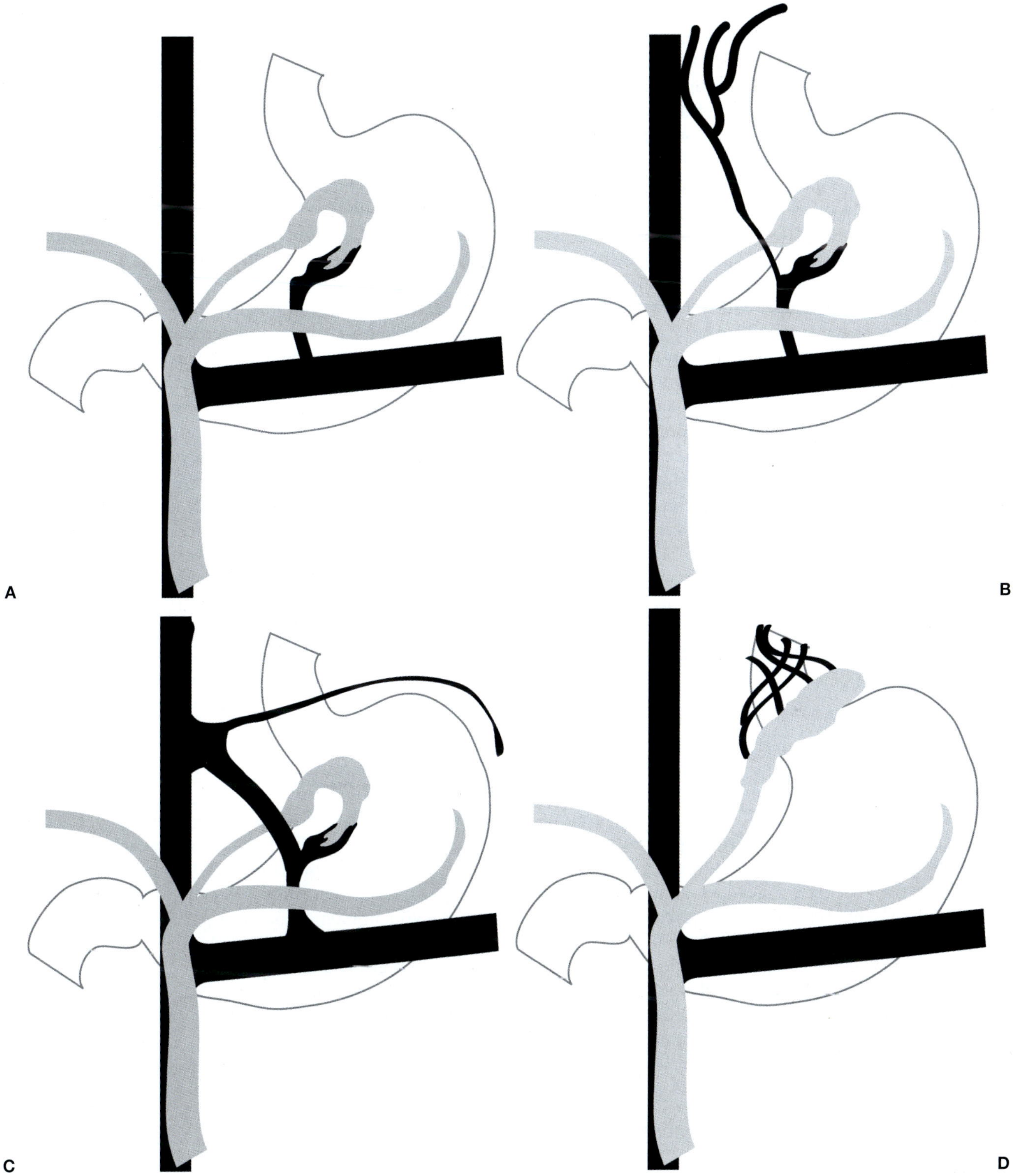

Figure 32.1 Classification based on venous drainage. **A:** Type A has a shunt with a single draining vein. **B:** Type B has a shunt with multiple collateral draining veins. **C:** Type C has both a gastrocaval and gastrorenal shunt. **D:** Type D has multiple small draining veins and no shunt. (From Sabri SS, Saad WEA. Balloon-occluded retrograde transvenous obliteration [BRTO]: technique and intraprocedural imaging. *Semin Intervent Radiol*. 2011;28:305.)

that a microcatheter be advanced as deeply as possible into the varix and sclerosing agent administered through the microcatheter. This allows the advantage of selective delivery of the sclerosant into the varix while minimizing the amount of volume (optimizing distribution of the sclerosant) used as well as minimizing the risk of balloon rupture when the sclerosant comes in contact with the balloon. Full opacification of gastric varices may be prevented by leaking collateral veins such as the inferior phrenic or paravertebral veins. Occlusion with coils or Gelfoam pledgets (Pfizer, New York, New York) through the microcatheter can help occlude these veins, allowing concentration of the sclerosant at the varix and minimize nontarget efflux of sclerosant into the portal system or systemic vasculature.

Following infusion of chosen sclerosant, the occlusion balloon(s) remain inflated for a minimum of 4 hours and a maximum of 24 hours. Although the balloon(s) may be left in place overnight and deflated under fluoroscopy the following day, this will likely increase access site bleeding, infection rates, and patient inconvenience. Research suggests that there is no observable change in obliteration rate or complication rate when leaving inflated for 4 hours as opposed to 24 hours.[13]

CLINICAL APPLICATIONS

Preprocedure Evaluation and Management

Clinical Management

A patient presenting with underlying liver disease and upper GI bleeding should be appropriately evaluated and closely monitored. When the patient is clinically stable, upper endoscopy is typically performed for first-line diagnostic and therapeutic purposes.[2] It is advised that aggressive volume resuscitation be avoided as variceal bleeding may be exacerbated by fluid overload. After identification of bleeding gastric varices, the management involves diagnostic and therapeutic considerations necessitating a multidisciplinary approach. A management protocol flowchart may be found in Figures 32.2 and 32.3. Although this will briefly be discussed in the following pages, a complete discussion regarding management of gastric varices is outside the scope of this chapter. The reader is referred to the current literature regarding indications and management of gastric varices.[27]

Endoscopic Evaluation and Treatment

As mentioned earlier, routine upper endoscopy is performed early in the clinical course of a patient presenting with melena or hematemesis. The endoscopic evaluation is essential for identification of which varices (if any) are bleeding in addition to identifying the types of underlying gastric varices. This is usually classified according to the Sarin endoscopic classification (Fig. 32.4). This classification helps to differentiate and triage the bleeding varices so that optimal therapy may be considered. Esophageal varices can often be controlled effectively by endoscopic-guided banding and sclerotherapy. Bleeding esophageal varices that cannot be controlled medically and endoscopically would warrant the creation of a TIPS. If gastric varices are identified on evaluation, then a different endoscopic and endovascular approach is warranted. In addition to etiologic identification, the stigmata of "high-risk gastric varices/impending bleeding" and/or stigmata of recent bleeding may be identified by endoscopy. If high-risk gastric varices with recent bleeding or actively bleeding cardiofundal varix is encountered in the course of that endoscopic evaluation, several clinical avenues may be considered. Conventional endoscopic therapy involves attempts at sclerosants and/or banding. However, studies have demonstrated relatively high failure rates for acute control and early rates of rebleeding.[28] Recent comparative trials of sclerotherapy versus banding demonstrate high rebleeding rates of 30% to 45% in both groups, underscoring the significant morbidity associated with such endoscopic methods and enforcing the need for alternative treatment techniques.[29] Cyanoacrylate injection may also be considered as a hemostatic agent for gastric variceal bleeding. Although its use in the United States has been limited, several trials have emerged as its use has been established as a primary means of achieving gastric varix obliteration. Although demonstrating improvement when compared with conventional techniques, cyanoacrylate maintains rebleeding rates from 15% to 27%.[30,31] The elevated rebleeding rate of both conventional TIPS and endoscopic treatments have only served to increase interest in alternative treatment techniques such as BRTO.

Preprocedure Imaging

Both three-phase contrast-enhanced computed tomography (CECT) and contrast-enhanced magnetic resonance angiography/venography (MRA/MRV) may be used for preprocedural evaluation and are equally effective at providing optimal visualization of the main portal vein and its tributaries.[2] Advantages of CECT include availability, multiplanar reconstructions, and speed. When protocoling a CECT for BRTO, it is important to not give oral contrast as this may obscure visualization of the varices. Water may be used as it provides gastric distension and acts as a negative contrast agent for the contrast-enhanced gastric varices. In addition, it is recommended that images be acquired from the level of the midchest through the pelvis so as to fully evaluate the extent of existing portosystemic shunts.[32] Advantages of MRA/MRV include lack of ionizing radiation, decreased nephrotoxicity, and evaluation of portal hemodynamics. It is important that images be acquired in the coronal plane and include dynamic postcontrast sequences. In addition, rapid sequences, such as the vastly undersampled isotropic projection reconstruction (VIPR) sequence (GE Healthcare, Milwaukee, Wisconsin), are promising in evaluating portal hemodynamics.[2]

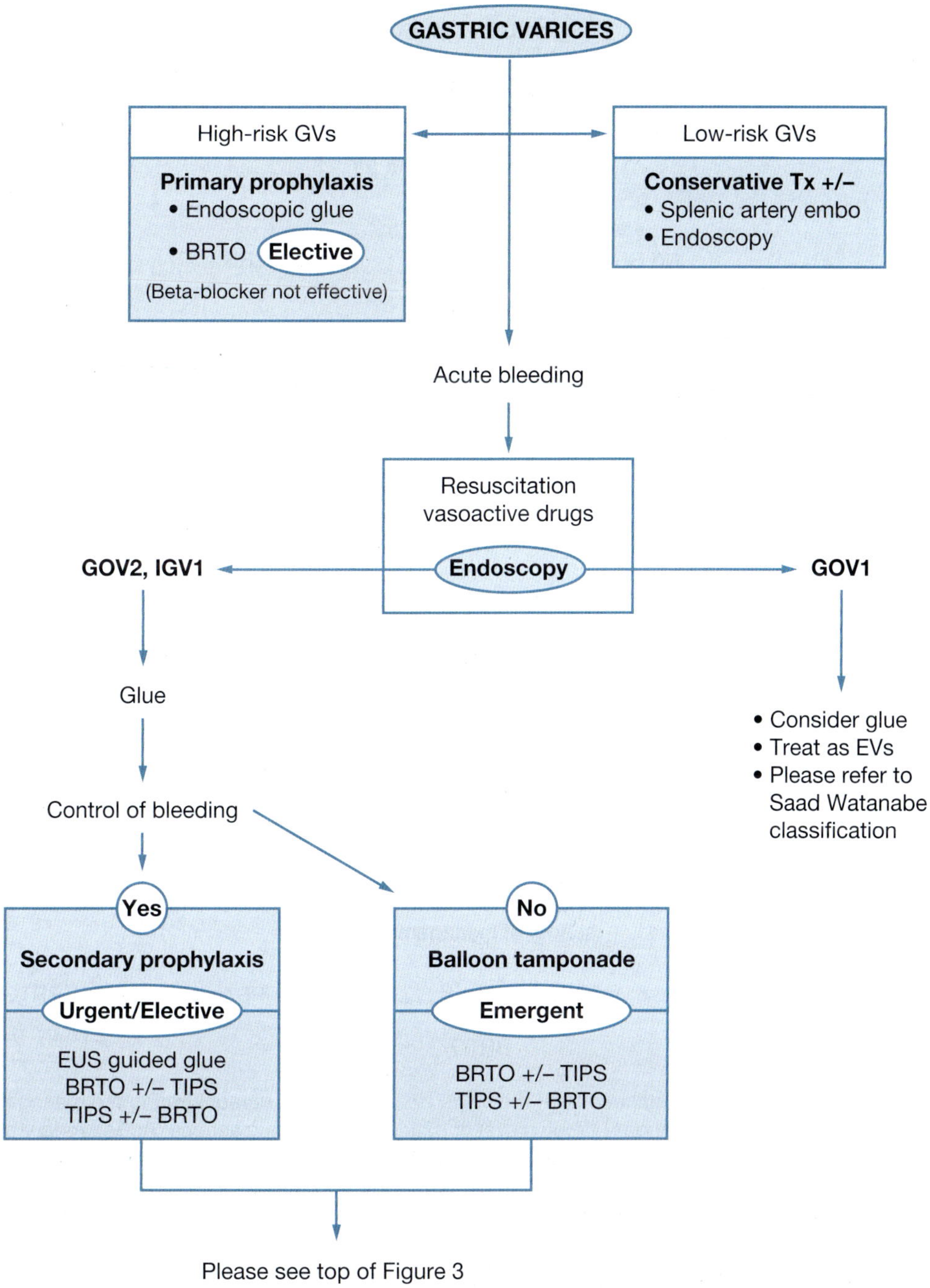

Figure 32.2 Flowchart demonstrating the management protocol (including primary and secondary prophylaxis) of patients with gastric varices. GVs, gastric varices; EVs, esophageal varices; splenic A embo, splenic artery embolization; glue, direct cyanoacrylate injection into gastric varices; conservative Tx, conservative treatment; endoscopic Tx, endoscopic treatment; GOV1: Sarin classification, gastroesophageal varices type 1; GOV2: Sarin classification, gastroesophageal varices type 2; IGV1: Sarin classification, isolated gastric varices type-1; EUS, endoscopic ultrasound. (From Saad WE, Kitanosono T, Koizumi J, et al. The conventional balloon-occluded retrograde transvenous obliteration procedure: indications, contraindications, and technical applications. *Tech Vasc Interv Radiol*. 2013;16:107.)

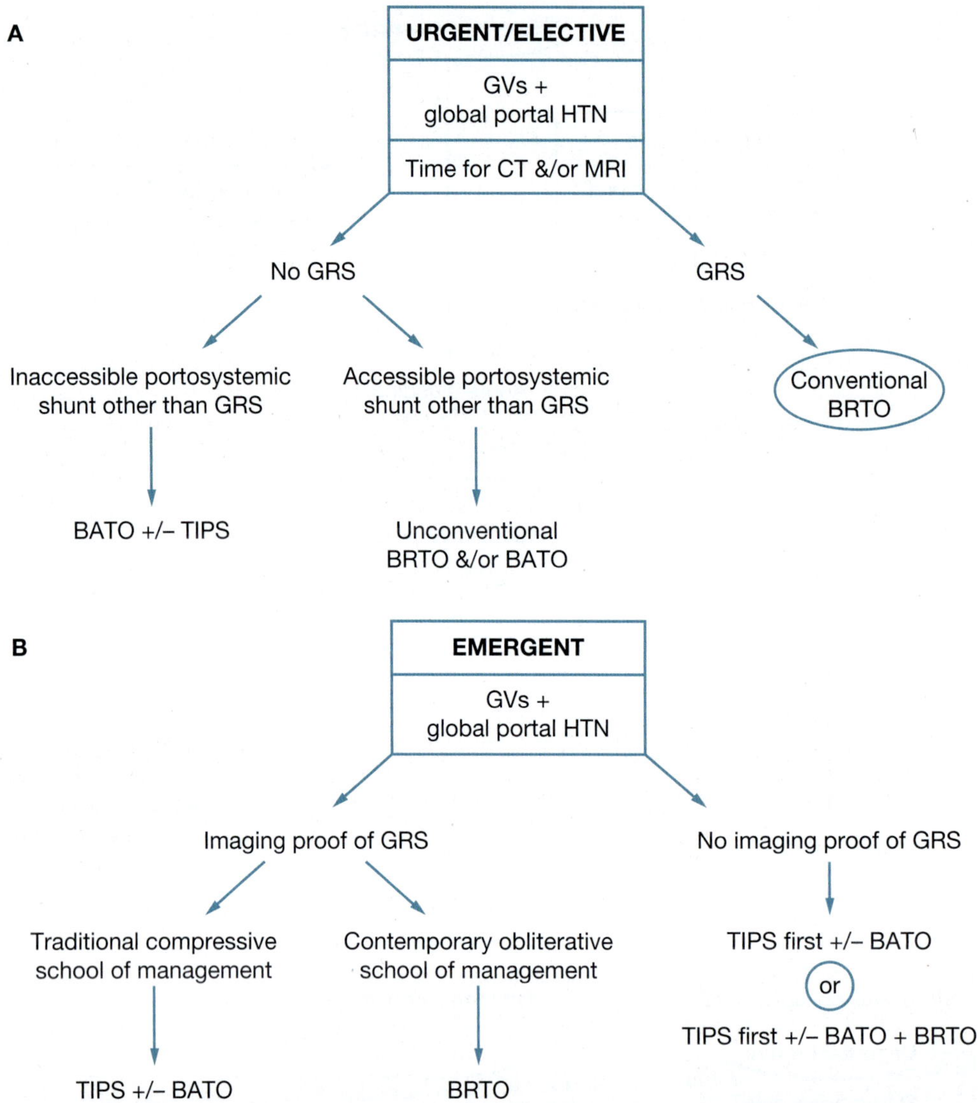

Figure 32.3 Continuation flowcharts (continued from the flowchart in Fig. 32.2) demonstrating the management protocol (including primary and secondary prophylaxis) of patients with gastric varices. **A:** Secondary prophylaxis of gastric varices (urgent or elective). **B:** Emergent management of gastric varices. GVs, gastric varices; portal HTN, portal hypertension (global hypertension or general hypertension); CT, computed tomography; MRI, magnetic resonance imaging; GRS, gastrorenal shunt; BATO, balloon-occluded antegrade transvenous obliteration; TIPS, transjugular intrahepatic portosystemic shunt; BRTO, balloon-occluded retrograde transvenous obliteration. (From Saad WE, Kitanosono T, Koizumi J, et al. The conventional balloon-occluded retrograde transvenous obliteration procedure: indications, contraindications, and technical applications. *Tech Vasc Interv Radiol*. 2013;16:108.)

Following image acquisition, many variables must be weighed when evaluating a patient for a possible BRTO and technical planning of the procedure. Several anatomic and hemodynamic factors to consider before performing a BRTO include splenic vein (SpV) patency, portal vein patency, and presence and size of the portosystemic shunt. In addition, for unconventional BRTO, one should note the presence and size of alternative portosystemic shunts and leading supradiaphragmatic and infradiaphragmatic systemic veins that can be seen traversing the diaphragm to reach the subphrenic gastric variceal complex. These include the left phrenic, left pericardiac vein, and the azygo-esophago venous/variceal axis (Fig. 32.5).[2]

Assessing SpV patency allows differentiation between segmental (sentinel) and generalized (global) portal hypertension. This differentiation is critical for the management of gastric varices. Segmental portal hypertension involves thrombosis of the entirety of the SpV in the absence of portal vein thrombosis. Alternatively, segmental portal hypertension may be caused by acute or chronic pancreatitis

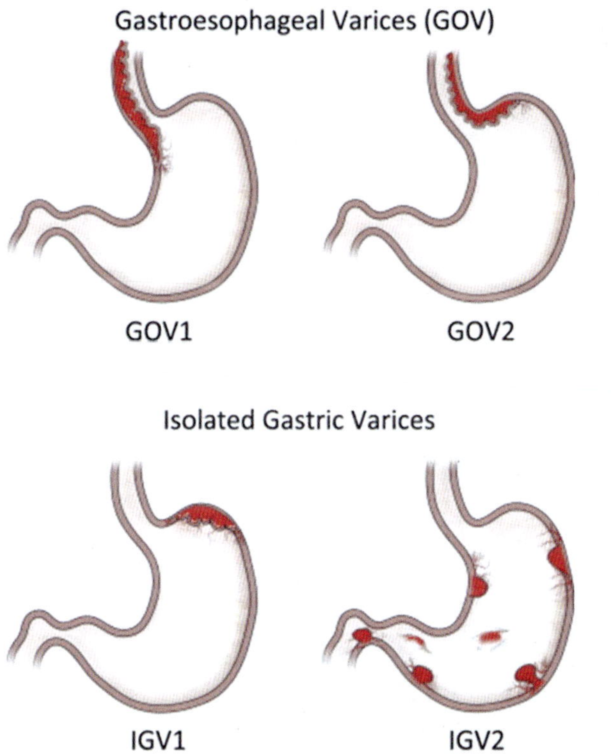

Figure 32.4 Illustration of the endoscopic classification of gastric and gastroesophageal varices by Sarin. Basic outline of various parts of the gastric anatomy and first part of the duodenum. GOV, gastroesophageal varices (type 1 and type 2); IGV, isolated gastric varices (type 1 and type 2). (From Saad WE. Vascular anatomy and the morphologic and hemodynamic classifications of gastric varices and spontaneous portosystemic shunts relevant to the BRTO procedure. *Tech Vasc Interv Radiol*. 2013;16:61.)

with focal occlusion of the distal SpV. Generalized portal hypertension may be differentiated by classically showing secondary signs of a hepatic etiology (i.e., cirrhosis). Radiographic signs of portal hypertension include portal vein diameter greater than 14 mm, occasional portal vein thrombosis (partial or complete), cavernous transformation of the portal vein, and the presence of right-sided portosystemic collaterals (e.g., recanalized paraumbilical vein and esophageal varices along the left gastric and hemiazygous venous axis).[2]

The presence or absence of portal vein thrombosis, although a potential sequelae of a GRS, should also be noted in preprocedural imaging. GRSs and splenorenal shunts are portosystemic collaterals that have hepatofugal flow and may promote hepatofugal flow in the SpV and even the main portal vein. A complex set of hemodynamic variables will determine to the extent that the portal circulation is affected by a GRS, including size of the GRS, presence of TIPS, patency of the main portal vein, resistance of the sinusoidal bed, etc.[26,33] As one would imagine, in the presence of main portal vein thrombosis, the GRS will act as a main outflow for the splenic and mesenteric veins. Occlusion of the GRS through a BRTO procedure would potentially cause mesenteric venous hypertension and mesenteric ischemia with possible thrombosis of the entire splanchnic portal venous circulation.[2] However, the hemodynamics of the portal circulation is incompletely understood and the risk may be somewhat diminished in the presence of cavernous transformation of the portal vein. These risks should be carefully weighed against any potential benefits before a proposed BRTO.[32]

Last, for a conventional BRTO procedure, one must assess for the presence of a large infradiaphragmatic (i.e., left-sided) portosystemic collateral/shunt. These shunts include the splenorenal, gastrorenal (combine gastrosplenorenal), gastrocaval, gastrophrenic, and gastrogonadal portosystemic shunts.[26] The most common shunt that is found and occluded during a conventional BRTO is a GRS, which provides portal venous outflow to the gastric varices in 90% of patients with gastric varices. The shunts may be classified according to the venous drainage pattern into A, B, C, or D (see Fig. 32.1).[12,25] In addition, the diameter of the shunt is usually measured to plan for the BRTO and select for the appropriate equipment. The diameter of the shunt is typically measured at the distal shunt near the renal vein and is frequently the location where the interventional radiologist will attempt to occlude the shunt with the occlusive balloon for the BRTO procedure. It should be noted that the distal shunt may not correspond to the narrowest point of the shunt and it is for this reason that a thorough evaluation throughout the extent of the shunt is warranted. Further, attention must be paid to the presence of venous webs that may cause additional narrowing within the shunt and may aid in occlusion balloon catheter placement. On occasion, the size of a GRS on cross-sectional imaging will preclude a BRTO procedure; however, one may be attempted as computed tomography (CT) and magnetic resonance imaging (MRI) frequently underestimate the presence of webs. Only after cannulation and balloon occlusion can the true diameter and ability to safely occlude the GRS be tested with the balloon occlusion catheter available.

In the absence of a GRS or gastrocaval shunt (required for a conventional BRTO), alternative portosystemic collaterals/routes may be evaluated for the possibility of an unconventional BRTO. These routes may include gastrophrenic, pericardiogastric (left pericardiac vein), and azygous/hemiazygous to left gastric vein axis. Additionally, these routes may be present with a coexisting GRS, which may hinder the BRTO and allow escape of sclerosant into the systemic circulation.

Treatment Modifications According to Draining Venous Pattern

As detailed earlier and outlined in Figure 32.1, shunts may be classified according to the venous drainage pattern into

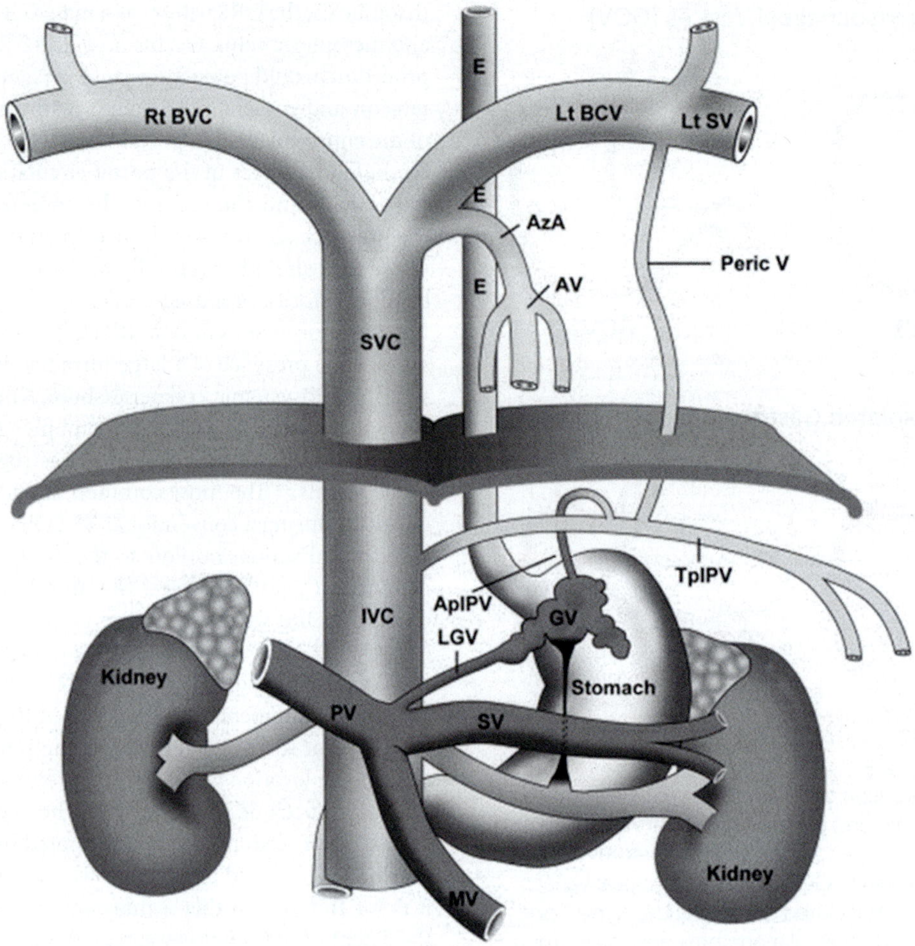

Figure 32.5 An illustration of a gastric variceal system without a gastrorenal shunt. The depicted portal venous feeder to the gastric varices (*GV*) is the left gastric vein (*LGV*). The systemic venous efferent drainage, as depicted, is the ascending portion of the inferior phrenic vein (*ApIPV*), which arcs over the transverse portion of the inferior phrenic vein (*TpIPV*) and into the inferior vena cava (*IVC*). Supradiaphragmatic systemic venous drainers of GVs may include the pericardial vein (*Peric V*) and azygos vein (*AV*) off the azygos arch (*AzA*). The Peric V usually comes off the junction of the left subclavian vein (*Lt SV*) and the left brachiocephalic vein (*Lt BCV*) and runs down the left heart border to anastomose with the TpIPV. Rt BCV, right brachiocephalic vein; E, esophagus; PV, portal vein; SV, splenic vein; MV, mesenteric vein. (From Saad WE. Vascular anatomy and the morphologic and hemodynamic classifications of gastric varices and spontaneous portosystemic shunts relevant to the BRTO procedure. *Tech Vasc Interv Radiol*. 2013;16:85.)

A, B, C, or D.[5] Treatment of gastric varices may require modification on the basis of the draining venous pattern.

Type A varices are contiguous with a single draining shunt. This is most commonly a GRS and less commonly a gastrocaval shunt draining through an enlarged inferior phrenic vein directly into the IVC. This type of drainage pattern is the easiest to treat given the absence of leaking collateral veins or additional shunts. Further, the entire varix can be visualized during balloon-occluded retrograde venography. As detailed earlier, the microcatheter can then be advanced through the balloon occlusion catheter as deep as possible into the varix and sclerosant administered to embolization end point of minimal filling of the afferent vein/portal vasculature (Fig. 32.6).[34]

Type B varices are contiguous with a single shunt (most commonly a GRS) and one or more collateral veins. These collaterals drain through a plexus of vessel back to the right atrium or IVC without formation of a definable shunt. These draining veins may include the pericardiophrenic, ascending lumbar, intercostal, perivertebral, or rarely the azygous. Unlike the type A drainage pattern, full opacification of the varices is not achieved on retrograde venography secondary to preferential flow of contrast into the leaking collateral veins. If the collateral veins are able to be catheterized, then embolization may be performed with coils or Gelfoam pledgets (Fig. 32.7). However, if the veins are unable to be catheterized due to size and/or number, several different treatment strategies exist. The occlusion balloon

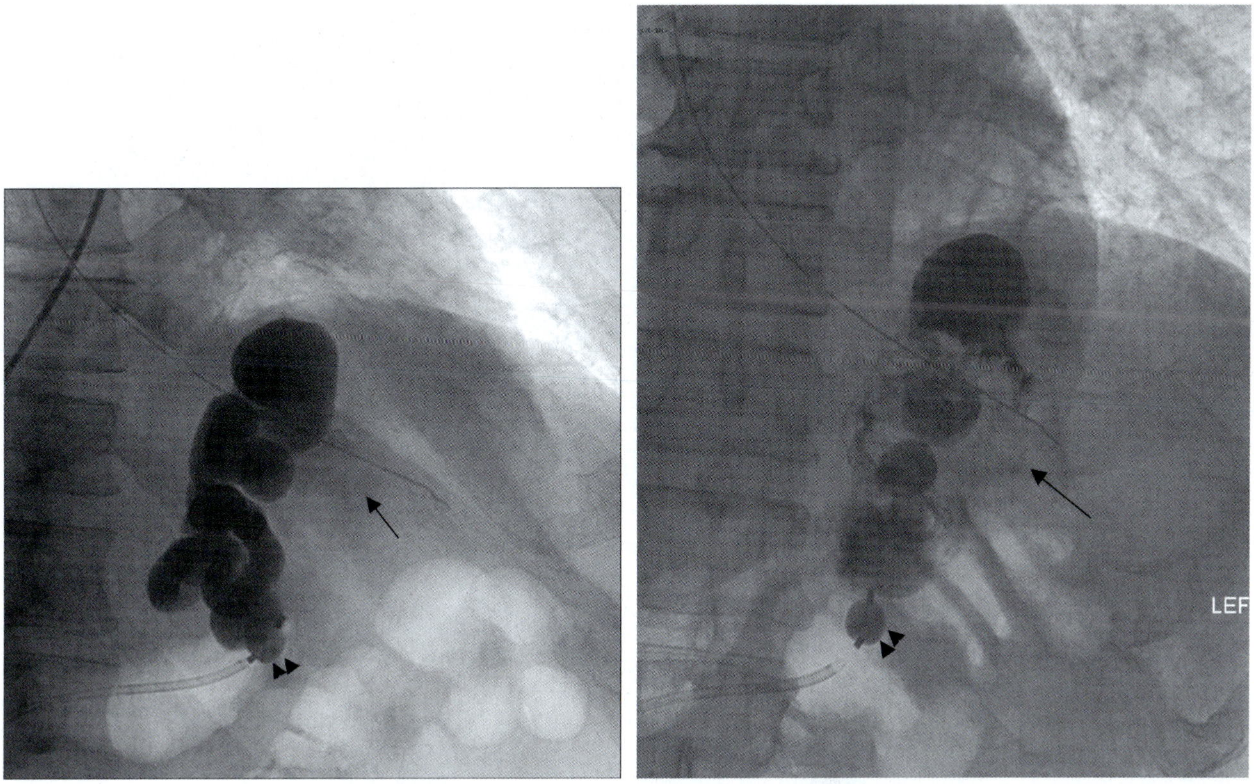

A B

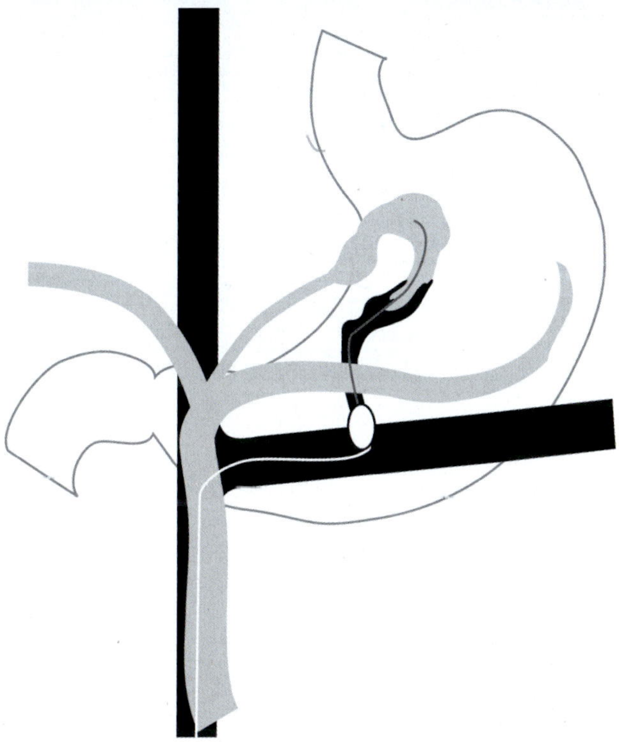

C

Figure 32.6 Type A venous outflow. **A:** With the occlusion balloon (*arrowheads*) positioned at the base of the gastrorenal shunt, balloon-occluded retrograde venography shows filling of the gastric varices as well as the afferent vein (*arrow*). **B:** With the occlusion balloon (*arrowheads*) inflated, the sclerosant was administered with minimal filling of the afferent vein (*arrow*). **C:** Overview of type A venous outflow treatment. (From Sabri SS, Saad WEA. Balloon-occluded retrograde transvenous obliteration [BRTO]: technique and intraprocedural imaging. *Semin Intervent Radiol*. 2011;28:307.)

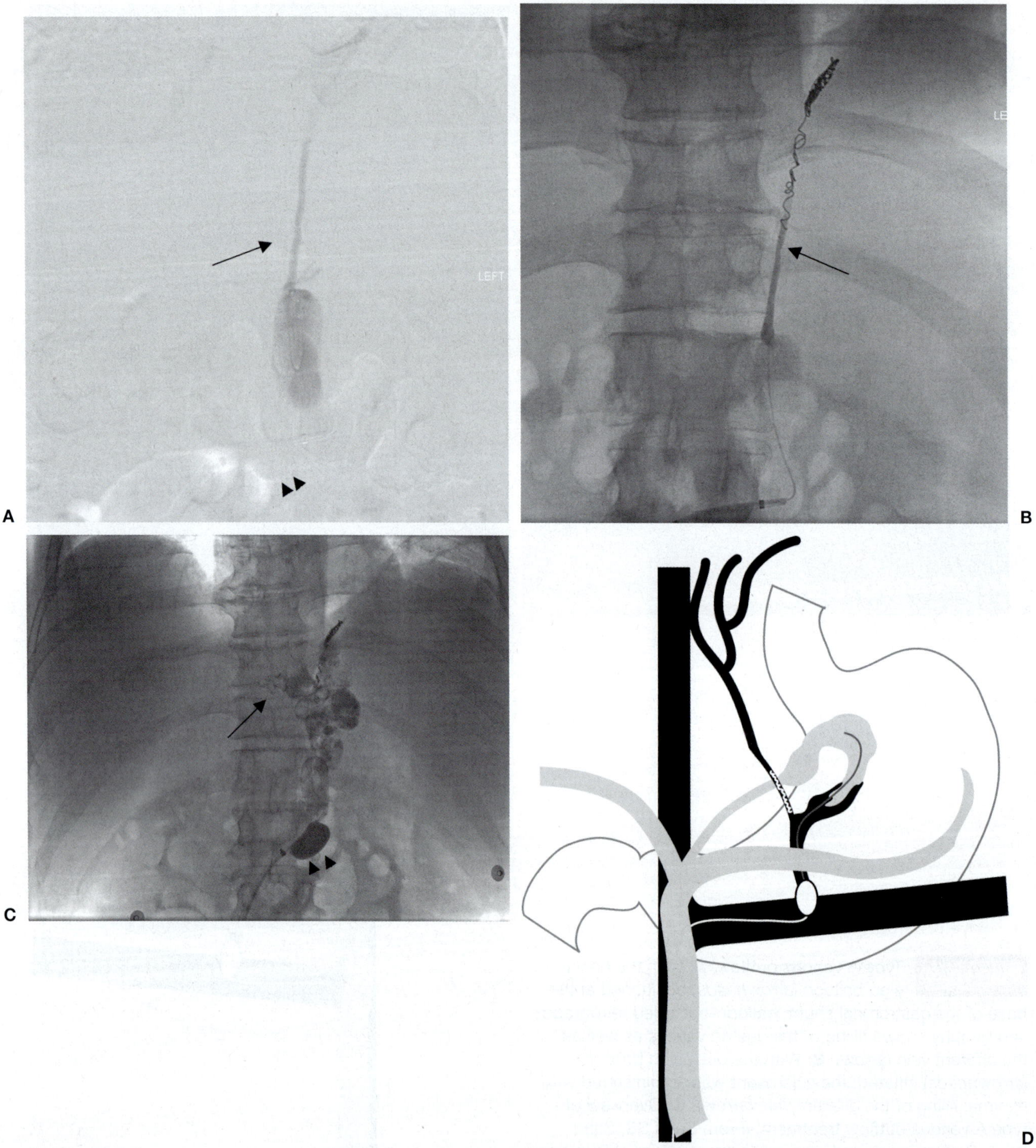

Figure 32.7 Type B venous outflow. **A:** With the occlusion balloon (*arrowheads*) positioned at the base of the gastrorenal shunt, balloon-occluded retrograde venography shows filling of the inferior phrenic vein (*arrow*). **B:** Using a microcatheter (*arrow*), the vein was catheterized and embolized using metallic coils. **C:** With the occlusion balloon (*arrowheads*) inflated, the sclerosant was administered with minimal filling of the afferent vein (*arrow*). **D:** Overview of type B venous outflow using metallic coils. (From Sabri SS, Saad WEA. Balloon-occluded retrograde transvenous obliteration [BRTO]: technique and intraprocedural imaging. *Semin Intervent Radiol*. 2011;28:309.)

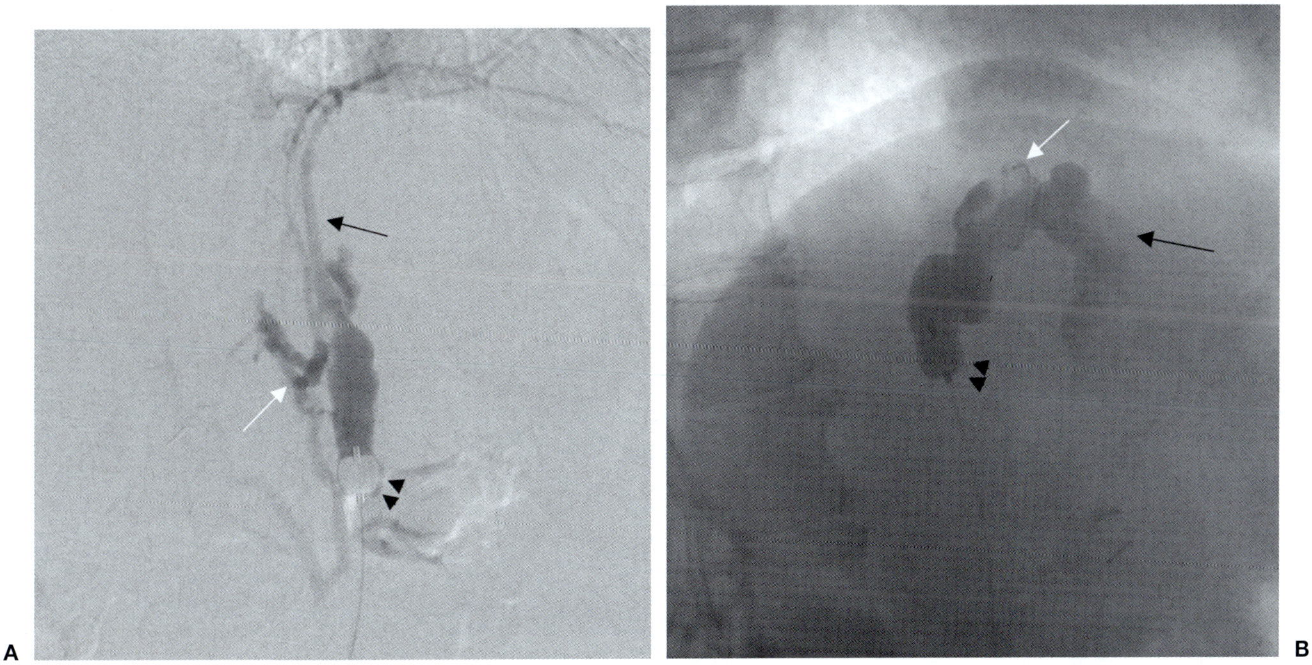

Figure 32.8 Type B venous outflow. **A:** With the occlusion balloon (*arrowheads*) positioned at the base of the gastrorenal shunt, balloon-occluded retrograde venography shows filling of multiple "leaking" collateral veins including inferior phrenic (*black arrow*) and perivertebral veins (*white arrow*). **B:** After the occlusion balloon (*arrowheads*) was advanced beyond the leaking collateral veins, venography through a microcatheter (*white arrow*) now shows opacification of the gastric varices (*black arrow*). (From Sabri SS, Saad WEA. Balloon-occluded retrograde transvenous obliteration [BRTO]: technique and intraprocedural imaging. *Semin Intervent Radiol*. 2011;28:308.)

may be advanced beyond the leaking collateral vessels and repeat venography performed. If this is able to fully opacify the varix without evidence of additional leaking collateral, sclerosant may safely be administered from this location (Fig. 32.8). This technique may be challenging due to shunt tortuosity and balloon catheter maneuverability. This limitation may be overcome by advancing the balloon over the microcatheter as deeply as possible into the varix. Fukuda et al. reported success in 87% of cases using this technique.[21] Alternatively, flow-directed embolization of the collaterals may be performed from the shunt using sclerosant, Gelfoam pledgets, or absolute alcohol in a stepwise fashion until repeat venography demonstrates full varix opacification. Last, the microcatheter may be advanced beyond the collateral and repeat venography performed. If this is able to fully opacify the varix without evidence of leaking collateral, the sclerosant may be administered from this location.[34]

Type C varices are contiguous with both gastrocaval and a gastrorenal shunt. If one of the shunts is small in size and can be catheterized using a microcatheter, the shunt may be coil embolized before sclerosant infusion through the remaining shunt. If the gastrocaval shunt is large enough to be catheterized with an occlusion balloon, then a second occlusion balloon may be advanced via a second access site (e.g., internal jugular). Repeat venography will then show full varix opacification and administration of the sclerosant can be performed (Fig. 32.9).[34]

Treatment Modification Based on Afferent Vein Anatomy

Gastric varices may also be categorized based on afferent vein anatomy (Fig. 32.10). Type 1 are supplied by a single afferent gastric vein and is most commonly the left or posterior gastric vein. As the outflow vein(s) are appropriately occluded, the sclerosant will reflux into the gastric variceal complex and stagnate secondary to the high pressure from the portal venous circulation. This allows slow minimal reflux into the afferent vein, signaling the critical end point of embolization. Any additional forceful injection can overcome the portal pressures and cause further reflux into the portal system.

Gastric varices are more frequently supplied by multiple afferent gastric veins.[34] In type 2, there are two separate afferent veins (left and posterior gastric veins). When the draining vein or veins are appropriately occluded, the sclerosant will stagnate in the gastric varices and minimally reflux into one or both afferent veins. However, the pressure in one of the afferent veins is commonly lower than in the other afferent vein. Reflux will be noted in the lower pressure vein, signaling the end point of embolization, and the procedure

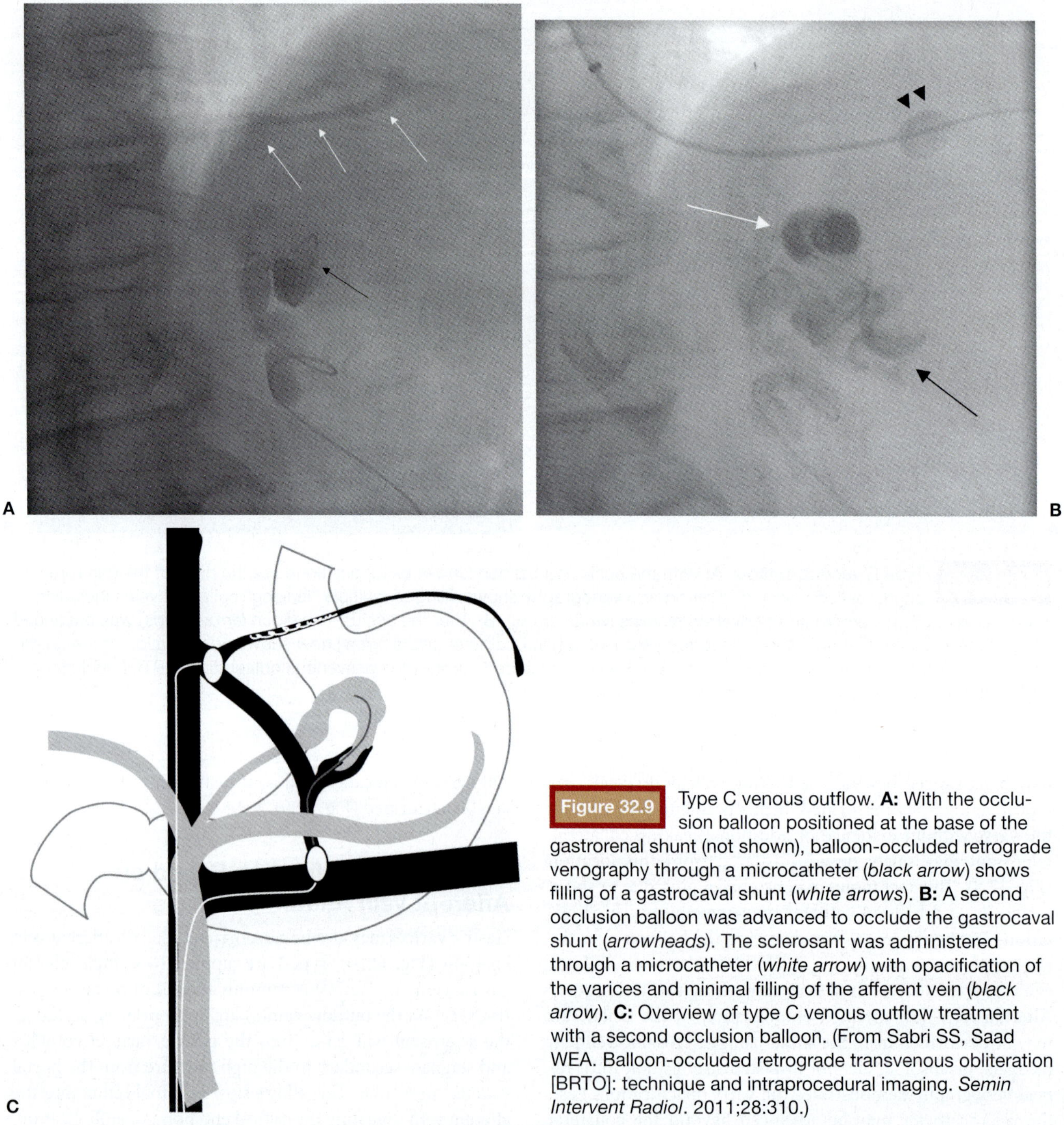

Figure 32.9 Type C venous outflow. **A:** With the occlusion balloon positioned at the base of the gastrorenal shunt (not shown), balloon-occluded retrograde venography through a microcatheter (*black arrow*) shows filling of a gastrocaval shunt (*white arrows*). **B:** A second occlusion balloon was advanced to occlude the gastrocaval shunt (*arrowheads*). The sclerosant was administered through a microcatheter (*white arrow*) with opacification of the varices and minimal filling of the afferent vein (*black arrow*). **C:** Overview of type C venous outflow treatment with a second occlusion balloon. (From Sabri SS, Saad WEA. Balloon-occluded retrograde transvenous obliteration [BRTO]: technique and intraprocedural imaging. *Semin Intervent Radiol*. 2011;28:310.)

is typically completed at that point. This will typically result in only partial obliteration of the varices because the other, higher pressure afferent vein will remain patent and supply a portion of the gastric varices, resulting in the necessity of a second BRTO procedure.[34] Preprocedure imaging may or may not identify both afferent veins and, unless both veins have similar pressures so that reflux into both veins is documented on balloon-occluded venography, the typical result is partial obliteration. Given the complication associated with excessive administration of sclerosant and untoward reflux into the portal venous system, it is appropriate to stage the procedure and plan on a repeat BRTO after several weeks to allow the sclerosed afferent vein to thrombose and allow for embolization of the higher pressure afferent vein at the second session.

Type 3 gastric varices have a separate afferent vein that drains directly into the shunt and does not communicate to the gastric varices. During BRTO, this will cause a challenge

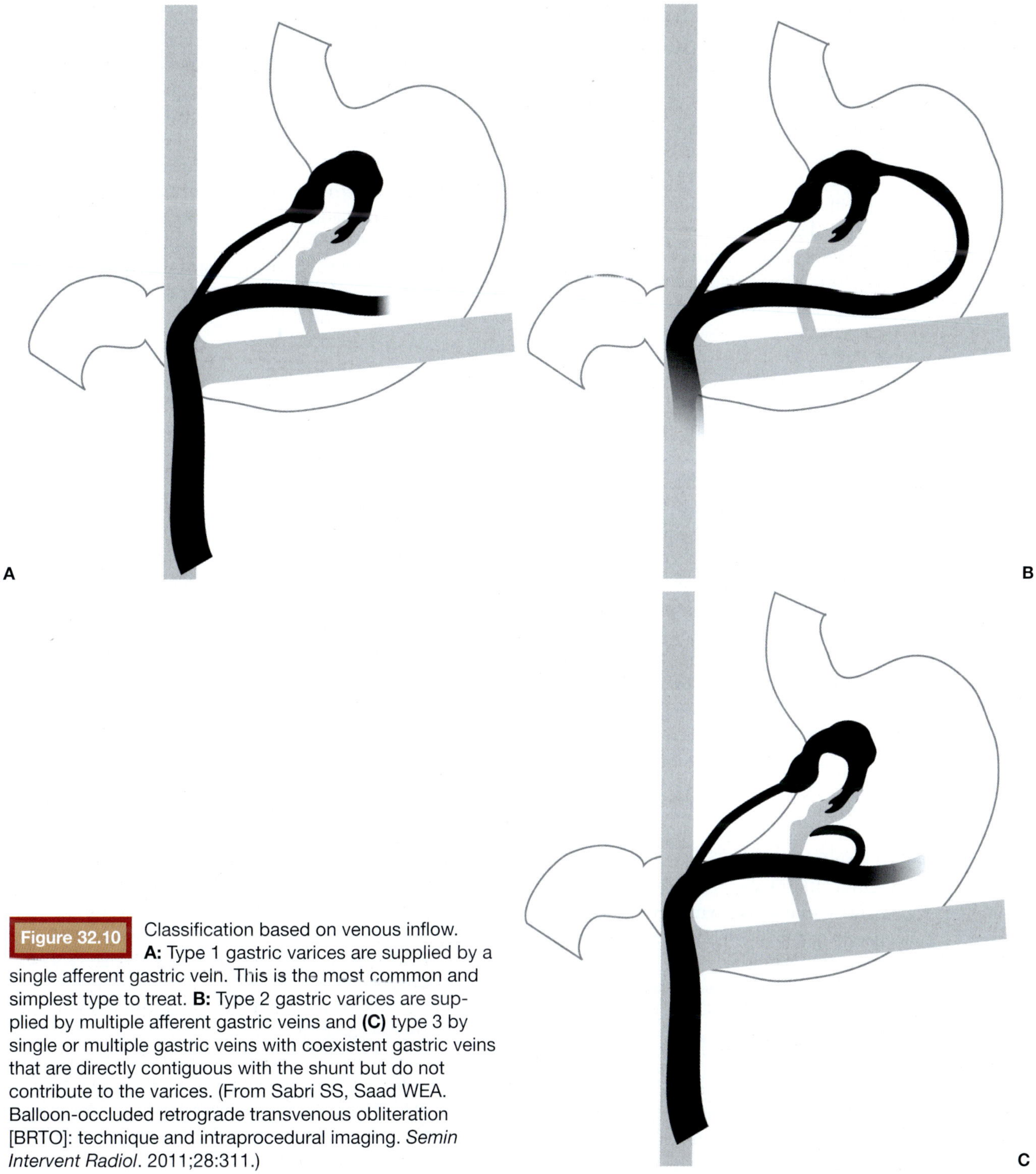

Figure 32.10 Classification based on venous inflow. **A:** Type 1 gastric varices are supplied by a single afferent gastric vein. This is the most common and simplest type to treat. **B:** Type 2 gastric varices are supplied by multiple afferent gastric veins and **(C)** type 3 by single or multiple gastric veins with coexistent gastric veins that are directly contiguous with the shunt but do not contribute to the varices. (From Sabri SS, Saad WEA. Balloon-occluded retrograde transvenous obliteration [BRTO]: technique and intraprocedural imaging. *Semin Intervent Radiol*. 2011;28:311.)

as sclerosant will typically flow into this separate afferent vein rather than the gastric varices and will cause reflux into the portal venous system.[34] It is essential to advance a microcatheter deeply into the gastric varices for a planning venogram to document the ability to achieve stagnation within the varices and reflux into the afferent veins feeding the gastric varices. If this cannot be achieved through the microcatheter, then the separate afferent vein must be embolized by a percutaneous transhepatic or transjugular route to eliminate it from the circuit.

Transjugular Intrahepatic Portosystemic Shunt and Portal Venous Modulators

In the United States, TIPS placement is still more frequently performed for bleeding gastric varices. Although TIPS has been reported as effective in the treatment of bleeding gastric varices, it has higher rates of encephalopathy when compared with endoscopic therapy and BRTO.[11,35,36] Further, large gastric varices will frequently continue at lower portal pressures because of the decompressive effect on the portal venous system. In addition, gastric varices are more likely to bleed at lower pressures when compared with esophageal varices.[11,13,37] Despite having a functioning TIPS, patients may still have recurrence of gastric variceal bleeding and require alternative treatments such as BRTO.[13] Many clinical and anatomic factors must be considered when deciding on treatment of bleeding gastric varices. As such, Saad and Darcy[3] have argued for combining BRTO and TIPS for patients with baseline substantial ascites or hydrothorax or uncontrolled esophageal varices who have reasonable hepatic reserve (Model for End-Stage Liver Disease [MELD] score <19). Alternatively, other portal venous modulators such as splenic artery embolization have been found to offset the increasing portal venous pressures after BRTO by the reduced development and bleeding rate of esophageal varices.[10] This has been substantiated by a recent study demonstrating superior results for combining BRTO with TIPS compared to BRTO only.[38] Rebleeding at 6, 12, and 24 months after the procedure(s) for BRTO and TIPS versus BRTO only was 0%, 0%, and 0% compared to 9%, 9%, and 21%, respectively.[38]

POTENTIAL COMPLICATIONS

Most described complications are often transient and self-limited. When compared with endoscopic *N*-butyl cyanoacrylate glue injection, BRTO shows similar incidence of complications.[39] Epigastric and back pain, fever, and hematuria are most common and found in large percentage of patients.[4,40–45] Less commonly, nausea, elevated blood pressure, and changes in laboratory values may be present.[42,45]

There are varying degrees and rates of new or worsened ascites and hydrothorax. Given the resultant elevated portal pressures following a BRTO, this is not unexpected, and some studies show ascites to increase in 44% of patients and worsened hydrothorax in 72% of patients.[45] Most of these patients frequently return to baseline a few months after the procedure.[46] The incidence of ascites after BRTO at 6, 12, and 24 months after BRTO is 43%, 57%, and 71%, respectively.[38] Portal vein and renal vein thrombosis may be found in a small number of patients but is typically clinically silent.[13,45] Pulmonary embolism has been a reported complication and can be symptomatic. However, the embolus has not been described as containing high-density material to suggest an origin from treated gastric varices.[13,45,47] Although rare, potentially life-threatening complications include ventricular fibrillation, pulmonary edema, and anaphylaxis to EO.[13,19,45,47] Careful respiratory monitoring is warranted as changes in pulmonary function parameters after BRTO may not be accompanied by clinical symptoms.[48] Although not frequently reported as a complication, balloon rupture can occur and may result in antegrade transit of sclerosant into the systemic vasculature.[49] Last, the use of foam sclerosant prepared with room air has been associated with air embolism to the lungs or the systemic arterial circulation in the presence of a patent foramen ovale.[21,22] This has not been reported with transcatheter variceal obliteration but has been associated with lower extremity vein sclerotherapy. The rate of this complication may theoretically be reduced by the use of CO_2 rather than room air.[50,51]

TIPS AND TRICKS

- Careful evaluation of preprocedural CECT or MRI is very important for preprocedural evaluation and planning. Coronal reformats are the most important and most informative.
- CECT or MRI usually overlook, if not underestimate, vascular weblike narrowings in the GRS, thus estimates of required balloon sizes before the procedure maybe serendipitously overestimated.
- Foam sclerosant (sclerosant is a foam state by mixing the sclerosant with air or CO_2) reduces the sclerosant dose-to-volume ratio and is probably safer from a systemic toxicity standpoint.
- The objectives of balloon-occluded retrograde venography are to (1) identify decompressive collaterals (potential escape routes for sclerosant), (2) familiarize the operator with shunt and variceal anatomy, and (3) familiarize the operator with the portal venous feeders.
- The technical end point of the BRTO procedure is to fill the entire gastric variceal system with sclerosant and partly fill/visualize the portal venous feeders.
- If you cannot pass a microcatheter coaxially through the balloon occlusion catheter, the microcatheter can be passed adjacent to the compliant balloon occlusion catheter.
- The ideal feature of a balloon occlusion catheter for BRTO is one that does not have the catheter tip extend beyond the compliant balloon. Moreover, a catheter that invaginates within the balloon is better.
- The negative aspect of the BRTO procedure is that the spontaneous GRS is obliterated as well as the gastric varices.
- The obliteration of the spontaneous GRS (a portosystemic shunt) potentially diverts portal blood flow (which commonly escapes portosystemically) back into the portal circulation, commonly increasing portal flow to the liver and increasing portal pressure.

- Increased portal pressure after BRTO is associated with negative hemodynamic effects such as worsening ascites, esophageal variceal bleeding, and splenomegaly.
- Increased hepatopetal portal blood flow after BRTO is associated with positive hemodynamic effects such as reduction in hepatic encephalopathy and improved synthetic function.

OUTCOMES

Technical success as defined by successful filling of gastric varices with sclerosant is reported to occur in 77% to 100% of patients.[52] Complete obliteration of the gastric varices is reported to occur in 82% to 100% of patients. Although some studies required repeat BRTO to achieve such high percentages, large volumes of sclerosants are often required.[4,7,11,53] Short and midterm follow-up periods are typically reported in the literature, and reported rebleeding rates are as high as 15%.[39] However, most studies report bleeding rates below 5%.[46] Long-term rebleeding from gastric varices at 12 and 24 months after BRTO were 0%.[38] When compared with endoscopic *N*-butyl cyanoacrylate injection in a recent prospective study, BRTO demonstrated a significantly higher probability of bleeding-free survival.[39] Further, this study showed increased survival rates in patients with transcatheter therapy or rescue transcatheter therapy after failed endoscopic therapy versus endoscopic therapy alone in the acute phase. Additionally, transcatheter obliteration frequently requires fewer treatment sessions, has higher eradication rates, and is associated with shorter hospital stays when compared with endoscopic sclerotherapy.

Given that the purpose of BRTO is to embolize a decompressive shunt, it is not unexpected that 10% to 68% of patients experience worsening esophageal varices. This is more likely to occur when the esophageal varices are present before the BRTO.[47,54] These are most often successfully treated endoscopically.[45] Further, although shunt embolization may cause an increase in portal pressures and worsening of esophageal varices, it may also cause redirection of portal blood flow toward the liver and result in clinical improvement. Resolution or marked decrease in degree of encephalopathy has been reported.[4,53] In addition, significant decreases in serum ammonia,[40,53] improved serum albumin,[41,55] resolution of ascites,[4] and improved hepatic reserved was reflected by improved Child-Pugh and/or MELD scores.[4,40,56]

FUTURE DIRECTIONS

The ideal management of a patient with bleeding gastric varices heavily depends on many factors such as patient anatomy, hemodynamic stability, and institutional availability. Furthermore, although BRTO will remain an effective treatment technique in this patient population, the combination of BRTO with portal venous modulating procedures (i.e., TIPS and splenic artery embolization) may be required in a select group of patients.[3,8,10] Determining defined parameters for both the clinical and imaging presentation of this patient population is an area of ongoing research. Additional research is being performed on the application of this technique to nontraditional varices such as small bowel varices,[57–59] spontaneous mesenteric portosystemic shunts,[54,60] and parastomal varices.[61] BRTO from unconventional venous routes is also being performed in greater numbers.[62–65] Combined techniques are also being evaluated. For example, a technique has been described that combines endoscopic and percutaneous approaches for balloon-occluded endoscopic injection sclerotherapy.[65] This method allows gastric variceal obliteration in patients without large draining veins.

CONCLUSIONS

BRTO is a well-established technique for treating gastric varices. Although the technique was popularized in Asia, it has been slow to be adopted in Western countries. However, the technique is rapidly being incorporated into the management of cirrhotic patients with bleeding gastric varices. Further investigation and research is needed to determine defined clinical and imaging parameters for patients presenting with bleeding gastric varices. In addition, more research into the combination of variceal obliteration with portal vein modulating treatments is needed. Although BRTO may cause aggravation of esophageal varices or exacerbation of transudative complications, the clinical weight of these consequences is yet to be determined. Despite these unknowns, BRTO has become and will remain a key component in the management of patients with bleeding gastric varices.

REFERENCES

1. Al-Osaimi AMS, Caldwell SH. Medical and endoscopic management of gastric varices. *Semin Intervent Radiol.* 2011;28: 273–282.
2. Al-Osaimi AMS, Sabri SS, Caldwell SH. Balloon-occluded retrograde transvenous obliteration (BRTO): preprocedural evaluation and imaging. *Semin Intervent Radiol.* 2011;28:288–295.
3. Saad WEA, Darcy MD. Transjugular intrahepatic portosystemic shunt (TIPS) versus balloon-occluded retrograde transvenous obliteration (BRTO) for the management of gastric varices. *Semin Intervent Radiol.* 2011;28:339–349.
4. Fukuda T, Shozo H, Sugimura K. Long-term results of balloon-occluded retrograde transvenous obliteration for the treatment of gastric varices and hepatic encephalopathy. *J Vasc Interv Radiol.* 2001;12:327–336.
5. Kiyosue H, Mori H, Matsumoto S, et al. Transcatheter obliteration of gastric varices: part 2. Strategy and techniques based on hemodynamic features. *Radiographics.* 2003;23:921–937.
6. Ibukuro K, Sugihara T, Tanaka R, et al. Balloon-occluded retrograde transvenous obliteration (BRTO) for a direct shunt

between the inferior mesenteric vein and the inferior vena cava in a patient with hepatic encephalopathy. *J Vasc Interv Radiol.* 2007;18:121–125.

7. Ninoi T, Nishida N, Kaminou T, et al. Balloon-occluded retrograde transvenous obliteration of gastric varices with gastrorenal shunt: long-term follow-up in 78 patients. *AJR Am J Roentgenol.* 2005;184:1340–1346.
8. Saad WE. The history and evolution of balloon-occluded retrograde transvenous obliteration (BRTO): from the United States to Japan and back. *Semin Intervent Radiol.* 2011;28:283–287.
9. Roossle M, Siegerstetter V, Olschewski M, et al. How much reduction in portal pressure is necessary to prevent variceal rebleeding? A longitudinal study in 225 patients with transjugular intrahepatic portosystemic shunts. *Am J Gastroenterol.* 2001; 96:3379–3383.
10. Ryan BM, Stockbrugger RW, Ryan JM. A pathophysiologic, gastroenterologic, and radiologic approach to the management of gastric varices. *Gastroenterology.* 2004;126:1175–1189.
11. Tripathi D, Therapondos G, Jackson E, et al. The role of the transjugular intrahepatic portosystemic stent shunt (TIPSS) in the management of bleeding gastric varices: clinical and haemodynamic correlations. *Gut.* 2002;51:270–274.
12. Kiyosue H, Mori H, Matsumoto S, et al. Transcatheter obliteration of gastric varices. Part 1. Anatomic classification. *Radiographics.* 2003;23:911–920.
13. Sabri SS, Swee W, Turba UC, et al. Bleeding gastric varices obliteration with balloon-occluded retrograde transvenous obliteration using sodium tetradecyl sulfate foam. *J Vasc Interv Radiol.* 2011;22:309–316.
14. Demagny A. Comparative study into the efficacy of a sclerosant product in the form of liquid or foam in echo- guided of arches of the long and short saphenous veins. *Phlebology.* 2002;55: 133–137.
15. Coleridge Smith P. Sclerotherapy and foam sclerotherapy for varicose veins. *Phlebology.* 2009;24:260–269.
16. Gandini R, Chiocchi M, Konda D, et al. Transcatheter foam sclerotherapy of symptomatic female varicocele with sodium-tetradecyl-sulfate foam. *Cardiovasc Intervent Radiol.* 2008;31: 778–784.
17. Gandini R, Konda D, Reale CA, et al. Male varicocele: transcatheter foam sclerotherapy with sodium tetradecyl sulfate—outcome in 244 patients. *Radiology.* 2008;246:612–618.
18. Tan KT, Kirby J, Rajan DK, et al. Percutaneous sodium tetradecyl sulfate sclerotherapy for peripheral venous vascular malformations: a single-center experience. *J Vasc Interv Radiol.* 2007;18:343–351.
19. Yamaki T, Nozaki M, Sakurai H, et al. Prospective randomized efficacy of ultrasound-guided foam sclerotherapy compared with ultrasound-guided liquid sclerotherapy in the treatment of symptomatic venous malformations. *J Vasc Surg.* 2008;47: 578–584.
20. Orsini C, Brotto M. Immediate pathologic effects on the vein wall of foam sclerotherapy. *Dermatol Surg.* 2007;33:1250–1254.
21. Ceulen RP, Sommer A, Vernooy K. Microembolism during foam sclerotherapy of varicose veins. *N Engl J Med.* 2008;358: 1525–1526.
22. Forlee MV, Grouden M, Moore DJ, et al. Stroke after varicose vein foam injection sclerotherapy. *J Vasc Surg.* 2006;43: 162–164.
23. Saad WE, Nicholson D, Koizumi J. Inventory used for balloon-occluded retrograde (BRTO) and antegrade (BATO) transvenous obliteration: sclerosants and balloon occlusion devices. *Tech Vasc Interv Radiol.* 2012;15:226–240.
24. Saad WE, Kitanosono T, Koizumi J, et al. The conventional balloon-occluded retrograde transvenous obliteration procedure: indications, contraindications, and technical applications. *Tech Vasc Interv Radiol.* 2013;16:101–151.
25. Saad WE, Simon PO Jr, Rose SC. Balloon-occluded retrograde transvenous obliteration of gastric varices. *Cardiovasc Intervent Radiol.* 2014;37:299–315.
26. Saad WE. Vascular anatomy and the morphologic and hemodynamic classifications of gastric varices and spontaneous portosystemic shunts relevant to the BRTO procedure. *Tech Vasc Interv Radiol.* 2013;16:60–100.
27. Saad WEA, Al-Osaimi AM, Caldwell S, et al. *ACR Appropriateness Criteria®: Radiologic Management of Gastric Varices.* Reston, VA: American College of Radiology; 2012.
28. Sarin SK. Long-term follow-up of gastric variceal sclerotherapy: an eleven-year experience. *Gastrointest Endosc.* 1997;46:8–14.
29. Jutabha R, Jensen DM, Kovacs TO, et al. Initial results of a prospective study of combination banding & sclerotherapy compared to sclerotherapy alone for bleeding gastric varices. *Gastrointest Endosc.* 1998;47:AB86
30. Lo GH, Lai KH, Cheng JS, et al. A prospective, randomized trial of butyl cyanoacrylate injection versus band ligation in the management of bleeding gastric varices. *Hepatology.* 2001;33: 1060–1064.
31. Tan PC, Hou MC, Lin HC, et al. A randomized trial of endoscopic treatment of acute gastric variceal hemorrhage: N-Butyl-2-Cyanoacrylate injection versus band ligation. *Hepatology.* 2006;43:690–697
32. Saad WE, Al-Osaimi A, Caldwell SH. Pre- and post-balloon-occluded retrograde transvenous obliteration clinical evaluation, management, and imaging: indications, management protocols, and follow-up. *Tech Vasc Interv Radiol.* 2012;15:165–202.
33. Saad WE, Lippert A, Saad NE, et al. Ectopic varices: anatomical classification, hemodynamic classification, and hemodynamic-based management. *Tech Vasc Interv Radiol.* 2013;16:158–175.
34. Sabri SS, Saad WEA. Balloon-occluded retrograde transvenous obliteration (BRTO): technique and intraprocedural imaging. *Semin Intervent Radiol.* 2011;28:303–313.
35. Khan S, Tudur Smith C, Williamson P, et al. Portosystemic shunts versus endoscopic therapy for variceal rebleeding in patients with cirrhosis. *Cochrane Database Syst Rev.* 2006;(4): CD000553.
36. Azoulay D, Castaing D, Majno P, et al. Salvage transjugular intrahepatic portosystemic shunt for uncontrolled variceal bleeding in patients with decompensated cirrhosis. *J Hepatol.* 2001;35:590–597.
37. Watanabe K, Kimura K, Matsutani S, et al. Portal hemodynamics in patients with gastric varices: a study in 230 patients with esophageal and/or gastric varices using portal vein catheterization. *Gastroenterology.* 1988;95:434–440.
38. Saad WE, Wagner CC, Lippert A, et al. Protective value of TIPS against the development of hydrothorax/ascites and upper gastrointestinal bleeding after balloon-occluded retrograde transvenous obliteration (BRTO). *Am J Gastroenterol.* 2013;108: 1612–1619.

39. Hong CH, Kim HJ, Park JH, et al. Treatment of patients with gastric variceal hemorrhage: endoscopic N-butyl-2-cyanoacrylate injection versus balloon-occluded retrograde transvenous obliteration. *J Gastroenterol Hepatol.* 2009;24:372–378.
40. Takuma Y, Nouso K, Makino Y, et al. Prophylactic balloon-occluded retrograde transvenous obliteration for gastric varices in compensated cirrhosis. *Clin Gastroenterol Hepatol.* 2005;3:1245–1252.
41. Hiraga N, Aikata H, Takaki S, et al. The long-term outcome of patients with bleeding gastric varices after balloon-occluded retrograde transvenous obliteration. *J Gastroenterol.* 2007;42:663–672.
42. Arai H, Abe T, Shimoda R, et al. Emergency balloon-occluded retrograde transvenous obliteration for gastric varices. *J Gastroenterol.* 2005;40:964–971.
43. Cho SK, Shin SW, Lee IH, et al. Balloon-occluded retrograde transvenous obliteration of gastric varices: outcomes and complications in 49 patients. *AJR Am J Roentgenol.* 2007;189:1523.
44. Kitamoto M, Imamura M, Kamada K, et al. Balloon-occluded retrograde transvenous obliteration of gastric fundal varices with hemorrhage. *AJR Am J Roentgenol.* 2002;178:1167–1174.
45. Sonomura T, Sato M, Kishi K, et al. Balloon-occluded retrograde transvenous obliteration for gastric varices: a feasibility study. *Cardiovasc Intervent Radiol.* 1998;21:27–30.
46. Kanagawa H, Mima S, Kouyama H, et al. Treatment of gastric fundal varices by balloon-occluded retrograde transvenous obliteration. *J Gastroenterol Hepatol.* 1996;11:51–58.
47. Akahoshi T, Hashizume M, Tomikawa M, et al. Long-term results of balloon-occluded retrograde transvenous obliteration for gastric variceal bleeding and risky gastric varices: a 10-year experience. *J Gastroenterol Hepatol.* 2008;23:1702–1709.
48. Arai H, Abe T, Takayama H, et al. Respiratory effects of balloon occluded retrograde transvenous obliteration of gastric varices: a prospective controlled study. *J Gastroenterol Hepatol.* 2011;26:1389–1394.
49. Park SJ, Chung JW, Kim HC, et al. The prevalence, risk factors, and clinical outcome of balloon rupture in balloon-occluded retrograde transvenous obliteration of gastric varices. *J Vasc Interv Radiol.* 2010;21:503–507.
50. Morrison N, Neuhardt DL, Rogers CR, et al. Comparisons of side effects using air and carbon dioxide foam for endovenous chemical ablation. *J Vasc Surg.* 2008;47:830–836.
51. Peterson JD, Goldman MP. An investigation into the influence of various gases and concentrations of sclerosants on foam stability. *Dermatol Surg.* 2011;37:12–17.
52. Patel A, Fischman AM, Saad WE. Balloon-occluded retrograde transvenous obliteration of gastric varices. *AJR Am J Roentgenol.* 2012;199(4):721–729.
53. Hirota S, Matsumoto S, Tomita M, et al. Retrograde transvenous obliteration of gastric varices. *Radiology.* 1999;211:349–356.
54. Minamiguchi H, Kawai N, Sato M, et al. Balloon occlusion retrograde transvenous obliteration for inferior mesenteric vein-systemic shunt. *J Vasc Interv Radiol.* 2011;22:1039–1044.
55. Hirota S, Kobayashi K, Maeda H, et al. Balloon-occluded retrograde transvenous obliteration for portal hypertension. *Radiat Med.* 2006;24:315–320.
56. Saad WE, Wagner CC, Al-Osaimi A, et al. The effect of balloon-occluded transvenous obliteration of gastric varices and gastrorenal shunts on the hepatic synthetic function: a comparison between Child-Pugh and model for end-stage liver disease scores. *Vasc Endovascular Surg.* 2013;47:281–287.
57. Tsurusaki M, Sugimoto K, Matsumoto S, et al. Bleeding duodenal varices successfully treated with balloon-occluded retrograde transvenous obliteration (B-RTO) assisted by CT during arterial portography. *Cardiovasc Intervent Radiol.* 2006;29:1148–1151.
58. Zamora CA, Sugimoto K, Tsurusaki M, et al. Endovascular obliteration of bleeding duodenal varices in patients with liver cirrhosis. *Eur Radiol.* 2006;16:73–79.
59. Hashimoto N, Akahoshi T, Yoshida D, et al. The efficacy of balloon-occluded retrograde transvenous obliteration on small intestinal variceal bleeding. *Surgery.* 2010;148:145–150.
60. Hayashi S, Baba Y, Senokuchi T, et al. Successful portal-systemic shunt occlusion of a direct shunt between the inferior mesenteric vein and inferior vena cava with balloon-occluded retrograde transvenous obliteration following recanalization after placing a covered stent in the portal and superior mesenteric veins. *Jpn J Radiol.* 2009;27:180–184.
61. Minami S, Okada K, Matsuo M, et al. Treatment of bleeding stomal varices by balloon-occluded retrograde transvenous obliteration. *J Gastroenterol.* 2007;42:91–95.
62. Araki T, Hori M, Motosugi U, et al. Can balloon-occluded retrograde transvenous obliteration be performed for gastric varices without gastrorenal shunts? *J Vasc Interv Radiol.* 2010;21:663–670.
63. Kageyama K, Nishida N, Matsui H, et al. Successful balloon-occluded retrograde transvenous obliteration for gastric varix mainly draining into the pericardiophrenic vein. *Cardiovasc Intervent Radiol.* 2012;35:180–183.
64. Minamiguchi H, Kawai N, Sato M, et al. Balloon-occluded retrograde transvenous obliteration for gastric varices via the intercostal vein. *World J Radiol.* 2012;28:121–125.
65. Shiba M, Higuchi K, Nakamura K, et al. Efficacy and safety of balloon-occluded endoscopic injection sclerotherapy as a prophylactic treatment for high-risk gastric fundal varices: a prospective, randomized, comparative clinical trial. *Gastrointest Endosc.* 2002;56:522–528.

33

Transcatheter Arterial Embolization of Benign Liver Disease

Chang Jin Yoon • Jae Hyung Park

Transcatheter arterial embolization (TAE) has been commonly used in treatment of malignant liver tumors. Although rare, however, it can be indicated in various benign liver diseases including benign liver tumors, iatrogenic vascular injury, polycystic liver disease, and congenital vascular lesions.

Owing to the widespread use of imaging analyses, either routinely or to evaluate symptomatic patients, benign liver tumors are diagnosed with increasing frequency.[1] Most benign liver tumors are incidentally discovered in otherwise healthy individuals. However, some of them are associated with serious complications, which require prompt treatments. Surgical resection has been considered a standard treatment for large or symptomatic lesions. TAE has been used as an alternative treatment for patients who cannot undergo surgery due to poor clinical conditions. It is also indicated to achieve hemostasis in cases of tumor rupture or as a preoperative procedure before surgical resection.[2–6]

TAE also plays an essential role in treatment of focal vascular abnormality of the liver. They are most commonly caused by iatrogenic injury following radiologic or surgical liver interventions.[7–9] Recently, as percutaneous transhepatic procedures are more frequently carried out, such vascular lesions are becoming more prevalent. Common vascular lesions include arterial pseudoaneurysm, arterioportal fistula, and arteriobiliary fistula. Small lesions are asymptomatic and may not need any specific treatment. However, a large aneurysm or fistulas with large amount of blood flows can lead to hemobilia, gastrointestinal bleeding, and portal hypertension. Congenital portosystemic shunt or vascular malformations are rare but can be associated with serious and potentially fatal complications.[10] In the past, most symptomatic vascular lesions required surgical treatment, but TAE has currently emerged as a valuable minimally invasive treatment option.[11]

TECHNIQUES AND EMBOLIC MATERIALS

Angiographic access is gained on either a femoral or a left axillary artery using Seldinger technique. Visceral arteriography is performed using a preshaped 4-Fr or 5-Fr angiographic catheter. In the liver, arterial anatomic variations are common. Selective examination of the celiac and superior mesenteric arteries is often necessary. Common variants include the left hepatic artery arising from the left gastric artery and the right hepatic artery replaced to the superior mesenteric artery. It is important to scrutinize the arteriogram for defects in hepatic parenchymal enhancement, which might alert one to the presence of anatomic variants or accessory vessels. Two or more projection hepatic angiograms including the portal venous phase may be required to identify the location of lesion and feeding vessels identified. The vessels to be embolized are catheterized as selectively as possible with use of a 2-Fr or 3-Fr microcatheter.

The liver is well suited to TAE because of its dual blood supply. Arterial embolization is unlikely to result in tissue infarction unless there is concomitant injury to the portal venous system. To minimize normal hepatic parenchyma, it is preferable to place the embolic agent as close to the target lesions as possible. The major considerations for selecting an embolic agent are lesion type and location, individual vascular anatomy, reliability of delivery, and preservation of normal tissue. For benign liver tumors, particulate embolic agents such as polyvinyl alcohol (PVA) and gelatin sponge particles have been frequently employed.[12] However, PVA particles are known to clump, resulting in more proximal vessel occlusion. Recently, calibrated microspheres (trisacryl gelatin microspheres) are used to achieve distal vessel blockade, leading to ischemic tumor necrosis.[13] For embolization of hepatic vascular injury such as arterioportal/arteriobiliary fistulas and pseudoaneurysms, microcoils, gelatin sponge pledgets, and *N*-butyl cyanoacylate (NBCA) are typically used either alone or in combination.[7–9] Coils are ideal for precise single-vessel occlusion. They provide controlled delivery with rapid occlusion and are available in various sizes. When using coils, they should be tightly packed without interstices to avoid late recanalization and coil migration. When treating arterial pseudoaneurysm, coils should not be placed inside the aneurysmal sac because there is risk of late rupture. The proximal and distal vessels to the pseudoaneurysm should be embolized so that revascularization by backflow may not occur (sandwich technique). Recently, NBCA has been gaining interest as a useful embolic material for TAE. It occludes target vessels rapidly and completely, which results in more reliable embolization and may reduce fluoroscopic and procedure time. By adjusting the ratio of NBCA and iodized oil, polymerization time and, accordingly, the level of embolization within target vessels can be controlled. This unique character of NBCA is especially useful when a microcatheter is not able to be advanced to desirable intravascular position due to tortuous vascular anatomy or arterial stenosis. In spite of these advantages, the use of liquid embolic agents including NBCA has been limited in TAE because of the concern that they carry a high risk for severe complications such as tissue necrosis and nontarget embolization secondary to uncontrolled reflux.[14] In embolization of a large, high-flow arteriovenous shunt, a more durable embolic device with large diameter such as Amplatzer Vascular Plug (St. Jude Medical, Inc., St. Paul, Minnesota) may be required to prevent migration.

CLINICAL APPLICATIONS

Benign Liver Tumors

Hepatocellular Adenoma

Hepatocellular adenoma (HA) is a rare hepatic tumor that is strongly associated with use of oral contraceptives or anabolic steroids and glycogen storage disease.[15] Unlike other benign liver tumors, approximately 80% of patients with HA have clinical symptoms; of these, half present with acute-onset abdominal pain due to hemorrhage and half present with symptoms related to mass effect. Only 20% of HAs are found as incidental findings.[16] Malignant transformation of HA is rare and associated with β-catenin mutations that are also found in hepatocellular carcinoma.[17] There are controversies with regard to the optimal treatment for HA because the potential for hemorrhage or malignant transformation of tumor is difficult to estimate. The patients with lesions smaller than 5 cm and normal α-fetoprotein levels are typically treated conservatively. Discontinuation of oral contraceptives may lead to regression of the tumor.[18] Patients with lesions larger than 5 cm should be considered for surgical resection because lesion size is an important indicator of potentials for hemorrhage or progression to hepatocellular carcinoma.[19] However, surgery carries an increased risk of postoperative morbidity and a longer recovery time and may not be practical in patients with multiple bilateral HAs.[20]

TAE, on the contrary, is minimally invasive. It can be applied to multiple and bilateral tumors. It can safely be repeated and is effective in decreasing the lesion size (Fig. 33.1). The data from literatures on embolization of HAs are summarized in Table 33.1. Currently, TAE is commonly indicated in patients presenting with acute hemorrhage from HAs. In several studies, TAE has been successfully performed to obtain adequate hemostasis without the need for urgent laparotomy.[5,21,22] Stoot et al.[21] treated 11 patients with ruptured HAs. Ten of the patients were stabilized after a single TAE, whereas one other patient needed three TAE sessions. No emergency resections were needed and only minor complications were found. In all patients, tumor size decreased after follow-up, with secondary resection being indicated only in a minority of patients. Because an emergency surgical resection inevitably involves considerable morbidity and mortality, TAE is proposed as the first treatment in hemodynamically unstable patients with ruptured HAs. In addition to the emergency indication, several reports have focused on the elective use of TAE for HAs larger than 5 cm with the aim of reducing the tumor mass by complete cessation of the arterial blood flow.[13,23,24] Kim et al.[23] performed TAE in 7 patients with large HAs and achieved tumor regression more than 50% in 6 patients. Complete resolution of the tumor was seen in 2 patients. No serious complication was reported except self-limiting postembolization syndrome. In past several years, TAE has been increasingly used in patients with unruptured HAs.[25] A randomized controlled study comparing surgical resection versus selective TAE is now going on.[26]

Focal Nodular Hyperplasia

Focal nodular hyperplasia (FNH) is the second most common benign liver tumor next to hemangioma and usually affects women of childbearing or middle age.[27] It is more often a solitary subcapsular lesion measuring less than 5 cm in size.

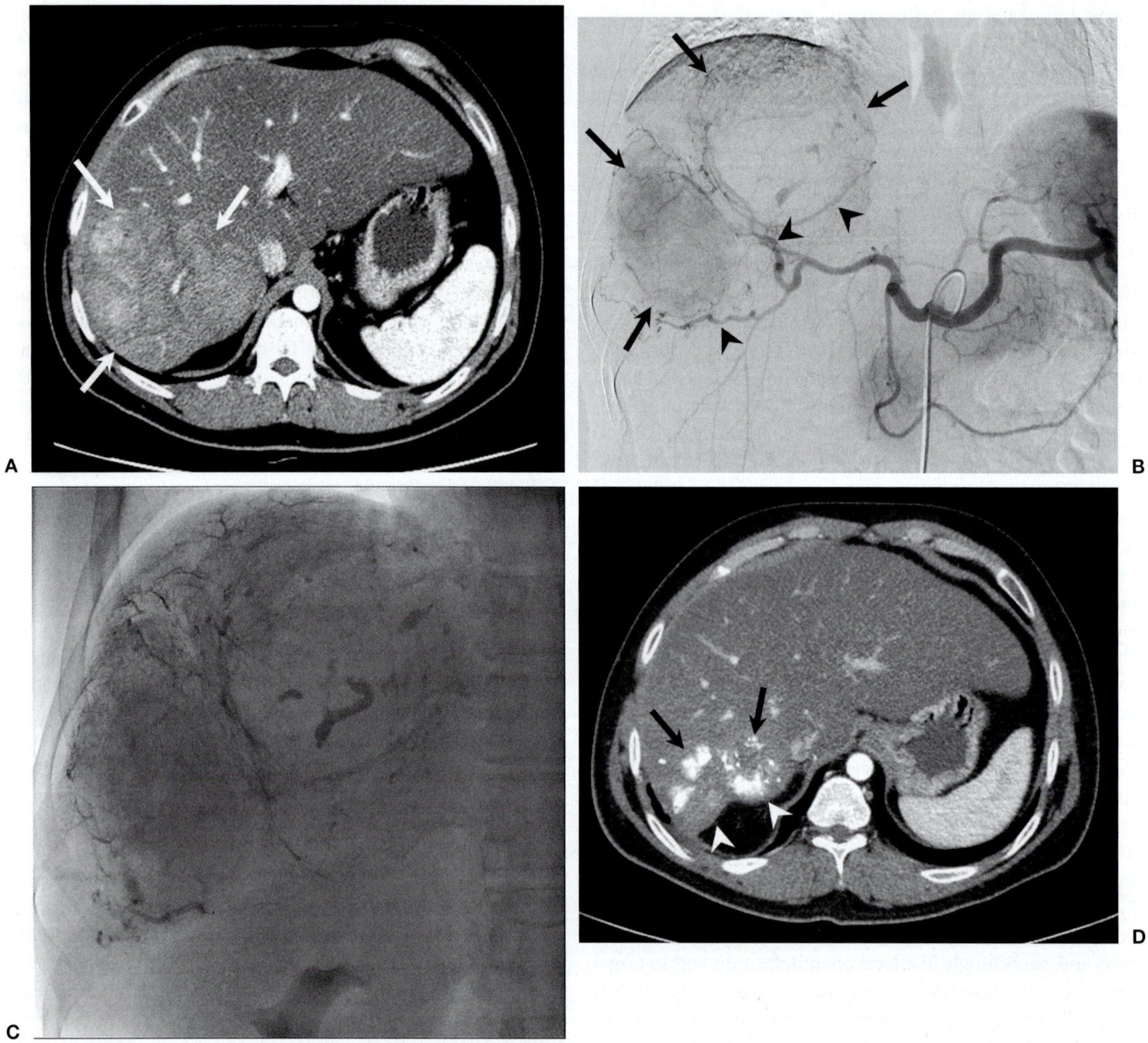

Figure 33.1 A 29-year-old patient with HA associated with glycogen storage disease. The patient underwent embolization for abdominal pain and increasing size of the liver tumor. **A:** An enhanced liver computed tomography (CT) obtained before embolization shows heterogeneously enhanced liver tumor in right posterior section (*arrows*). **B:** Celiac angiogram shows hypervascular tumor (*arrows*) with engorged tumor-feeding hepatic arteries (*arrowheads*). Embolization was performed with doxorubicin-iodized oil emulsion and gelatin sponge particles. **C:** A radiograph obtained immediately after embolization shows iodized oil accumulation in the tumor. The patient underwent two sessions of embolization with a 6-month interval. **D:** A follow-up CT obtained 12 months after initial embolization revealed near-complete regression of the tumor (*arrows*) with hepatic parenchymal atrophy (*arrowheads*).

Histologically, FNH is composed primarily of Kupffer cells and hepatocytes. It is believed to result from the response to a preexisting vascular abnormality. Patients with FNH are typically asymptomatic and may be managed conservatively because there is no predisposition to hemorrhage or malignant transformation. However, up to 30% of patients present with a vague abdominal pain due to mass effect, hepatomegaly, and/or abdominal mass.[28] Treatment should be considered in cases with a progressive increase in size or compressive symptoms. Surgical resection is currently the treatment of choice for FNH when indicated. TAE is considered to be an alternative to surgery when there is considerable surgical risk because of localization or poor clinical condition. Given FNH's genesis in abnormal arterial flow, embolization is a

Table 33.1 Recent Literature Case Series on Transcatheter Arterial Embolization of Hepatocellular Adenomas

Reference	Patients/ Tumors, n	Emergency/ Elective TAE	Embolic Materials	Mean Follow-up (month)	Outcomes
Deodhar et al.[13]	8/16	0/8	Trisacryl gelatin microspheres	24	Tumor regression in 13 tumors (81%)
Stoot et al.[21]	11/25	11/0	PVA particle, microcoils, NBCA	19	Hemostasis in 11 patients (100%) Tumor regression in 25 tumors (100%)
Erdogan et al.[22]	6/9	4/2	PVA particle, microcoils, gelatin sponge particle	NA	Hemostasis in 4 patients (100%) Tumor regression in 8 tumors (89%)
Kim et al.[23]	7/9	1/6	Doxorubicin-iodized oil emulsion, gelatin sponge particle	88	Hemostasis in 1 patient (100%) Tumor regression in 8 tumors (89%)

PVA, polyvinyl alcohol; NBCA, *N*-butyl cyanoacrylate; NA, not available.

feasible strategy.[29] Angiographic findings are fairly characteristic. Hepatic angiogram shows a hypervascular mass with dense tumor blush in the capillary and portal venous phases. Lucent septations can be seen within the blush corresponding with the fibrous septations. A single central feeding artery penetrating the tumor mass is usually seen in a large FNH, which makes TAE more feasible. When the lesion is supplied by multiple small feeding vessels, the need for repeat TAE should be anticipated.[29] Several small case series reported successful application of TAE in patients with symptomatic FNHs. Microspheres 150 to 750 μm were the most commonly employed embolic agent. TAE relieved symptoms in most patients and led to substantial shrinkage of the tumors (20% to 90%).[12,29,30]

Cavernous Hemangioma

Cavernous hemangioma is the most common benign tumor affecting the liver, with an estimated prevalence of 3% to 20%.[27] It occurs in all age groups but is more frequently discovered between the third and fifth decade, with a mean age of 50 years at diagnosis and is seen more often in females (female-to-male ratio 6:1).[27] Most hemangiomas are small, asymptomatic, and usually require no treatment or follow-up. However, giant hemangiomas (diameter >4 cm) may present with abdominal pain or discomfort (23% to 57%) caused by displacement of other organs, capsular stretch, partial infarction, or intralesional hemorrhage. A spontaneous or traumatic rupture is rare (1% to 4%), but mortality in this patient group is high (36% to 39%).[3] Kasabach-Merritt syndrome is also a rare but well-known complication of giant hemangiomas. It is characterized by the combination of a vascular tumor and consumptive coagulopathy, which can progress to disseminated coagulopathy. There is no consensus regarding the optimal management of giant hemangiomas, but presence of established complications, diagnostic uncertainty, and incapacitating symptoms are generally considered indications for surgical enucleation or resection.

TAE has been suggested as a good alternative treatment of symptomatic hemangiomas, either alone or as a preoperative procedure before surgical resection.[31–34] TAE can be successfully applied in tumors with extensive hilar involvement that makes surgical procedures difficult,[34] in patients with ruptured hemangiomas,[33] or to reduce blood loss at the time of surgery.[31] TAE rapidly and safely corrects the coagulopathy caused by Kasabach-Merritt syndrome, which is essential because these patients are poor surgical candidates.[35] Various embolic materials are being used, such as gelatin particle, steel coils, PVA particles, and NBCA. Typically, vascular interstices within the lesion are first embolized with PVA particles, followed by embolization of the principal arteries with steel coils.[36] In a multicenter study from China, hepatic hemangiomas of 98 patients were treated with chemoembolization using pingyangmycin-Lipiodol emulsion. Pingyangmycin has been found, like bleomycin, to reduce the DNA synthesis of cancer cells and cut off the DNA chain. The presumable mechanism of this treatment relies on pingyangmycin's ability to destroy the endothelial cells, resulting in the formation of microthrombi in sinuses and causing atrophy and fibrosis of the tumor. The tumor diameters decreased significantly from 9.7 to 3.0 cm at 12 months follow-up. Clinical symptoms were relieved in all patients. The most severe potential complication caused by pingyangmycin is pulmonary fibrosis. However, no pulmonary fibrosis has been observed in used dosage (8 to 24 mg).

Iatrogenic Vascular Injury

Iatogenic hepatic vascular injury is by far most commonly caused by radiologic transhepatic procedures including percutaneous liver biopsy, percutaneous transhepatic biliary drainage (PTBD), transjugular intrahepatic portosystemic shunt (TIPS), and radiofrequency ablation (RFA).[37] The incidence of clinically significant vascular injury following RFA and liver biopsy is estimated to be 0% to 0.5% and 0.06% to 1%, respectively. PTBD carries a higher risk (2% to 10%) because of the use of larger catheters and the presence of bile stasis.[38–40] Most common clinical presentation is gastrointestinal bleeding due to hemobilia.[41] This is due to close proximity of the hepatic arteriole and portal venule along with the biliary radical in the portal triad. Thus, an injury to the artery and vein makes the adjacent biliary duct prone to injury. In up to 90% of the patients with iatrogenic hemobilia, a vascular abnormality is found on angiography.[41] The most common finding is a pseudoaneurysm, followed by an arteriobiliary or an arterioportal fistula. Some arterioportal fistulas may remain quiescent for long periods, up to many years, but a large arterioportal fistula can lead to dynamic portal hypertension with gastroesophageal varices, ascites, or mesenteric ischemia.[42]

Nowadays, TAE is the preferred method to treat intrahepatic iatrogenic vascular injuries, which gives satisfactory results; success rates of 80% to 100% have been reported in the literature.[9,43–48] An overview of the embolization results for iatrogenic hepatic vascular injuries in the literature is presented in Table 33.2. Surgery is usually employed secondarily for unsuccessful embolization and complex lesions. The aim of embolization is to achieve selective and complete thrombosis of pseudoaneurysm or fistula closure with preservation of the adjacent normal vasculature. To achieve this, a microcatheter should be positioned as close as possible to the lesion site to limit hepatic devascularization. For hepatic arterial pseudoaneurysm, microcoils are most commonly used to embolize hepatic arteries just distal and proximal to the lesion, which allows for thrombosis (Fig. 33.2). When embolizing the right or left hepatic arteries, contralateral peripheral vascular bed is filled through intrahepatic collateral vessels immediately; thus, hepatic infarction is unlikely to occur. For embolization of arterioportal fistulas, the embolic agents should be chosen according to the size of the vascular communication. For high-flow fistulas, microcoils are most commonly selected embolic agent.[8,9,49] However, the use of microcoils has a potential risk of migration of the coil into the portal vein, especially when fistula is larger than 8 mm.[37] Detachable coils, such as the interlocking detachable coil or Guglielmi detachable coil, can avoid the risk of coil migration, but they may not cause thrombosis in high-flow fistula. Hirakawa et al.[8] suggested the use of detachable coil as a first anchoring coil and subsequent fibered coils to avoid coil migration and to achieve complete occlusion of large, high-flow fistula. Liquid embolic agent such as NBCA has not been widely used due to its higher risk of migration into the portal venous system. However, it can be a useful embolic agent when there is the presence of multiple small fistulae, all of which had to be embolized,[7] or proper placement of a microcatheter at the desirable intra-arterial position is impossible.[8] Particles such as gelatin sponge or PVA can be used in small, slow-flow fistulas.[11]

Miscellaneous Benign Liver Diseases

Polycystic Liver Disease

Polycystic liver is the most common extrarenal manifestation associated with autosomal dominant polycystic kidney disease (ADPKD), presenting in 80% of all ADPKD patients.[50] Most patients are asymptomatic and require no treatment. However, because of lengthened lifespan of ADPKD patients, recent patients often suffer from hepatic symptoms including abdominal discomfort, dyspepsia, or dyspnea. Surgical interventions to relieve these symptoms include laparoscopic or open cyst fenestration, partial hepatectomy, and hepatic transplantation.[51,52] However, these treatments are associated with significant morbidity and mortality, reported as high as 42%.[53] Recently, Ubara et al.[54] suggested that TAE may be an option for symptomatic patients who are not candidates for surgical treatment. Hepatic cysts in ADPKD patients are mostly supplied from hepatic arteries; therefore, embolization of hepatic artery branches that supply major hepatic cysts may lead to shrinkage of the cyst (Fig. 33.3). Thereafter, several investigators embolized the hepatic arteries supplying the dominant hepatic segments replaced by cysts using microcoils[55,56] or NBCA[57] and achieved symptomatic relief in 50% to 86% of their patients. Total liver volume and intrahepatic cyst volume substantially decreased. No serious complications were reported except mild transient elevation of the liver enzyme.[55–57]

Infantile Hemangioendothelioma

Infantile hemangioendothelioma (IHE) is the most frequent liver tumor in infants, which can occur as solitary or multifocal lesions. Although it is a benign tumor, potentially fatal complications can result from congestive heart failure and consumptive coagulopathy (Kasabach-Merritt-Syndrome). The mortality rate of untreated symptomatic IHE is reported up to 90%.[58] In these cases, immediate treatment is crucial for the outcome of the patients. Medical treatment consists of steroids, α-interferon, and symptomatic treatments. Surgical procedures include ligation of feeding vessels, hepatic resection, and liver transplantation. TAE has been considered an important alternative treatment because the patients are often at high surgical risk.[59–61] As the procedure involves percutaneous arterial access in infants, there is a risk of thrombotic occlusion of the femoral artery.

Table 33.2 Case Series Reporting the Use of Transcatheter Arterial Embolization for Iatrogenic Hemobilia

Reference	Patients	Causal Procedure	Angiographic Findings	Major Adverse Event	Success Rate
Rivera-Sanfeliz et al.[48]	8	PTBD	Pseudoaneurysm (n = 4) AB fistula (n = 3) AP fistula (n = 1)	None	7/8 (88%)
Croutch et al.[45]	8	PTBD	Pseudoaneurysm (n = 3) AB fistula (n = 4) AP fistula (n = 1)	None	8/8 (100%)
Hidalgo et al.[47]	7	Cholecystectomy (n = 1) PTBD (n = 1) Hepaticojejunostomy (n = 2) Liver biopsy (n = 3)	Pseudoaneurysm (n = 6) AP fistula (n = 2)	Biliary sepsis	6/7 (86%)
Savader et al.[46]	13	PTBD	Pseudoaneurysm (n = 8) AB fistula (n = 4) AP fistula (n = 1)	Liver abscess (n = 2) Hepatic infarction (n = 1)	13/13 (100%)
Nicholson et al.[43]	9	Cholecystectomy	Pseudoaneurysm (n = 9)	Liver abscess (n = 1)	9/9 (100%)
Okazaki et al.[44]	10	PTBD (n = 6) Operative biliary drainage (n = 1) Hepaticojejunostomy (n = 1) Hepatic angiography (n = 1) Liver biopsy (n = 1)	Pseudoaneurysm (n = 7) AB fistula (n = 2)	None	10/10 (100%)
Marynissen et al.[9]	12	Cholecystectomy (n = 1) PTBD (n = 2) Liver biopsy (n = 6) ERCP (n = 2) RFA (n = 1)	Pseudoaneurysm (n = 4) AB fistula (n = 1) AP fistula (n = 4) Contrast extravasation (n = 2)	None	12/12 (100%)

PTBD, percutaneous transhepatic biliary drainage; AB fistula, arteriobiliary fistula; AP fistula, arterioportal fistula; ERCP, endoscopic retrograde cholangiopancreatography; RFA, radiofrequency ablation.

This can be avoided if a venous approach is used with passage to the arterial side via the persistent ductus arteriosus or the oval foramen of right atrium.[61] In newborns, feeding vessels from the portal venous system can be embolized via the umbilical vein.[59] Warmann et al.[61] performed coil embolization in four patients with symptomatic IHE and achieved good clinical outcomes in three patients. Signs of heart failure resolved within 8 days after TAE and tumor size was reduced from a mean of 544 mL to 4 mL. Even in cases with incomplete regression of the tumors, the clinical improvement can be achieved shortly after embolization in most patients. Thus, if necessary, a surgical resection might follow after cardiopulmonary stabilization with reduced tumor size.[61]

Congenital Portosystemic Shunt

Congenital portosystemic shunts are rare (1/30,000) anomalies that result from developmental abnormalities of the portal venous system. They are classified into two types: extrahepatic (type I) and intrahepatic (type II, including patent ductus venosus). Intrahepatic type may be also divided into four different findings: single large tube connecting right portal vein to inferior vena cava, segmental peripheral portal and hepatic venous connection, aneurysmal connection, and diffuse con-

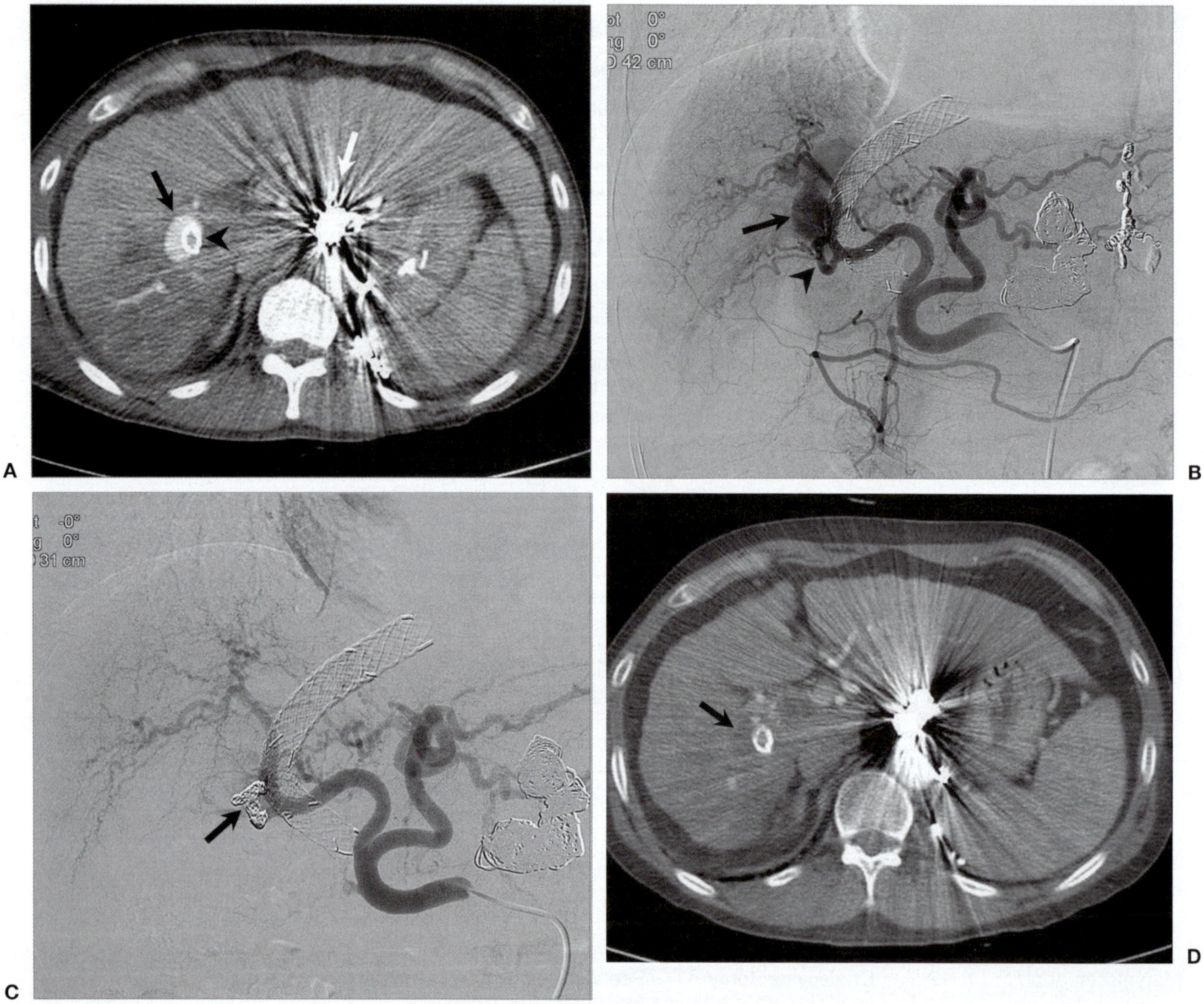

Figure 33.2 A 57-year-old patient who underwent TIPS for gastric variceal bleeding. **A:** A liver CT revealed a pseudoaneurysm (*black arrow*) adjacent to TIPS stent (*arrowhead*). Artifact is caused by coils in the left gastric vein placed at TIPS procedure (*white arrow*). **B:** Common hepatic angiogram shows the pseudoaneurysm (*arrow*) arisen from the right posterior hepatic artery (*arrowhead*). **C:** Embolization was performed with microcoils (*arrow*) to exclude the pseudoaneurysm. **D:** A follow-up CT demonstrates complete thrombosis of the pseudoaneurysm (*arrow*).

nection in both lobes.[62] The clinical course is determined by the diameter of the shunt. Patients with large shunts may have severe related complications including hypoxia owing to hepatopulmonary syndrome, dyspnea caused by pulmonary arterial hypertension, heart failure, encephalopathy, neonatal cholestasis, or liver tumor,[63] whereas those with small shunts may develop recurrent episodes of portosystemic encephalopathy that initiate in adulthood.[64]

Treatment in symptomatic patients consists of surgical or laparoscopic ligation of the shunt or endovascular embolization. Although surgical ligation prevailed for managing most cases in the past, with modern technologic advances of intravascular devices and radiologic techniques, it has been largely replaced by radiologic intervention.[65,66] However, because of the anatomical proximity of the vascular structures involved (portal vein and hepatic vein or vena cava), stable placement of a large embolic device inside of a short-length fistulous tract can be challenging. In addition, shunt closure can lead to acute portal hypertension when the hypoplastic portal system does not adapt rapidly. Therefore, an occlusion test with temporary balloon occlusion of the shunt with recording of the portal pressure is recommended before complete closure of the shunts. When portal pressure rises above 30 mm Hg with shunt occlusion test, shunt closure should be avoided, and an alternative two-step procedure (surgical or radiologic) or liver transplantation should be considered.[67] Steel coils has been successfully

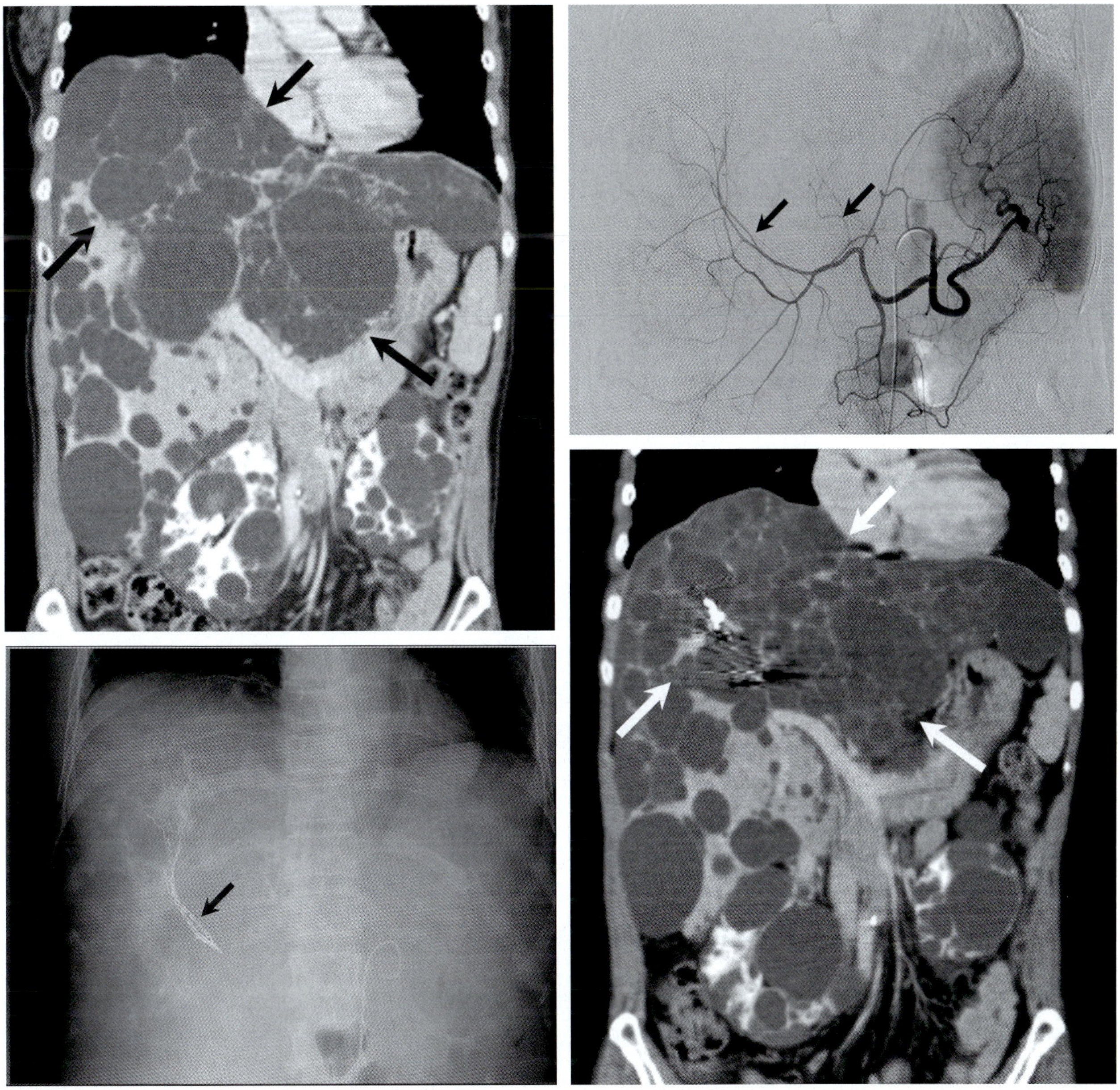

Figure 33.3 A 60-year-old patient with ADPKD. The patient underwent embolization for abdominal pain and dyspepsia. **A:** A contrast-enhanced CT obtained before embolization demonstrates innumerable liver cysts. Largest cysts predominantly involve hepatic segments 8 and 4, which are presumable cause of patient's symptoms (*arrows*). **B:** A celiac angiogram shows displacement of the hepatic arteries by the liver cysts (*arrows*). **C:** Selective embolization of two segmental hepatic arteries using PVA particles and microcoils (*arrow*). **D:** A 2-year follow-up CT revealed decreased size of the liver cysts in segments 8 and 4 (*arrows*).

used for shunt closure but carries the risk of migration.[63,65] In the case of large, high-flow fistula, an Amplatzer Vascular Plug with a diameter 30% to 50% larger than the shunt is recommended to reduce the risk of device migration[68] (Fig. 33.4).

POTENTIAL COMPLICATIONS

The procedures of TAE for benign liver disease are essentially same as those of TAE for malignant liver tumors. Therefore, theoretically, TAE for benign liver disease can be associated with all complications that occur following TAE for malignant liver tumors. Major complications include liver abscess, parenchymal infarction, intrahepatic aneurysm, ischemic cholecystitis or gallbladder infarction, and gastric or duodenal ulcerations. There are well-known predisposing factors for these complications, including major portal vein obstruction, compromised hepatic functional reserve, biliary obstruction, and previous biliary surgery. However, as

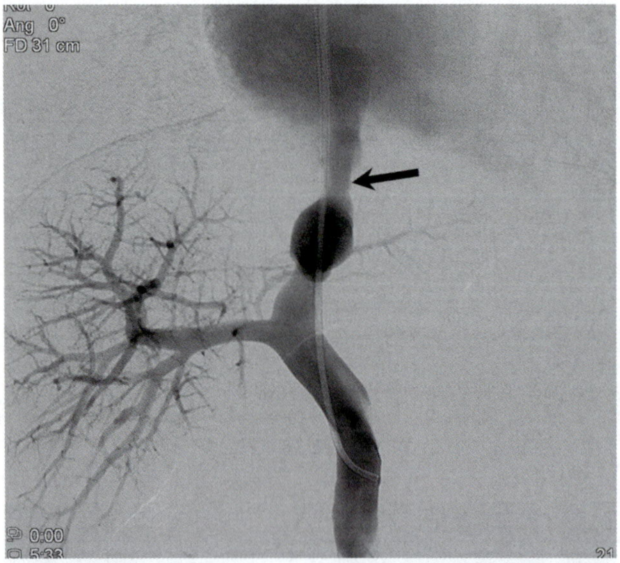
A

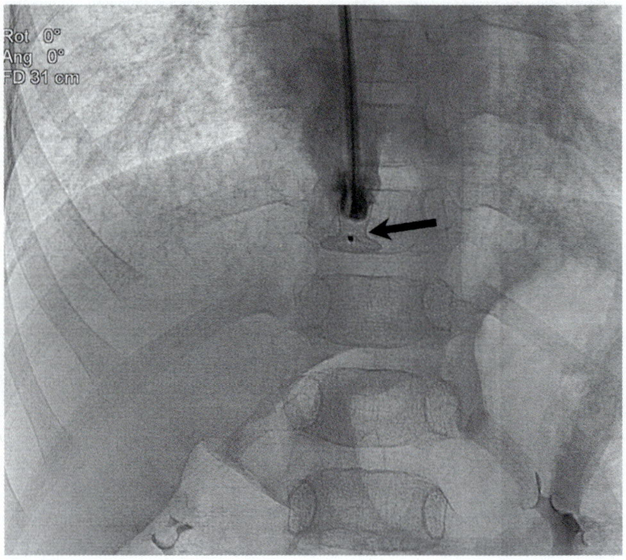
B

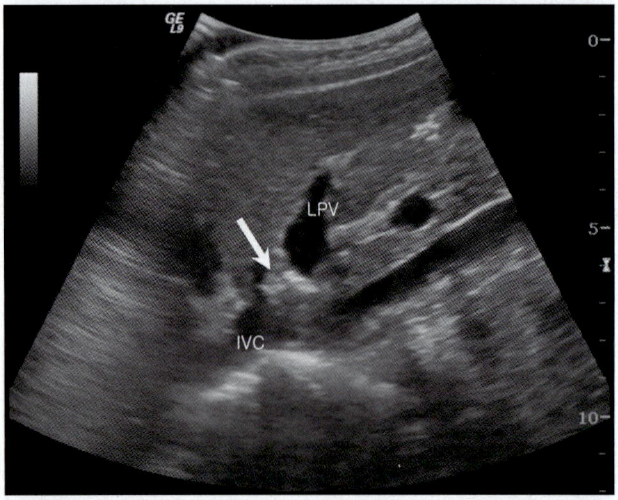

C

Figure 33.4 A 5-year-old patient with patent ductus venosus complicated with severe pulmonary hypertension and cognitive dysfunction. **A:** Direct portography obtained with jugular venous approach demonstrates an intrahepatic portosystemic shunt between the left portal vein and inferior vena cava (*arrow*). **B:** The shunt was embolized using Amplatzer occluder (*arrow*). **C:** Follow-up ultrasonography revealed the occluder precisely positioned within the shunt (*arrow*). Color Doppler examination confirmed complete embolization of the shunt. LPV, left portal vein; IVC, inferior vena cava.

the patients with benign liver disease usually have a good liver function and unlikely to have the predisposing factors, complications following TAE in benign liver diseases are rare and mostly consist of postembolization syndrome, vascular injury from catheter manipulation, and complications from use of contrast medium.

The postembolization syndrome is the most common complication that occurs in approximately 80% of patients after TAE. It is characterized by pain at the site of embolization, nausea and vomiting, malaise, fever, and leukocytosis, which usually occurs within 24 to 48 hours of embolization and lasts 3 to 7 days. Severity depends on the extent of the embolized liver tissue. Possible causes of the pain are acute ischemia of liver parenchyma, distension of the liver capsule, and/or gallbladder ischemia due to inadvertent embolization of the cystic artery. It is essentially a self-limited condition, which hardly requires any specific treatment. Nevertheless, it may be considered an important complication because it prolongs hospitalization and postpones additional treatment. The relevant systemic symptoms can be controlled by antiemetics, analgesics, antipyretics, and hydrocortisone.

Liver abscess and infarction rarely develops after TAE for benign liver diseases; only a few case series reported these complications. Savader et al.[46] experienced two liver abscesses and one infarction following 12 TAE procedures for iatrogenic hemobilia. Liver abscess is usually successfully managed with parenteral antibiotics and percutaneous drainage, but in some cases, it may result in fatal outcome if it is detected too late or managed inappropriately. As biliary-enteric bypass surgery is a well-known predisposing factor, aggressive prophylactic antibiotics administration before TAE is recommended in case of previous bile duct surgery or systemic disorders vulnerable to infection.

Nontarget embolization is the most dreaded complication of hepatic embolization but occurs infrequently if diagnostic angiogram has been carefully evaluated and the appropriate technique of embolization has been followed. The gallbladder is the most common "nontarget" organ because the cystic artery is often not opacified on arteriogram. Inadvertent embolization of the cystic artery causes prolonged postembolization syndrome with fever, pain, and nausea/vomiting. Most cases have self-limited clinical course, but more serious conditions have been reported such as gallbladder perforation and gangrenous or emphysematous cholecystitis, in which cholecystectomy or percutaneous cholecystostomy is required.[69] Gastroduodenal ulcer can occur due to inadvertent embolization of the accessory left gastric arteries that arise from the left hepatic artery and the right gastric artery that arises from the proper hepatic artery.[70] If these gastric branches are not recognized before the procedure, and appropriate protective measures are not taken, gastric complications are unavoidable. Embolization of gastric branches with coil or balloon occlusion of proper hepatic artery can redirect the blood flow.

When performing embolization for arterioportal fistula, there is a potential risk of the migration of embolic agents to the portal veins. This may cause the blockage of portal vein branches, leading to subsequent thrombosis. Hirakawa et al.[8] reported four cases in which portal vein thrombosis developed after TAE. Although portal vein thrombosis is frequently asymptomatic and hepatopetal portal flow maintained by cavernous transformation, this complication should be kept in mind when embolizing a large and high-flow fistula.

During hepatic embolization procedure, iatrogenic arterial injury, such as dissection, may occur in the visceral arteries. The two most common sites of dissection are the celiac artery and the proper hepatic artery. Although iatrogenic dissection of the arteries heals spontaneously in most patients, it may result in complete obstruction or pseudoaneurysm formation.[71–73]

TIPS AND TRICKS

Benign Liver Tumors

- To minimize damage of normal hepatic parenchyma, hepatic arterial embolization should be as close to the target lesions as possible.
- Particulate embolic agents are commonly used. Typically, vascular interstices within the lesion are first embolized with PVA particles, followed by embolization of the principal arteries with steel coils.
- When using coils, they should be tightly packed without interstices to avoid late recanalization.

Iatrogenic Vascular Injury

- In patients with iatrogenic hemobilia, vascular abnormalities such as pseudoaneurysm and arteriobiliary or arterioportal fistula can be demonstrated on angiography in most cases.
- When treating hepatic arterial pseudoaneurysm, coils should not be placed inside the aneurysmal sac because there is risk of late rupture. The proximal and distal vessels to the pseudoaneurysm should be embolized so that revascularization by backflow may not occur.
- When treating large, high-flow fistulas, the use of pushable microcoils has a potential risk of migration. Consider use of detachable coil as a first anchoring coil to prevent coil migration and subsequent pushable fibered coils to achieve complete occlusion of fistula.
- When a microcatheter is not able to be advanced to desirable intravascular position, consider use of NBCA. By adjusting the ratio of NBCA and iodized oil, the level of embolization within target vessels can be controlled.

Miscellaneous Benign Liver Diseases

- Hepatic cysts in ADPKD patients are mostly supplied from hepatic arteries; therefore, embolization of hepatic artery branches that supply major hepatic cysts may lead to shrinkage of the cyst.
- When the procedure involves percutaneous arterial access in infants, consider venous approach with passage via the persistent ductus arteriosus or the oval foramen of right atrium to avoid risk of arterial access related complications.
- When congenital portosystemic shunt is large, high-flow, with short-length fistulous tract, the use of coil carries risk of migration. Amplatzer Vascular Plug with a diameter 30%–50% larger than the shunt is recommended.

REFERENCES

1. Mezhir JJ, Fourman LT, Do RK, et al. Changes in the management of benign liver tumours: an analysis of 285 patients. *HPB (Oxford)*. 2013;15(2):156–163.
2. Pulvirenti E, Toro A, Di Carlo I. An update on indications for treatment of solid hepatic neoplasms in noncirrhotic liver. *Future Oncol.* 2010;6(8):1243–1250.
3. Hoekstra LT, Bieze M, Erdogan D, et al. Management of giant liver hemangiomas: an update. *Expert Rev Gastroenterol Hepatol.* 2013;7(3):263–268.
4. Sharpe EE III, Dodd GD III. Percutaneous radiofrequency ablation of symptomatic giant hepatic cavernous hemangiomas: report of two cases and review of literature. *J Vasc Interv Radiol.* 2012;23(7):971–975.
5. Huurman V, Schaapherder A. Management of ruptured hepatocellular adenoma. *Dig Surg.* 2010;27(1):56–60.
6. Kobayashi S, Sakaguchi H, Takatsuka M, et al. Two cases of hepatocellular adenomatosis treated with transcatheter arterial embolization. *Hepatol Int.* 2009;3(2):416–420.
7. Kumar A, Ahuja CK, Vyas S, et al. Hepatic arteriovenous fistulae: role of interventional radiology. *Dig Dis Sci.* 2012;57(10): 2703–2712.

8. Hirakawa M, Nishie A, Asayama Y, et al. Clinical outcomes of symptomatic arterioportal fistulas after transcatheter arterial embolization. *World J Radiol.* 2013;5(2):33–40.
9. Marynissen T, Maleux G, Heye S, et al. Transcatheter arterial embolization for iatrogenic hemobilia is a safe and effective procedure: case series and review of the literature. *Eur J Gastroenterol Hepatol.* 2012;24(8):905–909.
10. Gallego C, Miralles M, Marin C, et al. Congenital hepatic shunts. *Radiographics.* 2004;24(3):755–772.
11. Srivastava DN, Sharma S, Pal S, et al. Transcatheter arterial embolization in the management of hemobilia. *Abdom Imaging.* 2006;31(4):439–448.
12. Vogl TJ, Own A, Hammerstingl R, et al. Transarterial embolization as a therapeutic option for focal nodular hyperplasia in four patients. *Eur Radiol.* 2006;16(3):670–675.
13. Deodhar A, Brody LA, Covey AM, et al. Bland embolization in the treatment of hepatic adenomas: preliminary experience. *J Vasc Interv Radiol.* 2011;22(6):795–799; quiz 800.
14. Woo S, Yoon CJ, Chung JW, et al. Bronchial artery embolization to control hemoptysis: comparison of N-butyl-2-cyanoacrylate and polyvinyl alcohol particles. *Radiology.* 2013;269:594–602.
15. Giannitrapani L, Soresi M, La Spada E, et al. Sex hormones and risk of liver tumor. *Ann N Y Acad Sci.* 2006;1089:228–236.
16. Heeringa B, Sardi A. Bleeding hepatic adenoma: expectant treatment to limit the extent of liver resection. *Am Surg.* 2001; 67(10):927–929.
17. Grazioli L, Federle MP, Brancatelli G, et al. Hepatic adenomas: imaging and pathologic findings. *Radiographics.* 2001;21(4): 877–892; discussion 892–874.
18. Terkivatan T, de Wilt JH, de Man RA, et al. Treatment of ruptured hepatocellular adenoma. *Br J Surg.* 2001;88(2):207–209.
19. Deneve JL, Pawlik TM, Cunningham S, et al. Liver cell adenoma: a multicenter analysis of risk factors for rupture and malignancy. *Ann Surg Oncol.* 2009;16(3):640–648.
20. Toso C, Majno P, Andres A, et al. Management of hepatocellular adenoma: solitary-uncomplicated, multiple and ruptured tumors. *World J Gastroenterol.* 2005;11(36):5691–5695.
21. Stoot J, Van Der Linden E, Terpstra O, et al. Life-saving therapy for haemorrhaging liver adenomas using selective arterial embolization. *Br J Surg.* 2007;94(10):1249–1253.
22. Erdogan D, van Delden OM, Busch OR, et al. Selective transcatheter arterial embolization for treatment of bleeding complications or reduction of tumor mass of hepatocellular adenomas. *Cardiovasc Intervent Radiol.* 2007;30(6):1252–1258.
23. Kim YI, Chung JW, Park JH. Feasibility of transcatheter arterial chemoembolization for hepatic adenoma. *J Vasc Interv Radiol.* 2007;18(7):862–867.
24. Meirowitz RF, Tobin KD, Elias EG, et al. Resolution of inferior vena cava syndrome after embolization of a hepatic adenoma. *Gastroenterology.* 1990;99(5):1502–1506.
25. Karkar AM, Tang LH, Kashikar ND, et al. Management of hepatocellular adenoma: comparison of resection, embolization and observation. *HPB (Oxford).* 2013;15(3):235–243.
26. de Jong M, Stoot J, Coelen R, et al. Selective arterial embolisation versus resection of hepatocellular adenomas. In: Stoot J, ed. *Improving the Outcome of Liver Surgery.* Maastricht, The Netherlands: Universitaire Pers Maastricht; 2012:223.
27. Chamberlain RS, Oelhafen K. Benign hepatic neoplasms. In: Abdeldayem H, ed. *Hepatic Surgery.* Intech: Rijeka, Croatia; 2013.
28. Bioulac-Sage P, Balabaud C, Wanless IR. Diagnosis of focal nodular hyperplasia: not so easy. *Am J Surg Pathol.* 2001;25(10): 1322–1325.
29. Amesur N, Hammond JS, Zajko AB, et al. Management of unresectable symptomatic focal nodular hyperplasia with arterial embolization. *J Vasc Interv Radiol.* 2009;20(4):543–547.
30. Terkivatan T, Hussain SM, Lameris JS, et al. Transcatheter arterial embolization as a safe and effective treatment for focal nodular hyperplasia of the liver. *Cardiovasc Intervent Radiol.* 2002;25(5):450–453.
31. Seo HI, Jo HJ, Sim MS, et al. Right trisegmentectomy with thoracoabdominal approach after transarterial embolization for giant hepatic hemangioma. *World J Gastroenterol.* 2009; 15(27):3437–3439.
32. Zhou JX, Huang JW, Wu H, et al. Successful liver resection in a giant hemangioma with intestinal obstruction after embolization. *World J Gastroenterol.* 2013;19(19):2974–2978.
33. Lupinacci RM, Szejnfeld D, Farah JF. Spontaneous rupture of a giant hepatic hemangioma. Sequential treatment with preoperative transcatheter arterial embolization and conservative hepatectomy. *G Chir.* 2011;32(11–12):469–472.
34. Althaus S, Ashdown B, Coldwell D, et al. Transcatheter arterial embolization of two symptomatic giant cavernous hemangiomas of the liver. *Cardiovasc Intervent Radiol.* 1996;19(5): 364–367.
35. Malagari K, Alexopoulou E, Dourakis S, et al. Transarterial embolization of giant liver hemangiomas associated with Kasabach-Merritt syndrome: a case report. *Acta Radiol.* 2007; 48(6):608–612.
36. Vassiou K, Rountas H, Liakou P, et al. Embolization of a giant hepatic hemangioma prior to urgent liver resection. Case report and review of the literature. *Cardiovasc Intervent Radiol.* 2007; 30(4):800–802.
37. Isik FF, Greenfield AJ, Guben J, et al. Iatrogenic arterioportal fistulae: diagnosis and management. *Ann Vasc Surg.* 1989;3(1): 52–55.
38. Green MH, Duell RM, Johnson CD, et al. Haemobilia. *Br J Surg.* 2001;88(6):773–786.
39. Srivastava D, Gandhi D, Seith A, et al. Transcatheter arterial embolization in the treatment of symptomatic cavernous hemangiomas of the liver: a prospective study. *Abdom Imaging.* 2001;26(5):510–514.
40. Rhim H, Lim HK, Kim YS, et al. Hemobilia after radiofrequency ablation of hepatocellular carcinoma. *Abdom Imaging.* 2007;32(6):719–724.
41. Tessier DJ, Fowl RJ, Stone WM, et al. Iatrogenic hepatic artery pseudoaneurysms: an uncommon complication after hepatic, biliary, and pancreatic procedures. *Ann Vasc Surg.* 2003;17(6): 663–669.
42. Tanaka H, Iwai A, Sugimoto H, et al. Intrahepatic arterioportal fistula after blunt hepatic trauma: case reports. *J Trauma.* 1991; 31(1):143–146.
43. Nicholson T, Travis S, Ettles D, et al. Hepatic artery angiography and embolization for hemobilia following laparoscopic cholecystectomy. *Cardiovasc Intervent Radiol.* 1999;22(1): 20–24.
44. Okazaki M, Ono H, Higashihara H, et al. Angiographic management of massive hemobilia due to iatrogenic trauma. *Gastrointest Radiol.* 1991;16(3):205–204.

45. Croutch KL, Gordon RL, Ring EJ, et al. Superselective arterial embolization in the liver transplant recipient: a safe treatment for hemobilia caused by percutaneous transhepatic biliary drainage. *Liver Transpl Surg.* 1996;2(2):118–123.
46. Savader SJ, Trerotola SO, Merine DS, et al. Hemobilia after percutaneous transhepatic biliary drainage: treatment with transcatheter embolotherapy. *J Vasc Interv Radiol.* 1992;3(2):345–352.
47. Hidalgo F, Narvaez JA, Rene M, et al. Treatment of hemobilia with selective hepatic artery embolization. *J Vasc Interv Radiol.* 1995;6(5):793–798.
48. Rivera-Sanfeliz GM, Assar OS, LaBerge JM, et al. Incidence of important hemobilia following transhepatic biliary drainage: left-sided versus right-sided approaches. *Cardiovasc Intervent Radiol.* 2004;27(2):137–139.
49. Kadir S, Athanasoulis CA, Ring EJ, et al. Transcatheter embolization of intrahepatic arterial aneurysms. *Radiology.* 1980;134(2):335–339.
50. Drenth JP, Chrispijn M, Nagorney DM, et al. Medical and surgical treatment options for polycystic liver disease. *Hepatology.* 2010;52(6):2223–2230.
51. van Keimpema L, Drenth JP. Polycystic liver disease: a critical appraisal of hepatic resection, cyst fenestration, and liver transplantation. *Ann Surg.* 2011;253(2):419; author reply 420.
52. Gruttadauria S, di Francesco F, Gridelli B. Liver transplantation for polycystic liver and massive hepatomegaly. *World J Gastroenterol.* 2010;16(11):1425–1426.
53. Torres VE, Harris PC, Pirson Y. Autosomal dominant polycystic kidney disease. *Lancet.* 2007;369(9569):1287–1301.
54. Ubara Y, Takei R, Hoshino J, et al. Intravascular embolization therapy in a patient with an enlarged polycystic liver. *Am J Kidney Dis.* 2004;43(4):733–738.
55. Takei R, Ubara Y, Hoshino J, et al. Percutaneous transcatheter hepatic artery embolization for liver cysts in autosomal dominant polycystic kidney disease. *Am J Kidney Dis.* 2007;49(6):744–752.
56. Park HC, Kim CW, Ro H, et al. Transcatheter arterial embolization therapy for a massive polycystic liver in autosomal dominant polycystic kidney disease patients. *J Korean Med Sci.* 2009;24(1):57–61.
57. Wang MQ, Duan F, Liu FY, et al. Treatment of symptomatic polycystic liver disease: transcatheter super-selective hepatic arterial embolization using a mixture of NBCA and iodized oil. *Abdom Imaging.* 2013;38(3):465–473.
58. Woltering MC, Robben S, Egeler RM. Hepatic hemangioendothelioma of infancy: treatment with interferon alpha. *J Pediatr Gastroenterol Nutr.* 1997;24(3):348–351.
59. Daller JA, Bueno J, Gutierrez J, et al. Hepatic hemangioendothelioma: clinical experience and management strategy. *J Pediatr Surg.* 1999;34(1):98–105.
60. Peuster M, Windhagen-Mahnert B, Fink C, et al. Interventional therapy for hemangioendothelioma of the liver in a newborn infant using a central venous approach [in German]. *Z Kardiol.* 1998;87(10):832–836.
61. Warmann S, Bertram H, Kardorff R, et al. Interventional treatment of infantile hepatic hemangioendothelioma. *J Pediatr Surg.* 2003;38(8):1177–1181.
62. Park JH, Cha SH, Han JK, et al. Intrahepatic portosystemic venous shunt. *AJR Am J Roentgenol.* 1990;155(3):527–528.
63. Franchi-Abella S, Branchereau S, Lambert V, et al. Complications of congenital portosystemic shunts in children: therapeutic options and outcomes. *J Pediatr Gastroenterol Nutr.* 2010;51(3):322–330.
64. Ortiz M, Cordoba J, Alonso J, et al. Oral glutamine challenge and magnetic resonance spectroscopy in three patients with congenital portosystemic shunts. *J Hepatol.* 2004;40(3):552–557.
65. Kim IO, Cheon JE, Kim WS, et al. Congenital intrahepatic portohepatic venous shunt: treatment with coil embolisation. *Pediatr Radiol.* 2000;30(5):336–338.
66. Grimaldi C, Monti L, Falappa P, et al. Congenital intrahepatic portohepatic shunt managed by interventional radiologic occlusion: a case report and literature review. *J Pediatr Surg.* 2012;47(2):e27–e31.
67. Murray CP, Yoo SJ, Babyn PS. Congenital extrahepatic portosystemic shunts. *Pediatr Radiol.* 2003;33(9):614–620.
68. Lee SA, Lee YS, Lee KS, et al. Congenital intrahepatic portosystemic venous shunt and liver mass in a child patient: successful endovascular treatment with an amplatzer vascular plug (AVP). *Korean J Radiol.* 2010;11(5):583–586.
69. Tarazov PG, Polysalov VN, Prozorovskij KV, et al. Ischemic complications of transcatheter arterial chemoembolization in liver malignancies. *Acta Radiol.* 2000;41(2):156–160.
70. Morante A, Romano M, Cuomo A, et al. Massive gastric ulceration after transarterial chemoembolization for hepatocellular carcinoma. *Gastrointest Endosc.* 2006;63(4):718–720.
71. Yoon DY, Park JH, Chung JW, et al. Iatrogenic dissection of the celiac artery and its branches during transcatheter arterial embolization for hepatocellular carcinoma: outcome in 40 patients. *Cardiovasc Intervent Radiol.* 1995;18(1):16–19.
72. Jang ES, Jeong SH, Kim JW, et al. A case of acute ischemic duodenal ulcer associated with superior mesenteric artery dissection after transarterial chemoembolization for hepatocellular carcinoma. *Cardiovasc Intervent Radiol.* 2009;32(2):367–370.
73. So YH, Chung JW, Park JH. Balloon fenestration of iatrogenic celiac artery dissection. *J Vasc Interv Radiol.* 2003;14(4):493–496.

34

Bland Embolization

Karen T. Brown

Because the hepatic artery provides most blood flow to hepatocellular carcinoma (HCC), with the portal vein providing trophic blood supply to the liver parenchyma,[1] and the paucity of other effective nonsurgical treatments, it is not surprising that transarterial methods of treating unresectable HCC have become a mainstay of therapy over the last four decades. One of the early reports of transcatheter management of HCC by Charnsangavej et al.[2] in 1983 described results following two methods of treatment. The first group received continuous hepatic arterial infusion (HAI) of floxuridine, doxorubicin, and mitomycin C in 14 patients requiring a 5-day hospital stay, with two courses of treatment given at 4- to 6-week intervals. The second group of 9 patients (2 of whom crossed over from the HAI group) was treated with hepatic artery embolization (HAE) using Ivalon (Unipoint Industries, High Point, North Carolina). Response rates in the two groups were similar: 71% in HAI group versus 67% in HAE group, with median survival of 12.3 months and 17.4 months, respectively. Later that year, Yamada et al.[3] described the use of gelatin sponge cut into 1- to 2-mm pieces and "permeated" with mitomycin C or doxorubicin to treat 120 patients with HCC, infusing this chemotherapy-soaked gelatin sponge into the artery feeding the tumor. The 1-, 2-, and 3-year cumulative survival rates were 44%, 29%, and 15%, respectively. Yamada et al.[3] noted that given the knowledge that HCC derives blood supply from "only the hepatic artery,"[1] embolization can be expected to result in selective necrosis of the tumor tissue. They also suggested that although the effect of the single dose of mitomycin or doxorubicin may have been enhanced, it is possible that ischemia might be the primary mechanism of tumoricidal effect.[3] In a 1987 study by Takayasu et al.,[4] patients with HCC were divided into three groups for intra-arterial treatment. Group A received intra-arterial Lipiodol (Guerbet USA, Bloomington, Indiana) alone; group B, an emulsion of Lipiodol with doxorubicin; and group C, the same emulsion followed by embolization with gelatin sponge. Group C showed the best therapeutic effect; there was no significant difference in response between groups A and B, with practically no therapeutic effect from Lipiodol alone. Although these results can be interpreted in several ways, the authors pointed out that the results achieved using the anticancer emulsion plus gelatin sponge were superior to those previously described for embolization with gelatin sponge and anticancer agents and posited that the combination of Lipiodol blocking small vessels and gelatin sponge occluding more proximal feeding arteries resulted in an anoxic state "independent of drug sensitivity of the tumor." They also noted an association between uptake of Lipiodol by the tumor and therapeutic effect. In 1989, Nakamura described a similar effect on survival, comparing 100 patients treated with doxorubicin, iodized oil, and gelatin sponge to 104 historical controls embolized with gelatin sponge and either doxorubicin (96) or mitomycin (8) achieving 1-, 2-, and 3-year survivals of 53%, 33%, and 18% in the iodized oil group and 45%, 16%, and 4% in those treated with only gelatin sponge plus chemotherapy. Taken together, these findings confirm that transcatheter treatment of HCC brought about a radiologic response; however, several questions remained unanswered. What was the primary driver of that therapeutic effect: chemotherapy or ischemia? Does Lipiodol indeed prolong the intratumoral dwell time of chemotherapy? And, finally, does an imaging response to treatment translate into improved survival?

Pharmacokinetic data supporting the use of intra-arterial chemotherapy or chemotherapy plus Lipiodol administered as an emulsion with an embolic agent, as commonly used today, is less than convincing. Studies clearly demonstrating high and prolonged concentration of chemotherapeutic agents within the tumor were performed using mitomycin C, doxorubicin, and aclarubicin dissolved in hydrocarbon solvents and then in Lipiodol[5] or using a lipophilic agent,[6] methods which are not used clinically. In the animal study by Konno,[5] when the chemotherapeutic agent was dissolved in water and then mixed with Lipiodol and administered as an emulsion, concentration of drug in the tumor was high immediately but low at 6 hours, 1 day, and 7 days. In a study of 18 patients by Raoul et al.,[7] doxorubicin was given to patients intra-arterially using three different methods: alone as an infusion, emulsified with Lipiodol, or with Lipiodol and gelatin sponge. There was no significant difference in total amount of doxorubicin released into the circulating blood, but patients in whom gelatin sponge was used had less released within the first hour of treatment. Another study evaluated intra-arterial doxorubicin versus doxorubicin with Lipiodol[8] and found no difference in the area under the concentration-time curve, or terminal half-life, and no difference in pharmacokinetic profile or systemic toxicity using the same dose schedule compared to administering the doxorubicin intravenously. Even if the pharmacokinetic profile was more encouraging, none of these anticancer agents had ever been demonstrated to have a significant effect on the survival of patients with HCC when administered intravenously, making it difficult to know which agent, or which combination of agents, to use clinically. There are many embolic agents available for embolization. This has led to myriad methods of transcatheter intra-arterial therapy for HCC, limiting the ability to compare results between different groups. Meta-analysis by Simonetti et al.[9] in 1997 failed to support the effectiveness of nonsurgical treatments for HCC, but some evidence of "moderate benefit" emerged from trial using tamoxifen and transcatheter arterial embolization (without iodized oil). Combining the heterogeneous population of patients with HCC who present with varied etiology and stage of underlying liver disease, size and number of tumors, and vascular invasion status, with the diverse methods used to treat them, made it even more difficult to compare results of treatment between diverse investigators, and there were no strong randomized trials.

The lingering question of whether reported radiologic response would translate into survival benefit was addressed with two randomized trials reported in 2002, which compared transarterial therapies to supportive care. Lo et al.[10] treated a group of 80 patients, most had underlying hepatitis B, with either transarterial chemoembolization (TACE) using an emulsion of cisplatin and Lipiodol (Lipiodol Ultra-Fluide; Guerbet, Bloomington, Indiana) with gelatin sponge particles or best supportive care, using survival as the primary end point. There were 40 patients in each group; the TACE group received a total of 192 courses of embolization, median 4.5 per patient. TACE was associated with a significantly better actuarial survival of 57%, 31%, and 26% at 1, 2, and 3 years compared to 32%, 11%, and 3% in the best supportive care group. Later that same month, Llovet et al.[11] published a randomized trial with three arms: chemoembolization with doxorubicin, lipiodol, and gelatin sponge; gelatin sponge alone; and best supportive care. Again, the primary end point was survival; response was a secondary end point. The study design was sequential; patients were assessed every 3 months and the trial was stopped when a significant survival advantage was demonstrated for the chemoembolization group. At the time the study was stopped, the Z value of the sequential triangular test for the embolization group remained within the triangular boundaries, indicating the need to recruit additional patients to achieve a valid conclusion. Survival probabilities at 1 and 2 years were 75% and 50% for embolization, 82% and 63% for chemoembolization, and 63% and 27% for symptomatic treatment, respectively. Although the authors believe that chemoembolization leads to a survival benefit compared to embolization alone, this could not be concluded statistically because the study was stopped before such a benefit could be demonstrated or refuted. Additional patients would have needed to be recruited into the embolization arm to reach a valid conclusion with regard to the impact of embolization versus symptomatic treatment. Of interest, 30 patients treated achieved an objective response by imaging: 16 were in the embolization group, despite the fact that only 35 patients in that group were treated, and the other 14 were among the 40 patients treated with chemoembolization. Although this study provides level 1 statistical evidence that chemoembolization offers a survival benefit compared to best supportive care, it does not allow for any statement regarding the effectiveness of chemoembolization versus embolization alone or embolization versus best supportive care.

That same year, Camma et al.[12] published a meta-analysis of randomized chemoembolization trials. There were 18 randomized controlled trials pooled for analysis. The authors concluded that "chemoembolization significantly reduced the overall 2-year mortality rate (odds ratio, 0.54; 95% CI: 0.33, 0.89; $P = .015$) compared with nonactive treatment . . . overall mortality was significantly lower in patients treated with transarterial embolization (TAE) than in those treated with transarterial chemotherapy (odds ratio, 0.72; 95% CI: 0.53, 0.98, $P = .39$) and that there is no evidence that transarterial chemoembolization is more effective than TAE (odds ratio 1.007; 95% CI: 0.79, 1.27; $P = .95$), which suggests that the addition of an anticancer drug did not improve the therapeutic benefit."[12]

If indeed the primary effect of transarterial treatment is from ischemia rather than a local chemotherapeutic effect, it follows that methods that maximize ischemia should be adopted. To that end, calibrated microspheres that are capable of occluding intratumoral vessels should be employed for HAE. In a very elegant study using iron oxide labelled Embosphere Microspheres (Merit Medical Systems, Inc., South Jordan, Utah) published in 2008, Lee and colleagues[13] looked at the distribution of 100- to 300-μm and 300- to 500-μm spheres after embolization of VX2 tumor in rabbits. They found that on both magnetic resonance and histology, only the smaller 100- to 300-μm particles penetrated the tumor, whereas the 300- to 500-μm particles were found outside the tumor. Presuming that occlusion of intratumoral vessels will result in the most pronounced ischemia and resultant coagulation necrosis, these finding suggests that 100- to 300-μm particles or smaller should be used for embolization of liver tumors. Indeed, in 2008, Maluccio et al.[14] described results obtained in 322 patients thus treated at Memorial Sloan Kettering Cancer Center using small particle embolization alone. Median survival was 21 months, with 1, 2, and 3 years overall survival of 66%, 46%, and 33%, respectively. When patients with extrahepatic disease or portal vein tumor were excluded, the overall survival in the 159 patients with liver-only disease rose to 84%, 66%, and 51% at 1, 2, and 3 years, respectively, with a median survival of 40 months. These results are surprisingly (or perhaps not so surprisingly) similar to the 1- and 2-year overall survival with chemoembolization described by Llovet et al.[11] (82% and 63%) and are some of the best results ever reported for transcatheter treatment of HCC.

DEVICE/MATERIAL DESCRIPTION

Small calibrated microspheres without chemotherapy or Lipiodol are used to embolize HCC and other hypervascular tumors. Embosphere Microspheres are preferred by the author because of a demonstrated low incidence of postembolization occlusion of hepatic vessels.[15] These particles are made from trisacryl cross-linked acrylic copolymer combined with gelatin and are hydrophilic and compressible. They received 510(k) clearance in the United States in 2000 and are U.S. Food and Drug Administration (FDA) approved for uterine fibroid embolization (UFE). Having been available for almost 15 years, these microspheres are some of the most studied embolic agents currently in use and are available in sizes ranging from 40 to 120 μm to 900 to 1,200 μm. There are other calibrated spherical embolics that can be used for HAE including Bead Block (Biocompatibles UK LTD), available in sizes ranging from 100 to 300 μm to 900 to 1,200 μm and produced from a biocompatible polyvinyl alcohol (PVA) hydrogel, and Embozene Microspheres (CeloNova BioSciences, Inc., San Antonio, Texas), available in sizes ranging from 40 to 900 μm and composed of a hydrogel core with a surface modification of Polyzene-F, a biocompatible polymer. Bead Block received 510(k) approval for neurovascular embolization in 2004 and is now cleared for use in hypervascular tumors. Embozene Microspheres are the most tightly calibrated microspheres currently available. Embozene Microspheres received 510(k) approval from the FDA in December 2008 for use in hypervascularized tumors.

TECHNIQUE

After performing celiac and superior mesenteric angiography to define the direction of portal blood flow, arterial anatomy, and primary blood supply to the tumor(s), a catheter is placed selectively into the vessel or vessels supplying the tumor to be treated. Embolization is performed as selectively as possible often using a coaxial catheter. The catheter is advanced into the vessel(s) to be treated (Fig. 34.1), and the microspheres suspended in contrast and maintained in suspension by admixing through a three-way stopcock (Fig. 34.2) are injected under constant fluoroscopic control until stasis is evident.

Embolization is begun with the smallest size particle; in the case of Embosphere Microspheres, 40- to 120-μm spheres are used except in situations where the risk of systemic embolization is felt to be high, in which case embolization is begun with 100- to 300-μm spheres. Death related to systemic embolization of these small particles to the pulmonary circulation has been described,[16] and use of these small particles is discouraged in the following situations: tumors larger than 10 cm, large tumors high in the dome adjacent to the hemidiaphragm, tumors invading the hepatic veins, or with unexpected early hepatic vein drainage demonstrated angiographically.

When a large tumor burden is being treated and there is persistent antegrade flow after 10 mL of the 40- to 120-μm spheres have been injected, embolization is continued with the next largest size, 100- to 300-μm spheres. In situations where there is persistent flow after 10 mL of the 100- to 300-μm spheres have been used, embolization is continued with the next largest size, 300- to 500-μm spheres. There are two reasons to upsize the particles used. In theory, the smallest particles occlude the smallest intratumoral vessels, and it should then be possible to move to the next size to occlude upstream vessels. In addition, it has been demonstrated that it takes a larger volume of smaller particles to occlude a given vascular bed.[17] Because the particles are mixed with contrast, embolization of large tumors can require administration of a significant amount of contrast if only small particles are used; moving to larger spheres limits the contrast load and duration of procedure. If more than one vessel supplies the tumor, the catheter is placed sequentially into the next vessels to be embolized and embolization begun again with the smallest 40- to 120-μm spheres. Once again, if there is persistent antegrade flow after 10 mL of the 40- to 120-μm spheres have been injected, embolization is continued with the next largest size, 100- to 300-μm spheres, and so on until all target vessels have been embolized to stasis. Stasis as a hard end point is defined as lack of antegrade flow observed for at least 5 heartbeats[18] with lack of opacification

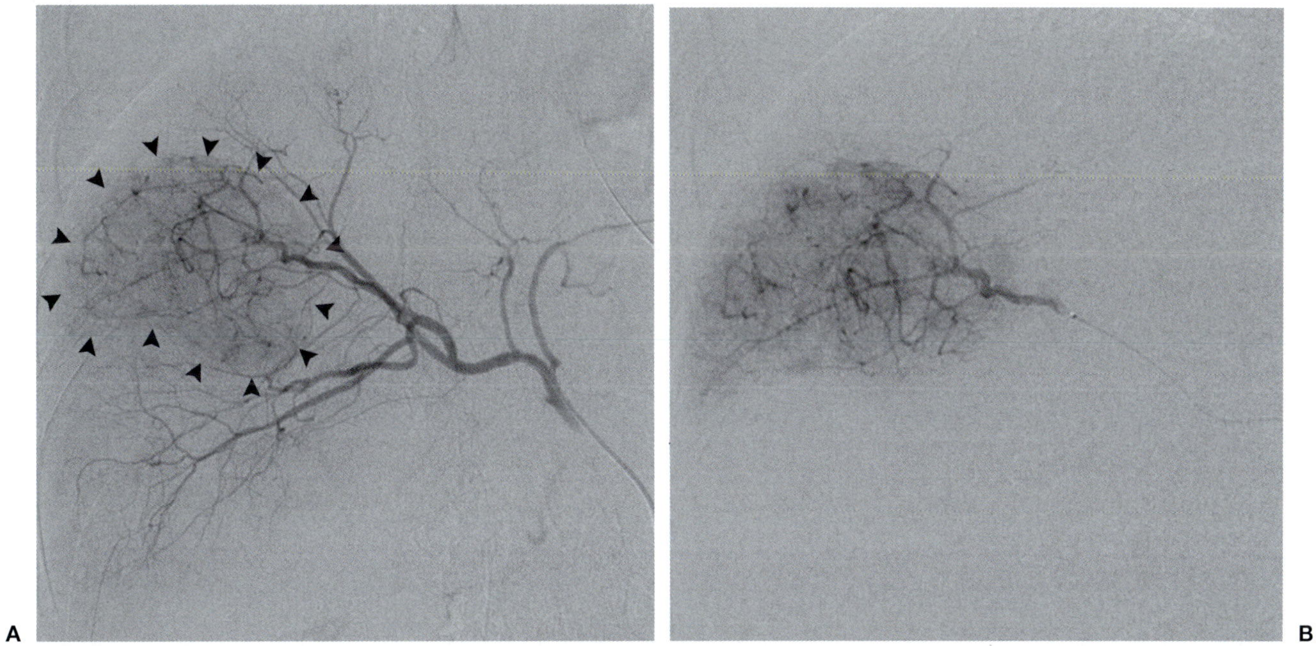

Figure 34.1 **A:** Selective injection into right hepatic artery demonstrates all branches of proper hepatic artery: left hepatic, middle (segment 4) hepatic, cystic, and right hepatic arteries. The hypervascular tumor is easily identified (*arrowheads*). **B:** Superselective injection into posterior division branch of right hepatic artery better delineating hypervascular tumor.

of the target vessel on postembolization digital angiography (Fig. 34.3). On occasion, antegrade flow is maintained by development of what have come to be called "embolization sinks," or spaces within the tumor where contrast pools despite the tumor vessels being completely occluded (Fig. 34.4).

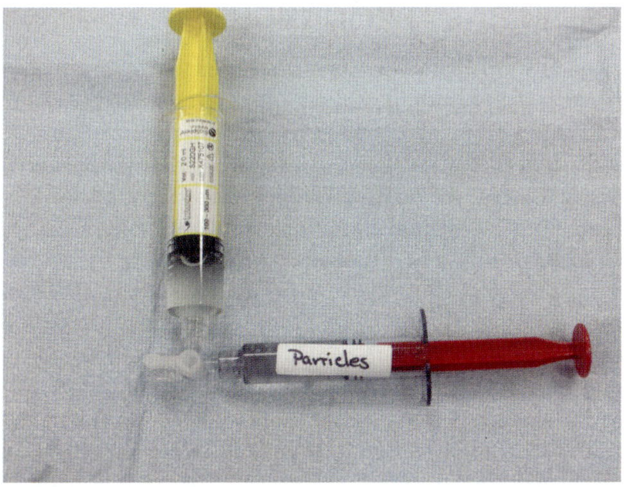

Figure 34.2 Demonstrates set up with Embosphere Microspheres in saline diluted 1:1 with contrast on one Luer connector and 6-mL red Medallion syringe attached to another that will be used to deliver embolic agent through catheter, which will be attached to available male Luer connector.

In this case, a small amount of PVA may be added to stabilize the end point.

The entire liver is never embolized at once because of the risk of hepatic failure. Patients who have multifocal disease necessitating treatment of both left and right hemilivers to treat the entire tumor burden have only one hemiliver embolized initially. They are brought back for the second embolization to complete the treatment cycle in 3 to 6 weeks depending on their recovery from the first embolization session. Embolization of individual segments on the right and left side of the liver during one embolization session is acceptable as long as the total volume of liver treated is not excessive. For example, one might treat a tumor in the anterior division of the right liver by embolizing segments 5 and 8 along with segment 4 on the left because tumors occurring on the anterior right/segment 4 border often have supply originating from both right and left hepatic arteries.

Noncontrast computed tomography (CT) performed immediately after HAE can provide information regarding the completeness of the embolization that is also prognostic. Contrast is retained within the treated tumor (Fig. 34.5) and both the degree of contrast retention as well as absence of defects in contrast retention have been shown to predict response to treatment.[19] This information is also useful for suggesting the presence of other blood supply to the tumor that has not been treated and might be treated either at the same time or planned for the future. This is particularly helpful in the case of supply from extrahepatic vessels because

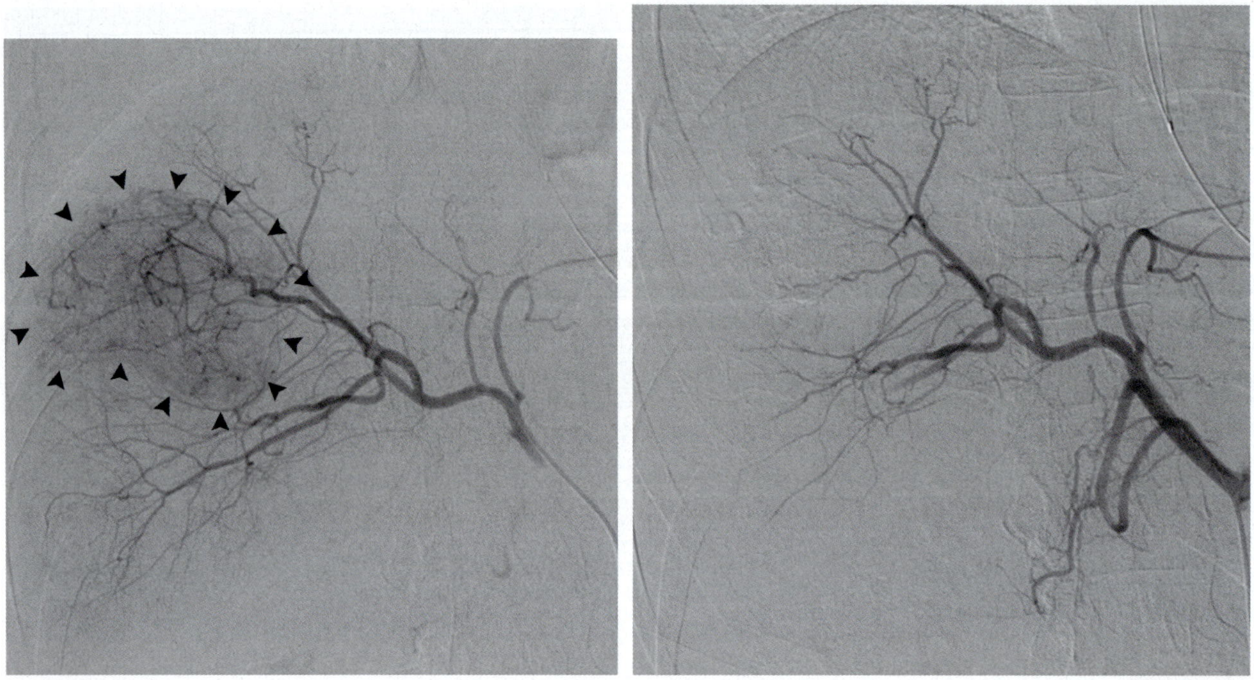

Figure 34.3 **A:**. Selective injection into right hepatic artery, same patient as in Figure 34.1. The hypervascular tumor is easily identified (*arrowheads*). **B:**. Same selective right hepatic artery injection following embolization demonstrating complete stasis within treated territory with complete lack of opacification of the target vessel and no evidence of tumor neovascularity.

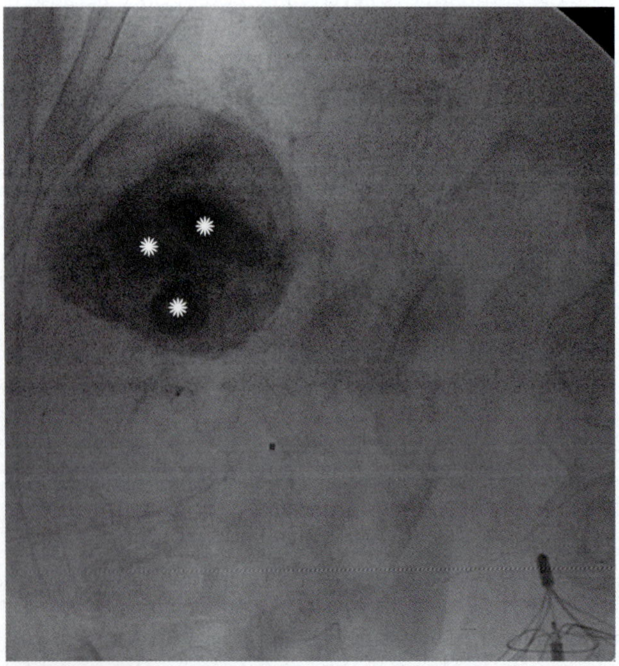

Figure 34.4 Photospot demonstrating appearance of "embolization sinks" that sometimes occur during the course of treatment. Note multiple "contrast pools" (*asterisks*).

supply from other hepatic arteries can often be demonstrated on the arteriogram obtained following embolization of the branch(es) already treated.

CLINICAL APPLICATIONS

Hepatic arterial embolization can be used to treat any hypervascular liver tumor, including but not limited to HCC and metastases from neuroendocrine tumor. HAE can also be used to treat hypervascular breast, sarcoma, renal cell carcinoma, thyroid, and ocular melanoma metastases. It has never been evaluated in gastrointestinal adenocarcinomas that are typically relatively hypovascular, such as hepatic metastases from colorectal cancer. It can be used in several different clinical settings. First, with curative intent, embolization can be used in an attempt to completely treat hepatic tumor in the case of patients with a single or a few small tumors limited to the liver without extrahepatic disease. Second, palliative embolization is useful for patients with pain related to tumor bulk or hormonal symptoms in the case of patients with metastatic neuroendocrine tumor, for instance. Finally, embolization can be used in an effort to prolong survival in patients who are not candidates for surgical resection, based on extent of disease or underlying cirrhosis/portal hypertension, by preventing progression of hepatic tumor. Embolization is indicated in patients with good performance status

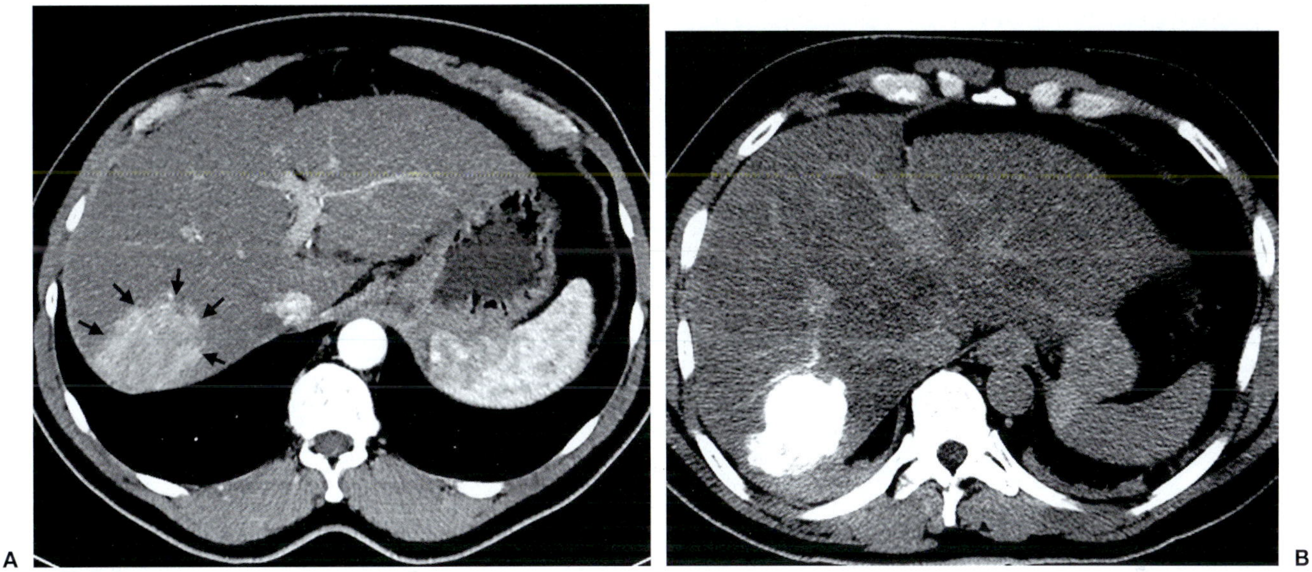

Figure 34.5 **A:** Pretreatment arterial phase CT from the same patient whose angiogram is shown in Figures 34.1 and 34.3. Note the hypervascular tumor located in the segment 7 right liver (*arrows*). **B:** Noncontrast CT performed immediately after embolization demonstrates contrast retention within the treated tumor with excellent retention of and good coverage with contrast; no defects in contrast retention are seen.

(0 or 1) and should not be employed in patients with significant comorbidities or underlying liver disease such as in patients with Child-Pugh class C cirrhosis/portal hypertension whose overall survival is typically dictated by their liver disease and not their tumor. Patients with poor liver function are also at increased risk for postembolization liver failure and other complications.[20,21]

After HAE, follow-up multiphase CT or magnetic resonance imaging is obtained approximately 4 weeks after complete treatment of the initial tumor burden. The treated tumor should be completely nonenhancing on the arterial phase scans (Fig. 34.6) and low density on the portal venous phase (Fig. 34.7); they are typically smaller as well. This scan serves as the new baseline scan for making future treatment decisions.

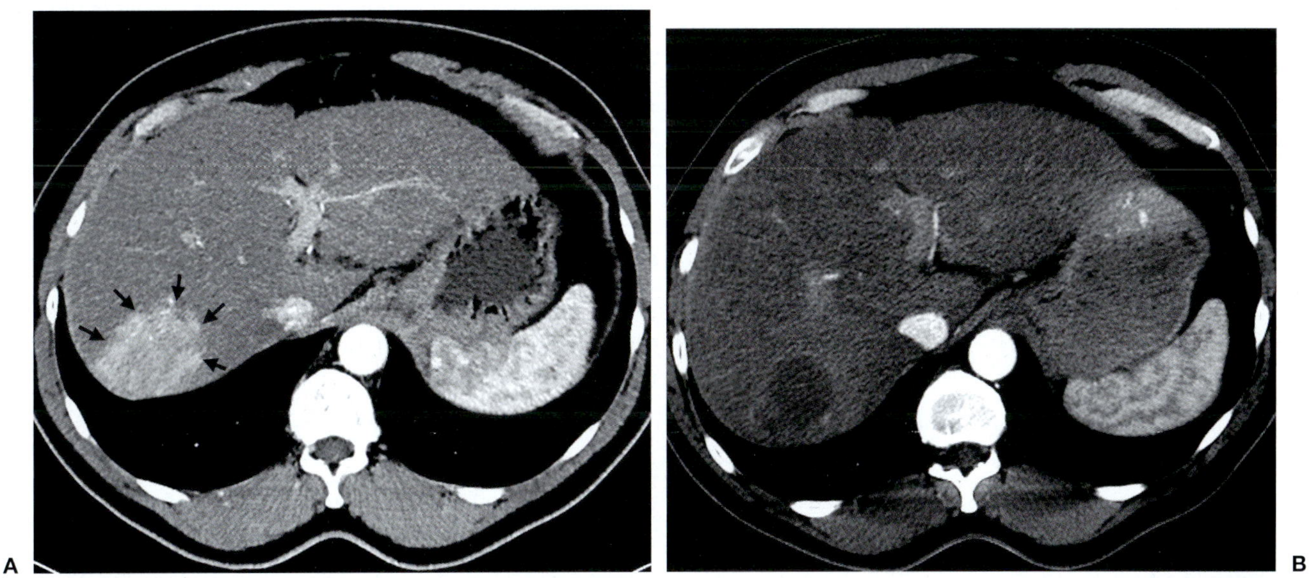

Figure 34.6 **A:** Pretreatment arterial phase CT from the same patient in Figures 34.1, 34.3, and 34.5. **B:** Posttreatment arterial phase CT 4.5 weeks following embolization at comparable level with complete lack of enhancement and decrease in size of tumor.

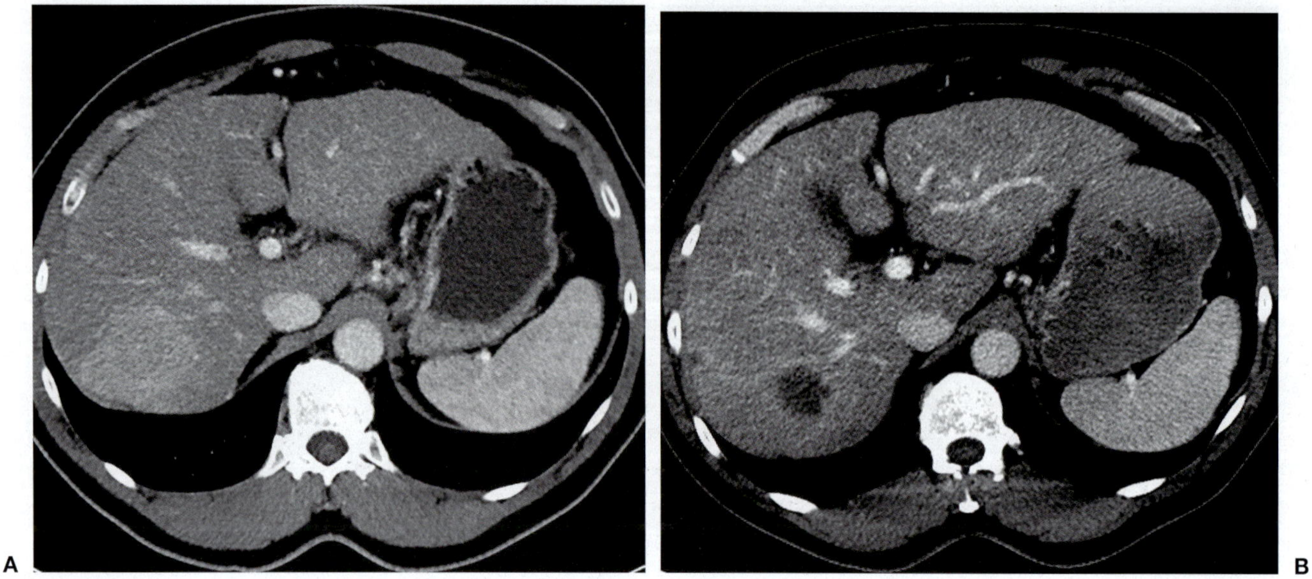

Figure 34.7 **A:** Pretreatment portal venous phase CT. **B:** Posttreatment portal venous phase CT 4.5 weeks following embolization at comparable level demonstrates decrease in size of tumor.

POTENTIAL COMPLICATIONS

Most patients develop postembolization syndrome (PES) consisting of some combination of pain, nausea/vomiting, and fever. PES symptoms usually abate over 24 to 48 hours. Elevation of liver enzymes is seen beginning the day after embolization but peaking on the second or third day posttreatment. The liver enzymes usually return to baseline with 1 month. Complications related to angiography such as vessel dissection and groin hematoma can also occur. Liver abscess is a rare but serious complication of HAE that is seen most commonly in patients with previous bilioenteric anastomosis (BEA) or any reason for compromise of the sphincter of Oddi, including preexisting biliary drainage catheter, biliary stent, or previous sphincterotomy. In a review of over 2,000 embolization procedures in 971 patients, Mezhir[22] found that 33% (11/34) of patients with BEA developed a postprocedure liver abscess compared to 1 of 916 (0.1%) patients with an intact sphincter. Liver abscess can occur in this setting despite a prolonged course of antibiotics in the periprocedural period. Postembolization liver failure or death are exceedingly rare, occurring in less than 1% of patients with proper patient selection.[21] Embolization of small particles into the pulmonary circulation via shunting to systemic veins, one of the most dreaded complications of this procedure given its often fatal outcome, can occur[23] and is best avoided by upsizing microsphere size in tumors larger than 10 cm, large tumors high in the dome adjacent to the hemidiaphragm, tumors invading the hepatic veins, or with unexpected early hepatic vein drainage demonstrated angiographically as outlined previously.

TIPS AND TRICKS

Objective or Problem	Tip or Trick
How to avoid surprises during embolization procedure?	Carefully review recent multiphase CT/MRI prior to procedure: identify target, know the arterial anatomy, and anticipate nonhepatic arterial supply.
Completely evaluate arterial anatomy angiographically, even with excellent pretreatment multiphase imaging.	Always begin with celiac and superior mesenteric artery angiography.
Do not underestimate underlying liver disease.	Get good portal phase angiographic imaging for direction of portal flow; cannot get that from CT.
Difficult celiac?	Start with Cobra (Angiodynamics, Latham, New York), then use Simmons 2 catheter, which will usually reach into common hepatic artery so at least seated in "parent" vessel.

Objective or Problem	Tip or Trick
Where to reform Simmons?	Avoid cerebrovascular accident territory; use 65 cm Simmons 2 catheter and reform over aortic bifurcation.
How to save contrast?	Use road mapping or blend mask.
How not to mix up syringes used for embolization with those used for control angiography?	Use color-coded syringes for embolization material, flush, and contrast during embolization (Fig. 34.8).

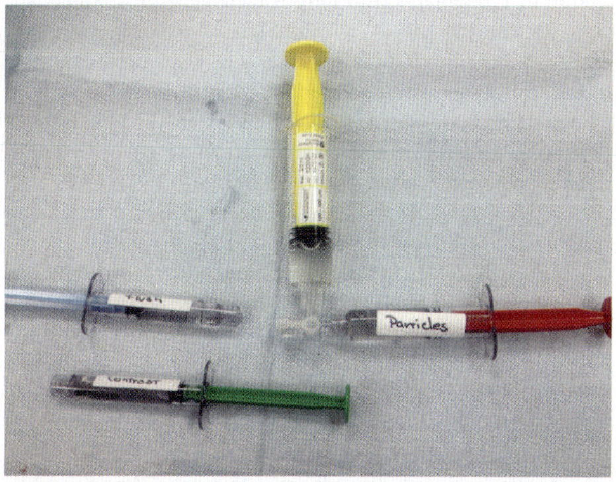

Figure 34.8 Color-coded and labelled syringes used for embolization. Embolization agent is delivered using *red syringe*, whereas flush is in *blue syringe* and contrast in *green syringe*. The microspheres come prepackaged in 20-mL syringes and color of those syringes varies depending on size microsphere being used but are easily distinguished by 20-mL size.

Objective or Problem	Tip or Trick
How to maximize intratumoral embolization?	Begin with smallest microspheres and move to next largest size after using 10 mL in any vessel.
Avoid dissection of or bubbles in vessel to be embolized.	Always advance catheters over guidewires and make sure you have blood return or backbleeding from catheter before you inject.
Persistent antegrade flow after tumor vessels occluded?	Stabilize embolization end point (get to "stasis") using 100-μm PVA.
Continued flow into embolization "sink"?	Get to stasis with 100-μm PVA.
How to mix PVA?	Add 10-mL full-strength contrast to vial (1 mL) of PVA; shake/mix. May need to add more contrast for small inner diameter coaxial catheters to avoid catheter occlusion.
Tumor in "watershed area" like 8/4 border?	Even if tumor appears to be totally supplied by one vessel, always study the "other" vessel before quitting.
Tumor located adjacent to hemidiaphragm or high in dome of liver?	Always study phrenic artery selectively.
Do you see prominent intercostal vessels on preembolization arterial phase CT?	Study those intercostals.
How do you find phrenic artery?	Find on preprocedure arterial phase imaging. Phrenic can arise from left of aorta or be reconstituted from renal or adrenal arteries.

REFERENCES

1. Breedis C, Young G. The blood supply of neoplasms in the liver. *Am J Pathol.* 1954;30(5):969–977.
2. Charnsangavej C, Chuang VP, Wallace S, et al. Work in progress: transcatheter management of primary carcinoma of the liver. *Radiology.* 1983;147(1):51–55.
3. Yamada R, Sato M, Kawabata M, et al. Hepatic artery embolization in 120 patients with unresectable hepatoma. *Radiology.* 1983;148(2):397–401.
4. Takayasu K, Shima Y, Muramatsu Y, et al. Hepatocellular carcinoma: treatment with intraarterial iodized oil with and without chemotherapeutic agents. *Radiology.* 1987;163(2):345–351.
5. Konno T. Targeting cancer chemotherapeutic agents by use of lipiodol contrast medium. *Cancer.* 1990;66(9):1897–1903.
6. Egawa H, Maki A, Mori K, et al. Effects of intra-arterial chemotherapy with a new lipophilic anticancer agent, estradiol-chlorambucil (KM2210), dissolved in lipiodol on experimental liver tumor in rats. *J Surg Oncol.* 1990;44(2):109–114.
7. Raoul JL, Heresbach D, Bretagne JF, et al. Chemoembolization of hepatocellular carcinomas. A study of the biodistribution and pharmacokinetics of doxorubicin. *Cancer.* 1992;70(3):585–590.
8. Johnson PJ, Kalayci C, Dobbs N, et al. Pharmacokinetics and toxicity of intraarterial adriamycin for hepatocellular carcinoma: effect of coadministration of lipiodol. *J Hepatol.* 1991; 13(1):120–127.
9. Simonetti RG, Liberati A, Angiolini C, et al. Treatment of hepatocellular carcinoma: a systematic review of randomized controlled trials. *Ann Oncol.* 1997;8(2):117–136.
10. Lo CM, Ngan H, Tso WK, et al. Randomized controlled trial of transarterial lipiodol chemoembolization for unresectable hepatocellular carcinoma. *Hepatology.* 2002;35(5):1164–1171.
11. Llovet JM, Real MI, Montana X, et al. Arterial embolisation or chemoembolisation versus symptomatic treatment in patients with unresectable hepatocellular carcinoma: a randomised controlled trial. *Lancet.* 2002;359(9319):1734–1739.
12. Camma C, Schepis F, Orlando A, et al. Transarterial chemoembolization for unresectable hepatocellular carcinoma: meta-analysis of randomized controlled trials. *Radiology.* 2002; 224(1):47–54.
13. Lee KH, Liapi E, Vossen JA, et al. Distribution of iron oxide-containing Embosphere particles after transcatheter arterial embolization in an animal model of liver cancer: evaluation with MR imaging and implication for therapy. *J Vasc Interv Radiol.* 2008;19(10):1490–1496.
14. Maluccio MA, Covey AM, Porat LB, et al. Transcatheter arterial embolization with only particles for the treatment of unresectable hepatocellular carcinoma. *J Vasc Interv Radiol.* 2008; 19(6):862–869.
15. Erinjeri JP, Salhab HM, Covey AM, et al. Arterial patency after repeated hepatic artery bland particle embolization. *J Vasc Interv Radiol.* 2010;21(4):522–526.
16. Brown KT. Fatal pulmonary complications after arterial embolization with 40-120- micro m tris-acryl gelatin microspheres. *J Vasc Interv Radiol.* 2004;15(2, pt 1):197–200.
17. Stampfl S, Bellemann N, Stampfl U, et al. Arterial distribution characteristics of Embozene particles and comparison with other spherical embolic agents in the porcine acute embolization model. *J Vasc Interv Radiol.* 2009;20(12):1597–1607.
18. Chrisman HB, Minocha J, Ryu RK, et al. Uterine artery embolization: a treatment option for symptomatic fibroids in postmenopausal women. *J Vasc Interv Radiol.* 2007;18(3):451–454.
19. Wang X, Erinjeri JP, Jia X, et al. Pattern of retained contrast on immediate postprocedure computed tomography (CT) after particle embolization of liver tumors predicts subsequent treatment response. *Cardiovasc Intervent Radiol.* 2013;36(4): 1030–1038.
20. Chung JW, Park JH, Han JK, et al. Hepatic tumors: predisposing factors for complications of transcatheter oily chemoembolization. *Radiology.* 1996;198(1):33–40.
21. Raoul JL, Sangro B, Forner A, et al. Evolving strategies for the management of intermediate-stage hepatocellular carcinoma: available evidence and expert opinion on the use of transarterial chemoembolization. *Cancer Treat Rev.* 2011;37(3):212–220.
22. Mezhir JJ. Pyogenic abscess after hepatic artery embolization: a rare but potentially lethal complication. *J Vasc Interv Radiol.* 2011;22(2):177–182.
23. Brown KT. Re: Fatal pulmonary complications after arterial embolization with 40-120-microm tris-acryl gelatin microspheres. *J Vasc Interv Radiol.* 2004;15(8):887–888.

35

Oil-Based Chemoembolization

Marcus Presley • Daniel B. Brown

Hepatocellular carcinoma (HCC) remains a uniformly lethal disease process in the absence of curative procedures such as transplantation or resection. Okuda et al.[1] described a median survival of 1.6 months for untreated patients in 1984. The dismal prognosis for patients with HCC is largely unchanged, with a median survival of 3 months reported in a prospectively evaluated group in 2005.[2] For decades, no systemic therapies were available and resection remains largely infeasible given the nearly universal presence of cirrhosis. In 1975, a series of 14 patients treated with systemic doxorubicin for HCC with 3 responders was reported.[3] A similar 16.6% response rate was identified in a 42-patient cohort in 1977.[4] Intra-arterial doxorubicin was then studied, and when infusion was performed with embolization, survival was extended to 19 months.[5,6] These reports spurred interest in further development of chemoembolization of HCC.

Several randomized trials were performed in the 1990s without evidence of benefit from chemoembolization. These studies had various flaws in their construction, including treatment of patients at timed intervals rather than based on imaging findings, poor patient selection, limited sample size unlikely to demonstrate statistical benefit, and inappropriate choice of embolic agents such as coils which limited the ability to retreat patients.[7–10]

In 2002, two prospective randomized trials were published demonstrating that in appropriately selected patient populations, chemoembolization resulted in superior survival compared to symptomatic treatment. Lo et al.[11] randomized 80 patients to either chemoembolization with cisplatin, Lipiodol, and gelfoam or best supportive care with survival as the primary end point. Patients were carefully selected with exclusion of individuals with advanced cirrhosis or macroscopic vascular invasion. Survival rates at 1, 2, and 3 years following chemoembolization were 57%, 31%, and 26%, respectively, compared to 32%, 11%, and 3% for supportive care (P = .002). Llovet et al.[12] performed a three-arm trial comparing chemoembolization, bland embolization, and best supportive care in a total of 112 patients with a primary end point of survival. The trial was halted when the chemoembolization group reached superiority versus supportive care with 1- and 2-year survivals of 82% and 63%, respectively, compared to 63% and 27% (P = .025). The outcomes from these two studies lent significant credibility to the practice of chemoembolization.

DEVICE/MATERIAL DESCRIPTION

Oily chemoembolization is one of the most cost-effective treatment options in all of interventional oncology. The cost of the chemotherapy, Lipiodol, and embolic is much less than drug-eluting beads or yttrium 90 (^{90}Y) microspheres. A challenge when comparing outcomes from different studies is the tremendous variation in embolics, chemotherapeutic agents, and how these tools are combined in a given procedure. This issue is further clouded by the absence from the marketplace of some of the widely reported agents over the last decade. At various times, Ethiodol, powdered cisplatin, and powdered doxorubicin have been unavailable. As a result of the mentioned variables, standardization of chemoembolization has been difficult to achieve.

The embolic agent of choice varies by study. In the previously mentioned randomized trials of Lo et al.[11] and Llovet et al.,[12] gelfoam was the embolic agent. Other authors have used polyvinyl alcohol with a transition to use of calibrated embolic microspheres as they became available.[13–15] However, direct comparisons of outcomes in oily chemoembolization with different embolic agents are sparse. One review compared gelfoam powder with polyvinyl alcohol and Ethiodol and resulted in nearly identical survival: 519 ± 80 days for gelfoam powder versus 511 ± 75 days for polyvinyl alcohol (P = .93).[16]

Literature comparing different chemotherapy regimens is more plentiful. Of note, no prospective randomized trial has identified a statistically significant difference in targeted outcomes when comparing regimens[17–23] (Table 35.1). One

Table 35.1 Findings in Trials Comparing Chemotherapy Drugs for Chemoembolization

Reference	Study Type	Drugs	Total Patients	Outcome Measures	Findings
Nonsignificant Findings ($P > .05$ between regimens)					
Kawai et al.[24]	Prospective randomized	Epirubicin/Ethiodol versus DE	415 patients	Overall survival	1-, 2-, 3-y survival: Epirubicin/Ethiodol: 69%, 44%, 33% DE: 73%, 54%, 37% ($P = .2296$)
Lammer et al.[18]	Prospective randomized	DEB versus DE	201 total: 93 DEB 108 doxorubicin	6-mo response	Complete response: 27% DEB versus 22% DE Partial response: 25% DEB versus 21% DE Disease control: 63% DEB versus 52% DE ($P = .11$)
Sahara et al.[19]	Prospective randomized	Epirubicin, cisplatin, mitomycin C, 5-fluorouracil (multidrug) versus epirubicin	51 total: 24 multidrug versus 27 epirubicin	1- and 2-y survival Time to progression Radiographic response	1- and 2-y survival: Multidrug: 95% and 65% Epirubicin: 85% and 76% Time to progression: Multidrug: 6.1 mo Epirubicin: 8.7 mo Radiographic response: Multidrug: 54% Epirubicin: 48%
Significant Findings ($P < .05$ between regimens)					
Yodono et al.[17]	Retrospective	Epirubicin versus cisplatin	202 total: 96 cisplatin 106 epirubicin	Overall survival	1-, 2-, 3-y survival: Cisplatin: 88.5%, 71.8%, 62.4% Epirubicin: 83.0%, 57.9%, 36.5% ($P = .0052$)
Song et al.[20]	Case-control matched	DEB versus DE or epirubicin/Ethiodol	40 total: 20 DEB 20 DE or epirubicin/Ethiodol	Objective tumor response by mRECIST	85% response for DEB 30% response for DE or epirubicin/Ethiodol ($P = .001$)
Kamada et al.[22]	Retrospective	Cisplatin versus DE	133 total: 108 cisplatin 26 DE	Overall survival	1-, 3-, 5-y survival Cisplatin: 81%, 41%, 19% DE: 67%, 18%, 0% ($P < .05$)
Lammer et al.[18]	Prospective randomized subgroup	DEB versus DE	135 total	Disease control at 6 mo with ECOG 1, Child-Pugh B, recurrent disease, or bilobar disease	DEB 63% versus DE 32% ($P = .026$)
Iwazawa et al.[41]	Retrospective	Miriplatin versus epirubicin	111 total: 64 epirubicin 47 miriplatin	Local control at 6 and 12 mo	Epirubicin: 83.4% and 69.2% Miriplatin: 70.7% and 44.8% ($P < .001$)
Dhanasekaran et al.[21]	Retrospective	DEB versus CDM	71 total: 45 DEB 26 cisplatin/doxorubicin/mitomycin C	Overall survival	DEB: 610 d median CDM: 284 d median ($P = .03$)

Continued

Table 35.1 Findings in Trials Comparing Chemotherapy Drugs for Chemoembolization *(continued)*

Reference	Study Type	Drugs	Total Patients	Outcome Measures	Findings
Significant Findings ($P < .05$ between regimens)					
Petruzzi et al.[23]	Retrospective	DE versus CDM versus DEB	122 total: 59 DE 30 CDM 33 DEB	Tumor response Progressive disease	Tumor response: DE: 51% CDM: 84% ($P = .003$) DEB: 82% ($P = .004$) Progressive disease: Doxorubicin: 37% CDM: 13% ($P = .02$) DEB: 9% ($P = .004$)

DE, doxorubicin and Ethiodol; DEB, drug-eluting beads; mRECIST, modified Response Evaluation Criteria In Solid Tumors; ECOG, Eastern Cooperative Oncology Group; CDM, cisplatin, doxorubicin, mitomycin C, and Ethiodol.
Reprinted with permission from Petruzzi NJ, Frangos AJ, Fenkel JM, et al. Single-center comparison of three chemoembolization regimens for hepatocellular carcinoma. *J Vasc Interv Radiol*. 2013;24(2):266–273. Copyright 2013, with permission from Elsevier.

prospective study compared epirubicin to doxorubicin without any difference in survival identified at 1, 2, or 3 years.[24] Given the intermittent unavailability of powdered doxorubicin, this finding suggests that epirubicin could be an adequate alternative.

A final consideration is timing the addition of embolics to the chemotherapy/oil mixture. A comparison of various approaches was compared by Geschwind et al.[25] They studied the percentage of intended chemotherapy that could be infused as well as the subsequent arterial patency in a treated area. Patients received one of three regimens: chemotherapy, oil, and polyvinyl alcohol particles simultaneously; chemotherapy and oil followed by polyvinyl alcohol; or chemotherapy and oil followed by gelfoam. When the embolic was mixed simultaneously with the chemotherapy and oil, both the intended percentage of chemotherapy to be infused as well as the subsequent arterial patency was lower than when embolics were added following oil/chemotherapy infusion. Outcomes for polyvinyl alcohol and gelfoam were similar regarding percentage of chemotherapy delivery (75.3% polyvinyl alcohol vs. 80.6% gelfoam) and subsequent arterial patency (74% polyvinyl alcohol vs. 81% gelfoam).

The delivery equipment is relatively standard for interventional radiology laboratories and includes arterial sheaths, selective catheters, and microcatheters. For patients with HCC, selection of segmental and subsegmental arteries is typically performed, making microcatheters a necessity for most, if not all, procedures. Microcatheters with 0.027-in lumens can perform diagnostic angiography as well, tolerating power injection rates up to 4 mL per second. The ability to perform high-quality angiography via the microcatheter is supplemented by the expanding use of C-arm computed tomography for targeting in this patient population. The viscosity of the chemotherapy and oil can make injection through smaller lumen catheters challenging, another reason to use larger bore devices. The mixture of oil and chemotherapy is toxic and can melt the junction of standard stopcocks and syringes with potential leakage of contents. At the advent of the procedure, glass syringes and metal stopcocks were used to avoid this issue. Currently, we use syringes and stopcocks made of polycarbonate. Although polycarbonate has made chemoembolic suspension less cumbersome, there is still potential for leakage and operators should operate with great care.

TECHNIQUE

Preprocedure Considerations

Patients should have either a dynamically enhanced computed tomography (CT) or magnetic resonance (MR) scan within 4 weeks of treatment. We hydrate patients with approximately 100 mL per hour of normal saline unless there is a history of congestive heart failure or other cardiac disease in which case lower rates are given. Patients are given midazolam and fentanyl for moderate sedation and ondansetron to control nausea. Labs are reviewed the morning of the procedure. When treating HCC, elevated bilirubin is a common scenario secondary to underlying cirrhosis. Historically, patients with total serum bilirubin greater than 2 mg/dL were approached with great caution. With a superselective approach, treatment of a small portion of the liver is possible, allowing for safe treatment in patients with liver dysfunction. Thrombocytopenia is also commonly present in cirrhotics as a consequence of portal hypertension. We do not routinely transfuse platelets as consumption by the engorged spleen will frequently limit the response. Preprocedure antibiotics are not required in patients with intact biliary anatomy (see complications section).

Procedural Considerations

Access to the femoral artery is obtained using the Seldinger technique, and a 6-Fr sheath is placed and connected to a pressurized flush. A 5-Fr selective catheter is used to select the superior mesenteric and celiac arteries and diagnostic arteriography performed. With advances in cross-sectional imaging, aberrant anatomy is frequently identified preprocedure that allows for targeted angiography with smaller volume contrast injections. Following selective angiography of the mesenteric artery, subselection with a microcatheter is performed over a hydrophilic microwire. Repeat digital subtraction angiography (DSA) is performed at the lobar or segmental level depending on the tumor location. If there is concern regarding complete tumor coverage in the selected area, we will perform C-arm CT with the reconstructed images compared to the preprocedure imaging. Once we confirm that the targeted area has been selected, the oil and chemotherapy mixture is suspended via a three-way stopcock. We use 1 mL of oil for each centimeter of tumor diameter up to 15 mL. Following injection of 4 to 6 mL of intra-arterial lidocaine, the suspended mixture is slowly infused using 3-mL syringes under fluoroscopic guidance, ensuring that antegrade flow is maintained. Once the entire mixture is infused, gelfoam slurry is added until the segmental artery reaches near stasis. If stasis is achieved before infusion of the entire slurry of chemotherapy, the gelfoam is added at that time. Final DSA is performed to evaluate for residual tumor enhancement. Our preference is to use closure devices in this patient group to decrease recumbency time due to postprocedural nausea and vomiting and the common incidence of thrombocytopenia. In our experience, success rates with closure devices are not adversely affected in the presence of thrombocytopenia.

Postprocedure Considerations

Patients are admitted overnight for hydration and pain control. Empiric ondansetron (8 mg) is given every 8 hours and a patient-controlled analgesia (PCA) pump is ordered, using Dilaudid 0.1 mg demand dose every 6 minutes without a basal rate. This level of analgesia is sufficient for over 90% of patients. Patients are started on a clear diet that is advanced as tolerated. Labs are rechecked overnight to ensure liver functions remain stable. The key components to discharge the next morning are the ability to tolerate oral intake and pain control with oral medications. During morning rounds, the PCA usage and patient pain scale is assessed. The PCA is discontinued if appropriate and the patient can be discharged following breakfast. We provide instructions on maintaining hydration following discharge and patients are asked to call interventional oncology if they are struggling with oral intake. Many times, early intervention with intravenous fluids in the clinic can avoid readmission. Patients are discharged with oral pain medication when appropriate as well as antiemetics. An appointment is made for follow-up imaging 4 weeks from treatment to assess treatment response.

CLINICAL APPLICATIONS

Chemoembolization is one of the most widely performed procedures for HCC because most patients present with cirrhosis too advanced to consider resection. Additionally, the number of patients requiring liver transplantation far outstrips the available supply of organs. To separate patients by disease status and prognosis, the Barcelona Clinic for Liver Cancer (BCLC) guidelines (Fig. 35.1) have been developed.[26] In a review of over 1,700 patients, BCLC was a better predictor of survival than both alternative scoring systems and serum biomarkers.[27] Survival was also relatively predictable by BCLC stage, with 5-year survival decreasing significantly with each advance in stage (Fig. 35.2).

Applying the criteria, patients without portal hypertension and with normal performance status and small solitary tumor (stage 0) may undergo resection safely, whereas transplantation is used for individuals with up to three tumors when all three are less than 3 cm (stage A). Patients with either larger tumors or a greater numerical burden are referred for chemoembolization (stage B). In the setting of a patient with a lesser performance status, portal venous invasion, and/or metastatic disease (stage C), targeted biologic therapy or a clinical trial may be offered. However, despite these recommendations, in clinical practice, chemoembolization remains widely performed with disease of lesser and greater severity than stage B (Fig. 35.2). Chemoembolization was used in 63% of stage 0, 54% of stage A, and 35.7% of stage C patients.[27] For patients with a lesser burden of disease, treatments such as ablation may be infeasible due to challenging targeting, whereas in advanced disease, the cost of treatments such as sorafenib are considerable. Additionally, studies in patients with advanced disease have raised questions about the value added from biologic therapy.

The cost of biologic therapies is a significant consideration. Considering this factor, Kim et al.[28] reviewed outcomes with sorafenib in advanced disease (BCLC stage C) and compared them to other treatments. There was no difference in overall survival between patients treated with sorafenib (8.4 months) and other therapies (8.2 months; $P > .05$). Sorafenib did provide better survival in patients with extrahepatic disease and infiltrative tumors. Similarly, Pinter et al.[29] described similar time to progression with chemoembolization versus sorafenib (5.3 months vs. 3.8 months; $P = .737$). Overall survival was also not significantly different between treatments (9.2 months for chemoembolization vs. 7.4 months for sorafenib; $P = .377$). Patients with macroscopic portal vein invasion treated with sorafenib did not have improved survival compared to chemoembolization, despite this imaging finding serving as an indication for biologic therapy using the BCLC criteria.

Chemoembolization is frequently used to treat patients to facilitate transplantation. Patients who are within Milan criteria can receive treatment as a bridge to transplantation. Without therapy, the average drop-off rate for

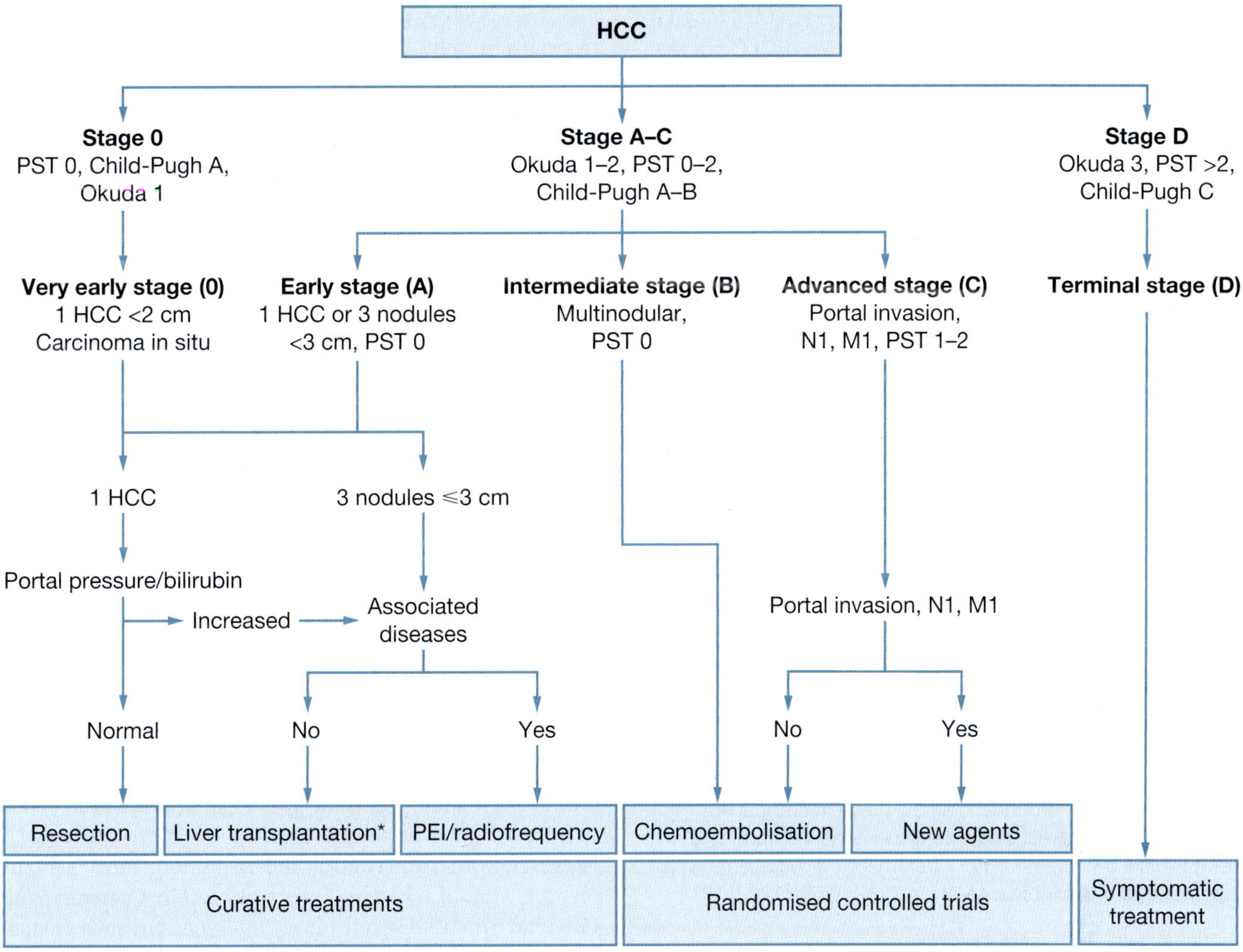

Figure 35.1 The Barcelona Clinic Liver Cancer staging criteria. (Reprinted with permission from Llovet JM, Burroughs A, Bruix J. Hepatocellular carcinoma. *Lancet*. 2003;362[9399]:1907–1917. Copyright 2003, with permission from Elsevier.)

patients diagnosed with HCC within Milan criteria is 17% at 6 months and 32% at 1 year.[30] For patients with prolonged wait times related to wait lists or documentation of sobriety, tumor treatment can potentially decrease the risk of progression and drop-off from the transplant list. Comparing chemoembolized patients to untreated matched controls, Frangakis et al.[31] found an 80% decrease in the drop-off rate from the transplant list.

Chemoembolization has also been used to induce tumor necrosis in patients beyond the Milan criteria to allow listing for transplantation, an approach commonly referred to as *downstaging*. Chapman et al.[32] described successful downstaging in over one-third of stage III patients with eventual liver transplant. Only 1 of 17 transplanted patients developed recurrent disease after surgery, a solitary lung metastasis that was resected. This outcome is comparable to the 31% success rate with chemoembolization described by Lewandowski et al.[33]

Given the relative shortage of donor organs for liver transplantation, chemoembolization ultimately acts as definitive therapy for a great number of patients. Outside of clinical studies, patients treated with chemoembolization are frequently more ill. The study by Llovet et al.[12] included just over 11% (112/908) of screened patients, and the study by Lo et al.[11] enrolled only 21% of potential patients (80/387). Their trials excluded individuals with moderate liver dysfunction and any vascular invasion. Although these criteria are reasonable for a clinical trial, in day-to-day practice, many patients have significantly greater comorbidities. Several retrospective reviews (Table 35.2) provide insight into the expected survival of patients with HCC treated with oily chemoembolization.[13–15,34] These trials produced survivals ranging from 13 to 16 months but included "all comers" such as Child-Pugh B patients or those with vascular invasion. This outcome is not dissimilar to ^{90}Y radioembolization. The largest nonrandomized trial evaluating ^{90}Y included 291 patients.[35] Survival

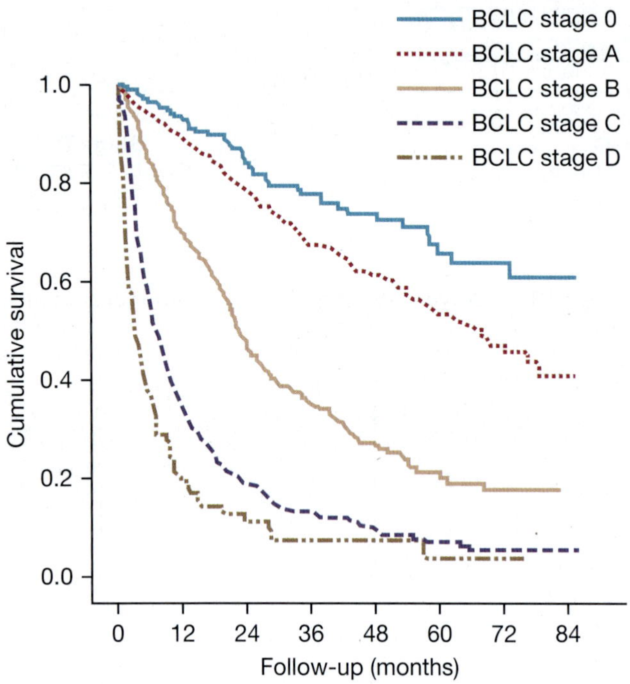

Figure 35.2 Survival of patients with hepatocellular carcinoma distributed by stage using the Barcelona Clinic Liver Cancer criteria. (Reprinted with permission from Kim BK, Kim SU, Park JY, et al. Applicability of BCLC stage for prognostic stratification in comparison with other staging systems: single centre experience from long-term clinical outcomes of 1717 treatment-naïve patients with hepatocellular carcinoma. *Liver Int*. 2012;32[7]:1120–1127.)

for Child-Pugh A and B patients was 17.2 and 7.7 months, respectively, with a time to progression of 7.9 months for the entire group. Two retrospective trials comparing ^{90}Y and chemoembolization have been performed.[36,37] No significant difference in survival was found in either trial. Lance et al.[37] reported 8-month survival with radioembolization versus 10.3 months with chemoembolization in a 73-patient cohort. In 245 treated patients, Salem et al.[36] reported 20.5 months survival for radioembolization versus 17.4 months for chemoembolization. Both trials suggested less toxicity for the patients treated with radioembolization, a factor that may help determine the best route of therapy for patients with lesser performance status at presentation.

POTENTIAL COMPLICATIONS

Complications occur in approximately 10% of patients.[38] Fortunately, most of these are minor. Death is reported following 2% to 3% of all chemoembolizations for all tumor types. The two most common complications in patients with HCC are liver failure, which occurs in 2.3% of patients, and readmission with prolonged postembolization syndrome, which is expected in 2% to 5% of patients.[38] Less common complications include gastrointestinal ulceration, arterial dissection, pulmonary artery oil embolus, or surgical cholecystitis (all $<1\%$). If the oily contrast mixture is inadvertently injected into the cystic artery, patients are more likely to present with prolonged postembolization syndrome.[39] However, with pain control and hydration, most patients recover without requiring intervention. Most patients with HCC have not undergone biliary interventions such as stent

Table 35.2 Survival of Patients Treated with Oily Chemoembolization with Comparison to Outcomes with Yttrium 90 Radioembolization.

Trial	N	Overall Survival	Time to Tumor Progression
Chemoembolization			
Solomon et al.[13]	38	15.5 mo	13.5 mo
Buijs et al.[14]	190	16 mo	
Gomes et al.[15]	124	15.8 mo	
Brown et al.[34]	201	13 mo	9 mo
	132 Child-Pugh A	16 mo	9 mo
	65 Child-Pugh B	9 mo	9 mo
Radioembolization			
Salem et al.[35]	291		7.9 mo
	116 Child-Pugh A	17.2 mo	10.8 mo
	122 Child-Pugh B	7.7 mo	8.4 mo

placement or sphincterotomy that violates the sphincter of Oddi, resulting in colonized bile. In such patients, the risk of abscess formation following treatment is exponentially higher than in those without previous biliary interventions. In this setting, periprocedural antibiotics are universally prescribed and some operators include bowel preparation as well. Our approach is to use moxifloxacin, a fourth-generation fluoroquinolone which is excreted through the bile. Using this approach, Khan et al.[40] reported no abscesses following 25 infusions.

TIPS AND TRICKS

Scenario	Management
A patient with stable chronic borderline liver function has sudden elevation the day of procedure.	Labs in cirrhotic patients can be sensitive to minimal dehydration. If performance status and other labs are unchanged, we will often treat as scheduled and hydrate aggressively. If other labs have worsened or if performance has decreased, proceed with caution (if at all).
A patient with chronic stable borderline liver functions has sudden bilirubin elevation and worsening of other labs the day of the procedure.	This may still be related to hydration issues. Although the procedure for that day may need to be rescheduled, recheck labs in a week when the patient is not on nothing by mouth status.
My patient was treated with chemoembolization and has residual disease at the margin of the tumor. I cannot find the enhancement via DSA or C-arm CT via the hepatic artery.	Strongly consider that an extrahepatic collateral may be the source of the residual enhancement. Common arteries: locations of enhancement include the following: • Inferior phrenic: dome • Intercostal: posterior/lateral • Internal mammary: anterior
The patient I treated yesterday has no pain but cannot eat at rounds.	Continue hydration throughout the morning and reassess at lunch. If tolerated, turn off the intravenous fluids and watch for 2 more hours, then discharge if OK.
A treated patient is calling from home with difficulty eating but is tolerating oral liquids.	Encourage continued hydration. This can include some sports drinks that have added electrolytes.
I was referred a patient with segmental portal vein thrombosis. Can chemoembolization be performed?	Segmental chemoembolization can be safely performed in the setting of normal liver functions.
A patient with tumor treated near the liver dome is calling with intractable pain.	Pain is often caused by capsular distension from postprocedural edema. Consider prescribing low-dose steroids for several days. Our preference is to use a methylprednisolone dose pack.
A patient with tumor treated near the liver dome is calling with intractable hiccups.	Consider prescribing haloperidol as an outpatient. Many patients are hesitant to take this medication, which can be used as a way to determine the severity of symptoms.
Following chemoembolization, a patient calls with excruciating right upper quadrant pain. CT in the emergency room demonstrates oily contrast in the gallbladder lumen.	Nontarget embolization of the gallbladder is typically managed with pain control and hydration. In most cases, nonoperative/noncatheter drainage management is adequate.
During chemoembolization, a branch of the left hepatic artery extends inferiorly and to the left, outside the apparent liver edge.	This finding likely represents a falciform artery. Treatment of this artery may result in skin erythema or necrosis. Options to prevent this include embolization of the branch or placement of an ice pack on the patient's abdomen to induce vasospasm.

REFERENCES

1. Okuda K, Obata H, Nakajima Y, et al. Prognosis of primary hepatocellular carcinoma. *Hepatology*. 1984;4(S1):3S–6S.
2. Yeung YP, Lo CM, Liu CL, et al. Natural history of untreated nonsurgical hepatocellular carcinoma. *Am J Gastroenterol*. 2005;100(9):1995–2004.
3. Olweny CL, Toya T, Katongole-Mbidde E, et al. Treatment of hepatocellular carcinoma with Adriamycin. Preliminary communication. *Cancer*. 1975;36(4):1250–1257.
4. Ihde DC, Kane RC, Cohen MH, et al. Adriamycin therapy in American patients with hepatocellular carcinoma. *Cancer Treat Rep*. 1977;61(7):1385–1387.
5. Wheeler PG, Nunnerley H, Melia WM, et al. The use of therapeutic embolisation at the time of hepatic arteriography in the management of primary tumours of the liver. *Ann Acad Med Singapore*. 1980;9(2):269–273.
6. Bern MM, McDermott W, Cady B, et al. Intraaterial hepatic infusion and intravenous Adriamycin for treatment of hepatocellular carcinoma: a clinical and pharmacology report. *Cancer*. 1978;42(2):399–405.
7. Bruix J, Llovet JM, Castells A, et al. Transarterial embolization versus symptomatic treatment in patients with advanced hepatocellular carcinoma: results of a randomized, controlled trial in a single institution. *Hepatology*. 1998;27(6):1578–1583.
8. Madden MV, Krige JE, Bailey S, et al. Randomised trial of targeted chemotherapy with lipiodol and 5-epidoxorubicin compared with symptomatic treatment for hepatoma. *Gut*. 1993;34(11):1598–1600.
9. Pelletier G, Roche A, Ink O, et al. A randomized trial of hepatic arterial chemoembolization in patients with unresectable hepatocellular carcinoma. *J Hepatol*. 1990;11(2):181–184.
10. Pelletier G, Ducreux M, Gay F, et al. Treatment of unresectable hepatocellular carcinoma with lipiodol chemoembolization: a multicenter randomized trial. Groupe CHC. *J Hepatol*. 1998;29(1):129–134.
11. Lo C-M, Ngan H, Tso W-K, et al. Randomized controlled trial of transarterial lipiodol chemoembolization for unresectable hepatocellular carcinoma. *Hepatology*. 2002;35(5):1164–1171.
12. Llovet JM, Real MI, Montaña X, et al. Arterial embolisation or chemoembolisation versus symptomatic treatment in patients with unresectable hepatocellular carcinoma: a randomised controlled trial. *Lancet*. 2002;359(9319):1734–1739.
13. Solomon B, Soulen MC, Baum RA, et al. Chemoembolization of hepatocellular carcinoma with cisplatin, doxorubicin, mitomycin-c, ethiodol, and polyvinyl alcohol: prospective evaluation of response and survival in a U.S. Population. *J Vasc Interv Radiol*. 1999;10(6):793–798.
14. Buijs M, Vossen JA, Frangakis C, et al. Nonresectable hepatocellular carcinoma: long-term toxicity in patients treated with transarterial chemoembolization—single-center experience. *Radiology*. 2008;249(1):346–354.
15. Gomes AS, Rosove MH, Rosen PJ, et al. Triple-drug transcatheter arterial chemoembolization in unresectable hepatocellular carcinoma: assessment of survival in 124 consecutive patients. *AJR Am J Roentgenol*. 2009;193(6):1665–1671.
16. Brown DB, Pilgram TK, Darcy MD, et al. Hepatic arterial chemoembolization for hepatocellular carcinoma: comparison of survival rates with different embolic agents. *J Vasc Interv Radiol*. 2005;16(12):1661–1666.
17. Yodono H, Matsuo K, Shinohara A. A retrospective comparative study of epirubicin-lipiodol emulsion and cisplatin-lipiodol suspension for use with transcatheter arterial chemoembolization for treatment of hepatocellular carcinoma. *Anticancer Drugs*. 2011;22(3):277–282.
18. Lammer J, Malagari K, Vogl T, et al. Prospective randomized study of doxorubicin-eluting-bead embolization in the treatment of hepatocellular carcinoma: results of the PRECISION V study. *Cardiovasc Intervent Radiol*. 2010;33(1):41–52.
19. Sahara S, Kawai N, Sato M, et al. Prospective evaluation of transcatheter arterial chemoembolization (TACE) with multiple anti-cancer drugs (epirubicin, cisplatin, mitomycin c, 5-fluorouracil) compared with TACE with epirubicin for treatment of hepatocellular carcinoma. *Cardiovasc Intervent Radiol*. 2012;35(6):1363–1371.
20. Song MJ, Park CH, Kim JD, et al. Drug-eluting bead loaded with doxorubicin versus conventional lipiodol-based transarterial chemoembolization in the treatment of hepatocellular carcinoma: a case-control study of Asian patients. *Eur J Gastroenterol Hepatol*. 2011;23(6):521–527.
21. Dhanasekaran R, Kooby DA, Staley CA, et al. Comparison of conventional transarterial chemoembolization (TACE) and chemoembolization with doxorubicin drug eluting beads (DEB) for unresectable hepatocelluar carcinoma (HCC). *J Surg Oncol*. 2010;101(6):476–480.
22. Kamada K, Nakanishi T, Kitamoto M, et al. Long-term prognosis of patients undergoing transcatheter arterial chemoembolization for unresectable hepatocellular carcinoma: comparison of cisplatin lipiodol suspension and doxorubicin hydrochloride emulsion. *J Vasc Interv Radiol*. 2001;12(7):847–854.
23. Petruzzi NJ, Frangos AJ, Fenkel JM, et al. Single-center comparison of three chemoembolization regimens for hepatocellular carcinoma. *J Vasc Interv Radiol*. 2013;24(2):266–273.
24. Kawai S, Tani M, Okamura J, et al. Prospective and randomized trial of lipiodol-transcatheter arterial chemoembolization for treatment of hepatocellular carcinoma: a comparison of epirubicin and doxorubicin (second cooperative study). The Cooperative Study Group for Liver Cancer Treatment of Japan. *Semin Oncol*. 1997;24(2)(suppl 6):38–45.
25. Geschwind JF, Ramsey DE, Cleffken B, et al. Transcatheter arterial chemoembolization of liver tumors: effects of embolization protocol on injectable volume of chemotherapy and subsequent arterial patency. *Cardiovasc Intervent Radiol*. 2003;26(2):111–117.
26. Llovet JM, Burroughs A, Bruix J. Hepatocellular carcinoma. *Lancet*. 2003;362(9399):1907–1917.
27. Kim BK, Kim SU, Park JY, et al. Applicability of BCLC stage for prognostic stratification in comparison with other staging systems: single centre experience from long-term clinical outcomes of 1717 treatment-naïve patients with hepatocellular carcinoma. *Liver Int*. 2012;32(7):1120–1127.
28. Kim HY, Park J-W, Nam B-H, et al. Survival of patients with advanced hepatocellular carcinoma: sorafenib versus other treatments. *J Gastroenterol Hepatol*. 2011;26(11):1612–1618.
29. Pinter M, Hucke F, Graziadei I, et al. Advanced-stage hepatocellular carcinoma: transarterial chemoembolization versus sorafenib. *Radiology*. 2012;263(2):590–599.
30. Freeman RB, Edwards EB, Harper AM. Waiting list removal rates among patients with chronic and malignant liver diseases. *Am J Transplant*. 2006;6(6):1416–1421.

31. Frangakis C, Geschwind J-F, Kim D, et al. Chemoembolization decreases drop-off risk of hepatocellular carcinoma patients on the liver transplant list. *Cardiovasc Intervent Radiol.* 2011;34(6):1254–1261.
32. Chapman WC, Majella Doyle MB, Stuart JE, et al. Outcomes of neoadjuvant transarterial chemoembolization to downstage hepatocellular carcinoma before liver transplantation. *Ann Surg.* 2008;248(4):617–625.
33. Lewandowski RJ, Kulik LM, Riaz A, et al. A comparative analysis of transarterial downstaging for hepatocellular carcinoma: chemoembolization versus radioembolization. *Am J Transplant.* 2009;9(8):1920–1928.
34. Brown DB, Chapman WC, Cook RD, et al. Chemoembolization of hepatocellular carcinoma: patient status at presentation and outcome over 15 years at a single center. *AJR Am J Roentgenol.* 2008;190(3):608–615.
35. Salem R, Lewandowski RJ, Mulcahy MF, et al. Radioembolization for hepatocellular carcinoma using yttrium-90 microspheres: a comprehensive report of long-term outcomes. *Gastroenterology.* 2010;138(1):52–64.
36. Salem R, Lewandowski RJ, Kulik L, et al. Radioembolization results in longer time-to-progression and reduced toxicity compared with chemoembolization in patients with hepatocellular carcinoma. *Gastroenterology.* 2011;140(2):497–507.e2.
37. Lance C, McLennan G, Obuchowski N, et al. Comparative analysis of the safety and efficacy of transcatheter arterial chemoembolization and yttrium-90 radioembolization in patients with unresectable hepatocellular carcinoma. *J Vasc Interv Radiol.* 2011;22(12):1697–1705.
38. Brown DB, Nikolic B, Covey AM, al. Quality improvement guidelines for transhepatic arterial chemoembolization, embolization, and chemotherapeutic infusion for hepatic malignancy. *J Vasc Interv Radiol.* 2012;23(3):287–294.
39. Leung DA, Goin JE, Sickles C, et al. Determinants of postembolization syndrome after hepatic chemoembolization. *J Vasc Interv Radiol.* 2001;12(3):321–326.
40. Khan W, Sullivan KL, McCann JW, et al. Moxifloxacin prophylaxis for chemoembolization or embolization in patients with previous biliary interventions: a pilot study. *AJR Am J Roentgenol.* 2011;197(2):W343–W345.
41. Iwazawa J, Ohue S, Hashimoto N, et al. Local tumor progression following lipiodol-based targeted chemoembolization of hepatocellular carcinoma: a retrospective comparison of miriplatin and epirubicin. *Cancer Manag Res.* 2012;4:113–119.

36

Chemoembolization with Drug-Eluting Beads

Julius Chapiro • Rafael Duran • Jean-François Geschwind

Primary liver cancer is the third most common cause of cancer-related death worldwide. Asia continues to be the region with the most cases of hepatocellular carcinoma (HCC), but increasing incidences have been reported in Europe and North America, primarily due to the concomitant rise in hepatitis C infection.[1] As most patients are diagnosed at advanced stages, therapeutic options remain limited and represent an oncologic challenge with a dismal prognosis. Over the past three decades, the importance of catheter-based intra-arterial therapies in the management of primary liver cancer patients with more advanced disease (intermediate to advanced) has continued to grow. This trend is mainly due to their tremendous advantages over systemic chemotherapy. The dual benefit of reduced systemic toxicity combined with effective local tumor control helped to include some procedures into the National Comprehensive Cancer Network treatment guidelines. Moreover, the success of intra-arterial therapies contributed to the formation of interventional oncology, a new subdiscipline within interventional radiology, unifying specialists in multidisciplinary teams of physicians from multiple specialities bound by the same desire to tackle primary liver cancer.[2] In this regard, transarterial chemoembolization (TACE) is one of the most frequently used and most exhaustively studied modalities.

A fairly recent development of advanced drug delivery systems such as drug-eluting beads (DEBs) provided an additional option for controlling drug release to tumors and paved the way for the DEB-TACE procedure. This technique was introduced to the majority of interventional radiologists less than 10 years ago. In DEB-TACE, the oily medium used for conventional TACE (cTACE) has been substituted for a polymer-based microsphere, which results in enhanced drug delivery to the tumor and further reduction in systemic drug exposure.[3] As a result, there has been a growing interest in using DEB-TACE to treat patients with HCC, and some trials combine this modality with systemically administered targeted agents to maximize the benefits of both therapies. This development has led to a shift away from cTACE toward DEB-TACE in the treatment of patients with HCC, especially in the United States and Europe.[3,4] In this chapter, we will describe the scientific rationale for DEB-TACE, discuss materials and techniques used for this procedure, and show the most recent clinical evidence for safety and efficacy of this modality. Finally, we will touch on the combination of DEB-TACE with systemically administered targeted agents.

MATERIALS

The general concept of TACE was originally introduced by Yamada et al.,[5] who exploited HCC's preferential blood supply from the hepatic artery for the local delivery of chemotherapy. The advent of DEBs further improved on the ability of cTACE to deliver higher concentration of drugs directly to liver tumors while significantly reducing the serum concentration of chemotherapy and thereby minimizing systemic toxicities.[6] Two major types of drug-eluting microsphere, LC Beads (DC Beads in Europe; Biocompatibles UK Ltd., Farnham, Surrey, United Kingdom) and QuadraSpheres (HepaSpheres in Europe; Merit Medical Systems, Inc., South Jordan, Utah), are available clinically in the United States. However, neither of the products is approved as a drug-delivery microsphere by the U.S. Food and Drug Administration (FDA) but rather as embolic material.

Most of the clinical data has been generated with the LC Beads. These beads are made of nonbiodegradable materials, such as polyvinyl alcohol (PVA) hydrogel that has been modified by the addition of sulfonic acid–containing components. The microspheres are soft, compressible, spherical particles that can be loaded with doxorubicin or irinotecan.[7,8] When polymerized, they can formulate different sizes, ranging from 75 to 900 μm. The smaller bead diameters achieve a more distal embolization and more extensive necrosis as compared with larger beads and are more commonly used.[9] The manufacturer defines the maximum loading capacity for doxorubicin as 40 mg/mL hydrated LC Beads, yet a loading of 25 mg/mL was recommended out of technical considerations.[10] Pharmacokinetic studies have demonstrated that drug elution occurs gradually and only in an ionic environment once the microspheres are delivered to the targeted tumor, which further underlined the pharmacokinetic difference between this targeted therapy and cTACE. Beads with larger diameters (700 to 900 μm) seem to release doxorubicin more slowly than the smaller beads.[11] The continuous release of doxorubicin from LC Beads to the tumor tissue has been demonstrated in several animal experiments.[6,12] Furthermore, histopathologic analysis described the high efficiency of DEB-mediated drug delivery and release to the tumor tissue, causing local coagulative necrosis and an inflammatory fibrotic tissue.[13]

The other types of microspheres (QuadraSphere/HepaSphere microspheres) consist of superabsorbent polymer (SAP), a nonbiodegradable material which is hydrophilic and highly absorbent. These spheres have the ability to absorb fluids up to 64 times their dry state volume and thus to expand their volume to a size of up to 800 μm. These microspheres can be loaded with doxorubicin, epirubicin, and cisplatin for drug delivery.[14] In summary, it is safe to say that the technical evidence clearly is in favor of the use of DEBs, but its general acceptance worldwide as a possible replacement for cTACE has not yet been officially endorsed.

PATIENT SELECTION/ CONTRAINDICATIONS

To date, DEB-TACE has been used in various clinical settings for palliative treatment of patients with unresectable primary liver cancer. Furthermore, it has been successfully used as an adjunctive option before tumor resection or as a bridge to orthotopic liver transplantation[15] (Fig. 36.1). In general, DEB-TACE can be indicated in patients with liver-dominant, unresectable HCC. However, the selection of patients must be based on the presence of adequate liver function, sufficient performance status (Karnofsky index, Eastern Cooperative Oncology Group performance status [ECOG]), and the absence of extrahepatic spread.[16] Table 36.1 summarizes the most important and universally valid contraindications for TACE procedures, which includes DEB-TACE. Because DEB-TACE is still relatively new and lacks sufficient clinical data, the list of exclusion criteria is more extensive as compared to cTACE.

TECHNIQUE AND RECOMMENDATIONS

All TACE procedures share a common approach. Following, we describe the Johns Hopkins Hospital technique for DEB-TACE using LC Bead microspheres, which is in agreement with the results of a consensus meeting held during the European Conference on Interventional Oncology[17] in 2012:

1. Evaluation: Initially, multiple diagnostic angiographic steps are performed to define the hepatic arterial anatomy, assess the blood supply to the tumor, and determine portal venous patency.
2. Catheter positioning: According to the latest recommendations, whenever possible, a 2-Fr microcatheter is placed for selective (fourth-order branch) to superselective (segmental or even subsegmental) injection (Fig. 36.2). DEBs (LC Beads), which have been preloaded with 100 mg of doxorubicin in the central oncology pharmacy, are suspended in equal volume of nonionic contrast medium (1:1) and left for 2 to 3 minutes to become homogeneously distributed within the syringe.
3. Injection: Up to 4 mL of the DEBs (loaded with 25 to 37.5 mg of doxorubicin per milliliter of beads) are administered by alternating injections of aliquots of the beads and contrast until complete delivery or when the blood flow of the feeding artery slowed down. The injection of DEBs should be performed slowly under fluoroscopic guidance to ensure that there is no reflux. Rotation of the syringe is also recommended to prevent sedimentation of the material. No injection of iodized oil (Lipiodol or Ethiodol) is required.
4. Embolization end point: Substantial arterial flow reduction to the tumor is the technical end point, whereas complete occlusion is avoided. This is essential to maintain the arterial pathway for retreatment. Repeated DEB-TACE sessions are recommended, and in our institution, an average of two treatments per target lesion is usually necessary to complete a cycle.

POTENTIAL COMPLICATIONS

Various clinical trials confirmed the overall safety of TACE procedures. The reported systemic adverse effects include nausea, vomiting, bone marrow aplasia, renal failure, and, potentially, cardiac toxicity. The self-limiting postembolization syndrome (PES) includes nausea, vomiting, fever, right upper quadrant pain, and increased white blood cell count. These symptoms reflect the effects of tumor necrosis, acute cytokine release, and systemic exposure to chemotherapeutic

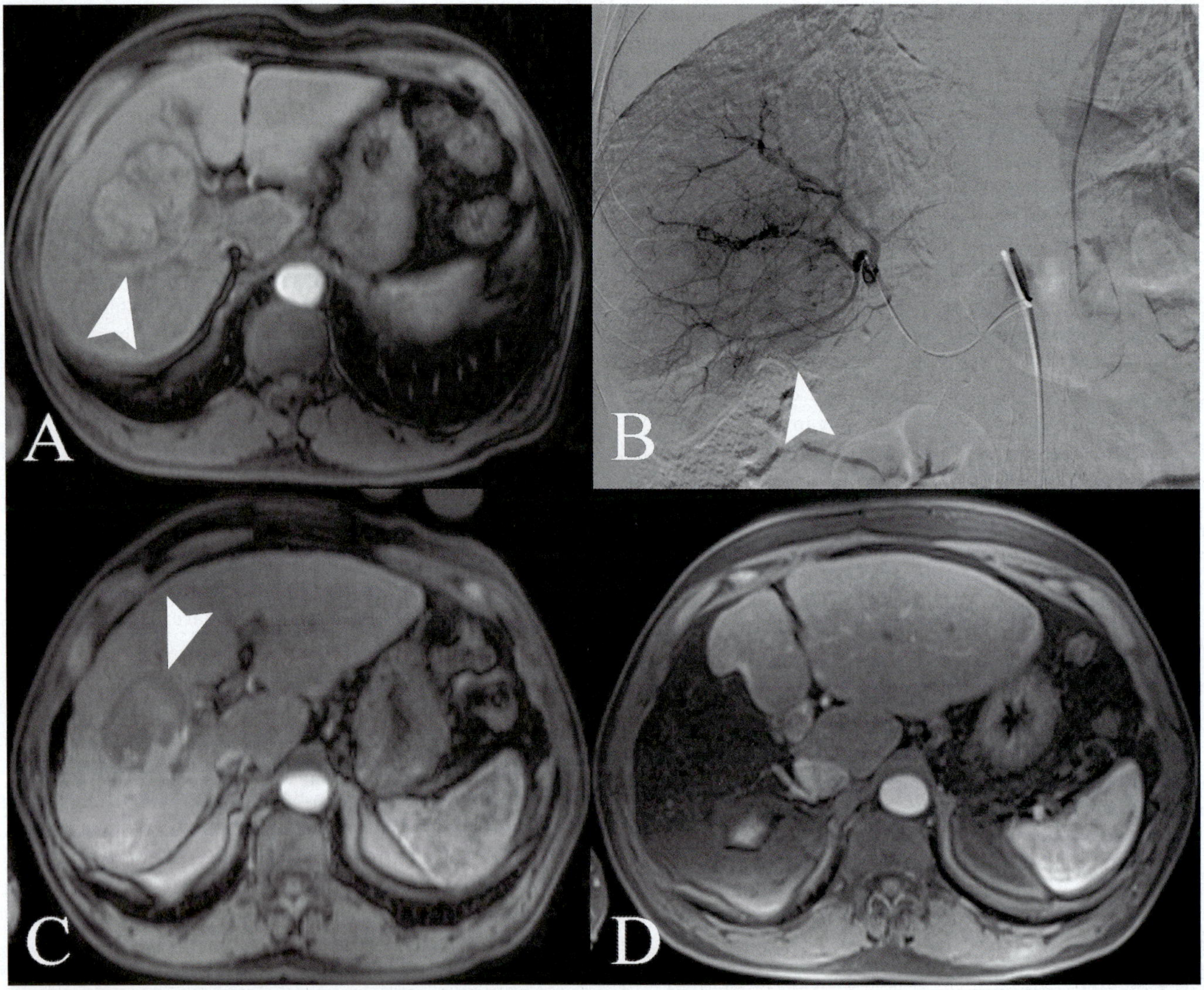

Figure 36.1 DEB-TACE before surgical resection (downstaging). A patient with a 7-cm HCC lesion in the right lobe of the liver. **A:** Baseline MRI shows a homogenous enhancement of the target lesion (*arrowhead*). **B:** Angiogram of the right hepatic artery shows a tumor blush (*arrowhead*). **C:** Follow-up MRI 1 month after treatment shows a largely necrotic lesion (*arrowhead*). **D:** MRI after surgical resection of the right lobe.

agents.[18,19] The use of DEBs has contributed to a significant decrease in systemic toxicities after TACE, and the PES following DEB-TACE is not as intense as following cTACE. The systemic side effects of DEB-TACE using doxorubicin range from alopecia and skin discoloration to mucositis and bone marrow suppression. Cholecystitis and liver abscess may occur less frequently. Periprocedural mortality is seen in less than 1% of cases.[20]

In one of the few studies of its kind, a prospective, randomized single-center phase II trial from Belgium thoroughly investigated plasma peak concentrations of doxorubicin after DEB-TACE using SAP microspheres in comparison with cTACE. As a result, patients treated with SAP microspheres showed significantly lower plasma peak concentrations and less systemic toxicities.[21] These results were confirmed for LC Beads by a multicenter, randomized, prospective phase II trial, which compared the safety and toxicity of DEB-TACE to that of cTACE in HCC patients. Here, the DEB-TACE procedure showed a significantly better toxicity profile than cTACE. This was true in terms of the overall frequency of treatment-related adverse effects as well as the toxicity grades and the severity of the adverse events. Analysis of true toxicity incidence revealed the presence of significant events only in 11.8% of patients treated with DEB-TACE versus 25.9% of patients treated with cTACE. More importantly, major liver toxicities were also lower in DEB-TACE as compared

Table 36.1 Absolute and Relative Contraindications for Transarterial Chemoembolization

Absolute Contraindications	Relative Contraindications[a]
■ Tumor resectability	■ Biliary obstruction
■ Intractable systemic infection	■ Serum bilirubin >3 mg/dL
■ Uncorrectable bleeding disorder	■ **BCLC stage C (vascular invasion including segmental portal obstruction)**
■ Uncorrectable contrast sensitivity	■ Lactate dehydrogenase >425 U/L
■ Leukopenia (white blood cell count <1,000/μL)	■ Aspartate aminotransferase >5 times higher than the upper limit of normal
■ Cardiac or renal insufficiency	■ **Tumor burden involving >50% of the liver**
■ Hepatic encephalopathy	■ Extrahepatic metastases
■ ECOG performance status >3	■ **Mild or severe ascites**
	■ Recent variceal bleeding
	■ Thrombocytopenia
	■ Intractable arteriovenous fistula
	■ Surgical portocaval anastomosis

[a]Specific contraindication for DEB-TACE in bold.

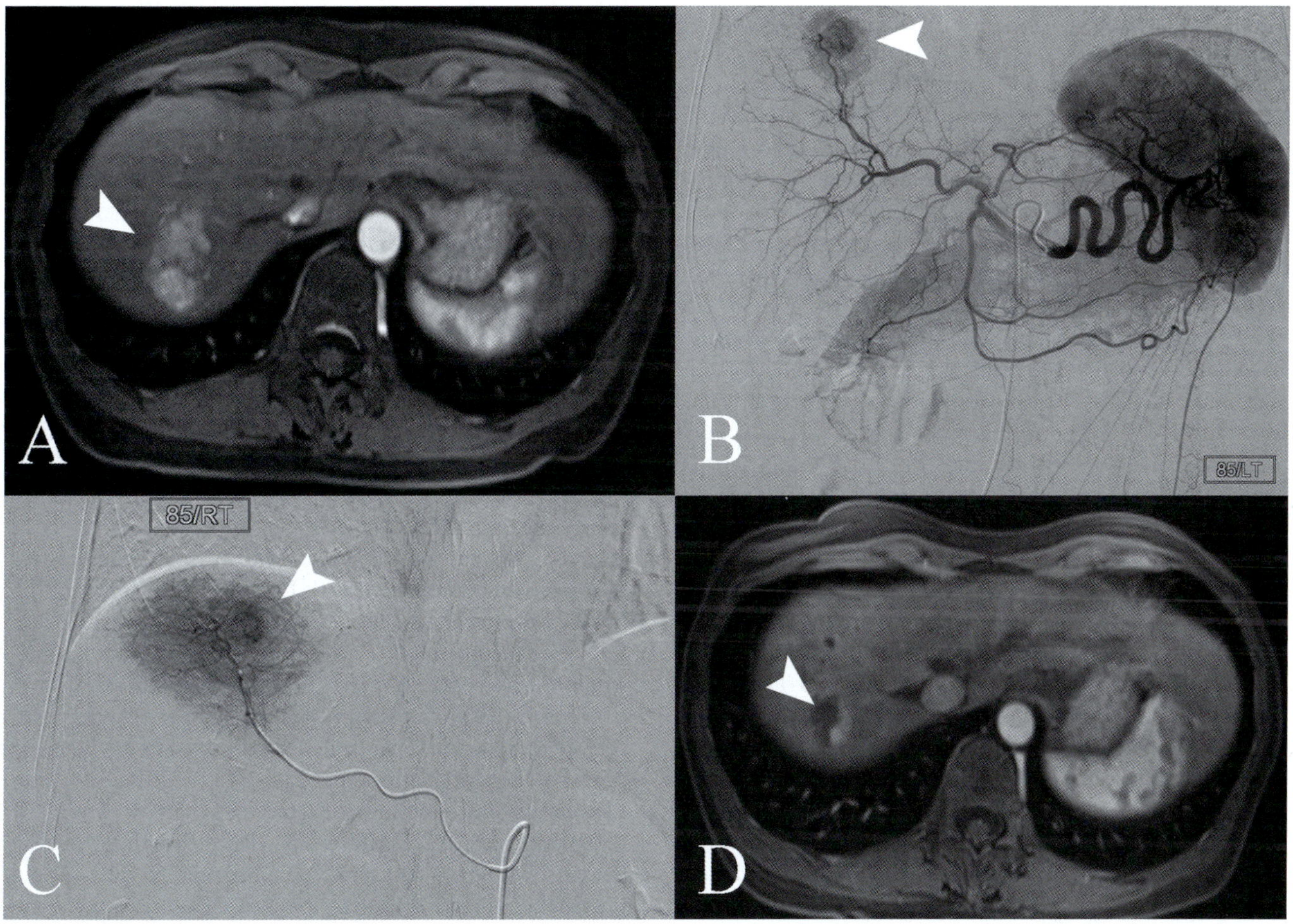

Figure 36.2 Superselective DEB-TACE. A patient with an HCC of the right liver lobe. **A:** Baseline MRI shows a well-enhancing lesion on arterial-phase images (*arrowhead*). **B:** Angiogram of the celiac trunk shows a tumor blush (*arrowhead*) of the target lesion with a well-contrasted tumor-feeding artery. **C:** Superselective angiogram of the tumor-feeding artery before embolization. The superselective angiographic run demonstrates the tumor blush (*arrowhead*). **D:** Follow-up MRI shows good tumor response after treatment (*arrowhead*).

to cTACE.[3] In conclusion, both studies confirmed that DEB-TACE is both safe and generally better tolerated by patients than cTACE.

OUTCOMES

The advent of DEBs has led to a number of trials using this new drug delivery system for TACE procedures. The first FDA-sanctioned experience with DEB-TACE in the United States was designed as a prospective phase II pilot study with the goal to evaluate safety, efficacy, as well as progression-free survival and overall survival in 20 mostly cirrhotic (80%) patients with unresectable HCC. Most of the treated patients were staged as Child-Pugh A (75%), whereas 12 patients (60%) were classified as Barcelona Clinic Liver Cancer (BCLC) stage C. According to the European Association for the Study of the Liver (EASL) criteria, 64% of the patients were classified as responders and 30% achieved complete response after an overall 34 sessions. As for safety, only modest toxicities were reported in all patients, once again confirming the advantages of DEB-TACE over cTACE. After 6 months, only 1 patient showed progressive disease according to the Response Evaluation Criteria In Solid Tumors (RECIST). The median overall survival of 26 months in most advanced patients (BCLC stage C) confirmed the potential of DEB-TACE as a better alternative than cTACE.[4]

The important PRECISION V study included 15 international centers and enrolled a large number of patients for a prospective, randomized phase II trial. The goal of this trial was to directly compare the safety and efficacy of cTACE to those of DEB-TACE. A total of 212 patients were randomized 1:1 and 201 patients received treatment according to standardized protocols. The two treatment groups were stratified according to ECOG performance status and the Child-Pugh class. As a result, patients in the DEB-TACE group showed better imaging response to treatment according to EASL criteria than those in the cTACE group. Although at the 6-month follow-up time point (the end point of the study) the complete response rate was nearly identical between the two groups (26.6% and 22.2% complete response in the DEB-TACE and cTACE groups, respectively), the rate of progressive disease was significantly lower in the DEB-TACE than in the cTACE group (32.3% vs. 40.7%).[3] Of note, this trial was not designed to compare overall survival between the two groups of patients, which is required to fully confirm the potential of DEB-TACE as a true alternative to cTACE.

The lack of survival studies in DEB-TACE was addressed by one of the longest follow-up studies available to date with DEB-TACE. Confirming the great promise of DEB-TACE, a prospective multicenter study from Greece included 173 unresectable HCC patients to assess long-term clinical outcome. Results revealed a 5-year survival of 29.4% and 12.8% for Child-Pugh class A and B, respectively.[22] These latest data on DEB-TACE clearly show the potential of that therapy. In an attempt to compare overall survival in patients treated with DEB-TACE with outcomes after cTACE, a retrospective trial included a total of 71 patients with unresectable HCC, 63% of whom received DEB-TACE and 37% cTACE treatment. As a result, median overall survival of patients treated with DEB-TACE was 610 days versus 284 days in the cTACE group, suggesting a survival advantage of DEB-TACE over cTACE. However, the results of this study must be interpreted with great caution because of the highly inhomogeneous groups and a lack of strict inclusion criteria. In summary, prospective randomized trials will be needed to deliver definitive data on patient survival before fully including DEB-TACE in the official guidelines. As of today, it is safe to say that DEB-TACE is better tolerated than cTACE with a clearly better toxicity profile.

DEB-TACE IN COMBINATION WITH SYSTEMIC TREATMENT

The main antitumor effects of both cTACE and DEB-TACE are due to a combination of ischemia and direct chemotherapy-induced cytotoxicity. The capability of chemoembolization to cause massive tumor destruction has been well demonstrated in multiple radiopathologic correlation studies[23]; however, tumor recurrence is frequently encountered. It has been postulated that the reason for tumor recurrence is the stimulation of neoangiogenic pathways that are significantly upregulated within 36 hours of TACE. The molecular mechanism behind this reaction is likely triggered by hypoxia within the tumor tissue caused by embolization of the tumor-feeding arteries. Indeed, molecular surrogate markers of tumor hypoxia including hypoxia-inducible factor-1 alpha (HIF-1α) as well as vascular endothelial growth factor (VEGF) are upregulated after TACE procedures, suggesting direct stimulation of angiogenesis.[24,25] As a result of these findings, inhibiting the angiogenic pathway during treatment with TACE seems to be logical. Multiple approaches to target this mechanism have been discussed. One such approach uses the drug sorafenib, a multikinase inhibitor with strong antiangiogenic properties, in combination with DEB-TACE. In this way, the proangiogenic changes induced by embolization within the tumor would possibly be counterbalanced by sorafenib, which would be used as a "partner" for TACE.[26] Of note, sorafenib has shown to significantly prolong patient survival over placebo in a randomized controlled trial that led to the FDA approval of the drug for patients with HCC, making sorafenib the very first systemically applicable drug to improve survival in patients with HCC.[27] Given this scientific rationale and the demonstrated impact of sorafenib on patient survival, several prospective clinical trials have been designed (and many are still underway) to assess the potential of this truly unique combination. The following paragraphs will summarize the results of the most important trials.

In one of the first FDA-sanctioned experiences with the combination of DEB-TACE and sorafenib in the United States, a single-center prospective phase II trial was conducted to evaluate the safety and efficacy of concurrent sorafenib and DEB-TACE therapy. A total of 35 individuals with unresectable HCC were enrolled. Major inclusion criteria were an ECOG performance status of 0 to 1, Child-Pugh liver function up to B7, and patients with segmental portal vein thrombosis (BCLC stage C). Patients were treated on a 6-week cycle regimen, in which one cycle consisted of 400 mg sorafenib twice daily, initiated 7 days before the first DEB-TACE. The 35 patients were treated with a total of 128 cycles of therapy. All patients received DEB-TACE and the mean dose of doxorubicin decreased over time: cycle one, 75 mg; two, 60 mg; three, 49 mg. Safety and toxicity were defined as the primary end points of this study, whereas efficacy was the secondary end point. All patients experienced at least one treatment-related toxicity during cycle one. However, most toxicities were minor and only 17% of all toxicities were grade 3 to 4. According to EASL criteria, 58% of the patients showed objective tumor response and the disease control rate was 100%, with no patient showing progression. This study was the first to confirm the safety profile of the DEB-TACE/sorafenib combination.[26] It must be noted that sorafenib was given continuously through the planned DEB-TACE treatments, making the treatment protocol of this trial truly unique. Most other trials used sorafenib either in an interrupted or sequential manner with TACE. As for the secondary end point of this trial, the published data also demonstrated promising survival outcomes and follow-up studies will answer more questions.

An international attempt to investigate the role of the combination of DEB-TACE with sorafenib was the first multicenter phase II randomized, double-blind, placebo-controlled clinical trial ("SPACE" = Sorafenib or Placebo in Combination with DEB-TACE for Intermediate-Stage HCC). This comprehensive trial, which enrolled patients across 85 centers in Europe, North America, and Asia, was recently presented (not yet published). Here, a total of 307 eligible patients were randomized to receive either sorafenib (n = 154) or placebo (n = 153) in combination with DEB-TACE. The dosage was similar to the trial described earlier and patients received a dose of 400 mg sorafenib twice daily or a matching placebo continuously on cycle duration of 4 weeks. All patients received DEB-TACE within the first week after the first dose of sorafenib/placebo and subsequently on day 1 of cycle 3, 7, and 13, respectively. The primary end points of this study were efficacy (specifically, the time to tumor progression [TTP]) and safety. The secondary end points were overall survival, time to vascular invasion, as well as other surrogate markers of tumor progression. As a result, median TTP was 169 days in the sorafenib group and 166 days in the placebo group, itself a rather unexpectedly moderate result. When further stratified, TTP at the 25th and 75th percentile was 112 days/88 days and 285 days/224 days in the sorafenib and placebo groups, respectively. Interestingly, the hazard ratios were low, favoring the combination treatment over the placebo arm. However, the overall preliminary results were somewhat disappointing as no statistically significant benefits regarding overall survival and TTP were shown.[28]

Multiple further trials are underway combining DEB-TACE as well as cTACE with sorafenib. It might be very well possible that the answer about the combination of sorafenib and TACE will be provided by the only phase III trial that is already underway in the United States. This randomized, double-blind, controlled multicenter trial which was proposed by one of the cooperative oncology groups (E1208) will compare the outcomes of DEB-TACE with or without sorafenib in HCC patients with or without vascular invasion (NCT01004978). The results of this trial should be available at the end of 2014.

TIPS AND TRICKS

- Preference is to use a glide Simmons 1 (Terumo, Tokyo, Japan) for selective catheterization of the superior mesenteric artery (SMA) and celiac axis. In most instances, there is no need for a flush aortogram. One can proceed directly to the visceral angiograms.
- Do the SMA run first to identify possible arterial supply to the liver from the SMA and confirm portal vein patency.
- It is critically important to recognize the arterial anatomy and make sure selective catheter placement is performed distal to potentially "dangerous" vessels such as omental or peritoneal branches, right gastric artery, and other small gastric or periduodenal arteries. Inadvertent administration of beads to any of these vessels may cause significant complications, hence the extra care in identifying and avoiding them.
- For centrally located liver tumors, evaluate bilateral blood supply by performing contrast runs from both hepatic arteries.
- Be aware that tumors identified on cross-sectional imaging (magnetic resonance imaging [MRI] or computed tomography [CT]) as being in the right or left lobe may not be supplied by the corresponding arteries; for example, a tumor located in segment 8 may actually be supplied by the segment 4 branch.
- Always perform a pretreatment dual-phase cone-beam CT as selective microcatheter placement in close proximity to the tumor is essential.
- If available, try to use a dedicated three-dimensional analysis software to help identify the appropriate tumor-feeding arteries and create a road map.
- While attempting to place the microcatheter superselectively by manipulating the guidewire, always make sure to carefully watch the Simmons catheter as well so it does not get displaced back into the aorta (Fig. 36.2C).

- When injecting the DEBs, make sure to suspend the beads frequently to prevent the beads from settling down. Preference is to use a 10-mL syringe and inject the DEBs slowly. The beads should be mixed with contrast in a 1:3–4 ratio for greater visibility once the beads leave the microcatheter. The injection should also be done slowly to ensure forward flow and prevent reflux of the beads along the catheter shaft.
- Always avoid stasis of the main artery to allow retreatment if it is necessary. The end point of the embolization should be 2–5 heartbeats to clear the contrast column or administration of the entire dose. Never add additional bland particles.
- Perform a cone-beam CT scan immediately after DEB-TACE so contrast retention within the tumor(s) can be readily identified. This scan must be done before hemostasis of the common femoral artery is obtained.

CONCLUSION

The use of the DEB-TACE technique in patients with unresectable HCC can be considered as a valuable alternative to cTACE and a potent palliative option. Initial data including several prospective randomized studies that focused on safety as well as phase II trials with efficacy as their end point have shown the benefits of DEB-TACE. It is clear that DEB-TACE is superior to cTACE in terms of local tumor response and the rate of systemic toxicities; however, the results regarding potential survival benefits over cTACE are yet to be reported. As for the combination of DEB-TACE with systemic and targeted therapies, initial trials are inconclusive and more data is needed to answer the innumerous open questions.

REFERENCES

1. Forner A, Llovet JM, Bruix J. Hepatocellular carcinoma. *Lancet.* 2012;379(9822):1245–1255.
2. Schumacher PA, Powell JJ, MacNeill AJ, et al. Multimodal therapy for hepatocellular carcinoma: a complementary approach to liver transplantation. *Ann Hepatol.* 2010;9(1):23–32.
3. Lammer J, Malagari K, Vogl T, et al. Prospective randomized study of doxorubicin-eluting-bead embolization in the treatment of hepatocellular carcinoma: results of the PRECISION V study. *Cardiovasc Intervent Radiol.* 2010;33(1):41–52.
4. Reyes DK, Vossen JA, Kamel IR, et al. Single-center phase II trial of transarterial chemoembolization with drug-eluting beads for patients with unresectable hepatocellular carcinoma: initial experience in the United States. *Cancer J.* 2009;15(6):526–532.
5. Yamada R, Sato M, Kawabata M, et al. Hepatic artery embolization in 120 patients with unresectable hepatoma. *Radiology.* 1983;148(2):397–401.
6. Hong K, Khwaja A, Liapi E, et al. New intra-arterial drug delivery system for the treatment of liver cancer: preclinical assessment in a rabbit model of liver cancer. *Clin Cancer Res.* 2006;12(8):2563–2567.
7. Constantin M, Fundueanu G, Bortolotti F, et al. Preparation and characterisation of poly(vinyl alcohol)/cyclodextrin microspheres as matrix for inclusion and separation of drugs. *Int J Pharm.* 2004;285(1–2):87–96.
8. Qian J, Truebenbach J, Graepler F, et al. Application of poly-lactide-co-glycolide-microspheres in the transarterial chemoembolization in an animal model of hepatocellular carcinoma. *World J Gastroenterol.* 2003;9(1):94–98.
9. Gonzalez MV, Tang Y, Phillips GJ, et al. Doxorubicin eluting beads-2: methods for evaluating drug elution and in-vitro:in-vivo correlation. *J Mater Sci Mater Med.* 2008;19(2):767–775.
10. Lewis AL, Gonzalez MV, Leppard SW, et al. Doxorubicin eluting beads - 1: effects of drug loading on bead characteristics and drug distribution. *J Mater Sci Mater Med.* 2007;18(9):1691–1699.
11. Liapi E, Lee KH, Georgiades CC, et al. Drug-eluting particles for interventional pharmacology. *Tech Vasc Interv Radiol.* 2007;10(4):261–269.
12. Lewis AL, Gonzalez MV, Lloyd AW, et al. DC bead: in vitro characterization of a drug-delivery device for transarterial chemoembolization. *J Vasc Interv Radiol.* 2006;17(2, pt 1):335–342.
13. Namur J, Citron SJ, Sellers MT, et al. Embolization of hepatocellular carcinoma with drug-eluting beads: doxorubicin tissue concentration and distribution in patient liver explants. *J Hepatol.* 2011;55(6):1332–1338.
14. de Luis E, Bilbao JI, de Ciercoles JA, et al. In vivo evaluation of a new embolic spherical particle (HepaSphere) in a kidney animal model. *Cardiovasc Intervent Radiol.* 2008;31(2):367–376.
15. Burrel M, Reig M, Forner A, et al. Survival of patients with hepatocellular carcinoma treated by transarterial chemoembolisation (TACE) using drug eluting beads. Implications for clinical practice and trial design. *J Hepatol.* 2012;56(6):1330–1335.
16. Georgiades CS, Liapi E, Frangakis C, et al. Prognostic accuracy of 12 liver staging systems in patients with unresectable hepatocellular carcinoma treated with transarterial chemoembolization. *J Vasc Interv Radiol.* 2006;17(10):1619–1624.
17. Lencioni R, de Baere T, Burrel M, et al. Transcatheter treatment of hepatocellular carcinoma with doxorubicin-loaded DC Bead (DEBDOX): technical recommendations. *Cardiovasc Intervent Radiol.* 2012;35(5):980–985.
18. Brown DB, Nikolic B, Covey AM, et al. Quality improvement guidelines for transhepatic arterial chemoembolization, embolization, and chemotherapeutic infusion for hepatic malignancy. *J Vasc Interv Radiol.* 2012;23(3):287–294.
19. Dhand S, Gupta R. Hepatic transcatheter arterial chemoembolization complicated by postembolization syndrome. *Semin Intervent Radiol.* 2011;28(2):207–211.
20. Liapi E, Geschwind JF. Transcatheter arterial chemoembolization for liver cancer: is it time to distinguish conventional from drug-eluting chemoembolization? *Cardiovasc Intervent Radiol.* 2011;34(1):37–49.
21. van Malenstein H, Maleux G, Vandecaveye V, et al. A randomized phase II study of drug-eluting beads versus transarterial chemoembolization for unresectable hepatocellular carcinoma. *Onkologie.* 2011;34(7):368–376.

22. Malagari K, Pomoni M, Moschouris H, et al. Chemoembolization with doxorubicin-eluting beads for unresectable hepatocellular carcinoma: five-year survival analysis. *Cardiovasc Intervent Radiol.* 2012;35(5):1119–1128.
23. Mannelli L, Kim S, Hajdu CH, et al. Assessment of tumor necrosis of hepatocellular carcinoma after chemoembolization: diffusion-weighted and contrast-enhanced MRI with histopathologic correlation of the explanted liver. *AJR Am J Roentgenol.* 2009;193(4):1044–1052.
24. Sergio A, Cristofori C, Cardin R, et al. Transcatheter arterial chemoembolization (TACE) in hepatocellular carcinoma (HCC): the role of angiogenesis and invasiveness. *Am J Gastroenterol.* 2008;103(4):914–921.
25. Scartozzi M, Faloppi L, Bianconi M, et al. The role of LDH serum levels in predicting global outcome in HCC patients undergoing TACE: implications for clinical management. *PLoS One.* 2012;7(3):e32653.
26. Pawlik TM, Reyes DK, Cosgrove D, et al. Phase II trial of sorafenib combined with concurrent transarterial chemoembolization with drug-eluting beads for hepatocellular carcinoma. *J Clin Oncol.* 2011;29(30):3960–3967.
27. Llovet JM, Ricci S, Mazzaferro V, et al. Sorafenib in advanced hepatocellular carcinoma. *N Engl J Med.* 2008;359(4):378–390.
28. Lencioni R, LLovet JM, Han G. Sorafenib or placebo in combination with transarterial chemoembolization (TACE) with doxorubicin-eluting beads (DEBDOX) for intermediate-stage hepatocellular carcinoma (HCC): phase II, randomised, double-blind SPACE trial. *J Clin Oncol.* 2012;30(suppl 4; abstr LBA154).

37

Radioembolization

Ryan M. Hickey • Robert J. Lewandowski • Riad Salem

Radioembolization refers to the transcatheter, intra-arterial injection of micrometer-sized embolic particles loaded with the high-dose radioisotope yttrium 90. Radioembolization combines the selective angiographic techniques essential to all embolization procedures with an understanding of radiation administration and safety, including radiation dosimetry and radiation dose modification based on tumor characteristics and the patient's clinical profile.

Radioembolization delivers an internal radiation source and is therefore considered brachytherapy. Whereas the radiosensitive nature of normal liver tissue has limited the role of external beam radiation in the treatment of primary and metastatic hepatic malignancies, radioembolization allows for the safe administration of high and therapeutic doses of radiation. More specifically, the likelihood of developing severe radiation-induced liver disease may exceed 50% for external beam radiation doses greater than 35 to 40 Gy, whereas radiation doses greater than 150 Gy have been safely administered with radioembolization.[1–4]

The high tumoral radiation doses achieved with radioembolization rely on the selective intra-arterial injection of the radioactive particles and the preferential deposition of these particles within tumor as opposed to normal liver tissue due to differences in normal and tumor tissue perfusion. Whereas normal liver parenchyma receives most (75%) of its blood supply from the portal vein, hepatic malignancies, particularly hypervascular tumors such as hepatocellular carcinoma (HCC), derive most of their blood supply from the hepatic arteries.[5,6]

The radioisotope yttrium 90 is irreversibly incorporated into glass or resin microspheres that range in size from 20 to 30 μm (glass) or 20 to 60 μm (resin). Yttrium 90 is a pure beta emitter with a half-life of 64.2 hours and tissue penetration ranging from 2.5 to 11 mm.[7–11] Glass microspheres (TheraSphere; Nordion, Kanata, Ontario, Canada) were approved in 1999 by the U.S. Food and Drug Administration (FDA) under a humanitarian device exemption (HDE) for the treatment of unresectable HCC.[12] Resin microspheres (SIR-Spheres; SIRTeX Medical Limited, New South Wales, Australia) were granted full premarketing approval in 2002 by the FDA for the treatment of unresectable colorectal metastases in conjunction with intrahepatic floxuridine.[13]

PATIENT SELECTION

The patient selection process for yttrium 90 (Y90) radioembolization is multifactorial and involves an assessment of the patient's burden of disease, biochemical profile, and performance status. Ideally, patients should have liver-only disease with a tumor burden comprising less than 70% of the liver volume. There should be adequate hepatic reserve, as indicated by the patient's liver function tests with a bilirubin less than or equal to 2 mg/dL and albumin greater than 3 g/dL. The prothrombin time is a sensitive indicator of hepatic synthetic function and should correspond to a normal international normalized ratio (INR). Cancer-related symptoms should be minimal, corresponding to an Eastern Cooperative Oncology Group (ECOG) score of 0 to 2. Although the presence of portal vein thrombosis (PVT) has been traditionally considered a contraindication to hepatic arterial embolization procedures, radioembolization has been shown to be safe and effective in the setting of partial and branch PVT.[14,15] Radioembolization should be performed with caution in patients who have had intervention or surgery involving the ampulla of Vater due to the risk of developing hepatic abscesses. These patients should receive aggressive antibiotic coverage at the time of the procedure that is continued into the postprocedural period.

TECHNIQUE

Y90 radioembolization is performed on an outpatient basis and involves two separate angiography procedures. An initial mapping angiography is performed, at which time a radioisotope lung shunt fraction is also determined. Y90 microspheres are then administered during a separate treatment angiography.

Due to the frequency of hepatic arterial variants and the propensity of hepatic tumors to exhibit arteriovenous shunting, the mapping angiography and lung shunt fraction calculation are integral to radioembolization. Meticulous visceral and hepatic angiography is required to establish the planned treatment volumes that will be used for radiation dosimetry as well as to identify extrahepatic arterial pathways that could result in devastating toxicities and complications from nontarget radioembolization.

HCC is associated with a relatively high incidence of direct arteriovenous shunts that bypass the tumor capillary bed.[16] The administration of microspheres smaller than these shunts could therefore result in direct shunting of the radioactive microspheres to the lungs, which can cause radiation pneumonitis at sufficient doses.[17]

^{99m}Tc-macroaggregated albumin (MAA) is of similar size to the Y90 microspheres and expected to mirror their distribution, including in pulmonary shunting. ^{99m}Tc-MAA 2 to 4 mCi is administered via the proper, right, or left hepatic artery, depending on the planned treatment site, at the conclusion of the initial angiography. The patient is then transferred to nuclear medicine for acquisition of planar and/or single-photon emission computed tomography (SPECT) gamma camera images that are used to calculate the fraction of administered ^{99m}Tc-MAA activity to arrive in the lungs. It is worth mentioning that the time required to transfer patients from the angiography suite to nuclear medicine is an important factor, as the normal, time-dependent degradation of ^{99m}Tc-MAA over a prolonged period can result in a falsely increased calculation of lung shunting.[18] For the most accurate calculation of lung shunting, it is recommended that the ^{99m}Tc-MAA be administered at the end of the mapping angiography and patients be transferred to nuclear medicine as soon as hemostasis has been achieved at the femoral access site. When lung shunting is identified, the cumulative pulmonary dose must be calculated along with the hepatic treatment doses. Pulmonary doses greater than 30 Gy per treatment or greater than 50 Gy cumulatively have been associated with the development of radiation pneumonitis.[19]

Hepatic arterial anatomy and corresponding treatment volumes are determined with the mapping angiography. Because the administered radiation dose depends on the activity of Y90 administered to a volume of tissue, common variants of hepatic vasculature can significantly alter the treatment plan. For example, in a patient with multinodular HCC limited to the right hepatic lobe, standard anatomy may allow for Y90 administration via the right hepatic artery. However, in the presence of an accessory hepatic artery, which typically perfuses the posterior segments 6 and 7, one injection must be performed via the accessory right hepatic artery according to the volume of segments 6 and 7 while a separate injection must be delivered via the right hepatic artery according to the volume of segments 5 and 8. The target lobar and/or segmental volumes corresponding to the angiographic anatomy are measured from the patient's preceding CT or magnetic resonance imaging (MRI) on a three-dimensional (3-D) workstation.

In addition to treatment planning, the mapping angiography provides a critical opportunity to identify extrahepatic arterial flow, particularly to the gastrointestinal tract, that could result in nontarget radioembolization. These vessels can either be eliminated with coil embolization during the mapping angiography or avoided by alterations in the treatment plan. A left gastric artery may have to be embolized to avoid reflux of Y90 to the stomach during treatment via a replaced or accessory left hepatic artery. The gastroduodenal and right gastric arteries are often prophylactically embolized, particularly when using the more embolic resin microspheres. The relative location of the cystic, supraduodenal, retroduodenal, falciform, and phrenic arteries should also be considered in determining the site of Y90 injection. An in-depth review of angiographic considerations and relevant variant anatomy has been previously published.[20]

A simplified matrix has been described for the treatment planning of patients with unresectable HCC based on the extent of disease and the patient's total bilirubin level.[18] For patients with uninodular disease and a normal bilirubin, Y90 can be administered via a lobar or segmental injection. For patients with uninodular disease but elevated bilirubin, treatment should only proceed if a segmental perfusing vessel can be isolated, resulting in high-dose radiation to the tumor and minimal distribution to the normal liver parenchyma. For patients with multinodular and/or bilobar disease and a normal bilirubin level, staged lobar treatments may be performed. In the setting of abnormal bilirubin and multinodular/bilobar disease, the risk of Y90 treatment may be unacceptably high.

DOSIMETRY

Y90 radiation dosimetry uses volumetric calculations of liver tissue (glass microspheres) or tumor burden and body surface area (resin microspheres). Several different software packages are available to calculate 3-D tissue volumes from triphasic CT or multiphasic contrast-enhanced MRI. Volumetric calculation and treatment planning require a sound understanding of the Couinaud hepatic segments and their anatomic landmarks on cross-sectional imaging.

For glass microsphere (TheraSphere) dosimetry, the volume that is measured and used in the dosimetry calculation is the volume of liver tissue that is perfused by the vessel infused. In other words, it is the volume of the liver segments being perfused by the vessel of interest.

Glass microspheres (TheraSphere) are available in vials of several different activities that are dispensed weekly on Wednesday by the manufacturer (Nordion) and calibrated at 12:00 noon (Eastern Standard Time) of the following Sunday. The microspheres have an approximate activity of 2,500 Bq per sphere.[1]

The recommended activity that should be administered to a tumor-containing hepatic lobe should correspond to a dose between 80 and 150 Gy. Patients with significant cirrhosis should be treated conservatively with doses between 80 and 100 Gy, whereas patients without cirrhosis may be treated at higher doses between 100 and 150 Gy. The most commonly used dose range at our institution is between 100 and 120 Gy. Activity required to deliver the desired dose can be calculated according to the equation:

$$A = \frac{D \times M}{50 \times \left(1 - \frac{\%LSF}{100}\right) \times \left(1 - \frac{\%R}{100}\right)}$$

Activity is measured in GBq infused to the target liver, *D* is the absorbed dose (Gy) to the target liver mass, M (kg). Liver volume (mL) is calculated with 3-D software and converted to mass using a conversion factor of 1.03 mg/mL. Lung shunt fraction (%LSF) is calculated from nuclear medicine images acquired following the initial mapping angiography. Residual activity within the vial (%R) is measured after Y90 administration and approximated to be 2% for pretreatment dosing calculations.[18]

Resin microspheres (SIR-Spheres) are available in 3 GBq vials dispensed three times per week and calibrated at 6:00 pm EST on the date of treatment. Each vial contains 40 to 80 million microspheres with an activity per sphere of 50 Bq.[1]

Resin microsphere dosimetry can be calculated using body surface area and estimates of tumor burden according to the equation:

$$A = BSA - 0.2 + \frac{\%Tumor\ involvement}{100}$$

Activity is GBq infused and BSA is the body surface area in square meters.

For resin microsphere dosimetry calculation, activity is decreased depending on the degree of LSF: less than 10% LSF, no reduction; 10% to 15% LSF, 20% reduction; 15% to 20% LSF, 40% reduction; greater than 20% LSF, no treatment.[18]

CLINICAL OUTCOMES

Several large studies have recently been published describing long-term outcomes following radioembolization in patients with intermediate and advanced stage HCC. Table 37.1 provides a summary of these findings. For context of the natural disease of HCC, meta-analysis of the reported survival rates of untreated HCC patients included in randomized controlled trials revealed 1-year survival rates for intermediate (Barcelona Clinic Liver Cancer [BCLC B]) and advanced (BCLC C) stage HCC of approximately 50% and 25%, respectively[21] (Table 37.1).

The long-term outcomes of a comprehensive, 291-patient cohort of intermediate and advanced stage HCC patients

Table 37.1 Clinical Outcomes following Yttrium 90 Radioembolization for Hepatocellular Carcinoma

	Salem et al[22]	Hilgard et al.[23]	Sangro et al.[24]	Salem et al.[26]	Mazzaferro et al.[25]
Purpose	To assess clinical outcomes of patients treated with Y90	To assess clinical outcomes of patients treated with Y90 in Europe	To evaluate prognostic factors of survival after Y90 in European patients	To compare the effectiveness of Y90 versus cTACE	To provide a prospective assessment of safety and efficacy for Y90 treatment of patients with intermediate and advanced disease
Patients	291	108	325	Y90: 123 TACE: 122	52
Response rate	WHO: 42% EASL: 57%	EASL: 40%	—	Y90: 49% TACE: 36%	WHO: 40% EASL: 40%
TTP (months)	7.9	10	—	Y90: 13.3 TACE: 8.4	11
Survival (months)	Child-Pugh A: 17.2 Child-Pugh B: 7.7	16.4	BCLC A: 24.4 BCLC B: 16.9 BCLC C: 10.0	Y90: 20.5 TACE: 17.4	15

Y90, yttrium 90; cTACE, conventional transarterial chemoembolization; TACE, transarterial chemoembolization; WHO, World Health Organization; EASL, European Association for the Study of Liver; BCLC, Barcelona Clinic Liver Cancer.
Adapted from Salem R, Lewandowski RJ. Chemoembolization and radioembolization for hepatocellular carcinoma. *Clin Gastroenterol Hepatol*. 2013;11:604–611.

were recently reported and is the first study to describe toxicity, imaging, and survival outcomes stratified according to BCLC staging, United Network for Organ Sharing (UNOS) tumor stage, and Child-Pugh classification.[22] Response rates to radioembolization were 42% and 57% according to World Health Organization (WHO) and European Association for the Study of Liver (EASL) criteria, respectively. Time to tumor progression (TTP) was 7.9 months. Child-Pugh A patients benefitted most from radioembolization, whereas Child-Pugh B patients with PVT had poor outcomes. Child-Pugh A patients had better response rates than Child-Pugh B patients, with median survival of 17.2 months and 7.7 months, respectively ($P = .002$). Child-Pugh B patients with PVT had a median survival of 5.6 months.

These outcomes were validated by a subsequent study of 108 patients with advanced HCC, confirming both the reproducibility of Y90 treatment in advanced HCC as well as outcomes equivalent to conventional transarterial chemoembolization (cTACE) and TACE with drug-eluting beads (DEB-TACE).[23] The response rate according to EASL criteria was 40%. TTP was 10.0 months, with median overall survival of 16.4 months.

A 325-patient study has further confirmed long-term survival outcomes stratified by BCLC stages.[24] Median overall survival was 12.8 months, which varied across BCLC stages (BCLC A, 24.4 months; BCLC B, 16.9 months; BCLC C, 10.0 months). The strongest independent prognostic factors for survival on multivariate analysis were ECOG status, tumor burden (>5 nodules), INR greater than 1.2, and extrahepatic disease.

A phase 2 study of 52 patients prospectively evaluated the efficacy of Y90 radioembolization using TTP as the primary end point for patients with intermediate and advanced stage HCC, the findings of which have led to a randomized phase 3 trial comparing radioembolization to sorafenib.[25] Overall response rate was 40.4%. TTP was 11 months, with no significant difference between patients with and without PVT. Median overall survival was 15 months.

Although there has been no randomized study comparing radioembolization to chemoembolization, a comparative effectiveness report described outcomes following radioembolization and cTACE in a 245-patient cohort. The authors determined that adverse events, clinical toxicities, response rate, and TTP were improved with radioembolization compared to cTACE. Overall survival was no different between radioembolization and cTACE, although likely as a result of the competing risks of death of HCC and cirrhosis. Post hoc analyses concluded that a sample size larger than 1,000 patients would be required to establish survival equivalence between cTACE and radioembolization.[26]

Radioembolization has shown favorable rates of downstaging HCC patients to transplantation, resection, or ablation and superior rates of downstaging to transplantation when compared to cTACE. In one study, 66% of patients who were initially not candidates for transplantation, resection, or ablation were successfully downstaged to transplantation, resection, or ablation following radioembolization.[27] In another study, 58% of patients with UNOS T3 disease (outside transplant criteria) treated with radioembolization were downstaged to T2 disease, compared to 31% of patients treated with cTACE.[28]

Diversion of portal venous flow away from the liver parenchyma with a transjugular intrahepatic portosystemic shunt (TIPS) has raised concern about the use of embolic transarterial therapies in patients with TIPS due to further reduction in liver perfusion resulting in hepatic ischemia. A retrospective comparison of patients with and without TIPS undergoing chemoembolization reported significantly higher rates of severe hepatotoxicity in patients with TIPS.[29] Radioembolization, however, is minimally embolic and has previously been shown to be safe and effective in the setting of partial and branch PVT.[14,15] Additionally, a recent report of Y90 radioembolization in the presence of TIPS indicated rates of hepatotoxicity comparable to those previously reported for Y90 in patients without TIPS. The authors concluded that radioembolization may be safely performed in patients with unresectable HCC and TIPS, particularly as a bridge to liver transplantation.[30]

SIDE EFFECTS AND COMPLICATIONS

The most common side effect of Y90 radioembolization is fatigue, which occurs in 50% to 60% of patients during 1 to 2 weeks following treatment. Approximately 20% of patients experience low-grade abdominal pain or nausea/vomiting, both of which are typically well controlled with oral medications.[22]

Meticulous angiographic technique and careful identification of potential routes of extrahepatic flow are absolutely essential to avoid gastrointestinal (GI) ulcers from nontarget radioembolization. Radiation-induced GI ulcers generally do not respond to proton pump inhibitors and therefore may require surgical resection in patients who are poor surgical candidates.

Biliary complications of Y90 include biliary dyskinesia, radiation cholecystitis, biliary stricture, and biliary necrosis. Biliary dyskinesia presents with postprandial abdominal pain without fever or leukocytosis and is usually self-limited. In the largest reported series evaluating biliary sequelae after Y90 radioembolization for the treatment of HCC as well as metastatic disease to the liver, 10% of patients demonstrated imaging findings related to the biliary tree, of which 1.8% required an unplanned interventional or surgical procedure. Findings included biliary necrosis (3.9%), biloma (1%), biliary stricture (2.4%), gallbladder wall enhancement (1.8%), and gallbladder wall disruption (0.9%).[31]

Radiation-induced liver disease (RILD), previously referred to as *radiation hepatitis*, was first described in patients undergoing external beam radiation and is the most severe potential hepatotoxicity to result from radioembolization. Sinusoidal congestion, venous occlusion, and hepatic fibrosis are the pathologic findings of RILD. The clinical manifestations include nausea, vomiting, abdominal pain, jaundice, and ascites, typically presenting 4 to 8 weeks after radiation exposure. Greater than twofold elevation of alkaline phosphatase is the most specific of liver chemistry abnormalities. Outcomes are variable, with a minority of patients dying of fulminant hepatic failure during the acute phase and most patients surviving with chronic liver failure. Rates of RILD following radioembolization have been reported between 4% and nearly 7%, which include patients with metastatic disease to the liver previously treated with chemotherapy.[32,33] There is no predictive model for the development of RILD following radioembolization. The use of an empiric model in the calculation of resin microspheres dosimetry, which is no longer recommended, has been associated with RILD.[32] Pathologically confirmed RILD has not been reported in patients receiving glass microsphere radioembolization for unresectable HCC.[34] Nonetheless, careful patient selection and appropriate radiation dosimetry are critical to minimize the risk of radiation injury to the liver.

POSTTREATMENT IMAGING

Imaging evaluation following Y90 radioembolization includes assessing tumor response as well as distinguishing benign from more worrisome imaging findings. Anatomic response assessment is based on changes in tumor size (WHO, Response Evaluation Criteria In Solid Tumors [RECIST]) and degree of necrosis as indicated by tumor tissue enhancement (EASL, modified RECIST). Because changes in tumor size alone often underestimate the actual response rate and outcomes following locoregional liver therapies, many clinical trials use the EASL criteria and modified RECIST (mRECIST) to assess residual viable tumor. Indeed, EASL response has been shown to be more consistent than WHO in predicting survival outcomes for HCC following locoregional therapy.[35] Functional imaging with diffusion-weighted MRI (DWI) can provide evidence of metabolic tumor responses on early posttreatment imaging that correlate with anatomic responses on subsequent imaging.[36]

Several benign incidental findings may be seen on imaging after Y90 radioembolization as a result of local radiation effects, including peritumoral edema, ring enhancement, perivascular edema, perihepatic fluid, and pleural effusion. Over time, atrophy of the treated lobe with hypertrophy of the untreated lobe, liver capsular retraction, fibrosis, and evidence of portal hypertension may be seen. More worrisome findings such as hepatic abscess, biloma, radiation cholecystitis, or radiation hepatitis warrant appropriate clinical investigation.[37]

REFERENCES

1. Kennedy AS, Nutting C, Coldwell D, et al. Pathologic response and microdosimetry of (90)Y microspheres in man: review of four explanted whole livers. *Int J Radiat Oncol Biol Phys.* 2004;60(5):1552–1563.
2. Emami B, Lyman J, Brown A, et al. Tolerance of normal tissue to therapeutic irradiation. *Int J Radiat Oncol Biol Phys.* 1991;21(1):109–122.
3. Ingold JA, Reed GB, Kaplan HS, et al. Radiation hepatitis. *Am J Roentgenol Radium Ther Nucl Med.* 1965;93:200–208.
4. Lawrence TS, Robertson JM, Anscher MS, et al. Hepatic toxicity resulting from cancer treatment. *Int J Radiat Oncol Biol Phys.* 1995;31(5):1237–1248.
5. Gyves JW, Ziessman HA, Ensminger WD, et al. Definition of hepatic tumor microcirculation by single photon emission computerized tomography (SPECT). *J Nucl Med.* 1984;25(9): 972–977.
6. Bierman HR, Byron RL Jr, Kelley KH, et al. Studies on the blood supply of tumors in man. III. Vascular patterns of the liver by hepatic arteriography in vivo. *J Natl Cancer Inst.* 1951;12(1):107–131.
7. Geschwind JF, Salem R, Carr BI, et al. Yttrium-90 microspheres for the treatment of hepatocellular carcinoma. *Gastroenterology.* 2004;127(5)(suppl 1):S194–S205.
8. Andrews JC, Walker SC, Ackermann RJ, et al. Hepatic radioembolization with yttrium-90 containing glass microspheres: preliminary results and clinical follow-up. *J Nucl Med.* 1994;35(10):1637–1644.
9. Sarfaraz M, Kennedy AS, Cao ZJ, et al. Physical aspects of yttrium-90 microsphere therapy for nonresectable hepatic tumors. *Med Phys.* 2003;30(2):199–203.
10. Dancey JE, Shepherd FA, Paul K, et al. Treatment of nonresectable hepatocellular carcinoma with intrahepatic 90Y-microspheres. *J Nucl Med.* 2000;41(10):1673–1681.
11. Salem R, Thurston KG, Carr BI, et al. Yttrium-90 microspheres: radiation therapy for unresectable liver cancer. *J Vasc Interv Radiol.* 2002;13(9, pt 2):S223–S229.
12. TheraSphere Yttrium-90 microspheres [package insert]. Kanata, Canada: Nordion; 2004.
13. SIR-Spheres Yttrium-90 microspheres [package insert]. New South Wales, Australia: SIRTeX Medical; 2004.
14. Kulik LM, Carr BI, Mulcahy MF, et al. Safety and efficacy of 90Y radiotherapy for hepatocellular carcinoma with and without portal vein thrombosis. *Hepatology.* 2008;47(1):71–81.
15. Iñarrairaegui M, Thurston KG, Bilbao JI, et al. Radioembolization with use of yttrium-90 resin microspheres in patients with hepatocellular carcinoma and portal vein thrombosis. *J Vasc Interv Radiol.* 2010;21(8):1205–1212.
16. Chen JH, Chai JW, Huang CL, et al. Proximal arterioportal shunting associated with hepatocellular carcinoma: features revealed by dynamic helical CT. *AJR Am J Roentgenol.* 1999;172(2):403–407.
17. Ho S, Lau, WY, Leung TW, et al. Partition model for estimating radiation doses from yttrium-90 microspheres in treating hepatic tumours. *Eur J Nucl Med.* 1996;23(8):947–952.
18. Salem R, Thurston KG. Radioembolization with 90Yttrium microspheres: a state-of-the-art brachytherapy treatment for primary and secondary liver malignancies. Part 1: technical and methodologic considerations. *J Vasc Interv Radiol.* 2006;17(8):1251–1278.
19. Ho S, Lau WY, Leung TW, et al. Clinical evaluation of the partition model for estimating radiation doses from yttrium-90 microspheres in the treatment of hepatic cancer. *Eur J Nucl Med.* 1997;24(3):293–298.

20. Lewandowski RJ, Sato KT, Atassi B, et al. Radioembolization with 90Y microspheres: angiographic and technical considerations. *Cardiovasc Intervent Radiol.* 2007;30(4):571–592.
21. Cabibbo G, Enea M, Attanasio M, et al. A meta-analysis of survival rates of untreated patients in randomized clinical trials of hepatocellular carcinoma. *Hepatology.* 2010;51(4):1274–1283.
22. Salem R, Lewandrowski RJ, Mulcahy MF, et al. Radioembolization for hepatocellular carcinoma using yttrium-90 microspheres: a comprehensive report of long-term outcomes. *Gastroenterology.* 2010;138(1):52–64.
23. Hilgard P, Hamami M, Fouly AE, et al. Radioembolization with yttrium-90 glass microspheres in hepatocellular carcinoma: European experience on safety and long-term survival. *Hepatology.* 2010;52(5):1741–1749.
24. Sangro B, Carpanese L, Cianni R, et al. Survival after yttrium-90 resin microsphere radioembolization of hepatocellular carcinoma across Barcelona clinic liver cancer stages: a European evaluation. *Hepatology.* 2011;54(3):868–878.
25. Mazzaferro V, Sposito C, Bhoori S, et al. Yttrium-90 radioembolization for intermediate-advanced hepatocellular carcinoma: a phase 2 study. *Hepatology.* 2013;57(5):1826–1837.
26. Salem R, Lewandowski RJ, Kulik L, et al. Radioembolization results in longer time-to-progression and reduced toxicity compared with chemoembolization in patients with hepatocellular carcinoma. *Gastroenterology.* 2011;140(2):497–507.e2.
27. Kulik LM, Atassi B, van Holsbeeck L, et al. Yttrium-90 microspheres (TheraSphere) treatment of unresectable hepatocellular carcinoma: downstaging to resection, RFA and bridge to transplantation. *J Surg Oncol.* 2006;94(7):572–586.
28. Lewandowski RJ, Kulik LM, Riaz A, et al. A comparative analysis of transarterial downstaging for hepatocellular carcinoma: chemoembolization versus radioembolization. *Am J Transplant.* 2009;9(8):1920–1928.
29. Kohi MP, Fidelman N, Naeger DM, et al. Hepatotoxicity after transarterial chemoembolization and transjugular intrahepatic portosystemic shunt: do two rights make a wrong? *J Vasc Interv Radiol.* 2013;24(1):68–73.
30. Donahue LA, Kulik L, Baker T, et al. Yttrium-90 radioembolization for the treatment of unresectable hepatocellular carcinoma in patients with transjugular intrahepatic portosystemic shunts. *J Vasc Interv Radiol.* 2013;24(1):74–80.
31. Atassi B, Bangash AK, Lewandowski RJ, et al. Biliary sequelae following radioembolization with yttrium-90 microspheres. *J Vasc Interv Radiol.* 2008;19(5):691–697.
32. Kennedy AS, McNellie P, Dezarn WA, et al. Treatment parameters and outcome in 680 treatments of internal radiation with resin 90Y-microspheres for unresectable hepatic tumors. *Int J Radiat Oncol Biol Phys.* 2009;74(5):1494–1500.
33. Sangro B, Gil-Alzugaray B, Rodriguez J, et al. Liver disease induced by radioembolization of liver tumors: description and possible risk factors. *Cancer.* 2008;112(7):1538–1546.
34. Goin JE, Salem R, Carr BI, et al. Treatment of unresectable hepatocellular carcinoma with intrahepatic yttrium 90 microspheres: factors associated with liver toxicities. *J Vasc Interv Radiol.* 2005;16(2, pt 1):205–213.
35. Memon K, Kulik L, Lewandowski RJ, et al. Radiographic response to locoregional therapy in hepatocellular carcinoma predicts patient survival times. *Gastroenterology.* 2011;141(2): 526–535, 535.e1–535.e2.
36. Rhee TK, Naik NK, Deng J, et al. Tumor response after yttrium-90 radioembolization for hepatocellular carcinoma: comparison of diffusion-weighted functional MR imaging with anatomic MR imaging. *J Vasc Interv Radiol.* 2008;19(8):1180–1186.
37. Atassi B, Bangash AK, Bahrani A, et al. Multimodality imaging following 90Y radioembolization: a comprehensive review and pictorial essay. *Radiographics.* 2008;28(1):81–99.

38

Combined Therapies

Riccardo Lencioni • Marcelo Guimaraes

Hepatocellular carcinoma (HCC) is the second leading cause of cancer-related death worldwide.[1] Unlike most solid cancers, future incidence and mortality rates for HCC were projected to largely increase in several regions around the world over the next 20 years.[2,3] A careful multidisciplinary assessment of tumor characteristics, liver function, and physical status is required for proper therapeutic management of patients with HCC.[4–7] Candidates for resection must be carefully selected to minimize the risk of postoperative liver failure and improve long-term results. Access to liver transplantation has to be balanced between precise estimation of survival contouring individual tumor characteristics and organ availability. When surgical options are precluded, interventional locoregional treatments are recommended as the most appropriate therapeutic choice for patients whose disease is limited to the liver.[4–7]

Image-guided tumor ablation is the first-line treatment for nonsurgical patients with early-stage HCC and is considered a potentially radical therapy in properly selected candidates.[8–10] Several reports have shown that the long-term survival of patients with compensated cirrhosis and small solitary tumors who received radiofrequency ablation (RFA) as the sole first-line anticancer therapy is similar to that reported in surgical series.[11,12] For patients presenting with more advanced or multinodular HCC—a common scenario due to the propensity of HCC to invade portal vein branches and to produce intrahepatic metastases—and relatively preserved liver function, transcatheter arterial chemoembolization (TACE) is the current standard of care. TACE is actually the most popular treatment for HCC worldwide.[13] Radioembolization with yttrium 90 microspheres is attracting increasing attention as a potential alternate treatment that seems to have potential to provide clinical benefit even in the complex setting of patients presenting with macroscopic vascular invasion.[14]

Despite their leading role in the clinical management of HCC, locoregional interventional therapies have limitations. The ability of image-guided ablation techniques to achieve complete tumor eradication appears to strongly depend on tumor size and location.[15] Even in those patients in whom successful tumor ablation has been achieved, the rate of tumor recurrence due to the emergence of new HCC lesions exceeds 80% at 5 years, similar to postresection figures.[16] On the other hand, in patients with large or multinodular tumor at the intermediate-stage HCC who received TACE, tumor recurrence or progression is almost inevitable. In randomized controlled trials, a sustained response lasting more than 3 to 6 months was observed in only 28% to 35% of the patients who received conventional TACE; in nonresponders, no survival benefit was identified compared to best supportive care.[17,18] Even in those patients in whom initial response was achieved, the 3-year cumulative rate of intrahepatic recurrence reached 65%, with recurrent tumor showing significantly shorter median doubling time.[19]

Several combined treatment strategies have been used in an attempt to overcome some of these limitations. These include various combinations of locoregional interventions as well as the association of locoregional and systemic therapies. This chapter is focused on discussing the potential synergies of TACE with either local ablation or molecular targeted agents, which have been the most extensively described combination approaches. Despite combined treatments are widely used in clinical practice, unequivocal evidence of clinical benefit associated with such strategies is still lacking as no robust phase III randomized clinical trials have been completed so far.

COMBINED TRANSCATHETER ARTERIAL CHEMOEMBOLIZATION AND LOCAL ABLATIVE THERAPY

RFA is currently established as the standard ablative modality for early-stage HCC.[20,21] Randomized trials comparing RFA versus the seminal percutaneous technique—ethanol injection—showed that RFA has higher local anticancer effect, leading to a better control of the disease and improved survival.[22-26] Nevertheless, histologic studies performed in liver specimens of patients who underwent RFA as bridge treatment for transplantation showed that the rate of complete tumor eradication highly depends on tumor size and presence of large (≥3 mm) abutting vessels. In fact, vessels adjacent to the target tumor cause heat loss due to perfusion-mediated tissue cooling within the area to be ablated. In one study, the rate of complete tumor necrosis was 50% or less in tumor exceeding 3 cm in diameter or in perivascular location.[15]

Several attempts have been made to increase the effect of RFA in HCC treatment. Because heat efficiency is the difference between the amount of heat produced and the amount of heat lost, most investigators devoted their attention to strategies that aim primarily at minimizing heat loss due to perfusion-mediated tissue cooling.[27] When a laparotomy or a laparoscopy approach is used to perform RFA, heat loss can be minimized by performing a Pringle maneuver.[27] In percutaneous procedures, given that HCC is mostly nourished by the hepatic artery, a combination of RFA and balloon catheter occlusion of the tumor arterial supply or prior transcatheter arterial embolization or chemoembolization has been used to increase heat efficiency.[28-31] The combination of TACE and RFA did not show significant clinical benefit when applied to the treatment of small (≤3 cm) HCC. In a randomized study, the rates of local tumor progression and overall survival did not differ between the combined treatment group as compared to the RFA-alone treatment group.[32] However, such an approach did show significant advantages both in terms of local tumor control and survival when used in intermediate-sized (3 to 5 cm) HCC[33,34] as well as in recurrent HCC after prior hepatectomy.[35]

The largest randomized clinical trials conducted so far included 189 patients with HCC less than 7 cm. Patients were randomly assigned to receive TACE combined with RFA (TACE–RFA; n = 94) or RFA alone (n = 95). The primary end point was overall survival. The secondary end point was recurrence-free survival, and the tertiary end point was adverse effects. The 1-, 3-, and 4-year overall survivals for the TACE–RFA group and the RFA group were 92.6%, 66.6%, and 61.8% and 85.3%, 59%, and 45.0%, respectively. The corresponding recurrence-free survivals were 79.4%, 60.6%, and 54.8% and 66.7%, 44.2%, and 38.9%, respectively. Patients in the TACE–RFA group had better overall survival and recurrence-free survival than patients in the RFA group (hazard ratio, 0.525; 95% CI, 0.335 to 0.822; $P = .002$; hazard ratio, 0.575; 95% CI, 0.374 to 0.897; $P = .009$, respectively). On logistic regression analyses, treatment allocation, tumor size, and tumor number were significant prognostic factors for overall survival, whereas treatment allocation and tumor number were significant prognostic factors for recurrence-free survival.[36]

The strategy of performing TACE first followed by RFA has the advantages of cutting the arterial blood supply, which reduces the "heat sink effect" during the RFA. Also, it is expected to have an increase in the size of the RFA ablation zone. This can be beneficial to guarantee a good surgical margin post ablation, but it can also be dangerous in case the ablation is performed close to a liver structure (confluence of the bile ducts) and to an adjacent organ (gallbladder, diaphragm, stomach, colon) in which undesired heat-induced injury may occur. TACE first also allows the delivery of high concentration of the chemotherapeutic agent to the entire tumor. In addition, it has been reported that the heat generated by the RFA post TACE could sensitize the chemotherapeutic agent.[37]

Currently, there is no evidence determining if conventional or drug-eluting bead (DEB) TACE is better when used in combination with RFA. However, if the RFA is performed under computed tomography (CT) guidance, the use of TACE with Lipiodol is helpful in identifying the nodule location (Fig. 38.1A–C). It also delineates the tumor border precisely (which is key to plan a 1-cm surgical margin around the tumor) and increases accuracy for RFA needle deployment and for multiple overlapping ablations planning. This feature is especially important for tumors larger than 2 or 3 cm and for those in risky locations. In this case, percutaneous thermal protective techniques may be used (Figs. 38.2A–C and 38.3A–F).

Another debatable question is the time interval between TACE and RFA. In theory, the time between the two procedures should be minimized to prevent hypoxia-induced neoangiogenesis. Typically, the tumor recruitment of existing and/or the formation of new arterial blood supply takes place between 2 and 3 weeks. One of this chapter authors (M.G.) routinely performs conventional TACE procedure followed by CT-guided RFA in the next day ("back-to-back technique"). This strategy has been well tolerated by Child-Pugh A and B patients. Also, it has optimized resources and minimized patient's dislocations and hospital admission time. These data, not published yet, have demonstrated encouraging results including large HCCs (Figs. 38.4A–F and 38.5A–G) with less than 1% tumor recurrence rate, increased patient's survival, and without major complications. Although TACE followed by RFA has been the most popular combination, alternate strategies have been investigated. In particular, DEB-TACE has been performed after RFA, rather than before, following a different rationale.[38] In a standard RFA, one can take advantage of only those temperatures that

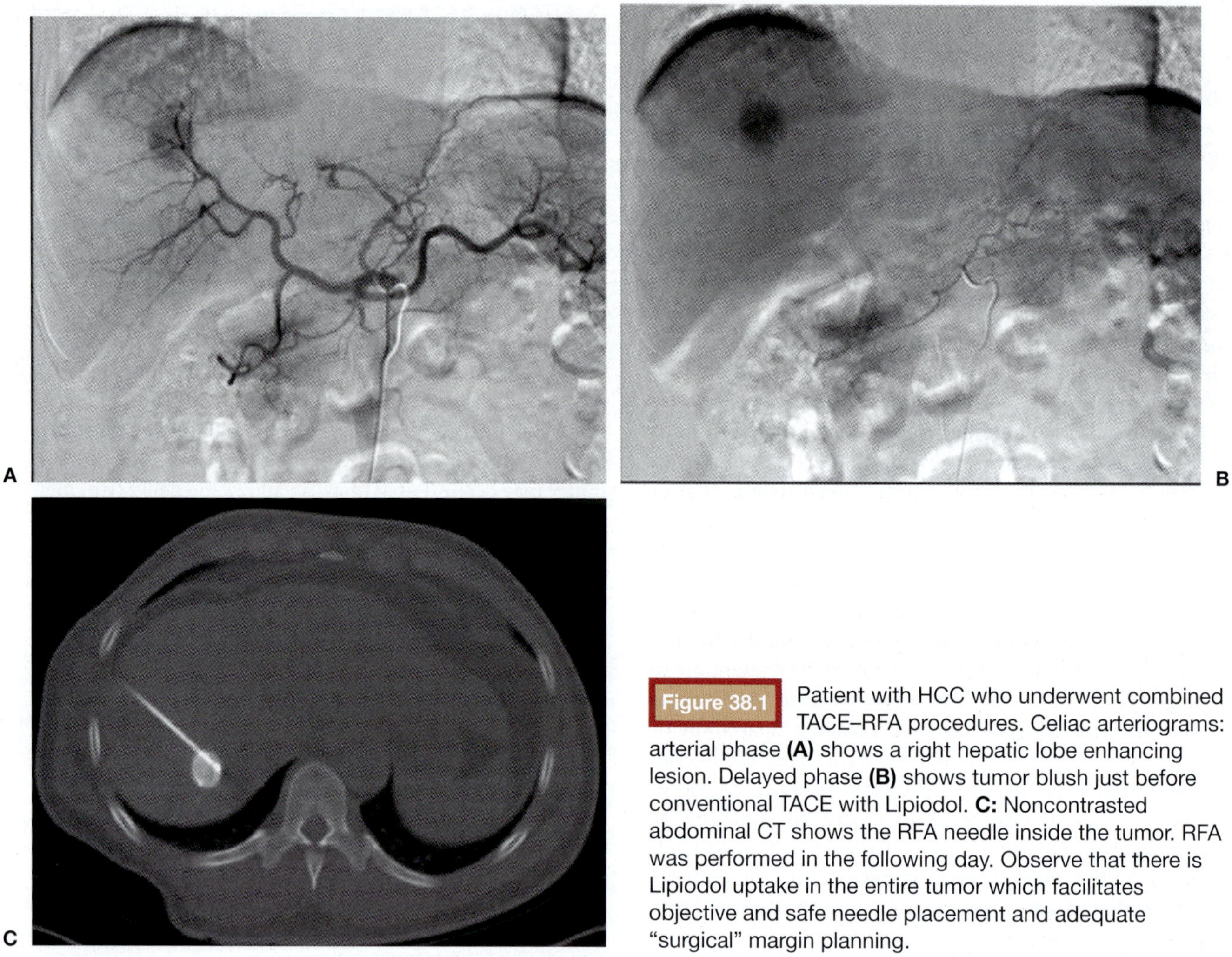

Figure 38.1 Patient with HCC who underwent combined TACE–RFA procedures. Celiac arteriograms: arterial phase **(A)** shows a right hepatic lobe enhancing lesion. Delayed phase **(B)** shows tumor blush just before conventional TACE with Lipiodol. **C:** Noncontrasted abdominal CT shows the RFA needle inside the tumor. RFA was performed in the following day. Observe that there is Lipiodol uptake in the entire tumor which facilitates objective and safe needle placement and adequate "surgical" margin planning.

are sufficient by themselves to induce coagulative necrosis (>50° to 55°C). However, there are large zones of sublethal heating created during radiofrequency (RF) application in tissues surrounding the electrode that are not being used to achieve sustained treatment effect. Experimental studies in animal tumor models have shown that lowering the temperature threshold at which cell death occurs by combining sublethal temperature with cell exposure to chemotherapeutic agents increases tumor necrosis, apparently occurring in tissues heated to 45° to 50°C.[39,40] It has been hypothesized that the administration of DEB to tumors incompletely killed by RFA could increase the anticancer effect as a result of both the delivery of highly concentrated doxorubicin into a relatively small volume of residual viable neoplastic tissue and the reduced cell resistance to the drug caused by the exposure to sublethal heating.[38]

In a pilot clinical study, DEB-TACE was performed within 24 hours of RFA to take advantage of the reactive hyperemia induced by RF application to facilitate delivery of the microspheres to the tumor-bearing area. In fact, marked periablational hypervascularity was observed at the time of the angiographic study. DEB administration resulted in substantial increase in tissue destruction, leading to confirmed complete response of the target lesion in 12 (60%) of 20 patients bearing large tumors refractory to standard RF treatment.[38] DEB-enhanced RFA was well tolerated, with no major complications associated with the technique. This pilot clinical study provided the first evidence of the synergy between RFA and local delivery of a chemotherapeutic agent in cancer treatment, supporting the findings from previous experimental work. Nevertheless, after this initial evaluation of efficacy and safety, further clinical investigation is warranted to prove the clinical benefit of this approach.

COMBINED TRANSCATHETER ARTERIAL CHEMOEMBOLIZATION AND SYSTEMIC THERAPY

Angiogenesis plays a pivotal role in the development, progression, and prognosis of HCC due to the vascularity of

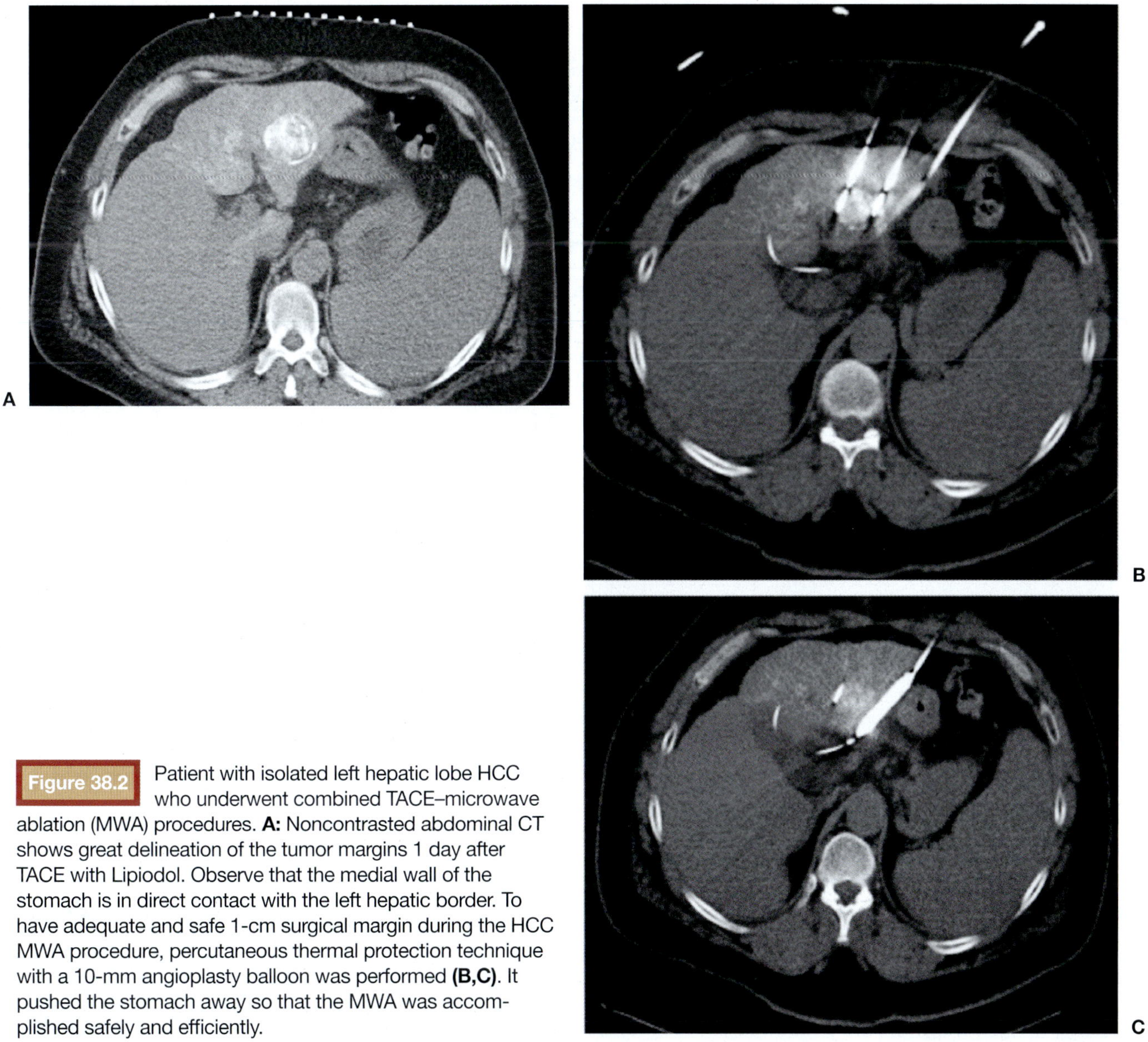

Figure 38.2 Patient with isolated left hepatic lobe HCC who underwent combined TACE–microwave ablation (MWA) procedures. **A:** Noncontrasted abdominal CT shows great delineation of the tumor margins 1 day after TACE with Lipiodol. Observe that the medial wall of the stomach is in direct contact with the left hepatic border. To have adequate and safe 1-cm surgical margin during the HCC MWA procedure, percutaneous thermal protection technique with a 10-mm angioplasty balloon was performed **(B,C)**. It pushed the stomach away so that the MWA was accomplished safely and efficiently.

these tumors. Upregulation of angiogenesis is first detected in dysplastic nodules, whereas malignant transformation leads to arterialization of its blood supply and sinusoidal capillarization. Vascular endothelial growth factor (VEGF) plays a critical role in this process. Growth factor signal receptors and their downstream transduction pathways play a central role in the development and progression of HCC. Among the most prominent contributors are the Ras/Raf/MEK/ERK, PI3/AKT/mTOR, and JAK/STAT receptor tyrosine kinase–activated pathways.[41] Signal transduction via the Ras/Raf/MEK/ERK pathway, which includes several ubiquitous enzymes, is involved in the development, progression, and maintenance of HCC. These pathways can be activated by binding of growth factors such as epidermal growth factor (EGF), hepatocyte growth factor (HGF), platelet-derived growth factor (PDGF), and VEGF, which are secreted in an autocrine or paracrine fashion by the tumor or surrounding tissues. These findings suggested that inhibitors of these pathways, particularly of the tyrosine kinases bound by growth factors, may inhibit the progression of HCC.

The first tyrosine kinase inhibitor developed for the treatment of HCC was sorafenib. This small-molecule multikinase inhibitor was shown to significantly inhibit the activity of Raf-1, wild-type and oncogenic BRAF, VEGFR-1 and -2, PDGFR, Flt-3, and c-Kit, as well as the phosphorylation of MEK and ERK, both in vivo and in vitro.[41,42] Moreover, its antitumor activity in human HCC xenografts in nude

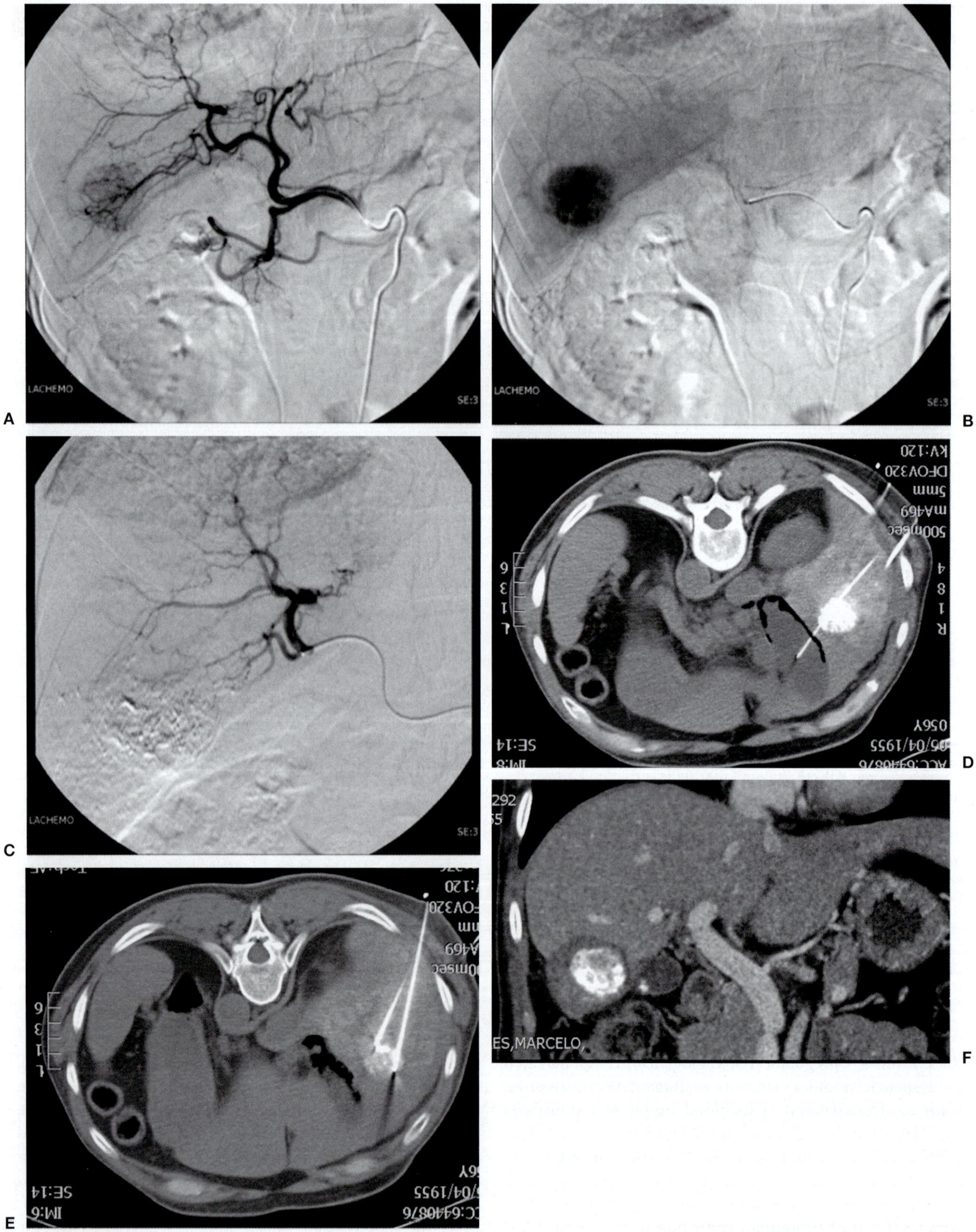

Figure 38.3 Patient with HCC who underwent combined TACE–RFA procedures. Common hepatic arteriograms: arterial phase **(A)** shows a right hepatic lobe enhancing lesion. Delayed phase **(B)** shows tumor blush. **C:** Final right hepatic angiogram demonstrates no tumor vascularization post superselective TACE. **D:** Noncontrasted abdominal CT shows a 21-gauge Chiba needle introduced in the gallbladder for thermal protection. After bile aspiration, chilled D5 infusion was kept throughout the case. **E:** Tumor uptake or Lipiodol helped adequate and safe RFA needle placement for surgical margin planning. **F:** Thirty-day liver contrasted CT demonstrates no viable tumor, adequate hypodense rim around the tumor, and no gallbladder complications.

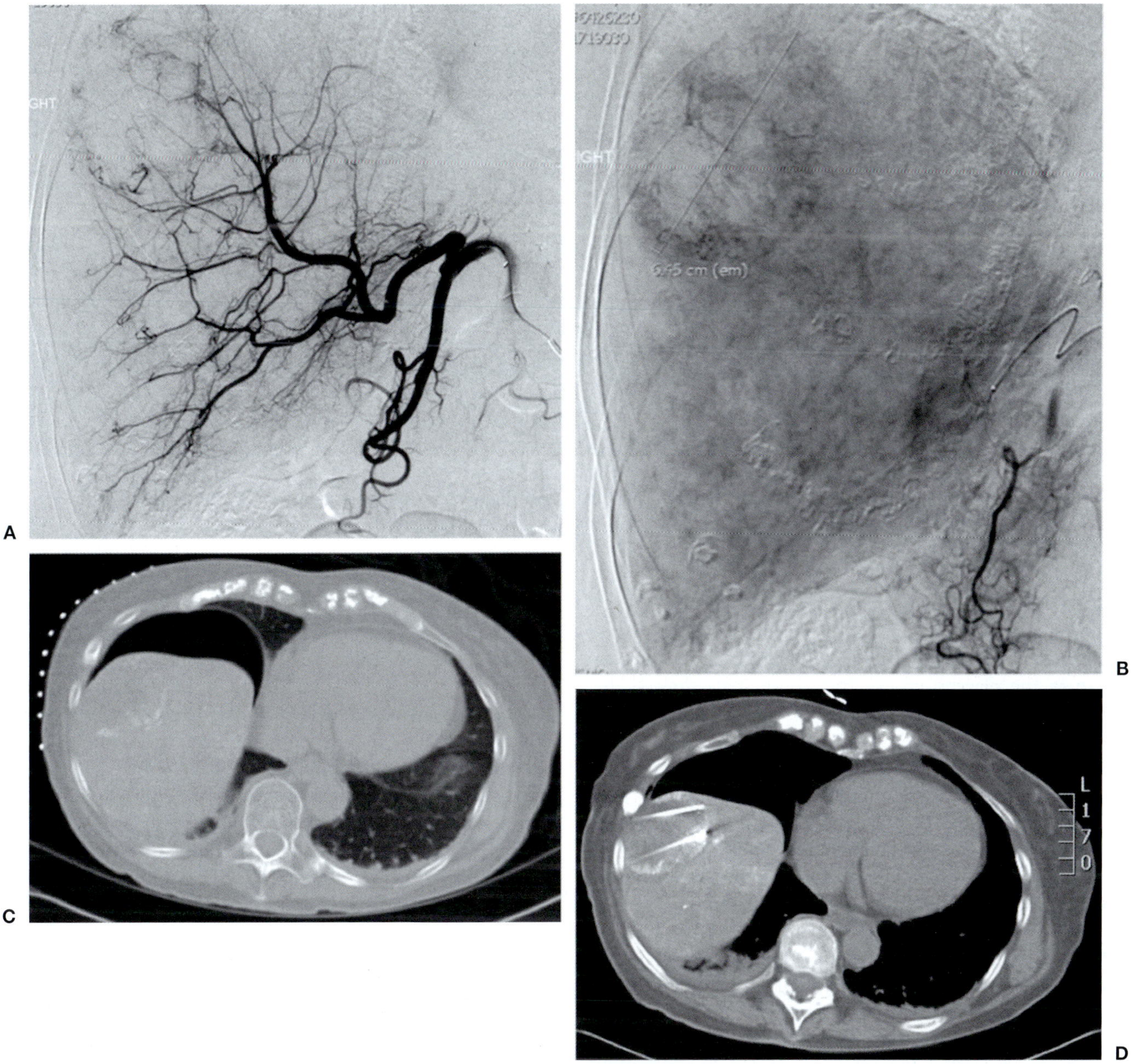

Figure 38.4 Patient with HCC in the dome of the right hepatic lobe who underwent combined TACE–RFA procedures. Common hepatic arteriograms: arterial phase **(A)** shows a right hepatic dome peripherally enhancing lesion. Delayed phase **(B)** shows a 6.45-cm tumor blush. **C:** Noncontrasted abdominal CT (lung window) shows the creation of CO_2 pneumoperitoneum for thermal protection of the diaphragm. **D:** Once diaphragmatic dislocation was confirmed, two RFA needles were advanced into the tumor (noncontrasted abdominal CT, mediastinal window). Note precise needle placement due to tumor Lipiodol uptake. *(Continued)*

mice correlated with its inhibition of MAP signaling.[41,42] Two large, phase III, randomized, placebo-controlled clinical trials have evaluated the efficacy and safety of sorafenib in patients with advanced HCC. In one study, the Sorafenib HCC Assessment Randomized Protocol (SHARP) trial, 602 previously untreated patients with advanced HCC were randomized 1:1 to receive either sorafenib 400 mg or matching placebo twice daily on a continuous basis.[43] Both median overall survival and median time to disease progression were significantly longer in the sorafenib group than in the placebo group. In the sorafenib Asia Pacific trial, 271 patients from the Asia Pacific region with advanced HCC were randomized 2:1 to receive either sorafenib 400 mg or matching placebo twice daily on a continuous basis.[44] As in the SHARP

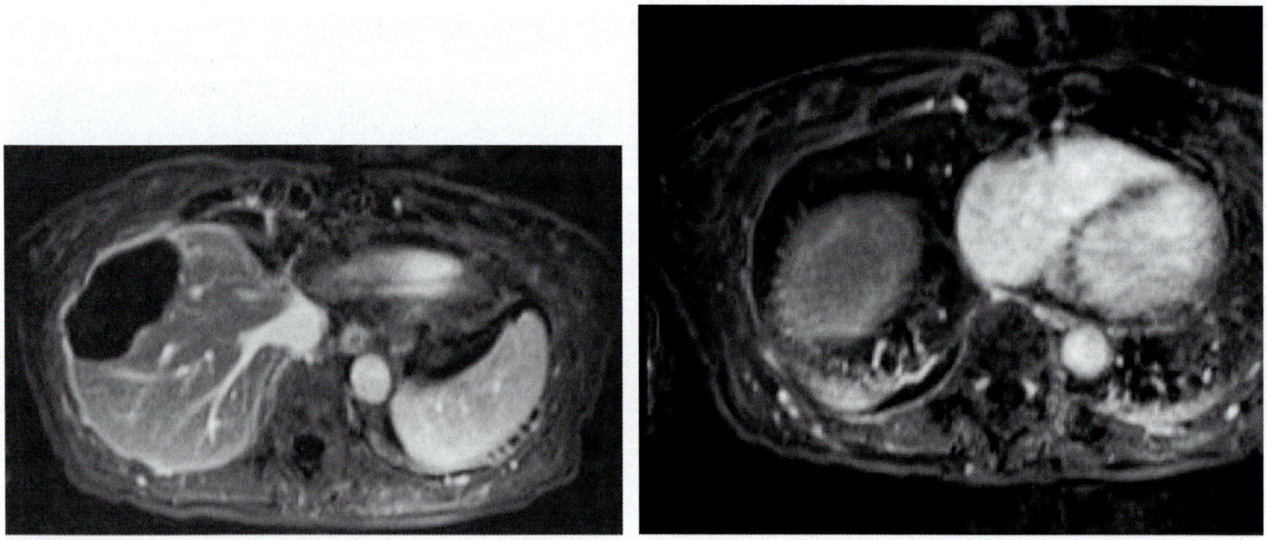

E F

Figure 38.4 *(Continued)* **E,F:** Three-month follow-up abdominal magnetic resonance imaging (MRI) shows adequate surgical margin, no tumor viability, and preservation of the diaphragm.

trial, median overall survival and median time to disease progression were significantly longer in the sorafenib group than in the placebo group. Thus, both trials showed that sorafenib is an appropriate option for the systemic treatment of patients with advanced HCC.

To date, studies of sorafenib have demonstrated its efficacy in advanced HCC; however, there may also be a role for this agent—or other molecular targeted drugs—in earlier stage disease in combination with TACE. Because the amount of oxygen supplied to a tumor is a function of the distance of the tumor cells from the local blood vessel, hypoxia in tumor cells that remain and are distant from the feeding blood vessel increases following TACE.[45] Surrogate markers of tissue hypoxia that increase after TACE include hypoxia-inducible factor 1 alpha and both plasma and hepatic VEGF.[46,47] Hypoxia in HCC can lead to neoangiogenesis, suggesting that inhibition of angiogenesis may be synergistic with TACE in patients with HCC.[48]

Treatment with an antiangiogenic agent such as sorafenib may therefore complement TACE. An antiangiogenic agent may inhibit TACE-induced angiogenesis and the development of tumor-feeding vessels associated with tumor cell proliferation. In addition, antiangiogenic agents may target lesions distant from the site of TACE. The availability of DEB, which ensures a minimal systemic exposure to the chemotherapeutic agent at the time of the TACE, is appealing for combination regimens based on mechanisms that are theoretically synergistic.

In a prospective single-center phase 2 study, safety and response of a combined protocol involving sorafenib 400 mg twice per day and DEB-TACE were assessed in 35 patients.[49] Although most patients experienced at least one grade 3 to 4 toxicity, most toxicities were minor (grade 1 to 2, 83% versus grade 3 to 4, 17%), and preliminary efficacy data were promising. The phase 2 randomized, double-blind, placebo-controlled SPACE study (Sorafenib or Placebo in Combination with DEB-TACE for intermediate-stage HCC) was conducted to evaluate the efficacy and safety of sorafenib in combination with DEB-TACE in patients with intermediate-stage HCC across Europe, North America, and the Asia Pacific region.[50] Of 452 patients screened, 307 were randomized to sorafenib (n = 154) or placebo (n = 153). The hazard ratio (HR) for time to progression (TTP) was 0.797 (95% CI, 0.588, 1.080; P = .072). Median TTP (50th percentile) was 169 days/166 days in the sorafenib and placebo groups, respectively; TTP at the 25th and 75th percentiles (preplanned) was 112 days/88 days and 285 days/224 days in the sorafenib and placebo groups, respectively.[50] There were no unexpected safety findings. The findings of the SPACE study were supported by recently published prospective, single-arm, phase 2 studies conducted in Asian patients with unresectable HCC.[51] Nevertheless, the encouraging signal captured by the SPACE trial requires confirmation with data from ongoing phase 3 trials.

Several questions remain as we attempt to improve treatment outcome in HCC patients. The pathophysiologic complexity of HCC, balanced with a goal of providing effective tumor therapy with preservation of organ function, makes optimal treatment choice a clinical challenge.[52] An understanding of exactly which features of HCC and patient health may predict the clinical outcome of combination regimens is essential for prescribing individualized, evidence-based therapeutic strategies.

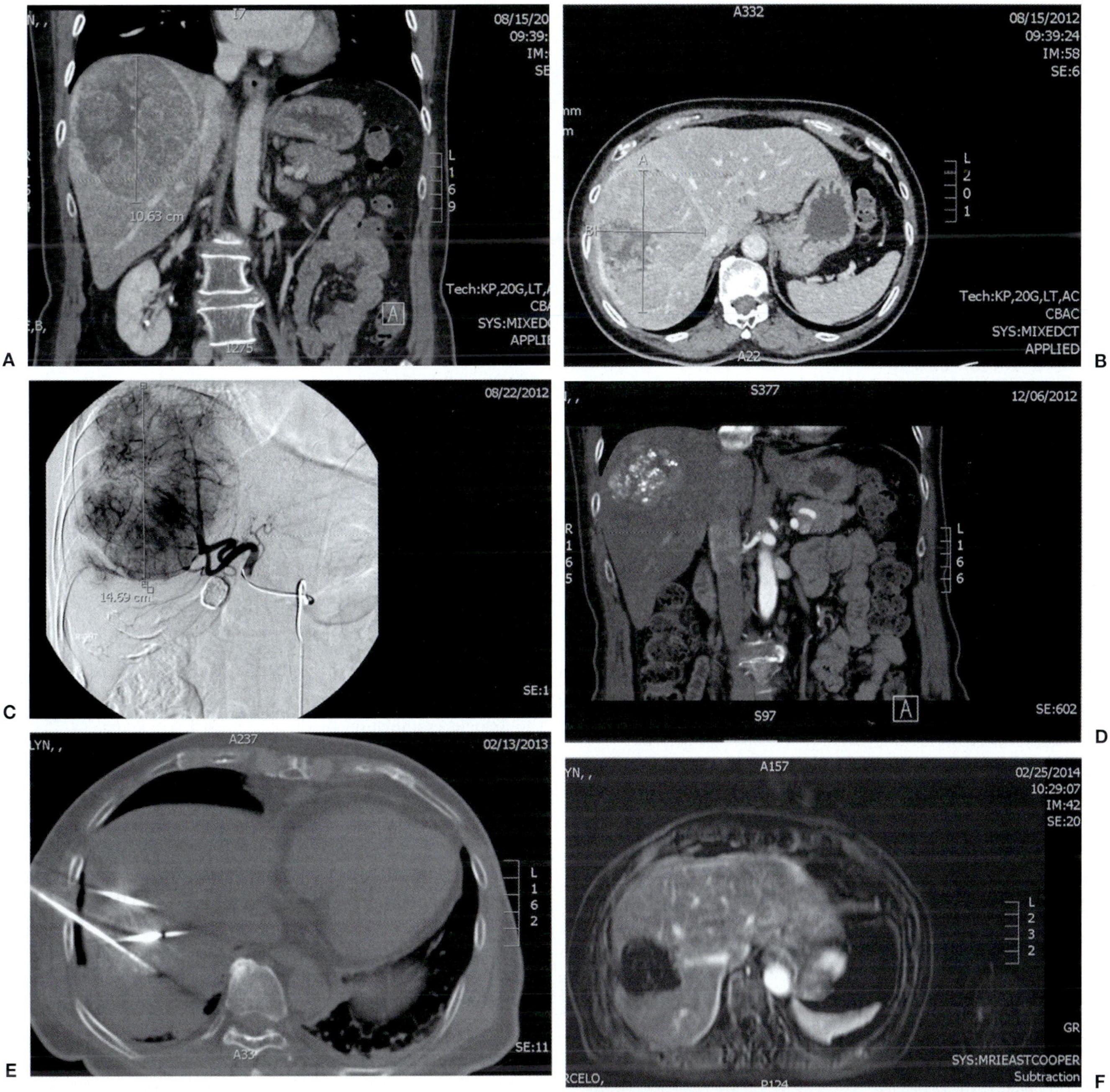

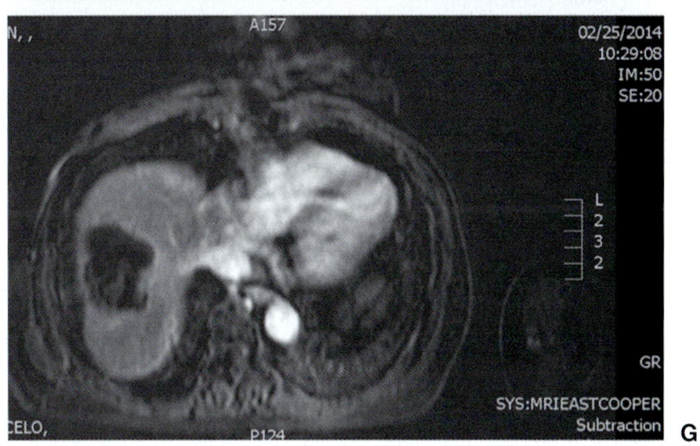

Figure 38.5 Patient with symptomatic HCC who underwent four sessions of TACE followed by CT-guided RFA. Coronal **(A)** and axial **(B)** views: venous phase of a contrasted abdominal CT shows a large HCC occupying most of the right hepatic lobe. **C:** Propria hepatic arteriogram shows a 14.7-cm tumor blush in the right hepatic lobe. After four TACE procedures, coronal contrasted abdominal CT **(D)** shows Lipiodol uptake and residual contrast enhancement in the tumor, at this point reduced to 7.2 cm. **E:** Noncontrasted abdominal CT shows three microwave needles used for the HCC ablation. Again, precise needle placement and surgical margin planning were facilitated by previous tumor Lipiodol uptake. **F,G:** Twelve-month follow-up abdominal MRI (subtraction images) demonstrates no evidence of residual, recurrent, or new tumor.

TIPS AND TRICKS

- Combination therapy including TACE and RFA has shown similar long-term survival and recurrence-free rates to hepatectomy in tumors up to 7 cm. However, randomized controlled trials comparing combined therapy and surgery have not been completed so far.
- Patient's selection is key to success in combination therapy and requires careful consideration of tumor stage, size, and location as well as patient's performance status and liver function.
- Consider performing the combined therapies (TACE and RFA) either in the same admission or in a few days apart.
- Consider the use of thermal protection techniques (such as hydrodissection with chilled D5, gallbladder puncture and aspiration followed by infusion of chilled D5, carbon dioxide [CO_2] pneumoperitoneum, infusion of chilled D5 in the bile ducts through a nasogastric tube, balloon angioplasty catheter interposition) as appropriate.
- Lipiodol retention within the tumor helps delineating the target well in CT-guided RFA and is helpful for precise needle placement and for planning multiple overlapping ablations aimed at providing a 1-cm surgical margin.
- Combined treatment of HCC with TACE and systemic molecular targeted therapy is a promising alternative; ongoing phase 3 clinical trials are expected to provide evidence of clinical benefit.

REFERENCES

1. International Agency for Research on Cancer. GLOBOCAN 2012: estimated cancer incidence, mortality and prevalence worldwide in 2012. http://globocan.iarc.fr. Accessed January 17, 2014.
2. Olsen AH, Parkin DM, Sasieni P. Cancer mortality in the United Kingdom: projections to the year 2025. *Br J Cancer.* 2008;99:1549–1554.
3. Davis GL, Alter MJ, El-Serag H, et al. Aging of the hepatitis C virus (HCV)-infected persons in the United States: a multiple cohort model of HCV prevalence and disease progression. *Gastroenterology.* 2010;138:513–521.
4. Bruix J, Sherman M. Management of hepatocellular carcinoma: an update. *Hepatology.* 2011;53:1020–1022.
5. Han KH, Kudo M, Ye SL, et al. Asian consensus workshop report: expert consensus guideline for the management of intermediate and advanced hepatocellular carcinoma in Asia. *Oncology.* 2011;81(suppl 1):158–164.
6. European Association for the Study of the Liver, European Organisation for Research and Treatment of Cancer. EASL–EORTC clinical practice guidelines: management of hepatocellular carcinoma. *J Hepatol.* 2012;56:908–943.
7. Verslype C, Rosmorduc O, Rougier P; ESMO Guidelines Working Group. Hepatocellular carcinoma: ESMO-ESDO clinical practice guidelines for diagnosis, treatment and follow-up. *Ann Oncol.* 2012;23(suppl 7):vii41–vii48
8. Lencioni R. Loco-regional treatment of hepatocellular carcinoma. *Hepatology.* 2010;52:762–773.
9. Lencioni R, Crocetti L. Loco-regional treatment of hepatocellular carcinoma. *Radiology.* 2012;262:43–58.
10. Colombo M, Raoul JL, Lencioni R, et al. Multidisciplinary strategies to improve treatment outcomes in hepatocellular carcinoma: a European perspective. *Eur J Gastroenterol Hepatol.* 2013;25:639–651.
11. Feng K, Yan J, Li X, et al. A randomized controlled trial of radiofrequency ablation and surgical resection in the treatment of small hepatocellular carcinoma. *J Hepatol.* 2012;57:794–780.
12. Pompili M, Saviano A, de Matthaeis N, et al. Long-term effectiveness of resection and radiofrequency ablation for single hepatocellular carcinoma ≤3 cm. Results of a multicenter Italian survey. *J Hepatol.* 2013;59:89–97.
13. Lencioni R, Kudo M, Ye SL, et al. GIDEON (Global Investigation of therapeutic DEcisions in hepatocellular carcinoma and Of its treatment with sorafeNib): second interim analysis. *Int J Clin Pract.* 2014;68:609–617.
14. Salem R, Mazzaferro V, Sangro B. Yttrium 90 radioembolization for the treatment of hepatocellular carcinoma: biological lessons, current challenges, and clinical perspectives. *Hepatology.* 2013;58:2188–2197.
15. Lu DS, Yu NC, Raman SS, et al. Radiofrequency ablation of hepatocellular carcinoma: treatment success as defined by histologic examination of the explanted liver. *Radiology.* 2005;234:954–960.
16. Lencioni R, Cioni D, Crocetti L, et al. Early-stage hepatocellular carcinoma in cirrhosis: long-term results of percutaneous image-guided radiofrequency ablation. *Radiology.* 2005;234:961–967.
17. Lo CM, Ngan H, Tso WK, et al. Randomized controlled trial of transarterial lipiodol chemoembolization for unresectable hepatocellular carcinoma. *Hepatology.* 2002;35:1164–1171.
18. Llovet JM, Real MI, Montana X, et al. Arterial embolisation or chemoembolisation versus symptomatic treatment in patients with unresectable hepatocellular carcinoma: a randomised controlled trial. *Lancet.* 2002;359:1734–1739.
19. Woo HY, Jang JW, Choi JY, et al. Tumor doubling time after initial response to transarterial chemoembolization in patients with hepatocellular carcinoma. *Scand J Gastroenterol.* 2010;45:332–339.
20. Gervais DA, Goldberg SN, Brown DB, et al. Society of Interventional Radiology position statement on percutaneous radiofrequency ablation for the treatment of liver tumors. *J Vasc Interv Radiol.* 2009;20(7)(suppl):S342–S347.
21. Crocetti L, De Baere T, Lencioni R. Quality improvement guidelines for radiofrequency ablation of liver tumours. *Cardiovasc Intervent Radiol.* 2010;33:11–17.
22. Lencioni R, Allgaier HP, Cioni D, et al. Small hepatocellular carcinoma in cirrhosis: randomized comparison of radiofrequency thermal ablation versus percutaneous ethanol injection. *Radiology.* 2003;228:235–240.
23. Lin SM, Lin CJ, Lin CC, et al. Radiofrequency ablation improves prognosis compared with ethanol injection for hepatocellular carcinoma < or = 4 cm. *Gastroenterology.* 2004;127:1714–1723.

24. Shiina S, Teratani T, Obi S, et al. A randomized controlled trial of radiofrequency ablation versus ethanol injection for small hepatocellular carcinoma. *Gastroenterology*. 2005;129:122–130.
25. Lin SM, Lin CJ, Lin CC, et al. Randomised controlled trial comparing percutaneous radiofrequency thermal ablation, percutaneous ethanol injection, and percutaneous acetic acid injection to treat hepatocellular carcinoma of 3 cm or less. *Gut*. 2005;54:1151–1156.
26. Brunello F, Veltri A, Carucci P, et al. Radiofrequency ablation versus ethanol injection for early hepatocellular carcinoma: a randomized controlled trial. *Scand J Gastroenterol*. 2008;43:727–735.
27. Goldberg SN, Hahn PF, Tanabe KK, et al. Percutaneous radiofrequency tissue ablation: does perfusion-mediated tissue cooling limit coagulation necrosis? *J Vasc Interv Radiol*. 1998; 9:101–111.
28. Rossi S, Garbagnati F, Lencioni R, et al. Percutaneous radiofrequency thermal ablation of nonresectable hepatocellular carcinoma after occlusion of tumor blood supply. *Radiology*. 2000;217:119–126.
29. Veltri A, Moretto P, Doriguzzi A, et al. Radiofrequency thermal ablation (RFA) after transarterial chemoembolization (TACE) as a combined therapy for unresectable non-early hepatocellular carcinoma (HCC). *Eur Radiol*. 2006;16:661–669.
30. Helmberger T, Dogan S, Straub G, et al. Liver resection or combined chemoembolization and radiofrequency ablation improve survival in patients with hepatocellular carcinoma. *Digestion*. 2007;75:104–112.
31. Yamasaki T, Kurokawa F, Shirahashi H, et al. Percutaneous radiofrequency ablation therapy for patients with hepatocellular carcinoma during occlusion of hepatic blood flow. Comparison with standard percutaneous radiofrequency ablation therapy. *Cancer*. 2002;95:2353–2360.
32. Shibata T, Isoda H, Hirokawa Y, et al. Small hepatocellular carcinoma: is radiofrequency ablation combined with transcatheter arterial chemoembolization more effective than radiofrequency ablation alone for treatment? *Radiology*. 2009;252:905–913.
33. Morimoto M, Numata K, Kondou M, et al. Midterm outcomes in patients with intermediate-sized hepatocellular carcinoma: a randomized controlled trial for determining the efficacy of radiofrequency ablation combined with transcatheter arterial chemoembolization. *Cancer*. 2010;116:5452–5460.
34. Kim JH, Won HJ, Shin YM, et al. Medium-sized (3.1-5.0 cm) hepatocellular carcinoma: transarterial chemoembolization plus radiofrequency ablation versus radiofrequency ablation alone. *Ann Surg Oncol*. 2011;18:1624–1629.
35. Takaki H, Yamakado K, Sakurai H, et al. Radiofrequency ablation combined with chemoembolization: treatment of recurrent hepatocellular carcinomas after hepatectomy. *AJR Am J Roentgenol*. 2011;197:488–494.
36. Peng ZW, Zhang YJ, Chen MS, et al. Radiofrequency ablation with or without transcatheter arterial chemoembolization in the treatment of hepatocellular carcinoma: a prospective randomized trial. *J Clin Oncol*. 2013;31:426–432.
37. Goldberg SN, Saldinger PF, Gazelle GS, et al. Percutaneous tumor ablation: increased necrosis with combined radio-frequency ablation and intratumoral doxorubicin injection in a rat breast tumor model. *Radiology*. 2001;220:420–427.
38. Lencioni R, Crocetti L, Petruzzi P, et al. Doxorubicin-eluting bead-enhanced radiofrequency ablation of hepatocellular carcinoma: a pilot clinical study. *J Hepatol*. 2008;49:217–222.
39. Goldberg SN, Girnan GD, Lukyanov AN, et al. Percutaneous tumor ablation: increased necrosis with combined radiofrequency ablation and intravenous liposomal doxorubicin in a rat breast tumor model. *Radiology*. 2002;222:797–804.
40. Ahmed M, Liu Z, Lukyanov AN, et al. Combination radiofrequency ablation with intratumoral liposomal doxorubicin: effect on drug accumulation and coagulation in multiple tissues and tumor types in animals. *Radiology*. 2005;235:469–477.
41. Wilhelm SM, Adnane L, Newell P, et al. Preclinical overview of sorafenib, a multikinase inhibitor that targets both Raf and VEGF and PDGF receptor tyrosine kinase signaling. *Mol Cancer Ther*. 2008;7:3129–3140.
42. Liu L, Cao Y, Chen C, et al. Sorafenib blocks the RAF/MEK/ERK pathway, inhibits tumor angiogenesis, and induces tumor cell apoptosis in hepatocellular carcinoma model PLC/PRF/5. *Cancer Res*. 2006;66:11851–11858.
43. Llovet JM, Ricci S, Mazzaferro V, et al. Sorafenib in advanced hepatocellular carcinoma. *N Engl J Med*. 2008;359:378–390.
44. Cheng AL, Kang YK, Chen Z, et al. Efficacy and safety of sorafenib in patients in the Asia-Pacific region with advanced hepatocellular carcinoma: a phase III randomised, double-blind, placebo-controlled trial. *Lancet Oncol*. 2009;10:25–34.
45. Carmeliet P, Jain RK. Angiogenesis in cancer and other diseases. *Nature*. 2000;407:249–257.
46. Rhee TK, Young JY, Larson AC, et al. Effect of transcatheter arterial embolization on levels of hypoxia-inducible factor-1 alpha in rabbit VX2 liver tumors. *J Vasc Interv Radiol*. 2007;18: 639–645.
47. Li X, Feng GS, Zheng CS, et al. Expression of plasma vascular endothelial growth factor in patients with hepatocellular carcinoma and effect of transcatheter arterial chemoembolization therapy on plasma vascular endothelial growth factor level. *World J Gastroenterol*. 2004;10:2878–2882.
48. Wang B, Xu H, Gao ZQ, et al. Increased expression of vascular endothelial growth factor in hepatocellular carcinoma after transcatheter arterial chemoembolization. *Acta Radiol*. 2008;49:523–529.
49. Pawlik TM, Reyes DK, Cosgrove D, et al. Phase II trial of sorafenib combined with concurrent transarterial chemoembolization with drug-eluting beads for hepatocellular carcinoma. *J Clin Oncol*. 2012;29:3960–3967.
50. Lencioni R, Llovet JM, Han G, et al. Sorafenib or placebo in combination with transarterial chemoembolization (TACE) with doxorubicin-eluting beads (DEBDOX) for intermediate-stage hepatocellular carcinoma (HCC): phase II, randomized, double-blind SPACE trial. *J Clin Oncol*. 2012;30(suppl 4; abstr LBA154).
51. Park JW, Koh YH, Kim HB, et al. Phase II study of concurrent transarterial chemoembolization and sorafenib in patients with unresectable hepatocellular carcinoma. *J Hepatol*. 2012;56:1336–1342.
52. Gish RG, Lencioni R, Di Bisceglie AM, et al. Role of the multidisciplinary team in the diagnosis and treatment of hepatocellular carcinoma. *Expert Rev Gastroenterol Hepatol*. 2012;6: 173–185.

39

Transcatheter Arterial Chemoembolization (Conventional and with Drug-Eluting Beads) and Radioembolization

Julius Chapiro • Rafael Duran • Jean-François Geschwind

Intrahepatic cholangiocarcinoma (IHC) is the second most common primary hepatic neoplasm after hepatocellular carcinoma.[1] With an annual incidence of 5,000 new cases in the United States and similar rates in Europe, it remains a rare cancer, although rates are considerably higher in Japan and other Asian countries.[2] At the time of diagnosis, patients with IHC usually present with advanced stage disease, thus only 30% of the patients are candidates for surgical treatment.[3] The overall prognosis in this disease is dismal, and not even surgical candidates achieve survival rates much higher than 30% at 5 years after resection with curative intent.[4] Systemic chemotherapy has been disappointing regarding survival benefits for patients, and most regimens resulted in a median survival of no more than 12 months.[5] Most regimen include gemcitabine and various combinations of 5-fluorouracil with cisplatin. However, until today, no randomized phase III trial exists to evaluate different chemotherapy regimen in IHC, and there has been great interest in exploring other modalities of treatment. In particular, multiple catheter-based intra-arterial therapies are possible to effectively treat patients with unresectable IHC. Unlike surgical or ablative approaches, intra-arterial techniques are not limited by tumor size, number of lesions, or proximity of major sensitive structures. Although mostly hypovascular, IHC still derives its blood supply from hepatic arteries, making intra-arterial delivery of anticancer agents (chemotherapeutic drugs or radiation) a potentially attractive therapy. The following describes the most commonly used intra-arterial therapies for IHC and discusses the available clinical evidence.

DISCLOSURES: J.C. No potential conflicts of interest to disclose. **R.D.** No potential conflicts of interest to disclose. **J.F.G.** Financial activities related to the present article: none to disclose. Financial activities not related to the present article: paid consultant to Nordion, Biocompatibles/BTG, Bayer HealthCare, and Guerbet; institution has grants/grants pending from the National Institutes of Health, U.S. Department of Defense (DOD), Biocompatibles/BTG, Bayer HealthCare, Philips Medical, Nordion, ContextVision, Society of Interventional Radiology, and the Radiological Society of North America. Other relationships: none to disclose.

CONVENTIONAL TRANSARTERIAL CHEMOEMBOLIZATION

Background

Of all the intra-arterial therapies used in the treatment of unresectable IHC, conventional transarterial chemoembolization (cTACE) is the most commonly used (Fig. 39.1). During this procedure, a mixture of chemotherapeutic agents combined with an oil-based contrast medium (Lipiodol or Ethiodol) is selectively delivered to the tumor-feeding artery. Lipiodol has unique properties and functions as an embolizing agent as well as an emulsion carrier for chemotherapeutic drugs.[6] Doxorubicin is the most widely used single chemotherapeutic agent worldwide, yet the mix of doxorubicin, cisplatin, and mitomycin is the preferred combination in the United States and Europe.[7] After injection of the drug-containing emulsion, embolic materials (such as gelfoam, polyvinyl alcohol [PVA] particles, or trisacryl gelatin [TG] microspheres) are administered with the purpose to cause stasis in segmental and subsegmental arteries, thus preventing washout of the previously deposited material.[8]

Clinical Evidence

One of the very first prospective trials designed to evaluate feasibility, safety, and overall survival after cTACE enrolled 17 patients with pathologically proven, mass-forming unresectable IHC. Eleven patients (65%) received cTACE as the first-line therapy, whereas 6 patients (35%) had received previous treatment including systemic chemotherapy and radiation therapy. On this protocol, chemotherapeutic agents used for most patients were 100 mg cisplatin, 50 mg doxorubicin hydrochloride, and 10 mg mitomycin-C. Most patients (82%) tolerated the procedure well and no life-threatening events were reported. In terms of efficacy, two of the patients were bridged to successful surgical resection after cTACE, and the median overall survival (OS) was 23 months.[9] Another more recent single-center study from Germany retrospectively analyzed a larger cohort of 115 IHC patients treated with cTACE and confirmed the previously described results. Patients were repeatedly treated with cTACE (mean of 7.1 sessions per patient), yielding good tumor response rates (57.4% with Stable Disease [SD]). After a total of 819 TACE procedures, the overall safety profile and tolerability was exceptionally good for the entire cohort. However, it must be noted that no homogeneous treatment protocol was applied and various drugs and their combinations (mitomycin-C, gemcitabine, and cisplatin) were injected. Finally, the mean OS was 20.8 months with a 3-year survival of 10%, which is in agreement with the previously reported results.[10] Another important two-center experience demonstrated the synergistic potential of cTACE with systemic chemotherapy. Here, a total of 62 patients with unresectable IHC (37 of which were pathologically proven) underwent repetitive

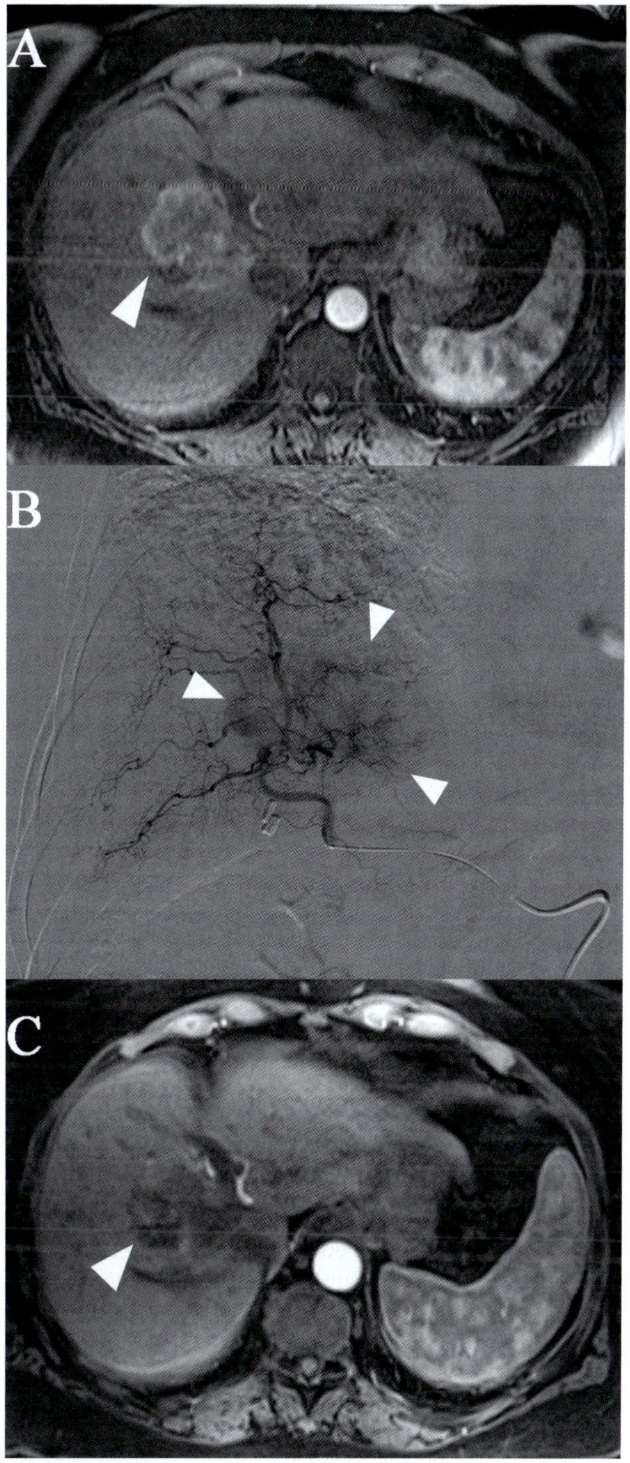

Figure 39.1 TACE in cholangiocarcinoma. A 67-year-old patient who presented for chemoembolization of a centrally located 6.5-cm intrahepatic cholangiocarcinoma. **A:** Demonstrates the lesion (*arrowhead*) on an arterial-phase contrast-enhanced MRI before the procedure. **B:** Demonstrates the tumor blush (*arrowheads*). **C:** Shows extensive tumor necrosis (*arrowhead*) on postprocedural MRI 4 weeks after treatment.

cTACE treatment, and the used drug combination consisted of mitomycin-C, doxorubicin, and cisplatin. With only minor systemic toxicities and no disease-specific mortality 30 days after the initial treatment, cTACE was safe. Interestingly, the most important finding of this study was the significantly higher median survival rate in patients who received systemic chemotherapy when compared with those who did not receive any (28 months vs. 16 months, respectively). Furthermore, cTACE can also play an important role as an alternative adjuvant therapy for patients who underwent radical surgery. To explore this setting, a retrospective analysis included 125 IHC patients who underwent radical surgery with curative intent. A total of 53 patients (42%) received cTACE with various drug combinations (fluorouracil, carboplatin, epirubicin and hydroxycamptothecin, gemcitabine). A comparison of this group of patients with 72 nontreated individuals revealed no significant difference in the tumor recurrence rate. However, patients treated with TACE showed some survival benefits as compared to the nontreated group (1-, 3-, and 5-year OS of 69.8%, 37.7%, and 28.3% and 54.2%, 25.0%, and 20.8%, respectively). Of note, the results of this retrospective study must be interpreted with great caution primarily because of a highly inhomogeneous treatment protocol.[11]

TRANSARTERIAL CHEMOEMBOLIZATION WITH DRUG-ELUTING BEADS

Background

The advent of drug-eluting beads (DEBs) provided an additional therapeutic option for patients with unresectable IHC. Instead of the oily medium, DEB-TACE delivers polymer-based microspheres to achieve three aims at once: embolization, controlled local drug release, and reduced systemic toxicity.[12] Two major types of drug-eluting microspheres are available clinically in the United States: LC Beads (Biocompatibles UK Ltd., Farnham, Surrey, United Kingdom) that can be loaded with doxorubicin (DEBDOX) or irinotecan (DEBIRI)[13,14] and QuadraSpheres/HepaSpheres (Merit Medical Systems, Inc., South Jordan, Utah) that can be loaded with various drugs including doxorubicin, epirubicin, irinotecan, or cisplatin.[15,16] Initially designed for the use in HCC, these products are increasingly used for the treatment of IHC.

Clinical Evidence

One of the very first studies to investigate the safety and feasibility of DEB-TACE in IHC patients used oxaliplatin-eluting microspheres to treat a small collective of nine patients. Patients were prospectively enrolled to receive DEB-TACE associated with continued systemic chemotherapy with oxaliplatin and gemcitabine. A total of 30 DEB-TACE procedures were performed. To assess the true procedure-related toxicity, a retrospective comparison with a group of patients treated only with systemic chemotherapy (N = 11) was performed. As a result, no patient in the DEB-TACE group experience grade 4 toxicities and only very few adverse effects were reported. According to the Response Evaluation Criteria In Solid Tumors (RECIST), 44% of patients achieved partial response and 56% showed stable disease. Most importantly, patients who received both intra-arterial and systemic chemotherapies showed significant survival benefits when compared to chemotherapy alone (OS of 30 and 12.7 months, respectively).[17] However, this result must be interpreted with great caution, particularly because of the small sample size. Furthermore, this study was not designed as a prospective randomized trial and patients in the chemotherapy-only group were likely not eligible for intra-arterial therapies because of the very advanced stage of their disease. One of the first true prospective trials, designed to evaluate the safety and efficacy of DEB-TACE in patients with IHC, recruited a total of 11 patients who received a total of 29 individual TACE procedures. Here, each patient received 100 to 150 mg doxorubicin, which appeared to be safe, and no major toxicities were reported. Imaging follow-up was available in all patients, and according to RECIST criteria, all patients were responders and one case demonstrated complete response. The very important aspect of quality of life was addressed, and in 90% of the cases, an improvement was achieved when assessed using the Edmonton Symptom Assessment System questionnaire. As in previous trials and because of the low overall incidence of IHC, the small number of patients in this trial was a significant limitation with regard to survival analysis. Another prospective trial of DEB-TACE in this disease enrolled 26 consecutive patients and was designed to assess feasibility, safety, and efficacy of this approach. Here, irinotecan was used for the loading of DEBs. In addition to the slightly larger number of enrolled patients, the outcome of this trial was retrospectively compared to two independent trials, where a similar cohort of patients received cTACE or systemic chemotherapy. As a result, progression-free survival (PFS) and OS in the DEB-TACE group were 3.9 months and 11.7 months, respectively. When compared with the cTACE cohort (PFS of 1.8 months and OS 5.7 months), DEB-TACE safe and well tolerated and provided a slightly better local tumor control than the other therapies.[18] In summary, the data on the use of DEB-TACE for IHC are growing, especially in view of a stronger tumor response when compared to cTACE. However, no prospective randomized trial is available to show clear evidence of survival benefits for DEB-TACE over cTACE. Furthermore, because patients treated with TACE and systemic therapy are living longer, there is now a strong interest in designing prospective randomized trials that would combine TACE with systemic therapy, specifically gemcitabine and cisplatin.

RADIOEMBOLIZATION

Background

Radioembolization exploits the same scientific rationale as TACE and uses the arterial pathway to deliver the payload directly to the tumor. Instead of chemotherapy, however, this modality uses small embolic particles loaded with yttrium 90, a pure β-particle–emitting radionuclide with a half-life of 64.1 hours.[19] Currently, there are two types of particles available for clinical use in the United States and Europe: the resin-based SIR-Spheres (SIRTeX Medical Limited, New South Wales, Australia) and the glass-based TheraSpheres (Nordion, Kanata, Ontario, Canada).[20] Because of the extremely small size of these particles (ranging from 20 to 60 μm), radioembolization bears the risk of extrahepatic distribution of the aggressive payload via hepatopulmonary shunts. Thus, all patients must be subjected to angiographic evaluation as well as shunt studies using a test injection of ^{99m}Tc-labeled macroaggregated albumin (tc-MAA) before the actual procedure.[21] The use of radioembolization in liver cancer patients was initially approved in Canada, and only in 1999, the U.S. Food and Drug Administration (FDA) approved this procedure in the United States under the humanitarian device exemption for patients with hepatocellular carcinoma. For most other liver cancer patients including IHC, case-by-case institutional review board approval must be obtained.[22]

Clinical Evidence

The clinical evidence on radioembolization for IHC is not as comprehensive as the one using cTACE or DEB-TACE. However, a few studies have demonstrated promising results with radioembolization regarding safety and disease control. For instance, a prospective single-center pilot study investigated the feasibility as well as efficacy of radioembolization in 24 patients. All patients had histologically proven diagnosis of IHC. Patients with an Eastern Cooperative Oncology Group (ECOG) performance status of 0 to 2 were eligible for treatment. At the time of the first radioembolization procedure, 38% had imaging signs of portal vein thrombosis (PVT) and a total of 13 patients had multifocal disease. No major life-threatening events were recorded. However, 17% of patients developed grade 3 albumin toxicities and 1 patient developed a refractory gastroduodenal ulcer, itself a characteristic complication of radioembolization. According to EASL response criteria, radioembolization yielded excellent tumor control. Nine percent of the patients achieved complete response and 77% showed partial response on magnetic resonance imaging (MRI). The initial median OS of the entire group was 14.9 months. When stratified according to ECOG performance status, patients with ECOG 0 showed the strongest survival benefits (31.8 months vs. 1 month for ECOG 2).[22] This result underlined the impact of the initial patient performance not only for radioembolization but also for all intra-arterial therapies in general. A recently published follow-up study from the same center provided more data and expanded the number of patients to a total of 46. This analysis revealed the potential of radioembolization, showing successful downstaging of the disease to resectable status in 5 patients. The overall median OS in patients without PVT was 14.4 months (5.3 months with PVT).[23] Currently, the presence of PVT in candidates for intra-arterial therapies is being discussed, and some evidence indicates slight benefits of radioembolization over TACE in this subgroup of patients.[24] However, no final data is available as of today. The results of both studies[22,23] were confirmed by another prospective single-center study designed to show the beneficial effects of radioembolization in patients with unresectable IHC. Here, similar survival data (14.7 months for ECOG 1 patients) and comparable toxicity profiles in a cohort of 19 patients were demonstrated.[25] Therefore, it is safe to say that radioembolization may also play a beneficial role in the treatment of patients with IHC; however, more prospective randomized trials are needed.

TIPS AND TRICKS

- Use cross-sectional imaging with delayed phases to evaluate the lesions before treatment due to the fibrotic character of the lesions.
- Cholangiocarcinomas are notoriously difficult to visualize angiographically. As a result, it is extremely important to perform cone-beam computed tomography (CT) imaging from various locations to confirm appropriate targeting. This may mean performing several cone-beam CTs during the procedure, especially if the tumor is centrally located and has more than one feeding artery.
- Because most IHC lesions are centrally located, both hepatic arteries must be evaluated even if 90% of the flow is provided by one artery. Angiograms from the right and left hepatic arteries must therefore be performed.
- For radioembolization, inject from a proximal localization and treat in a lobar fashion.
- Use cone-beam CT after the procedure to assess Lipiodol deposition within the tumor after conventional TACE.
- It is better to handle the wire with your fingers rather than a dedicated torque device as they provide true tactile feedback.
- In patients with coagulopathy, closure devices should be considered to reduce the risk of bleeding and hematoma at the puncture site.

CONCLUSION

Intra-arterial therapies provide a valuable alternative for patients with unresectable IHC. Based on the data presented here, the level of evidence for the use of cTACE is sufficient, and it can be concluded that this modality significantly contributes to an improved survival and preserves quality of life in patients with an otherwise dismal prognosis. As for DEB-TACE, most studies provide enough data on safety and show efficient tumor control; however, no clear evidence for survival benefits over cTACE is available. The data for radioembolization is growing, and more studies are needed for a sound assessment of this modality in patients with IHC.

REFERENCES

1. Tyson GL, El-Serag HB. Risk factors for cholangiocarcinoma. *Hepatology*. 2011;54(1):173–84.
2. Hong K, Geschwind JF. Locoregional intra-arterial therapies for unresectable intrahepatic cholangiocarcinoma. *Semin Oncol*. 2010;37(2):110–117.
3. Scheuermann U, Kaths JM, Heise M, et al. Comparison of resection and transarterial chemoembolisation in the treatment of advanced intrahepatic cholangiocarcinoma—a single-center experience. *Eur J Surg Oncol*. 2013;39(6):593–600.
4. Poultsides GA, Zhu AX, Choti MA, et al. Intrahepatic cholangiocarcinoma. *Surg Clin North Am*. 2010;90(4):817–837.
5. Dodson RM, Weiss MJ, Cosgrove D, et al. Intrahepatic cholangiocarcinoma: management options and emerging therapies. *J Am Coll Surg*. 2013;217:736–750.e4.
6. Yamada R, Nakatsuka H, Nakamura K, et al. Hepatic artery embolization in 32 patients with unresectable hepatoma. *Osaka City Med J*. 1980;26(2):81–96.
7. Kiefer MV, Albert M, McNally M, et al. Chemoembolization of intrahepatic cholangiocarcinoma with cisplatinum, doxorubicin, mitomycin C, ethiodol, and polyvinyl alcohol: a 2-center study. *Cancer*. 2011;117(7):1498–1505.
8. Brown DB, Gould JE, Gervais DA, et al. Transcatheter therapy for hepatic malignancy: standardization of terminology and reporting criteria. *J Vasc Interv Radiol*. 2009;20(7)(suppl):S425–S434.
9. Burger I, Hong K, Schulick R, et al. Transcatheter arterial chemoembolization in unresectable cholangiocarcinoma: initial experience in a single institution. *J Vasc Interv Radiol*. 2005;16(3):353–361.
10. Vogl TJ, Naguib NN, Nour-Eldin NE, et al. Transarterial chemoembolization in the treatment of patients with unresectable cholangiocarcinoma: results and prognostic factors governing treatment success. *Int J Cancer*. 2012;131(3):733–740.
11. Shen WF, Zhong W, Liu Q, et al. Adjuvant transcatheter arterial chemoembolization for intrahepatic cholangiocarcinoma after curative surgery: retrospective control study. *World J Surg*. 2011;35(9):2083–2091.
12. Lammer J, Malagari K, Vogl T, et al. Prospective randomized study of doxorubicin-eluting-bead embolization in the treatment of hepatocellular carcinoma: results of the PRECISION V study. *Cardiovasc Intervent Radiol*. 2010;33(1):41–52.
13. Constantin M, Fundueanu G, Bortolotti F, et al. Preparation and characterisation of poly(vinyl alcohol)/cyclodextrin microspheres as matrix for inclusion and separation of drugs. *Int J Pharm*. 2004;285(1–2):87–96.
14. Qian J, Truebenbach J, Graepler F, et al. Application of poly-lactide-co-glycolide-microspheres in the transarterial chemoembolization in an animal model of hepatocellular carcinoma. *World J Gastroenterol*. 2003;9(1):94–98.
15. Seki A, Hori S, Kobayashi K, et al. Transcatheter arterial chemoembolization with epirubicin-loaded superabsorbent polymer microspheres for 135 hepatocellular carcinoma patients: single-center experience. *Cardiovasc Intervent Radiol*. 2011;34(3):557–565.
16. Huppert P, Wenzel T, Wietholtz H. Transcatheter arterial chemoembolization (TACE) of colorectal cancer liver metastases by irinotecan-eluting microspheres in a salvage patient population. *Cardiovasc Intervent Radiol*. 2014;37:154–164.
17. Poggi G, Amatu A, Montagna B, et al. OEM-TACE: a new therapeutic approach in unresectable intrahepatic cholangiocarcinoma. *Cardiovasc Intervent Radiol*. 2009;32(6):1187–1192.
18. Kuhlmann JB, Euringer W, Spangenberg HC, et al. Treatment of unresectable cholangiocarcinoma: conventional transarterial chemoembolization compared with drug eluting bead-transarterial chemoembolization and systemic chemotherapy. *Eur J Gastroenterol Hepatol*. 2012;24(4):437–443.
19. Chakravarty R, Dash A, Pillai MR. Availability of yttrium-90 from strontium-90: a nuclear medicine perspective. *Cancer Biother Radiopharm*. 2012;27(10):621–641.
20. Salem R, Thurston KG. Radioembolization with 90Yttrium microspheres: a state-of-the-art brachytherapy treatment for primary and secondary liver malignancies. Part 1: technical and methodologic considerations. *J Vasc Interv Radiol*. 2006;17(8):1251–1278.
21. Gil-Alzugaray B, Chopitea A, Inarrairaegui M, et al. Prognostic factors and prevention of radioembolization-induced liver disease. *Hepatology*. 2013;57(3):1078–1087.
22. Ibrahim SM, Mulcahy MF, Lewandowski RJ, et al. Treatment of unresectable cholangiocarcinoma using yttrium-90 microspheres: results from a pilot study. *Cancer*. 2008;113(8):2119–2128.
23. Mouli S, Memon K, Baker T, et al. Yttrium-90 radioembolization for intrahepatic cholangiocarcinoma: safety, response, and survival analysis. *J Vasc Interv Radiol*. 2013;24:1227–1234.
24. Lau WY, Sangro B, Chen PJ, et al. Treatment for hepatocellular carcinoma with portal vein tumor thrombosis: the emerging role for radioembolization using yttrium-90. *Oncology*. 2013;84(5):311–318.
25. Rafi S, Piduru SM, El-Rayes B, et al. Yttrium-90 radioembolization for unresectable standard-chemorefractory intrahepatic cholangiocarcinoma: survival, efficacy, and safety study. *Cardiovasc Intervent Radiol*. 2013;36(2):440–448.

40

Neuroendocrine Tumors

Joseph J. Zechlinski • William S. Rilling

Neuroendocrine tumors (NETs) represent a broad spectrum of tumors arising from neuroendocrine (NE) cells throughout the body, often secreting peptides which cause characteristic hormonal syndromes. Classically, this manifests as diarrhea, flushing, wheezing, abdominal cramping, and/or peripheral edema, the constellation of symptoms known as *carcinoid syndrome*. In contrast, most pancreatic NETs (pNETs) are nonfunctioning, although they can secrete various peptide hormones and are named as such, including insulinoma, gastrinoma, glucagonoma, and vasoactive intestinal peptide (VIPoma).

NE carcinoma was classically described as a more indolent neoplasm; however, tumor biology is variable and can be aggressive. To this point, a large proportion of patients with NETs have liver metastases at the time of diagnosis and often have a high disease burden, with only 10% of patients being candidates for surgical resection at presentation.[1] These patients have the best chance for long-term survival following surgical resection, with 5-year survival approaching 60% to 80%.[2] In contrast, chemotherapy generally has a more limited role, with disease control lasting only 8 to 10 months.[3] Given this disparity, various other treatment modalities are employed in the multidisciplinary care of NETs, including liver-directed therapies and targeted molecular therapies.

CLASSIFICATION

Traditionally considered a rare neoplasm, analysis of the Surveillance, Epidemiology, and End Results (SEER) database in contemporary reviews reveals that NETs have a similar incidence as testicular cancer, cervical cancer, multiple myeloma, Hodgkin lymphoma, and cancers of the central nervous system. Furthermore, the prevalence of NETs is increasing—365% in the last 30 years—now being more common than esophageal cancer, gastric cancer, pancreatic cancer, and hepatobiliary cancer in the United States.[4,5]

NETs can arise from many tissues in the body, but gastrointestinal, pancreatic, lung, and thymic origins have been most extensively studied with regard to classification. Several systems exist, with the World Health Organization (WHO) classification most commonly used for tumors of the gastrointestinal tract.[6] Recently updated in 2010, it divides NETs into low grade, NE neoplasm grade 1; intermediate grade, NE neoplasm grade 2; and high grade, NE carcinoma grade 3. Tumor differentiation, referring to the histologic similarity of the tumor to the tissue of origin, and tumor grade, based on mitotic count and Ki 67 index (a measure of proliferative rate), are principle determinants of tumor aggressiveness and act as prognostic factors. Generally, high-grade tumors have an elevated mitotic rate (>10 to 20 mitoses per 10 high-power fields), high Ki 67 index (>20%), extensive necrosis, and pleomorphism.[7] Staging is based on the tumor, node, metastasis (TNM) system, using cytologic grade, proliferative index (Ki 67), tumor size, degree of metastases, and the primary site.

CURATIVE TREATMENTS

Surgical resection and/or intraoperative ablation offers the best curative treatment for neuroendocrine liver metastases (NLMs), with 5-year survival estimated at 70.5% for resectable lesions based on a recent systematic review.[8] Aggressive pursuit of the primary tumor is a critical part of the surgical treatment algorithm. The goal of curative surgery is a macroscopically complete (R0/R1) resection and/or ablation. Palliative surgical "debulking" is somewhat controversial and may be considered appropriate if greater than 90% of the tumor burden can be resected or surgically ablated.[9,10] Despite the demonstrated survival benefit, disease recurrence is extremely common following resection and/or intraoperative ablation. In a recent review of 339 patients, 94% had recurrent disease at 5 years.[11] Survival can be improved with liver-directed therapies performed in patients with progressive disease following initial resection.[12] As stated earlier, a minority (~10%) of patients are candidates for resection at initial presentation.[2] For the remaining majority of patients, liver-directed therapies and/or systemic and targeted molecular therapies are considered.

Orthotopic liver transplantation (OLT) is a potential curative treatment of NLMs; however, prognosis is worse relative to all other liver transplant recipients (5-year survival 57.8% vs. 74% among 185 patients transplanted in the United States),[1] and postoperative mortality is relatively high. Similar data were observed in a European series of 103 patients across 23 institutions (overall survival of 47% and recurrence-free survival of 24% at 5 years).[13] Nevertheless, some centers will consider patients with NLMs for transplantation.

Systemic and Targeted Molecular Therapies

Systemic chemotherapy has varied success in the treatment of NLMs and depends on primary tumor site and histologic tumor grade. Regimens for well-differentiated pNET generally include combinations of streptozotocin, doxorubicin, and 5-fluorouracil (5-FU). Midgut NET has been treated with similar regimens with the addition of cyclophosphamide, and etoposide/cisplatin has been studied in poorly differentiated gastroenteropancreatic NET.[3] Systemic chemotherapy for carcinoid tumors has been less successful.

Somatostatin analogues (SSA) have been used extensively, especially for symptom control. Many other targeted therapies are under review, acting on the mTOR, VEGF, EGFR, IGF-1R, histone deacetylase, protein degradation, immunomodulating, c-kit, and PDGFR pathways.[14] To date, bevacizumab, sunitinib, and everolimus are the most promising available agents and have been studied in phase III clinical trials.[15]

Somatostatin functions as an inhibitor of endocrine activity, reducing portal venous blood flow, decreasing gastrointestinal secretions, inhibiting peristalsis, and downregulating gastrointestinal hormone production. Native human somatostatin peptides have a short half-life of approximately 1 minute,[16] but synthetic analogues have been developed with half-lives of 2 hours—chiefly among these are octreotide and lanreotide. These work exceptionally well for symptom control and reduction of urine 5-hydroxyindoleacetic acid levels[17–21] and also have antiproliferative effects. Side effects are generally mild, including nausea, bloating, and steatorrhea.[7] The PROMID study, a randomized phase III trial using octreotide long-acting repeatable (LAR) versus supportive care in gastroenteropancreatic NETs, reported a median time to progression of 14.3 months for octreotide versus 6 months for placebo (P = .000072), but there was no significant difference in survival.[22] Additionally, this benefit was most pronounced in patients with low tumor burden, well-differentiated tumors, and resected primary tumor.

The mTOR inhibitors temsirolimus and everolimus have been studied in NETs. In the RADIANT 1 trial, everolimus monotherapy (n = 115) had a response rate and median progression-free survival (PFS) of 9% and 9.7 months, respectively, and everolimus plus octreotide (n = 45) demonstrated a 4% response rate and PFS of 16.7 months.[23] In a subsequent phase III trial of metastatic functional carcinoid tumors (RADIANT 2), increased PFS of 16.4 months versus 11.3 months was observed when 10 mg oral everolimus daily was added to 30 mg intramuscular octreotide LAR every 28 days, compared to octreotide LAR alone. This result was borderline significant (P = .026).[24] The RADIANT 3 trial randomized 410 patients with PNETs to everolimus versus supportive care, showing PFS of 11.0 months versus 4.6 months for placebo.[25]

Inhibition of the VEGF pathway has been promising, as increased circulating levels of VEGF are associated with NET progression. A monoclonal antibody to VEGF, bevacizumab, showed a 95% PFS at 18 weeks versus 68% for pegylated interferon (PEG-IFN).[26] Another agent, sunitinib, a tyrosine kinase receptor inhibitor, was also studied in patients with PNET. This phase III study including 171 patients demonstrated median PFS of 11.4 months versus 5.5 months, favoring sunitinib 37.5 mg daily to placebo.[27]

Liver-Directed Transarterial Therapies

Interventional approaches to NET include but are not limited to transarterial techniques of tumor embolization and radioembolization. Embolization can be further subdivided into transarterial embolization (TAE), transarterial chemoembolization (TACE), and drug-eluting bead chemoembolization (DEB-TACE). NETs are typically hypervascular within the liver, receiving greater than 90% of their blood supply from the hepatic artery, compared to normal liver parenchyma which receives 75% to 80% of its blood supply from the portal vein and only 20% to 25% from the hepatic artery.[28–30] This provides a rationale for embolic, chemoembolic, or radioembolic material to concentrate with hepatic metastases when administered via selective or superselective catheter angiography. Liver-directed therapies are generally indicated for patients with symptomatic unresectable disease. The timing of integrating liver-directed therapy in asymptomatic patients is somewhat controversial, but given the high response rates in general, many centers favor integrating liver-directed therapies earlier in the disease course.

Hepatic Arterial Embolization and Transarterial Chemoembolization

First proven in the treatment of hepatocellular carcinoma, bland embolization and chemoembolization are gaining traction as palliative treatment of NLMs, particularly in cases of high metastatic tumor burden in the liver. Occasionally, patients are successfully rendered surgically resectable following this type of liver-directed therapy (Fig. 40.1). Administration of embolic material via the hepatic artery, with or without coadministration of chemotherapy, has shown generally high response rates both in tumor control and symptom palliation. Although it is

A B C D

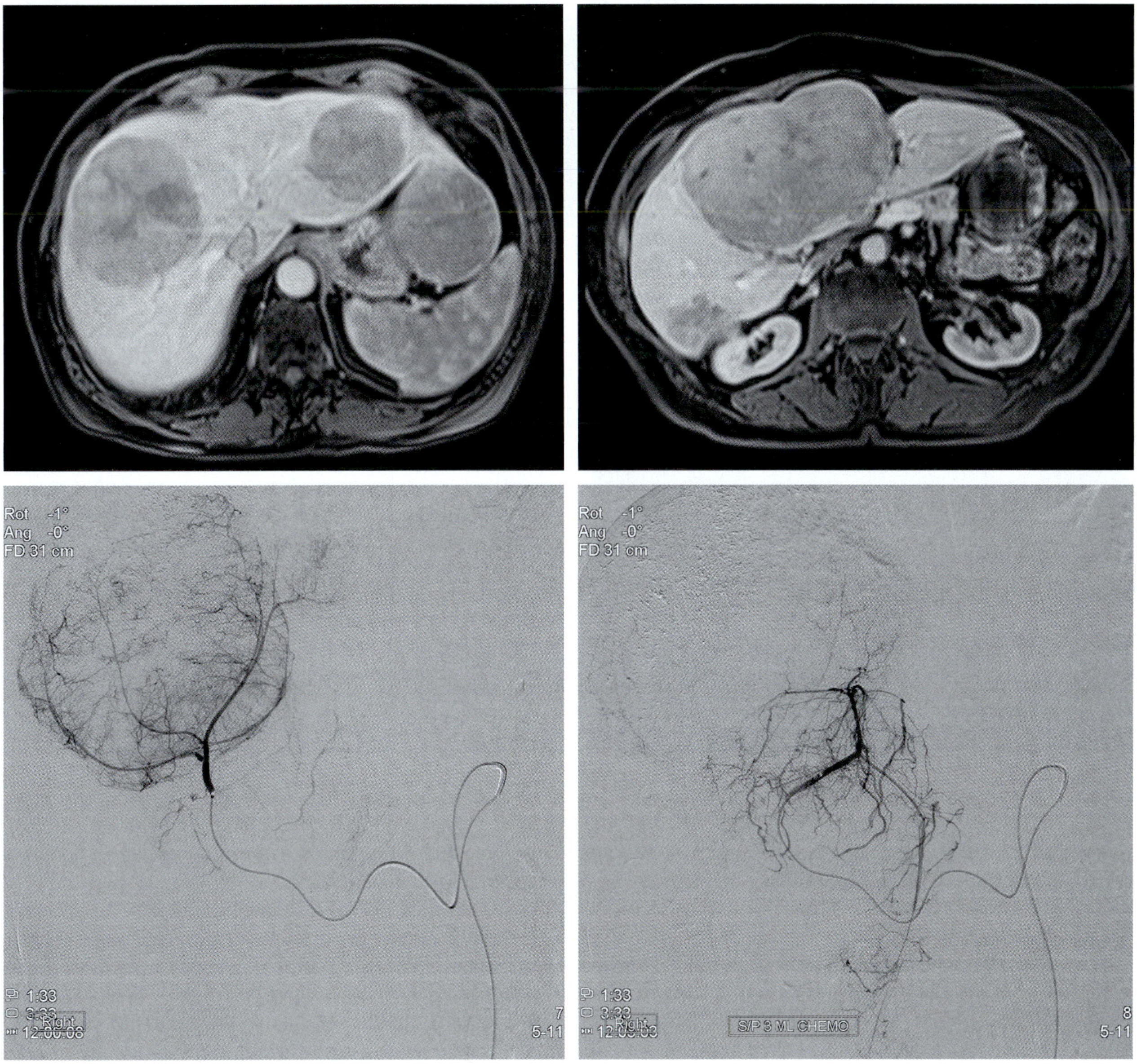

Figure 40.1 A 69-year-old woman initially presented to her primary care physician with cramping abdominal pain. An abdominal ultrasound was obtained after her symptoms recurred despite initial improvement with initiation of a proton pump inhibitor. This demonstrated multiple hepatic lesions, which were confirmed on CT and further characterized with multiphase magnetic resonance imaging (MRI) (**A** and **B**; postcontrast T1 weighted images) confirming bulky bilobar disease. Subsequent liver biopsy confirmed metastatic NE carcinoma with a Ki 67 proliferation index of 12%. Additional workup including octreoscan revealed no primary tumor. The patient was evaluated for surgical resection but ultimately referred for liver directed therapy. **C,D:** Selective angiography of the right hepatic lobe demonstrating tumoral neovascularity and tumoral blush. The patient subsequently underwent a total of five TACE procedures over the course of a year with excellent response. *(Continued)*

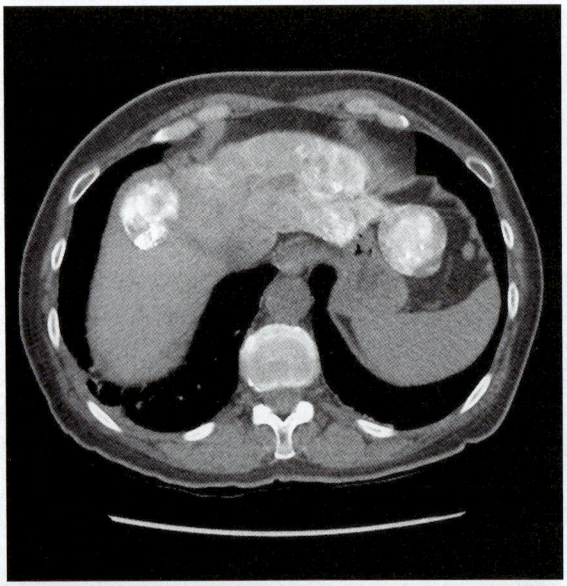

E

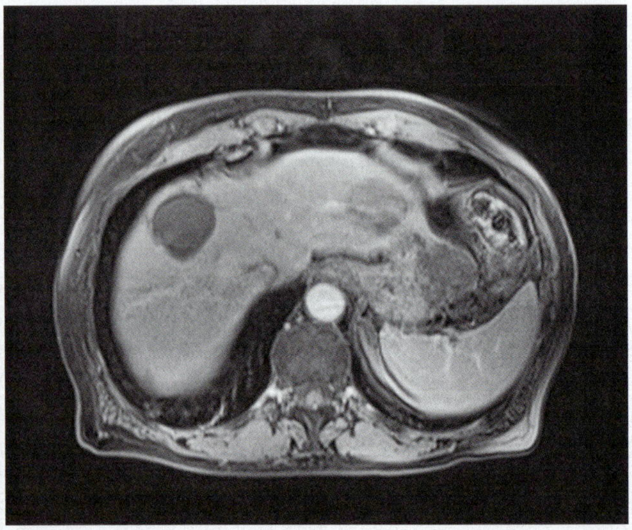

F

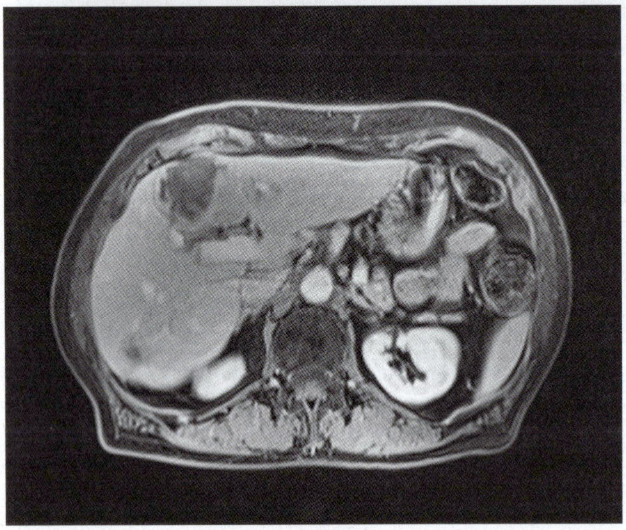

G

Figure 40.1 *(Continued)* **E:** Dense Ethiodol deposition within segment 8 tumor is noted on noncontrast abdominal CT. **F,G:** Follow-up MRI in the portal venous phase demonstrating significantly decreased size of dominant lesions within the liver. The patient underwent left trisegmentectomy liver resection and microwave ablation of the two lesions in the right lobe 1 year after initiation of liver-directed therapy. Pathology demonstrated 95% tumor necrosis and negative resection margins. Additional TACE was performed 8 months following surgery for small hypervascular lesions in segment 7 (measuring <2 cm) with excellent response (not shown). Resolving postoperative changes and no suspicious hepatic lesions were noted on follow-up MRI performed 2 years after initial diagnosis (not shown). Clinically, the patient continues to do well, with slowly resolving fatigue and a dull ache in the right upper quadrant. She no longer requires pain medications, and she is considering returning to work at the age of 71 years.

known that chemotherapy accumulates up to a 20-fold greater concentration when coadministered with an embolic agent,[1] the choice of TAE versus TACE in this setting remains controversial.[31]

TAE and TACE have been studied in NLMs for over three decades (Table 40.1). Carrasco et al.[32] treated 25 patients with carcinoid syndrome using TAE consisting of Ivalon particles (Unipoint Industries, High Point, North Carolina) delivered from the main hepatic artery or a branch vessel, taking care to maintain vessel patency to allow for repeat embolization procedures; a total of 79 embolizations were performed. Symptom improvement was dramatic among 20 of the 23 patients who were followed, with over two-thirds reporting excellent symptom control and a median response duration of 20 months. Among 52 patients with carcinoid tumors treated with either TAE or TACE, 63% had an improvement in symptoms in a study by Gupta et al.[33] Carcinoid crisis was observed following 12.3% of procedures, which was managed in part with octreotide.

In contrast, in a study of 69 patients with metastatic carcinoid, patients treated with TAE were actually six times more likely to respond radiographically than those treated with TACE (81% vs. 44.4%; $P = .002$); however, overall survival was similar between the two treatments.[34] Given the relative resistance of carcinoid tumors to systemic chemotherapy, this result is not necessarily unexpected. In contrast, patients with islet cell tumors showed a trend toward improved response (50% vs. 25%) and prolonged survival (31.5 months vs. 18.2 months) with TACE compared to TAE, but the differences were not statistically significant. Ruutiainen et al.[35] reviewed the results of 219 embolizations in 67 patients with NLMs.[35] Twenty-three patients had TAE, whereas 44 patients had triple drug TACE. Overall, 30-day mortality was 1.4%, with no difference in grade 3 or greater

Table 40.1 Current Series of Transarterial Embolization, Transarterial Chemoembolization, and Drug-Eluting Bead Chemoembolization

Investigators	Device/ Material	No. of Patients	Symptom Improvement	Outcome	Median PFS (months)	Overall Survival (months)	5-Y Survival
Carrasco et al.[32]	TAE	23 carcinoid	87%	87% responders; median duration of response 11+ mo			
Ruszniewski et al.[52]	TACE	18 carcinoid	73%	CR 11%, PR 33%; median duration of effect 14 mo			
Eriksson et al.[53]	TAE	29 carcinoid 12 pNET		52% OR, median duration of effect 12 mo 50% OR, median duration of effect 10 mo		120 20 (from TAE), 60 (from diagnosis)	83% 50%
Schell et al.[54]	TAE	24 carcinoid	64.3% became asymptomatic	Decreased 79.2%, stable 16.7%			72% (predictive)
Gupta et al.[33]	TAE and TACE	81 carcinoid	63%	PR 67%, MR 8.7%, SD 16%, PD 8.7%			24% (predictive)
Loewe et al.[55]	TAE	23 small bowel		CR 18%, PR 55%, SD 22.7%, PD 4.5%			65%
Gupta et al.[34]	TAE and TACE	69 carcinoid 54 pNET		PR 67%, MR 8.7%, SD 16%, PD 8.7% PR 35%, MR 2%, SD 59%, PD 4%	22.7 16.1		29% 14%
Ruutiainen et al.[35]	TAE TACE	44 23	93% 92%	PR 50%, SD 38%, PD 13% at 1 mo PR 66%, SD 22%, PD 12% at 1 mo	6 12		39% 49%
Kamat et al.[56]	TAE and TACE	38	65%	PR or MR 27%	9.2	17.9	
Maire et al.[36]	TAE and TACE	26		PR or MR 30%, SD 35%, PD 1%	19.2 and 23.6		
Hur et al.[57]	TACE	24 npNET 22 pNET		CR or PR 50%, SD or PD 50% CR or PR 66.7%, SD or PD 33.3%	17.4 15.3	55.0 27.6	
de Baere et al.[39]	DEB-TACE	20	81%	PR 80%, SD 15%, PD 5% at 3 mo	15 (TTP)		
Gaur et al.[40]	DEB-TACE	18		PR 36%, SD 43%, PD 21% at >3 mo	13.8 (TTP)		
Bhagat et al.[41a]	DEB-TACE	13		92% stable disease at 1 mo by RECIST, 90% control rate at 6 mo by RECIST			

[a]Trial ended prematurely due to biloma formation.
TAE, transarterial embolization; TACE, transarterial chemoembolization; CR, complete response; PR, partial response; OR, objective response; pNET, pancreatic neuroendocrine tumor; MR, minimal response; SD, stable disease; PD, progressive disease; npNET, nonpancreatic neuroendocrine tumor; DEB-TACE, drug-eluting bead chemoembolization; TTP, time to progression; RECIST, Response Evaluation Criteria In Solid Tumors.

toxicity or hospital stay (1.5 days) between the two groups. Mean duration of symptom control was 15 months for TACE and 7.5 months for TAE. There was no significant difference in survival between the two groups.

A small prospective randomized study was recently published by Maire et al.[36] Twenty-six patients with unresectable NLM were randomized to TAE versus TACE. Two-year PFS was not significantly different (38% TACE, 44% TAE), with no significant difference in 2-year overall survival. An extensive review comparing TAE and TACE for treatment of metastatic carcinoid and islet cell carcinomas concluded that the therapeutic advantage of adding chemotherapy to the embolization regimen is questionable and that the regimens vary widely in the literature such that a consensus on ideal chemotherapy has not been established.[31]

Transarterial Chemoembolization with Drug-Eluting Beads

Although coadministration of chemotherapy with an embolic agent effectively increases drug concentration within liver metastases, the pharmacokinetics are variable and not optimized. Drug-eluting beads (DEBs) are a relatively new local drug delivery platform that can allow for much slower and reproducible drug release. In vitro study of an emulsion of doxorubicin and Lipiodol demonstrated complete release of the chemotherapeutic agent within 4 hours, whereas only 15% of the doxorubicin eluded from 100- to 300-μm DC beads in 24 hours.[37] Theoretically, DEBs can therefore maximize drug delivery to hepatic metastases and minimize systemic toxicity. Plasma levels of circulating chemotherapy are diminished up to 70% to 85% with use of DEBs versus conventional TACE in a rabbit hypervascular tumor model.[38]

Initial experience with DEB-TACE in NETs has shown high response rates, but there are concerns regarding increased incidence of biliary toxicity. de Baere et al.[39] treated 20 patients with well-differentiated gastroenteropancreatic tumors with DEBs (500 to 700 μm) loaded with doxorubicin. After 3 months, partial response was seen in 16 of 20 patients (80%), and only 1 patient (5%) had progressive disease. Mean time to progression was 15 months. Five patients (25%) developed subsegmental regions of liver necrosis identified on follow-up computed tomography (CT) scans located peripheral to the tumors targeted for embolization. In another study of 18 patients with metastatic NETs, an objective response was observed in 17 of 26 (65%) procedures at intermediate-term (>3 months) follow-up.[40] Two patients developed biliary injuries, one of whom required placement of a percutaneous internal/external biliary drainage catheter and the other noted incidentally on routine follow-up imaging and did not require additional treatment. In a more recent study of 13 patients with metastatic NETs, an objective response rate of 78% was observed in the targeted lesions; however, 7 patients (54%) developed bilomas following DEB-TACE (100- to 300-μm beads loaded with doxorubicin).[41] Four of them required percutaneous drainage.

Guiu et al.,[42] expanding on the initial report by de Baere et al.,[39] analyzed 278 patients with NETs who underwent either conventional TACE (n = 152) or DEB-TACE (n = 126), compared to patients with hepatocellular carcinoma (HCC) who underwent conventional TACE (n = 142) or DEB-TACE (n = 56). Liver/biliary injuries were defined as either a dilated bile duct, portal vein narrowing or thrombosis, or a biloma/liver infarct (grouped together given the difficulty in discriminating between these two entities at contrast-enhanced CT). Liver/biliary injuries occurred with a frequency of 35.7% for NET and 30.4% for HCC after DEB-TACE sessions, whereas frequencies of 7.2% and 4.2% were observed following conventional TACE for treatment of NET and HCC, respectively. On multivariate analysis, the risk of liver/biliary injury was 6.63 times greater with DEB-TACE than with conventional TACE.

Radioembolization

External beam radiation therapy has a limited role in the treatment of hepatic metastases due to the sensitivity of normal hepatic parenchyma relative to the doses required to treat metastatic lesions. However, use of a microsphere platform to deliver localized radiotherapy has been used with success in HCC and has subsequently been used to treat hepatic metastases.[43] Selective internal radiation therapy (SIRT) consists of yttrium 90 (^{90}Y) microspheres delivered via the hepatic artery typically to a target dose of 120 Gy. ^{90}Y is a pure β emitter with a tissue penetration of approximately 2.5 mm. Similar to the preferential uptake of Lipiodol emulsions with TACE procedures, hypervascular NE metastases preferentially accumulate ^{90}Y microspheres relative to normal liver parenchyma. Two devices are currently available: glass microspheres (TheraSphere; Nordion, Ottawa, Ontario, Canada) and resin microspheres (SIR-Spheres; SIRTeX Medical Limited, New South Wales, Australia). Several trials have investigated their use for NLMs (Table 40.2).

Use of ^{90}Y microspheres to treat NLMs was first reported in 1968 in a series of five patients using various percutaneous approaches and laparotomy-assisted procedures with delivery of 15-μm carbonized microspheres suspended in dextran.[44] Distribution of ^{90}Y radioactivity was assessed postprocedurally with Bremsstrahlung scanning. Three of the five patients experienced significant improvement in symptoms following radioembolization. In two patients, however, higher than expected levels of radioactivity were administered to the stomach. Both patients experienced poor outcomes due to gastric ulceration and severe upper gastrointestinal hemorrhage, illustrating the critical importance of preventing nontarget delivery of ^{90}Y microspheres.

More recently, King et al.[45] treated 34 patients with progressive unresectable NETs with SIR-Spheres administered concurrent with a radiosensitizing agent (consisting of 5-FU given intravenously for 7 days, beginning the day before SIRT). The mean dose of ^{90}Y was 1.99 GBq (range 0.92 to

Table 40.2 Current Series of Yttrium 90 Radioembolization

Investigators	Device/Material	No. of Patients	Symptom Improvement	Outcome	Overall Survival (months)	5-Y Survival
Simon et al.[44]	Carbonized microspheres	5	57%			
King et al.[45]	SIR-Spheres + 5-FU	34	55% at 3 mo, 50% at 6 mo	CR 18%, PR 32%, SD 15%, PD 32%	27.6	
Kennedy et al.[46]	SIR-Spheres	148		CR 2.7%, PR 60.5%, SD 22.7%, PD 4.9%	70	
Murthy et al.[58]	SIR-Spheres	8		PR 12.5%, SD 50%, PD 37.5%	14	
Rhee et al.[47]	SIR-Spheres	20		PR 50%, SD 43.8%, PD 6.3% at 6 mo	28 (projected)	
	TheraSphere	22		PR 54%, SD 38.4%, PD 7.7% at 6 months	22 (projected)	
Kalinowski et al.[59]	SIR-Spheres	9	86% at 6 mo	PR 66.7%, SD 33.3% at 6 mo		57% (3-y)
Saxena et al.[48]	SIR-Spheres	48		CR 15%, PR 40%, SD 23%, PD 23%	35	46%
Memon et al.[49]	TheraSphere	40	84%	CR 1.2%, PR 62.7%, SD 32.5%, PD 3.6%	34.4	45% (3-y)
Paprottka et al.[50]	SIR-Spheres	42	95% at 3 mo	CR 0%, PR 22.5%, SD 75%, PD 2.5% at 3 mo	95% alive at 16.2 mo	

5-FU, 5-fluorouracil; CR, complete response; PR, partial response; SD, stable disease; PD, progressive disease.

2.80 GBq) delivered as a whole liver treatment using separate infusions via the right and left hepatic artery for bilobar disease. Mean survival was 27.6 months; a complete or partial response was seen in 50% of the cohort. In the largest series to date, Kennedy et al.[46] reported a retrospective, multi-institutional review encompassing 148 patients with various NETs, the majority arising from the midgut or pancreas, predominantly of carcinoid histology. The mean dose per procedure was 1.31 GBq. Mean survival was 70 months, with nearly two-thirds of the cohort demonstrating a complete or partial response at 3 months.

The TheraSphere and SIR-Spheres devices have shown similar efficacy in a multicenter study by Rhee et al.[47] treating patients with carcinoid and pancreatic islet tumors, demonstrating overall response rates of 92% and 94%, respectively, despite the inherent differences in relative embolic and radiation effects between these two devices. Grade 3 hepatic toxicities were more common among patients treated with the TheraSphere device, but this was largely attributed to the early experience with glass microspheres and possibly greater exposure to prior TAE and TACE treatments among this cohort. Use of more stringent patient selection criteria led to fewer toxicities with both glass- and resin-based microsphere devices in subsequent treatment sessions of this phase II trial. Several more recent single institution series continue to demonstrate excellent symptom control and tumor response rates, and reasonable overall survival, using both devices among various tumors.[48-50] Paprottka et al.[50] treated 42 patients with treatment-refractory NET liver metastases using SIR-Spheres and demonstrated symptomatic improvement in 36 of 38 patients at 3 months. Partial response or stable disease was observed in 97.5% of the cohort, and 95.2% of patients remained alive at the mean follow-up (16.2 months). Memon et al.[49] demonstrated satisfactory 1-, 2-, and 3-year overall survival rates (72.5%, 62.5%, and 45%, respectively) using the TheraSphere device in 40 patients, a cohort with predominantly low hepatic tumor burden (<25% in 32 of 40 patients) and good performance status (Eastern Cooperative Oncology Group [ECOG] 0 in 30 patients), although most patients had received prior systemic therapy. By WHO guidelines, complete response in 1.2% of lesions and partial response in 62.7% was observed, whereas using European Association for the Study of Liver (EASL) criteria, complete response (100% lesion necrosis) was seen in 20.5% of lesions, with a median time to response of 4.9 months. On multivariate analysis, ECOG performance status of 0 and bilirubin less than 1.2 mg/dL were identified as good prognostic indicators.

Choice of Therapy

Despite the multitude of trials using liver-directed therapies, fewer studies have directly compared surgical, intra-arterial, and systemic therapies for NLMs. Given the broad spectrum of primary tumor site and tumor aggressiveness, this is particularly problematic when appraising the current literature to make patient-specific treatment decisions. Guidelines from the National Comprehensive Cancer Network (NCCN) recommend complete resection when possible for metastatic carcinoid tumors and pNETs and observation with markers and scans every 3 to 12 months for asymptomatic, low-volume unresectable disease.[51] For symptomatic disease, the approach is patient-specific and may include cytoreductive surgery/ablative therapy, liver-directed therapy, or cytotoxic chemotherapy. Often, a combination of therapies may be employed (Fig. 40.2).

Interestingly, a multicenter international study demonstrated no discernible benefit from surgery over intra-arterial therapy for asymptomatic, high-volume (>25%) hepatic disease, concluding that liver-directed therapies may hence be a more appropriate therapy for this patient population.[2] Added to this milieu are targeted molecular therapies (namely octreotide, everolimus, and sunitinib), more of which are likely to become available in the future. Further prospective studies will be essential to compare these various therapies and help guide decision making in the multidisciplinary care of NE hepatic metastases.

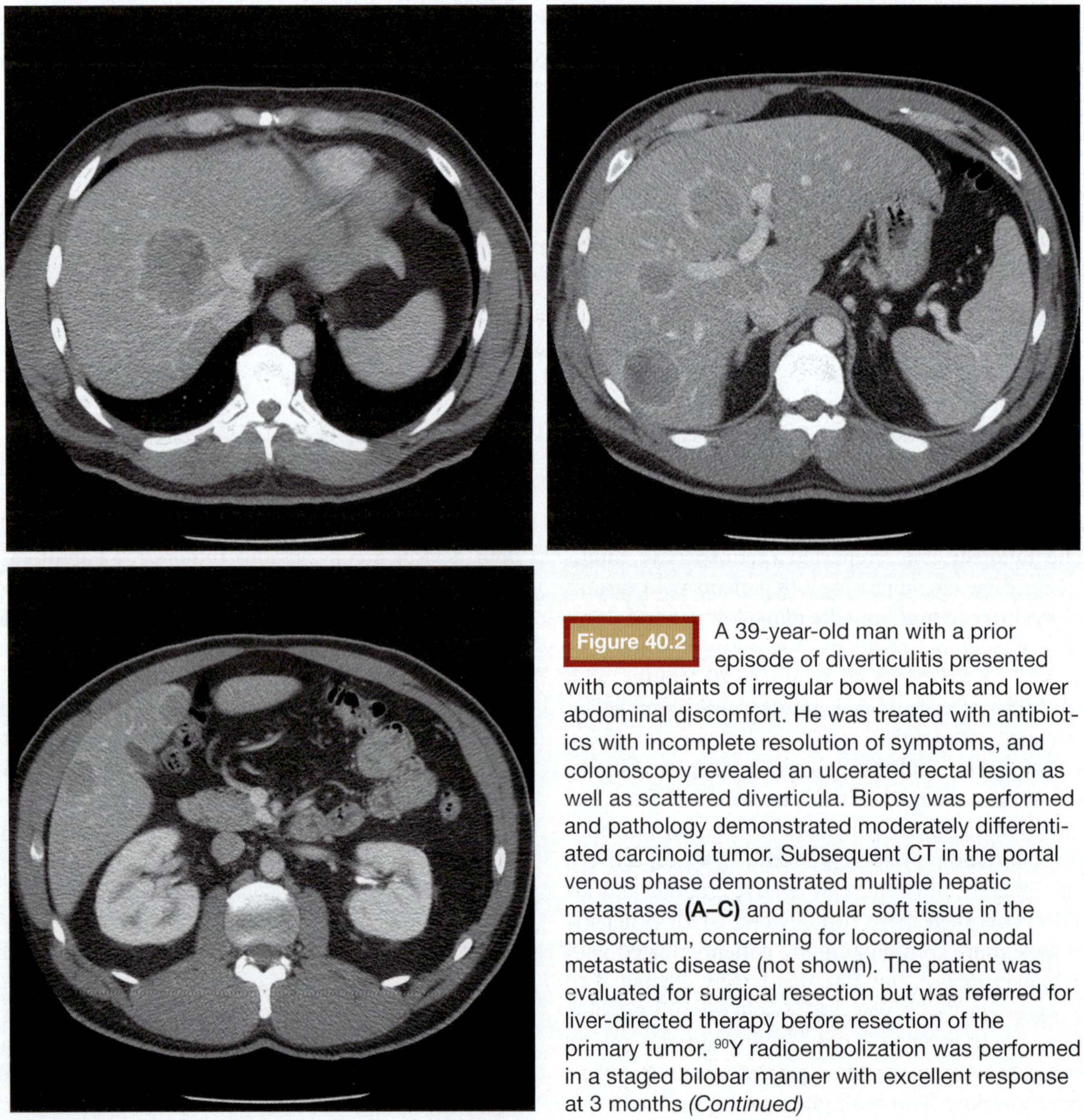

A B C

Figure 40.2 A 39-year-old man with a prior episode of diverticulitis presented with complaints of irregular bowel habits and lower abdominal discomfort. He was treated with antibiotics with incomplete resolution of symptoms, and colonoscopy revealed an ulcerated rectal lesion as well as scattered diverticula. Biopsy was performed and pathology demonstrated moderately differentiated carcinoid tumor. Subsequent CT in the portal venous phase demonstrated multiple hepatic metastases **(A–C)** and nodular soft tissue in the mesorectum, concerning for locoregional nodal metastatic disease (not shown). The patient was evaluated for surgical resection but was referred for liver-directed therapy before resection of the primary tumor. ^{90}Y radioembolization was performed in a staged bilobar manner with excellent response at 3 months *(Continued)*

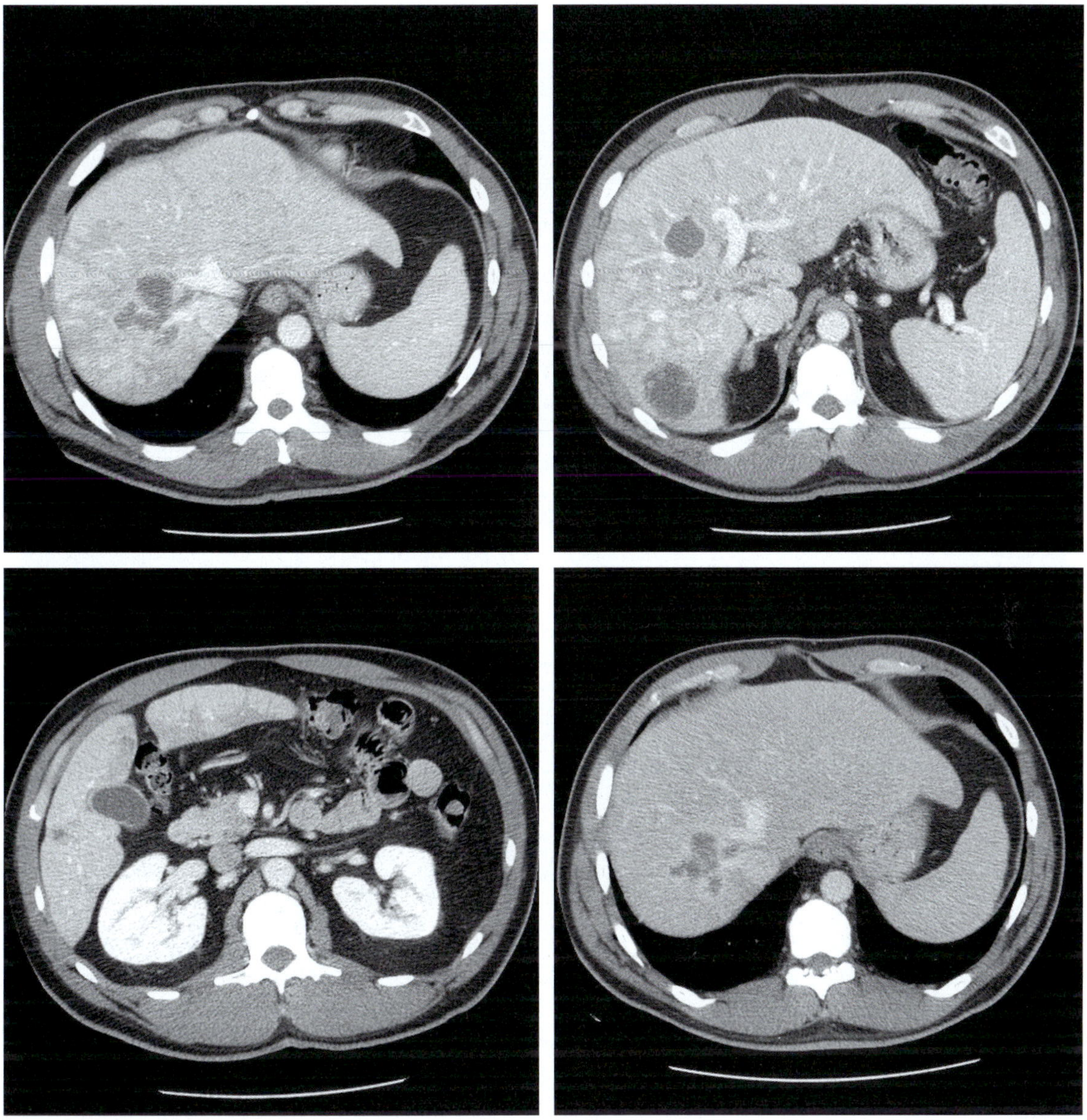

D E F G

Figure 40.2 *(Continued)* **(D–F)** such that the patient underwent a low anterior resection with J-pouch anal anastomosis and diverting loop ileostomy. Continued response was observed at 6 months *(Continued)*

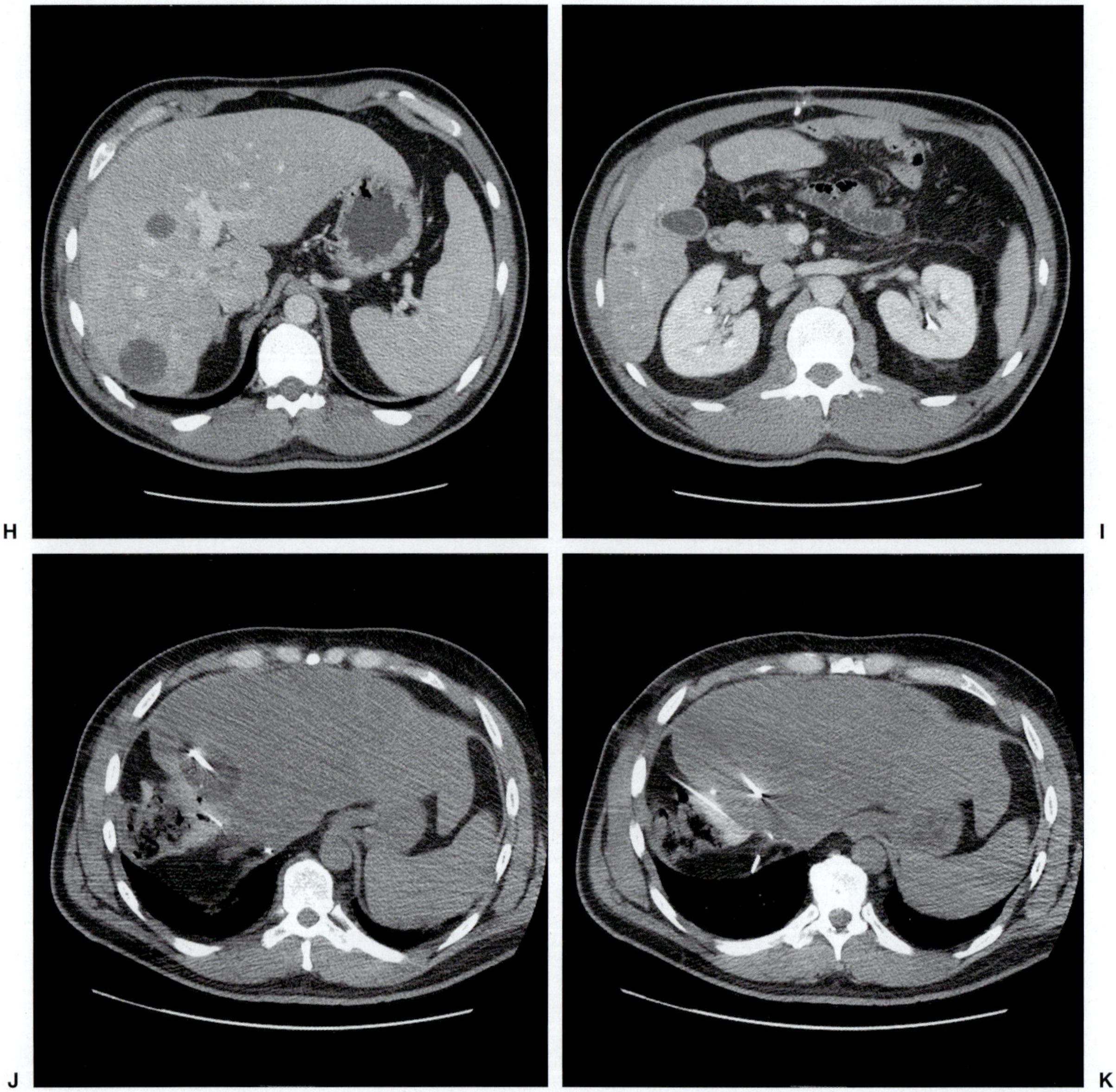

Figure 40.2 *(Continued)* **(G–I)**, and the patient ultimately underwent right hepatic lobectomy and intraoperative microwave ablation of multiple liver tumors 1 year after radioembolization. Multiple recurrences over the next 5 years have necessitated a combination of operative and interventional treatments, with the patient undergoing three additional operative procedures (including intraoperative ultrasound, microwave ablation, and resection of a tumor in the caudate lobe), three percutaneous cryoablation procedures (**J,K**; hydrodissection-assisted cryoablation to the periphery of the hypertrophied left hepatic lobe near the surgical resection margin), and two TACE procedures (not shown). The patient is currently undergoing evaluation for possible liver transplantation.

SUMMARY

NETs are a heterogeneous group of malignancies with a range of biologic behavior and increasing incidence. Relative to other solid organ tumors, prognosis is generally good, with many patients surviving long enough to receive many different types of therapy. Liver-directed interventional therapies play a key role in the multidisciplinary and multimodality management of these patients. Further prospective studies will be required to refine patient selective criteria, compare different liver-directed therapies, and study combinations of systemic and locoregional approaches.

REFERENCES

1. Harring TR, Nguyen NT, Goss JA, et al. Treatment of liver metastases in patients with neuroendocrine tumors: a comprehensive review. *Int J Hepatol.* 2011;2011:154541.

2. Mayo SC, de Jong MC, Bloomston M, et al. Surgery versus intra-arterial therapy for neuroendocrine liver metastasis: a multicenter international analysis. *Ann Surg Oncol.* 2011;18(13):3657–3665.
3. O'Toole D, Hentic O, Corcos O, et al. Chemotherapy for gastro-enteropancreatic endocrine tumours. *Neuroendocrinology.* 2004;80(suppl 1):79–84.
4. Yao JC, Hassan M, Phan A, et al. One hundred years after "carcinoid": epidemiology of and prognostic factors for neuroendocrine tumors in 35,825 cases in the united states. *J Clin Oncol.* 2008;26(18):3063–3072.
5. Lawrence B, Gustafsson BI, Chan A, et al. The epidemiology of gastroenteropancreatic neuroendocrine tumors. *Endocrinol Metab Clin North Am.* 2011;40(1):1–18, vii.
6. Klimstra DS, Modlin IR, Coppola D, et al. The pathologic classification of neuroendocrine tumors: a review of nomenclature, grading, and staging systems. *Pancreas.* 2010;39(6):707–712.
7. Strosberg JR, Cheema A, Kvols LK. A review of systemic and liver-directed therapies for metastatic neuroendocrine tumors of the gastroenteropancreatic tract. *Cancer Control.* 2011;18(2):127–137.
8. Saxena A, Chua TC, Perera M, et al. Surgical resection of hepatic metastases from neuroendocrine neoplasms: a systematic review. *Surg Oncol.* 2012;21(3):e131–e141.
9. McEntee GP, Nagorney DM, Kvols LK, et al. Cytoreductive hepatic surgery for neuroendocrine tumors. *Surgery.* 1990;108(6):1091–1096.
10. Sarmiento JM, Heywood G, Rubin J, et al. Surgical treatment of neuroendocrine metastases to the liver: a plea for resection to increase survival. *J Am Coll Surg.* 2003;197(1):29–37.
11. Mayo SC, de Jong MC, Pulitano C, et al. Surgical management of hepatic neuroendocrine tumor metastasis: results from an international multi-institutional analysis. *Ann Surg Oncol.* 2010;17(12):3129–3136.
12. Saxena A, Chua TC, Zhao J, et al. Liver-directed therapy for neuroendocrine neoplasm hepatic metastasis prolongs survival following progression after initial surgery. *J Surg Oncol.* 2012;105(4):342–350.
13. Lehnert T. Liver transplantation for metastatic neuroendocrine carcinoma: an analysis of 103 patients. *Transplantation.* 1998;66(10):1307–1312.
14. Naraev BG, Strosberg JR, Halfdanarson TR. Current status and perspectives of targeted therapy in well-differentiated neuroendocrine tumors. *Oncology.* 2012;83(3):117–127.
15. Yim KL. Role of biological targeted therapies in gastroenteropancreatic neuroendocrine tumours. *Endocrine.* 2011;40(2):181–186.
16. Bousquet C, Puente E, Buscail L, et al. Antiproliferative effect of somatostatin and analogs. *Chemotherapy.* 2001;47(suppl 2): 30–39.
17. Kvols LK, Moertel CG, O'Connell MJ, et al. Treatment of the malignant carcinoid syndrome. evaluation of a long-acting somatostatin analogue. *N Engl J Med.* 1986;315(11):663–666.
18. di Bartolomeo M, Bajetta E, Buzzoni R, et al. Clinical efficacy of octreotide in the treatment of metastatic neuroendocrine tumors. A study by the italian trials in medical oncology group. *Cancer.* 1996;77(2):402–408.
19. Maton PN, Gardner JD, Jensen RT. Use of long-acting somatostatin analog SMS 201-995 in patients with pancreatic islet cell tumors. *Dig Dis Sci.* 1989;34(3)(suppl):28S–39S.
20. Rubin J, Ajani J, Schirmer W, et al. Octreotide acetate long-acting formulation versus open-label subcutaneous octreotide acetate in malignant carcinoid syndrome. *J Clin Oncol.* 1999;17(2):600–606.
21. O'Toole D, Ducreux M, Bommelaer G, et al. Treatment of carcinoid syndrome: a prospective crossover evaluation of lanreotide versus octreotide in terms of efficacy, patient acceptability, and tolerance. *Cancer.* 2000;88(4):770–776.
22. Rinke A, Muller HH, Schade-Brittinger C, et al. Placebo-controlled, double-blind, prospective, randomized study on the effect of octreotide LAR in the control of tumor growth in patients with metastatic neuroendocrine midgut tumors: a report from the PROMID study group. *J Clin Oncol.* 2009;27(28): 4656–4663.
23. Yao JC, Lombard-Bohas C, Baudin E, et al. Daily oral everolimus activity in patients with metastatic pancreatic neuroendocrine tumors after failure of cytotoxic chemotherapy: a phase II trial. *J Clin Oncol.* 2010;28(1):69–76.
24. Pavel ME, Hainsworth JD, Baudin E, et al. Everolimus plus octreotide long-acting repeatable for the treatment of advanced neuroendocrine tumours associated with carcinoid syndrome (RADIANT-2): a randomised, placebo-controlled, phase 3 study. *Lancet.* 2011;378(9808):2005–2012.
25. Yao JC, Shah MH, Ito T, et al. Everolimus for advanced pancreatic neuroendocrine tumors. *N Engl J Med.* 2011;364(6): 514–523.
26. Yao JC, Phan A, Hoff PM, et al. Targeting vascular endothelial growth factor in advanced carcinoid tumor: a random assignment phase II study of depot octreotide with bevacizumab and pegylated interferon alpha-2b. *J Clin Oncol.* 2008;26(8): 1316–1323.
27. Raymond E, Dahan L, Raoul JL, et al. Sunitinib malate for the treatment of pancreatic neuroendocrine tumors. *N Engl J Med.* 2011;364(6):501–513.
28. Breedis C, Young G. The blood supply of neoplasms in the liver. *Am J Pathol.* 1954;30(5):969–977.
29. Venook AP. Embolization and chemoembolization therapy for neuroendocrine tumors. *Curr Opin Oncol.* 1999;11(1):38–41.
30. Vogl TJ, Naguib NN, Zangos S, et al. Liver metastases of neuroendocrine carcinomas: interventional treatment via transarterial embolization, chemoembolization and thermal ablation. *Eur J Radiol.* 2009;72(3):517–528.
31. Madoff DC, Gupta S, Ahrar K, et al. Update on the management of neuroendocrine hepatic metastases. *J Vasc Interv Radiol.* 2006;17(8):1235–1249; quiz 1250.
32. Carrasco CH, Charnsangavej C, Ajani J, et al. The carcinoid syndrome: palliation by hepatic artery embolization. *AJR Am J Roentgenol.* 1986;147(1):149–154.
33. Gupta S, Yao JC, Ahrar K, et al. Hepatic artery embolization and chemoembolization for treatment of patients with metastatic carcinoid tumors: the M.D. Anderson experience. *Cancer J.* 2003;9(4):261–267.
34. Gupta S, Johnson MM, Murthy R, et al. Hepatic arterial embolization and chemoembolization for the treatment of patients with metastatic neuroendocrine tumors: variables affecting response rates and survival. *Cancer.* 2005;104(8):1590–1602.
35. Ruutiainen AT, Soulen MC, Tuite CM, et al. Chemoembolization and bland embolization of neuroendocrine tumor metastases to the liver. *J Vasc Interv Radiol.* 2007;18(7):847–855.

36. Maire F, Lombard-Bohas C, O'Toole D, et al. Hepatic arterial embolization versus chemoembolization in the treatment of liver metastases from well-differentiated midgut endocrine tumors: a prospective randomized study. *Neuroendocrinology.* 2012;96(4):294–300.
37. Lewis AL, Gonzalez MV, Lloyd AW, et al. DC bead: in vitro characterization of a drug-delivery device for transarterial chemoembolization. *J Vasc Interv Radiol.* 2006;17(2, pt 1):335–342.
38. Hong K, Khwaja A, Liapi E, et al. New intra-arterial drug delivery system for the treatment of liver cancer: preclinical assessment in a rabbit model of liver cancer. *Clin Cancer Res.* 2006;12(8):2563–2567.
39. de Baere T, Deschamps F, Teriitheau C, et al. Transarterial chemoembolization of liver metastases from well differentiated gastroenteropancreatic endocrine tumors with doxorubicin-eluting beads: preliminary results. *J Vasc Interv Radiol.* 2008;19(6):855–861.
40. Gaur SK, Friese JL, Sadow CA, et al. Hepatic arterial chemoembolization using drug-eluting beads in gastrointestinal neuroendocrine tumor metastatic to the liver. *Cardiovasc Intervent Radiol.* 2011;34(3):566–572.
41. Bhagat N, Reyes DK, Lin M, et al. Phase II study of chemoembolization with drug-eluting beads in patients with hepatic neuroendocrine metastases: high incidence of biliary injury. *Cardiovasc Intervent Radiol.* 2013;36(2):449–459.
42. Guiu B, Deschamps F, Aho S, et al. Liver/biliary injuries following chemoembolisation of endocrine tumours and hepatocellular carcinoma: Lipiodol vs. drug-eluting beads. *J Hepatol.* 2012;56(3):609–617.
43. Memon K, Lewandowski RJ, Riaz A, et al. Chemoembolization and radioembolization for metastatic disease to the liver: available data and future studies. *Curr Treat Options Oncol.* 2012;13(3):403–415.
44. Simon N, Warner RR, Baron MG, et al. Intra-arterial irradiation of carcinoid tumors of the liver. *Am J Roentgenol Radium Ther Nucl Med.* 1968;102(3):552–561.
45. King J, Quinn R, Glenn DM, et al. Radioembolization with selective internal radiation microspheres for neuroendocrine liver metastases. *Cancer.* 2008;113(5):921–929.
46. Kennedy AS, Dezarn WA, McNeillie P, et al. Radioembolization for unresectable neuroendocrine hepatic metastases using resin 90Y-microspheres: early results in 148 patients. *Am J Clin Oncol.* 2008;31(3):271–279.
47. Rhee TK, Lewandowski RJ, Liu DM, et al. 90Y radioembolization for metastatic neuroendocrine liver tumors: preliminary results from a multi-institutional experience. *Ann Surg.* 2008;247(6):1029–1035.
48. Saxena A, Chua TC, Bester L, et al. Factors predicting response and survival after yttrium-90 radioembolization of unresectable neuroendocrine tumor liver metastases: a critical appraisal of 48 cases. *Ann Surg.* 2010;251(5):910–916.
49. Memon K, Lewandowski RJ, Mulcahy MF, et al. Radioembolization for neuroendocrine liver metastases: safety, imaging, and long-term outcomes. *Int J Radiat Oncol Biol Phys.* 2012; 83(3):887–894.
50. Paprottka PM, Hoffmann RT, Haug A, et al. Radioembolization of symptomatic, unresectable neuroendocrine hepatic metastases using yttrium-90 microspheres. *Cardiovasc Intervent Radiol.* 2012;35(2):334–342.
51. Kulke MH, Benson AB III, Bergsland E, et al. Neuroendocrine tumors. *J Natl Compr Canc Netw.* 2012;10(6):724–764.
52. Ruszniewski P, Rougier P, Roche A, et al. Hepatic arterial chemoembolization in patients with liver metastases of endocrine tumors. A prospective phase II study in 24 patients. *Cancer.* 1993;71(8):2624–2630.
53. Eriksson BK, Larsson EG, Skogseid BM, et al. Liver embolizations of patients with malignant neuroendocrine gastrointestinal tumors. *Cancer.* 1998;83(11):2293–2301.
54. Schell SR, Camp ER, Caridi JG, et al. Hepatic artery embolization for control of symptoms, octreotide requirements, and tumor progression in metastatic carcinoid tumors. *J Gastrointest Surg.* 2002;6(5):664–670.
55. Loewe C, Schindl M, Cejna M, et al. Permanent transarterial embolization of neuroendocrine metastases of the liver using cyanoacrylate and lipiodol: assessment of mid- and long-term results. *AJR Am J Roentgenol.* 2003;180(5): 1379–1384.
56. Kamat PP, Gupta S, Ensor JE, et al. Hepatic arterial embolization and chemoembolization in the management of patients with large-volume liver metastases. *Cardiovasc Intervent Radiol.* 2008;31(2):299–307.
57. Hur S, Chung JW, Kim HC, et al. Survival outcomes and prognostic factors of transcatheter arterial chemoembolization for hepatic neuroendocrine metastases. *J Vasc Interv Radiol.* 2013;24(7):947–956.
58. Murthy R, Kamat P, Nunez R, et al. Yttrium-90 microsphere radioembolotherapy of hepatic metastatic neuroendocrine carcinomas after hepatic arterial embolization. *J Vasc Interv Radiol.* 2008;19(1):145–151.
59. Kalinowski M, Dressler M, Konig A, et al. Selective internal radiotherapy with yttrium-90 microspheres for hepatic metastatic neuroendocrine tumors: a prospective single center study. *Digestion.* 2009;79(3):137–142.

41

Colorectal Liver Disease

C. T. Sofocleous • P. Sideras • Elena N. Petre

Intra-arterial therapies directed to the liver take advantage of the dual hepatic blood supply and specifically the fact that liver tumors are fed by the hepatic artery, whereas the normal liver parenchyma gets its supply primarily from the portal vein.[1] Surgery confers the best treatment option for colorectal liver metastases (CLM) but, unfortunately, only 20% of patients are eligible. Even more unfortunate is the 70% rate of patients developing new liver metastases after resection.[1] There is, therefore, a tremendous need for nonsurgical therapies targeting liver metastases in patients with colorectal cancer. When using intra-arterial therapies in the setting of liver metastases, a drug (or radiation) injected in the hepatic artery will preferentially reach the tumor. Intra-arterial therapies to the liver include radioembolization or selective internal radiation therapy (SIRT), hepatic arterial chemotherapy (HAC), and transarterial chemoembolization (TACE) with oil or drug-eluting beads (DEB-TACE).[2] Such treatments have been used as salvage therapies to manage progression after systemic therapies or other local or locoregional therapies.[3–5] Intra-arterial therapies have also been used earlier in the course of the disease to achieve maximal response aiming to convert a candidate from nonsurgical to surgical. HAC with different chemotherapeutic agents allows 90% response rates and conversion to surgery up to 40% to 50% of initially inoperable patients.[6] TACE and, in particular, DEB-TACE with irinotecan-loaded beads (DEBIRI) have been used for CLM with promising response rates and oncologic outcomes.[7–9] Radioembolization or SIRT is a unique way of delivering a high tumoricidal dose of radiation to the tumor via the arterial pathway while minimizing toxicity to uninvolved liver. This therapy received original U.S. Food and Drug Administration approval when the use of resin microspheres in combination with HAC proved superior in terms of response and liver tumor control when compared to HAC alone.[10] Subsequent results of SIRT were promising enough and led to further randomized control trials in the salvage setting as well as an ongoing trial with the use of SIRT with first-line chemotherapy (SIRFLOX).[11–14] With these new techniques, as well as the much better established percutaneous thermal ablation, interventional oncology has emerged as an integral part of the colon cancer patient management in a multidisciplinary and tailored manner along with radiation, surgical, and medical oncology. Such tailored and multidisciplinary approach can achieve the best possible oncologic outcomes and specifically improve disease progression-free and patient overall survivals. In this chapter, we will discuss the indications for and the use of arterially directed liver therapies and we will review the literature with their respective expected outcomes.

INDICATIONS

Arterially directed liver therapies (ATs) are local or regional treatments that are most often used in patients suffering from colon cancer liver metastases without or with limited and controlled extrahepatic disease. Such therapies have been used as salvage treatments after failure of intravenous (IV) standard of care chemotherapy. Interestingly, the response rates were improved even in cases where the AT was administered with a drug that previously failed.[12] Candidates for intra-arterial therapies are generally patients with a life expectancy of more than 3 months, ideally with Eastern Cooperative Oncology Group (ECOG) status of 2 or better and with a sufficient functional liver reserve. There is no uniform agreement on what is considered sufficient liver function, but a bilirubin level of greater than 3 mg/dL, an albumin level of less than 3 g/dL, and an international normalized ratio of 1.6 or higher are often deemed contraindications for any AT. Biliary obstruction should be corrected before any AT to prevent biliary necrosis and rapid deterioration of liver function, which can be fatal. Furthermore, patients with insufficient sphincter of Oddi are at increased risk of hepatic abscess formation, and in these cases, preprocedural and postprocedural biliary excreted antibiotic coverage is mandatory.[15]

Whenever such therapies are used as first-line treatments, also called *induction treatments*, their goal is to obtain the highest response as early as possible in the disease to convert a nonsurgical to a surgical candidate. Indeed, it has been shown that there is a linear correlation between the response rate and the resection rate when ATs were used as induction therapies.[16] It is necessary to indicate that ATs are commonly used in patients who cannot undergo surgery or ablation. As such, most patients will have more than three tumors in the liver or larger tumors that cannot be resected or ablated with clear margins.[17]

HEPATIC ARTERIAL CHEMOTHERAPY

Intra-arterial hepatic chemotherapy has the goal of increasing drug concentrations in the metastatic deposits resulting in significant increase in response rates. The advantage of this route is proportional to the first-pass extraction of the drug by the liver and inversely proportional to body clearance. One drug that has been extensively used is floxuridine (FUDR), having a 95% liver extraction with liver exposures ranging from 100 to 300 times higher than with systemic administration.[2] Also, the advantage of HAC applied with other chemotherapeutic agents was that exposure was several-fold increased by this method rather than IV perfusion alone. This allows intermittent administration with repeated course of chemotherapy over few weeks through the peripheral arterial access where a permanent subcutaneous port is linked to the intra-arterial catheter. This affords a better quality of life.

HAC requires placement of permanent intra-arterial catheter linked to a port usually placed surgically,[1,18,19] although percutaneous placement is also feasible.[20,21] During placement, the surgeon skeletonizes the hepatic arteries around the tip of the catheter that is placed in the gastroduodenal artery. This is done to prevent any extrahepatic delivery of the chemotherapeutic agent in the gastrointestinal tract. Often, the placement of the hepatic arterial infusion pump (HAIP) is performed while the patient is under general anesthesia for resection of the primary and/or a liver metastasis. At the same type, cholecystectomy is routinely performed.[1] When no resection is anticipated, the HAIP can be placed through minimal invasive techniques, replacing largely the need for open surgery or repeated catheterizations.[21] Similarly to the surgical ligation of arterial branches during intra-arterial hepatic pump placement, interventional radiologists ensure remodeling of flow before the insertion of the indwelling catheter so that there is only hepatopetal flow from the catheter's tip where chemotherapy is released in a distribution that covers all the intrahepatic metastases, preventing the extrahepatic delivery of cytotoxic agents. First, any arterial branches that may cause delivery of the chemotherapy outside the liver should be occluded with coil percutaneously.[22] Arteries that do not feed the liver such as right gastric and gastroduodenal are routinely coil-embolized to avoid gastrointestinal toxicity of extrahepatic drug perfusion resulting in gastroduodenal ulceration due to perfusion of chemotherapy in an extrahepatic vessel that remains patent beyond the tip.[23] This can still occur when a small branch was not detected or recanalized after surgical ligation or coil embolization. A Tc-99m macroalbumin aggregate (MAA) study after pump placement is routinely performed to indicate that there is only hepatopetal flow without extrahepatic accumulation of tracer. In the event of extrahepatic accumulation of tracer, angiographic embolization may still be needed to correct the flow and salvage the intra-arterial pump/catheter for safe chemotherapy administration.[24,25] Historically when combination of 5-fluorouracil (5-FU) and folinic acid was the standard regimen for IV chemotherapy in CLM, all clinical trials using 5-FU or FUDR demonstrated a better response rate for HAC than for IV treatments alone, with a few trials demonstrating survival benefit.[26,27] In a more recent study, intra-arterial oxaliplatin combined with IV 5-FU demonstrated an overall response rate of 62% among the 39 assessable patients, including 17, 12, and 12 patients who had failed to respond to prior systemic chemotherapy with FOLFIRI, FOLFOX, or both, respectively.[28] Of note, in the same report, an R0 surgical resection was performed afterward in 18% of initially nonresectable patients and ablation with clear margins (A0) in 2%. More combined chemotherapy schemes including a single intra-arterial agent such as FUDR plus two IV agents such as oxaliplatin and irinotecan allowed as high as 90% tumor response rates.[29] In another study involving 36 patients with extensive nonresectable liver metastases (i.e., ≥4 metastases in 86% and bilobar disease in 91% of patients), HAC was used with oxaliplatin (100 mg/m^2 in 2 hours) plus IV 5-FU and leucovorin (leucovorin 400 mg/m^2 in 2 hours; 5-FU 400 mg/m^2 bolus then 2,500 mg/m^2 in 46 hours) and cetuximab (400 mg/m^2 then 250 mg/m^2/week or 500 mg/m^2 every 2 weeks) as first-line treatment. Overall response rate (ORR) was 90% and disease control rate was 100%. Forty-eight percent of patients were downstaged enough to undergo an R0 resection and/or ablation.[2]

TRANSARTERIAL CHEMOEMBOLIZATION AND DRUG-ELUTING BEADS

There are several different techniques under the acronym TACE. The most common procedure is the intra-arterial injection of chemotherapy emulsified with Lipiodol Ultra-Fluide (LUF; Guerbet, Aulnay-sous-Bois, France) followed by injection of embolic material.[30–34] Lipiodol was first injected into the hepatic arteries in the early 1980s because of its capacity to target and remain fixed in tumors; LUF was first used as a diagnostic tool for the evaluation of disseminated hepatocellular carcinoma[30] and then emulsified with various drugs for the treatment of liver tumors.[31] The emulsion produces oil drops in the arterial flow, and these drops have a propensity to go through the largest arteries (which are the tumor feeders) without entering the small ones due to the surfactant properties of the oil drops.[32] With Lipiodol-TACE, ratio of drug concentration in the tumor compared to the healthy liver and to peripheral blood levels can be as high as 10 and 1,000 times, respectively.[33] Embolization after chemo-Lipiodol increases the efficacy of treatment by prolonging contact of chemotherapy to the tumor cells and by adding ischemia to the highly hypervascularized tumor usually targeted with this treatment. Such embolization has been reported to induce failure of the transmembrane pump, thus increasing drug retention inside of cells.[34]

Regimens used to deliver TACE included (1) cisplatin, doxorubicin, mitomycin C, Ethiodol, and polyvinyl alcohol that had shown an ORR of 43% in one study[35]; median survivals of 33 months from initial diagnosis, 27 months from the time of liver metastases, and 9 months from the start of chemoembolization were documented, suggesting a possible improvement over reported survival time for systemic therapies alone[35]; and (2) mitomycin C alone (52.5%), mitomycin C with gemcitabine (33%), or mitomycin C and irinotecan (14.5%) showing an ORR of 63%.[9]

In 2006, the development of DEB loaded with irinotecan (DEBIRI) came for the first time in clinical practice for the management of CLM.[36] DEBIRI loaded with irinotecan had a 75% reduced systemic plasma level compared with intra-arterial irinotecan alone.[37]

In a randomized study of two courses of DEBIRI (36 patients) compared with eight courses of IV irinotecan, 5-FU, and leucovorin (FOLFIRI; 38 patients) used to treat 74 patients who failed at least two lines of chemotherapy, the DEBIRI arm was met with statistically significant improvement of all oncologic outcomes including patient survival.[38] Specifically, the response rates were 69% for the DEBIRI group compared with 30% for the systemic FOLFIRI group. Similarly, the 2-year overall survival (OS) was 56% compared with 32%, and the median OS was 22 months compared with 15 months for DEBIRI versus FOLFIRI groups.

Improvement in quality of life was of longer duration for the DEBIRI group (8 months) compared to the FOLFIRI group (3 months, $P = .0002$). Finally, overall cost was lower for the DEBIRI treatment arm.

In a multicenter, single-arm study of 55 patients who underwent DEBIRI after failing systemic chemotherapy, response rates were 66% at 6 months and 75% at 12 months, with an OS of 19 months and a progression-free survival of 11 months.[5]

A recent comparison study of DEBIRI versus radioembolization for salvage therapy for liver-dominant CLM including series of 36 patients reported similar survival for both treatments as salvage therapy, with median survival times of 7.7 months for the DEBIRI group and 6.9 months for the radioembolization (SIRT) group. The 1-, 2- and 5-year survival rates were 43%, 10%, and 0%, respectively, in the DEBIRI group and 34%, 18%, and 0%, respectively, in the SIRT group.[4]

Around 30% of TACE sessions are associated with adverse events during or after the treatment. The factors predictive of adverse events and significantly greater hospital length of stay are lack of pretreatment with hepatic arterial lidocaine ($P = .005$), more than three treatments ($P = .05$), achievement of complete stasis ($P = .04$), treatment with greater than 100 mg DEBIRI in one session ($P = .03$), and bilirubin greater than 2.0 μg/dL with more than 50% liver replaced by tumor ($P = .05$).[39] Table 41.1 displays results of studies using TACE for the treatment of CLM.

RADIOEMBOLIZATION/SELECTIVE INTERNAL RADIATION THERAPY

Traditional external beam radiation therapy in patients with diffuse hepatic malignancy does not improve overall survival[40] because liver tolerance for developing radiation-induced injury is low compared with the doses required for tumoricidal effect.[41] The usual dose of normal liver tissue tolerance to radiation is 30 Gy, whereas the dose required to induce a tumoricidal effect of a solid tumor is 70 Gy or higher.[42] These facts resulted in the idea of selective internal transarterial radiation with the delivery of radiotherapy yttrium 90 (Y90)–impregnated microspheres. Currently, two different Y90 microsphere products with a mean diameter of 20 to 35 μm are available: TheraSpheres (Nordion, Ottawa, Ontario, Canada), which are glass microspheres, and SIR-Spheres (SIRTeX Medical Limited, New South Wales, Australia), which are resin microspheres.

Radioembolization delivers targeted radiation therapy to unresectable liver metastases by the injection of β-emitting isotope Y90, which is bound to nondegradable microspheres into the arterial supply of the liver. These microspheres are unable to pass through the vasculature of the liver due to their relatively large size in comparison to the capillaries and are therefore trapped in the tumor capillaries.

The physical properties of this radioactive isotope are a half-life of 64 hours and no γ-energy emission, thus allowing immediate release of the patient after treatment. The average range of radiation penetration in tissues is 2.5 mm to 1 cm. This allows delivery of high dose of ionizing radiation to the tumor with minimal radiation to surrounding tissue and thus causing considerably less toxicity to the normal liver.[43] Criteria for radioembolization include patients with unresectable (and noneligible for ablation) CLM, patients with liver-only or liver-dominant disease, life expectancy of at least 3 months, and acceptable liver reserve. As a matter of fact, in a recent phase I trial, we demonstrated that SIRT

Table 41.1 Embolotherapies for the Treatment of Metastatic Liver Disease

Authors/Series	Study Type	Type of Embolization	Type of Chemotherapy Agent	Number of Patients	Median Overall Survival (months)
Pohlen et al.[8]	Prospective/ single arm	Starch microspheres	5-FU, interferon-α, folinic acid (arterial pump)	95	24
Vogl et al.[9]	Prospective/ nonrandomized	Starch microspheres	Mitomycin C, mitomycin C plus gemcitabine, mitomycin C plus irinotecan	463	14
Martin et al.[5]	Prospective/ single arm	Drug-eluting beads	Irinotecan	95	19
Albert et al.[35]	Retrospective	Lipiodol plus polyvinyl alcohol	Cisplatin plus doxorubicin plus mitomycin C	121	9
Aliberti et al.[56]	Prospective/ phase II	Drug-eluting beads	Irinotecan	82	25
Fiorentini et al.[38]	Prospective/ phase III	Drug-eluting beads	Irinotecan versus systemic FOLFIRI	36	22
Tellez et al.[57]	Prospective/ phase II	Collagen	Cisplatin, doxorubicin, mitomycin C	30	8.6
Wasser et al.[58]	Retrospective	Starch microspheres	Mitomycin C	21	13.8
Salman et al.[59]	Prospective/ phase II	Polyvinyl alcohol	Polyvinyl alcohol only versus polyvinyl alcohol + interferon + 5-FU	50	15 versus 10

5-FU, 5-fluorouracil; FOLFIRI, 5-fluorouracil, leucovorin, irinotecan.

can be safely used as a salvage therapy in heavily pretreated patients who progressed after multiple lines of systemic chemotherapy and HAC as well as resection (Fig. 41.1). Provided that the bilirubin level is low (≤1.5 mg/dL), the risk of radiation-induced liver failure is extremely low even in the most heavily pretreated population.[44]

Once the patient is selected for radioembolization, pretreatment angiography (mapping) is performed. Considering the highly variable hepatic arterial anatomy and the potential hazardous effects of a nontarget delivery of radioactive microspheres into extrahepatic sites, one has to ensure that there is no hepatofugal flow from the point of sphere injection. Preparation before radioembolization, similarly to the previously described preparation for HAIP placement, requires either embolization of vessels such as the gastroduodenal, right gastric, falciform, and pancreaticoduodenal arteries or placement of an infusion catheter distal enough to all vessels with potential hepatofugal flow and nontarget sphere delivery.[45] Another particular feature of tumor vessels is arteriovenous shunting. Because the highest tolerable dose to the lung is around 30 Gy for a single application, one has to assess the fraction of the lung shunting before radioembolization by means of lung scanning after the intra-arterial infusion of 200 to 400 MBq (4 to 10 mCi) Tc-99m MAA (Fig. 41.2). The *lung shunting fraction* is defined as the percent shunt fraction of microspheres from liver to lung. The dose of radioactive microspheres should be adapted according to the lung shunting fraction. It is also important to correlate the Tc-99m MAA scan with angiographic findings by using single-photon emission computed tomography (SPECT) or even SPECT/CT to identify potential extrahepatic accumulations.[46] Y90 delivery should aim to treat all the lesions with as selective approach as possible, allowing more precise tumor targeting while minimizing the radiation exposure to healthy uninvolved hepatic parenchyma. At the same time, this selective approach eliminates the need of prophylactic embolization of vessels that will no longer be a source of extrahepatic delivery of radioactive spheres due to reflux. For patients with bilobar disease, the lobe with the most lesions should be treated first, and administration to the contralateral lobe should be performed in a separate session 4 to 6 weeks later. New developments now allow the safe delivery of Y90 spheres without the need for coil embolization. These include recent unpublished expertise indicating that it is safe to mix resin microspheres with iodinated contrast. This allows immediate visualization and very early detection of reflux that further

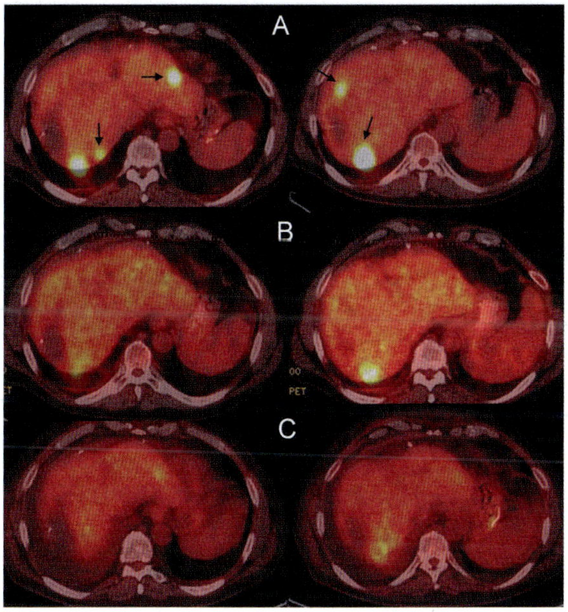

Figure 41.1 A 63-year-old-male with metastatic colon cancer previously treated with systemic as well as pump chemotherapy, prior hepatic resection, and ablation of liver metastases presented with several hypermetabolic lesions **(A)** in segment 2, segment 7, and segment 8 (*arrows*). Patient underwent Y90 radioembolization in two sessions administered 6 weeks apart with partial response as seen on fused PET/CT scans at 8 weeks **(B)** that continued to improve up to 7 months **(C)** after SIRT.

increases the safety of Y90 administration. Finally, the use of antireflux catheters also allows the delivery of the entire dose without the need of coil embolization.

Radioembolization has initially had large application in chemorefractory disease. Overall response of 17% to 35% and stable disease rates of 24% to 61% have been described.[47,48] Median survival after radioembolization has been from 6.7 to 17 months.[49] Table 41.2 represents overall patient survival after SIRT treatment.

Modest effects of radioembolization were seen when it was used as a salvage monotherapy after complete chemotherapy failure. Radioembolization alone in this setting showed an overall response of 24%, a progression-free survival of 3.7 months, and 1- and 2-year OS rates of 50.4% and 19.6%, respectively.[50]

The major contribution of radioembolization were documented when it was used together with systemic chemotherapy.[12,51] The concept behind this combined treatment was that tumors were sensitized by one treatment for the other and thus a synergistic effect of SIRT with chemotherapy was seen with better response rates.[52]

As a matter of fact, in a randomized controlled trial,[12] it was shown that the combination of SIRT with protracted 5-FU had a significantly better progression-free survival when compared to protracted 5-FU alone in patients who had previously failed 5-FU–containing regimens. Table 41.3 represents median overall patient survival with combination chemotherapy and SIRT.

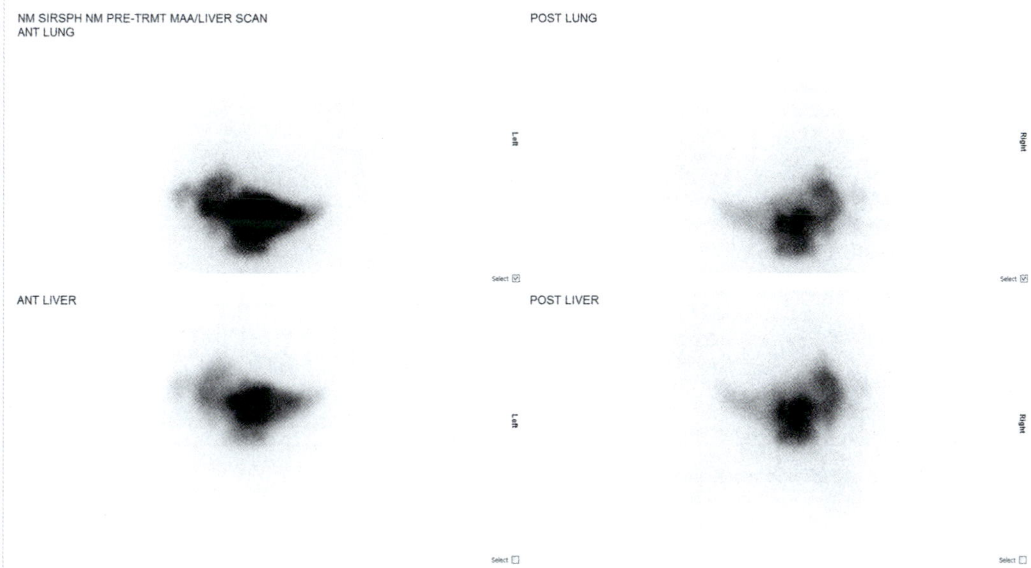

Figure 41.2 Liver–lung scintigram for the evaluation of lung shunting or extrahepatic tracer deposition after injection of 4 mCi of Tc 99m MAA in the left hepatic artery in a patient with CLM progressing in the remnant left hemiliver post right hepatectomy. The calculated lung shunting fraction was 6%, requiring no adjustment of the radioactive microspheres activity. There is only hepatic distribution without evidence of extrahepatic tracer delivery.

Table 41.2 Overall Median Survival after Selective Internal Radiation Therapy for Colorectal Liver Metastases Progressing after Several Lines of Chemotherapy

Study/Series	Study Type	Number of Patients	Response (%) By CT	Response (%) By PET	Median Overall Survival after Yttrium Treatment (months)
Lewandowski et al.[60]	Prospective/phase II	27	35	88	9.3
Kennedy et al.[47]	Retrospective	208	35	NA	10.5[a]
Jakobs et al.[48]	Retrospective	36	17	91	10.5
Mulcahy et al.[61]	Prospective/single arm	72	40	77	14.5
Cianni et al.[62]	Retrospective	41	46	NA	11.6
Sofocleous et al.[44]	Prospective/phase I	19	58	53	14.9
Evans et al.[3]	Retrospective	140	NA	NA	7.9

Disease control rates include patients with complete response, partial response, or stable disease.
[a]In responders (vs. 4.5 months in nonresponders).
CT, computed tomography; PET, positron emission tomography; NA, not available.

Table 41.3 Median Overall Patient Survival with Combination Chemotherapy and Selective Internal Radiation Therapy in Patients Previously Treated with Chemotherapy

Authors/Series	Study Type	Number of Patients	Study Design	Median Overall Survival (months)	Median Progression-Free Survival (months)
van Hazel et al.[51]	Prospective/ randomized/phase II	21	5-FU/LV with/ without Y90	29.4 versus 12.8 ($P = .02$)	18.6 versus 3.6 ($P < .0005$)
Gray et al.[10]	Prospective/ randomized/phase III	74	Floxuridine HAC with/without Y90	17 versus 15.9[a] ($P = .18$)	15.9 versus 9.7[b] ($P = .001$)
Hendlisz et al.[63]	Prospective/ randomized/phase III	46	5-FU with/without Y90	10 versus 7.3 ($P = .8$)	5.5 versus 2.1[b] ($P = .003$)
Sharma et al.[14]	Prospective/ nonrandomized/ phase I	20	FOLFOX plus Y90, oxaliplatin dose escalation	NA	9.3 (14.2 for liver-confined disease)
van Hazel et al.[64]	Prospective/phase I	25	Irinotecan with Y90	12.2	6.0
Kosmider et al.[13]	Retrospective	19	5-FU/LV or FOLFOX plus Y90	29.4 (37.8 vs. 13.4 for liver-confined disease vs. EHD; $P = .03$)	10.4

[a]Patients who survived more than 15 months had improvement in survival ($P = .06$).
[b]Liver progression.
5-FU, 5-fluorouracil; LV, leucovorin; HAC, hepatic arterial chemotherapy; FOLFOX, folinic acid, fluorouracil, and oxaliplatin (systemic chemotherapy regimen); NA, not available; EHD, extrahepatic disease.

TIPS AND TRICKS

Tips

- Use CT angiography or cone-beam CT to optimally delineate segmental anatomy and arterial tumor supply.
- Selective Y90 infusion (sectoral or segmental) allows more precise tumor targeting while minimizing the radiation exposure to healthy uninvolved liver tissue and eliminates the need of prophylactic embolization of vessels that will no longer be a source of extrahepatic delivery of radioactive spheres due to reflux.
- Follow-up imaging with PET/CT might be a more sensitive indicator of early tumor response (PET response criteria in solid tumors; PERCIST) compared to dynamic CT.

Tricks

- Prophylactic transcatheter embolization of the right gastric artery (RGA) in preparation for radioembolization/HAC can be more easily achieved in retrograde approach via left gastric artery (LGA).
- Decrease the need for prophylactic embolization of extrahepatic vessels by performing selective Y90 delivery with the catheter tip more than 3 cm away from any vessel that could cause nontarget delivery.
- Consider using iodinated contrast material when pushing resin microspheres and 5% dextrose for flushing the catheter in between administrations.

DISCUSSION

In the last 30 years, the natural history of colorectal cancer has been significantly improved due to the development of several chemotherapeutic agents.[53] As described in a review in the mid-1980s, solitary CLM, if left untreated, had survival rates of about 70% and 45% at 1 and 2 years, respectively.[54] Thirty years later, in 2011, survival rates have dramatically improved to more than 60% at 2 years and 35% at 5 years. This improvement is attributed to the availability of new chemotherapeutic agents along with improved imaging for early tumor detection as well as aggressive surgical debulking and locoregional therapies including AT.

Although the National Comprehensive Cancer Network (NCCN) guidelines[53] support the value of systemic chemotherapy in the management of CLM, they do not support the widespread use of intra-arterial locoregional therapies largely because of their lower level of evidence (mostly level 3, small numbers of level 2, and sparse numbers of level 1 evidence). Despite the relative lack of endorsement by the NCCN guidelines regarding the use of intra-arterial therapies (mostly attributed to the small number of randomized controlled trials), these methods show improved progression-free survivals and provide a very promising research ground especially in combination with different chemotherapeutic agents.

Tumor control and decrease in tumor load in metastatic disease is achieved with systemic treatment. Although the mainstay of treatment of CLM is by IV administration of oxaliplatin and irinotecan, targeted chemotherapies with administration through the hepatic artery achieve higher response rates than does IV therapy.[27,28]

Transarterial therapies have the advantage of preferentially reaching metastases because their vascularization is nearly 100% arterial, whereas the vascularization of liver parenchyma is 30% arterial and 70% portal. In addition, if the drug injected in the hepatic artery is selectively retained in the liver during embolization, systemic passage and therefore systemic toxicity of the drug will be reduced as well.

TACE and radioembolization are two techniques commonly used for treating liver metastases from different tumor entities. Intra-arterial–directed therapies such as HAC, TACE, DEB-TACE, and SIRT have shown high response rates and can now be used as an adjunct to the initial chemotherapy agent that failed[12] or as induction chemotherapy to downsize unresectable liver metastases to resection.[35,55]

Particularly, HAC and SIRT have reported a fraction of treated patients being downsized to resection. Both HAC and SIRT have also been associated with best oncologic outcomes when combined with earlier lines of systemic chemotherapy.[10]

Earlier series of TACE with several chemotherapeutic agents indicated that chemoembolization might offer some benefit in the control of CLM, particularly for those patients who progressed through prior lines of systemic chemotherapy.[35,36]

The recent development of DEBIRI shows initial promise. A very recent randomized controlled trial by Fiorentini et al.[38] demonstrated that DEBIRI in combination with FOLFIRI offered a statistically significant prolongation of the progression-free survival and, more importantly, the overall survival of patients with CLM. This study sets the stage for more and larger similarly designed trials to prove the value of arterially directed therapies for patients with nonresectable CLMs.

SIRT with Y90-impregnated beads is another new therapy that essentially delivers very high doses of radiation directly in the tumor via the arterial tree. Several series have shown the safety and efficacy of this treatment even in the most heavily and compromised patients with colon cancer hepatic metastases.[44] SIRT is now accepted in the salvage setting when systemic chemotherapy has failed to control CLM.[50,60]

Similarly to DEBIRI, several series have indicated that SIRT in combination with different systemic chemotherapy regimens prolongs the progression-free survival and may prolong overall survival.[13,51]

These data show that currently, there are several intra-arterial therapies for the patient with CLM who cannot undergo resection or ablation. The selection of the best therapy for each patient certainly requires multidisciplinary discussion and cooperation. SIRT has the advantage of a limited recovery time, allowing the patient to be discharged the same day. It carries a risk, however, for radiation-induced liver disease that has been reported as late as 4 months after therapy.[11] To prevent this risk, a careful selection of even heavily pretreated patients is required for effective and safe treatment.[44]

In addition, SIRT requires a preparatory arteriogram for hepatic arterial flow evaluation and redistribution, lung shunt, and detailed dose calculation. On the other hand, TACE with or without DEBIRI is associated with postembolization syndrome, requiring a short stay in the hospital for supportive care. One point that should be kept in mind is that one type of therapy does not preclude the use of another treatment. Therefore, if local progression is documented at short time interval after one arterially directed therapy, one might consider the use of a different arterially directed treatment.

This chapter was undertaken with the intention to give an overview of the interventional arterial therapies available for the treatment of hepatic metastases. As such, we performed a relatively concise description and discussions of the most commonly used image-guided intra-arterial interventional embolotherapies and have provided most of the relevant references. We would like to close by stating that we, like many others in the field, aspire that interventional oncology may have reached the point to be considered the fourth pillar in oncology along with medical, surgical, and radiation oncology. This is in particular the case when it comes to the management of hepatic metastases and in those originating from colorectal cancer.

REFERENCES

1. Cohen AD, Kemeny NE. An update on hepatic arterial infusion chemotherapy for colorectal cancer. *Oncologist*. 2003;8:553–566.
2. de Baere T, Deschamps F. Arterial therapies of colorectal cancer metastases to the liver. *Abdom Imaging*. 2011;36:661–670.
3. Evans KA, Richardson MG, Pavlakis N, et al. Survival outcomes of a salvage patient population after radioembolization of hepatic metastases with yttrium-90 microspheres. *J Vasc Interv Radiol*. 2010;21:1521–1526.
4. Hong K, McBride JD, Georgiades CS, et al. Salvage therapy for liver-dominant colorectal metastatic adenocarcinoma: comparison between transcatheter arterial chemoembolization versus yttrium-90 radioembolization. *J Vasc Interv Radiol*. 2009;20:360–367.
5. Martin RC, Joshi J, Robbins K, et al. Hepatic intra-arterial injection of drug-eluting bead, irinotecan (DEBIRI) in unresectable colorectal liver metastases refractory to systemic chemotherapy: results of multi-institutional study. *Ann Surg Oncol*. 2011;18:192–198.
6. Kemeny NE, Melendez FD, Capanu M, et al. Conversion to resectability using hepatic artery infusion plus systemic chemotherapy for the treatment of unresectable liver metastases from colorectal carcinoma. *J Clin Oncol*. 2009;27:3465–3471.
7. Martin RC, Joshi J, Robbins K, et al. Transarterial chemoembolization of metastatic colorectal carcinoma with drug-eluting beads, irinotecan (DEBIRI): multi-institutional registry. *J Oncol*. 2009;2009:539795.
8. Pohlen U, Mansmann U, Berger G, et al. Multicenter pilot study of 5-fluorouracil, folinic acid, interferon alpha-2b and degradable starch microspheres via hepatic arterial infusion in patients with nonresectable colorectal liver metastases. *Anticancer Res*. 2004;24:3275–3282.
9. Vogl TJ, Gruber T, Balzer JO, et al. Repeated transarterial chemoembolization in the treatment of liver metastases of colorectal cancer: prospective study. *Radiology*. 2009;250:281–289.
10. Gray B, Van Hazel G, Hope M, et al. Randomised trial of SIR-Spheres plus chemotherapy vs. chemotherapy alone for treating patients with liver metastases from primary large bowel cancer. *Ann Oncol*. 2001;12:1711–1720.
11. Sato KT, Lewandowski RJ, Mulcahy MF, et al. Unresectable chemorefractory liver metastases: radioembolization with 90Y microspheres—safety, efficacy, and survival. *Radiology*. 2008;247:507–515.
12. Hendlisz A, Van den Eynde M, Peeters M, et al. Phase III trial comparing protracted intravenous fluorouracil infusion alone or with yttrium-90 resin microspheres radioembolization for liver-limited metastatic colorectal cancer refractory to standard chemotherapy. *J Clin Oncol*. 2010;28:3687–3694.
13. Kosmider S, Tan TH, Yip D, et al. Radioembolization in combination with systemic chemotherapy as first-line therapy for liver metastases from colorectal cancer. *J Vasc Interv Radiol*. 2011;22:780–786.
14. Sharma RA, Van Hazel GA, Morgan B, et al. Radioembolization of liver metastases from colorectal cancer using yttrium-90 microspheres with concomitant systemic oxaliplatin, fluorouracil, and leucovorin chemotherapy. *J Clin Oncol*. 2007;25:1099–1106.
15. Geschwind JF, Kaushik S, Ramsey DE, et al. Influence of a new prophylactic antibiotic therapy on the incidence of liver abscesses after chemoembolization treatment of liver tumors. *J Vasc Interv Radiol*. 2002;13:1163–1166.
16. Folprecht G, Grothey A, Alberts S, et al. Neoadjuvant treatment of unresectable colorectal liver metastases: correlation between tumour response and resection rates. *Ann Oncol*. 2005;16:1311–1319.
17. Wang X, Sofocleous CT, Erinjeri JP, et al. Margin size is an independent predictor of local tumor progression after ablation of colon cancer liver metastases. *Cardiovasc Intervent Radiol*. 2013;36:166–175.
18. Kemeny M. Hepatic artery infusion of chemotherapy as a treatment for hepatic metastases from colorectal cancer. *Cancer J*. 2002;8(suppl 1):S82–S88.
19. Kemeny MM. The surgical aspects of the totally implantable hepatic artery infusion pump. *Arch Surg*. 2001;136:348–352.
20. Tanaka T, Arai Y, Inaba Y, et al. Radiologic placement of side-hole catheter with tip fixation for hepatic arterial infusion chemotherapy. *J Vasc Interv Radiol*. 2003;14:63–68.
21. Arai Y, Takeuchi Y, Inaba Y, et al. Percutaneous catheter placement for hepatic arterial infusion chemotherapy. *Tech Vasc Interv Radiol*. 2007;10:30–37.
22. Sofocleous CT, Petre EN, Gonen M, et al. CT-guided radiofrequency ablation as a salvage treatment of colorectal cancer hepatic metastases developing after hepatectomy. *J Vasc Interv Radiol*. 2011;22:755–761.
23. Deschamps F, Elias D, Goere D, et al. Intra-arterial hepatic chemotherapy: a comparison of percutaneous versus surgical implantation of port-catheters. *Cardiovasc Intervent Radiol*. 2011;34:973–979.

24. Sofocleous CT, Schubert J, Kemeny N, et al. Arterial embolization for salvage of hepatic artery infusion pumps. *J Vasc Interv Radiol.* 2006;17:801–806.
25. Bloom AI, Gordon RL, Ahl KH, et al. Transcatheter embolization for the treatment of misperfusion after hepatic artery chemoinfusion pump implantation. *Ann Surg Oncol.* 1999;6:350–358.
26. Reappraisal of hepatic arterial infusion in the treatment of nonresectable liver metastases from colorectal cancer. Meta-Analysis Group in Cancer. *J Natl Cancer Inst.* 1996;88:252–258.
27. Kemeny NE, Niedzwiecki D, Hollis DR, et al. Hepatic arterial infusion versus systemic therapy for hepatic metastases from colorectal cancer: a randomized trial of efficacy, quality of life, and molecular markers (CALGB 9481). *J Clin Oncol.* 2006;24:1395–1403.
28. Boige V, Malka D, Elias D, et al. Hepatic arterial infusion of oxaliplatin and intravenous LV5FU2 in unresectable liver metastases from colorectal cancer after systemic chemotherapy failure. *Ann Surg Oncol.* 2008;15:219–226.
29. Kemeny N, Jarnagin W, Paty P, et al. Phase I trial of systemic oxaliplatin combination chemotherapy with hepatic arterial infusion in patients with unresectable liver metastases from colorectal cancer. *J Clin Oncol.* 2005;23:4888–4896.
30. Nakakuma K, Tashiro S, Hiraoka T, et al. Hepatocellular carcinoma and metastatic cancer detected by iodized oil. *Radiology.* 1985;154:15–17.
31. Konno T, Maeda H, Iwai K, et al. Selective targeting of anticancer drug and simultaneous image enhancement in solid tumors by arterially administered lipid contrast medium. *Cancer.* 1984;54:2367–2374.
32. de Baere T, Dufaux J, Roche A, et al. Circulatory alterations induced by intra-arterial injection of iodized oil and emulsions of iodized oil and doxorubicin: experimental study. *Radiology.* 1995;194:165–170.
33. Egawa H, Maki A, Mori K, et al. Effects of intra-arterial chemotherapy with a new lipophilic anticancer agent, estradiol-chlorambucil (KM2210), dissolved in lipiodol on experimental liver tumor in rats. *J Surg Oncol.* 1990;44:109–114.
34. Kruskal JB, Hlatky L, Hahnfeldt P, et al. In vivo and in vitro analysis of the effectiveness of doxorubicin combined with temporary arterial occlusion in liver tumors. *J Vasc Interv Radiol.* 1993;4:741–747.
35. Albert M, Kiefer MV, Sun W, et al. Chemoembolization of colorectal liver metastases with cisplatin, doxorubicin, mitomycin C, ethiodol, and polyvinyl alcohol. *Cancer.* 2011;117:343–352.
36. Aliberti C, Tilli M, Benea G, et al. Trans-arterial chemoembolization (TACE) of liver metastases from colorectal cancer using irinotecan-eluting beads: preliminary results. *Anticancer Res.* 2006;26:3793–3795.
37. Taylor RR, Tang Y, Gonzalez MV, et al. Irinotecan drug eluting beads for use in chemoembolization: in vitro and in vivo evaluation of drug release properties. *Eur J Pharm Sci.* 2007;30:7–14.
38. Fiorentini G, Aliberti C, Tilli M, et al. Intra-arterial infusion of irinotecan-loaded drug-eluting beads (DEBIRI) versus intravenous therapy (FOLFIRI) for hepatic metastases from colorectal cancer: final results of a phase III study. *Anticancer Res.* 2012;32:1387–1395.
39. Martin RC, Howard J, Tomalty D, et al. Toxicity of irinotecan-eluting beads in the treatment of hepatic malignancies: results of a multi-institutional registry. *Cardiovasc Intervent Radiol.* 2010;33:960–966.
40. Russell AH, Clyde C, Wasserman TH, et al. Accelerated hyperfractionated hepatic irradiation in the management of patients with liver metastases: results of the RTOG dose escalating protocol. *Int J Radiat Oncol Biol Phys.* 1993;27: 117–123.
41. Emami B, Lyman J, Brown A, et al. Tolerance of normal tissue to therapeutic irradiation. *Int J Radiat Oncol Biol Phys.* 1991;21:109–122.
42. Dawson LA, McGinn CJ, Normolle D, et al. Escalated focal liver radiation and concurrent hepatic artery fluorodeoxyuridine for unresectable intrahepatic malignancies. *J Clin Oncol.* 2000;18:2210–2218.
43. Kennedy AS, Nutting C, Coldwell D, et al. Pathologic response and microdosimetry of (90)Y microspheres in man: review of four explanted whole livers. *Int J Radiat Oncol Biol Phys.* 2004;60:1552–1563.
44. Sofocleous CT, Garcia AR, Pandit-Taskar N, et al. Phase I trial of selective internal radiation therapy for chemorefractory colorectal cancer liver metastases progressing after hepatic arterial pump and systemic chemotherapy. *Clin Colorectal Cancer.* 2014;13:27–36.
45. Liu DM, Salem R, Bui JT, et al. Angiographic considerations in patients undergoing liver-directed therapy. *J Vasc Interv Radiol.* 2005;16:911–935.
46. Ahmadzadehfar H, Sabet A, Biermann K, et al. The significance of 99mTc-MAA SPECT/CT liver perfusion imaging in treatment planning for 90Y-microsphere selective internal radiation treatment. *J Nucl Med.* 2010;51:1206–1212.
47. Kennedy AS, Coldwell D, Nutting C, et al. Resin 90Y-microsphere brachytherapy for unresectable colorectal liver metastases: modern USA experience. *Int J Radiat Oncol Biol Phys.* 2006;65:412–425.
48. Jakobs TF, Hoffmann RT, Dehm K, et al. Hepatic yttrium-90 radioembolization of chemotherapy-refractory colorectal cancer liver metastases. *J Vasc Interv Radiol.* 2008;19:1187–1195.
49. Vente MA, Wondergem M, van der Tweel, I et al. Yttrium-90 microsphere radioembolization for the treatment of liver malignancies: a structured meta-analysis. *Eur Radiol.* 2009;19: 951–959.
50. Cosimelli M, Golfieri R, Cagol PP, et al. Multi-centre phase II clinical trial of yttrium-90 resin microspheres alone in unresectable, chemotherapy refractory colorectal liver metastases. *Br J Cancer.* 2010;103:324–331.
51. Van Hazel G, Blackwell A, Anderson J, et al. Randomised phase 2 trial of SIR-Spheres plus fluorouracil/leucovorin chemotherapy versus fluorouracil/leucovorin chemotherapy alone in advanced colorectal cancer. *J Surg Oncol.* 2004;88:78–85.
52. Nicolay NH, Berry DP, Sharma RA. Liver metastases from colorectal cancer: radioembolization with systemic therapy. *Nat Rev Clin Oncol.* 2009;6:687–697.
53. Benson AB III, Bekaii-Saab T, Chan E, et al. Metastatic colon cancer, version 3.2013: featured updates to the NCCN Guidelines. *J Natl Compr Canc Netw.* 2013;11:141–152; quiz 152.
54. Wagner JS, Adson MA, Van Heerden, JA et al. The natural history of hepatic metastases from colorectal cancer. A comparison with resective treatment. *Ann Surg.* 1984;199:502–508.
55. Goere D, Deshaies I, de Baere T, et al. Prolonged survival of initially unresectable hepatic colorectal cancer patients treated with hepatic arterial infusion of oxaliplatin followed by radical surgery of metastases. *Ann Surg.* 2010;251:686–691.

56. Aliberti C, Fiorentini G, Muzzio PC, et al. Trans-arterial chemoembolization of metastatic colorectal carcinoma to the liver adopting DC Bead(R), drug-eluting bead loaded with irinotecan: results of a phase II clinical study. *Anticancer Res.* 2011;31:4581–4587.
57. Tellez C, Benson AB III, Lyster MT, et al. Phase II trial of chemoembolization for the treatment of metastatic colorectal carcinoma to the liver and review of the literature. *Cancer.* 1998;82:1250–1259.
58. Wasser K, Giebel F, Fischbach R, et al. Transarterial chemoembolization of liver metastases of colorectal carcinoma using degradable starch microspheres (Spherex): personal investigations and review of the literature [in German]. *Radiologe.* 2005;45:633–643.
59. Salman HS, Cynamon J, Jagust M, et al. Randomized phase II trial of embolization therapy versus chemoembolization therapy in previously treated patients with colorectal carcinoma metastatic to the liver. *Clin Colorectal Cancer.* 2002;2:173–179.
60. Lewandowski RJ, Thurston KG, Goin JE, et al. 90Y microsphere (TheraSphere) treatment for unresectable colorectal cancer metastases of the liver: response to treatment at targeted doses of 135-150 Gy as measured by [18F]fluorodeoxyglucose positron emission tomography and computed tomographic imaging. *J Vasc Interv Radiol.* 2005;16:1641–1651.
61. Mulcahy MF, Lewandowski RJ, Ibrahim SM, et al. Radioembolization of colorectal hepatic metastases using yttrium-90 microspheres. *Cancer.* 2009;115:1849–1858.
62. Cianni R, Urigo C, Notarianni E, et al. Radioembolisation using yttrium 90 (Y-90) in patients affected by unresectable hepatic metastases. *Radiol Med.* 2010;115:619–633.
63. Hendlisz A, Van den Eynde M, Peeters M, et al. Phase III trial comparing protracted intravenous fluorouracil infusion alone or with yttrium-90 resin microspheres radioembolization for liver-limited metastatic colorectal cancer refractory to standard chemotherapy. *J Clin Oncol.* 2010;28:3687–3694.
64. van Hazel GA, Pavlakis N, Goldstein D, et al. Treatment of fluorouracil-refractory patients with liver metastases from colorectal cancer by using yttrium-90 resin microspheres plus concomitant systemic irinotecan chemotherapy. *J Clin Oncol.* 2009;27:4089–4095.

42

Percutaneous Hepatic Perfusion

Krishna Kandarpa

Surgically unresectable metastases confined to the liver are the life-limiting component of disease for many patients with melanoma, whether ocular or cutaneous in origin. Hepatic metastases are present in 40% to 50% of patients at initial diagnosis with ocular melanoma, and there is subsequent liver involvement in up to 95% of individuals who develop ocular melanoma metastases.[1] Ocular melanoma, although rare, is the most common primary ocular malignancy in adults. The mean age-adjusted incidence of ocular melanoma in the United States is approximately 4.3 new cases per million population per year.[2] However, liver involvement occurs in only about 15% to 20% of patients with metastatic cutaneous melanoma.[3,4] Median survival for patients with hepatic melanoma metastasis is less than 6 months. Most therapies, whether systemic or regional, have low response rates and limited efficacy.[5–8]

New systemic therapies have recently been approved for cutaneous melanoma (i.e., ipilimumab and vemurafenib). However, ipilimumab is only effective in 25% of cutaneous melanoma patients and it often has a delayed time to response of 3 to 6 months, which is too long to benefit many patients.[9] Vemurafenib is an option for only the 50% of patients with cutaneous melanoma who have BRAF mutations, but almost all of these patients relapse within 6 to 8 months. Because BRAF mutations are not observed in patients with ocular melanoma, vemurafenib is not an option for them, and immunologic therapies, such as ipilimumab, have not shown benefit to date.

Surgical resection of melanoma liver metastases is limited by their numbers and location and is the only potentially curative option, albeit in fewer than 10% of patients.[10] As there is currently no treatment that can alter the course of the disease, there remains a critical unmet need for these patients.

RATIONALE FOR PERCUTANEOUS HEPATIC PERFUSION

Intense nonsurgical regional treatment of the liver aims to provide maximal efficacy while limiting systemic exposure to toxic drug effects. Focal cryotherapy, radiofrequency heating, or ethanol injection are approaches to ablating tumors while minimizing injury to surrounding normal liver. Lesion visibility, numbers, size, and the proximity to vital structures limit the use of these treatments.[11] They are a suboptimal option if occult micrometastases are present.

The liver possesses unique anatomic characteristics that allow it to be completely isolated from the rest of the systemic circulation, facilitating high-dose infusion of chemotherapy to the liver via the hepatic artery. Unlike local ablation or embolization that only treat selected visible tumors, hepatic perfusion treats the entire liver, including occult micrometastases, potentially limiting recurrence and improving efficacy while minimizing systemic drug exposure and toxicity. An open-abdominal surgical approach known as *isolated hepatic perfusion* (IHP) isolates the liver's vasculature and creates a closed circuit within which a high dose of melphalan is circulated though the liver parenchyma. The small volume of blood confined within the circuit never mixes with the systemic circulation and is discarded after the procedure. IHP has been reported to control disease and extend survival for patients with unresectable hepatic metastases.[12–16] IHP has had limited adoption because of its technical complexity, invasiveness, high morbidity, and the development of intra-abdominal adhesions that limit it to a one-time-only treatment.

In part to overcome the limitations of IHP, percutaneous hepatic perfusion (PHP) was developed as a minimally invasive alternative. It is an investigational drug (melphalan hydrochloride)/device combination product in the United States (not approved by the U.S. Food and Drug Administration [FDA]), but the device component has European Union CE mark approval to be used in combination with independently procured melphalan. The device consists of several sterile, single-use components, including catheters and an extracorporeal circuit with hemofiltration cartridges (Delcath Systems, Inc., New York, New York). A high dose of melphalan is delivered to the liver via a hepatic artery catheter, and the hepatic venous return is captured and filtered extracorporeally to minimize systemic exposure before it is returned to the systemic circulation (Fig. 42.1). This is achieved by creating an extracorporeal venovenous bypass circuit following adequate anticoagulation with heparin. A double-balloon catheter is placed across the retrohepatic inferior vena cava to isolate the hepatic venous blood. The procedure takes approximately 3 hours (in-room) and is performed under general anesthesia and uses standard interventional radiology techniques.

ROLE OF THE INTERVENTIONAL RADIOLOGIST

The decision to treat with PHP is generally made during interdisciplinary rounds that include oncologists, surgeons, interventional radiologists, and possibly other specialists. Once the decision is made to treat with PHP, the interventional radiologist becomes the designated procedural leader, but the oncologist remains the primary managing physician. The interventional radiologist manages the medical imaging and performs the necessary catheter placements and arterial embolization to redirect the vasculature as needed.[16,17]

Embolization is preferably completed during an earlier session at least a week ahead of the planned PHP procedure. Although embolization may be performed during the

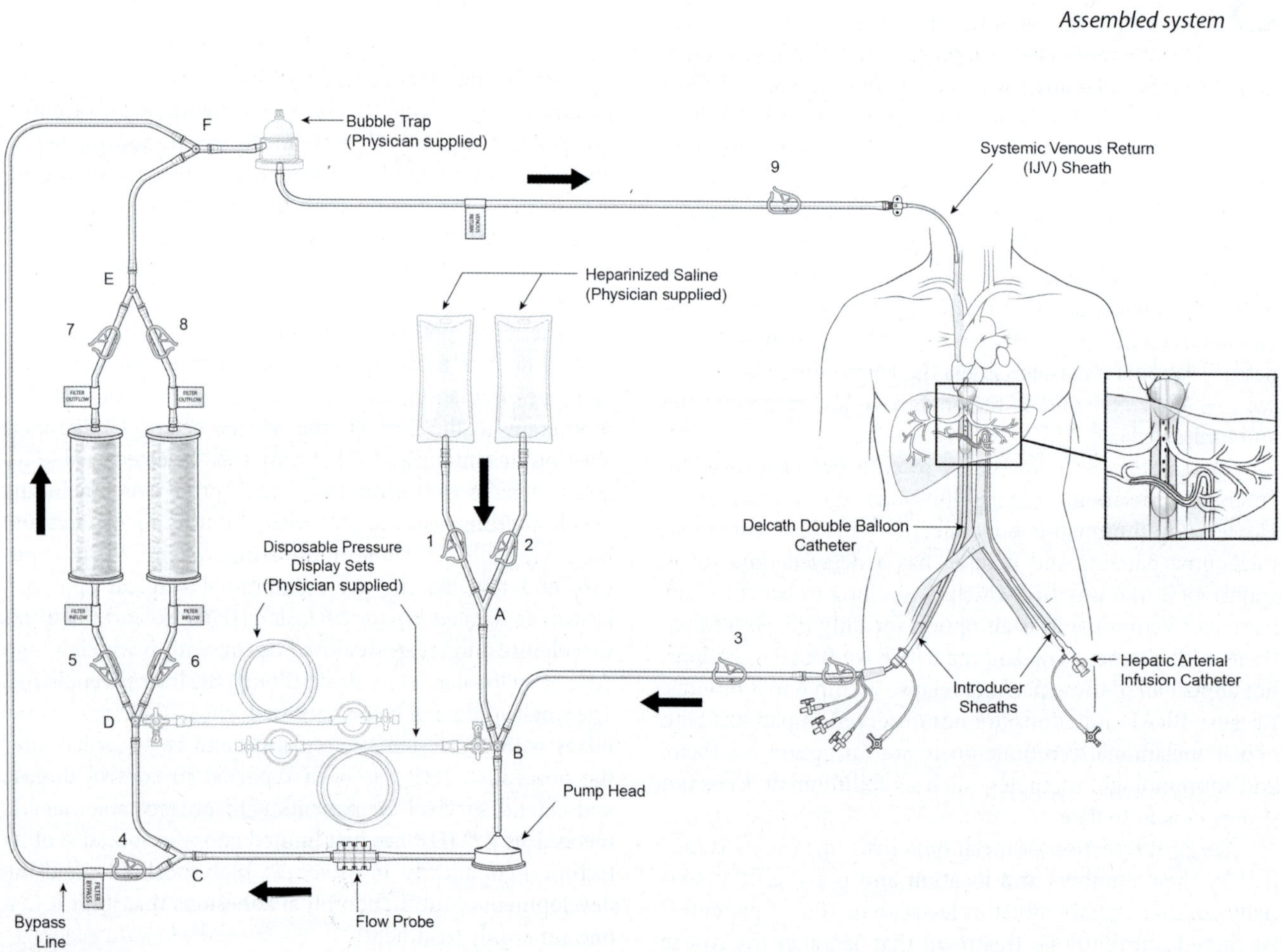

Figure 42.1 Schematic of the perfusion circuit including intravascular and extracorporeal components. A double-balloon catheter is deployed to capture hepatic venous blood (*inset at right*).

procedure, it is generally not advised as the intraprocedural use of large quantities of heparin may preclude adequate occlusion of the acutely embolized branches. This practice also allows the arterial access site to heal, if one does not use a closure device after embolization, and it reduces the duration of general anesthesia and the PHP procedure.

In addition to the other imaging required, the interventional radiologist must perform complete visceral angiography (celiac and superior mesenteric arteries with visualization of the portal vein to assess flow and patency). All gastrointestinal (GI) branches arising from the hepatic arteries are assessed for potential misperfusion, whether directly by antegrade flow or by retrograde reflux into branches proximal to the site of infusion. In an analysis of patients who randomized primarily to PHP in the phase 3 trial discussed in the following text, Stedman et al.[18] reported 91 embolization procedures in 42 patients. These included 64 gastroduodenal, 12 right gastric, and 5 left gastric branches. An additional 10 embolizations included phrenic, supraduodenal, gastrohepatic, aberrant left gastric arising from hepatic, and other less common branches. Patients who crossed over from the control to the treatment arm (n = 28) had a similar pattern of embolization. Most embolizations were performed before the first PHP cycle, with far fewer performed before cycles 2 to 4 and none during cycle 5 or 6 (up to 6 cycles of PHP were allowed for qualifying patients). This practice of hepatic vascular "redistribution" is familiar to interventional radiologists, but unlike some other liver-directed therapies, lung shunting studies have not been needed.

On the day of PHP, the interventional radiologist places the femoral arterial, femoral venous, and internal jugular venous sheaths and catheters and actively directs the team during the procedure, working with the anesthesiologist and perfusionist (B. McCormick et al., unpublished data, 2014) to safely establish the extracorporeal (EC) circuit, to perform hepatic arterial infusion, and to terminate the EC circuit once the procedure is completed. The actual percutaneous hepatic perfusion procedure takes 1 hour: during the first half hour, melphalan is infused into the hepatic artery with simultaneous filtration, and during the second half hour, infusion is stopped, but an additional 30 minutes of washout filtration is continued. When the extracorporeal blood flow is initiated, profound hypotension can occur, and the anesthesiologist should manage the depth of the BP drops through the use of prophylactic corticosteroid and vasopressors as well as additional intraprocedural vasopressors as needed. The use of vasopressors may be accompanied by peripheral vasospasm. Thus, during the procedure, the interventional radiologist must check frequently for hepatic arterial vasospasm and relieve it using intra-arterial (IA) nitroglycerin. Stedman et al.[18] reported a median IA dose of 230 μg (range 50 to 1,200 μg). Once the procedure is completed and EC circuit terminated, the anesthesiologist reverses the anticoagulation and provides the needed postprocedural support for the patient (C.M. Chen et al., unpublished data, 2014). The interventional radiologist removes the catheters and sheaths and works with the anesthesiologist and intensive care unit (ICU) physicians until the patient has recovered from procedure-related side effects overnight. The patient is moved to the general wards the next day at which time the oncologist takes over the subsequent management of the patient. Seamless communication and cooperation between all team members is crucial for the safe administration of PHP treatments.

CLINICAL DEVELOPMENT PROGRAM

All of the U.S. clinical trials discussed in the following sections were all conducted with an older generation device (Gen 1). The (Gen 1) filter melphalan removal efficiency was consistent across the trials, with overall means ranging from 71.2% to 76.4%. A completely redesigned device (Gen 2) is currently approved (CE mark) and marketed in the European Union. It has been employed during compassionate use cases in the United States. The new filters have experimental in vitro and in vivo porcine model efficiencies of 98% or better for melphalan removal. Nearly 130 clinical procedures have been performed worldwide with the new Gen 2 device for treating various tumor metastases in the liver. Neither the Gen 1 nor Gen 2 device has FDA approval.

An open-label, phase 1, single-center, sequential, dose escalation study was used to determine the maximum tolerated dose of melphalan administered by PHP to patients with unresectable hepatic metastases from melanoma (cutaneous and ocular, n = 16) and assorted other tumors (n = 18). This study established a maximum tolerated dose of melphalan of 3.0 mg/kg ideal body weight (IBW).[19] A phase 2, open-label, single-center, nonrandomized study was conducted (simultaneously with the phase 3 multicenter trial) to examine the efficacy of PHP in patients with unresectable primary hepatic malignancies and unresectable metastatic hepatic malignancies from other tumor types (GI, adenocarcinoma, neuroendocrine, and cutaneous or ocular melanoma). This study included four patients with melanoma who were not candidates for the phase 3 trial.

The Phase 3 Trial

The phase 3 study was a randomized, controlled, multicenter trial to evaluate the efficacy, safety, and tolerability of PHP treatment versus best alternative care (BAC) in patients with unresectable hepatic metastases from cutaneous or ocular melanoma. This study used the aforementioned Gen 1 device. The primary end point was hepatic progression-free survival. Notably, this was the first randomized, controlled, phase 3 clinical trial to include patients with ocular melanoma and was conducted following special protocol assessment review by the FDA.

In the phase 3 study, patients in the BAC group were allowed to cross over to PHP treatment at the time of documented hepatic progression provided they continued to meet the eligibility criteria for the study at the time of crossover. The crossover study design was agreed with FDA because of (1) the lack of any standard or effective therapy for metastatic melanoma with liver-dominant disease, particularly for ocular melanoma, and (2) it would be unethical to not allow for crossover to a potentially active and lifesaving therapy that had shown positive results in a phase 1 study. It was anticipated that the crossover design would confound analyses of survival. Phase 2 and phase 3 study patients are being followed for survival.

Study Population

This clinical trial was conducted in the United States at the National Cancer Institute and nine additional sites. The demographic and baseline characteristics of patients enrolled in the PHP clinical trials were representative of the target indication of unresectable metastatic melanoma in the liver. There were no statistically significant differences between the PHP (n = 44) and BAC (n = 49) groups for any demographic or baseline disease characteristic in the phase 3 study, with the exception of Eastern Cooperative Oncology Group (ECOG) performance status which was statistically significantly worse in the PHP group, with more ECOG status 1 patients, than in the BAC group. In all of the studies, most of the patients were white and younger than 65 years of age.

Most patients (n = 83) in the phase 3 study had ocular melanoma with five or more hepatic lesions at baseline. All 4 patients in the melanoma subset in the phase 2 study had ocular melanoma, and of the 16 patients in the phase 1, 12 had ocular melanoma and 4 had cutaneous melanoma. The median time since diagnosis of the primary tumor across the studies ranged between 38.1 months and 55.7 months, and the median time since diagnosis of hepatic metastasis ranged between 1.9 months and 6.5 months for the phase 3 study and the phase 1 study, respectively, indicating recent life-threatening disease relative to the overall length of disease; this was not evaluated for the phase 2 study. In the phase 3 study, patients who received PHP had a median of three cycles of treatment (range 1 to 6).

Efficacy

In all three studies, both hepatic and extrahepatic lesions were evaluated using the Response Evaluation Criteria In Solid Tumors (RECIST); however, only the presence or absence of extrahepatic lesions was recorded and there was not a fixed schedule for the evaluation of extrahepatic lesions. In the phase 3 study, the primary efficacy end point, hepatic progression-free survival (hPFS), assessed by the independent review committee (IRC), was met. Investigator assessments were consistent with the IRC. Alexander[20] reported a median hPFS of 8.0 months for PHP compared to 1.6 months for BAC (HR = 0.35 [0.23−0.54]; $P < .001$) and an overall response rate of 32% for PHP versus 2% for BAC ($P = .001$). Fifty-five percent of patients had crossed over from BAC to PHP upon hepatic progression, and as anticipated, no significant difference in overall survival could be demonstrated.

A consistent treatment benefit was seen for PHP treatment across the primary and secondary efficacy end points in the phase 3 study. The exception was overall survival, which was confounded by the high number of BAC patients who crossed over to PHP treatment. To date, most patients still alive in the phase 3 study received PHP treatment (7/10 patients: 2 who were randomized to PHP and 5 who crossed over). Historically, only a rare patient with liver-dominant melanoma is a long-term survivor (approximately 2%). The results seen in the phase 3 study were reinforced by consistent results for hPFS and hepatic Overall Response (hOR) in the melanoma subset in the supportive phase 1 and phase 2 studies and may serve as surrogates for overall survival because the overwhelming cause of death in melanoma patients with liver-dominant disease is early liver progression and liver failure.

Safety

The safety profile of the melphalan/PHP system has been evaluated in three clinical studies in patients with unresectable hepatic metastases or primary liver tumors. A total of 155 patients received PHP treatment in these studies: 33 in the phase 1 study, 52 in the phase 2 study, and 70 in the phase 3 study (42 randomized to PHP and 28 who crossed over to PHP). Laboratory monitoring was conducted more frequently in the PHP group than in the BAC group.

In all three clinical studies, adverse events were analyzed by two procedural periods: the periprocedure and postprocedure periods (Fig. 42.2). The periprocedure period was defined as the period from the date of the planned procedure until the earlier of 3 days or patient discharge from the hospital. Adverse events reported during this period are more likely to be device/procedure-related adverse events. The postprocedure period was defined as the time from the end of the periprocedure period until the day before the date of the next treatment cycle. For the last treatment cycle, the end of the postprocedure period was the earlier of either the date of death or 30 days after the date of the final study dose. Adverse events reported during this period are more likely to be melphalan-related adverse events.

Adverse Events

The most frequent adverse events during the periprocedure period are consequences of the technical aspects of the PHP procedure, including the need for systemic anticoagulation and hemofiltration. Frequent periprocedural adverse events included thrombocytopenia, anemia, hypoalbuminemia, prolonged activated partial thromboplastin time (aPTT), elevated hepatic transaminases with or without hyperbilirubinemia, and hypocalcemia. Most of these events

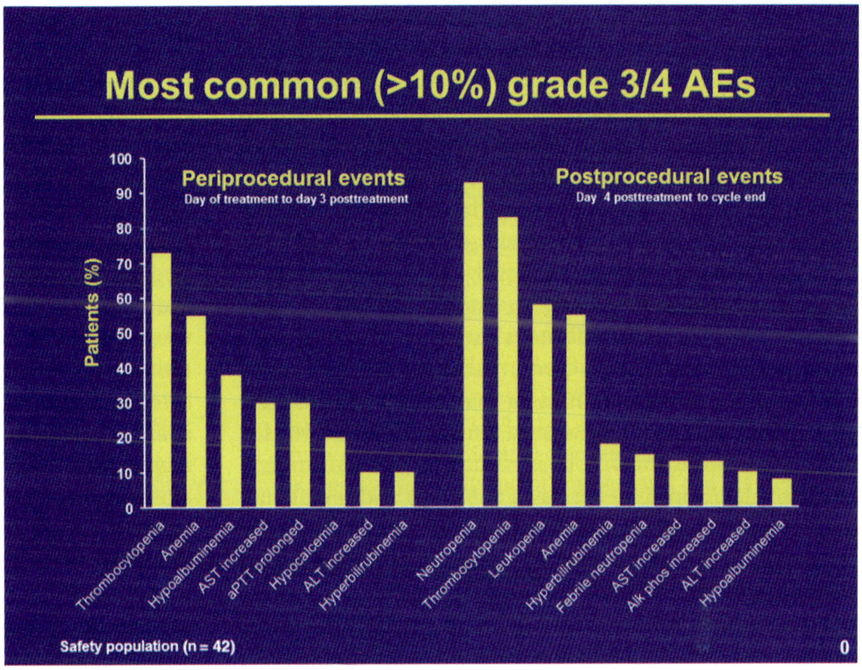

Figure 42.2 Grade ¾ periprocedure and postprocedure adverse events (AEs). AST, aspartate aminotransferase; aPTT, activated partial thromboplastin time; ALT, alanine aminotransferase; Alk phos, alkaline phosphatase.

were predictable, mitigated with appropriate treatment intervention before patient discharge from the hospital. The phase 1 and phase 2 periprocedural adverse event profiles were consistent with phase 3. Thrombocytopenia and anemia are a consequence of platelet and red blood cell (RBC) sequestration by the filters and were managed with transfusions as clinically indicated. Plasma proteins, such as albumin and certain coagulation factors, were also removed by the filters but were typically corrected by the administration of fresh frozen plasma and/or cryoprecipitate at the end of the procedure to reverse the intense anticoagulation required. Prolonged aPTT is an intended outcome from heparin anticoagulation during the PHP procedure. Because restoration of normal coagulation with protamine sulfate, fresh frozen plasma, and cryoprecipitate at the end of the procedure requires some time, there is an increased risk of bleeding during this period. Therefore, patients were monitored closely and vascular sheaths were not removed until coagulation was normalized.

Hepatic laboratory abnormalities occurred in 10% to 30% of patients. Elevated hepatic transaminases, with or without hyperbilirubinemia—known adverse effects associated with melphalan and with liver-directed procedures—were monitored for any clinical sequelae but typically resolved without intervention.

Hypotension is also frequently seen during the PHP procedure, and the patients should be monitored closely for possible related adverse events. Hypotension is thought to be the consequence of the removal of catecholamines by the filters and possibly a limited systemic inflammatory response to the device components. Hypotension was managed by intravenous hydration and the vigilant administration of pressor agents during the procedure. Recent modifications to the treatment protocol, such as premedication with corticosteroids, have further mitigated the depth and duration of hypotension and eased procedural management.

The safety profile during the postprocedure period of the phase 3 study was characterized predominantly by adverse events related to bone marrow suppression, a well-known and understood principal toxicity of melphalan. Frequent postprocedural adverse events included neutropenia, thrombocytopenia, and anemia. These events occurred in most patients in the PHP group because prophylactic growth factor administration was not required by the study protocol. Neutropenia recovery was seen in 10.5 days with secondary growth factor support (i.e., filgrastim, granulocyte-macrophage colony-stimulating factor). Thrombocytopenia had a median recovery time of 16 days; patients received platelet transfusions as needed. Anemia (<8 g/dL) occurred in over half the patients; recovery was seen in 5 days with packed RBC transfusions and, in some cases, epoetin administration. Although the bone marrow suppression events required treatment, the clinical sequelae associated with these events were predictable and relatively infrequent. The phase 1 and phase 2 postprocedural adverse event profiles were consistent with phase 3.

Deaths

Among the 155 PHP-treated patients in the melphalan/PHP clinical development program, there were five deaths (four in the phase 3 study and 1 in the phase 2 study) reported by the investigators to be a consequence of treatment-related adverse events. Three of the deaths (all in the phase 3 study) occurred within 30 days or less of the last treatment cycle; these deaths were attributed to hepatic failure, streptococcal sepsis, and gastric perforation. The remaining two deaths (one in the phase 3 study and one in the phase 2 study) occurred more than 30 days from the last treatment cycle; these deaths were attributed to neutropenia and upper GI hemorrhage. The death due to hepatic failure was related to underlying disease burden (>70% liver volume). After this event, the study protocol was amended to prevent a recurrence by requiring a liver biopsy to confirm normal liver tissue if the tumor burden was greater than 50% on imaging. The death due to gastric perforation was possibly related to the infusion of melphalan during hepatic artery spasm and melphalan reflux. After this event, the study protocol was amended by requiring the prophylactic administration of proton pump inhibitors, recommending the administration of nitroglycerin if hepatic artery spasm was seen during the procedure, and recommending that melphalan not be infused until the spasm resolved. The death due to upper GI hemorrhage in the phase 2 study was in a patient with a prior Whipple procedure and consequent abnormality in the architecture of the upper GI tract and biliary tree and the arterial anatomy. Following that death, the protocols were amended to no longer include patients with such prior surgery. Thus, to help to mitigate such treatment-related deaths, the ongoing study protocols were proactively amended to modify eligibility criteria and treatment techniques. There were no further same-cause deaths once each amendment was implemented.*

Serious Adverse Events

The melphalan/PHP clinical development program has clearly defined and characterized the periprocedural and postprocedural toxicities associated with melphalan/PHP treatment.

The most frequent adverse events during the periprocedure period are consequences of the technical aspects of the PHP procedure, including the need for systemic anticoagulation before hemofiltration. Frequent periprocedural events include thrombocytopenia, anemia, hypoalbuminemia, prolonged aPTT, elevated hepatic transaminases with or without hyperbilirubinemia, and hypocalcemia. Most of these events were mitigated with appropriate treatment interventions (i.e., transfusions, protamine administration, calcium infusions) before patient discharge from the hospital.

Overall, about a third of patients in the PHP group had a serious adverse event during the periprocedure period in the phase 3 study. In general, it is important to monitor for cardiovascular (stroke, myocardial infraction) and hepatic (enzyme elevations) risks potentially related to the procedure.

The safety profile during the postprocedure period was characterized predominantly by events related to bone marrow suppression, the known principal toxicity of melphalan. Frequent postprocedural adverse events included thrombocytopenia, neutropenia (including febrile neutropenia), and anemia, consistent with the known toxicities associated with melphalan noted in its product prescribing information. These events occurred in most patients and required treatment; however, the clinical sequelae associated with these events were predictable and infrequent. These events were manageable by a combination of supportive care and timing of the next treatment cycle.

Overall, about two-thirds of patients in the PHP group had a postprocedural serious grade 3/4 adverse events, which included neutropenia, thrombocytopenia, febrile neutropenia (18% in patients who did not receive prophylactic growth factors; this was not required by study protocol), and decreased hemoglobin as the most frequent serious adverse events reported. Similar results were seen in the supportive phase 1 and phase 2 studies.

CONCLUSION

Collectively, these data provide evidence of clinical benefit for PHP in patients with unresectable metastatic melanoma in the liver, for which there are no suitable alternative therapies for ocular melanoma and emerging therapies of limited effectiveness for cutaneous melanoma.

PHP treatment of this patient population is able to alter the disease course, as evidenced by the highly consistent, statistically significant, and clinically meaningful benefits seen with PHP treatment across efficacy end points in the pivotal phase 3 study. The most common grade 3/4 adverse events were thrombocytopenia and anemia. Postprocedure (in-cycle) neutropenia was common but can be mitigated by prophylactic use of growth factors. Recent improvements in the design of the device (Gen 2), procedural technique, and medical management indicate improved safety in European use that needs to be documented through registries and future randomized controlled clinical trials. The periprocedural and postprocedural toxicities associated with melphalan/PHP treatment need to be balanced against the natural course of metastatic melanoma with liver-dominant disease, the large unmet medical need for these patients, and the ability of PHP treatment to potentially alter the disease course.

*One patient death was reported in commercial use in Europe. The cause of death was spontaneous retroperitoneal bleeding confirmed by autopsy, a well-known complication of anticoagulation with heparin. There was no reported device malfunction. This is the first such death in nearly 500 procedures performed worldwide.

TIPS AND TRICKS

Tips

- Ensure adequate and acceptable cardiovascular, hepatic, renal, and hematologic functions.
- As with all interventions, proper patient selection is key: The life-limiting component of the disease must be confined to the liver. Liver tumor burden on imaging should be less than 50%; if greater, at least 30% of the liver parenchyma should be deemed disease-free.
- Minimal extrahepatic non–life-limiting metastases are permissible, especially if they are treatable with local interventions (e.g., radiation therapy or ablation).
- Exclude patients who have had prior extensive surgery that distorts hepatic vascular or biliary duct anatomy (e.g., Whipple procedure).
- Diligently preembolize GI arterial branches to prevent reflux into them during hepatic arterial perfusion.
- Preembolize parasitized collateral branches to prevent competing flow inflow to the tumor (e.g., phrenic branches).
- *Caution*: Embolization on the same day as PHP is not recommended. If unavoidable, heparinize the patient only after stable occlusion of the embolized branch has been achieved.
- Close communication and coordination with the treating team before and during the procedure is critical:
  - Anesthesiologist should expect intraprocedural hypotension and be prepared to manage it.
  - Because melphalan, as reconstituted for this purpose, has a half-life of about 90 min, the pharmacist should deliver the drug in a timely fashion.
  - The perfusionist manages all aspects of the EC circuit in close coordination with the anesthesiologist and interventional radiologist.
  - Coordinate the need for postprocedure blood products with the anesthesiologist and/or hematologist–oncologist.
- *Do not* start the EC bypass circuit until a stable activated clotting time (ACT) more than 400 s has been achieved.
- Check for hepatic arterial spasm and relieve with IA nitroglycerin before each administration of the drug into these vessels.
- Work with the ICU and/or anesthesiologist for overnight care.
- Work with the oncologist for outpatient care/management and planning of next PHP.

Tricks

- Premedicate with allopurinol if liver tumor burden is greater than 25% to prevent consequences of tumor lysis.
- Premedicate with prophylactic proton pump inhibitors in case of inadvertent reflux into GI arterial branches.
- Use prophylactic antibiotics for patients who have had prior biliary duct manipulations.
- Premedicate with prophylactic corticosteroids to minimize a systemic inflammatory response to the EC components and help mitigate intraprocedural hypotension.
- If there is an inadvertent suprainguinal puncture, postpone the procedure to another day because the required anticoagulation poses a serious risk of bleeding.
- Place the perfusion catheter in a stable position within the hepatic artery to assure maximal antegrade flow to distal branches while minimizing retrograde reflux.
- Minimize manipulations and use of microwires and microcatheters to minimize vascular spasm. Relieve with IA nitroglycerin if spasm is noted.
- Diligently check for proper placement of the double-balloon catheter (in the retrohepatic inferior vena cava) before initiation of treatment. There should be no evidence of leakage from this isolated segment.
- Reverse anticoagulation immediately upon termination of the 30-min washout phase and disconnection of EC circuit. Remove sheaths upon complete reversal of anticoagulation.

REFERENCES

1. Egan KM, Seddon JM, Glynn RJ, et al. Epidemiologic aspects of uveal melanoma. *Surv Ophthalmol*. 1988;32:239–251.
2. Singh AD, Turell ME, Topham AK. Uveal melanoma: trends in incidence, treatment, and survival. *Ophthalmology*. 2011;118: 1881–1885.
3. Leiter U, Meier F, Schittek B, et al. The natural course of cutaneous melanoma. *J Surg Oncol*. 2004;86:172–178.
4. Cohn-Cedermark G, Mansson Brahme E, Rutqvist LE, et al. Metastatic patterns, clinical outcome, and malignant phenotype in malignant cutaneous melanoma. *Acta Oncol*. 1999;38:549–557.
5. Gragoudas ES, Egan KM, Seddon JM, et al. Survival of patients with metastases from uveal melanoma. *Ophthalmology*. 1991;98:383–390.
6. Kath R, Hayungs J, Bornfeld N, et al. Prognosis and treatment of disseminated uveal melanoma. *Cancer*. 1993;72:2219–2223.
7. Korn EL, Liu PY, Lee SJ, et al. Meta-analysis of phase II cooperative group trials in metastatic stage IV melanoma to determine progression-free and overall survival benchmarks for future phase II trials. *J Clin Oncol*. 2008;26:527–534.
8. Unger JM, Flaherty LE, Liu PY, et al. Gender and other survival predictors in patients with metastatic melanoma on Southwest Oncology Group trials. *Cancer*. 2001;91:1148–1155.

9. Hodi FS, O'Day SJ, McDermott DF, et al. Improved survival with ipilimumab in patients with metastatic melanoma. *N Engl J Med.* 2010;363:711–723.
10. Sato T. Locoregional management of hepatic metastasis from primary uveal melanoma. *Semin Oncol.* 2010;37:127–138.
11. Lau WY, Leung TW, Yu SC, et al. Percutaneous local ablative therapy for hepatocellular carcinoma: a review and look into the future. *Ann Surg.* 2003;237:171–179.
12. Alexander HR, Libutti SK, Bartlett DL, et al. A phase III study of isolated hepatic perfusion using melphalan with or without tumor necrosis factor for patients with ocular melanoma metastatic to liver. *Clin Cancer Res.* 2000;6:3062–3070.
13. Alexander HR Jr, Libutti SK, Pingpank JF, et al. Hyperthermic isolated hepatic perfusion using melphalan for patients with ocular melanoma metastatic to liver. *Clin Cancer Res.* 2003;9:6343–6349.
14. Noter SL, Rothbarth J, Pijl ME, et al. Isolated hepatic perfusion with high-dose melphalan for the treatment of uveal melanoma metastases confined to the liver. *Melanoma Res.* 2004;14:67–72.
15. Rizell M, Mattson J, Cahlin C, et al. Isolated hepatic perfusion for liver metastases of malignant melanoma. *Melanoma Res.* 2008;18:120–126.
16. Yamamoto M, Zager JS. Isolated hepatic perfusion for metastatic melanoma. *J Surg Oncol.* 2014;109:383–388. doi:10.1002/jso.23474.
17. Deneve JL, Zager JS. Chemosaturation with percutaneous hepatic perfusion for unresectable hepatic metastases from sarcoma. *Cardiovasc Intervent Radiol.* 2012;35:1480–1487.
18. Stedman B, Moeslein FM, Nutting CW, et al. Chemosaturation with percutaneous perfusion: utilization of vasopressors, nitroglycerin and pre-embolization. Presented at the British Society of Interventional Radiology, BSIR 2012 Annual Meeting. November 12–16, Bournemouth, England UK.
19. Pingpank JF, Libutti SK, Chang R, et al. Phase I study of hepatic arterial melphalan infusion and hepatic venous hemofiltration using percutaneously placed catheters in patients with unresectable hepatic malignancies. *J Clin Oncol.* 2005;23:3465–3474.
20. Alexander HR. Hepatic perfusion (CHEMOSAT or CS-PHP) of melphalan versus best alternative care (BAC) in patients with hepatic metastases from melanoma: update of a randomized phase 3 study. Poster presented at: European Society for Medical Oncology 2012 Meeting; September 28–October 2, 2012; Vienna, Austria.

Section I Intravascular Delivery of Therapeutic Agents

43

Hepatopancreatic Disease

Ricardo Yamada • Christopher Hannegan
J. Bayne Selby • Marcelo Guimaraes

Cellular therapy has been used since late 1950s, when transplantation of hematopoietic cells was performed by E. Donnall Thomas[1] based on the previous work of Jean Dousset, who identified the first human leukocyte antigen on the surface of cells, leading to a better understanding of histocompatibility and rejection. Since then, cell therapy, in the form of bone marrow transplant, has become a well-established treatment modality for some hematologic disorders. Recently, this therapeutic approach has expanded to other organs and systems, including the central nervous system, liver, pancreas, and heart. This expansion relies on several factors, such as technical improvements in cell harvesting, tracking, delivery, and engraftment.

Cell delivery to the target organ is a key step in the whole process. Bone marrow transplant is done by delivering hematopoietic cells through systemic infusion via a central venous access. Because bone marrow is located within multiple sites, systemic infusion permits widespread cell colonization. However, for a specific target organ, such as brain, heart, or liver, systemic infusion is inadequate because most of the cells will be delivered away from their desired destination, leading to poor engraftment and increased cell loss. In this context, the catheter-based technique is extremely suitable as it provides the capability of selective delivery of transplanting cells to a specific organ in a minimally invasive fashion. Therefore, selective intravascular administration of therapeutic cells, either through arteries or veins, is a growing field yet to be fully explored.

DEVICE/MATERIAL DESCRIPTION

In contrast to other procedures described in this book, here, the embolic agents are live cells capable of altering the targeting organ function. The embolic effect is not the primary goal but rather a secondary result of the cell delivery process. Development of these techniques has expanded the usefulness of minimally invasive procedures beyond structural/anatomic corrections to also comprise specific cellular physiologic changes such as increased production of insulin and improved toxin clearance.

Unfortunately, the source of the "embolic agent" is a major limiting factor for widespread use of cellular therapy, as cell availability is limited by lack of donated organs. Currently, as described in the next sections, the pool of cells used for transplantation is obtained by isolating them from the donated organs of a different person (allogeneic transplant) or from the patient's organ itself (autotransplant).

To overcome this problem, another potential source for cells is under constant investigation—the so-called stem cells. There are two different types of stem cells: embryonic and adult. The embryonic stem cells are obtained from the inner cell mass of the blastocyst and have the capability of differentiation into any type of cell (pluripotent). On the other hand, adult stem cells are obtained from the bone marrow, adipose tissue, or umbilical cord and have less differentiation capability (multipotent).[2] Ethical and religious aspects limit embryonic stem cell research and clinical application, but adult stem cell use is not controversial and might become an unlimited cell source.

PANCREAS

Type 1 Diabetes Mellitus

Clinical Application

According to the World Health Organization's (WHO) last update on diabetes mellitus (DM), there are more than

34 million people worldwide affected by type 1 DM.[3] Those patients have poor quality of life and decreased life expectancy due to inadequate glycemic control, which leads to acute and chronic complications, including severe unawareness of hypoglycemic events, retinopathy, glomerulopathy, and neuropathy. Pathogenesis is based on autoimmune destruction of β-cells within the islet of Langerhans. These cells are responsible for insulin production and are the most predominant pancreatic islet cells, representing up to 75% of islet composition.[4]

Currently, the mainstay therapy is intensive exogenous insulin administration through multiple daily subcutaneous injections or continuous insulin infusion via an implanted pump. Despite all different insulin regimens available, control of glucose level is not ideal yet, and high incidence of hypoglycemic events is still a major concern. So far, the only treatment that has shown successful results in controlling disease progression without hypoglycemic events is total pancreas transplantation.[5,6] However, organ transplant is limited by lack of donors, in addition to associated comorbidities related to surgery and rejection.[7]

To overcome the unsatisfactory glucose level control with exogenous insulin therapy and surgical complications of whole pancreas transplant, a lot of effort has been put into developing an alternative therapy, which is β islet cell transplantation (ICT). This procedure gained a lot of attention after 2000, when Shapiro et al.[8] reported the results of the Edmonton series in which all seven patients were still insulin-independent after a median follow-up of 11.9 months. This result was based on the use of a glucocorticoid-free immunosuppressive regimen. Until that time, only 8.2% of patients were insulin-free 1 year after ICT.[9]

Most likely, the population that benefits the most from ICT is the group of patients who have labile diabetes and/or severe hypoglycemic events with sustained renal function because whole pancreas transplant alone has higher morbidity and mortality compared to ICT.[10] Patients with associated chronic renal insufficiency benefit more with kidney–pancreas transplant.

Labile diabetes is defined as inconsistent glucose levels that follow no predictable pattern, interfering with a patient's quality of life. To quantify that, a lability index (LI) was created based on glucose level measurements during a period of 4 weeks.[11] A severe hypoglycemic event is defined as a hypoglycemic episode that requires outside assistance to be treated; a composite hypoglycemic score, called HYPO, was also developed to quantify the frequency, severity, and degree of unawareness of hypoglycemia.[11] These measurement systems are important to promote an objective indication of the disease's severity and thus guide treatment choice.

Similar to whole-organ transplantation, ICT for type 1 DM requires lifelong immunosuppressive therapy, which is associated with frequent and severe side effects. In addition, despite its minimal invasiveness, the procedure carries some risk of serious complications, such as infection, bleeding, and portal vein thrombosis. Therefore, the procedure should be performed only in patients who present severe complications related to poor glycemic control and/or unacceptable quality of life. The patient should understand clearly that exogenous insulin therapy would be exchanged for an immunosuppressive therapy, and so the problems associated with type 1 DM must be severe enough to justify it.

Regardless of the increasing success rate that has been reported,[12] ICT is not yet considered a conventional therapy. Issues related to organ availability, cell extraction, delivery and engraftment, and also immunosuppressive regimen remain limiting factors. Hence, according to the American Diabetes Association,[10] ICT should be performed only in the setting of controlled research studies in a tertiary care center capable of managing all complex medical situations associated with transplanted patients.

According to the last Collaborative Islet Transplant Registry (CITR) annual report, insulin independence can be achieved in up to 80% to 90% of patients, especially in the presence of favorable predictive factors, such as lower baseline insulin requirement and age older than 35 years.[12] Unfortunately, sustained insulin independence decreases over time, and only 10% of patients remain insulin-independent 5 years after transplant.[12] Graft functionality is determined by any detection of serum C-peptide by local assay or stimulated serum C-peptide level greater than or equal to 3 ng/mL. Therefore, transplanted islet cells are categorized as fully functional (detectable C-peptide level and insulin independence), partially functional (insulin dependence but detectable C-peptide level), or nonfunctional (no detectable C-peptide).

Despite the low long-term insulin-independence rate, persistent C-peptide level greater than or equal to 3 ng/mL can be achieved in around 80% of patients even 5 years after transplant,[12] meaning that a significant number of patients will have at least a partially functioning graft. This has been proven clinically significant by the drop in both hypoglycemic score and lability index[13] seen also among insulin-dependent patients, representing improvement of glycemic control, which is the main goal of ICT. In addition, studies have demonstrated that ICT leads to stabilization and even some improvement of the long-term type 1 DM complications, including retinopathy,[14] glomerulopathy,[15] and neuropathy.[16]

Technique

The procedure is performed under moderate sedation, and preevaluation is focused on any conditions that increase sedation risk, such as airway compromise and cardiopulmonary dysfunction. If the patient has an increased risk for moderate sedation, general anesthesia should be considered. Blood workup includes serum creatinine, as the use of iodine contrast dye is necessary and these patients may have some degree of renal dysfunction. Platelets and prothrombin time are also needed because bleeding is the major procedure-related complication. For antibiotic prophylaxis, cefazolin sodium 1 mg intravenously 1 hour before the procedure and every 6 hours for 24 hours after the transplant has been typically used. Sulfamethoxazole/trimethoprim 400/80 mg is given orally twice a week for 24 weeks to prevent *Pneumocystis* pneumonia and valganciclovir 450 mg is prescribed orally once a day for 12 weeks to prevent cytomegalovirus infection.[17]

Under sterile technique and after local anesthesia, a 21-gauge Chiba needle is advanced into the liver parenchyma under fluoroscopic guidance at the level of the right midaxillary line, avoiding transpleural approach. The needle is advanced horizontally and with slight cephalic angulation (10 to 15 degrees). The abdominal midline should not be crossed. The needle is then slowly retracted while small amounts of contrast are injected, searching for portal vein branches. After finding a branch, a more forceful hand contrast injection is performed to confirm needle location within the portal system (Fig. 43.1). Use of ultrasound-guided puncture has been advocated as a safer approach, with less needle passages through the liver parenchyma and single-wall vein puncture.[18] Ideally, a second- or third-order branch should be punctured to decrease the risk of bleeding, as the access to the portal system is upsized to accommodate a larger catheter. After confirming the needle location within the portal system, a 0.018-in wire is advanced into the main portal vein under fluoroscopic guidance and a 4-Fr catheter is introduced. After access is secured, heparin is given intravenously according to the patient's weight. Baseline portal vein pressure is measured. Pressure above 20 mm Hg is a contraindication for cell infusion due to increased risk of portal vein thrombosis. Next, portography is performed through a power injector and a side-hole catheter, infusing 6 mL of iodine contrast per second and a total volume of 30 mL. Portal vein anatomy is delineated, confirming its patency and hepatopetal flow (Fig. 43.2).

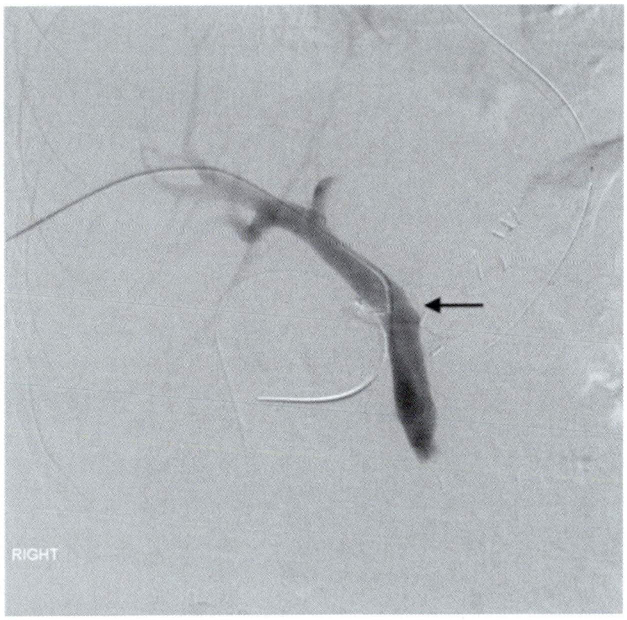

Figure 43.2 Catheter is positioned in the main portal vein (*black arrow*) and iodine contrast is infused through a power injector in a rate of 5 mL per second for 6 seconds. Portal vein patency and flow direction are confirmed before cell infusion.

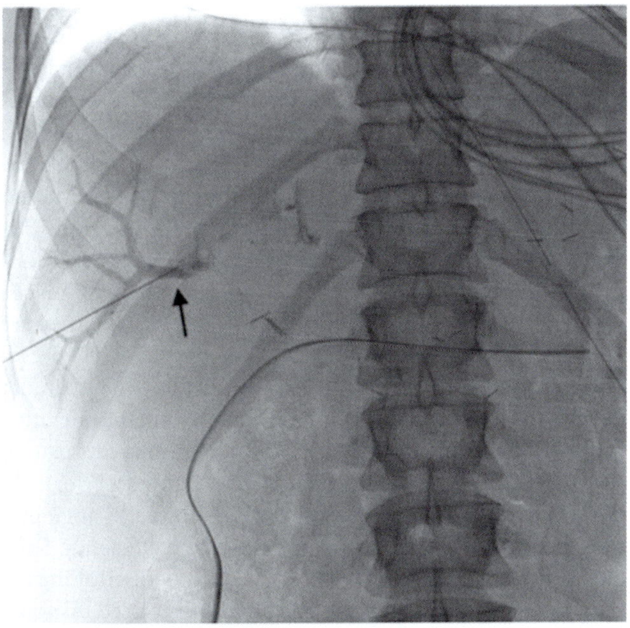

Figure 43.1 Along the midaxillary line, a 21-gauge Chiba needle is introduced into the hepatic parenchyma with slightly cephalic angulation. After slowly withdrawing the needle until access in the portal system is obtained, hand contrast injection is performed to confirm intraportal location and point of access. In this case, access was obtained in a secondary branch (*black arrow*).

A catheter with at least 700-μm inner diameter is recommended for infusion to avoid cell damage from possible shear forces or increased pressure; therefore, a 4-Fr catheter is more than appropriate.[19] The catheter tip is positioned beyond portal vein bifurcation to allow cell distribution in both hepatic lobes (Fig. 43.2). Harvested cell administration by gravity flow is preferred over direct syringe infusion because administration by gravity allows a safety mechanism of natural flow reduction that parallels any increase of portal vein pressure, avoiding precipitous pressure rise.[19] Direct syringe infusion seems to be associated with an increased risk of portal vein thrombosis. To avoid that, bag method infusion uses a closed gravity feeding bag system, consisting of a transfer bag and a rinse bag connected via sterile tubing (Fig. 43.3). During infusion, portal vein pressure is measured periodically, and an increase of more than double the baseline or above 22 mm Hg for more than 10 minutes should prompt interruption of the infusion due to increased risk of portal vein thrombosis. After infusion, a final portal vein pressure and portography are obtained.

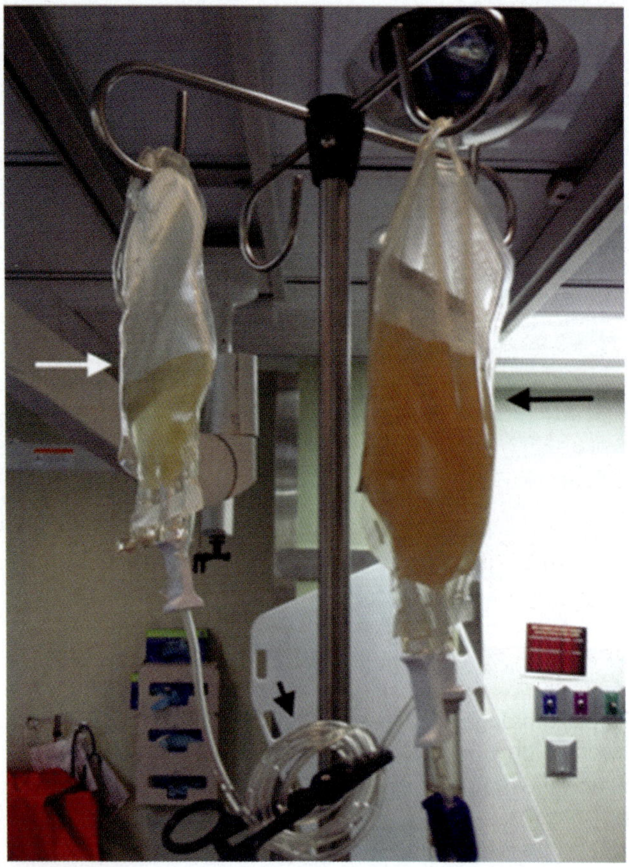

Figure 43.3 The bag method infusion technique by gravity. The larger bag on the right is the transfer bag, where the harvested cells are kept (*black arrow*). On the left, connected by sterile tubing, is the rinse bag, containing an albumin-based solution (*white arrow*). After interruption of cell infusion, the rinse bag solution is transferred to the cell-containing bag through a connecting tube (*short black arrow*) and used to wash out all remaining cells, and then the infusion is resumed. This aims to maximize the number of administered cells, avoiding waste within the system.

Despite the use of low-profile systems (4-Fr), embolization of the parenchymal track is performed at the end of the procedure as it is believed to substantially decrease the risk of postprocedure bleeding.[20] Under fluoroscopic guidance, the catheter is slowly withdrawn from the portal vein. Proper catheter location within the parenchymal track is confirmed with gentle hand injection of a small amount of iodine contrast. Embolization of the track can then be performed with different types of embolic agents, including gelfoam, coils, and *N*-butyl cyanoacrylate. The ideal embolic agent should promote a complete seal of the track with accurate deployment, avoiding intravascular embolization. Embolization is recommended for at least 5 to 7 cm of hepatic parenchyma to prevent postprocedure bleeding from the liver surface.[21]

After the procedure is terminated, the patient should be admitted to an intensive care unit, with close monitoring of vital signs and complete blood cell count measurement every 6 hours. If bleeding is not initially suspected, to prevent portal vein thrombosis, intravenous heparin infusion is started, aiming a thromboplastin time of 50 to 60 seconds. After 48 hours, intravenous heparin is switched to subcutaneous low-molecular-weight heparin for 1 week.

Chronic Pancreatitis

Clinical Application

Chronic pancreatitis (CP) is an important disabling entity that leads to significant detriment of life quality, mainly due to severe abdominal pain and opioid abuse. CP has a reported incidence of 3.5 to 10 per 100,000 people per year, and incapacitating pain is present in nearly 90% of these patients.[22] The primary treatment goal is pain alleviation, which can be associated with pancreatic duct dilation or not. When ductal dilation is present, endoscopic or surgical drainage is indicated. However, when dilation of the pancreatic duct is absent or drainage fails, total pancreatectomy (TP) should be considered.

In patients with established diabetes, the decision to proceed with pancreatic resection is more convenient because surgery is not adding a new comorbidity. On the other hand, nondiabetic patients submitted to pancreatectomy will have an incidence greater than 50% of postoperative diabetes, usually associated with more difficult glucose control and severe hypoglycemic events.[23,24]

To overcome this problem, islet cell autotransplantation (IAT) was first introduced in 1977 in the University of Michigan.[25] Since then, other centers in the United States have been performing this type of transplant successfully. In this process, the resected organ is sent to a cell laboratory, where a collagenase-based digestion process is started by pancreatic duct cannulation and enzymatic infusion. This will separate islet cells from the exocrine pancreas and connective tissue. Once islet cells are isolated, they are placed in a bag with albumin solution and antibiotic, and they are ready to be transplanted.

In the initially described technique, the patient (under general anesthesia) and the surgical team wait in the operating room (OR) while the cells are harvested. This process usually takes around 4 hours. More recently, we started performing the cell infusion at the interventional radiology (IR) angiography suite with the goal to maximize cost and efficiency. Soon after the pancreas is resected, the cells get processed at the cell therapy center while the patient's abdomen is closed. Alternatively, the patient may be sent to the intensive care unit for a few minutes in case there is any delay in pancreatic islet cell separation and preparation process[26] (Fig. 43.4).

In contrast to allogeneic ICT, IAT does not require immunosuppression, and therefore the patient is spared from its side effects. The long-term outcome is also better with IAT in comparison to allogeneic transplant as nearly 50% of IAT

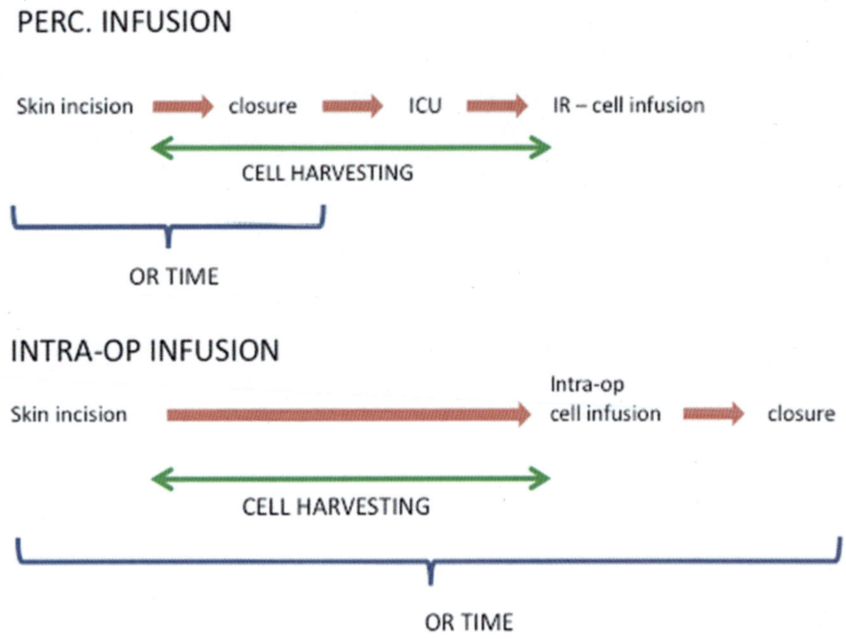

Figure 43.4 Diagram comparing intraoperative cell infusion and infusion done in the IR suite. Note the amount of OR time spared when the infusion process takes place in the IR department. (Reprinted with permission from Morgan KA, Nishimura M, Uflacker R, et al. Percutaneous transhepatic islet cell autotransplantation after pancreatectomy for chronic pancreatitis: a novel approach. *HPB [Oxford]*. 2011;13[7]:511–516.)

patients who achieved insulin independence remained insulin-free after 5 years.[27] As shown earlier, only 10% of patients were off insulin 5 years after allogeneic transplant.[13] Many reasons have been brought up to explain this discrepancy, including longer cold ischemia time, donor brain death, immunosuppression toxicity, and autoimmune deleterious effects.[27]

Technique

When cell preparation is finished, the patient is brought to the IR room for the infusion process, which can be performed via three different approaches: percutaneous transhepatic route,[26] surgically placed catheter in the portal system through a dissected mesenteric branch during pancreatecotmy, or through temporary exposure of an omental tongue containing a tributary vein.[28]

Infusion through a percutaneous transhepatic route requires the same technique described earlier for allogeneic ICT in patients with type 1 DM, with similar procedure-related complications, especially bleeding (see the following discussion). Using the two other techniques, bleeding is almost excluded, although a second small abdominal incision is performed to expose the omentum in the technique described by Nath et al.[28] Initially at our institution, the transhepatic route was the preferred one; however, recently, we have changed our practice by using the surgically placed catheter technique, which is believed to be safer. Percutaneous transhepatic infusion is now reserved for cases in which the surgical access is lost or not ideal.

For the surgically placed catheter technique, a mesenteric vein is cannulated and a glide wire is advanced distally into the portal vein, followed by a 5-Fr KMP (Cook Medical, Inc., Bloomington, Indiana) catheter placement. The wire is removed and the catheter is secured to the mesentery with silk sutures. The vein distal to the cannulation site is ligated and the catheter is brought out through the midline abdominal incision, which is closed with the standard surgical technique. The catheter is secured to the skin with silk sutures (Fig. 43.5).

The first step of the infusion process is to verify the catheter's tip location within the portal system by hand contrast injection. Most of the time, the catheter needs to be repositioned to a better location (Fig. 43.6). Less commonly, the access to the portal system is completely lost and percutaneous transhepatic access is required. After confirmation of the ideal position, pressure is measured and cell infusion by gravity gets started (Fig. 43.7). It is thought that active cell aspiration from the bag and then portal vein infusion by hand injection might damage the cells. A completion portogram is then performed to verify portal vein patency and absence of intraluminal filling defects within the main portal vein and its major branches. It is expected to see wedge-shaped filling defects in the periphery of the liver and delayed contrast washout of the secondary branches (Fig. 43.8).

Once infusion is terminated and before catheter removal, homeostasis of the mesenteric vein needs to be achieved to avoid intraperitoneal bleeding. Exposing the vein through the midline incision and ligation with surgical clips is one of the approaches that can be used. In situations where the vein cannot be externalized through the abdominal incision, the branch must be embolized. For this, the catheter is slowly retracted from the main portal vein until it reaches the mesenteric branch (Fig. 43.9). At this point, embolization can be performed through the 5-Fr catheter, or a microcatheter can be advanced coaxially. This can be extremely helpful when

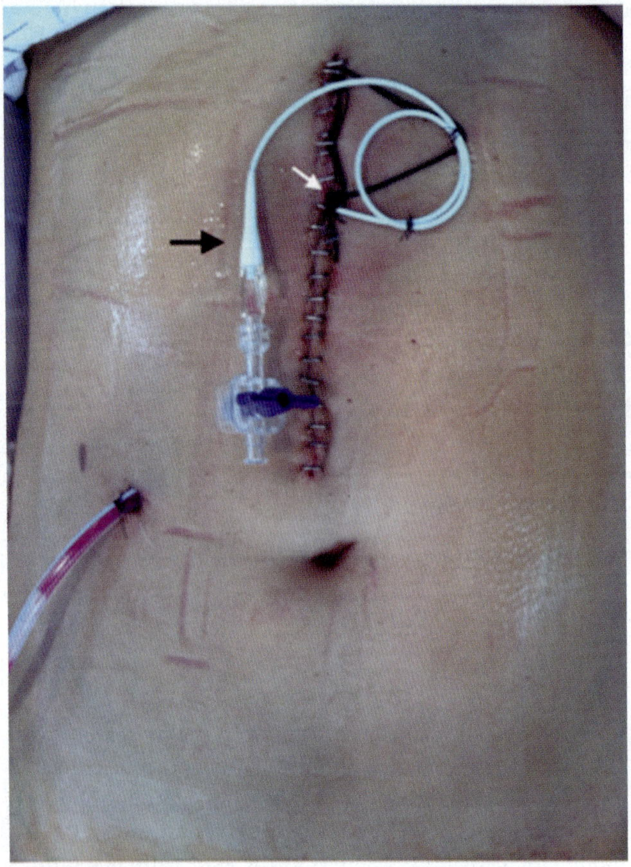

Figure 43.5 After abdominal closure, the 5-Fr KMP catheter (*black arrow*) is coiled and secured to the skin while the patient is transferred first to intensive care unit and then to the IR room. The *white arrow* demonstrates the catheter entry point into the mesenteric vein branch, which is surgically superficialized. On the right midquadrant is a surgical cavitary drain.

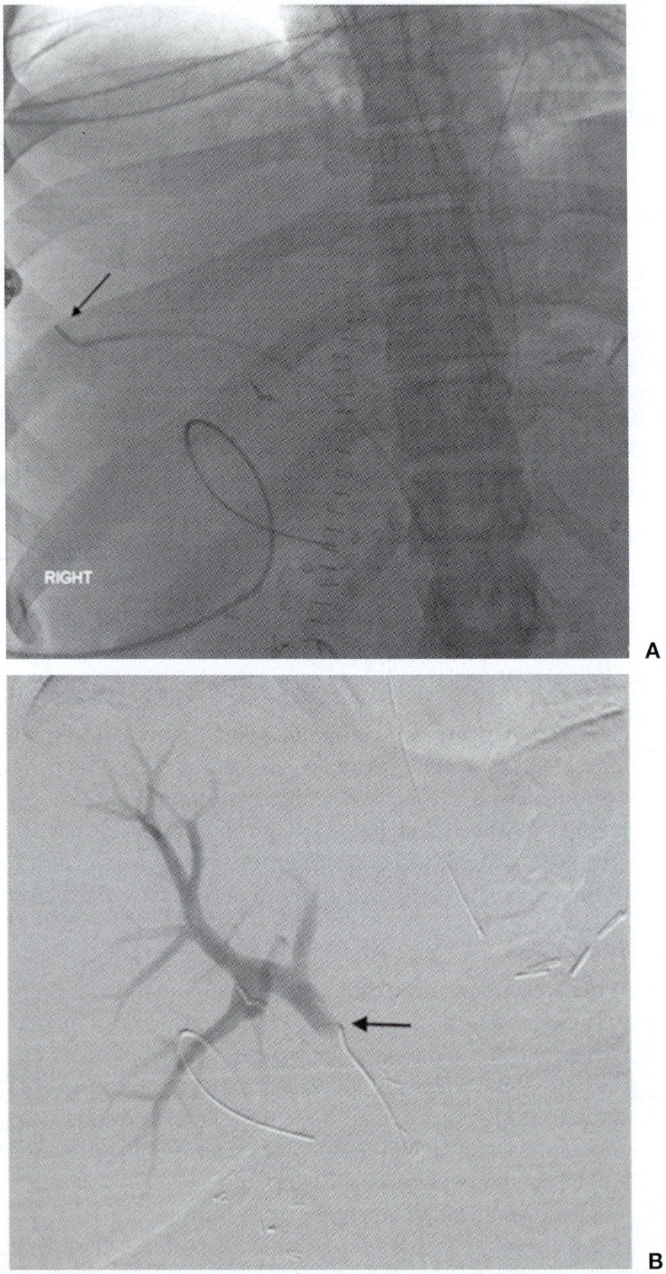

Figure 43.6 **A:** Scout film of the right upper quadrant shows the catheter distal within the portal system at the liver periphery (*arrow*). **B:** After catheter retraction, hand contrast injection demonstrated the catheter tip (*arrow*) in the main portal vein, below the bifurcation. That is the ideal location for cell infusion.

dealing with a very short vein segment, as access stability and more accurate embolization can be achieved. Use of low-profile devices in combination with a larger catheter usually promotes adequate support. Coils are the preferred embolic devices, but others can be used in combination, especially *N*-butyl cyanoacrylate. A postembolization venogram is performed to confirm complete sealing of the vein before the catheter is removed.

LIVER

Clinical Application

Currently, clinical use of hepatocyte transplantation (HCT) is limited to a few specialized centers worldwide and is still an evolving technique. Studies in HCT have been focused on three different clinical settings: chronic liver disease, inborn metabolic liver disease, and acute liver failure. In 1976, Matas et al.[29] published their successful experiment in a rat model for Crigler-Najjar syndrome type 1, showing reduction of serum bilirubin level after intraportal infusion of genetic modified hepatocytes. Then, in 1992, Mito et al.[30] reported the first human experience with hepatocyte infusion in 10 patients with chronic liver disease by direct splenic inoculation of harvested hepatocytes from patient's left hepatic lobe (autotransplantation). Although hepatocytes

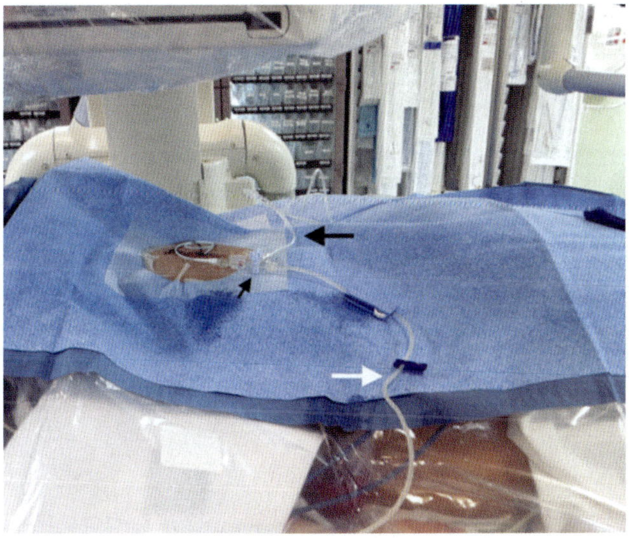

Figure 43.7 A three-way stopcock (*short black arrow*) is connected to the catheter. One port is connected to the infusion bag (*white arrow*), while the other one is connected to the pressure measurement system (*long black arrow*). Pressure monitoring is easily performed during cell infusion.

could be identified within the spleen up to 6 months after transplantation, clinical benefits were not achieved.[30] Subsequent studies with allotransplantation of hepatocytes from noncirrhotic liver donors showed more promising clinical results, promoting declined serum ammonia levels, improved encephalopathy, and successful "bridging" to whole-organ transplant.[31,32]

In 1994, Grossman et al.[33] reported the first human trial of genetically modified hepatocyte transfusion for familial hypercholesterolemia in a 29-year-old patient who achieved sustained reduction in the low-density lipoprotein-to-high-density lipoprotein ratio after intraportal hepatocyte transfusion.[33] Since then, reports of other human inborn metabolic diseases treated with HCT have been published with encouraging results, including Crigler-Najjar, α-1 antitrypsin deficiency, factor VII deficiency, glucose storage disease, and urea cycle defect.[34] For acute liver failure, Habibullah et al.[35] were the first to publish HCT in humans in 1994, and similar to chronic liver disease patients, it showed promising clinical results.

As noted, HCT can be a valuable tool in critical clinical scenarios in which satisfactory treatment is not yet established, such as inborn metabolic liver disease, or it is not fully available, as for acute/chronic liver disease, where the number of donated organs is not sufficient to meet the demand. In addition, the minimally invasive nature of the procedure is a huge advantage over conventional liver transplantation, which is a major open surgery.

Technique

Cell Source

The first human HCT experience was actually an autotransplant using hepatocytes from the resected left lobe of a patient's cirrhotic liver.[30] As mentioned before, clinical success was not accomplished, probably related to suboptimal function of the transplanted cells. Currently, hepatocytes come from the liver of noncirrhotic donors who are not suitable for orthotopic liver transplantation due to prolonged ischemia time, traumatic damage to the graft, capsular tear, blood group incompatibility, and/or vascular or biliary injury.[36] In addition to these criteria

A 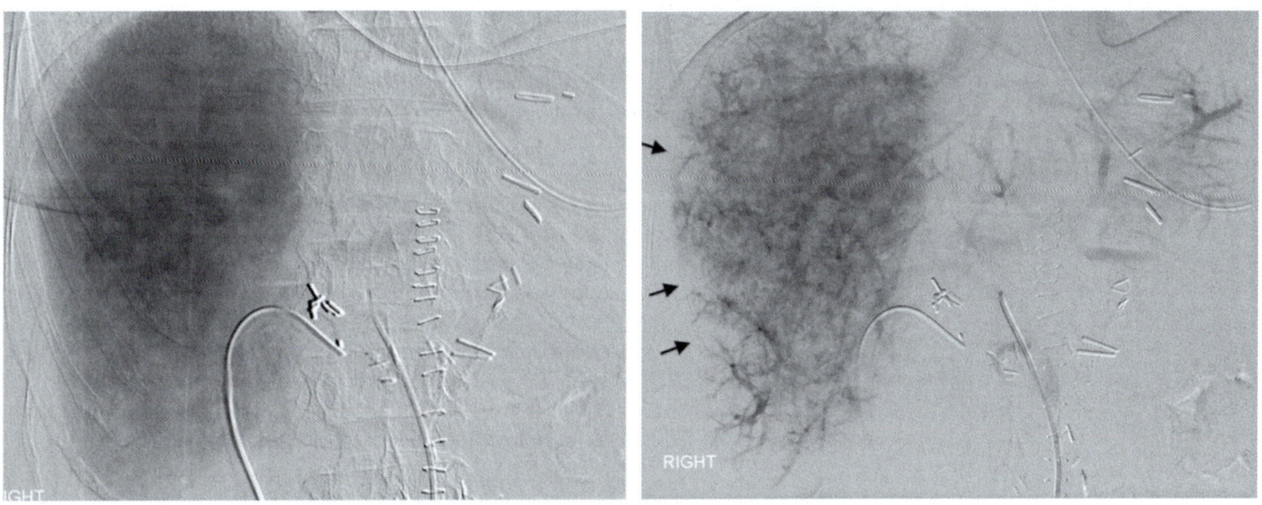 B

Figure 43.8 **A:** Preinfusion late-phase portogram showing homogeneous parenchymal opacification and complete contrast washout from the portal branches. **B:** Postinfusion late-phase portogram demonstrating multiple wedge-shaped peripheral filling defects (*black arrows*) and delayed contrast washout from secondary portal vein branches as a result of the embolic effect of the infused cells.

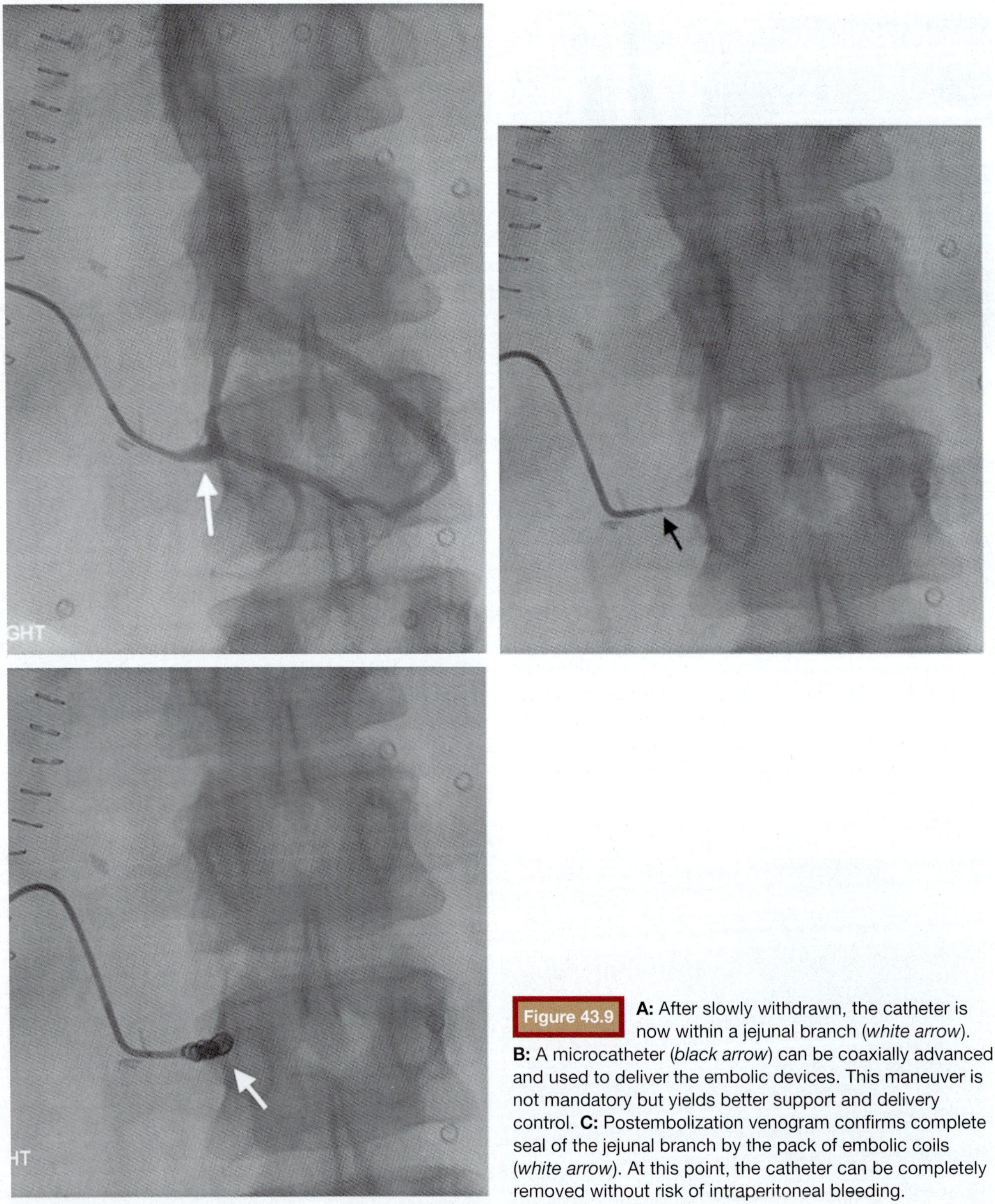

A

B

C

Figure 43.9 **A:** After slowly withdrawn, the catheter is now within a jejunal branch (*white arrow*). **B:** A microcatheter (*black arrow*) can be coaxially advanced and used to deliver the embolic devices. This maneuver is not mandatory but yields better support and delivery control. **C:** Postembolization venogram confirms complete seal of the jejunal branch by the pack of embolic coils (*white arrow*). At this point, the catheter can be completely removed without risk of intraperitoneal bleeding.

of nonsuitability for whole-organ transplant, the donor should also be free of sepsis, neoplasia, and viral infection (hepatitis C and B, HIV, human T-lymphotropic virus, and syphilis) and should present with less than 30% of steatosis. Studies have showed that fatty liver infiltration decreases cell viability.[37]

Once the organ is available, cell isolation is performed through an enzymatic digestion process that starts with cannulation of the hepatic arteries and portal veins, followed by parenchymal perfusion with a collagenase-based solution. Sequentially, mechanical disintegration, filtration, and centrifugation are performed, providing isolated hepatocytes. These cells are then tested for viability because at least 60% cell viability is recommended before transplantation. They are also tested for fungal, bacterial, mycoplasma, and endotoxin contamination.

At this point, the cells are ready to be infused or, in contrast to pancreatic ICT where solely fresh cells are administered, isolated hepatocytes can undergo a cryopreservation process, in which hepatocytes are frozen and preserved for later use. This storage process has the advantage of allowing a planned cell infusion and not only emergently and also permits creation of a cell bank, where hepatocytes can be preserved and readily available for transfusion. The drawback is the loss of viability after the frozen/thawing process, which can reach up to 50% of the cells.[38]

Route of Infusion

When first performed in humans, cell transplantation was done by direct splenic puncture.[30] Although animal lab research has shown that this route of infusion leads to a better hepatocytes engraftment,[39] this approach is rarely used nowadays due to increased potential risk of intraperitoneal bleeding, especially in the setting of coagulopathy and portal hypertension. Currently, two main routes have been used: intrahepatic–transportal and intrasplenic–transarterial.

The intrasplenic–transarterial route is the preferred one in patients with chronic liver disease and portal hypertension, as the embolic effect of transplanted cells can increase portal pressure and the risk of portal vein thrombosis, not to mention the possibility of having hepatofugal flow in cirrhotic patients with portal hypertension. In addition, the spleen in cirrhotic patients can be up to 8 to 10 times bigger than a normal spleen, allowing adequate accommodation of the cell load.[40] For this method, the common femoral artery (usually the right) is cannulated with Seldinger technique and a 5-Fr sheath is placed to secure the access. A 5-Fr Mickelson catheter (Boston Scientific, Marlborough, Massachusetts) is used to select the celiac trunk, and selective angiography is performed to delineate the vascular anatomy and confirm splenic artery patency (Fig. 43.10). Next, the splenic artery is catheterized selectively using a 0.035-in hydrophilic wire and the 5-Fr diagnostic catheter. Distal splenic angiography is performed to confirm the catheter tip location and to exclude vasospasm or dissection (Fig. 43.11). At this point, cell transfusion can begin and is carried on until all the cells are infused or flow stasis is achieved. A completion angiogram is performed, which typically will reveal multiple perfusion defects, similar to what is seen in the liver parenchyma after intraportal islet cell infusion (Fig. 43.12). The hemostasis at the femoral artery puncture site is obtained with a closure device or by 15 minutes of manual compression.

Access to the portal system for the intrahepatic–transportal infusion can be obtained through different techniques, including surgical access to a mesenteric vein, percutaneous liver

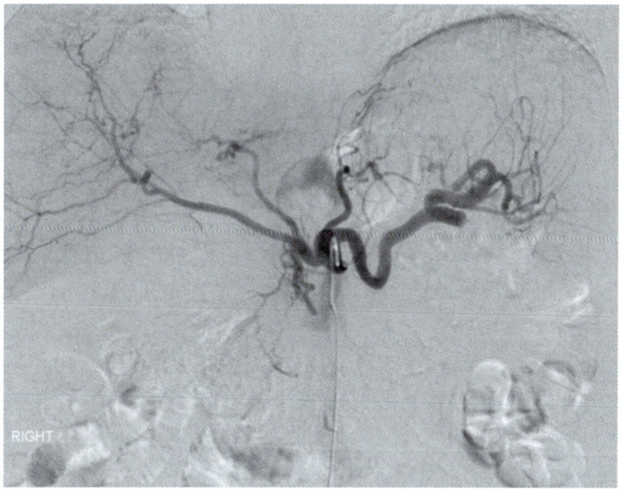

Figure 43.10 Celiac trunk arteriogram showing usual branching: common hepatic, left gastric, and splenic arteries. Note patent splenic artery and trifurcation of the common hepatic artery (anatomic variance).

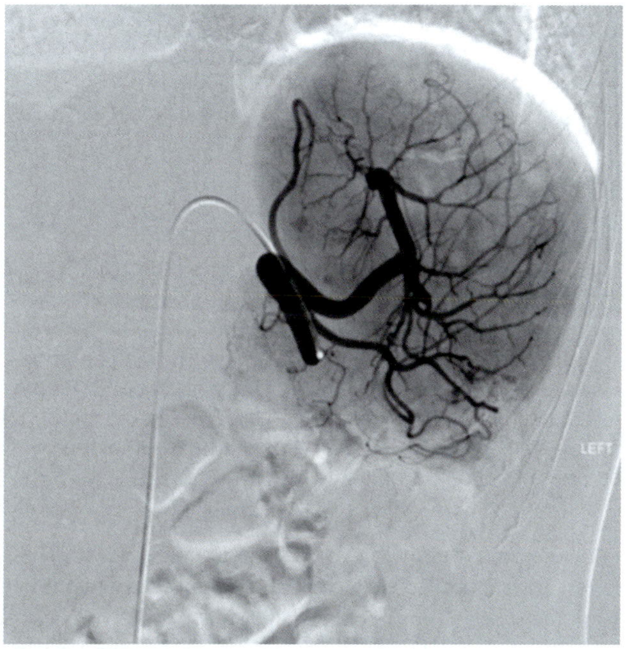

Figure 43.11 Superselective splenic arteriogram with the catheter tip placed distally confirms absence of vasospasm and dissection.

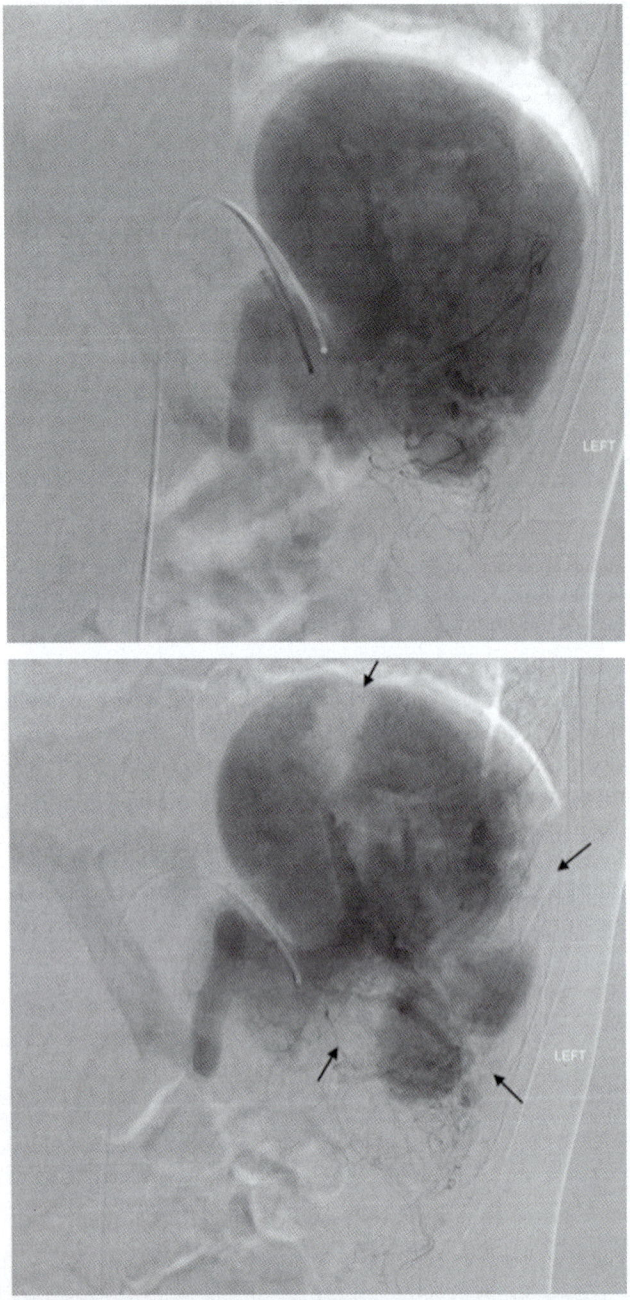

Figure 43.12 **A:** Preinfusion late phase showing homogeneous parenchymal opacification. **B:** Postinfusion late phase demonstrating multiple wedge-shaped peripheral filling defects (*black arrows*) as a result of the embolic effect of the infused cells.

puncture, and by umbilical vein catheterization in newborn patients. The surgical access technique to the portal system is beyond the scope of this book. Percutaneous transhepatic access is achieved with the same technique described earlier for pancreatic islet transplantation. A different percutaneous approach can also be used, as reported by Fox et al.[41] who performed HCT in a 10-year-old patient with Crigler-Najjar syndrome through the left portal vein. Under ultrasound guidance, the vein was punctured with a 21-gauge needle and a micropuncture introducer sheath was used to upsize the access, allowing the placement of a 5-Fr KMP catheter.

In newborns, during the first week of life, access to the portal system can be obtained through the umbilical vein (UV). UV catheterization is commonly used in critically ill infants as a way to obtain central venous access because the ductus venosus is still patent until the 20th day of life (Fig. 43.13).

Horslen et al.[42] reported multiple hepatocyte transfusions in a patient with a urea cycle disorder through the UV access. Transfusions were performed during the first 51 days of life, with the first transfusion done 10 hours after birth. Under fluoroscopic guidance, the originally placed UV catheter was manipulated into the portal vein. As the ductus venosus was still patent, placement of an occlusion balloon was performed to isolate the portal system from the systemic circulation.[42] Between transfusion sessions, the catheter was retracted into the distal UV to avoid portal vein thrombosis and secure the access for the next infusion.

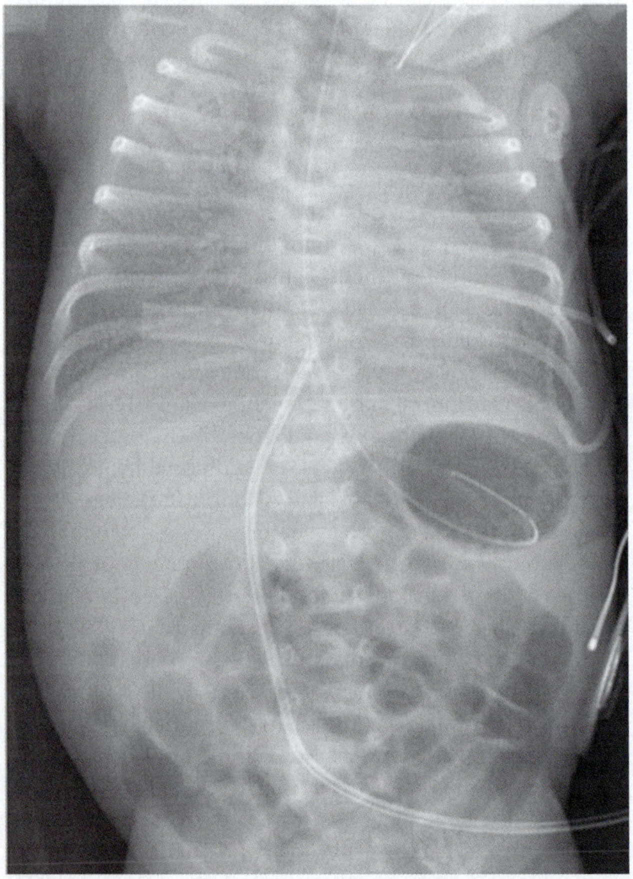

Figure 43.13 Newborn with a UV catheter. The UV connects to the left portal vein, and access to the inferior vena cava/right atrium is obtained through the ductus venosus. With this particular anatomy, access to the portal system in newborns is easily achieved.

Because multiple transfusions may be required in the same patient, a technique for long-term portal vein access has been advocated by Darwish et al.[43] The authors described surgical placement of an implantable port device in three patients. Through a small transverse left upper abdominal incision, the transverse colon is explored, allowing dissection of an appropriate colonic vein, which is cannulated with a 7-Fr catheter. The device is pulled through the left mesocolon, passed via abdominal muscles, and connected to the metallic chamber positioned in the subcutaneous tissue of the left upper quadrant along the anterior axillary line. The longest period of implantation was 5 months, and no complications were reported, especially portal vein thrombosis. One patient had catheter displacement after 30 days of implantation and required a second laparotomy to correct its location. According to the authors, special attention must be paid to correctly secure the catheter to avoid catheter migration outside the vein and potential risk of intraperitoneal bleeding.

POTENTIAL COMPLICATIONS

As these procedures are considered new techniques under constant development, complication rates should be analyzed with caution. For example, the complication profile of ICT for type 1 DM has changed because operators have gained more experience over time. Use of a more refined technique with smaller devices has helped decrease the incidence of adverse events. This has been confirmed by the CITR Seventh Annual Report, which demonstrated that life-threatening events occurred in 26% of cases performed during 1999 to 2003, whereas during 2007 to 2009, those events involved 11% of patients.[12]

Therefore, it is important to consider the most recent set of data when analyzing the complication rate. It is also relevant to differentiate between complications related to the infusion process itself or to the immunosuppressive therapy. For instance, ICT for type 1 DM during 2007 to 2010 presented 9.6% of serious adverse events related to the infusion process and 13.3% related to the immunosuppressive regimen during the first 30 days after transplant. Of note, 90.7% of those patients who experienced a serious adverse event recovered completely or remained with minimal sequelae.[12] Table 43.1 depicts some common complications after ICT in type 1 DM patients.

As noticed, bleeding is the most common complication related to the percutaneous transhepatic infusion process. Villiger et al.[21] on their analysis of 132 islet cell transplants found that a cumulative number of transplantation procedures and intraprocedure heparin dose of greater than or equal to 45 units per kilogram were independent risk factors for bleeding complication. To eliminate this risk, IAT in postpancreatectomy patients has been performed through a surgically placed catheter, as mentioned earlier. Portal vein thrombosis, another procedure-related complication, occurred in 2.1% of the patients, with complete recovery in 83.3% of the cases.[12]

Table 43.1 Data Collected from Collaborative Islet Transplant Registry Seventh Annual Report

Complications	%
Granulocytes abnormalities	44.8
Altered liver enzymes	39.7
Ketoacidosis	19.2
Infection	17.1
Pain	13.8
Hypoglycemia	13.3
Bleeding complications	12.2
Portal vein thrombosis	2.1

From Collaborative Islet Transplant Registry. CITR seventh annual report. https://web.emmes.com/study/isl/reports/01062012_7thAnnualReport.pdf. Accessed June 4, 2013.

Percutaneous intraportal hepatocyte infusion has the same potential complications of ICT, including portal vein thrombosis and bleeding. So far, human experience has not showed any major adverse event, although mild complications such as transient elevation of aspartate aminotransferase (AST)/alanine aminotransferase (ALT) and hypoxemia have been reported.[44] Transarterial intrasplenic cell infusion carries the same complication risks of any arterial puncture, including hematoma, pseudoaneurysm, dissection, and thrombosis, because the procedure is performed through a femoral artery access.

TIPS AND TRICKS

- Multiple sticks in the liver, while attempting to get access to the portal vein, is associated to significant bleeding complication. Consider ultrasound guidance, especially useful for the left hepatic lobe.
- Consider using micropuncture kit (0.021-in wire) that may be converted to a 0.035-in system (AccuStick system; Boston Scientific Corporation, Natick, Massachusetts).
- Any cell therapy should be infused by gravity. Avoid hand injection, which may damage the cells.
- Portal vein pressure measurement preinfusion, at one-half of the infusion, and postinfusion should be performed. The few cases of portal vein thrombosis occurred when the portal vein pressure increased above 30 mm Hg. If the initial portal pressure is above 25 mm Hg, consider performing very slow cell infusion.
- To decrease the chance of bleeding through the transparietohepatic access, access track

embolization with gelfoam torpedo/coils should be always considered.

- The arterial hepatocyte infusion into the spleen can be challenging due to the increased tortuosity of the splenic artery. The combination of a soft diagnostic catheter and a glide wire can facilitate selective distal catheterization of the splenic artery.
- In coagulopathic patients, the radial artery puncture should be considered as an alternative as it has been demonstrated to reduce bleeding-related complications in comparison to femoral approach.
- Percutaneous access to the portal system can be associated with significant bleeding complication, and the use of a micropuncture can decrease this risk. Multiple passages of the 21-gauge needle through the liver parenchyma can be performed without much concern.
- A second method to decrease the risk of bleeding is accessing the portal system through the left lobe under ultrasound guidance. To decrease the chances of bleeding through the transparietohepatic access, access track embolization should be always considered.
- Hemostasis postpancreatectomy ICT can be achieved by embolization of the mesenteric vein branch in which the catheter was surgically inserted. A microcatheter can be used coaxially to deploy the embolic agent precisely. This technique is helpful when working with a very short vein segment because adequate support and stability can be obtained (Fig. 43.9).
- The arterial hepatocyte infusion into the spleen can be challenging due to the increased tortuosity of the splenic artery. In this situation, combination of a soft diagnostic catheter and a glide wire can facilitate selective distal catheterization of the splenic artery.
- These patients very often have at least some degree of coagulation dysfunction, which increases arterial access risk. Therefore, common femoral artery puncture can be performed under ultrasound guidance with a micropuncture kit to guarantee a single-wall puncture above the femoral bifurcation.

REFERENCES

1. Thomas ED, Lochte HL Jr, Lu WC, et al. Intravenous infusion of bone marrow in patients receiving radiation and chemotherapy. *N Engl J Med*. 1957;257(11):491–496.
2. Nikolic B, Faintuch S, Goldberg SN, et al. Stem cell therapy: a primer for interventionalists and imagers. *J Vasc Interv Radiol*. 2009;20(8):999–1012.
3. World Health Organization. Diabetes. Diabetes: fact sheet no. 312, August 2011. http://www.who.int/mediacentre/factsheets/fs312/en/. Accessed May 16, 2013.
4. Brissova M, Fowler MJ, Nicholson WE, et al. Assessment of human pancreatic islet architecture and composition by laser scanning confocal microscopy. *J Histochem Cytochem*. 2009;53(9):1087–1097.
5. Morel P, Chau C, Brayman K, et al. Quality of metabolic control at 2 to 12 years after a pancreas transplant. *Transplant Proc*. 1992;24:835–838.
6. Sutherland DER, Gruessner RWG, Dunn DL, et al. Lessons learned from more than 1,000 pancreas transplants at a single institution. *Ann Surg*. 2001;233(4):463.
7. Gruessner AC, Sutherland DE. Pancreas transplant outcomes for United States (US) and non-US cases as reported to the United Network for Organ Sharing (UNOS) and the International Pancreas Transplant Registry (IPTR) as of June 2004. *Clin Transplant*. 2005;19:433–455.
8. Shapiro AM, Lakey JR, Ryan EA, et al. Islet transplantation in seven patients with type 1 diabetes mellitus using a glucocorticoid-free immunosuppressive regimen. *N Engl J Med*. 2000;343:230–238.
9. Brendel MD, Hering B, Schultz AO, et al. *International Islet Transplant Registry: Newsletter 8*. Giessen, Germany: Justus-Liebig-University of Giessen; 2001.
10. Ryan EA, Bigam D, Shapiro AM. Current indications for pancreas or islet transplant. *Diabetes Obes Metab*. 2006;8(1):1–7.
11. Ryan EA, Shandro T, Green K, et al. Assessment of the severity of hypoglycemia and glycemic lability in type 1 diabetic subjects undergoing islet transplantation. *Diabetes*. 2004;53(4):955–962.
12. Collaborative Islet Transplant Registry. CITR seventh annual report. https://web.emmes.com/study/isl/reports/01062012_7thAnnualReport.pdf. Accessed June 4, 2013.
13. Ryan EA, Paty BW, Senior PA, et al. Five-year follow-up after clinical islet transplantation. *Diabetes*. 2005;54(7):2060–2069.
14. Thompson DM, Begg IS, Harris C, et al. Reduced progression of diabetic retinopathy after islet cell transplantation compared with intensive medical therapy. *Transplantation*. 2008;85(10):1400–1405.
15. Fiorina P, Folli F, Zerbini G, et al. Islet transplantation is associated with improvement of renal function among uremic patients with type I diabetes mellitus and kidney transplants. *J Am Soc Nephrol*. 2003;14(8):2150–2158.
16. Lee TC, Barshes NR, O'Mahony CA, et al. The effect of pancreatic islet transplantation on progression of diabetic retinopathy and neuropathy. *Transplant Proc*. 2005;37(5):2263–2265.
17. Gaba RC, Garcia-Roca R, Oberholzer J. Pancreatic islet cell transplantation: an update for interventional radiologists. *J Vasc Interv Radiol*. 2012;23(5):583–594.
18. Venturini M, Angeli E, Maffi P, et al. Technique, complications, and therapeutic efficacy of percutaneous transplantation of human pancreatic islet cells in type 1 diabetes: the role of US. *Radiology*. 2005;234(2):617–624.
19. Daly B, O'Kelly K, Klassen D. Interventional procedures in whole organ and islet cell pancreas transplantation. *Semin Intervent Radiol*. 2004;21(4):335–343.
20. Baidal DA, Froud T, Ferreira JV, et al. The bag method for islet cell infusion. *Cell Transplant*. 2003;12(7):809–813.
21. Villiger P, Ryan EA, Owen R, et al. Prevention of bleeding after islet transplantation: lessons learned from a multivariate analysis of 132 cases at a single institution. *Am J Transplant*. 2005;5(12):2992–2998.

22. Thuluvath PJ, Imperio D, Nair S, et al. Chronic pancreatitis. Long-term pain relief with or without surgery, cancer risk, and mortality. *J Clin Gastroenterol.* 2003;36(2):159–165.
23. Park JW, Jang JY, Kim EJ, et al. Effects of pancreatectomy on nutritional state, pancreatic function and quality of life. *Br J Surg.* 2013;100(8):1064–1070.
24. Barbier L, Jamal W, Dokmak S, et al. Impact of total pancreatectomy: short- and long-term assessment [published online ahead of print January 29, 2013]. *HPB (Oxford).*
25. Sutherland DE, Matas AJ, Najarian JS. Pancreatic islet cell transplantation. *Surg Clin North Am.* 1978;58(2):365–382.
26. Morgan KA, Nishimura M, Uflacker R, et al. Percutaneous transhepatic islet cell autotransplantation after pancreatectomy for chronic pancreatitis: a novel approach. *HPB (Oxford).* 2011;13(7): 511–516.
27. Sutherland DE, Gruessner AC, Carlson AM, et al. Islet autotransplant outcomes after total pancreatectomy: a contrast to islet allograft outcomes. *Transplantation.* 2008;86(12): 1799–1802.
28. Nath DS, Kellogg TA, Sutherland DE. Total pancreatectomy with intraportal auto-islet transplantation using a temporarily exteriorized omental vein. *J Am Coll Surg.* 2004;199(6): 994–995.
29. Matas AJ, Sutherland DER, Steffes MW, et al. Hepatocellular transplantation for metabolic deficiencies: decrease plasma bilirubin in Gunn rats. *Science.* 1976;1992:897.
30. Mito M, Kusano M, Kawaura Y. Hepatocyte transplantation in man. *Transplant Proc.* 1992;24(6):3052–3053.
31. Soriano HE, Wood RP, Kang DC, et al. Hepatocellular transplantation (HCT) in children with fulminant liver failure. *Hepatology.* 1997;30:239A.
32. Strom SC, Fisher RA, Thompson MT, et al. Hepatocyte transplantation as a bridge to orthotopic liver transplantation in terminal liver failure. *Transplantation.* 1997;63(4):559–569.
33. Grossman M, Raper SE, Kozarsky K, et al. Successful ex vivo gene therapy directed to liver in a patient with familial hypercholesterolaemia. *Nat Genet.* 1994;6(4):335–341.
34. Fisher RA, Strom SC. Human hepatocyte transplantation: worldwide results. *Transplantation.* 2006;82(4):441–449.
35. Habibullah CM, Syed IH, Qamar A, et al. Human fetal hepatocyte transplantation in patients with fulminant hepatic failure. *Transplantation.* 1994;58(8):951–952.
36. Pareja E, Martinez A, Cortes M, et al. Hepatic cell transplantation. Technical and methodological aspects. *Cir Esp.* 2010;87(3):139–147.
37. Donato MT, Lahoz A, Jimenez N, et al. Potential impact of steatosis on cytochrome P450 enzymes of human hepatocytes isolated from fatty liver grafts. *Drug Metab Dispos.* 2006;34(9):1556–1562.
38. Terry C, Dhawan A, Mitry RR, et al. Cryopreservation of isolated human hepatocytes for transplantation: state of the art. *Cryobiology.* 2006;53(2):149–159.
39. Nagata H, Ito M, Shirota C, et al. Route of hepatocyte delivery affects hepatocyte engraftment in the spleen. *Transplantation.* 2003;76(4):732–734.
40. Sterling RK, Fisher RA. Liver transplantation. Living donor, hepatocyte, and xenotransplantation. *Clin Liver Dis.* 2001;5(2):431–460.
41. Fox IJ, Chowdhury JR, Kaufman SS, et al. Treatment of the Crigler-Najjar syndrome type I with hepatocyte transplantation. *N Engl J Med.* 1998;338(20):1422–1426.
42. Horslen SP, McCowan TC, Goertzen TC, et al. Isolated hepatocyte transplantation in an infant with a severe urea cycle disorder. *Pediatrics.* 2003;111:1262–1267.
43. Darwish AA, Sokal E, Stephenne X, et al. Permanent access to the portal system for cellular transplantation using an implantable port device. *Liver Transpl.* 2004;10:1213–1215.
44. Smets F, Najimi M, Sokal EM. Cell transplantation in the treatment of liver diseases. *Pediatr Transplant.* 2008;12(1):6–13.

44

Vascular Disease

Mark D. Iafrati • Joseph Zuniga

INTRAVASCULAR DELIVERY OF THERAPEUTIC AGENTS

Peripheral arterial disease (PAD) is a chronic condition that primarily arises from atherosclerosis and ultimately results in the occlusion of arteries to the limbs. It affects millions of Americans and is responsible for a significant burden of mortality, loss of limb, and decreased functional capacity and quality of life. Epidemiologic studies have estimated the prevalence to be at least 10% in the general population, with an almost twofold increase observed in people older than 70 years of age (approximately 15% to 20%).[1,2]

As PAD evolves, it causes progressive impedance in blood flow to distal tissues and subsequent ischemia. In severe cases, it causes critical limb ischemia (CLI), a condition characterized by rest pain, impaired wound healing, ulceration, and gangrene. CLI has classically been managed surgically via bypass procedures. Unfortunately, a large fraction of these procedures have proved unsuccessful due to the inadequacy of autologous veins for use as a bypass conduit, the occlusion of downstream arteries (poor "runoff"), or concurrent microvascular disease which impairs wound healing despite a successful bypass procedure. Ultimately, limb amputation remains the only option for several patients. Major limb amputation, however, is itself associated with significant (15% to 20%) perioperative mortality. For one-third of amputation survivors, amputation of the remaining limb will eventually be required.[3]

The need for safe and effective treatment cannot be overemphasized. The last 10 years have been witness to a dramatic shift to less invasive therapeutic approaches for PAD. In a study done by Goodney and associates[4] in 2009, a threefold increase in endovascular procedures was documented alongside a 42% decrease in bypass surgery. This shift to less invasive therapy was accompanied by a 25% decrease in major lower extremity amputations and a decrease in overall mortality.[4] Although other factors including improved medical management and wound care have undoubtedly played a role in this decline, the change appears to be at least partially driven by the successful use and safety of endovascular lower extremity revascularization.

Despite the tremendous progress made in the medical management and endovascular treatment of PAD, a significant number of patients referred to as *no option critical limb ischemia* (NO-CLI) patients have exhausted their conventional therapeutic options. Mechanical revascularization techniques, both bypass and endovascular, require an inflow source, an outflow target, and a conduit. For patients lacking any of these components, an alternative treatment approach using percutaneous or catheter-based delivery of pharmaceutical or biologic agents may offer the next best hope for symptom relief and limb salvage. This chapter will present a review of some of the more promising minimally invasive therapeutic options.

THERAPEUTIC AGENTS

Growth Factors

Angiogenesis is the formation and growth of new blood vessels from a previously existing vascular bed. This complex process entails disruption of vascular basement membranes, subsequent migration and proliferation of endothelial cells, and formation and maturation of blood vessels, all occurring under the strict regulation of growth and inhibitory factors.

Normally in adults, angiogenesis is a dormant process. The presence of angiogenesis in the setting of limb ischemia is of biologic interest as the ability to form new vessels to provide collateral arterial circulation may prove beneficial in the amelioration of ischemia caused by chronic arterial occlusion.

Multiple growth factors are involved in promoting formation of new blood vessels. Vascular endothelial growth factor (VEGF), in particular, plays a crucial role in angiogenesis mainly because its receptors are predominantly localized in the endothelial cells of blood vessels. Studies have also revealed lower levels of VEGF in the affected leg of CLI patients,[5] hence supplementation with this growth factor has been hypothesized to assist in arterial collateralization.

Animal and clinical studies have shown that administration of VEGF either systemically or locally stimulates therapeutic angiogenesis.[3,6,7] Its delivery, however, remains a big challenge. With a short half-life of about 1 hour, high dosages may be required to achieve desired effects.[7] Systemic administration may also result in new vessel growth in undesired locations, such as in the retina, and raises the possibility of carcinogenesis.[8]

In 2008, the U.S. Food and Drug Administration reviewed the potential for carcinogenesis with prolonged use of the topical platelet-derived growth factor becaplermin. It was concluded that the increase in the risk of death from cancer in patients with prolonged exposure to topical becaplermin was five times higher than in those patients who did not use the product.[9]

Given the nonspecificity of delivering growth factors via infusion catheters, several delivery systems have been developed to limit systemic effects and improve target specificity. The introduction of a delivery vehicle made of cross-linked DNA–gelatin nanospheres greatly increased the stability of DNA, transfection efficiency, and target specificity.

Animal studies have shown the use of intra-arterial gene transfer via angioplasty using balloons coated with plasmid VEGF in improving blood supply to the ischemic limb.[10–12] Isner et al.[13] in 1996 reported that this method worked on a 71-year-old patient with limb ischemia and tissue loss. They administered human plasmid VEGF to the popliteal artery using a hydrogel-coated angioplasty balloon and reported increased collateral vessel formation on follow-up angiography at 4 weeks. Adverse events directly related to angiogenesis included the development of spider angiomas on the ankle and foot of the same extremity that was treated. Transient peripheral edema was also observed in the treated extremity likely due to the increased vascular permeability induced by VEGF. This was treated with diuretics and resolved by 4 weeks. Despite improvement in collateral flow, the gangrene could not be reversed and the patient eventually required a major amputation about 5 months after the procedure.[8,13] Multiple randomized controlled trials (RCTs) using intra-arterial as well as intramuscular transfer of growth factor genes have been subsequently been reported.

Hammer and Steiner[14] in 2013 analyzed 12 RCTs studying local administration of growth factors (VEGF, FGF, HGF, Del-1, HIF-1 alpha) using plasmid or viral gene transfer by intra-arterial or intramuscular injections. A total of 1,494 patients with the majority suffering from CLI (64 %) were included. This meta-analysis showed neither a significant benefit nor harm for gene therapy for all-cause mortality (odds ratio [OR] 0.88; 95% confidence interval [CI], 0.62 to 1.26), amputations (OR 0.64; 95% CI, 0.31 to 1.31), or ulcer healing (OR 1.79; 95% CI, 0.8 to 4.01). Despite the potential benefit seen from the individual clinical trials, no clear overall benefit was seen from gene therapy for PAD regardless of severity.[14]

Prostanoids

Prostaglandins are lipid compounds known to exert significant vasoactive effects. Specific types of prostaglandins are known to produce vasodilation, motivating researchers to explore the application of this property in the management of CLI.

When used either alone or in conjunction with angioplasty, intravenous or direct intra-arterial administration of prostaglandin E_1 (PGE_1) has been reported to markedly improve microcirculation.[15,16] This is evident through enhancement in efficacy parameters such as transcutaneous oxygen tension and ankle–brachial index (ABI). The effect of PGE_1 is attributed not only to its vasodilatory property but also to several other factors such as inhibition of ischemia-induced neutrophil activation, reduction of platelet activation, improvement in hemorheologic properties and cellular metabolism, reduction in the number of circulating endothelial cells, and inhibition of adhesion molecule expression.[15]

Heider and associates[16] discussed the role of PGE_1 post percutaneous transluminal angioplasty (PTA). They demonstrated that angiography causes significant impairment of peripheral microcirculation in patients with intermittent claudication. Peripheral oxygen tension is significantly reduced after PTA and remains decreased for the next 4 weeks. This impairment can be addressed with PGE_1 therapy by exploiting two of its pharmacologic effects: (1) the vasodilatory property, which diminishes angioplasty-caused vasoconstriction, and (2) its endothelial-protective effect, which has been shown to protect endothelial function after disturbance by nonionic contrast material.

In a recent meta-analysis by Ruffolo et al.[17] in 2010, 20 publications describing RCTs on the use of prostanoids on CLI were reviewed. Prostanoids were found to be effective in relief of rest pain (risk ratio [RR] 1.32; 95% CI 1.10 to 1.57, $P = .003$) and ulcer healing (RR 1.54; 95% CI, 1.22 to 1.96). Iloprost in particular showed favorable results in terms of preventing major amputations (RR 0.69; 95% CI, 0.52 to 0.93). Despite these positive results, however, the authors of the meta-analysis believe that there is no conclusive evidence with regard to long-term effectiveness and safety of different prostanoids in patients with CLI.

Stem Cell

The management of CLI from severe PAD is a challenge for the vascular medicine specialists. This is especially true for patients on whom conservative management has failed and who, at the same time, are not suitable for either surgical or endovascular revascularization due to existing comorbidities or anatomy.

A promising treatment strategy emerged about a decade ago for patients whose only other option in the past was to undergo limb amputation. The inspiration for this treatment arose from the observation that cells in the bone marrow or the peripheral blood that express CD34 surface markers have the capacity to transform into functional endothelial cells in vitro. [18,19] These stem cells have the capability of producing angiogenic factors and thus may play a potential role in the management of tissue ischemia by facilitating blood vessel development. Several studies done in the early 2000s reported remarkable outcomes when stem cell therapy was used to improve peripheral blood circulation in preclinical models. [20,21]

The Therapeutic Angiogenesis using Cell Transplantation (TACT) study was the first clinical trial to ascertain the feasibility of this concept. It demonstrated that the intramuscular implantation of autologous bone marrow cells into critically ischemic legs significantly improved ABI, transcutaneous oxygen pressures, and rest pain.[22] Multiple clinical trials have yielded similar encouraging results.[23,24] Although most cellular therapy for CLI has been administered intramuscularly, a few studies have reported intra-arterial injection of bone marrow aspirate either alone or in combination with an intramuscular injection produced no significant difference in treatment result when compared to intramuscular implantation. These studies claim that intra-arterial administration ensured that the stem cells would reach all targeted vessels in an antegrade manner, allowing perfused ischemic muscle regions to receive a high concentration of stem cells. However, concern remains about the possibility of arterial puncture site complications, downstream arterial thrombosis, and the possibility that the cells will not reach the intended tissues of interest in patients with extremely poor baseline perfusion.[25]

Current knowledge supports intramuscular administration of bone marrow cells as a relatively safe, feasible, and potentially effective treatment for the patient with CLI which may reduce the need for major amputations. A recent systematic review of RCTs reporting intramuscular administration of bone marrow mononuclear cell concentrates in 291 NO-CLI patients (treatment group: 149, control: 142) reported a reduction in major limb amputation risk from 25.4% to 14.8% ($P = .03$).[23] Furthermore, the treatment was found to be safe with few treatment-related complications. Pivotal studies are underway with the objective to verify the efficacy of this novel therapy.

Anti-inflammatory Agents

The process of restenosis after vessel injury is mainly thought to involve inflammatory cells located in the vessel adventitia such as macrophages, dendritic cells, lymphocytes, neutrophils, and mast cells. Within hours after injury, these cells initiate the release of other inflammatory modulators such as cytokines, growth factors, and reactive oxygen species, which contribute to smooth muscle and adventitial cell proliferation. This same inflammatory response has also been noted to occur after vascular procedures.[26,27]

In line with the hypothesis, Owens et al.[27] did a prospective, first-in-man study to determine the feasibility and safety of percutaneous perivascular delivery of dexamethasone after treatment of the femoral–popliteal segment. Using an over-the-wire microinfusion catheter, a microneedle was deployed into the vessel adventitia to deliver dexamethasone. Twenty patients with a mean age of 66 years with Rutherford category 2 to 5 were enrolled in this study. The range of lesion length treated was 8.9 ± 5.3 cm, half of which involved chronic total occlusions. Technical success of drug delivery was 100%, and no procedural or drug-related adverse events were noted. The preliminary results at 6 months suggest that perivascular dexamethasone treatment may improve outcomes following angioplasty to the femoral and popliteal arteries. The mean Rutherford score decreased from 3.1 ± 0.7 (median, 3.0) preoperatively to 0.5 ± 0.7 at the end of the study period (median, 0.0, $P < .00001$). The ABI index increased from 0.68 ± 0.15 to 0.89 ± .19 ($P = .0003$). Only two lesions reoccluded.[28] These preliminary results are encouraging.

Antiproliferative Agents

Another mechanism by which restenosis has been postulated to occur is through neointimal hyperplasia. In line with this, antiproliferative agents have been used to prevent restenosis after vascular procedures. Among these agents, paclitaxel, sirolimus, and everolimus have been well studied for this purpose. Their use was heightened with their incorporation into balloons and stents.[28,29] Because the function of these antiproliferative agents is intimately tied to their delivery techniques, a more detailed description of these agents is presented in the following sections describing device considerations.

DEVICES

In the modern era of endovascular interventions for PAD, multiple devices have been developed to deliver therapeutic agents as close as possible to problematic regions with the goal of localizing treatment to prevent undesirable systemic effects.

The standard endovascular technique of using guidewire and catheter has undergone very minimal change throughout the years, and improvements were primarily centered on modifying the physical attributes of the devices being used.

Porous Balloon Catheters

A porous balloon catheter is a variation of the standard balloon catheter used in percutaneous angioplasty. With its reservoir and peripheral perforations, it is well suited for the administration of various therapeutic agents during or after balloon angioplasty.

The porous balloon catheter was developed with the intent to create an instrument that could deliver high concentrations of therapeutic agents locoregionally to the involved segment of the vasculature, thus allowing medications to work without exposing the entire circulation to the agent's effects. Wolinsky and Thung,[30] through their work with canine arteries in 1990, pioneered the use of porous balloon catheters in local drug delivery. This technique has been particularly significant in the prevention of restenosis. By itself, balloon angioplasty causes vessel damage, which may produce restenosis of the treated segment in the long term. It has been shown that the addition of therapeutic agents, such as reviparin, decreases the incidence of restenosis.[31]

Several factors such as the size of the particles within the infusate, infusion pressure, and infusate volume should be considered when using porous balloon catheters. Large particles cause more severe vascular damage, incite an inflammatory reaction, and promote intimal thickening. Similar detrimental effects are seen when trying to force a large volume of infusate through the porous balloon catheter. The use of infusates containing nanoparticles has been proven to cause less vascular damage than an infusate containing microparticles. Also with smaller particles, less infusion pressure is required to achieve deeper agent penetration with potentially greater treatment effect.

Porous balloon catheters are also used in thrombolysis. Specifically, the ClearWay (Atrium Medical, Hudson, New Hampshire) balloon catheter (Fig. 44.1) allows direct administration of thrombolytic agents within the thrombus. Benefits observed with the use of this catheter included a decreased lytic requirement and reduced duration of thrombolysis,[32] thus reducing the potential for hemorrhagic complications related to prolonged exposure to the thrombolysis agent.

A more recent nonrandomized trial by Patrick Kelly (personal information) using the ClearWay infusion balloon catheter was done to determine if a single limited dose infusion of paclitaxel after standard endovascular revascularization would prevent recurrent stenosis due to intimal hyperplasia. A total of 42 limbs (16 limbs with 2 lesions, 2 limbs with 3 lesions) treated with angioplasty, stenting, and atherectomy individually or in combination with subsequent paclitaxel infusion were followed for 19 months. No adverse reaction was noted from paclitaxel administration. Six of the 42 (14%) limbs required additional revascularization (4 of 6 had total occlusion) during the study period. No amputations or bypass procedures were required. These early findings show favorable results. Long-term follow up studies are underway.

Iontophoresis Balloon Catheters

Another catheter-based system developed to deliver medications directly into the vessel wall involves manipulation of electric charges. Iontophoresis uses electric current to enhance the movement of charged molecules and thus facilitates the transfer of therapeutic agents from the source to surrounding tissues. It has proved valuable in a multitude of specialties, ranging from the delivery of chemotherapeutic agents to the transdermal administration of pain medications.

In PAD, iontophoresis is used for locoregional delivery of therapeutic agents. This technology has been incorporated into porous balloons. When the balloon is in the proper position during an endovascular procedure, it is expanded to occlude the vessel, thus allowing apposition of the porous membrane with the vessel wall. An electric field then drives the charged molecules of the agent into the arterial wall.

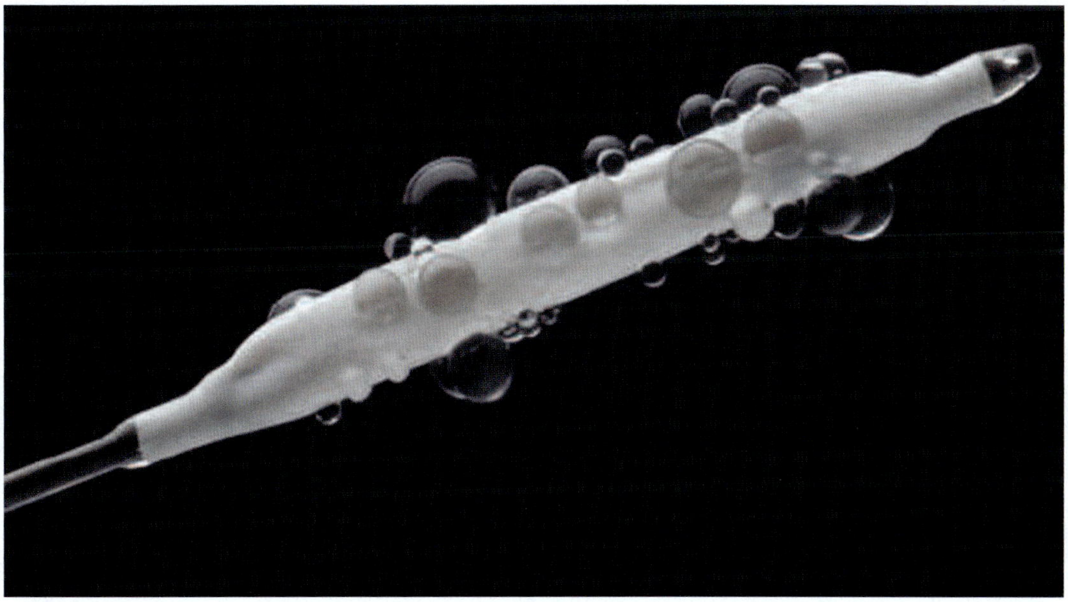

Figure 44.1 ClearWay infusion catheter (Atrium Medical, Hudson, New Hampshire).

The first study to investigate the iontophoresis balloons in enhancing medication delivery involved hirudin administration in a porcine carotid model.[33] Results showed that the concentration of hirudin was about 80-fold greater than would be anticipated when the same medication is administered via diffusion. Hirudin was also noted to have penetrated the entire circumference of the vessel wall. Predictably, the amount of hirudin within the vessel wall increased with the duration of administration. Increased duration of occlusion may be required to achieve desired effects with the balloon, thus raising the possibility of causing distal ischemia. A reperfusion lumen catheter may be required in this situation to reduce the ischemic risk. This study also showed that retention of the therapeutic agent is time-dependent, with approximately 80% of the drug eliminated from the arterial wall after 1 hour. A similar study demonstrated substantial intramural delivery of heparin using the same technology, and the results correlated with the observed therapeutic effects.[34]

Unfortunately, no further studies regarding the use of iontophoresis in PAD have been published since this report from 1997, as effort has been apparently been concentrated in other delivery techniques.

Drug-Eluting Balloons and Drug-Coated Balloons

Balloon angioplasty has been proven effective in the revascularization of extremities with stenosed or occluded arteries. However, prevention of restenosis due to neointimal hyperplasia remains a major challenge.

The drug-eluting balloon (DEB) (Fig. 44.2) platform has remained largely the same as that of standard PTA except for

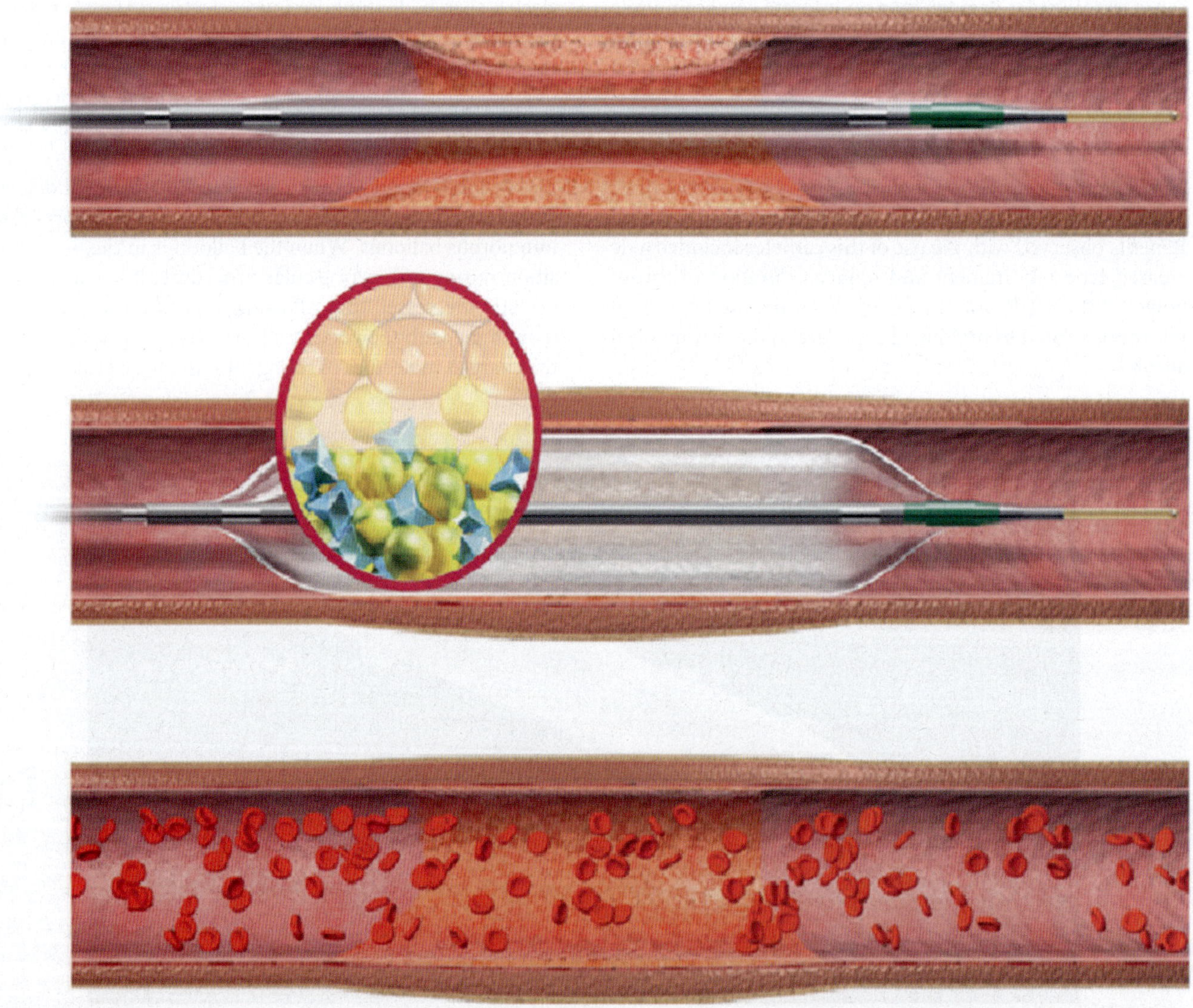

Figure 44.2 Drug-eluting balloon. (Borrowed from Fröhlich GM, Lansky AJ, Ko DT, et al. Drug eluting balloons for de novo coronary lesions—a systematic review and meta-analysis. *BMC Med.* 2013;11:123.)

its drug-eluting component. The most frequently used agent is paclitaxel, a cytotoxic drug which halts the cell cycle in the M phase of the mitotic cycle. It is well studied and is known to have hydrophobic–lipophilic properties, facilitating drug delivery and uptake.

To achieve lasting antiproliferative effects on the vessel wall, a sufficient drug dose must be delivered to the target site during angioplasty. The amount of drug absorbed by the vessel wall depends on the chemical properties of the drug, the dose, the transfer system, inflation time, and release pattern.

The Paclitaxel-coated Balloons in Femoral Indication to Defeat Restenosis (PACIFIER) trial by Werk et al.[29] in 2012 randomized 91 limbs (44 to DEB and 47 to uncoated balloons) to evaluate the safety and efficacy of DEB versus standard balloons in the revascularization of infrainguinal arteries. This revealed that use of DEB for femoropopliteal PTA is feasible and safe. This trial also showed significant reduction in restenosis rates in comparison with current conventional balloons with fewer binary restenoses (3 [8.6%] vs. 11 [32.4%], $P = .01$). The reduced restenosis rate also translated to fewer target lesion revascularization (TLR) (3 [7.1%] vs. 12 [27.9%], $P = .02$) at up to 1-year follow-up.[30]

Drug-Eluting Balloon in Peripheral Intervention for Below-the-Knee Angioplasty Evaluation (DEBATE-BTK) is another randomized study designed to evaluate the advantage of DEBs over standard PTA balloons in terms of 12-month restenosis and TLR, specifically in diabetic patients with CLI undergoing revascularization of arteries, this time below the knee. A total of 158 infrapopliteal lesions were treated (DEB: 74, control: 74). The 12-month restenosis rate was significantly reduced using DEBs, with a relative reduction of 64% with results independent of the length of lesion or the technique of revascularization. Clinically driven TLRs were also reduced (12 [18%] vs. 29 [43%], $P = .002$).[28]

Another advantage noted with DEB is the absence of a foreign body being left inside the artery as occurs with stent placement. Although stents, either bare metal or drug eluting, have provided superior results to standard PTA for femoropopliteal disease, they permanently change the structure of the vessel, cause local inflammatory reaction, and potentially hasten restenosis. It is also known that in-stent restenosis is more difficult to treat than restenosis in nonstented segments.

The use of DEB has been tested using various inflation and drug-coating techniques. Cremers et al.[35] found no difference in drug delivery when inflation times were varied (10 seconds, 60 seconds, and 2 × 60 seconds), suggesting that most of the drug was released on initial contact. Low inflation pressure (2 atm) was as effective as high pressure (12 atmospheres) in reducing late luminal loss (LLL) and intimal thickness.[36] Further demonstrating that more is not always better, Kelsch et al.[37] found 1 μg/mm^2 doses of paclitaxel to be as efficacious as 3 μg/mm^2, whereas 9 μg/mm^2 lead to excess thrombotic complications. Despite the demonstrated biologic activity with relatively low doses of paclitaxel, it should be noted that only a small percentage of the drug applied to the balloon is taken up by the target tissues. During the process of guiding the balloon to the target lesion, approximately 10% of the initial drug is lost. During inflation, approximately 80% of the drug dose is released, with 20% of that delivered to the target vessel wall. The remaining 10% of the initial dose remains on the balloon and is removed from the patient.[37,38] Although most of the drug is ultimately systemically circulated, the concentrations are low and by 24 hours have dropped to undetectable levels.[39] In contrast to the quick systemic clearance, paclitaxel is known to remain in vascular smooth muscle cells for up to a week.[40,41] Although the low circulating drug levels appear safe, there are ongoing efforts to improve the delivery kinetics. One promising approach is the use of "expedients," which increase the contact area between paclitaxel molecules and the vessel wall, thus enhancing local bioavailability. Agents currently under investigation including urea, butyryl-trihexyl citrate, and iopromide have shown promising initial results.[38,42]

Drug-Eluting Stents

Drug-eluting stents (Fig. 44.3) are the most popular and widely studied of the local agent delivery devices. They are

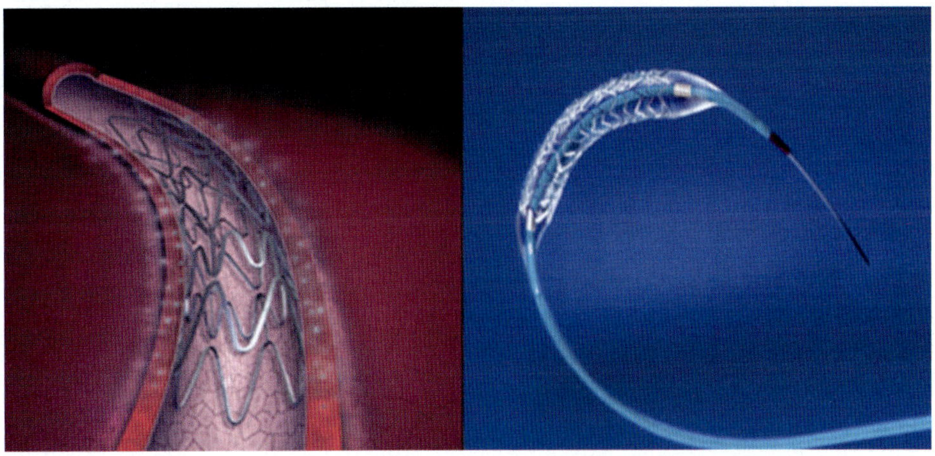

Figure 44.3 Drug-eluting stent. (Borrowed from Balghith M. Artery bypass versus PCI using new generation DES. In: Aronow WS, ed. *Artery Bypass*. InTech; 2013.)

well-established tools in the field of coronary artery disease due to their lower rate of restenosis and TLR as compared with bare metal stents (BMS).[43,44] This has prompted researchers to explore the possibility of using coronary balloon-expandable drug-eluting stents in other arterial beds such as the infrapopliteal region.

However, safety concerns surfaced with the new phenomena of late and very late stent thrombosis (ST) attributed to delayed endothelial healing, vessel wall inflammation, and impaired endothelial function.[45]

In 2011, the RCT by Rastan et al.[46] looked at the 1-year primary patency rate of sirolimus-eluting stents compared with BMS for focal infrapopliteal lesions in patients with either claudication or CLI. Primary patency was 80.6% for drug-eluting stent versus 55.6% for BMS ($P = .004$), with respective 1-year secondary patency rates of 91.9% and 71.4%, respectively ($P = .005$).[46]

The Drug-Eluting Stents in the Critically Ischemic Lower Leg (DESTINY) trial in 2012 by Bosiers et al.[47] showed in a randomized controlled study that for infrapopliteal disease in patients with CLI, everolimus-eluting stents had better primary patency compared to BMS. Seventy-four patients were treated with Xience V (Abbott, Santa Clara, California) everolimus-eluting stents, and 66 were treated with Vision BMS (Abbott, Santa Clara, California). At the end of 1 year, primary patency was 85% versus 54% ($P < .0001$) in favor of the Xience V stents. Freedom from TLR was also superior at 91% versus 66% ($P < .001$).[47] More recently, a meta-analysis by Fusaro et al.,[48] which included data from the two previous studies mentioned, revealed that in focal disease of infrapopliteal arteries, drug-eluting stent reduces the risk of reintervention and amputation compared with plain balloon angioplasty or BMS implantation at 1-year follow-up.

The use of metal implantable devices is not without limitations, however. Stent fractures or occlusions may occur, and patients need to be placed on long-term antiplatelet therapy, typically double antiplatelet therapy. Stent occlusions develop from neointimal formation and incomplete endothelialization brought on by the inflammatory response of the vessel wall to the continuous mechanical and chemical stimuli induced by the stent's metal mesh and polymeric coating. These occlusions are especially problematic because the endovascular options are very limited for retreatment of the lesion. In addition, stent placement is not recommended in very small vessels, vessel bifurcations, and specific anatomical locations such as the popliteal artery and the distal third of the anterior tibial artery.

TIPS AND TRICKS

Porous balloon catheters	The size of the particles within the infusate, infusion pressure, and infusate volume should be considered when using porous balloon catheters. Large particles cause more severe vascular damage, incite an inflammatory reaction, and promote intimal thickening. Similar detrimental effects are seen when trying to force a large volume of infusate through the porous balloon catheter.
Iontophoresis balloon catheters	Great potential to increase drug delivery while minimizing hydrostatic pressure and local wall trauma, but no recent development reported
Drug-eluting balloons	Ideally used for *long* lesions with high risk of recurrence
Drug-eluting stents	Ideally used for *short* lesions with high risk of recurrence
Stem cell therapy/bone marrow aspirate	Potentially ideal for patients lacking outflow targets Injection pattern proposed; "biologic bypass" by linear injection patterns of stem cells onto the potential site of a bypass graft if revascularization was possible. Monitored anesthesia care preferred over general anesthesia.[25]

CONCLUSION

The world of peripheral vascular therapy has undergone a tremendous evolution during the last two decades resulting from improved awareness, medical therapies, smoking reduction, and endovascular techniques. This concentration of effort has resulted in a general decrease in cardiovascular morbidity, including amputation risk. The next decade promises to bring additional great strides as localized delivery of medications and cellular therapy further pushes back the frontiers in PAD, promising a truly transformative approach to this daunting problem. Although much remains to be discovered, this chapter has outlined some of the more promising approaches, one or more of which are likely to play a role in the development of the therapies of the future.

REFERENCES

1. Criqui MH, Fronek A, Barrett-Connor E, et al. The prevalence of peripheral arterial disease in a defined population. *Circulation*. 1985;71:510–515.
2. Selvin E, Erlinger TP. Prevalence of and risk factors for peripheral arterial disease in the United States: results from the National Health and Nutrition Examination Survey, 1999-2000. *Circulation*. 2004;110:738–743.
3. Amsden BG, Timbart L, Marecak D, et al. VEGF-induced angiogenesis following localized delivery via injectable, low viscosity poly(trimethylene carbonate). *J Control Release*. 2010;145:109–115.
4. Goodney PP, Beck AW, Nagle J, et al. National trends in lower extremity bypass surgery, endovascular interventions, and major amputations. *J Vasc Surg*. 2009;50:54–60.
5. Palmer-Kazen U, Wariaro D, Luo F, et al. Vascular endothelial cell growth factor and fibroblast growth factor 2 expression in patients with critical limb ischemia. *J Vasc Surg*. 2004; 39:621–628.
6. Rajagopalan S, Mohler ER III, Lederman RJ, et al. Regional angiogenesis with vascular endothelial growth factor in peripheral arterial disease: a phase II randomized, double-blind, controlled study of adenoviral delivery of vascular endothelial growth factor 121 in patients with disabling intermittent claudication. *Circulation*. 2003;108:1933–1938.
7. Jiang H, Zhang T, Sun X. Vascular endothelial growth factor gene delivery by magnetic DNA nanospheres ameliorates limb ischemia in rabbits. *J Surg Res*. 2005;126:48–54.
8. Isner JM, Walsh K, Symes J, et al. Arterial gene therapy for therapeutic angiogenesis in patients with peripheral artery disease. *Circulation*. 1995;91:2687–2692.
9. U.S. Food and Drug Administration. Update of safety review: follow-up to the March 27, 2008, communication about the ongoing safety review of Regranex (becaplermin). 2008. http://www.fda.gov/Drugs/DrugSafety/PostmarketDrugSafetyInformationforPatientsandProviders/DrugSafetyInformationforHeathcareProfessionals/ucm072148.htm. Accessed August 5, 2014.
10. Nabel EG, Plautz G, Nabel GJ. Site-specific gene expression in vivo by direct gene transfer into the arterial wall. *Science*. 1990;249:1285–1288.
11. Unger EF, Banai S, Shou M, et al. Basic fibroblast growth factor enhances myocardial collateral flow in a canine model. *Am J Physiol*. 1994;266:H1588–H1595.
12. Takeshita S, Rossow ST, Kearney M, et al. Time course of increased cellular proliferation in collateral arteries after administration of vascular endothelial growth factor in a rabbit model of lower limb vascular insufficiency. *Am J Pathol*. 1995; 147:1649–1660.
13. Isner JM, Pieczek A, Schainfeld R, et al. Clinical evidence of angiogenesis after arterial gene transfer of phVEGF165 in patient with ischaemic limb. *Lancet*. 1996;348:370–374.
14. Hammer A, Steiner S. Gene therapy for therapeutic angiogenesis in peripheral arterial disease—a systematic review and meta-analysis of randomized, controlled trials. *Vasa*. 2013;42:331–339.
15. Schellong S, Altmann E, von Bilderling P, et al. Microcirculation and tolerability following i.v. infusion of PGE1 and iloprost: a randomized cross-over study in patients with critical limb ischemia. *Prostaglandins Leukot Essent Fatty Acids*. 2004;70:503–509.
16. Heider P, Wildgruber M, Wolf O, et al. Improvement of microcirculation after percutaneous transluminal angioplasty in the lower limb with prostaglandin E1. *Prostaglandins Other Lipid Mediat*. 2009;88:23–30.
17. Ruffolo AJ, Romano M, Ciapponi A. Prostanoids for critical limb ischaemia. *Cochrane Database Syst Rev*. 2010;(1):CD006544.
18. Fadini GP, Agostini C, Avogaro A. Autologous stem cell therapy for peripheral arterial disease meta-analysis and systematic review of the literature. *Atherosclerosis*. 2010;209:10–17.
19. Horie T, Onodera R, Akamastu M, et al. Long-term clinical outcomes for patients with lower limb ischemia implanted with G-CSF-mobilized autologous peripheral blood mononuclear cells. *Atherosclerosis*. 2010;208:461–466.
20. Hamano K, Li TS, Kobayashi T, et al. The induction of angiogenesis by the implantation of autologous bone marrow cells: a novel and simple therapeutic method. *Surgery*. 2001;130:44–54.
21. Iwase T, Nagaya N, Fujii T, et al. Adrenomedullin enhances angiogenic potency of bone marrow transplantation in a rat model of hindlimb ischemia. *Circulation*. 2005;111:356–362.
22. Tateishi-Yuyama E, Matsubara H, Murohara T, et al. Therapeutic angiogenesis for patients with limb ischaemia by autologous transplantation of bone-marrow cells: a pilot study and a randomised controlled trial. *Lancet*. 2002;360:427–435.
23. Benoit E, O'Donnell TF, Patel AN. Safety and efficacy of autologous cell therapy in critical limb ischemia: a systematic review. *Cell Transplant*. 2013;22:545–562.
24. Iafrati MD, Hallett JW, Geils G, et al. Early results and lessons learned from a multicenter, randomized, double-blind trial of bone marrow aspirate concentrate in critical limb ischemia. *J Vasc Surg*. 2011;54:1650–1658.
25. Franz RW, Parks A, Shah KJ, et al. Use of autologous bone marrow mononuclear cell implantation therapy as a limb salvage procedure in patients with severe peripheral arterial disease. *J Vasc Surg*. 2009;50:1378–1390.
26. Schillinger M, Haumer M, Schlerka G, et al. Restenosis after percutaneous transluminal angioplasty in the femoropopliteal segment: the role of inflammation. *J Endovasc Ther*. 2001; 8:477–483.
27. Owens CD, Gasper WJ, Walker JP, et al. Safety and feasibility of adjunctive dexamethasone infusion into the adventitia of the femoropopliteal artery following endovascular revascularization. *J Vasc Surg*. 2014;59(4):1016–1024.
28. Liistro F, Porto I, Angioli P, et al. Drug-eluting balloon in peripheral intervention for below the knee angioplasty evaluation (DEBATE-BTK): a randomized trial in diabetic patients with critical limb ischemia. *Circulation*. 2013;128:615–621.
29. Werk M, Albrecht T, Meyer DR, et al. Paclitaxel-coated balloons reduce restenosis after femoro-popliteal angioplasty: evidence from the randomized PACIFIER trial. *Circ Cardiovasc Interv*. 2012;5:831–840.
30. Wolinsky H, Thung SN. Use of a perforated balloon catheter to deliver concentrated heparin into the wall of the normal canine artery. *J Am Coll Cardiol*. 1990;15:475–481.
31. Oberhoff M, Baumbach A, Hermann T, et al. Local and systemic delivery of low molecular weight heparin following PTCA: acute results and 6-month follow-up of the initial clinical experience with the porous balloon (PILOT-study). Preliminary

Investigation of Local Therapy Using Porous PTCA Balloons. *Cathet Cardiovasc Diagn*. 1998;44:267–274.

32. Dakhil B, Lacal P, Abdesselam AB, et al. Evaluation of balloon catheter-guided intra-arterial thrombolysis for acute peripheral arterial occlusion. *Ann Vasc Surg*. 2013;27:781–784.
33. Fernandez-Ortiz A, Meyer BJ, Mailhac A, et al. A new approach for local intravascular drug delivery. Iontophoretic balloon. *Circulation*. 1994;89:1518–1522.
34. Mitchel JF, Azrin MA, Fram DB, et al. Localized delivery of heparin to angioplasty sites with iontophoresis. *Cathet Cardiovasc Diagn*. 1997;41:315–323.
35. Cremers B, Speck U, Kaufels N, et al. Drug-eluting balloon: very short-term exposure and overlapping. *Thromb Haemost*. 2009;101:201–206.
36. Cremers B, Kelsch B, Clever YP, et al. Inhibition of neointimal proliferation after bare metal stent implantation with low-pressure drug delivery using a paclitaxel-coated balloon in porcine coronary arteries. *Clin Res Cardiol*. 2012;101:385–391.
37. Kelsch B, Scheller B, Biedermann M, et al. Dose response to Paclitaxel-coated balloon catheters in the porcine coronary overstretch and stent implantation model. *Invest Radiol*. 2011;46:255–263.
38. Scheller B, Speck U, Abramjuk C, et al. Paclitaxel balloon coating, a novel method for prevention and therapy of restenosis. *Circulation*. 2004;110:810–814.
39. Freyhardt P, Zeller T, Kroncke TJ, et al. Plasma levels following application of paclitaxel-coated balloon catheters in patients with stenotic or occluded femoropopliteal arteries. *Rofo*. 2011;183:448–455.
40. Axel DI, Kunert W, Goggelmann C, et al. Paclitaxel inhibits arterial smooth muscle cell proliferation and migration in vitro and in vivo using local drug delivery. *Circulation*. 1997;96:636–645.
41. Herdeg C, Oberhoff M, Baumbach A, et al. Local paclitaxel delivery for the prevention of restenosis: biological effects and efficacy in vivo. *J Am Coll Cardiol*. 2000;35:1969–1976.
42. Scheller B, Speck U, Romeike B, et al. Contrast media as carriers for local drug delivery. Successful inhibition of neointimal proliferation in the porcine coronary stent model. *Eur Heart*. J 2003;24:1462–1467.
43. Stone GW, Ellis SG, Cannon L, et al. Comparison of a polymer-based paclitaxel-eluting stent with a bare metal stent in patients with complex coronary artery disease: a randomized controlled trial. *JAMA*. 2005;294:1215–1223.
44. Moses JW, Leon MB, Popma JJ, et al. Sirolimus-eluting stents versus standard stents in patients with stenosis in a native coronary artery. *N Engl J Med*. 2003;349:1315–1323.
45. Bhatt DL. Intensifying platelet inhibition—navigating between Scylla and Charybdis. *N Engl J Med*. 2007;357:2078–2081.
46. Rastan A, Tepe G, Krankenberg H, et al. Sirolimus-eluting stents vs. bare-metal stents for treatment of focal lesions in infrapopliteal arteries: a double-blind, multi-centre, randomized clinical trial. *Eur Heart J*. 2011;32:2274–2281.
47. Bosiers M, Scheinert D, Peeters P, et al. Randomized comparison of everolimus-eluting versus bare-metal stents in patients with critical limb ischemia and infrapopliteal arterial occlusive disease. *J Vasc Surg*. 2012;55:390–398.
48. Fusaro M, Cassese S, Ndrepepa G, et al. Drug-eluting stents for revascularization of infrapopliteal arteries: updated meta-analysis of randomized trials. *JACC Cardiovasc Interv*. 2013;6:1284–1293.

Section J Abdominal Aorta Aneurysm Endoleaks

45

Abdominal Aorta Aneurysm Endoleaks

Ajita Deodhar • John A. Kaufman

The goal of endovascular repair of an abdominal aortic aneurysm (AAA) is complete exclusion of the aneurysm sac so that it is no longer exposed to arterial pressure, thereby eliminating the risk of rupture. An *endoleak* is defined as persistent pressurization of the aneurysm sac post endovascular stent graft repair of the aneurysm (EVAR). This usually manifests on imaging studies as aneurysmal sac growth, but not always as sac contrast opacification. Endoleaks are reported in 4% to 30% of patients post EVAR[1,2] and carry the risk of subsequent increase in aneurysm sac size and rupture.[1,2]

Endoleaks may be early (within 30 days post procedure) or late (after 30 days), simple with only inflow, or complex with inflow and outflow. Endoleaks are classified into five types (Table 45.1). A type I endoleak originates at the stent graft seal site in the proximal aorta (IA), distal aorta (IB), or at the iliac occluder site in an aorto-uni-iliac graft (IC). Incomplete apposition of the stent graft with the aortic wall leads to direct communication between the aneurysm sac and the systemic arterial circulation. This type of endoleak is usually seen in the early postprocedural period. However, progressive remodeling of the aorta and aneurysm sac can lead to dilation of the aneurysm neck and iliac angulation, thereby affecting the longitudinal and lateral stability of the stent graft within the aorta.[3] This can lead to delayed device migration, kinking (type I endoleak), or component separation (type III). Factors that predispose to early type IA endoleak include a short, angulated, and thrombus-containing neck. Similarly, tortuous and dilated iliac arteries can predispose to an early type IB endoleak.

Type II endoleaks are the most common type of endoleaks encountered after an EVAR, accounting for approximately 40% of all endoleaks.[4] In this, there is retrograde flow through one or multiple aortic branches into the aneurysm sac. The inferior mesenteric artery, lumbar arteries, and median sacral and gonadal arteries are the usual culprits. Conceptually, most type II endoleaks are like arteriovenous malformations, with multiple inflow vessels that coalesce in a nidus (the aneurysm sac) and multiple outflow vessels.

Type III endoleaks occur with structural stent graft failure. This includes junctional separation of modular devices or disruption of the graft fabric. Type III endoleaks are fairly unusual, particularly in the early postprocedure setting. Component separation can result from the previously described aortic remodeling.

Type IV endoleaks are uncommon with current endograft technologies. These endoleaks, related to graft porosity, are usually seen during the immediate post stent graft deployment and resolve spontaneously within 48 hours.

Type V endoleak is enlargement of the AAA sac without identification of a distinct endoleak. With older devices that are now no longer in use (i.e., the first-generation Excluder; W. L. Gore & Associates, Flagstaff, Arizona), sac enlargement was due to ultrafiltration of blood by the graft material. This was not a true leak. With the newer devices, a type V endoleak is most likely due to an unidentified type I through III endoleak.

Table 45.1 Endoleaks Types and Management

Type	Endoleak Source	Management
I	Inadequate seal at graft ends ■ IA: Proximal end ■ IB: Distal end ■ IC: Iliac occluder with an aorto-uni-iliac graft	Coda angioplasty balloon Balloon-expandable Palmaz stent Overlapping stent graft cuff
II	Branch to branch: retrograde flow in branch vessels such as IMA, lumbar arteries, gonadal artery, median sacral artery ■ IIA: Simple – inflow vessel only ■ IIB: Complex – inflow and outflow vessels from sac	Obliteration of the patent lumen within the aneurysm sac and embolization of the feeding artery(ies) at the origin in the aorta. Coils, glue, and Onyx may be used individually or in combination.
III	Mechanical graft failure ■ IIIA: Junctional separation of modular components ■ IIIB: Fractures/defects in the fabric	New stent graft across the region of device disruption
IV	Porous graft material	Currently, it is a rare problem; typically self-limited
V	Endotension: continued sac expansion secondary to exposure to graft pulsations. Not a true leak.	No therapy is indicated. AAA sac fluid drainage is contraindicated because it tends to reaccumulate.

DIAGNOSIS OF ENDOLEAK

Routine surveillance of patients undergoing EVAR is essential. Surveillance modalities include radiography, ultrasound (US), computed tomography (CT), and magnetic resonance imaging (MRI). Endoleaks can also be diagnosed definitively on angiograms, but the invasive nature of the procedure precludes this from being a routine surveillance modality. In general, CT angiography (CTA) is the accepted standard of care.[5] Hence, most patients undergoing EVAR undergo CTA at 1 month, 6 months, and 12 months followed by yearly examinations thereafter, provided there are no complications. Follow-up strategies are in evolution with a tendency toward decreased use of CT. The stent material (stainless steel, nitinol, or Elgiloy), strut thickness, and geometry can affect the choice of follow-up imaging modality.[5] Patients with a nitinol endoprosthesis can undergo magnetic resonance angiography (MRA).[6] Abdominal US and radiography in combination are useful in patients who are unable to get a CT or magnetic resonance examination, usually due to high serum creatinine/low glomerular filtration rate. Abdominal radiographs are helpful in evaluating for stent graft migration, separation of modular components, or limb kinking. Color Doppler US can evaluate for aneurysm sac size as well as the presence of endoleaks, although the sensitivity is operator dependent and varies from 42% to 97%.[7] Recent use of second-generation US contrast agents has improved the sensitivity,[8] but these agents are not widely used.

CTA and MRA demonstrate endoleaks as contrast material within the aneurysm sac (Fig. 45.1). It is important to obtain delayed-phase images as an endoleak may not be visible on the arterial phase. On US, endoleaks manifest as Doppler signal within the aneurysm sac or to-and-fro waveform in the feeding vessel (Fig. 45.2).

Type I endoleaks are usually evident on the post stent graft deployment angiogram as continued sac opacification of contrast resulting from insufficient proximal or distal seal (Fig. 45.3). On CTA/MRA, they will be visualized as contrast adjacent to or in communication with the proximal or distal seal zone. With a type II endoleak, contrast is visualized within the aneurysm sac, usually at its periphery with retrograde opacification of the vessel responsible for the endoleak (Fig. 45.1). The location of the contrast suggests the vessel of origin: anterior opacification may be from the inferior mesenteric artery or a gonadal artery; posterior opacification may be from lumbar or median sacral arteries. Diagnostic angiograms typically demonstrate retrograde flow, filling the culprit vessel and opacifying the aneurysm sac (Fig. 45.4). The most common sources are collateral flow to the inferior mesenteric artery via an arc of Riolan (from the superior mesenteric artery), lumbar artery via the iliolumbar branch of the internal iliac artery, or the median sacral artery.

Endoleaks located around the stent graft and sparing the periphery of the sac on CTA/MRA may represent type III leaks. Angiography will demonstrate a leak through the graft material (Fig. 45.5). Abdominal CT, radiograph, or fluoroscopy can demonstrate separation of the modular components. Type IV and V leaks are diagnosis of exclusion. US, CT, and MRI all demonstrate sac size enlargement. In

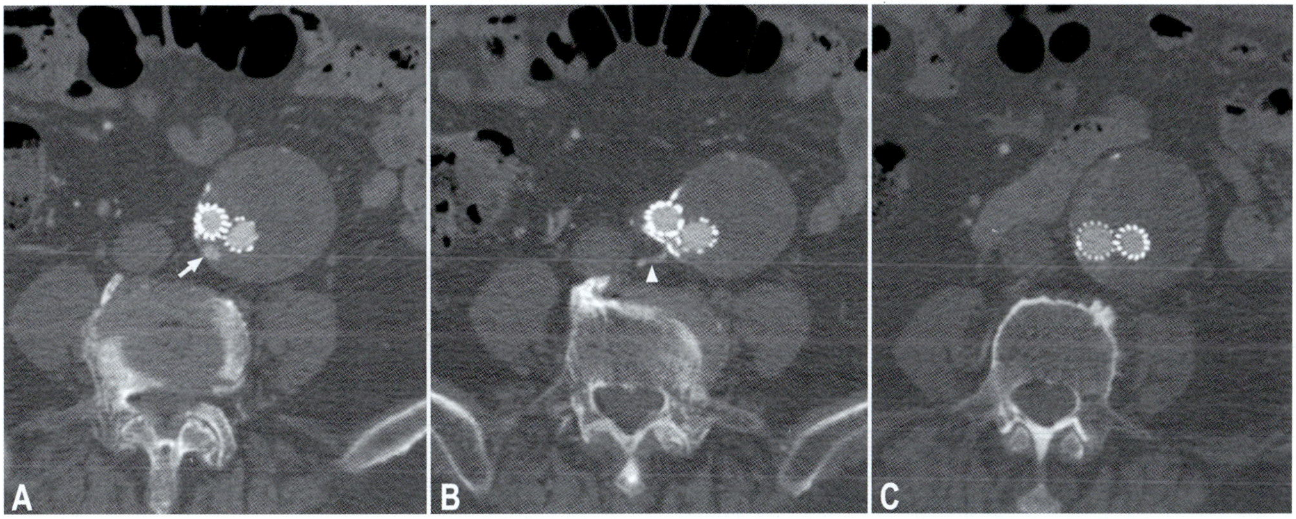

Figure 45.1 One month after EVAR. **A,B:** CT angiogram, arterial phase images demonstrate aneurysmal sac contrast blush (*arrow*) and its communication with the lumbar artery (*arrowhead*). **C:** Delayed image demonstrates continued opacification of the sac with contrast.

type IV, CTA or MRA will demonstrate contrast opacification of the aneurysm sac with no evident reason. In type V, there will be sac enlargement without contrast opacification of the sac on CTA or MRA. Diagnostic angiogram will confirm lack of a type I through III endoleak.

TREATMENT

Endoleaks can lead to continued growth in the aneurysm sac size and increase the risk of rupture. Type I and type III endoleaks should always be considered for repair soon after diagnosis. Type II endoleaks can be watched provided there is no growth in sac size and the patient is asymptomatic. Treatment options included endovascular repair and open surgical repair in the case of failed endovascular attempts. A type I

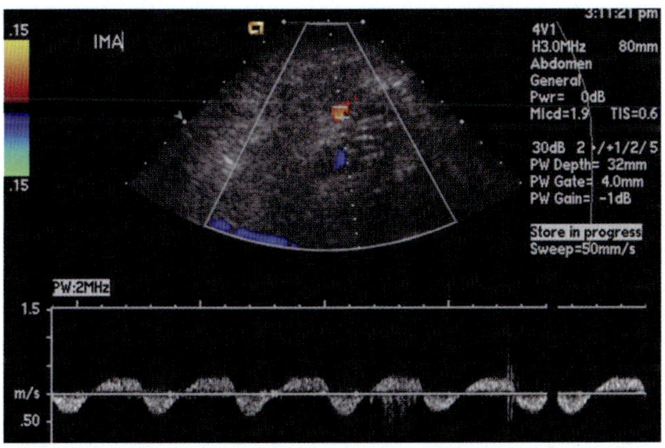

Figure 45.2 Doppler US of the inferior mesenteric artery demonstrates to-and-fro flow in the artery indicative of flow into the aneurysm sac.

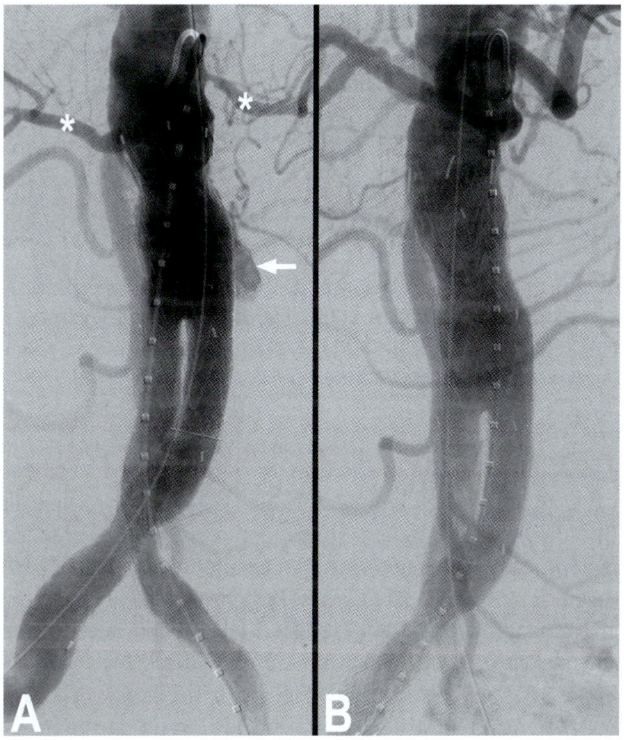

Figure 45.3 **A:** Angiographic images during stent graft placement for the repair of a 6.7-cm infrarenal aortic aneurysm. It demonstrates early sac opacification at the proximal seal zone consistent with a type I endoleak (*arrow*). The renal arteries are marked with an *asterisk*. **B:** Angiographic images postdeployment of an aortic cuff demonstrates resolution of the type I endoleak. Note that the cuff covers both renal arteries which was determined to be a reasonable strategy in this patient with chronic renal failure on dialysis.

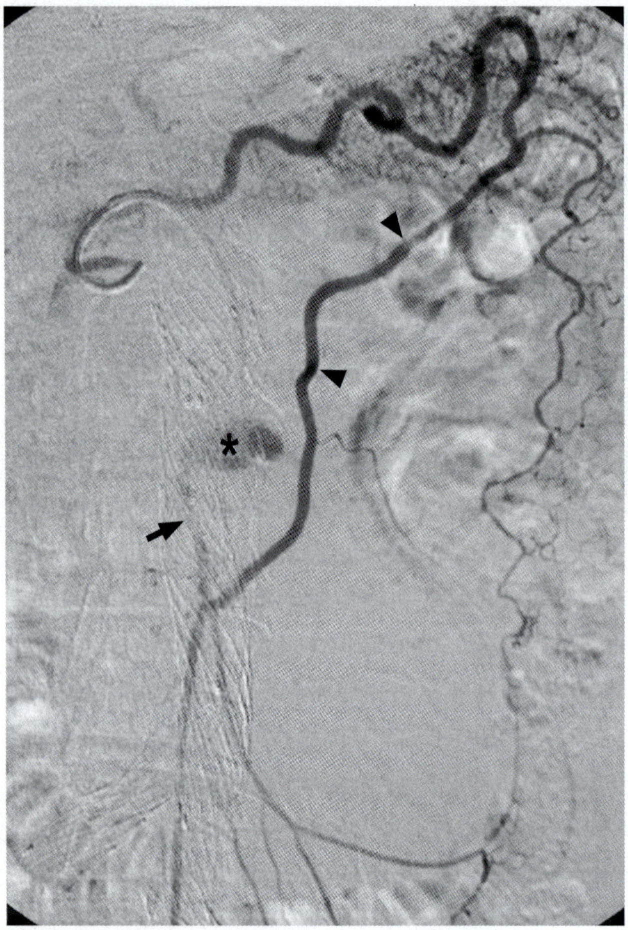

Figure 45.4 A 5-Fr diagnostic catheter in the SMA. Angiogram demonstrates retrograde opacification of the IMA (*arrow*) and the aneurysm sac (*asterisk*) via the arc of Riolan (*arrowheads*).

endoleak is repaired at the time of initial device placement using angioplasty balloon (e.g., Coda Balloon; Cook Medical, Inc., Bloomington, Indiana) to mold the existing stent graft for better fixation. If angioplasty fails, a balloon-expandable bare metal stent (Palmaz XL; Cordis, Bridgewater, New Jersey) or an overlapping stent graft (extension, cuff, or dedicated device such as the Zenith Renu from Cook Medical, Inc., Bloomington, Indiana) can be used (Fig. 45.3). The choice of a bare metal stent versus a stent graft depends largely on the proximity of visceral aortic branches such as the renal artery, superior mesenteric artery (SMA), or hypogastrics that may be occluded with a stent graft (Fig. 45.6). Endostaples (Aptus Endosystems, Inc., Sunnyvale, California) are available that can be used to approximate the endograft fabric to the wall of the aorta[9] (Fig. 45.7). To prevent a type I endoleak resulting from a hypogastric artery when the endograft must be extended into the external iliac artery, prophylactic embolization of the hypogastric artery should be performed either with coils or a vascular plug. With this approach, it is important to ensure

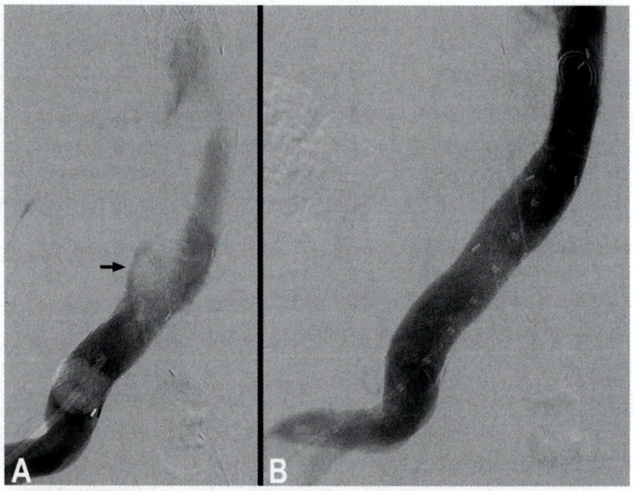

Figure 45.5 **A:** Occlusion balloon retrograde angiography of the right iliac limb of a bifurcated stent graft. Note that this is not the modular limb. This confirmed a type IIIB leak through the graft material (*arrow*), possibly due to angioplasty of the limb in an area of heavy calcification. **B:** Resolution of the type III endoleak post relining of the limb with an endograft.

that the contralateral internal iliac artery is patent to avoid pelvic and buttock ischemia. Similarly, type III and type V endoleaks are repaired by placing a stent graft across the region of device disruption (type III) or entire stent graft (type V).

Whether and when to repair a type II endoleak is an area of debate. Small type II endoleaks often thrombose spontaneously, particularly over time.[10] Hence, some interventionalists choose to follow these via imaging, whereas others will be more aggressive in repairing them as soon as they are diagnosed. Most interventionalists agree on treating type II leaks that are associated with an abdominal pain, increase in sac size, or with a large nonshrinking sac (>5.5 cm) to prevent rupture.

Type II endoleaks can be challenging to repair. The goal is to obliterate the patent lumen within the aneurysm sac as well as embolize the feeding vessels at their insertion from the aorta. Embolization of the feeding vessel without addressing the intra-aneurysmal component can lead to recruitment of other collateral vessels with continued flow to the sac. In essence, the aneurysm sac should be viewed like an arteriovenous malformation where it is of paramount importance to treat the nidus. Embolization can be achieved via a transarterial route, percutaneous translumbar or transcaval sac puncture, or perigraft access (see Fig. 45.6).[6] With a transarterial approach, a microcatheter is used to catheterize the culprit artery via the collateral feeding it (e.g., IMA via the arc of Riolan) and placed within the sac. The sac is embolized first followed by the feeding artery. In a direct sac puncture, an angiographic catheter is inserted in the supine position. Then, the patient is placed in a prone position to identify the optimal site for puncture. The sac is punctured

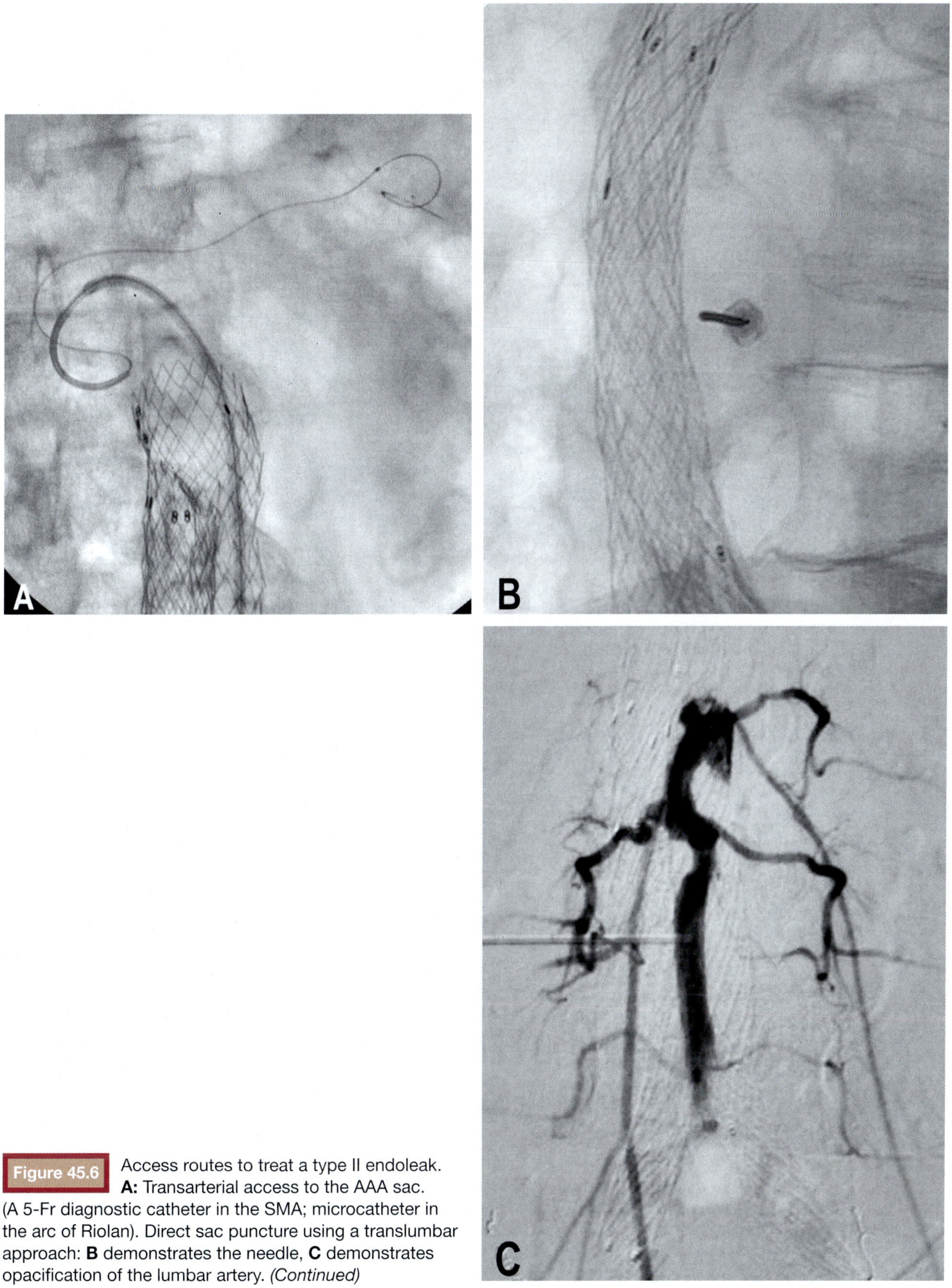

Figure 45.6 Access routes to treat a type II endoleak. **A:** Transarterial access to the AAA sac. (A 5-Fr diagnostic catheter in the SMA; microcatheter in the arc of Riolan). Direct sac puncture using a translumbar approach: **B** demonstrates the needle, **C** demonstrates opacification of the lumbar artery. *(Continued)*

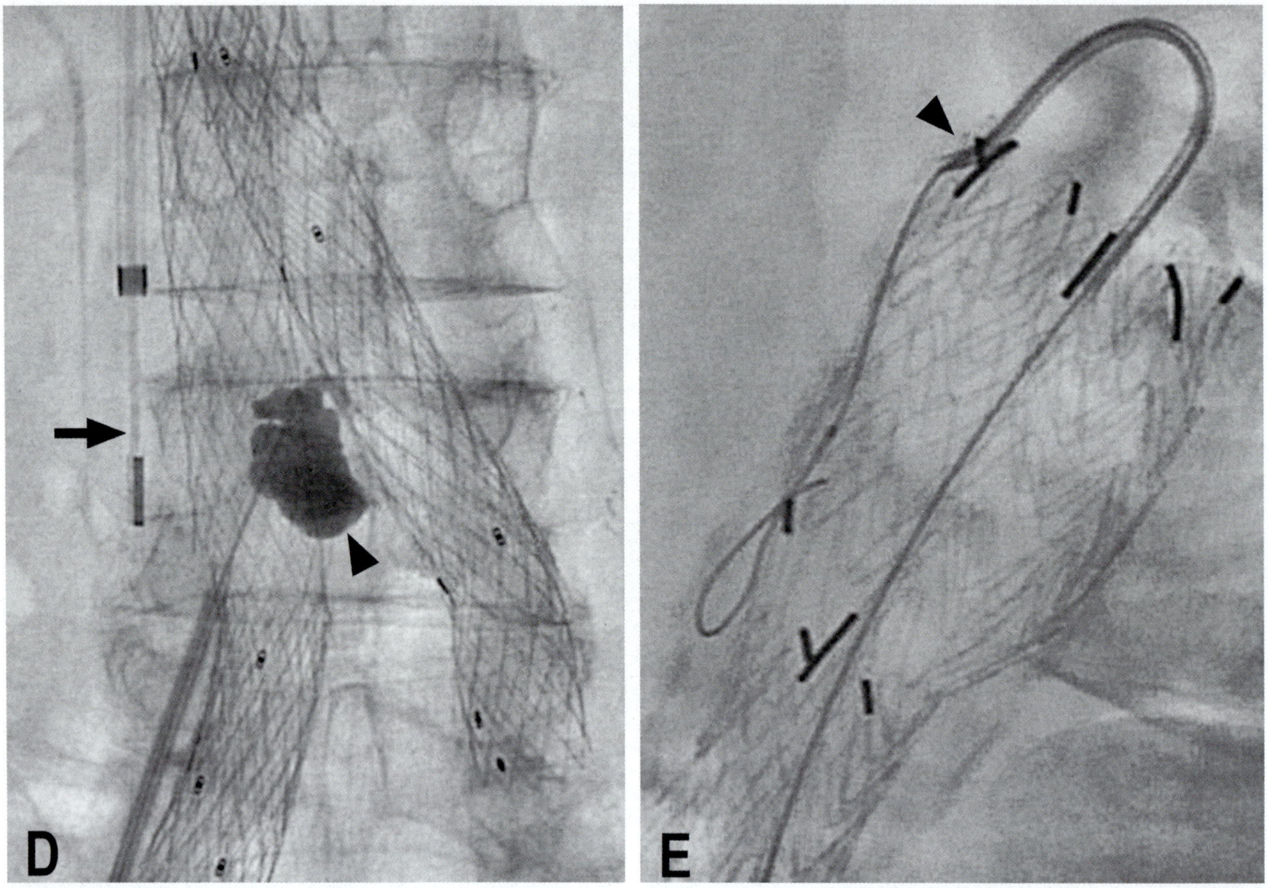

Figure 45.6 *(Continued)* **D:** Transcaval approach using intravascular ultrasound (IVUS) guidance (*arrow*). Liquid embolic agent, Onyx (Covidien, Irvine, California), is noted in the lumen of the aneurysm sac (*arrowhead*). **E:** Perigraft catheterization of the feeding vessel (*arrowhead*).

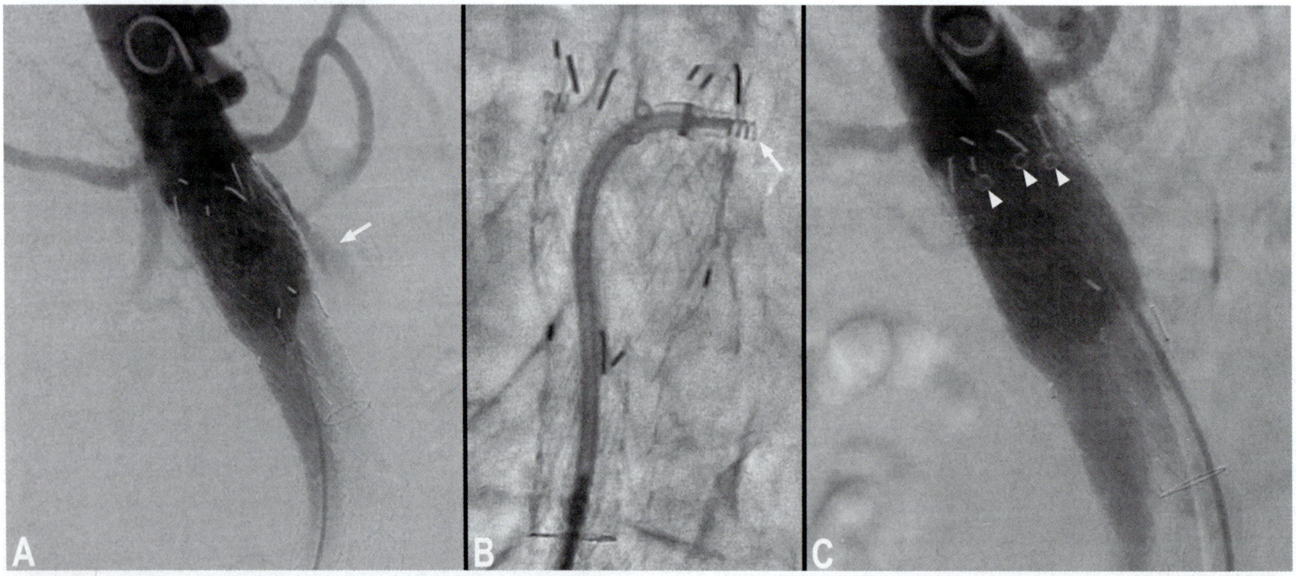

Figure 45.7 **A:** Angiographic images after stent graft placement for an infrarenal aortic aneurysm demonstrate early sac opacification at the proximal seal zone consistent with a type I endoleak (*arrow*). **B:** Fluoroscopic image demonstrates the Aptus deployment system (Aptus Endosystems, Inc., Sunnyvale, California) and the endograft. The EndoAnchor (staple) is marked with an *arrow*. **C:** Angiographic images postdeployment of the EndoAnchors demonstrate resolution of the type I endoleak. The EndoAnchors are marked with *arrowheads*.

under fluoroscopy or cone-beam CT guidance, usually via a left translumbar approach. Alternatively, the access site can be selected based on landmarks from the angiogram as well as diagnostic CT. A transcaval approach can also be used safely, usually with intravascular US guidance. Needle placement within the sac is confirmed by blood return and subsequent contrast injection, which will also demonstrate the feeding and draining vessels. The endoleak cavity and vessels can then be embolized using stainless steel or platinum coils or liquid embolics such as *N*-butyl cyanoacrylate (NBCA) (TruFill; Cordis Neurovascular, Miami Lakes, Florida) "glue" or Onyx (Covidien, Irvine, California) (Fig. 45.6D). Recent studies[11] have shown that the transarterial and translumbar approach are approximately equal and 70% to 75% effective in treating a type II endoleak.

Continued surveillance is recommended even after successful treatment of an endoleak as these can recur, particularly type I, due to sac remodeling and potential progression of the aneurysmal disease proximally and distally. In addition, continued sac expansion has been seen in the absence of an endoleak in patients who continue to smoke or are hyperlipidemic.[12]

PREVENTING ENDOLEAKS

Not all endoleaks can be prevented. However, appropriate patient selection and meticulous attention to planning before stent graft deployments can limit the incidence of endoleaks. Type I endoleaks can be avoided by selecting an appropriate seal zone. Manufacturers have different recommendations depending on the type of graft (e.g., minimum neck length). These instructions for use should be adhered to particularly when the operator has limited experience. Complete embolization of the internal iliac artery origin should be performed when extending the limbs into the external iliac artery. Some authors advocate pre-EVAR embolization of patent IMA[13,14] and lumbar arteries to prevent type II endoleaks. However, there is insufficient data to recommend this practice routinely pre-EVAR. Type III endoleaks can be prevented by ensuring adequate overlap between modular components. Endoleaks occurring due to fabric defects are materials' limitations that cannot be entirely prevented but are fortunately rare. However, aggressive angioplasty after deployment of the stent graft in a region of heavy calcification can lead to fabric disruption and a type III endoleak. Type IV endoleaks are device dependent and usually only seen during the EVAR procedure.

A new approach to endoleak prevention is the use of sac fillers (Nellix Endograft; Endologix, Irvine, California). This technology uses bags attached to the endograft that are filled with biostable polymer during placement of the stent graft. The polymer-filled bags are intended to fill the aneurysm sac, thereby eliminating types II, IV, and V endoleaks. This device is not approved for clinical use in the United States, although early results from international trials are promising.[15]

TIPS AND TRICKS

- Preoperative embolization to prevent a type II endoleak:
  - Coil embolization of accessory renal artery, prominent lumbar arteries,[13] and IMA
  - Coil or vascular plug embolization of ipsilateral internal iliac artery in case the stent graft landing zone is in the external iliac artery
- Stent graft: Careful sizing, adequate component overlap, and an AAA neck with good anatomy (correct patient selection) can help prevent an endoleak.
- Endoleak diagnosis: Performing selective angiograms of the superior mesenteric and internal iliac arteries will increase the chance of diagnosing an endoleak.
- Endoleak treatment: The AAA sac (endoleak cavity) must be seen as the nidus of an arteriovenous malformation when embolizing the source of a type II endoleak. The AAA sac and the feeding vessels must be adequately embolized.
- Never assume that there is only one type of an endoleak or that an endoleak will not recur.
- Repeat interventions are common, so long-term surveillance is needed.

CONCLUSION

Endoleaks remain an unsolved problem in the treatment of AAA with stent grafts. As endograft technology improves, more attention will shift to the prevention of endoleaks. The treatment of endoleaks begins with careful analysis of cross-sectional imaging and detailed angiography to appropriately characterize the endoleak and determine AAA size. A full range of endograft and embolization techniques are required to successfully treat endoleaks.

REFERENCES

1. Veith FJ, Baum RA, Ohki T, et al. Nature and significance of endoleaks and endotension: summary of opinions expressed at an international conference. *J Vasc Surg*. 2002;35(5):1029–1035.
2. van Marrewijk C, Buth J, Harris PL, et al. Significance of endoleaks after endovascular repair of abdominal aortic aneurysms: the EUROSTAR experience. *J Vasc Surg*. 2002;35(3):461–473.
3. Rafii BY, Abilez OJ, Benharash P, et al. Lateral movement of endografts within the aneurysm sac is an indicator of stent-graft instability. *J Endovasc Ther*. 2008;15(3):335–343.
4. Bashir MR, Ferral H, Jacobs C, et al. Endoleaks after endovascular abdominal aortic aneurysm repair: management strategies according to CT findings. *AJR Am J Roentgenol*. 2009;192(4):W178–W186.
5. Stavropoulos SW, Charagundla SR. Imaging techniques for detection and management of endoleaks after endovascular aortic aneurysm repair. *Radiology*. 2007;243(3):641–655.

6. Ayuso JR, de Caralt TM, Pages M, et al. MRA is useful as a follow-up technique after endovascular repair of aortic aneurysms with nitinol endoprostheses. *J Magn Reson Imaging*. 2004;20(5):803–810.
7. Raman KG, Missig-Carroll N, Richardson T, et al. Color-flow duplex ultrasound scan versus computed tomographic scan in the surveillance of endovascular aneurysm repair. *J Vasc Surg*. 2003;38(4):645–651.
8. Gilabert R, Bunesch L, Real MI, et al. Evaluation of abdominal aortic aneurysm after endovascular repair: prospective validation of contrast-enhanced US with a second-generation US contrast agent. *Radiology*. 2012;264(1):269–277.
9. Deaton DH, Mehta M, Kasirajan K, et al. The phase I multicenter trial (STAPLE-1) of the Aptus endovascular repair system: results at 6 months and 1 year. *J Vasc Surg*. 2009;49(4):851–857.
10. White SB, Stavropoulos SW. Management of endoleaks following endovascular aneurysm repair. *Semin Intervent Radiol*. 2009;26(1):33–38.
11. Stavropoulos SW, Park J, Fairman R, et al. Type 2 endoleak embolization comparison: translumbar embolization versus modified transarterial embolization. *J Vasc Interv Radiol*. 2009;20(10):1299–1302.
12. Sarac TP, Gibbons C, Vargas L, et al. Long-term follow-up of type II endoleak embolization reveals the need for close surveillance. *J Vasc Surg*. 2012;55(1):33–40.
13. Axelrod DJ, Lookstein RA, Guller J, et al. Inferior mesenteric artery embolization before endovascular aneurysm repair: technique and initial results. *J Vasc Interv Radiol*. 2004;15(11):1263–1267.
14. Marchiori A, von Ristow A, Guimaraes M, et al. Predictive factors for the development of type II endoleaks. *J Endovasc Ther*. 2011;18(3):299–305.
15. Krievins DK, Holden A, Savlovskis J, et al. EVAR using the Nellix sac-anchoring endoprosthesis: treatment of favourable and adverse anatomy. *Eur J Vasc Endovasc Surg*. 2011;42(1):38–46.

46

Splenic and Gastrointestinal Aneurysms

Daniel C. Brown • Constantino S. Peña • James F. Benenati

BACKGROUND

Visceral abdominal aneurysms (VAAs) are rare, accounting for less than 1% of all arterial aneurysms, but can be life threatening, with reports of morbidity and mortality ranging up to 100% in the setting of aneurysm rupture.[1,2] The treatment options vary depending on the vessels involved, aneurysm type (true aneurysm or pseudoaneurysm), etiology, and size.

The incidence of VAAs has been reported to be between 0.1% and 2% of the population, although autopsy studies have demonstrated much higher rates, up to 10%.[3–5] An increased incidence in visceral aneurysms in recent years likely corresponds to the detection of asymptomatic aneurysms seen on the simultaneously increased number of cross-sectional imaging (computed tomography [CT] and magnetic resonance imaging [MRI]) examinations obtained over this time. Additionally, the higher prevalence of interventional procedures in the treatment of various abdominal pathologies has led to a concomitant increase in the incidence of iatrogenic pseudoaneurysms.[1,3,4]

True aneurysms are defined as a vessel diameter expansion of at least 50% that involves all three vessel wall layers: the intima, media, and adventitia.[3] A pseudoaneurysm (or false aneurysm) fails to involve all three vessel layers but instead represents a form of vessel wall disruption allowing a plane of blood flow that is usually only contained by the adventitia[3] or surrounding tissues, explaining its higher mortality compared to true aneurysms. Pseudoaneurysms (PAs) are usually iatrogenic or related to trauma and inflammatory conditions such as pancreatitis.[6] Unfortunately, determining the type of aneurysm is not always possible from imaging characteristics alone, requiring a complete evaluation of the patient's history, physical, and other vascular anatomy. The splenic (60%) and hepatic (20%) arteries account for the largest distribution of visceral aneurysms followed by the superior mesenteric (5%) and celiac (4%) arteries[3,7] (Table 46.1). Interestingly, more than one visceral aneurysm is found in greater than a third of patients.

The possible etiologies of visceral aneurysms can be extensive (Table 46.2). However, attempting to determine their specific cause may be helpful in establishing the risk of rupture and developing successful treatment options. Degenerative and atherosclerotic aneurysms are commonly seen in the splenic, celiac, and superior mesenteric arteries. The presence of vessel wall calcifications usually suggests a stable, chronic process, whereas eccentric aneurysms without thrombus or calcification may be more concerning for rupture. In the setting of inflammatory or infectious processes, it may be best to ameliorate the process with systemic therapies before proceeding with nonemergent therapy.

As with other peripheral aneurysms, the strict use of a size criteria to guide the decision to treat is controversial and likely too simplistic. There are several factors that should determine the need for treatment. Several nonspecific guidelines have reported the use of a 2-cm threshold for the treatment of large vessel, asymptomatic visceral aneurysms such

Table 46.1 Incidence of Visceral Artery Aneurysms

Splenic artery	60%
Hepatic artery	20%
Right hepatic	16%
Left and middle hepatic	4%
Superior mesenteric artery (SMA)	5%
Celiac trunk	4%
Gastric arteries	4%
Gastroduodenal arteries	1.5%
SMA branches	3%
IMA branches	1%

IMA, inferior mesenteric artery.

as those associated with the hepatic and splenic arteries.[8,9] However, the decision to treat and how to do so should likely include many factors, including the patient's symptoms, aneurysm location and type, etiology, presence of calcification or thrombus, and particular visceral vessel hemodynamics. The potential treatment options will be based on these factors, and the possible complications from those various treatment options must also be considered. Generally speaking, PAs and symptomatic aneurysms should be treated regardless of their size. In contrast, over the last decade, most interventionalists have chosen to follow stable true visceral aneurysms that are less than 2.5 cm in diameter and lack concerning features, such as interval growth, which is considered a reason for treatment. It must be stated that the data on when to treat VAA is based on a limited experience primarily derived from single center and retrospective evaluations of ruptured aneurysms over the last three decades.

Table 46.2 Etiology of Visceral Artery Aneurysms

- Atherosclerosis
- Posttraumatic
- Iatrogenic
- High-flow states
  - Portal hypertension
  - Pregnancy
  - Vessel stenosis
- Fibromuscular dysplasia
- Cystic medial necrosis
- Vasculitis: polyarteritis nodosa
- Hereditary
  - Ehlers-Danlos syndrome
  - Marfan syndrome
- Idiopathic
- Pancreatitis
- Segmental arterial mediolysis
- Infectious/septic emboli

Treatment Options

Given the high morbidity and mortality observed with visceral aneurysm rupture, treatment to prevent rupture is paramount. Traditionally, surgical management was the primary treatment option, whereas endovascular options were initially only considered when patients were deemed too high risk for surgery. However, endovascular treatment offers a multitude of therapeutic options, with high technical success rates and minimal morbidity and mortality.[10–12] As a result, endovascular treatment is now the first option, with surgery typically reserved for instances of acute large vessel ruptures, rebleeding, or growth after intervention and aneurysms that are not amenable to primary or repeat endovascular therapy.

VAA treatment should begin with a careful assessment of the patient's history and physical examination to assess the etiology and chronicity of the aneurysm. The evaluation of cross-sectional imaging is also crucial for planning a successful treatment strategy. Computed tomography angiography (CTA) and magnetic resonance angiography (MRA) evaluation allows for the assessment of an aneurysm neck and the number and size of afferent and efferent vessels. The amount and extent of at-risk end organ tissue should also be evaluated. The presence of other visceral vessel stenosis and collateral pathways should be considered in deciding possible embolization techniques, locations, and agents. Additionally, thought and attention should be made to the endovascular access and treatment vessels to help determine potential treatment options, including puncture site location (femoral, upper extremity, direct puncture), sheath, catheter and microcatheter size, landing zone, coil or plug size, and delivery. Along with standard axial images, we also reformat CTA into thick (12×2 mm) maximum intensity projections (MIPs) in coronal and sagittal planes or used real time three-dimensional volume–rendered reconstructions to aid us in making these decisions before undertaking treatment.

Devices and Techniques

At an elementary level, VAA treatment involves prevention of subsequent aneurysm rupture by stopping blood flow to the aneurysmal or weakened portion of the artery. Treatment techniques attempt to prevent or minimize downstream or end organ effects by preserving collaterals or some form of end organ perfusion.[1] The use of embolization coils to block flow has been the primary treatment tool. Recent advances include retrievable and gel expanding coils that achieve great success in obstructing inflow and outflow vessels or in the filling of an aneurysm sac with coils. Additionally, metallic expandable plugs have been used to similarly block efferent and afferent vessels.[13] The use of liquid embolics (*N*-butyl cyanoacrylate [NBCA (glue)] and ethylene vinyl alcohol [Onyx; Covidien, Irvine, California]) to fill and mold to the size of the aneurysm sac has also been a useful technique in excluding flow to the aneurysm sac. However, although effective, these liquid embolics require delivery in an extremely controlled fashion.[14] In VAA, the collateral pathways can be a double-edged sword that may protect end organ flow but may also revascularize the aneurysm by providing collateral or backflow into the aneurysm from other vessels that were not initially evident. For this reason, careful evaluation of VAA hemodynamics must be performed. Additionally, these pathways may limit the use of particle embolics as the potential for end organ damage may be great.

The development of covered stents has allowed for the possibility of preventing vessel rupture by strengthening or reinforcing the weakened vessel segment but also allowing continued end organ flow. These devices allow for the traditional blood flow patterns to continue within the visceral vessels. Unfortunately, the size of the covered stent delivery systems relative to the treatment vessel size as well as vessel tortuosity have limited their application to proximal splenic and hepatic arteries. Additionally, the vessel diameter proximal and distal to the aneurysm must be relatively equivalent.[7] Stent-assisted coiling can also be performed to treat VAA. This is a technique that uses a bare metal stent by placing it across an aneurysm neck where it serves as a support or scaffold through which a catheter is then used to deploy coils into the aneurysm. The bare stent preserves distal flow while the coils are positioned through and around the stent into the aneurysm sac.

SPLENIC ARTERY ANEURYSMS

Splenic artery aneurysms (SAAs) are the most common true visceral artery aneurysm. They are most often saccular and located in the mid to distal splenic artery. The etiology of true SAA is varied including atherosclerosis, high-flow states such as pregnancy and portal hypertension, and liver transplantation.[4,15,16] Traditionally, the splenic artery represents the single inflow and the single outflow vessel. This allows for coil embolization of the outflow segment first, followed by the inflow segment, a technique known as the *sandwich technique*, the *isolation technique*, or the *coil-trapping* technique. This may or may not also involve coil packing of the aneurysm sac itself (Fig. 46.1). This technique can also be performed with vascular plugs. The potential for collateral flow back to the SAA should be excluded by occluding both the inflow and outflow vessels adjacent to the aneurysm.

The rich small gastric and gastroepiploic collaterals usually protect the spleen from infarction. However, the possibility of covering the SAA with a covered stent is another potential treatment option[2] that would preserve flow through the splenic artery (Fig. 46.2). As previously mentioned, the size of the splenic vessel and its tortuosity may limit this treatment. SAA with relatively small or narrow necks projecting from the splenic artery can be coiled primarily (Fig. 46.3) to maximize distal flow. In wide-necked aneurysms, bare metal stent–assisted aneurysm coiling may be employed; however, it is rarely used in the splenic artery as there is usually rich collateral blood flow.

Splenic artery PAs are rare and often associated with pancreatitis or trauma.[6] Intraparenchymal splenic artery PAs are often observed in the setting of blunt abdominal trauma. The injury to the spleen in these instances often includes parenchymal laceration in addition to PA formation. There is some variability in the techniques used to treat these types of splenic injuries. Distal arterial embolization with or without adjunctive proximal splenic artery embolization[17,18] has been described, whereas others have advocated that proximal splenic artery embolization may be an appropriate standalone option in hemodynamically stable patients, depending on severity of splenic injury.[19]

As with all embolization, consideration must be made to the possibility of collateral blood flow back into the PA as well as end organ perfusion when embolizing the splenic artery. Distal splenic artery coil embolization will result in focal parenchymal ischemia and/or infarction. In contrast, a small series demonstrated only a modest splenic artery pressure decrease after proximal balloon occlusion.[20] This is likely due to the vast collateral network present resulting in perfusion to the splenic hilum via short gastric and gastroepiploic arteries as well as superior mesenteric artery filling of the dorsal pancreatic, pancreatica magna, transverse pancreatic, and pancreaticoduodenal arteries.[21] In the setting of bleeding splenic PA, however, care must be taken to completely embolize the source of bleeding by excluding antegrade, retrograde, and collateral pathways (Fig. 46.4).

HEPATIC ARTERY ANEURYSMS

Hepatic artery aneurysms (HAAs) are the second most common type of VAA. Most occur in the extraparenchymal hepatic artery segment and are degenerative in nature, whereas intrahepatic aneurysms are mostly false aneurysms. Over the last two decades, there has been a rise in iatrogenic PA involving the hepatic arteries, gastroduodenal artery, and the vessels of the pancreaticoduodenal arcades, which are derived from the growth of percutaneous and surgical procedures in this area.[3,10]

The dual blood supply to the liver from the hepatic artery and the portal vein allows for aggressive treatment of HAA. However, the patency of the portal vein and its particular branches should be assessed before undergoing embolization of the hepatic artery. During treatment, the presence of transhepatic as well as extrahepatic collaterals should be considered. Treatment of these aneurysms typically includes the embolization of the outflow and inflow arteries (Fig. 46.5). Loss of distal perfusion is usually well tolerated because of portal venous flow, especially in patients who are free of underlying liver disease. Even with a dual blood supply to the liver, proximal HAA can be challenging to treat due to the amount of hepatic tissue placed at risk with complete arterial occlusion (Fig. 46.6).

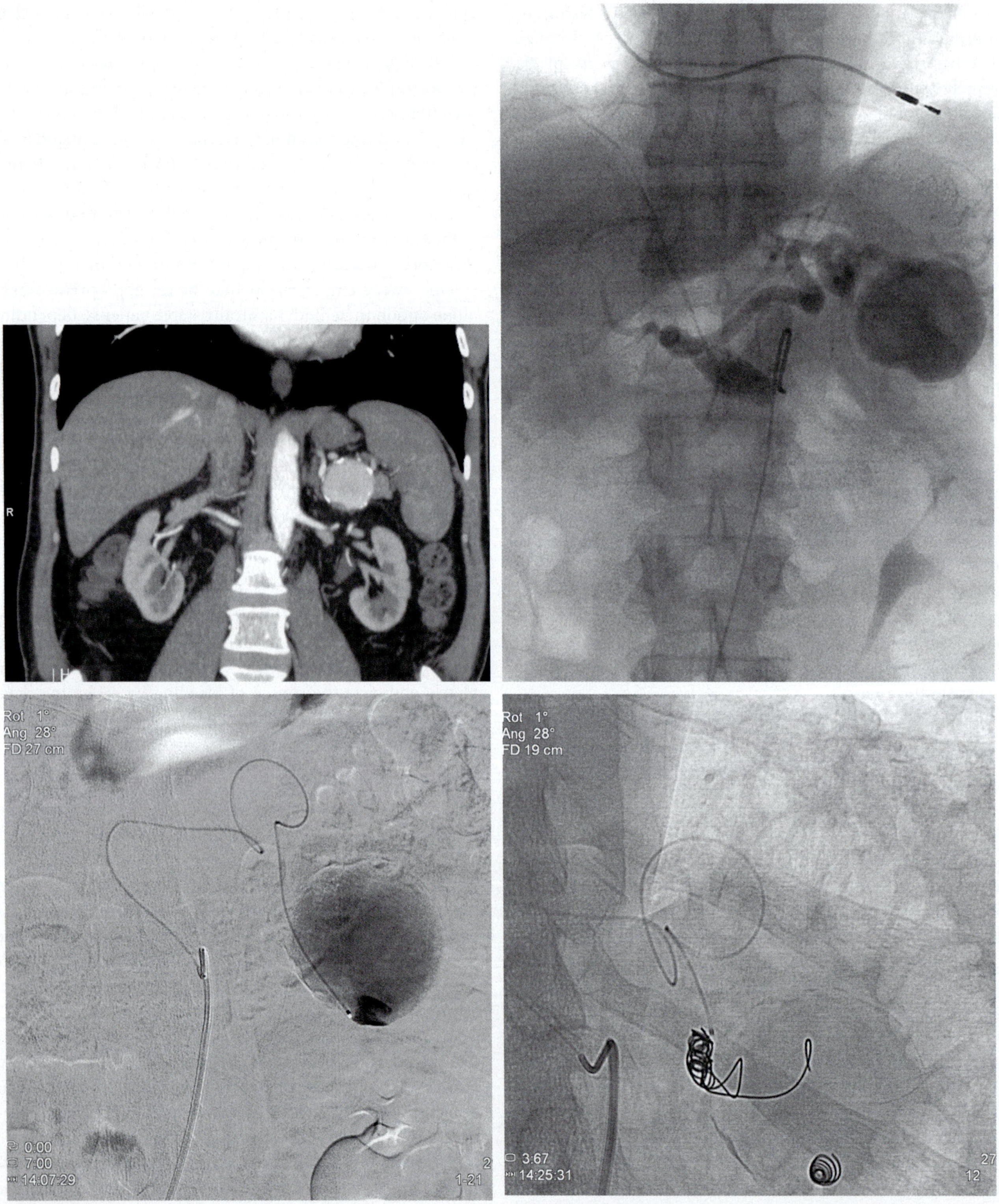

A B C D

Figure 46.1 SAA treated with a "sandwich" technique. A 56-year-old man with incidentally discovered 4.5-cm SAA. Coronal CTA image **(A)** demonstrates the aneurysm, while the preintervention angiogram **(B)** depicts the tortuosity of the splenic artery leading to the aneurysm. Given this tortuosity, a triaxial technique was employed to reach the aneurysm **(C)** using a 6-Fr left internal mammary artery (LIMA) guide catheter through which a 4-Fr Simmons 1 (Cook Medical Inc., Bloomington, Indiana) catheter was advanced into the proximal splenic artery and a microcatheter ultimately advanced to the aneurysm. Coil embolization across the proximal and distal neck of the aneurysm was achieved **(D)**. *(Continued)*

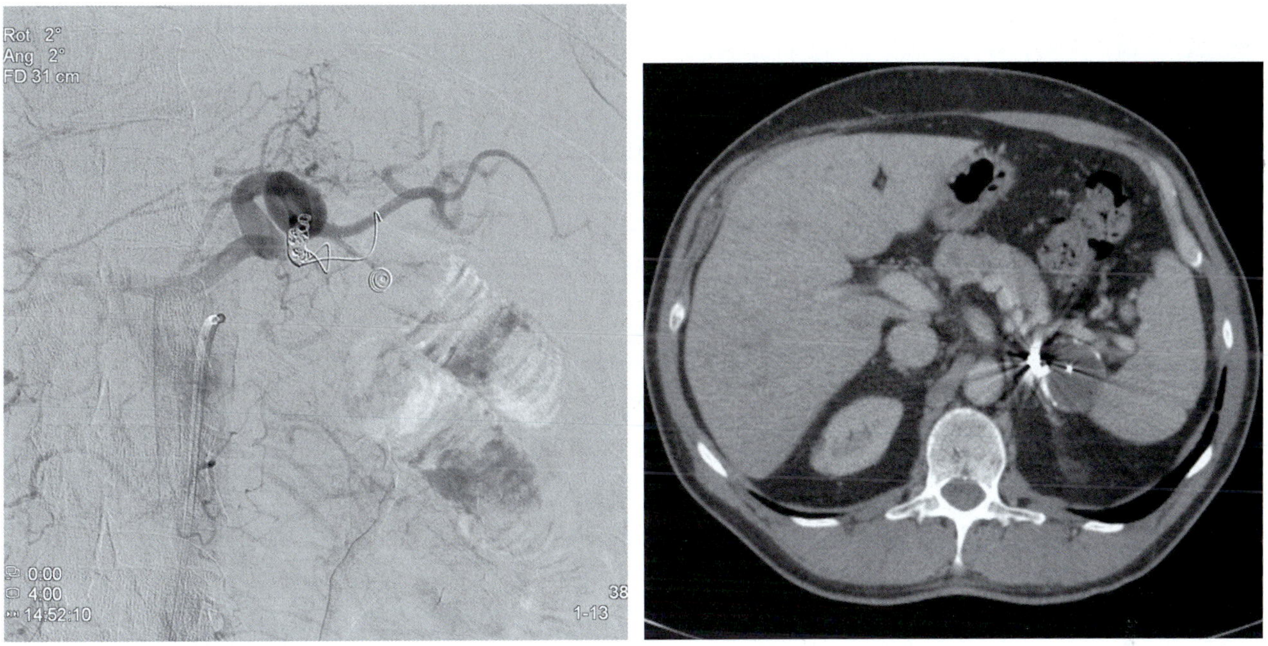

E F

Figure 46.1 *(Continued)* Completion angiogram confirms cessation of flow within the sac **(E)**. Follow-up CTA 3 months after embolization confirms lack of flow within the SAA sac **(F)**.

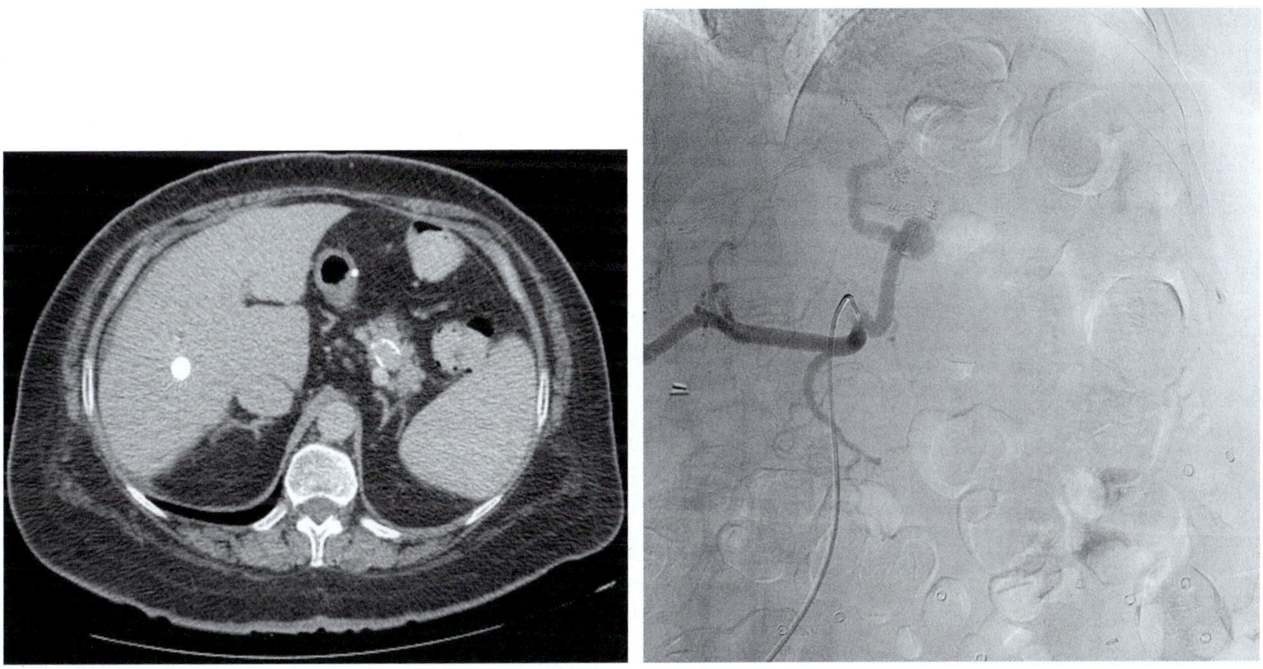

A B

Figure 46.2 SAA treated with a covered stent. A 58-year-old female with history of cirrhosis and prior transjugular intrahepatic portosystemic shunt (TIPS) procedure was found to have partially calcified approximately 2-cm SAA. The partially calcified SAA is seen, along with partially imaged TIPS on the axial **(A)** CT images acquired in the delayed phase. Celiac artery angiogram before intervention depicts the SAA **(B)**. *(Continued)*

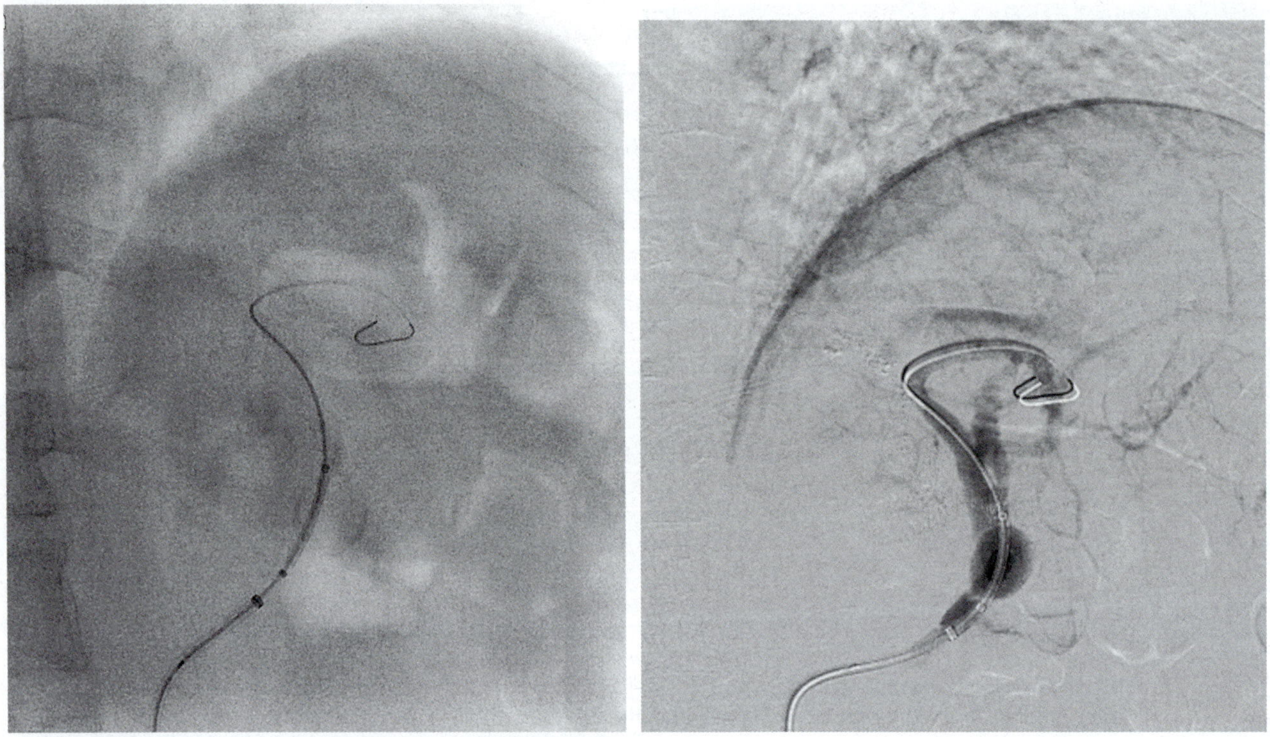

C

D

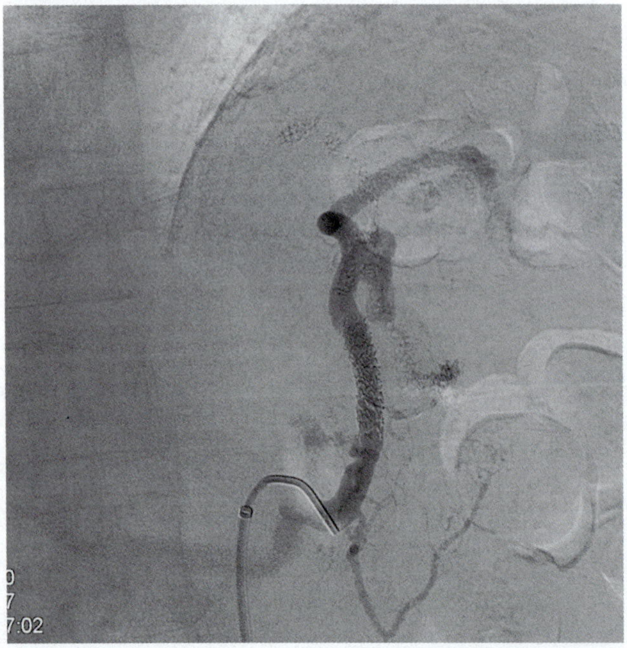

E

Figure 46.2 *(Continued)* A 6-Fr Shuttle sheath (Cook Medical Inc., Bloomington, Indiana) was advanced into the splenic artery and a 6- × 22-mm balloon-expanding covered stent was positioned across the neck of the aneurysm **(C)**. Once appropriate positioning was confirmed with angiogram **(D)**, the stent was deployed. Completion angiogram demonstrates successful exclusion of the aneurysm **(E)**.

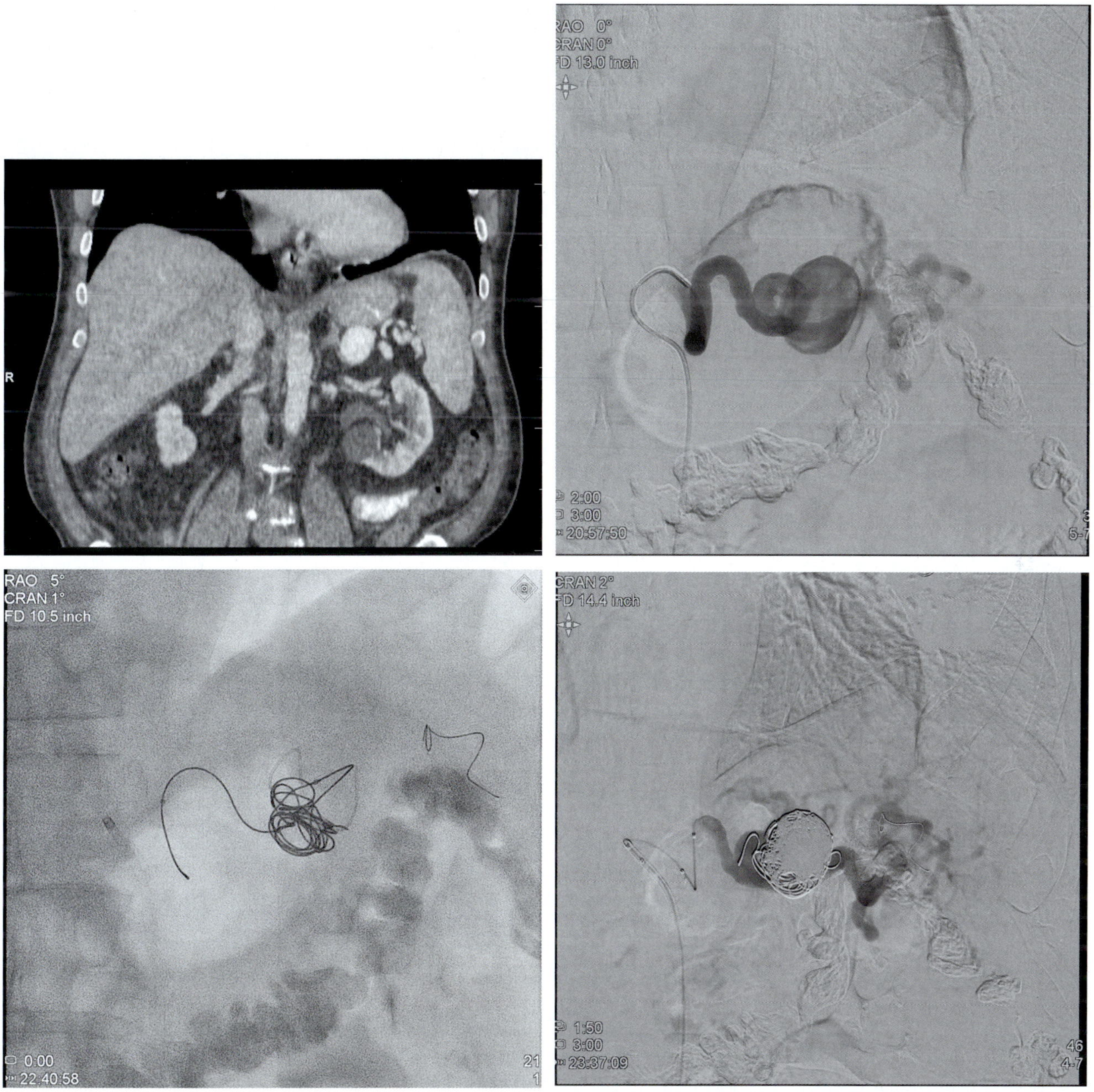

A B C D

Figure 46.3 Coil exclusion of an SAA sac. A 65-year-old male with an incidentally discovered 3.5-cm SAA. **A:** Coronal CTA reformation highlights superior to inferior extent of the splenic artery aneurysm. **B:** The preintervention angiogram emphasizes the proximal splenic artery tortuosity. Intraprocedural image demonstrates the treatment technique of a 6-Fr long sheath in the proximal splenic artery **(C)** with a 5-Fr Cobra 2 (Cook Medical, Inc., Bloomington, Indiana) catheter in the proximal splenic artery and a coaxial microcatheter. A half-deployed Nester coil (Cook Medical, Inc., Bloomington, Indiana) is seen within the micro catheter. **D:** The final angiogram confirms coils within the aneurysm sac with a patent distal splenic artery and no flow within the aneurysm sac.

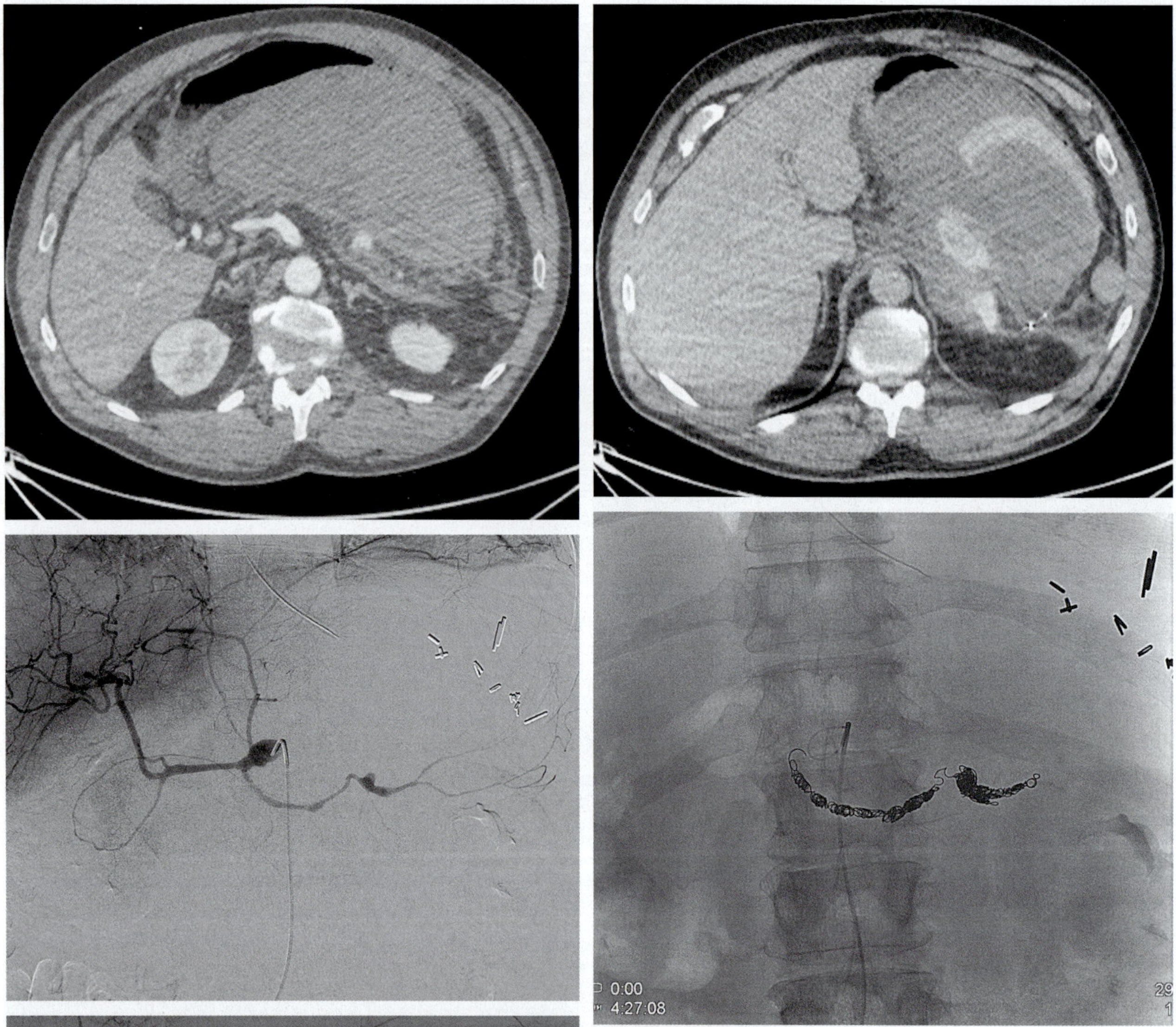

A B C D

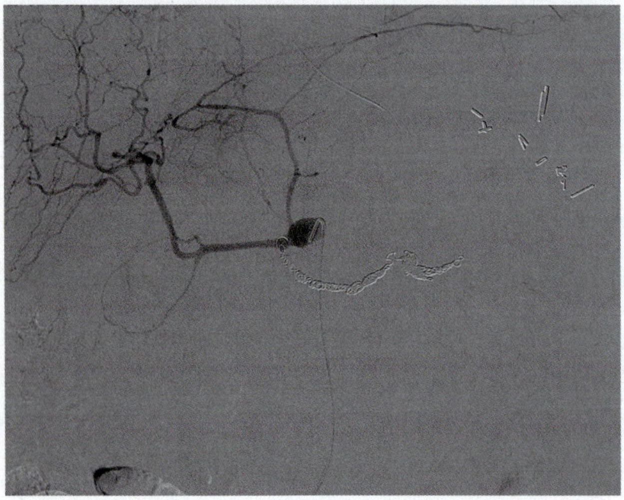

E

Figure 46.4 Treatment of a ruptured splenic artery stump PA. A 60-year-old male with history of splenectomy 10 years ago subsequent to a traumatic event presented with nontraumatic acute-onset left upper quadrant pain. He underwent CTA, which demonstrates a large intraperitoneal hematoma with arterial blush on the axial arterial phase **(A)**. There is marked expansion of the contrast extravasation seen on the subsequent axial portal venous phase **(B)**. Angiogram depicts irregularity of the entire length of the remnant splenic artery as well as midartery focal ectasia likely representing the PA **(C)**. Using a 5-Fr Cobra 2 as a base catheter, coaxial microcatheter technique was used to deliver Nester microcoils from the distal to proximal remnant splenic artery **(D)**. Completion angiogram demonstrates occlusion of flow through the remnant splenic artery **(E)**.

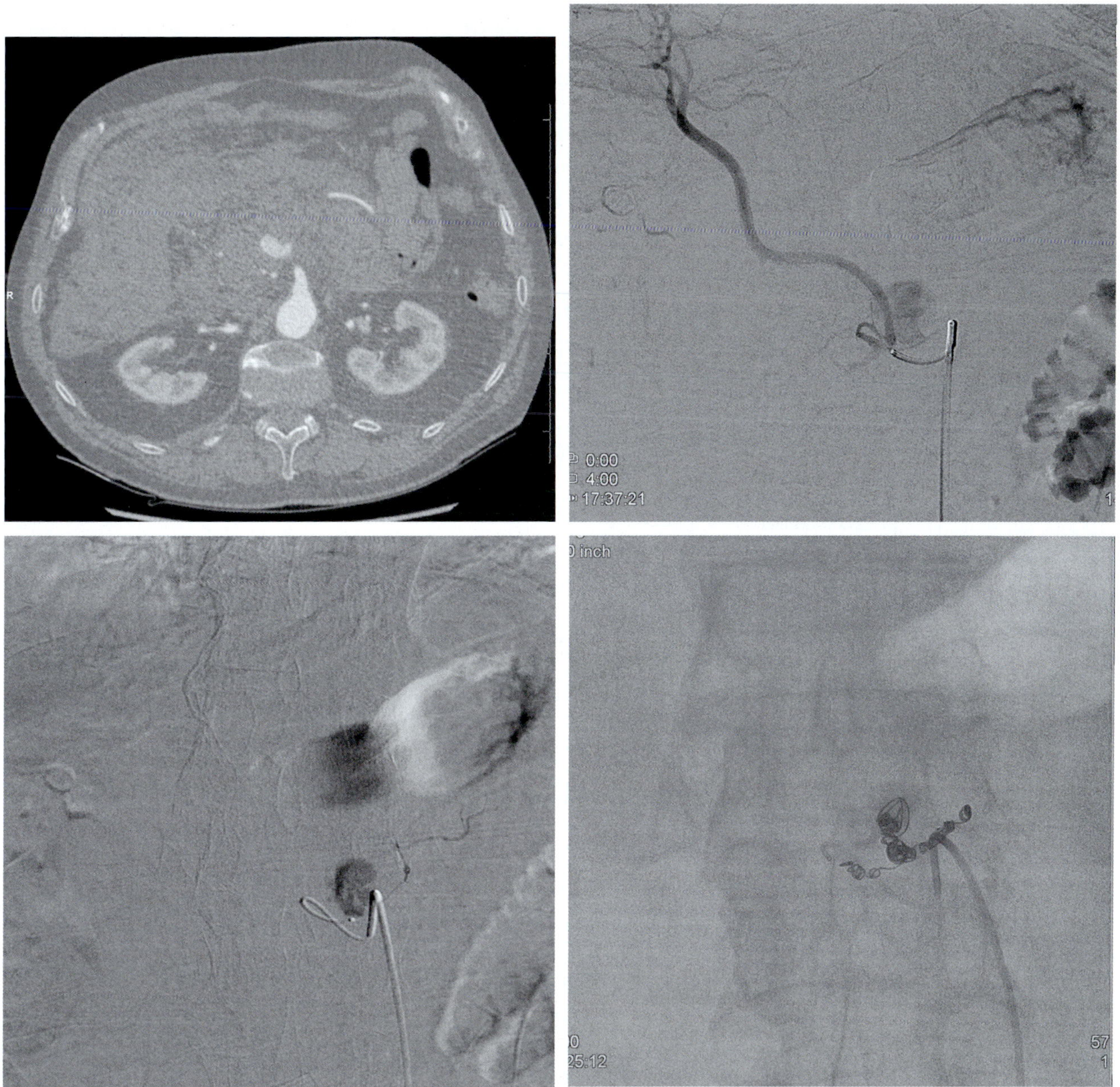

A B C D

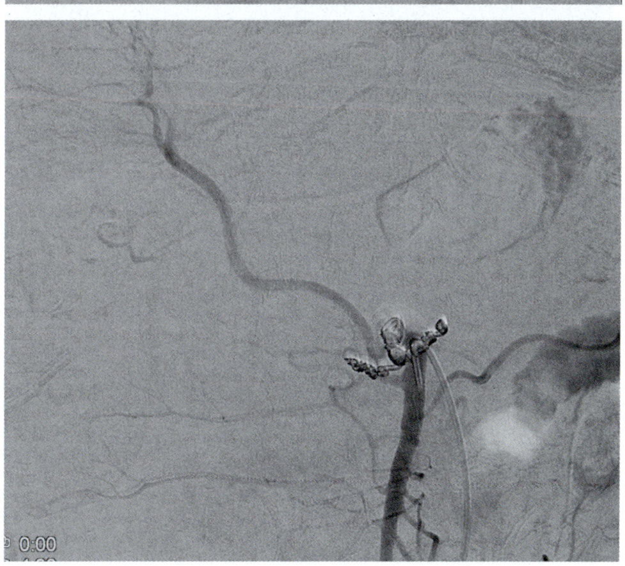

E

Figure 46.5 Aneurysm from a replaced right hepatic artery from the SMA. The patient is an 87-year-old male brought to the emergency department after he was found to be hypotensive subsequent to a witnessed syncopal episode. Axial CTA image depicts a ruptured 2-cm aneurysm arising from the proximal aspect of a replaced right hepatic artery arising from the superior mesenteric artery **(A)**. Angiogram depicts the extravasating aneurysm selected with the use of 5-Fr Cobra 2 catheter and coaxial microcatheter **(B,C)**. Coil embolization from distal to proximal across the site of active extravasation was achieved **(D)**. Completion angiogram **(E)** shows no residual active extravasation with preservation of flow within the replaced right hepatic artery and pancreaticoduodenal arcade.

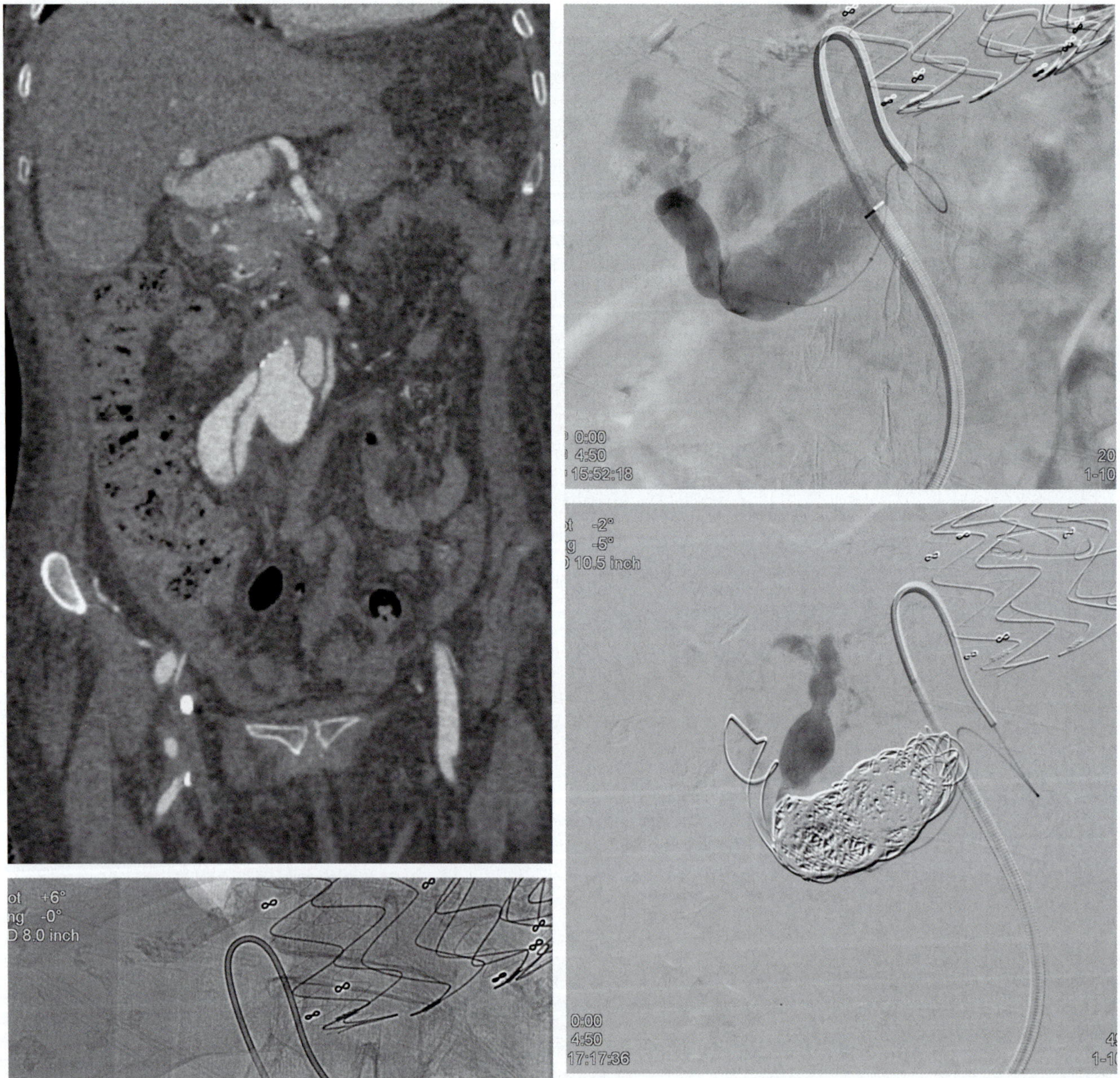

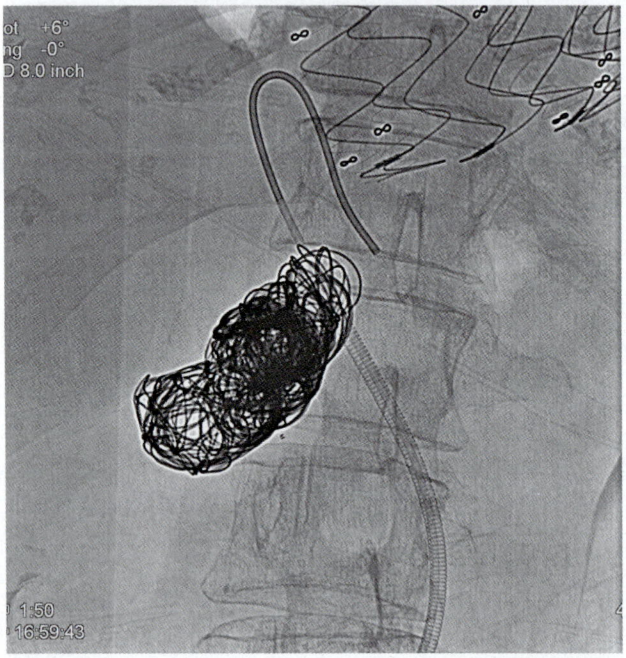

Figure 46.6 Proper hepatic artery aneurysm. The patient is a 72-year-old female with numerous visceral aneurysms as well as a history of repaired type A aortic dissection. Coronal CTA image depicts multiple proper HAAs including a large fusiform proper HAA measuring 4.7 × 2.4 cm **(A)**. Preintervention angiogram demonstrates the hepatic aneurysm **(B)**. With a supporting 6-Fr sheath, a Simmons 2 catheter was positioned in the celiac trunk and coil embolization of the aneurysm was performed via a coaxially placed microcatheter and multiple detachable coils **(C)**. Completion angiogram demonstrates exclusion of the HAA **(D)**.

SUPERIOR MESENTERIC ARTERY ANEURYSMS

In contrast to other VAA, superior mesenteric artery (SMA) aneurysms are usually symptomatic, presenting with abdominal pain.[22] The proximal SMA is more commonly associated with aneurysm formation. These are usually degenerative or atherosclerotic true aneurysms, whereas PAs occur mostly commonly from infectious (septic emboli), inflammatory, and hereditary causes.[22] Because of the number of essential vessels supplying the small bowel and right colon, treatment of these aneurysms can be difficult as maximal distal blood flow preservation is the goal. Unfortunately, these aneurysms have a high risk for rupture as well as a risk of distal embolization.[23] Treatment options include surgical ligation with distal revascularization or transcatheter embolization, usually using a covered stent or a bare stent to trap the coils within the aneurysm (stent-assisted coiling). Liquid embolics have been used, but the delicate distal bed favors larger, more controlled devices. There have been recent publications and accounts of using multilayered stents in this region to maintain distal flow while diverting flow away from the aneurysms.[21] This technology does not yet carry an "on label" indication in the United States.

CELIAC ARTERY ANEURYSMS

The short and angled nature of the celiac artery with its usual three main branches makes treatment of celiac artery aneurysms (CAAs) difficult. CAAs are usually of atherosclerotic etiology; however, infectious, traumatic, and inflammatory conditions such as polyarteritis nodosa, fibromuscular dysplasia, and Behcet disease also occur. CAAs are relatively rare, but the mortality from rupture has been reported at nearly 100%. These aneurysms are usually long saccular aneurysms that involve two or more of the distal celiac vessels. Traditional surgical treatment for these aneurysms has been resection or ligation with distal revascularization. In patients who are high risk for surgery, transcatheter embolization of the branches and the aneurysms can be considered as a treatment option. The development of collateral pathways between the SMA and celiac may favor stepwise occlusion to strengthen these collateral pathways and minimize distal bed ischemia. Additionally, the liver (dual blood supply), spleen, and stomach are protected by their rich collateral pathway; however, the distal extent of the aneurysms that need to be occluded to prevent retrograde perfusion of the aneurysm may be distal to these collateral pathways[24] (Fig. 46.7).

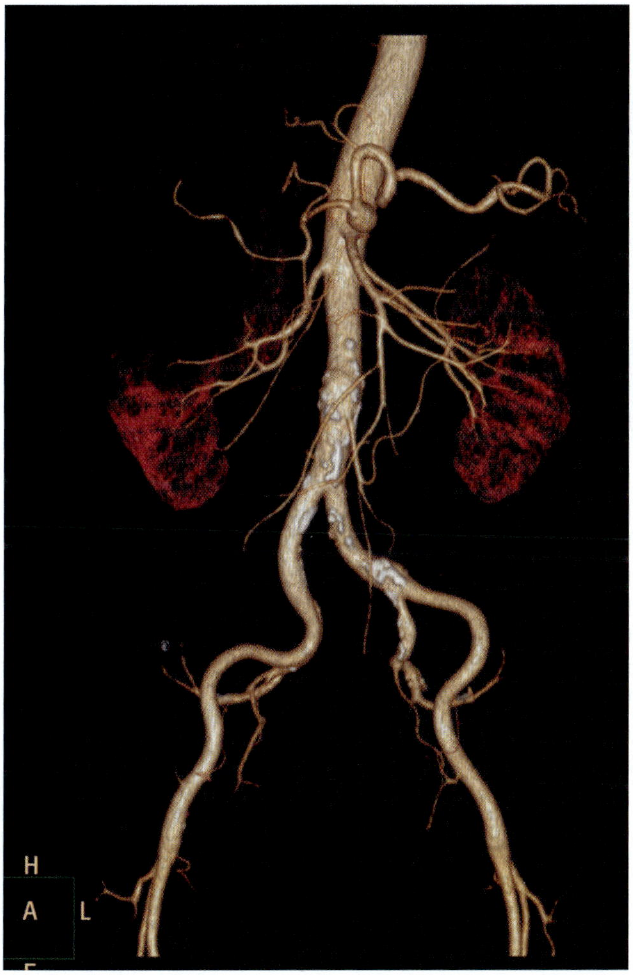

A

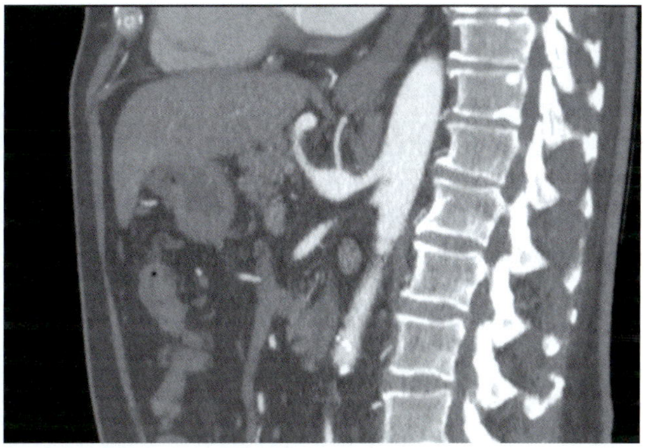

B

Figure 46.7 Celiac artery aneurysm. CTA demonstrates a CAA on volume-rendered images **(A)** and on sagittal reconstructions **(B)**, highlighting the difficulty of treating these lesions because of the involvement of several vessels and the short and acute access from the aorta. *(Continued)*

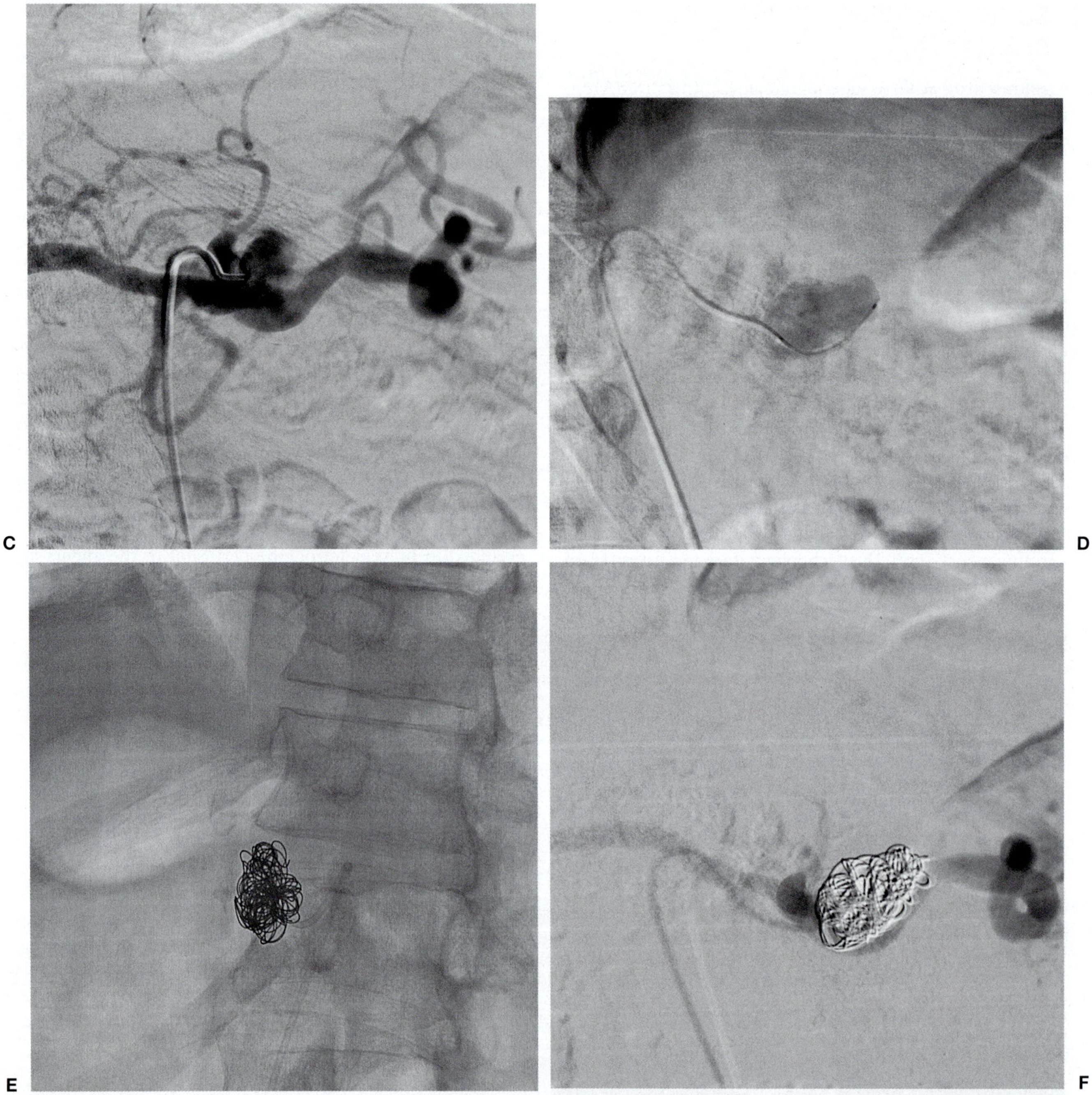

Figure 46.7 *(Continued)* In a different patient, celiac angiogram demonstrates a proximal CAA **(C)**. The aneurysm was selected using coaxial technique with a 5-Fr Simmons 2 diagnostic catheter and a microcatheter **(D)**. Effective treatment was accomplished with coil embolization **(E)**. Completion angiogram demonstrates nonfilling of the aneurysm with persistent flow into the common hepatic and splenic arteries **(F)**.

GASTRODUODENAL AND PANCREATICODUODENAL ARTERY ANEURYSMS

Aneurysms and PAs in this region are commonly related to prior procedures and pancreatitis. They usually present with bleeding and associated pain. The deep location of these small structures is usually seen in the setting of large hematomas, and pancreatitis-related collections makes transcatheter localization and embolization favorable. The rich collateral supply of the pancreaticoduodenal arcade makes these aneurysms difficult to treat without completely isolating the area of bleeding and carefully assessing for possible collateral flow (Fig. 46.8).

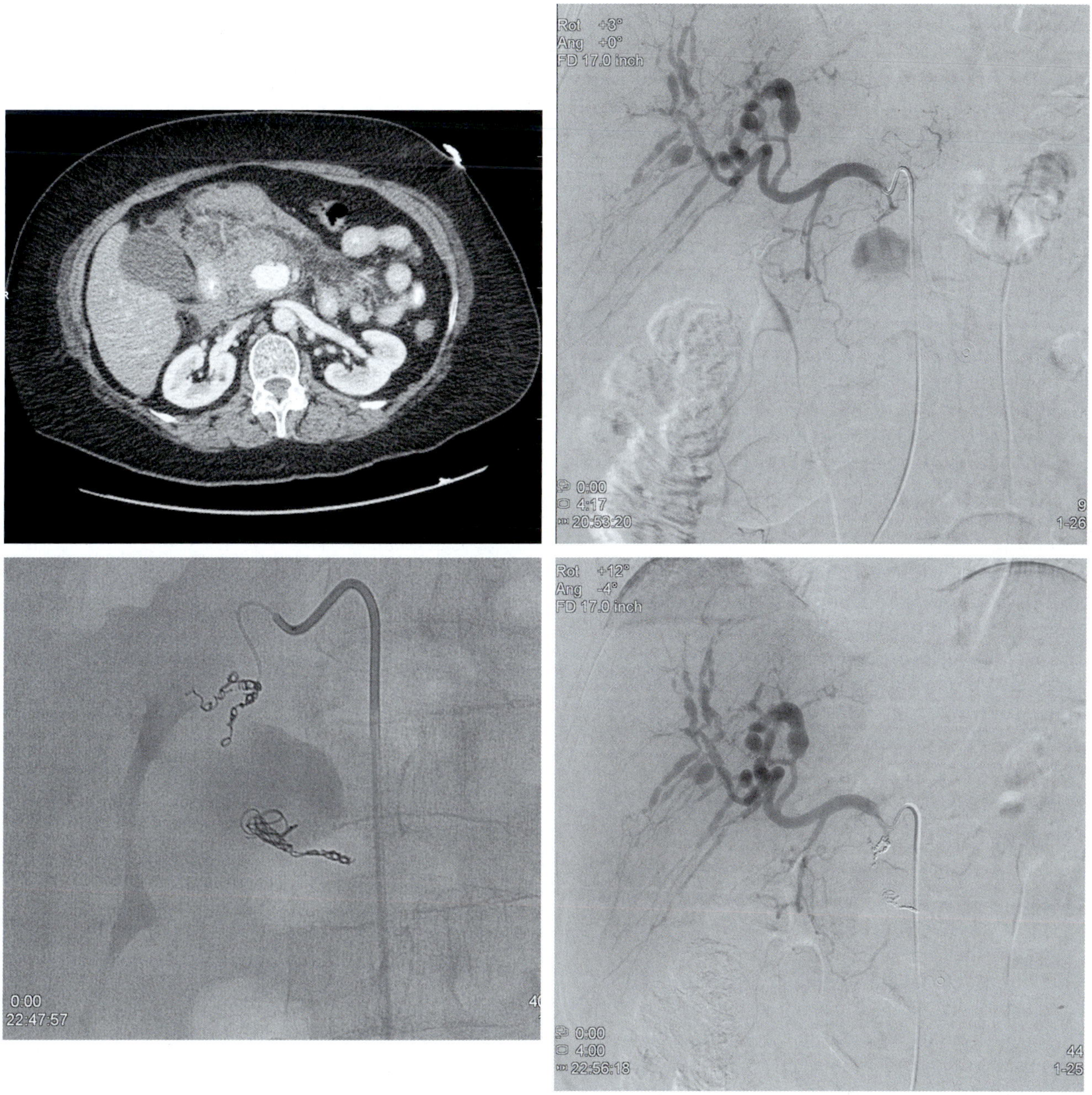

Figure 46.8 Pancreaticoduodenal arcade pseudoaneurysm. A 69-year-old female presents with acute abdominal pain. Axial CTA image depicts a 3-cm PA with significant surrounding hematoma **(A)**. Angiogram after selection of the common hepatic artery with a 5-Fr Sos 1 (Cook Medical Inc., Bloomington, Indiana) catheter demonstrates the PA as well as multifocal saccular aneurysms of the intrahepatic arteries secondary to an underlying vasculitis **(B)**. Using a coaxial microcatheter, the aneurysm was embolized by deploying coils into three separate branches identified supplying the PA **(C)**. Completion angiogram demonstrates no further opacification of the PA **(D)**.

FOLLOW-UP OF TREATED ANEURYSMS

The need for evaluation after treatment and continued follow-up is controversial. Usually, an initial follow-up is performed to document exclusion of the aneurysm sac. Unfortunately, the follow-up of treated VAA can be difficult because of the artifact created by coils as well as other agents. The final angiogram at the time of embolization is important to document sac exclusion as well as collateral flow. Doppler ultrasound and CTA may be limited in many patients, but it may help identify flow within the aneurysm and continued aneurysm growth prompting repeat treatment. Recently, the use of MRI in patients who have undergone treatment with platinum-based coils has been explored. The post gadolinium images have been helpful at identifying residual flow within the treated aneurysm sac.[25] The need for follow-up is necessary because of the risk for coil compaction and recanalization that may allow flow back into the visceral aneurysm sac. A single-site study of over 45 true VAA with a mean follow-up of 37 months found coil compaction and recanalization in almost 30% of patients. Larger aneurysms (>2 cm) typically had less coil density after their treatment; both factors were associated with an increased risk of recanalization of flow when compared to smaller VAA and those with a higher coil density.[26] Recurrent or persistent VAA flow may also occur from collateral vessels and partial thrombosis.

There is no accepted or mandated posttreatment imaging follow-up protocol; however, it can be performed at 3 months, 12 months, and annually thereafter. The need for an earlier imaging follow-up may be adapted especially when treating a PA or if occlusion was not clear on the final treatment angiogram.[3]

TIPS AND TRICKS

General

- When possible, optimize imaging to visualize aneurysm neck and inflow and outflow vessels. This may include both preintervention cross-sectional and angiographic imaging.
- Consider collateral circulation before beginning embolization. In many cases, it will be easier to cross aneurysm and treat distal and proximal.
- Ensure embolization catheter is well seated before attempting to deploy coils to ensure the coils do not back up and/or migrate to nontarget sites.
- Guide catheters can provide additional stability and more secure access for microcatheters in tortuous vessels or otherwise tenuous positions.

Techniques/Devices

- Large, detachable framing coils can shorten procedure time when coil embolizing an aneurysm sac.
- Use of vascular plugs can also shorten procedure time when embolizing an inflow and/or outflow vessel.
- Liquid embolics can be an excellent alternative to coils in select cases.
- Preserve distal flow to an end organ by using stent-assisted coiling. A bare metal stent is placed across an aneurysm neck where it serves as a support or scaffold through which a catheter is then used to deploy coils into the aneurysm.
- When preservation of distal flow is not as vital or not possible, the "sandwich" technique can be employed where coils are first placed in the distal vessel and then in then proximally, often across the PA neck to ensure no retrograde or collateral flow is maintained to the PA.
- When the anatomy allows, covered-stent placement across the aneurysm neck can provide a quick, durable treatment option.

REFERENCES

1. Etezadi V, Gandhi R, Benenati J, et al. Endovascular treatment of visceral and renal artery aneurysms. *J Vasc Interv.* 2011;22:1246–1253.
2. Rossi M, Rebonato A, Greco L, et al. Endovascular exclusion of visceral artery aneurysms with stent grafts: technique and long-term follow-up. *Cardiovasc Intervent Radiol.* 2008;31:36–42.
3. Spiliopoulos S, Sabharwal T, Karnabatidis D, et al. Endovascular treatment of visceral aneurysms and pseudoaneurysms: long-term outcomes from a multicenter European study. *Cardiovasc Intervent Radiol.* 2012;35:1315–1325.
4. Hossain A, Reis ED, Dave SP, et al. Visceral artery aneurysms: experience in a tertiary-care center. *Am Surg.* 2001;67:432–437.
5. Bedford PD, Lodge B. Aneurysm of the splenic artery. *Gut.* 1960;1:312–320.
6. Tessier DJ, Stone WM, Fowl RJ, et al. Clinical features and management of splenic artery pseudoaneurysm: case series and cumulative review of literature. *J Vasc Surg.* 2003;38:969–974.
7. Saltzberg SS, Maldonado TS, Lamparello PJ, et al. Is endovascular therapy the preferred treatment for all visceral aneurysms? *Ann Vasc Surg.* 2005;19(4):507–515.
8. Berceli SA. Hepatic and splenic artery aneurysms. *Semin Vasc Surg.* 2005;18:196–201.
9. Hirsch AT, Haskal ZJ, Hertzer NR, et al. ACC/AHA 2005 practice guidelines for the management of patients with peripheral arterial disease (lower extremity, renal, mesenteric, and abdominal aortic): a collaborative report from the American Association for Vascular Surgery/Society for Vascular Surgery, Society for Cardiovascular Angiography and Interven-

tions, Society for Vascular Medicine and Biology, Society of Interventional Radiology, and the ACC/AHA Task Force on Practice Guidelines (Writing Committee to Develop Guidelines for the Management of Patients With Peripheral Arterial Disease): endorsed by the American Association of Cardiovascular and Pulmonary Rehabilitation; National Heart, Lung, and Blood Institute; Society for Vascular Nursing; TransAtlantic Inter-Society Consensus; and Vascular Disease Foundation. *Circulation*. 2006;113:e463–e654.

10. Tulsyan N, Kashyap VS, Greenberg RK, et al. The endovascular management of visceral artery aneurysms and pseudoaneurysms. *J Vasc Surg*. 2007;45:276–283.
11. Hislop SJ, Patel SA, Abt PL, et al. Therapy of renal artery aneurysms in New York state: outcomes of patients undergoing open and endovascular repair. *Ann Vasc Surg*. 2009;23:194–200.
12. Sachdev-Ost Ulka. Visceral artery aneurysms: review of current management options. *Mt Sinai J Med*. 2010;77:296–303.
13. Pech M, Mohnike K, Wieners G, et al. Advantages and disadvantages of the Amplatzer Vascular Plug IV in visceral embolization: report of 50 placements. *Cardiovasc Intervent Radiol*. 2011;34:1069–1073.
14. Bratby MJ, Lehmann ED, Bottomley J, et al. Endovascular embolization of visceral artery aneurysms with ethylene-vinyl alcohol (Onyx): a case series. *Cardiovasc Intervent Radiol*. 2006;29(6):1125–1128.
15. Abbas MA, Stone WM, Fowl RJ. Splenic artery aneurysms: two decades experience at Mayo Clinic. *Ann Vasc Surg*. 2002;16:442–449.
16. Patel A, Weintraub J, Nowakowski S. Single-center experience with elective transcatheter coil embolization of splenic artery aneurysms: technique and midterm follow-up. *J Vasc Interv Radiol*. 2012;23:893–899.
17. Requarth JA, D'Agostino R, Miller P. Nonoperative management of adult blunt splenic injury with and without splenic artery embolotherapy: a meta-analysis. *J Trauma*. 2011;71:898–903.
18. Haan J, Bochicchio G, Kramer N, et al. Nonoperative management of blunt splenic injury: a 5-year experience. *J Trauma*. 2005;58:492–498.
19. Bessoud B, Denys A, Calmes J-M et al. Nonoperative management of traumatic splenic injuries: is there a role for proximal splenic artery embolization? *AJR Am J Roentgenol*. 2011;86:779–785.
20. Requarth JA. Distal splenic artery hemodynamic changes during transient proximal splenic artery occlusion in blunt splenic injury patients: a mechanism of delayed splenic hemorrhage. *J Trauma*. 2010;69:1423–1426.
21. Balderi A, Antonietti A, Pedrazzini F, et al. Treatment of visceral aneurysm using multilayer stent: two-year follow-up results in five patients. *Cardiovasc Intervent Radiol*. 2013;36:1256–1261.
22. Choo CH, Yen HH. Unusual upper gastrointestinal bleeding: ruptured superior mesenteric artery aneurysm in rheumatoid arthritis. *World J Gastroenterol*. 2013;19(28):4630–4632.
23. Nosher JL, Chung J, Brevetti LS, et al. Visceral and renal artery aneurysms: a pictorial essay on endovascular therapy. *Radiographics*. 2006;26:1687–1704.
24. Syed M, Shaikh A, Neravetla S. Celiac artery aneurysm embolization by coil occlusion. *Ann Vasc Surg*. 2005;19(1):113–119.
25. Koganemaru M, Abe T, Nonoshita M, et al. Follow-up of true visceral artery aneurysm after coil embolization by three-dimensional contrast-enhanced MR angiography. *Diagn Interv Radiol*. 2014;20(2):129–135. doi:10.5152/dir.2013.13236.
26. Yasumoto T, Osuga K, Yamamoto H, et al. Long-term outcomes of coil packing for visceral aneurysms: correlation between packing density and incidence of coil compaction or recanalization. *J Vasc Interv Radiol*. 2013;24(12):1798–1807.

47

Renal Artery Aneurysms

Carlos Abath • Romero Marques • Marcos Barbosa de Souza Júnior

Primary renal artery aneurysms (RAAs) are relatively rare, contributing to 1% of all aneurysms and 15% to 22% of visceral aneurysms.[1] They have an estimated incidence of 0.09% in the general population, 0.1% to 2.5% in angiographic series, and up to 9.7% in autopsy series.[2–4] However, the trend for more widespread investigation of the renal arteries with noninvasive methods has resulted in an increasing number of cases receiving medical attention.[5]

In most cases, the clinical relevance of the aneurysm is uncertain as the patient has no symptoms directly related to the aneurysm. Some patients may present arterial hypertension, renal ischemia, hematuria, or flank pain, but the cause-and-effect relationship is hardly established.[4,6,7] The natural history of RAA is poorly documented. Although rupture is rare, with an incidence reported at 5% to 10%, it may be associated with mortality rates as high as 80%. The risk of RAA rupture is significantly increased in pregnancy and polyarteritis nodosa (PAN) and is also related to the aneurysm size.[4,8–10]

The accepted indications for RAA treatment include symptomatic patients, women who are pregnant or in those contemplating pregnancy, PAN, and enlarging lesions. Currently, no consensus exists for the size at which an RAA should be repaired in an asymptomatic patient. It is recommended that the lesion should be treated when greater than 1.5 to 3 cm, although most use 2 cm as the reference size for treatment.[4,6,7,10,11]

The surgical management of RAA is relatively safe, with a low mortality rate ranging from 0% to 4%. Otherwise, in complex lesions, intentional nephrectomy occurs in up to 20% of cases and unplanned nephrectomy in 5% of cases.[1,6] With the progress of endovascular techniques and development of new devices, even very complex lesions can be selectively treated, sparing the normal vascular tree. Therefore, this less invasive procedure carries a much lower morbidity and mortality rate, assuring that a complete understanding of aneurysm angioarchitecture is achieved and a proper endovascular strategy is planned. In this chapter, we will describe our endovascular management of RAA, discussing the patient and endovascular technique selection criteria and determining the immediate and long-term anatomic results.

TECHNIQUE

Atherosclerosis and fibrous dysplasia are the most common causes of aneurysm formation. This can also be associated with some systemic diseases, such as PAN, neurofibromatosis, and tuberous sclerosis. Traumatic and iatrogenic renal artery pseudoaneurysms are frequent vascular lesions but represent another pathophysiologic entity.

Over the last decade, we have treated 21 cases of nontraumatic RAA. There were 16 females and 5 males, with a mean age of 51.2 years (range, 19 to 79 years). Six patients had hypertension, 2 of them with a solitary kidney. Five other patients presented flank pain related to the side where the aneurysms were located. Two other patients had hematuria. In the 8 remaining patients, the aneurysms were found incidentally.

Atherosclerosis, fibromuscular dysplasia, and tuberous sclerosis coexisted in 4, 14, and 3 patients, respectively. The mean aneurysm diameter was 26 mm (range, 15 to 38 mm). For the purposes of endovascular treatment strategy, the RAAs were classified according to their location[12,13] as type I, main renal artery (3 cases); type II, arterial bifurcations (14 cases); and type III, distal intrarenal (3 cases) (Fig. 47.1).

The endovascular treatment of RAA must be precise, safe, and durable, achieving complete aneurysm exclusion from the blood circulation and preserving, as much as possible, the arterial tree and renal parenchyma. To achieve these goals, the lesions can be treated by stent graft implant or

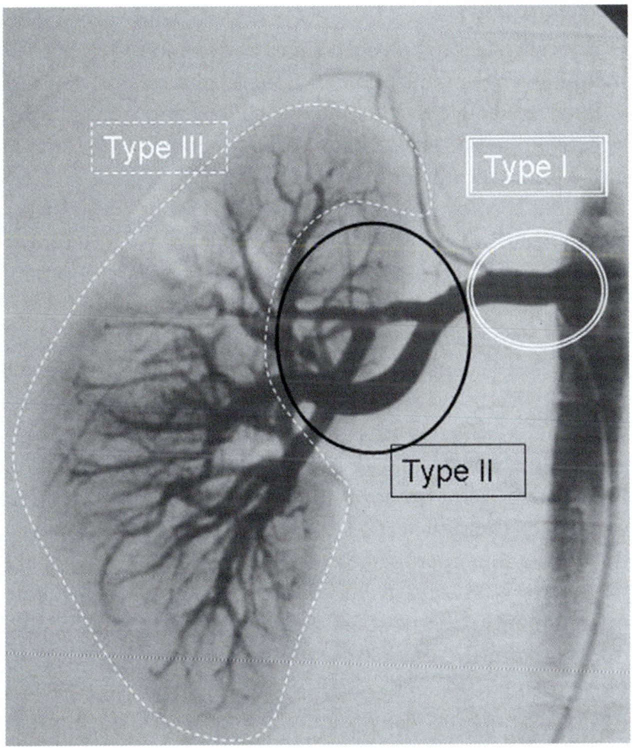

Figure 47.1 Topographic RAA classification.

selective embolization of the aneurysm sac. Unfortunately, both of these techniques have limitations and cannot be applied to every case. It is sometimes necessary to perform a parent vessel occlusion to treat the aneurysm, with some grade of renal parenchyma compromise. A full understanding of the arterial anatomy is needed for the recognition of challenging technical difficulties that will guide the choice of the best strategy and proper tools for each specific case. Complex and large lesions, broad-necked aneurysms, and bifurcation-located aneurysms, with arterial branch involvement, must be well identified and studied before the endovascular treatment. The noninvasive diagnostic methods, mainly the multidetector computed tomography, can provide valuable information regarding the aneurysm size, mural thrombus, wall calcification, and relationship with the parent vessel. Digital angiography with three-dimensional (3-D) reconstruction remains the best method for a pretreatment anatomic evaluation.

Angiography

As usual, the diagnostic angiography, via a femoral approach, begins with an aortography, unless there is an abnormal renal function. This initial study may show additional aneurysms or other lesions in the contralateral kidney, which can change the original treatment plan. It also can show the presence of accessory renal arteries. A selective renal angiography is then performed, in anteroposterior and oblique views, to demonstrate the aneurysm neck on profile. The distances from the aneurysm to renal artery ostium and renal artery bifurcation must be shown and are essential to the decision of placing a stent graft. The involvement of arterial branches by the aneurysm must also be disclosed. If the aneurysm is large or close to the renal bifurcation, it can be extremely difficult to obtain adequate visualization of the structures because the aneurysm sac is superposed over the renal vascular tree. Therefore, it is very useful to do a rotational angiography for 3-D image reconstruction. With the aid of a workstation, it is possible to play with the 3-D images to get the best views and to find the ideal working projection, where the neck is visualized on true profile. Once the working projection is found, the arch is positioned according to the angulations displayed in the workstation. Another advantage is the possibility of obtaining the vessel and aneurysm measurements with a minimal error margin. In our practice, we use Allura (Philips Healthcare, The Netherlands) or Artis zeego (Siemens Corporation, Malvern, Pennsylvania) equipment, doing the rotational angiography with 20 mL of nonionic contrast at a flow rate of 4 mL per second.

Stent Graft

Despite the development of new, more flexible, low-profile devices, the stent graft has restricted use in the treatment of RAA. It should not be applied in type II aneurysms because it would cover an important branch at the bifurcation, leading to a major renal infarction. It is not useful in type III distal lesions either because it does not have enough flexibility and low profile to navigate in tiny and tortuous vessels. The stent graft is a treatment option only in selected type I aneurysms, when the main renal artery is straight and the edges of the aneurysm neck are located at least 15 mm away from the renal ostium and hilar bifurcation. If these limits are not respected, there is a risk of technical failure, resulting in endoleak and persistent flow inside the aneurysm pouch. This occurred in the only case in which we tried to use a stent graft to seal a type I aneurysm, and the procedure had to be complemented by Onyx (Covidien, Irvine, California) embolization (Fig. 47.2).

Thromboembolism is another problem related to the use of stent graft in small-sized vessels such as the renal arteries, demanding a long-term administration of double antiplatelet therapy with acetylsalicylic acid and clopidogrel.

Flow-Diverter Stents

Flow-diverters stents have been developed for endovascular treatment of intracranial aneurysms, and today, two such stents are available: the Pipeline (Covidien, Plymouth, Minnesota) stent and the Silk stent (Balt Extrusion, Montmorency, France). Although they represent a safe, durable, and curative treatment of selected wide-necked, large, and giant intracranial aneurysms, important complications such

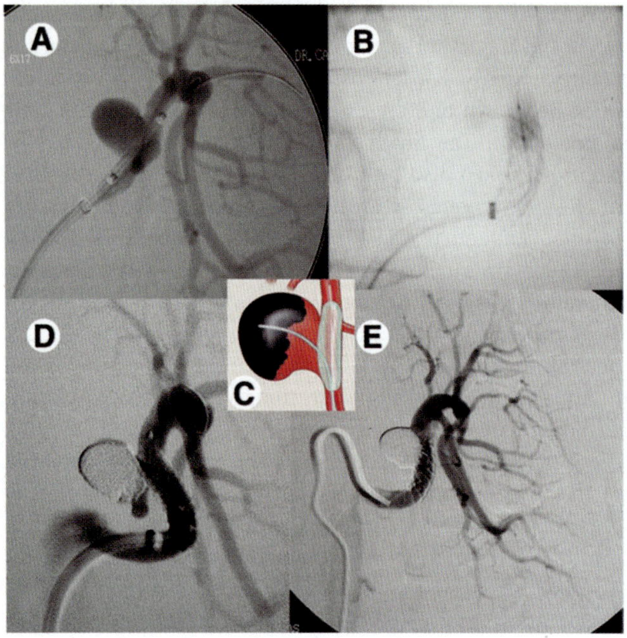

Figure 47.2 Type I RAA. **A:** Stent graft across the aneurysm neck. **B:** Distal leakage after stent delivery; sealing test before Onyx injection. **C:** Onyx injection with the balloon inflated across the neck. **D:** Angiographic control showing aneurysm occlusion. **E:** Angiographic durable result after 1 year.

as stent thrombosis, side branch occlusion, or postimplantation bleeding have been reported.[14]

The Cardiatis multilayer stent (Cardiatis, Isnes, Belgium) is a new type of flow-diverter stent consisting of two interconnected layers without any coverage, leading to decreased turbulent flow velocity in the aneurysm sac while improving laminar flow in the main artery and its branches. The stent is made of a biocompatible cobalt alloy wire, is available in diameters from 2 to 50 mm, and can be loaded in small (6-Fr) delivery systems.[15] Even though it is a promising tool for the endovascular treatment of some selected visceral and peripheral aneurysms, only few case reports and small series have been published.[15] At the moment, this technology should be restricted to the rare cases where the other options are not applicable until its clinical effectiveness and safety is proved in further studies with longer follow-up.

Selective Coil Embolization

The advent of microcatheter and guidewire systems and new embolic agents allowed a selective occlusion of the most RAAs regardless of the topographic localization. The best lesions for this endovascular approach are saccular aneurysms with a well-defined narrow neck, measuring less than 4 mm or presenting a dome-to-neck proportion equal or superior to 2:1, without arterial branches arising from the aneurysm.

Preference is given to perform the procedure under general anesthesia for controlled apnea and generous use of road mapping. The embolization is safer and quicker and contrast volume is reduced. After digital subtraction aortography, selective renal artery catheterization is done with a double curve guiding catheter 6-Fr (Mach 1, Boston Scientific Corporation, Natick, Massachusetts). Thereafter, superselective catheterization of the aneurysm is performed with the Excelsior 14 microcatheter (Boston Scientific Corporation, Natick, Massachusetts) over a platinum tip 0.0014-in steerable guidewire (Transcend; Boston Scientific Corporation, Natick, Massachusetts) under road mapping fluoroscopy. The microcatheter is advanced coaxially through the guiding catheter, which is fitted proximally with a rotating hemostatic valve. The coaxial system is continuously flushed with heparinized saline solution to prevent thrombus formation in between the catheters.

Once the microcatheter tip is inside the aneurysm, the cavity is progressively filled with multiple detachable microcoils. Currently, there are many types of detachable microcoils in the market from different manufacturers. In most of our cases, the Guglielmi detachable coil (GDC; Boston Scientific Corporation, Natick, Massachusetts) is used. GDCs are circular or multishaped soft platinum coils, varying in size and length. The coil is attached to a Teflon-coated stainless steel delivery wire by a short portion of uninsulated stainless steel. After the correct position of the implanted coil is confirmed angiographically, a positive direct electrical current is applied to the proximal end of the stainless delivery wire. The negative pole is connected to a needle positioned in the patient's skin. Within 1 minute, the current dissolves the uninsulated stainless steel section proximal to the platinum coil by electrolysis and the delivery wire is then withdrawn. The size of the first coil should equal the aneurysm size, achieving a basketlike configuration within the sac (Fig. 47.3B). The remaining cavity is filled with smaller coils, which are placed within the network of the first GDC, until the whole cavity of the aneurysm is densely packed with coils (Fig. 47.3C). Unfortunately, this technique alone cannot be applied to more complex lesions, such as large-neck aneurysms or when arterial branches arise from the aneurysm sac. In these cases, it is essential to perform associated remodeling techniques to protect the neck and avoid parent vessel or branch occlusion. This complication was observed early in our experience, when we did not protect the wide aneurysm neck in a type II lesion (Fig. 47.4).

REMODELING TECHNIQUES

Until the development of remodeling techniques, wide-necked aneurysms could not be treated by selective embolization without a significant risk of parent vessel occlusion caused by coil migration into the unprotected parent artery.

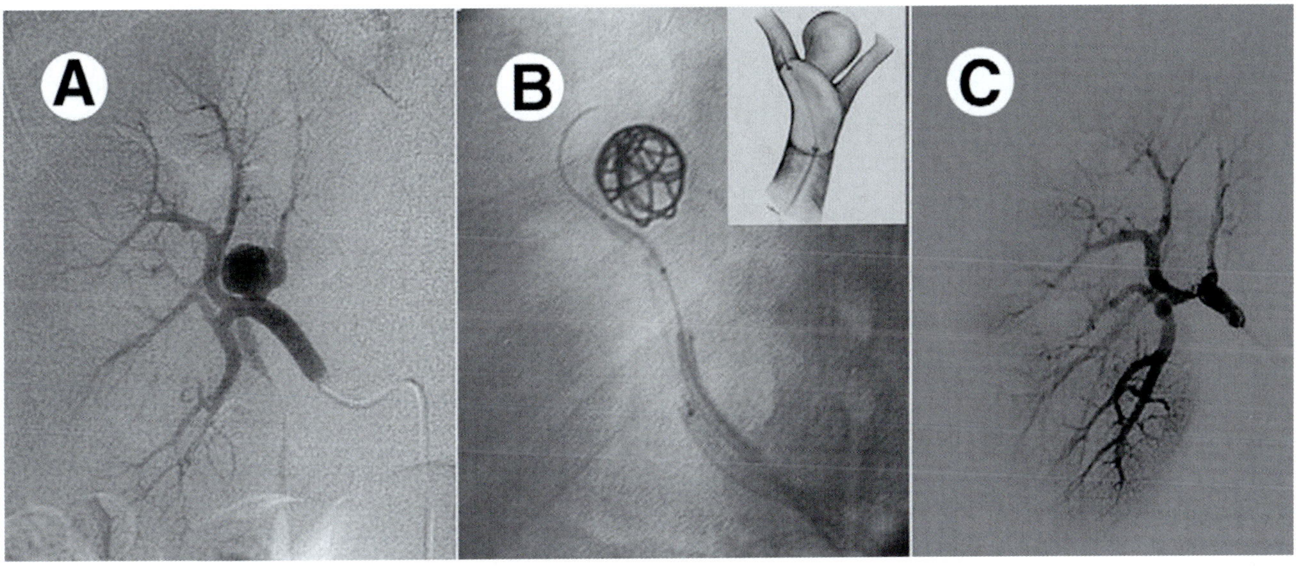

Figure 47.3 Balloon-assisted coil embolization. **A:** Selective renal artery angiography showing a type II RAA. **B:** Balloon-assisted coil embolization showing a basketlike configuration after the first GDC deployment. **C:** Dense packing with aneurysm exclusion in the control angiography.

In the remodeling technique, a temporary balloon is inflated intermittently at the aneurysmal neck while the microcoil or other embolic agents are deposited. Alternatively, a stent can be delivered to protect the neck, acting as a scaffold in the parent artery, while coils or other embolic materials are deposited into the aneurysmal lumen.

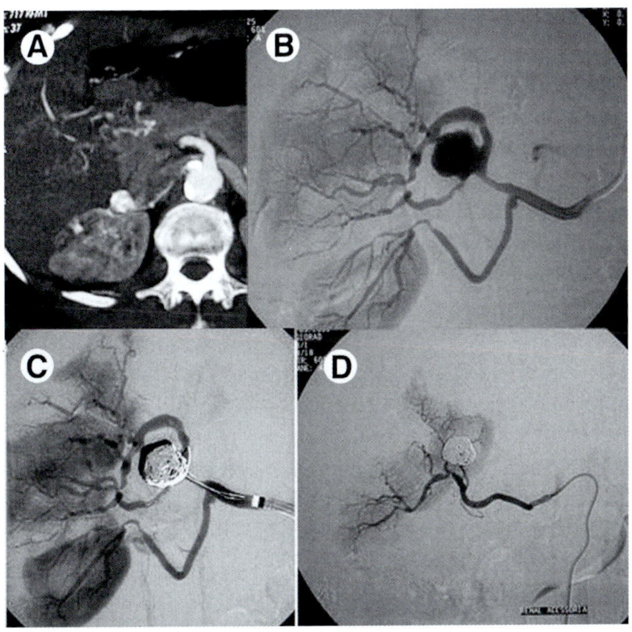

Figure 47.4 Selective coil embolization. **A:** CT: large RAA with calcified wall. **B:** Wide-necked type II RAA. **C:** Control angiography showing coil migration to the parent vessel. **D:** Accessory renal artery.

Balloon-Assisted Coiling

The balloon remodeling technique, first described by Moret and coworkers[16] in 1997, was the initial alternative to surmount the problem of wide-necked brain aneurysms. In this technique, a soft semicompliant or conformable balloon is positioned across the neck of an aneurysm and inflated during coiling. The balloon works as a mechanical barrier that allows tighter packing of the aneurysm while preventing coil herniation into the parent artery during coil delivery. Also, the balloon stabilizes the microcatheter during coil delivery and forces the coils to conform to the 3-D shape of the aneurysm. The best balloons, specially designed for this technique, are the flexible, very low profile, compliant balloons: HyperGlide and HyperForm (Covidien, Plymouth, Minnesota). We routinely use the HyperGlide, leaving the HyperForm for some aneurysms located in bifurcations. Unfortunately, in some cases, the size of these balloons, which reaches only 4 mm in diameter, does not fit the main renal artery diameter, which ranges from 5 to 7 mm. So, they must be replaced by regular peripheral balloons with the desired diameters (Aviator plus; Cordis Corporation, Somerville, New Jersey).

When the balloon remodeling technique is performed, it is necessary to use a larger 7-Fr guiding catheter (Mach 1, Boston Scientific Corporation, Natick, Massachusetts) or a 6-Fr renal sheath introducer (Flexor® Cook Medical, Inc., Bloomington, Indiana), allowing passage for a balloon and a microcatheter at same time. Alternatively, we can do bilateral femoral puncture, introducing one 6-Fr guiding catheter in each side for the balloon and microcatheter, respectively. Special attention must be paid to the heparinization, keeping the

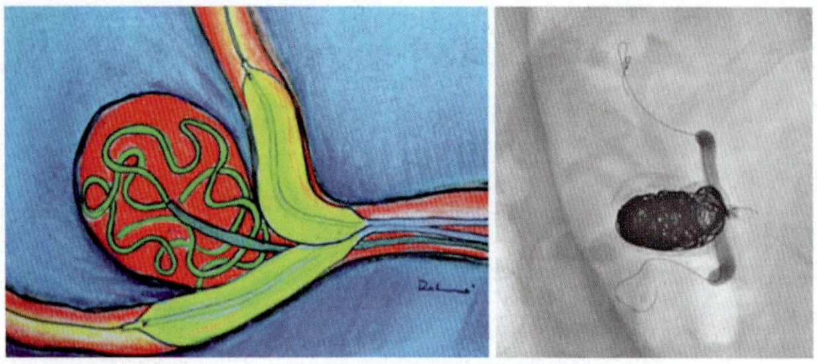

Figure 47.5 Double balloon protection technique.

activated coagulation time (ACT) three times the basal level. With the guiding catheter selectively placed in the main renal artery, the deflated balloon is positioned in the parent vessel, across the aneurysm neck. Selective microcatheterization of the aneurysm is then performed. Inflation of the balloon across the aneurysm neck temporarily occludes the neck and the parent vessel. Under balloon protection, coils are then delivered into the aneurysm. After placement of each coil into the aneurysm but before detachment, the balloon is deflated to test the stability of the coil. If no displacement of the coil is observed, the coil is detached. If movement is detected after balloon deflation, the coil is considered unstable and repositioned or removed. The procedure is repeated to obtain a dense and stable packing (Fig. 47.3).

Sometimes, when both branches are involved by a large-neck aneurysm located at the bifurcation, a double balloon protection technique is required to avoid occlusion of one of the branches by coil herniation (Fig. 47.5).

Stent-Assisted Coiling

Although the balloon technique constitutes an important method for the endovascular treatment of wide-necked aneurysms, the adjunctive use of stents may be an appealing alternative in RAA.

The implantation of a stent across the neck area serves as a buttress to the coil mass and contributes to changing the hemodynamic parameters locally by redirecting the flow and providing a substrate for endothelialization in that area, decreasing the chance of long-term aneurysm recanalization.

Similarly to the balloon-assisted embolization technique, the stent is positioned and deployed in front of the aneurysmal neck. Thereafter, selective microcatheterization of the aneurysmal lumen is done through the stent mesh or on parallel to it. The microcoils then are successively positioned and detached to achieve good packing.

Liquid Embolic Agents

Even when an aneurysm looks densely packed, there is a lot of space between the coils that may contribute to a significant number of recurrences after embolization, especially in large and giant wide-necked aneurysms. The use of a liquid agent that would be able to obliterate the aneurysm sac completely and seal the neck has significant advantages and has been examined for several years. The liquid nonadhesive embolic agent for this application is Onyx. Specifically designed for endovascular use, Onyx is an ethylene vinyl alcohol copolymer dissolved in an organic solvent, dimethyl sulfoxide (DMSO). When this liquid embolic agent comes in contact with an aqueous solution, it precipitates and initially forms an outer soft and spongy polymer cast with a semiliquid center. As further material is injected into the cast, it fills the space into which it is injected, and additional material then breaks out through the outer layer of the existing cast.

Despite the fact that Onyx has been developed to deal with cerebral aneurysm and that almost all scientific literature is related to neurointerventional procedures,[17,18] we think that the concepts can also be applied to RAA. We have performed Onyx renal artery embolization in patients with type I and type II aneurysms, under general anesthesia, via a right femoral approach.

A 7-Fr guiding catheter or a 6-Fr renal sheath introducer is selectively placed in the main renal artery. The technique of Onyx embolization begins with the placement of a highly compliant DMSO-compatible occlusion balloon (HyperGlide or HyperForm) within the parent vessel over the aneurysm neck. As the maximum sizes for these balloons are 5 × 20 mm and 7 × 7 mm, respectively, they may not fit to the main renal artery diameter in every case. In this case, we have to use a bigger regular peripheral balloon (Aviator plus), without any problem related to DMSO compatibility. The balloon is left deflated while a DMSO-compatible microcatheter (Rebar; Covidien, Plymouth, Minnesota) is placed within the aneurysm. A slow test injection of contrast material through the microcatheter is made with the balloon inflated to ensure that the neck is controlled and a satisfactory seal is achieved with stasis of contrast material within the aneurysm. The microcatheter is then purged with saline to clear any contrast residue and primed with DMSO with a volume to match the dead space within the microcatheter. Onyx (HD 500) is then injected through the microcatheter. After a volume of approximately 0.2 mL, the Onyx approaches the end of the microcatheter and the balloon is inflated to a predetermined volume (measured when testing the seal between the aneurysm neck and parent vessel, as mentioned previously). The balloon temporarily occludes the parent vessel during the procedure while the aneurysm is filled with the Onyx, which forms a cast that seals off the aneurysm from the circulation and, in effect, reconstructs the parent vessel wall (Fig. 47.6).

The Onyx is injected at a rate of approximately 0.1 mL per minute, during approximately 5 minutes, by using a special syringe, which operates by means of a screw thread. Because Onyx is a viscous material, it accumulates around

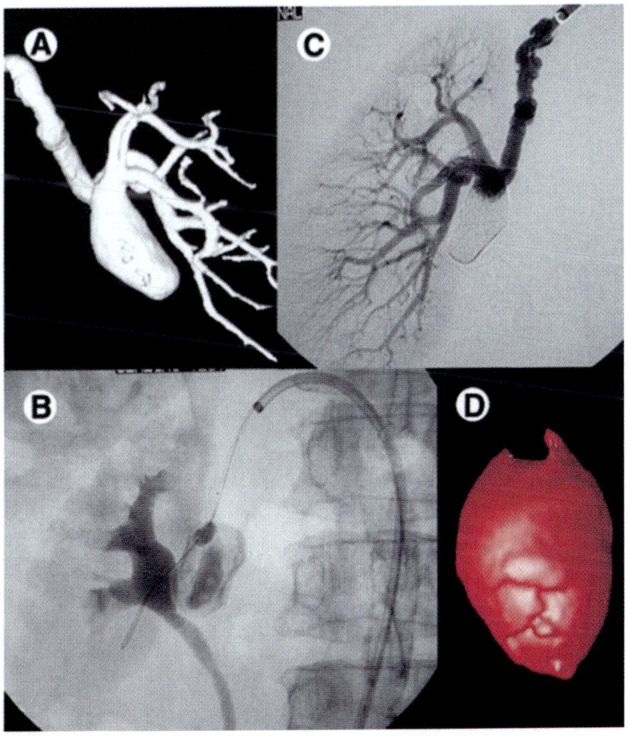

Figure 47.6 Type II RAA. **A:** 3-D angiography showing the vascular anatomy. **B:** Balloon-assisted Onyx embolization. **C:** Complete filling of the aneurysm cavity by the Onyx material. **D:** 3-D reconstruction of the Onyx casting.

the microcatheter tip and gradually enlarges to form a kernel that remains attached to the end of the microcatheter. After each injection, the balloon is left inflated for another 2 minutes and is then deflated to allow renal reperfusion for 2 additional minutes, and the cycle is repeated. With each injection, new portions of the aneurysm fill (Fig. 47.7); eventually, the material flows down to the margins of the balloon and occludes the aneurysm neck. When the material comes into contact with the balloon, the injection is slowed or stopped, with brief 15- to 30-second pauses, to minimize the risk of leakage into the parent artery and beyond the balloon. At this point, it is advisable to follow the Onyx injection by subtracted fluoroscopy, under apnea, for better visualization of the embolic agent. It is important to ensure that material covers the aneurysm neck to achieve complete and durable occlusion and reduce the risk of aneurysm regrowth. The microcatheter position is not adjusted once the injection has begun. After angiographic confirmation of complete or satisfactory occlusion of the aneurysm occurs, the catheter syringe is decompressed by aspiration of 0.2 mL of the material and a 10-minute pause is taken to allow complete solidification of the polymer with the balloon deflated. The balloon is then reinflated, and the microcatheter is removed by gentle traction.

Another liquid embolic agent used to treat RAA is the tissue adhesive agent *N*-butyl cyanoacrylate (NBCA) (Histoacryl; B Braun Melsungen AG, Melsungen, Germany), which immediately polymerizes when it contacts ionic fluids, such as blood, forming a cast within vessel lumen resulting in occlusion. The glue is used in mixture with the oil dye Lipiodol (Guerbet, Aulnay-sous-Bois, France) to become visible under x-ray and delay the polymerization time. We use a concentration of 20% to 50% of NBCA in the treatment of renal vascular lesions. Unlike the embolic agent Onyx, the polymerization behavior of the NBCA/Lipiodol mixture is something unforeseeable and can lead to inadvertent parent vessel occlusion. So we reserve this embolic agent to treat only distal type III renal aneurysms when it is possible to occlude the parent vessel, provoking an acceptable small area of renal parenchyma infarction (Fig. 47.8).

ASSOCIATION OF TECHNIQUES AND MATERIALS

The management of complex RAA sometimes demands association of different techniques and embolic agents to be successful and safe. If one technique or material fails to completely exclude an aneurysm from the circulation, another strategy is performed for total obliteration of the lesion. In our series, a type I renal aneurysm was initially treated with a stent graft (Jograft; Jomed, Rangendingen, Germany), but the lesion continued to be patent due to a leakage at the distal end of the stent graft. Therefore, the tip of a microcatheter was positioned within the aneurysm and Onyx was injected while a balloon was inflated over the aneurysm neck, achieving a complete occlusion of the aneurysm sac (Fig. 47.2).

On other occasions, different materials are associated to obtain better and durable results or expand the safety margin of the procedure. This was the case of a huge type I renal aneurysm, whose neck encompassed the parent vessel wall. First, we deployed a bare stent across the neck and then a microcatheter was placed within the aneurysm lumen through the mesh of the stent. A peripheral balloon was inflated in front of the aneurysm neck and 7.5 mL of Onyx were injected inside the lesion. As a small leakage of Onyx was noticed through the aneurysm neck and beyond the balloon, we stopped the liquid agent injection and finished the neck occlusion with detachable microcoils. This way, a complete aneurysm occlusion was achieved, reconstructing and keeping the parent vessel patent. Besides the dense compaction of the aneurysm lumen, the stent changed the local hemodynamic parameters, redirecting the flow and decreasing the chance of a long-term recanalization (Fig. 47.9).

In another complex lesion, a type III intrarenal aneurysm ruptured, leading to an arteriovenous fistula (AVF),

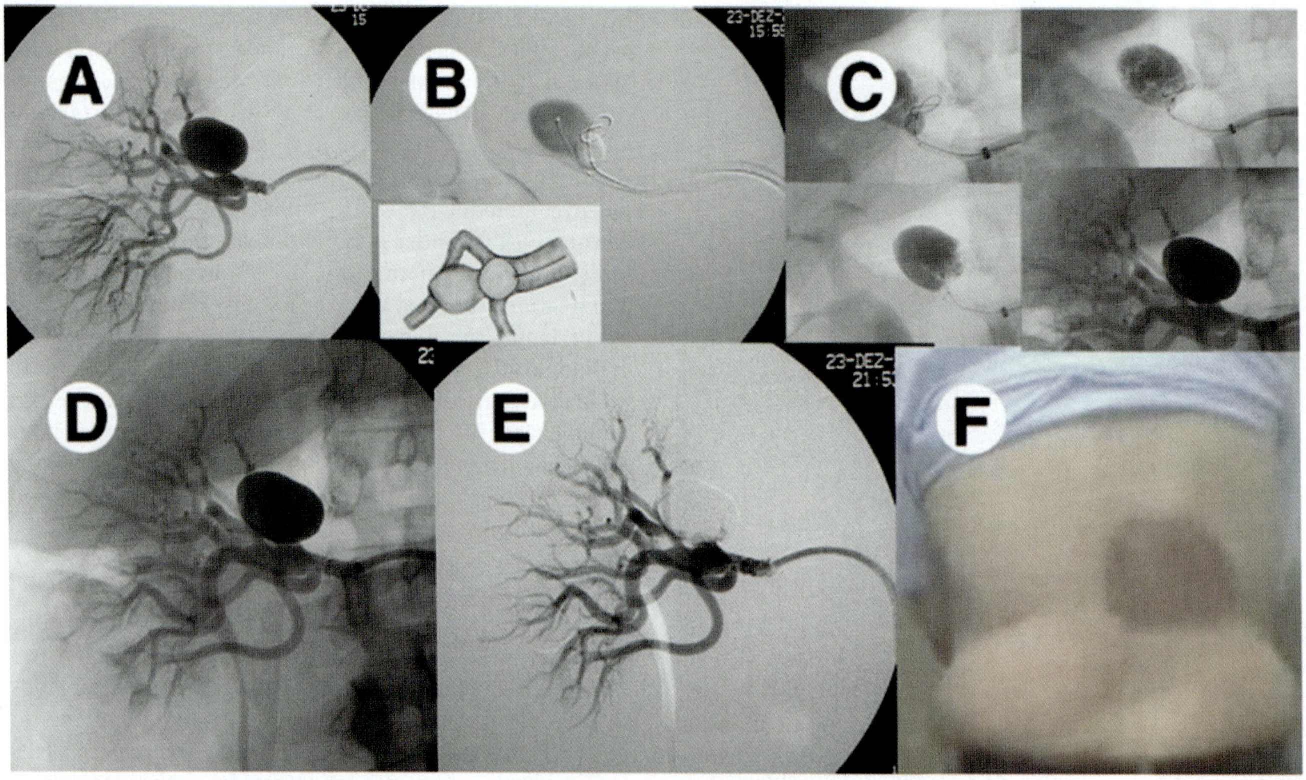

Figure 47.7 Type II RAA. **A:** Selective renal angiography. **B:** Balloon protection of the aneurysm neck during sealing test before Onyx injection. **C:** Onyx injection showing progressive filling of the aneurysm cavity. **D,E:** Complete obliteration of the aneurysm sac by the Onyx casting. **F:** Actinic dermatitis due to x-ray exposure.

associated with a venous dilation. Initially, a detachable microcoil was delivered within the arterial aneurysm to decrease the flow. Then, the embolization was concluded by injecting glue (⅔ lipiodol + ⅓ cyanoacrylate: 33%) to obliterate the AVF and fill the aneurysm cavity (Fig. 47.8).

RESULTS

Twenty-one large or giant RAAs were submitted to endovascular treatment in 21 patients, with complete occlusion of the aneurysm cavity in all of them (100% technical success).

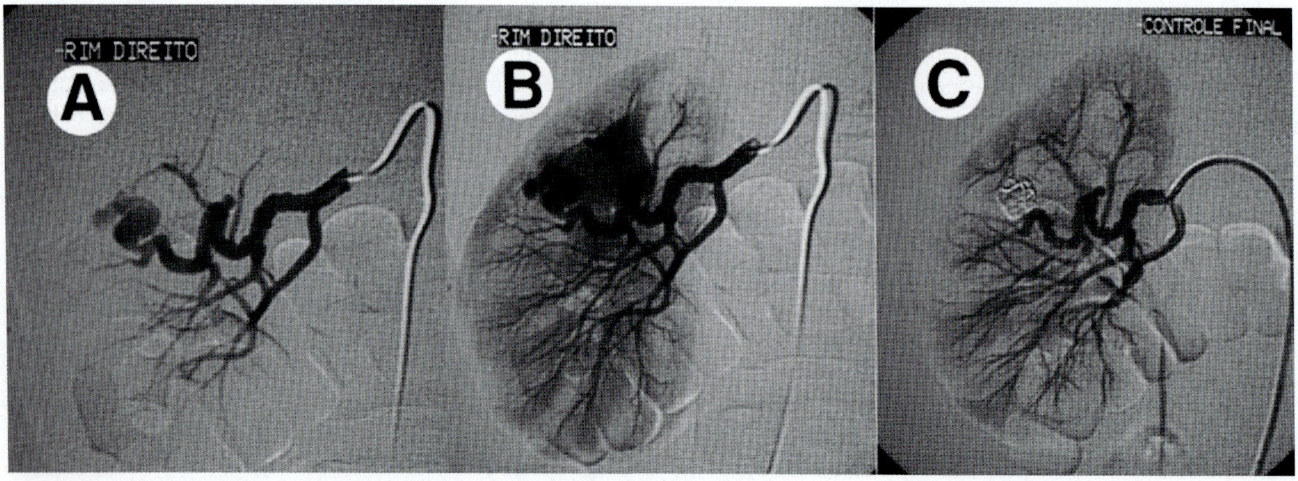

Figure 47.8 Type III RAA. **A,B:** Distal type III RAA with an associated AVF. **C:** A coil was deployed to decrease the flow, and definitive AVF and aneurysm occlusion was achieved by glue injection.

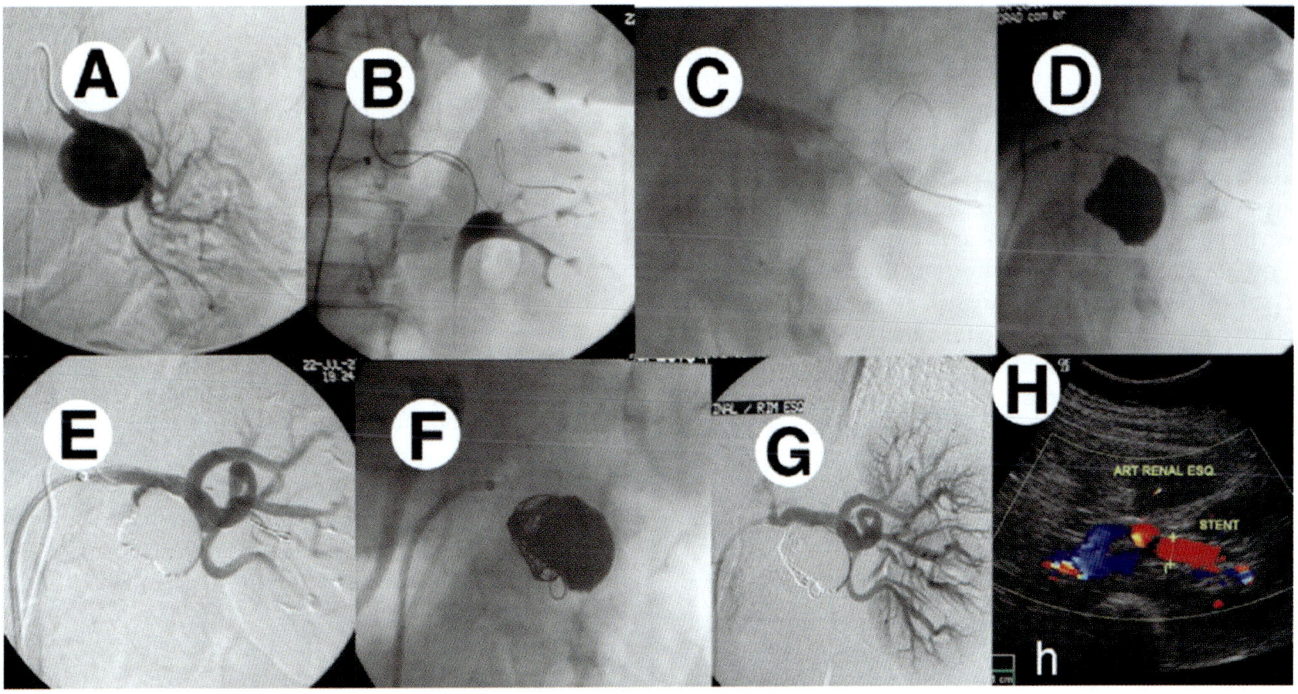

Figure 47.9 Type I RAA. **A:** Giant aneurysm without a well-defined neck. **B:** Bare stent before delivery across the aneurysm neck. The microcatheter tip is within the aneurysm sac. **C:** Peripheral balloon inflated within the stent to protect the parent vessel during Onyx injection. **D:** Onyx material approaching the neck with leakage risk. **E–G:** Residual neck after Onyx embolization, completely occluded with some coils. **H:** Doppler ultrasonography showing RAA exclusion after 6 months.

Two aneurysms were classified as type I lesions and 16 as type II. All of them but one were treated with remodeling technique coil or Onyx embolization. Unintentional branch occlusion occurred just in one type II lesion in which we did not use the remodeling technique, resulting in a small but clinically asymptomatic renal infarction (Fig. 47.4). In one large type I aneurysm, an association of techniques and materials was used, leading to a significant patient x-ray exposure. Clinical follow-up demonstrated a localized actinic dermatitis at the skin over the affected kidney (Fig. 47.7).

Three aneurysms were classified as type III lesions and were embolized with glue after distal superselective catheterization. Despite the occlusion of the tiny parent vessels, none or minimal renal parenchyma infarction was noted, with no clinical significance.

A clinical and diagnostic Doppler ultrasonography follow-up was performed in all patients (mean, 32.6 months; range, 9 to 75 months). Digital angiography was available in only one patient a year after the endovascular treatment. In two patients with hematuria, the bleeding disappeared immediately after embolization. The patients with arterial hypertension and flank pain presented total or partial improvement of their signs and symptoms. In all patients, the serum creatinine levels were normal, remaining unchanged after the procedure. Ultrasonography and angiography follow-up examinations confirmed successful and durable occlusion of all aneurysms, without any recurrence (Figs. 47.2 and 47.9).

DISCUSSION

The rare occurrence of RAAs has created a debate regarding the threshold for repair. There is general consensus that repair should be performed when meeting the following criteria: RAAs exceeding 2 or 2.5 cm, or documented enlarging aneurysm; symptomatic RAAs with flank pain, hematuria, or hypertension; RAAs with documented distal embolization; RAAs in pregnancy or in women of childbearing age; and RAAs with associated significant stenosis or renal malperfusion.[4,6,7,10,11,13]

Although surgical mortality of elective operation in experienced institutions is essentially nonexistent, morbidity and long recovery periods persist. Aortorenal bypass graft occlusions and unplanned nephrectomy occur even in the largest series.[6,19] With the advent of covered stents, lower profile endovascular devices, and new embolic agents, the technical feasibility of treating a larger number of RAA is now increased. Currently, the endovascular techniques allow the successful treatment of complex RAA despite of having complicating factors such as large size, wide neck, location near or at the bifurcation, branch involvement by the aneurysm, and association with AVF.

Rundback and coworkers[12] proposed an angiographic classification of RAAs that helps to establish treatment strategies. Type I lesions are saccular aneurysms that arise from the main artery or a large segmental branch and can be excluded with stent grafts. At the moment, the stent grafts present some limitations because the devices available are still rigid and high profile and have poor endovascular navigability.[20] Besides, the aneurysm neck is often situated close to the renal artery bifurcation, even in type I aneurysms, precluding a satisfactory seal. If the distance from the aneurysm to the renal artery bifurcation is less than 15 mm, the stent graft may not exclude the aneurysm sac from the circulation, as happened in one case of this series (Fig. 47.2). Another problem related to the stent graft is the need of long-term double antiplatelet therapy after the procedure. Selective coil or Onyx embolization, associated or not to remodeling technique, is a valuable alternative to treat type I RAA.

Type II RAAs are either fusiform or adjacent to a bifurcation and were generally treated with surgery or nephrectomy if required. These challenging lesions accounted for the most of our cases and were dealt with only endovascular approach. In this particular group of aneurysms, the use of remodeling technique, as an adjunct to selective coil or Onyx embolization, is strongly recommended to avoid inadvertent branch or parent vessel occlusion.

Type III RAA lesions arise from small segmental arteries that supply a small portion of the kidney and can be embolized by occlusion. Several embolic agents, such as microcoils and glue, can be used to obliterate these distal aneurysms.

Because of the reduced number of RAA cases, it is impossible to make a definitive comparison between coils and Onyx.[17–28] Being a liquid agent, the Onyx is able to better obliterate the aneurysm sac and, theoretically, would avoid aneurysm recurrence or regrowth. On the other hand, even with remodeling technique, it is difficult to avoid leakage of Onyx beyond the protection balloon at the end of the procedure, which could be responsible for thromboembolic events or late parent vessel occlusion. Certainly, it is much safer and easier to occlude the remnant aneurysm neck using microcoils instead of Onyx. Finally, the Onyx embolization procedure lasts longer and exposes the patient to more radiation.

However, it is important to say that the different embolic agents, such as coils and Onyx, should be used as complementary tools, and the interventional radiologist must take advantage of both to offer the best benefit for the patient. In very large aneurysms, it is possible to almost completely fill the aneurysm cavity with Onyx and finish the residual neck occlusion safely with microcoils. 3-D angiography is a very important technique for better understanding of the renal vascular anatomy. A complete comprehension of the renal aneurysm angioarchitecture is essential to choose the best therapeutic strategy planning.

TIPS AND TRICKS

- The selective embolization of complex RAA is a challenging procedure, demanding high-quality image, done on apnea, for a better understanding of the aneurysm angioarchitecture. So, do the cases under general anesthesia.
- To better control the embolic material deposition inside the aneurysm sac, it is essential to see the aneurysm neck on profile and to identify the origin of secondary branches involved by the aneurysm. This is not easy with plain angiography. Then, begin the procedure with a rotational angiography and 3-D reconstruction for a better definition of the working projections.
- Give preference for a preshaped sheath (Flexor® Ansel 6-Fr from Cook) instead of a preshaped guide catheter. The sheath has a larger internal lumen, with more space available for the microcatheter and remodelling balloon.
- Always use continuous pressurized heparinized saline solution on the guide sheath to avoid thromboembolic complications.
- When using Onyx to embolize RAAs, be sure to choose a microcatheter brand compatible with the Onyx solution because the DMSO can dissolve the microcatheter wall. You may use any of the DMSO-compatible microcatheters produced by Covidien.
- To deal with complex renal aneurysm, try to be familiar with the neurointervention tools, such as microcatheters, microwires, remodelling balloons, detachable microcoils, and Onyx.

CONCLUSION

The endovascular treatment of RAA is a feasible, safe, and effective procedure, which seems durable, even in complex lesions. Despite the good results, larger series with long-term follow-up are necessary to establish the real role of the endovascular techniques.

REFERENCES

1. Klein GE, Szolar DH, Breinl E, et al. Endovascular treatment of renal artery aneurysms with conventional non-detachable microcoils and Guglielmi detachable coils. *Br J Urol.* 1997;79:852–860.
2. Sahin S, Okbay M, Cinar B, et al. Wide-necked renal artery aneurysm: endovascular treatment with stent-graft. *Diagn Interv Radiol.* 2007;13:42–45.
3. Henke PK, Cardneau JD, Welling TH III, et al. Renal artery aneurysms: a 35-year clinical experience with 252 aneurysms in 168 patients. *Ann Surg.* 2001;234:454–462.

4. Ufberg JW, McNeil B, Swisher L. Ruptured renal artery aneurysm: an uncommon cause of acute abdominal pain. *J Emerg Med.* 2003;25:35–38.
5. Browne RF, Riordan EO, Roberts JA, et al. Renal artery aneurysms: diagnosis and surveillance with 3D contrast-enhanced magnetic resonance angiography. *Eur Radiol.* 2004;14:1807–1812.
6. English WP, Pearce JD, Craven TE, et al. Surgical management of renal artery aneurysms. *J Vasc Surg.* 2004;40:53–60.
7. Malacrida G, Dalainas I, Medda M, et al. Endovascular treatment of a renal artery branch aneurysm. *Cardiovasc Intervent Radiol.* 2007;30:118–120.
8. Soliman KB, Shawky Y, Abbas MM, et al. Ruptured renal artery aneurysm during pregnancy, a clinical dilemma. *BMC Urol.* 2006;31:6–22.
9. Schneidereit NP, Lee S, Morris DC, et al. Endovascular repair of a ruptured renal artery aneurysm. *J Endovasc Ther.* 2003;10: 71–74.
10. Mondek P, Zita Z, Sefranek V, et al. Kidney salvage after urgent repair of large ruptured renal artery aneurysm: case report and review of the literature. *Eur J Vasc Endovasc Surg.* 2003;6: 67–69.
11. Trocciola SM, Chaer RA, Lin SC, et al. Embolization of renal artery aneurysm and arteriovenous fistula-a case report. *Vasc Endovascular Surg.* 2005;39:525–529.
12. Rundback JH, Rizvi A, Rozenblit GN, et al. Percutaneous stent-graft management of renal artery aneurysms. *J Vasc Interv Radiol.* 2000;11:1189–1193.
13. Horesh L. RAA exclusion with a Viabahn stent graft. *Endovascular Today.* November 2004.
14. Lylyk P, Miranda C, Ceratto R, et al. Curative endovascular reconstruction of cerebral aneurysms with the pipeline embolization device: the Buenos Aires experience. *Neurosurgery.* 2009;64(4):632–642.
15. Meyer C, Verrel F, Weyer G et al. Endovascular management of complex renal artery aneurysms using the multilayer stent. *Cardiovasc Intervent Radiol.* 2011;34:637–641.
16. Moret J, Cognard C, Weil A, et al. Reconstruction technique in the treatment of wide-neck intracranial aneurysms: long-term angiographic and clinical results. Apropos of 56 cases. *J Neuroradiol.* 1997;24:30–44.
17. Levy EI, Guterman LR, Hopkins LN. Neuroendovascular surgery: techniques, indications, and patient selection. *Neurosurg Clin N Am.* 2005;16(2):xiii–xv.
18. Hopkins LN, Rosenwasser RH. Endovascular neurosurgery. *Neurosurgery.* 2006;59(suppl 5):93–102.
19. Bisschops RH, Popma JJ, Meyerovitz MF. Treatment of fibromuscular dysplasia and renal artery aneurysm with use of a stent-graft. *J Vasc Intervent Radiol.* 2001;12:757–760.
20. Andersen PE, Rohr N. Endovascular exclusion of renal artery aneurysm. *Cardiovasc Intervent Radiol.* 2005;28:665–667.
21. Lupattelli T, Abubacker Z, Morgan R, et al. Embolization of a renal artery aneurysm using ethylene vinyl alcohol copolymer (Onyx). *J Endovasc Ther.* 2003;10:366–370.
22. Tateno T, Kubota Y, Sasagawa I, et al. Successful embolization of a renal artery aneurysm with preservation of renal blood flow. *Intl Urol Nephrol.* 1996;28:283–287.
23. Karkos CD, D'Souza SP, Thomson GJ, et al. Renal artery aneurysm: endovascular treatment by coil embolisation with preservation of renal blood flow. *Eur J Vasc Endovasc Surg.* 2000;19:214–216.
24. Somani BK, Nabi G, McClinton S. Successful embolization of symptomatic renal artery aneurysm in solitary kidney. *Urology.* 2005;65:795–796.
25. McDonnell CO, Farrell NL, Kelly IMG, et al. Endovascular management of renal artery aneurysm. *Eur J Vasc Endovasc Surg.* 2004;8:81–82.
26. Dib M, Sedat J, Raffaelli C, et al. Endovascular treatment of a wide-neck renal artery bifurcation aneurysm. *J Vasc Intervent Radiol.* 2003;14:1461–1464.
27. Tshomba Y, Deleo G, Ferrari S, et al. Renal artery aneurysm: improved renal function after coil embolization. *J Endovasc Ther.* 2002;9:54–58.
28. Serter S, Oran I, Parildar M, et al. Fibromuscular dysplasia-related renal artery stenosis associated with aneurysm: successive endovascular therapy. *Cardiovasc Intervent Radiol.* 2007;30: 297–299.

Section L Genitourinary Embolization

L.1 Arterial Embolization

48 Renal Cell Carcinoma

Michael Darcy

The standard of care for managing renal cell carcinoma (RCC) is surgical resection, whereas in nonsurgical candidates, small RCCs are commonly treated with percutaneous ablation. So even though embolization of RCC has been around since the initial description in 1973,[1] its role is still relatively limited. However, in certain situations, it can be a very useful technique.

DEVICE DESCRIPTION

Catheters needed for embolization are generally not exotic. Standard 5-Fr catheters such as Cobra or Sos-shaped catheters are adequate to engage the main renal artery. If the RCC involves only a portion of the kidney, a microcatheter can be used to advance closer to the tumor's vasculature. Because coils are rarely used and particles or liquid embolics are favored, microcatheters with larger internal diameters can be useful. Occasionally, if the embolization is to be carried out from the main renal artery and the artery is short, a balloon occlusion catheter can be used to help prevent reflux of embolic materials.

The choice of embolic agent depends somewhat on the goal of the embolization. If you are simply providing preoperative devascularization, occluding the major arterial branches is adequate. Thus, large particles or even coils can be used to rapidly occlude the arteries. If embolization is the definitive therapy, then one wants to occlude very small peripheral branches to maximize the percentage of tumor tissue that undergoes necrosis. The fact that arteriovenous fistulae may sometimes be present in an RCC may guide the selection of embolic agents because particles or liquids could rapidly pass through the fistula.

Particles such as polyvinyl alcohol (PVA) are favored by some because they are readily available, relatively inexpensive, and easy to use. Suspending the PVA in contrast allows fluoroscopic monitoring to ensure that the particles are injected where intended. The size of the particles selected depends on the goal of embolization. Larger particles can easily occlude the major branches and reduce flow for preoperative devascularization. To achieve complete tissue necrosis for definitive therapy, smaller particles (100 to 300 μm) are a better choice.

Alcohol is favored by many because it will penetrate into peripheral small branches, thus reducing the chance of any collateral perfusion keeping the tumor alive. The problem is that alcohol is not radiopaque and therefore more difficult to use. As outlined in Chapter 9, mixing ethanol with Ethiodol provides opacification so the injections can be fluoroscopically monitored. It has an added benefit of allowing more peripheral embolization. Pure ethanol causes spasm, immediate protein denaturation, and thrombus formation. Mixing ethanol with Ethiodol blunts this effect and allows the ethanol to penetrate further into the precapillary arteries.[2] Although alcohol can be delivered through a peripherally positioned end-hole catheter, balloon occlusion catheters are favored when alcohol needs to be injected into the main renal artery. This is to prevent reflux from the renal artery into the abdominal aorta. Cyanoacrylate glue or Onyx (Covidien, Irvine, California) can also be used, but the expense of these agents cannot be justified given how easy it is to embolize an RCC with these other less expensive agents.

TECHNIQUE

There are several considerations before starting an embolization for RCC. Preoperative antibiotics are often used to reduce the chance of abscess formation in the necrotic tumor. Although renal embolization can be done with local anesthesia and sedation, general anesthesia should be considered if ethanol is going to be used (especially in larger volumes) because it can be painful. For large tumors extending into the renal vein or inferior vena cava (IVC), one concern is that embolization-induced necrosis will cause the tumor thrombus to become detached and embolize to the heart. Placing a suprarenal IVC filter has been used as a way to protect against embolization.[3] In some cases, the tumor thrombus may extend too far into the IVC and there may not be enough room to deploy a filter without extending into the right atrium. In that setting, we have still embolized the kidney and have not seen tumor embolization (Fig. 48.1), although that is still a concern. Use of a large self-expanding stent has been described to hold the tumor against the IVC wall to prevent embolization.[4] This has the added benefit of restoring caval patency. However, this technique would primarily be useful during palliative embolization because stenting across the tumor would interfere with a surgical resection. Finally, one may need to address a renal artery stenosis first to allow easier catheterization of the renal artery or to help preserve function of the normal parenchyma.[5]

An effective embolization always starts with a good diagnostic arteriogram. Although preprocedure cross-sectional imaging will often indicate the number of major renal arteries supplying the kidney, one can miss small accessory renal arteries that might supply the tumor. Also, RCCs can parasitize blood supply from surrounding structures. Thus, diagnostic arteriography is needed to discover all the potential sources

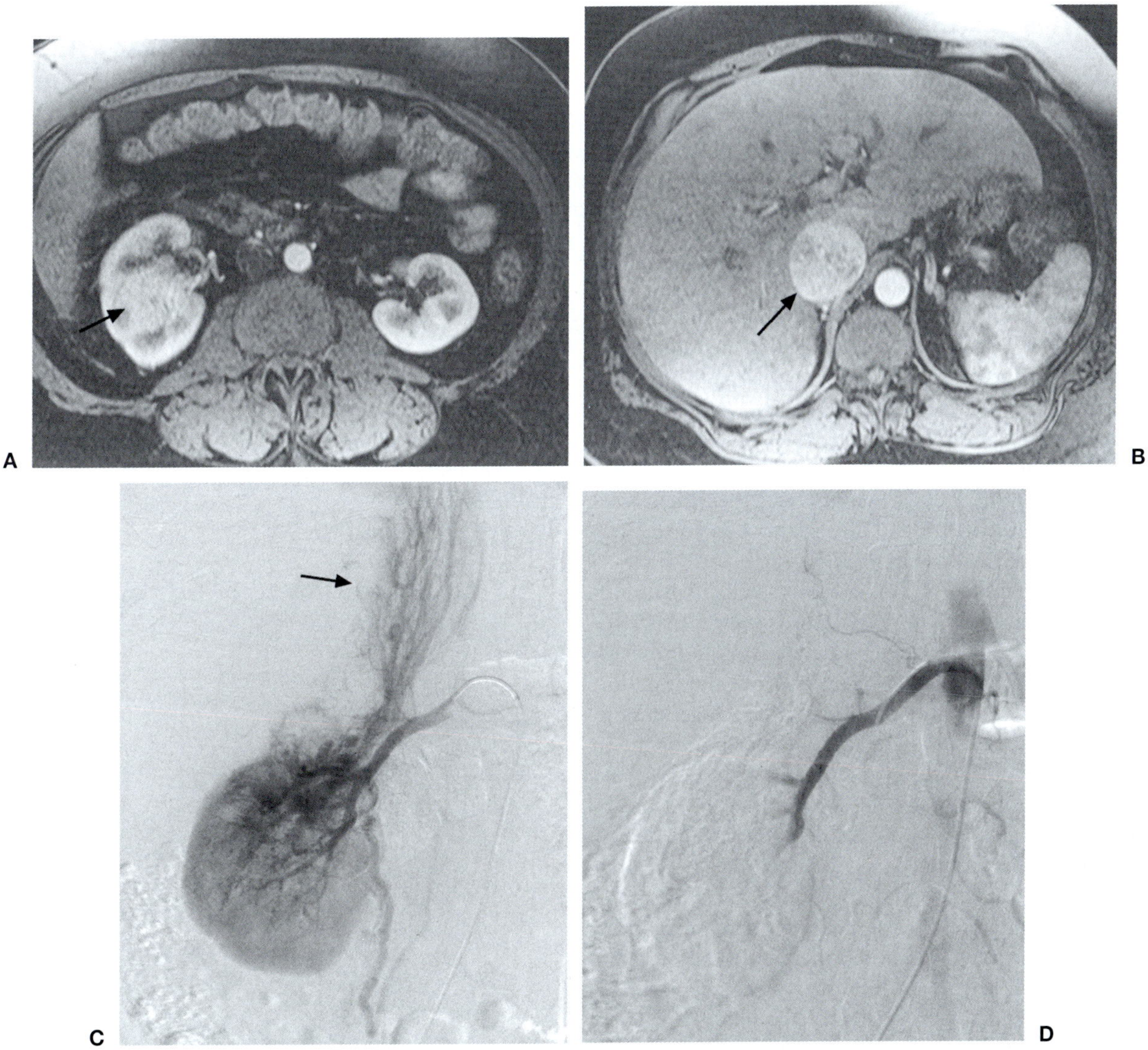

Figure 48.1 **A:** CT showing an RCC (*arrow*) centrally in the right kidney. **B:** More cephalad CT image shows the tumor extends into the intrahepatic portion of the IVC (*arrow*). **C:** Arteriogram showing the tumor vascularity (*arrow*) extending up the IVC. **D:** Arteriogram after preoperative alcohol embolization of the right kidney. In this case, there was no room to deploy an IVC filter above the tumor and the patient did not experience tumor embolization.

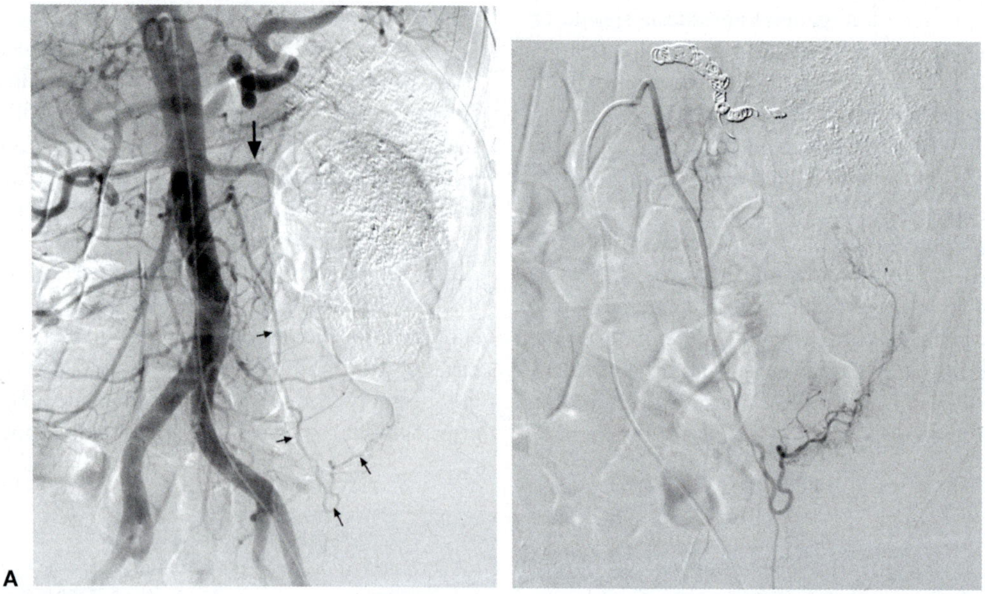

Figure 48.2 **A:** Aortogram in a patient with a left RCC who has persistent hematuria despite prior embolization of the main renal artery. The main renal artery (*large arrow*) only fills proximally, indicating the prior embolization was effective. However, a branch (*small arrows*) off the gonadal artery is seen heading to the lower pole of the kidney. **B:** Selective gonadal arteriogram showing parasitized blood supply to the left renal lower pole.

of blood supply to the tumor. This is best accomplished with a flush aortogram so that all vessels supplying the tumor will be opacified. Alternatively, in cases of very large RCCs with tortuous and distorted vascular anatomy, it may be difficult to see small arteries supplying the RCC because of overlapping larger vessels. Thus, it may be easier to identify smaller arteries supplying the RCC if you first embolize the major vessels supplying the tumor and then perform an aortogram to search for those vessels (Fig. 48.2).

Catheter choice depends on individual patient anatomy. For RCCs involving only a portion of the kidney, microcatheters are used for superselective catheterization to preserve as much normal renal parenchyma as possible. But even for large RCCs that will require embolizing the whole kidney, some prefer to use microcatheters because positioning them very peripherally in the kidney reduces the chance of reflux and nontarget embolization (Fig. 48.3). The downside to microcatheters for larger tumors is that you have to selectively catheterize multiple branches. When dealing with a large RCC that occupies most of the kidney, it is often more expeditious to embolize from a more proximal position in the main renal artery. It is important to make sure the catheter is positioned far enough into the main renal artery to avoid infusing embolic material into the adrenal arteries (Fig. 48.4), which could cause adrenal dysfunction or hypertensive crisis. When using a balloon occlusion catheter, an initial contrast injection is done with the balloon inflated to see what volume of contrast is needed to fill the renal artery. This is done to gauge how much ethanol needs to be injected.

For preoperative devascularization, some interventionalists prefer to just catheterize the main renal artery, inject some PVA peripherally, and then deposit coils in the main renal artery. One caveat is that coils should not be placed too proximally in the renal artery because that can interfere with effective clipping or ligation of the main renal artery during nephrectomy.

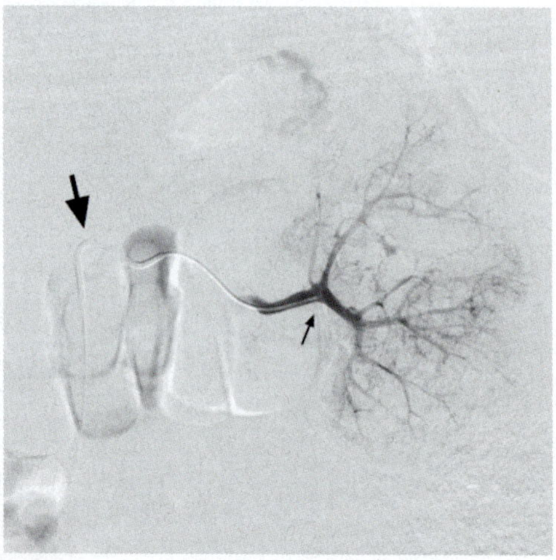

Figure 48.3 Left RCC being embolized through a microcatheter. The catheter tip (*small arrow*) is far away from the main renal artery ostium (*large arrow*) so reflux and nontarget embolization is very unlikely.

CLINICAL OUTCOMES

Embolization for Palliative Therapy of Renal Cell Carcinoma

With laparoscopic surgical techniques or percutaneous ablation, definitive therapy can be accomplished with relatively low risk in most patients. However, there are some patients for whom surgery is still too risky or the tumor is too large to be managed with percutaneous ablation alone. Embolization provides a reasonable alternative in these patients. In solitary kidneys, embolization can also be used as an alternative to surgery to limit loss of functioning parenchyma.

One of the main palliative uses of embolization is relief of symptoms. Serafin et al.[6] reported on 73 patients who underwent palliative embolization of advanced RCCs. In their study, 34% and 32% of patients presented with hematuria or flank pain, respectively. Embolization eliminated hematuria and flank pain in 100% and 72% of cases, respectively.

At least one study has shown that embolization can also significantly prolong survival even when distant metastases are present. Onishi et al.[7] compared matched cohorts with unresectable RCC and distant metastases. Patients who underwent embolization with ethanol had a median survival of 229 days and 1-, 2-, and 3-year survival rates of 29%, 15%, and 10%, respectively. Those not treated with embolization had median survival of 116 days and 1-, 2-, and 3-year survival rates of 13%, 7%, and 3%, respectively. There have been reports of metastases regressing after embolization of the primary tumor.[8] Significant increase in natural killer cell activity has been seen 48 hours after embolization of RCCs.[9] Thus, it has been postulated that embolization can upregulate the immune system's antitumor activity.

Embolization for Rupture of Bleeding

The incidence of spontaneous rupture of RCC is 0.3% to 0.6%. Although radical nephrectomy is typically required in this scenario, embolization may be used to arrest the hemorrhage.[10] Aside from stabilizing the patient by reducing blood loss, embolization also provides an important role by converting an emergent nephrectomy into an elective operation. This provides time to be able to medically prepare the patient for the nephrectomy, which is a major operation. For patients who are not surgical candidates, terminating hemorrhage by embolization can be an important lifesaving palliative procedure.

Embolization can also be used to control hemorrhage after radiofrequency ablation (RFA) of an RCC[11] or when patients develop pseudoaneurysms after partial nephrectomy. The main benefit here is that embolization can selectively occlude the bleeding vessel while preserving most of the normal renal parenchyma, which is particularly useful after surgery or RFA has already removed some of the functioning parenchyma.

When treating a ruptured RCC, a specific bleeding site is not often visible at angiography, thus embolization of the entire RCC is the preferred technique. However, for postoperative or post-RFA bleeding, the goal is to stop the bleeding and not provide any direct tumor therapy. In this setting, extravasation or pseudoaneurysm can often be seen angiographically. Therefore, superselective embolization through microcatheters is optimal.

Embolization before Nephrectomy

RCCs are highly vascular tumors and thus there is great potential for blood loss during resection. Thus, for larger tumors, preoperative embolization may facilitate surgical resection. Although some studies[12] have shown that there is no reduction in blood loss compared to nephrectomy without embolization, other studies have shown that preoperative embolization can significantly reduce intraoperative blood loss.[13]

As mentioned, infarction of RCCs can trigger an immunologic response, which can lead to spontaneous regression of metastases.[14] This has led to the hypothesis that embolization should be done before surgical nephrectomy for the immunologic benefits. However, the results have been somewhat mixed. A Southwest Oncology Group study of 30 patients with metastatic RCC treated by embolization followed by delayed nephrectomy reported no complete remissions and only one partial remission.[15] Also, 1-year survival and median survival was similar to studies in which no therapy was performed. However, more recently, a large study was done in which 118 patients who underwent embolization before nephrectomy were compared to a matched population of 116 patients who were treated with nephrectomy alone.[16] The 5- and 10-year survival rates for patients embolized before nephrectomy was 62% and 47%, respectively, compared to 35% and 23% in patients who were not embolized ($P = .01$).

Embolization as Adjunct to Percutaneous Ablation

Although data are limited, embolization has been used before RFA of RCC. The potential benefit is that devascularizing the tumor should reduce the heat sink effect, which may increase the size of the ablation zone and decrease the chance of local recurrence. It could also reduce the chance of postprocedural hemorrhage and improve visualization of the tumor during computed tomography (CT)–guided puncture. A small pilot[17] study of 10 patients reported no major complication and no recurrences during a mean follow-up of 47 months. Yamakado et al.[18] treated 12 RCCs all larger than 3.5 cm with RFA after arterial embolization. Even though tumor extended into the renal sinus in 10 of 12, tumor enhancement was completely eliminated after just one RFA session in 75% of tumors.[18]

POTENTIAL COMPLICATIONS

The largest series that specifically addressed complications of RCC embolization was the study by Lammer et al.[19] They noted

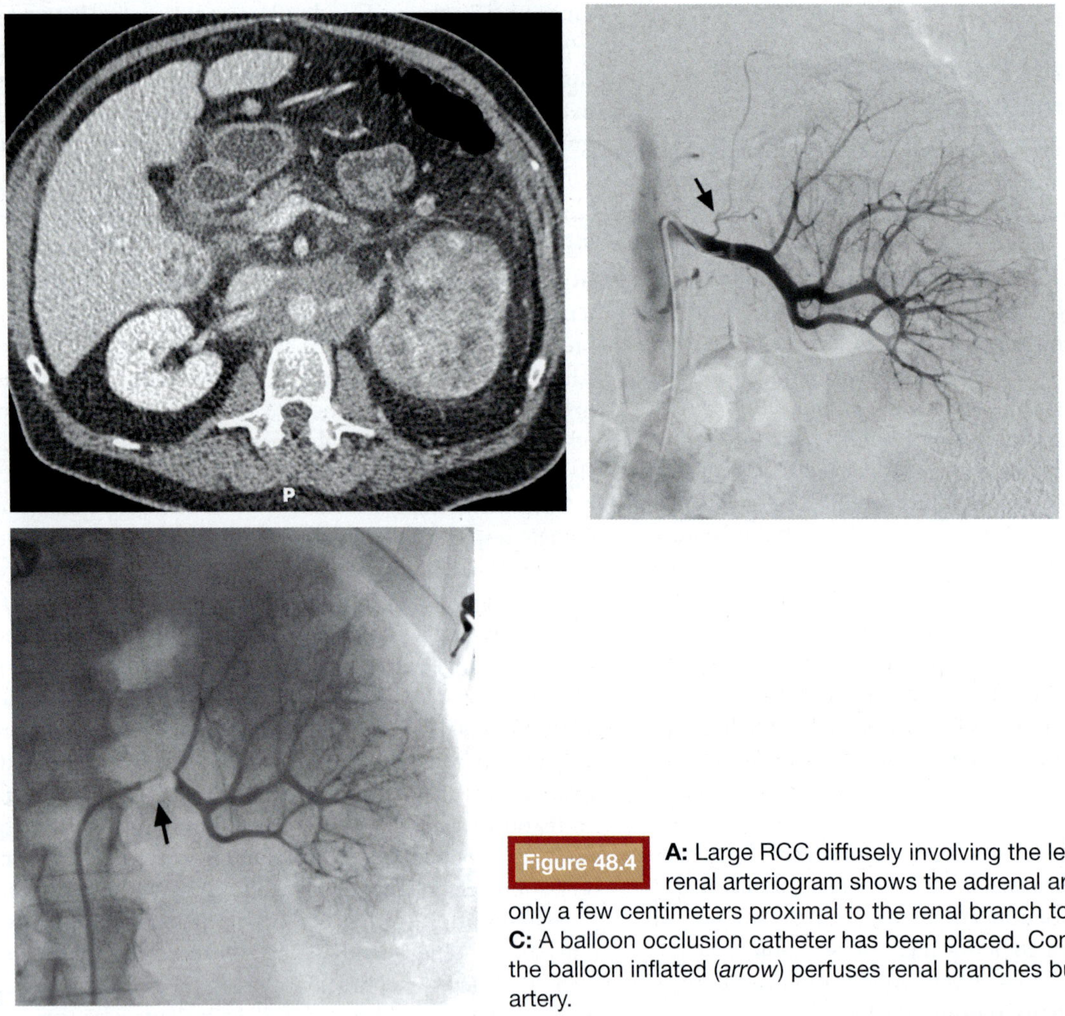

Figure 48.4 **A:** Large RCC diffusely involving the left kidney. **B:** Left renal arteriogram shows the adrenal artery (*arrow*) arising only a few centimeters proximal to the renal branch to the upper pole. **C:** A balloon occlusion catheter has been placed. Contrast injected with the balloon inflated (*arrow*) perfuses renal branches but not the adrenal artery.

an overall complication rate of 9.9%, with a mortality rate of 3.3%. An important finding was that the complication rate was five times higher (20% vs. 4.9%) in patients undergoing embolization for palliative therapy versus those undergoing preoperative embolization. This was attributed to the large mass of the tumors and the poor health of the patients in the palliative group. When combining embolization and RFA, minor complications have been reported in as many as 50% of cases.[17] These included back pain, subcapsular hematomas, hematuria, or nausea and were all self-limited.

Postembolization syndrome is nearly universal and consists predominantly of pain and fever. Fortunately, symptoms are typically limited to the first few days and are managed with supportive care alone. Transient hypertension is also occasionally seen and treated with short-term antihypertensive agents as needed.

One of the major complications is nontarget embolization, which has been seen in as many as 10% of cases, 4% of which were symptomatic embolization to the lower extremities in that series.[6] Two cases of colonic infarction were reported after left renal embolization with ethanol.[20] This was presumably due to reflux from the renal artery to the inferior mesenteric artery. The remarkable thing about this report was that large volumes of ethanol (25 and 20 mL) were injected at a fairly high rate (1.5 to 2 mL per second) without opacification of the ethanol or use of a balloon occlusion catheter.

Other major complications are rare. Although devitalized tumor could be a potential nidus for infection to develop, abscess formation requiring drainage has only rarely been reported.[18] As mentioned earlier, tumor embolization to the lungs can occur. Although rare, it can be catastrophic. Okuda et al.[21] reported a case of fatal massive tumor embolism to pulmonary arteries after an RCC embolization.

TIPS AND TRICKS

- Careful angiography is essential to defining all the arteries supplying the tumor.
- Ethanol is an excellent embolic agent but should either be opacified with Ethiodol or injected with a balloon occlusion catheter to prevent nontarget embolization.
- Embolization can be used as an adjunct to increase the efficacy of RFA.

REFERENCES

1. Almgard LE, Fernstrom I, Haverling M, et al. Treatment of renal adenocarcinoma by embolic occlusion of the renal circulation. *Br J Urol.* 1973;45(5):474–479.
2. Wright KC, Loh G, Wallace S, et al. Experimental evaluation of ethanol-ethiodol for transcatheter renal embolization. *Cardiovasc Intervent Radiol.* 1990;13(5):309–313.
3. Hirota S, Matsumoto S, Ichikawa S, et al. Suprarenal inferior vena cava filter placement prior to transcatheter arterial embolization (TAE) of a renal cell carcinoma with large renal vein tumor thrombus: prevention of pulmonary tumor emboli after TAE. *Cardiovasc Intervent Radiol.* 1997;20(2):139–141.
4. Zamora CA, Sugimoto K, Mori T, et al. Prophylactic stenting of the inferior vena cava before transcatheter embolization of renal cell carcinomas: an alternative to filter placement. *J Endovasc Ther.* 2004;11(1):84–88.
5. Mondshine RT, Owens S, Mondschein JI, et al. Combination embolization and radiofrequency ablation therapy for renal cell carcinoma in the setting of coexisting arterial disease. *J Vasc Interv Radiol.* 2008;19(4):616–620.
6. Serafin Z, Karolkiewicz M, Strzesniewski P, et al. Palliative percutaneous kidney embolization with enbucrilate in patients with renal cell carcinoma: safety and symptom control. *Med Sci Monit.* 2007;13(suppl 1):98–104.
7. Onishi T, Oishi Y, Suzuki Y, et al. Prognostic evaluation of transcatheter arterial embolization for unresectable renal cell carcinoma with distant metastasis. *BJU Int.* 2001;87(4):312–315.
8. Munro NP, Woodhams S, Nawrocki JD, et al. The role of transarterial embolization in the treatment of renal cell carcinoma. *BJU Int.* 2003;92(3):240–244.
9. Bakke A, Gothlin JH, Haukaas SA, et al. Augmentation of natural killer cell activity after arterial embolization of renal carcinomas. *Cancer Res.* 1982;42(9):3880–3883.
10. Watanabe S, Hama Y, Kaji T, et al. Pre-operative embolization for spontaneous rupture of renal cell carcinoma. *Ulster Med J.* 2005;74(1):66–67.
11. Roach H, Whittlestone T, Callaway MP. Life-threatening hematuria requiring transcatheter embolization following radiofrequency ablation of renal cell carcinoma. *Cardiovasc Intervent Radiol.* 2006;29(4):672–674.
12. Lanigan D, Jurriaans E, Hammonds JC, et al. The current status of embolization in renal cell carcinoma—a survey of local and national practice. *Clin Radiol.* 1992;46(3):176–178.
13. Bakal CW, Cynamon J, Lakritz PS, et al. Value of preoperative renal artery embolization in reducing blood transfusion requirements during nephrectomy for renal cell carcinoma. *J Vasc Interv Radiol.* 1993;4(6):727–731.
14. Mohr SJ, Whitesel JA. Spontaneous regression of renal cell carcinoma metastases after preoperative embolization of primary tumor and subsequent nephrectomy. *Urology.* 1979;14(1):5–8.
15. Gottesman JE, Crawford ED, Grossman HB, et al. Infarction-nephrectomy for metastatic renal carcinoma. Southwest oncology group study. *Urology.* 1985;25(3):248–250.
16. Zielinski H, Szmigielski S, Petrovich Z. Comparison of preoperative embolization followed by radical nephrectomy with radical nephrectomy alone for renal cell carcinoma. *Am J Clin Oncol.* 2000;23(1):6–12.
17. Nakasone Y, Kawanaka K, Ikeda O, et al. Sequential combination treatment (arterial embolization and percutaneous radiofrequency ablation) of inoperable renal cell carcinoma: single-center pilot study. *Acta Radiol.* 2012;53(4):410–414.
18. Yamakado K, Nakatsuka A, Kobayashi S, et al. Radiofrequency ablation combined with renal arterial embolization for the treatment of unresectable renal cell carcinoma larger than 3.5 cm: initial experience. *Cardiovasc Intervent Radiol.* 2006;29(3):389–394.
19. Lammer J, Justich E, Schreyer H, et al. Complications of renal tumor embolization. *Cardiovasc Intervent Radiol.* 1985;8(1):31–35.
20. Cox GG, Lee KR, Price HI, et al. Colonic infarction following ethanol embolization of renal-cell carcinoma. *Radiology.* 1982;145(2):343–345.
21. Okuda H, Toda F, Ito F, et al. A case of sudden death by pulmonary embolism after angio-embolization of renal cell carcinoma extending into the inferior vena cava [in Japanese]. *Hinyokika Kiyo.* 1999;45(1):49–51.

49

Renal Angiomyolipomas

Gregory Nadolski • S. William Stavropoulos

Angiomyolipomas (AMLs) are a benign neoplasm of the kidney composed of varying mixtures of adipose, muscle, and vascular tissues. Although benign, the vasculature within these tumors develops abnormally and may spontaneously hemorrhage. The incidence of massive spontaneous hemorrhage increases with the degree of vascularity and size of the AML. Spontaneous massive hemorrhage can be managed with emergent nephrectomy. More recently, transarterial embolization has emerged as a preferred nephron-sparing option. To prevent the complication of hemorrhage, renal AMLs have been historically removed using nephrectomy or partial nephrectomy. More recently, prophylactic embolization of AMLs has become the treatment of choice to prevent AML hemorrhage once the tumor has grown to a sufficient size. In this chapter, the surveillance and treatment of AMLs will be discussed with a focus on indications, techniques, and outcomes of percutaneous transarterial embolization.

BACKGROUND

Histopathology and Epidemiology

Originally believed to be hamartomas with abnormal proliferation of tissues normally present in the kidney, AMLs are now classified as neoplasms of adipose, vascular, and smooth muscle tissue.[1] These lesions arise from clonal proliferation of perivascular epithelioid cells, which first develop into small nodules of spindle cells within the capsule, cortex, or medulla of the kidney.[1] As these neoplasms grow, they may develop into one of two basic forms of AML: typical and epithelioid.

First described in 1900 by Grawitz, typical AMLs consist of varying amounts of adipose, vascular, and smooth muscle tissue.[2] The blood vessels within typical AMLs are structurally abnormal. They contain no internal elastic lamina, and the smooth muscle of their media is replaced by fibrous tissue. Thus, the vascular tissue of AMLs is tortuous, rigid, and prone to microaneurysm and macroaneurysm formation.[3] The epithelioid variant has little if any adipose tissue and few blood vessels. Instead, this variant is composed almost entirely of epithelioid cells and behaves more aggressively than typical AMLs.[2] Given the difficulty in differentiating epithelioid AMLs on imaging from other solid renal neoplasms such as renal cell carcinoma, epithelioid AMLs are almost exclusively managed surgically, and the diagnosis is often suspected clinically and confirmed postoperatively.[4] Because epithelioid AMLs are rare and the imaging features and biologic behavior are different from typical AMLs, the subsequent discussion of AMLs will refer only to the typical variety.

Renal AMLs may occur sporadically or in association with tuberous sclerosis complex or lymphangioleiomyomatosis (LAM).[2] The overall incidence of sporadic renal AMLs is now thought to be more common than once appreciated, with a frequency of about 13 per 10,000 adults (0.13%).[1] Autopsy data from individuals without stigmata of TSC has demonstrated frequencies of 0.02% of males and 0.29% of females in the total population.[5] Similarly, ultrasound screening of healthy individuals for incidental AMLs have demonstrated an incidence of 0.1% in males and 0.22% in females.[6] Although some speculate the differences in incidence between sexes may be related to fewer males in most studies, others suggest the consistently observed higher frequency in females may be related to hormonal differences, which has been supported by the frequent presence of estrogen and progesterone receptors within AMLs.[7]

Tuberous sclerosis, also known as *tuberous sclerosis complex* (TSC), is a rare autosomal dominantly inherited multisystem disease characterized by tumors in the brain, kidneys, heart, lungs, and skin, which classically presents in childhood with seizures, developmental delay, behavioral problems, and skin abnormalities. These patients are prone to forming cysts, AMLs, and malignant neoplasms in the kidney. AMLs can be detected in children with TSC, and the number and size of these lesions continue to progress as the patient ages. Autopsy data on patients with TSC suggest the incidence of AMLs in this population may approach 67%.[8]

Clinical Symptoms and Indications for Intervention

Although renal AMLs may be asymptomatic, they typically manifest clinically in one of two ways. First, patients may present with spontaneous, nontraumatic renal hemorrhage, which when confined to the subcapsular and perirenal space is referred to as *Wunderlich syndrome* (Fig. 49.1). Alternatively, and much less commonly, AMLs may slowly and progressively invade the normal renal parenchyma, resulting in renal failure.[9,10] The latter manifestation is usually confined to patients with syndromes resulting in numerous renal AMLs, whereas hemorrhage may occur in either sporadic or syndromic AMLs. Although benign, renal AMLs rarely can invade the renal vein and inferior vena cava, placing the individual at risk for caval thrombosis and pulmonary embolism.[4,11] This rare presentation of typical AMLs is most commonly associated with tumors measuring greater than 9.5 cm in diameter and found in women.

Hemorrhage within an AML results from rupture of microaneurysms and macroaneurysms within the tumor vasculature, which can subsequently bleed into the retroperitoneum. Other less common symptoms of AML include pain, flank mass, and hematuria.[12] Overall, symptoms occur in 73% of patients with sporadic AMLs and 64% of patients with TSC-related AMLs, and hemorrhage is the presenting symptom in 14% and 44% of patients with sporadic and TSC renal AMLs, respectively.[12]

The risk of hemorrhage within an AML has been associated with both overall size of the AML as well as the size of the aneurysms within them. Most clinicians use overall size greater than 4 cm as an indication for prophylactic embolization, which has been supported by several studies. In a review of 253 AMLs, Oesterling et al.[13] found 82% of AMLs with a diameter of 4 cm or larger were symptomatic, whereas only 23% of tumors smaller than 4 cm were symptomatic. Furthermore, of all symptomatic AMLs, 90% were at least 4 cm in diameter. Over half of AMLs 4 cm or larger bled, and one-third of the patients with acute hemorrhage presented in shock.[13] Similarly, based on retrospective review of computed tomography (CT) of 29 kidneys with AMLs, 8 with and 21 without hemorrhage, tumor size larger than 4 cm and aneurysm size equal to 5 mm or larger were present in all hemorrhagic lesions.[14] However, in this same study, aneurysm size of 5 mm or greater was more specific for tumor hemorrhage than overall size (86% vs. 38%), although both metrics had 100% specificity.[14] Other series have shown no difference in the size of AMLs in patients who were treated after presenting with flank pain compared to those presenting with hemorrhage, further supporting the theory that aneurysm size is more important than overall AML size in determining risk of hemorrhage.[15] Interestingly, size greater than 4 cm at presentation has been shown to correlate with a higher rate of subsequent growth (46% vs. 27%) and higher likelihood for eventual intervention (53.8% vs. 7%) compared to smaller AMLs, underscoring the value of the 4-cm threshold for intervening on asymptomatic AMLs.

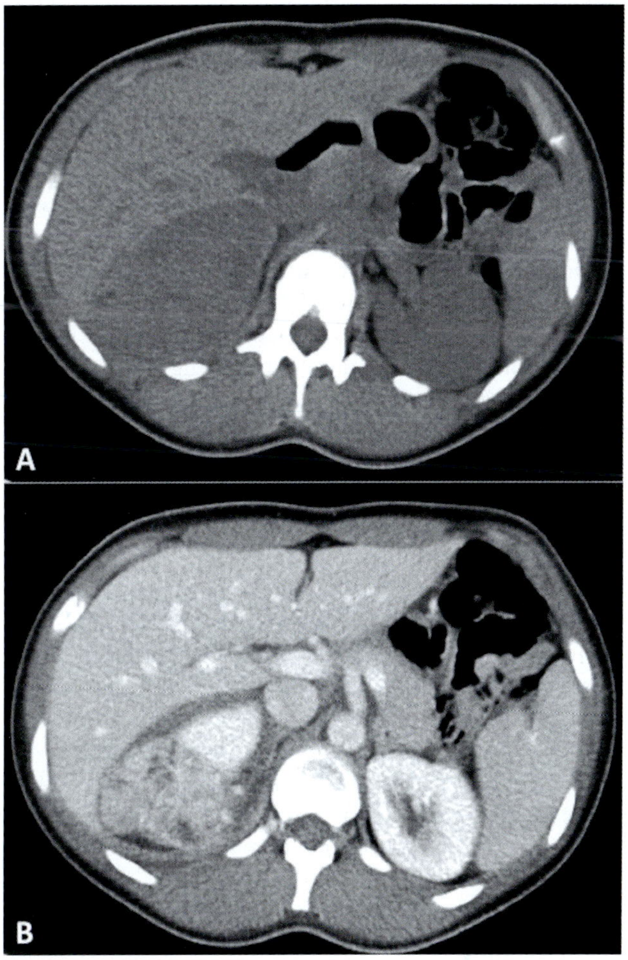

Figure 49.1 Spontaneous nontraumatic right perinephric hemorrhage secondary to angiomyolipoma. The perinephric space contains complex or high-attenuation fluid consistent with acute hemorrhage on unenhanced CT **(A)**. Following the administration of contrast, a heterogeneously enhancing mass containing macroscopic fat consistent with an AML is visualized **(B)**.

Management and Treatment Options

Whereas all symptomatic AMLs are treated to alleviate symptoms, asymptomatic AMLs can be managed with surveillance until growth in size or development of aneurysmal vascularity necessitates intervention because these neoplasms have no malignant potential. Regardless of the method of intervention, optimum treatment requires preservation of renal function.[15] Originally, surgical intervention, either total or partial nephrectomy, was employed to prevent hemorrhage. Subsequently, percutaneous embolization was developed to offer a minimally invasive nephron-sparing approach to management. Recently, oral medications targeting the mammalian target of rapamycin (mTOR) have shown promise in slowing or regressing the growth of AMLs. Following a discussion of imaging and imaging surveillance, medical and surgical options for treating AMLs will be discussed briefly, followed by detailed discussion of AML embolization technique and outcomes.

Diagnostic Imaging Techniques and Surveillance

When imaging a potential AML, the most important consideration is differentiating an AML from a malignant renal neoplasm. The distinction is particularly important for small masses because management of asymptomatic AMLs less than 4 cm involves imaging surveillance, whereas a malignancy would be managed with surgery or ablation. AMLs can be diagnosed using ultrasound, CT, or magnetic resonance imaging (MRI). In all three modalities, the diagnosis is primarily based on detection of macroscopic fat within a renal mass.

Classically on ultrasound, the fat-containing AMLs appear as a strongly hyperechoic mass with acoustic shadowing. However, lipid-poor AMLs are isoechoic and difficult to differentiate from adjacent parenchyma.[16–18] Furthermore, there is significant overlap in the ultrasound appearance of AMLs with that of renal cell carcinoma, particularly for lesions less than 3 cm, which limits its use in the surveillance of presumed AMLs.[18,19] Color and power Doppler have been used to improve the diagnostic accuracy of ultrasound for the detection of AMLs, but the diagnostic accuracy only approaches 83% for lesions measuring under 3 cm.[20] Although ultrasound can detect hemorrhage in the perinephric space with great sensitivity, it may not be able to definitively diagnose the presence of an AML in the acute setting, which would require further evaluation with CT or MRI.

Because there is significant overlap of the ultrasound features of AML and renal cell carcinoma, CT is often the preferred method of diagnosing AMLs. The diagnosis of AML by CT depends on visualizing macroscopic fat characterized by a negative Hounsfield unit (Fig. 49.1); however, other renal masses can contain fat, including renal cell carcinoma.[16] Classically, AMLs appear as predominantly fatty masses similar in attenuation to the subcutaneous or retroperitoneal fat with various amounts of soft tissue scattered within it. However, the exact appearance of an AML depends on the exact proportion of the adipose, vascular, and smooth muscle tissue.[13,16,21] If large areas of macroscopic fat cannot readily be visualized, use of thinner sections or pixel mapping can improve detection of fat within the mass.[22,23] Although renal cell carcinoma has been reported to rarely contain fat, this is believed to be either secondary to tumor necrosis or trapping of renal sinus fat.[24,25] Differentiating lipid-poor AMLs from renal cell carcinoma can be more challenging, but multiphase contrast-enhanced CT can be used to differentiate the two. The best predictor of a lipid-poor AML on CT is homogeneous prolonged enhancement, which has a positive predictive value of 91%.[18] Last, CT is particularly useful in the setting of acutely symptomatic AMLs as it can accurately detect perinephric hemorrhage, possibly identify aneurysms within the mass, and distinguish AMLs from other sources of flank pain such as urolithiasis and pyelonephritis.

MRI is particularly well suited at detecting both macroscopic and microscopic fat with high accuracy, making it an ideal imaging modality for diagnosing and following AMLs. Classically, the presence of macroscopic fat in the mass can be imaged by assessing differences in signal intensity between fat-suppressed and non–fat-suppressed sequences. Alternatively, opposed-phase imaging, which typically is used to detect intracellular lipid in adrenal adenomas, can be used to characterize AMLs and differentiate them from renal cell carcinoma (Fig. 49.2). In particular, when using opposed-phase imaging, an India ink or etching artifact occurs because the presence of fat and water protons within the same voxel results in signal loss at fat–water interfaces. In a retrospective study, Israel et al.[26] found 100% of the 23 AMLs studied demonstrated an India ink artifact between the AML and the adjacent normal renal parenchyma, allowing correct diagnosis in all cases while only mischaracterizing a single small renal cell carcinoma. Of note, the clear cell subtype of renal cell carcinoma is known to lose signal on opposed-phase imaging because of the presence of intracellular lipid; however, these lesions do not lose signal on fat-suppressed sequences. In their series, Israel et al.[26] examined two clear cell renal cell carcinomas, neither of which demonstrated India ink artifact. Last, although lipid-poor AMLs do not contain a focus of macroscopic fat, these tumors do contain enough fat to be detected using chemical-shift imaging even if fat could not be detected on CT.[27,28]

Although all three modalities are acceptable for diagnosing AML, at our institution MRI is typically used to confirm the diagnosis, to perform active surveillance of incidental AMLs less than 4 cm, and to assess treatment response. MRI is particularly useful in patients with TSC. Following multiple interventions on multiple AMLs, these patients may have baseline chronic kidney disease, making contrast-enhanced CT less feasible. Although there is no consensus on how frequently surveillance imaging should be performed, asymptomatic AMLs less than 4 cm tend to remain stable in size and may be observed; thus, yearly surveillance is sufficient.[29–31] This has been supported by additional investigations of a series of 91 patients with AML of which 73

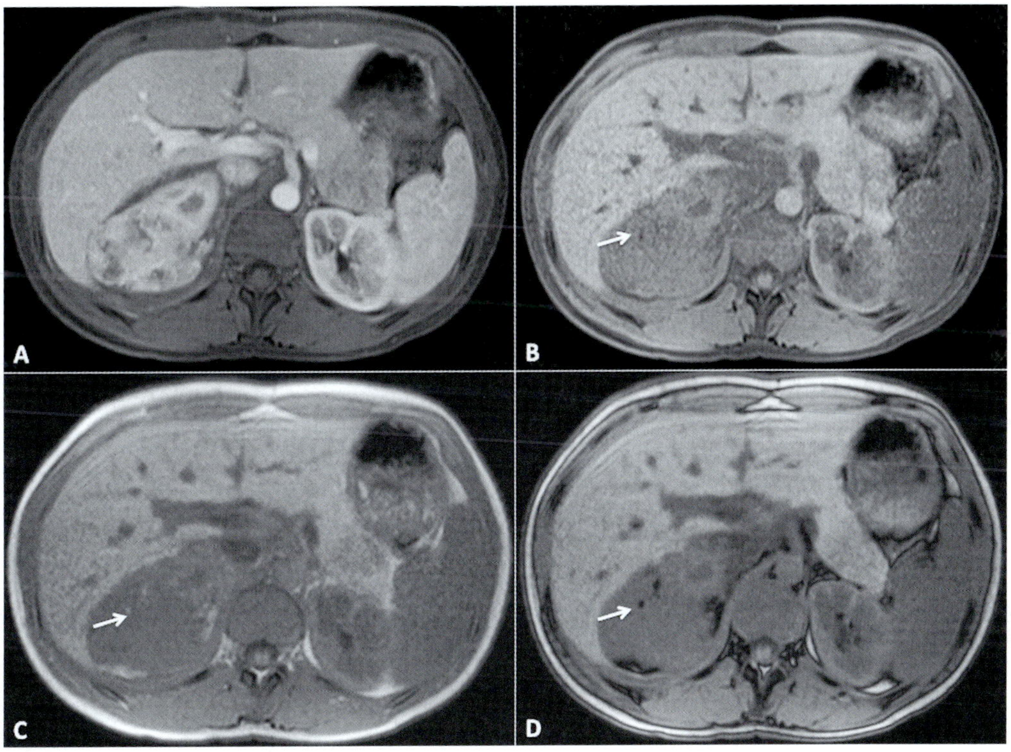

Figure 49.2 MRI of angiomyolipoma. Postcontrast T1 weighted sequences **(A)** show a hypervascular mass in the right kidney. Macroscopic fat is present in a right renal mass, which is seen as loss of signal intensity (*arrow*) between fat-suppressed precontrast T1 weighted image **(B)** and the in-phase non–fat-suppressed gradient echo sequence **(C)**. Alternatively, opposed-phase gradient echo imaging **(D)** shows an India ink or artifact at fat–water interface (*arrow*).

were incidentally identified.[32] In this series, 45 of the patients had small AMLs, which were observed with surveillance imaging. The mean AML growth rate was 0.09 cm per year.[32] Three patients failed surveillance and underwent intervention, two with spontaneous hemorrhage and one with rapid growth of 0.7 cm per year. Periodic surveillance imaging of asymptomatic AMLs less than 4 cm appears to have low risk of failure given the relative stability of small AMLs. However, failure can occur, and given the incidence of hemorrhage in larger AMLs, asymptomatic lesions greater than 4 cm should undergo prophylactic elective treatment, which will be discussed subsequently.

Surgical and Medical Management of Angiomyolipomas

Surgical options to manage AMLs include total and partial nephrectomy. Partial nephrectomy has shown a similar success rate (near 100%) as total nephrectomy in treating AMLs without increased incidence of local recurrence during follow-up.[12,32] Additionally, patients undergoing partial nephrectomy have been shown to have a significantly lower incidence of developing stage 3 or greater chronic kidney disease (defined as glomerular filtration rate <60 mL per minute) compared to those treated with total nephrectomy.[33] However, despite the improvements in postprocedure renal function with partial nephrectomy, this procedure carries a total complication rate ranging between 5% and 23%.[12,34] Additionally, the rate of conversion from partial to total nephrectomy may be higher when resecting AMLs compared to other lesions, although small series of laparoscopic partial nephrectomy showed no difference in complication rates or blood loss between AML and other renal neoplasms.[34,35] Last, some studies suggest embolization of AMLs is preferable to partial nephrectomy in cases of acute hemorrhage and multifocal disease because of more rapid symptom control and better preservation of renal function, respectively.[36] Alternatively, radiofrequency ablation (RFA), either laparoscopic or percutaneous image guided, has been employed as a less invasive nephron-sparing approach with outcomes similar to partial nephrectomy with possibly a reduction in complications.[37]

Although embolization or resection is the current standard of care for AMLs, which are symptomatic or greater than 4 cm, recent investigations of medical therapy using mTOR inhibitors have shown promise in causing regression of AML size. Additionally, investigators have begun employing multimodality therapy combining pretreatment with the mTOR inhibitor sirolimus followed by partial nephrectomy to further preserve posttreatment renal function.[38]

Once medical treatment is stopped, AMLs can continue to grow. In addition, long-term studies involving the effectiveness of medical therapy at decreasing the incidence of AML bleeding have not been done.

EMBOLIZATION MATERIALS AND TECHNIQUE

Renal Arteriography

Knowledge of the classic anatomy and variations of the renal vessels is important in the planning before AML embolization. Careful evaluation of preprocedural CT or MRI can be helpful in identifying variant anatomy.

Normally, the renal arteries arise from the abdominal aorta, below the origin of the superior mesenteric artery, typically at the level between the superior endplate of L1 and the inferior endplate of L2. Both renal arteries originate at the anterolateral aspect of the abdominal aorta, best profiled using a 10- to 30-degree left anterior oblique (LAO) projection. Near the renal hilum, each renal artery divides into an anterior and a posterior branch, which in turn divide into upper, middle, and lower pole segmental arteries. The segmental vessels bifurcate into lobar arteries, which penetrate the renal parenchyma and divide into the interlobar arteries. The interlobar arteries course between the renal pyramids and give rise to the arcuate arteries running parallel to the kidney surface. The arcuate arteries supply the interlobular arteries, which become the afferent arterioles entering the glomeruli.

Two types of variant renal arteries exist. Early division is a variant in which branching of the main renal arteries occurs more proximally than the hilum. The second type of variant is known as *extrarenal arteries* and can be further divided into two groups: accessory and aberrant arteries. Accessory arteries enter the kidney from the hilum along with the main renal artery, whereas aberrant arteries enter the kidney directly from the capsule, outside of the hilum. Accessory renal arteries are the most common and most clinically relevant vascular variant occurring in up to 30% of patient. Multiple renal arteries are unilateral in 30% of patients and bilateral in 10%. These accessory renal arteries usually arise from the aorta or iliac arteries anywhere from the level of T11 to the level of the L4 vertebra. In rare cases, these arteries can arise from other abdominopelvic or mesenteric arteries.[39]

Ethanol Plus Lipiodol Technique

Transarterial embolization of AML, performed under moderate sedation using fentanyl and midazolam, commonly employs the use of a mixture of ethiodized oil and ethanol mixed in a ratio of 3:7.[40,41] Before the procedure, intravenous antibiotics, such as cefazolin 1 g, are administered before the procedure. After obtaining arterial access and placing a 5-Fr vascular sheath, an abdominal aortogram is obtained using a flush catheter positioned immediately inferior to the superior mesenteric artery to define the renal arterial anatomy using a 20 mL per second injection for a total volume of 20 mL. After aortography, selective renal catheterization is performed typically with a 5-Fr Cobra 2 catheter (Boston Scientific, Marlborough, Massachusetts) or a 5-Fr Sos reverse curve catheter (Angiodynamics, Latham, New York). If engaging or maintaining access to the renal origin is difficult secondary to atherosclerotic disease at the renal artery origin, tortuosity of the iliac vessels, or the obliquity of the renal artery origin, a long curved vascular sheath or alternative catheters such as the RC-2 (Angiodynamics, Latham, New York), Simmons, or Levin catheters (Cook Medical, Inc., Bloomington, Indiana) may be used to engage the origin or to better support access.

Selective renal arteriography is then performed using a 5 to 6 mL per second rate to determine the number of vessels feeding the AML (Fig. 49.3). Through the 5-Fr catheter, a high-flow 3-Fr microcatheter is advanced over a wire into a vessel supplying the tumor so that the microcatheter is distal to any branches supplying normal renal parenchyma. The guidewire is removed, and contrast material is injected to verify position using digital subtraction imaging. Additionally, the rate of contrast material injection is used to estimate the rate of Ethiodol/ethanol mixture injection, which can be used without causing reflux and nontarget embolization. At a separate sterile table designated for the embolic materials, the Ethiodol is mixed with the ethanol in a 3:7 ratio of Ethiodol to ethanol using polycarbonate syringes and metal three-way stopcocks. The feeding artery is then embolized until stasis is achieved. Postembolization control angiography is performed to determine the degree of embolization with the goal end points of occluding the arterial branches supplying the tumor and nonopacification of the tumor itself (Fig. 49.4). If residual tumor vascularity is visualized, additional Ethiodol/ethanol can be injected in the manner described earlier until satisfactory stasis is achieved. Additional branches supplying the mass can be catheterized selectively and the process repeated until the entire tumor is embolized.

After embolization, patients are often admitted overnight for close monitoring, pain control, and observation for immediate complications. Some centers discharge patients after a 4-to 6-hour postprocedure observation period based on the degree of symptoms they are experiencing. After discharge, follow-up clinical evaluation and posttreatment imaging are performed 1 month, 6 months, 12 months, and 24 months after the procedure. At these visits, postprocedure labs including serum creatinine are obtained. Subsequent visits and imaging occur at 12-month intervals for patients with syndromic AMLs and 24-month intervals for sporadic AMLs, assuming the patient does not have a recurrence.

During posttreatment imaging, the AML may not decrease in overall size. Reduction in size is felt to depend on the volume of fat within the AML. The muscle and vascular tissues within the AML typically regress after embolization, whereas the hypovascular adipose tissue does not.[40,42,43] Thus, an AML with little fat would be expected to decrease in

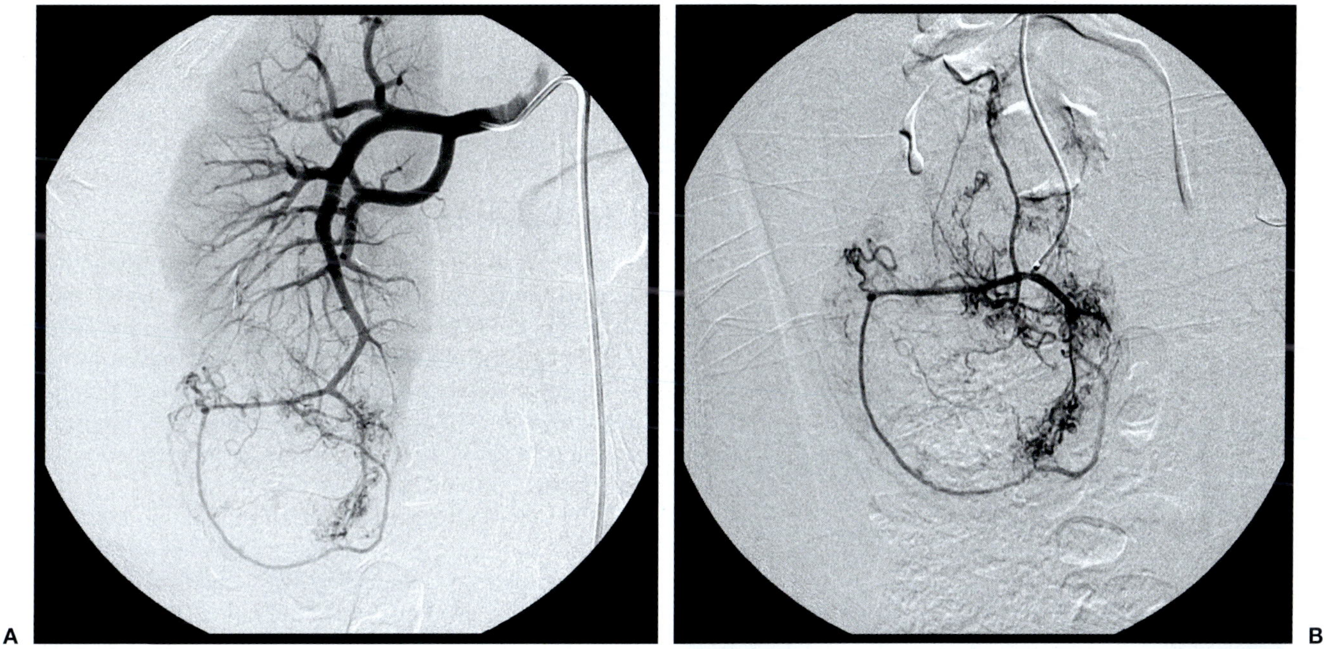

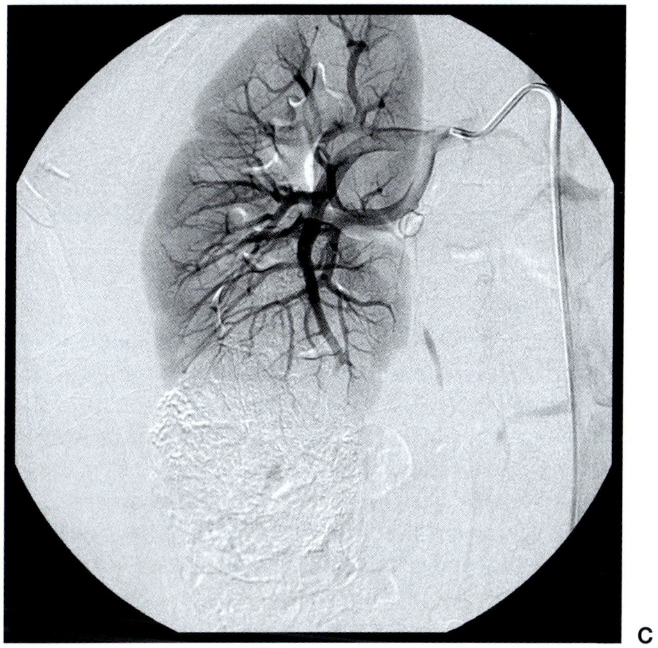

Figure 49.3 Selective renal arteriogram demonstrates the vascular supply to a left lower pole AML **(A)**. Selective arteriography of the feeding artery selected with 3-Fr high-flow microcatheter confirms a single artery that supplies the AML **(B)**. Tortuous, abnormal internal vasculature is demonstrated within the AML. From this position, 3:7 Ethiodol/ethanol mixture can be safely delivered while sparing normal renal parenchyma **(C)**.

size to a greater extent than a lipid-rich AML of equal size. Overall, on posttreatment imaging, approximately 43% to 70% of AMLs show a reduction in tumor size.[41,43–45]

OUTCOMES OF ETHANOL PLUS LIPIODOL

Ethanol Plus Lipiodol Technique

Sole treatment of AMLs with embolization is safe and effective. Early investigations suggested a clinical success rate of 90% in a group of patients with a mean follow-up period of 21 months.[46] In this study, no complications occurred at the authors' institution. However, review of the reported literature identified several serious periprocedural complications including two cases of aneurysm rupture and two necrotic tumors requiring percutaneous drainage.[46]

Subsequently, a review of selective arterial embolization using ethanol mixed with iodized oil to treat 30 AMLs in 19 patients, 10 of which had TSC, demonstrated the long-term efficacy of this technique, particularly in cases of sporadic AML.[40] Using the 3:7 Ethiodol/ethanol mixture, all tumors were completely embolized to vascular stasis. AML recurrence, defined as an increase in tumor size of greater than 2 cm on follow-up imaging and/or recurrent symp-

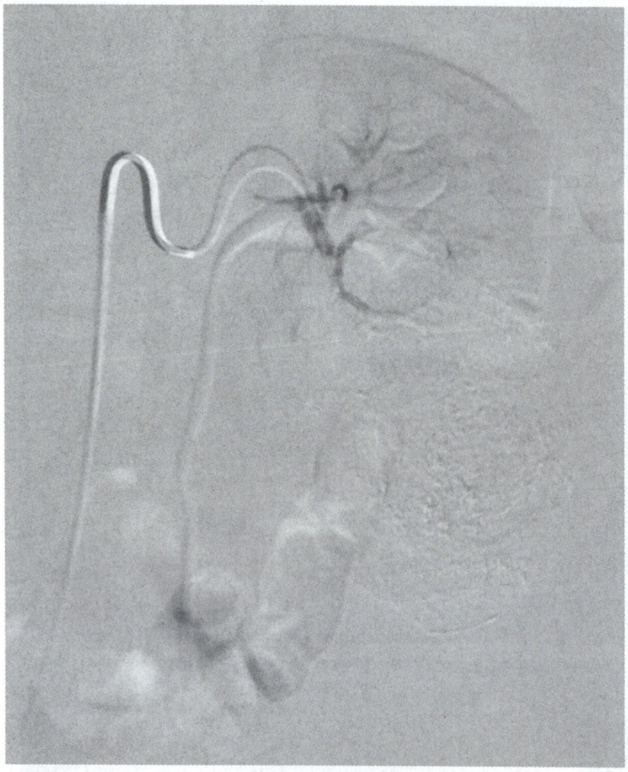

Figure 49.4 Selective postembolization control arteriography of the feeding artery selected with 3-Fr high-flow microcatheter confirms stasis in the feeding artery and nonopacification of the AML.

toms, occurred in 30% of lesions overall. Importantly, all of the recurrences occurred in patients with TSC, whereas no recurrences occurred in the patients with sporadic AML. In the 10 patients with TSC, there was a total of 21 AMLs, and the overall tumor recurrence rate was 42.9%. Six of these lesions had to be reembolized for recurrent symptoms, including one hemorrhage, and three lesions in two patients required repeat embolization because of a greater than 2 cm increase in size. The median time interval from embolization to recurrence was 78.7 months (range, 13 to 132 months). Statistical analysis revealed patients with TSC were significantly more likely to develop recurrence after embolization than those without TSC.[40] Thus, the authors concluded Ethiodol/ethanol mixture is safe and effective therapy for AMLs, and lifelong surveillance for recurrence after AML embolization is essential in patients with TSC.

Likewise, investigation of using the 3:7 Ethiodol/ethanol mixture to embolize giant AMLs, those greater than 10 cm, demonstrated similar efficacy.[41] Embolization was technically successful in all cases in the 16 patients treated, 6 of whom underwent planned staged embolizations in multiple sessions to initially treat the AML. During follow-up, only one AML recurred with an increase in size by 2 cm.[41] Overall, 2 of the 16 patients in this series required repeat embolization, 1 for regrowth and 1 for reperfusion seen on surveillance imaging. Last, only 1 of the 16 patients had an AML hemorrhage, which occurred 59 months after AML embolization, supporting the efficacy of this technique in managing giant AMLs.[41]

Alternative Embolic Materials

Alternatives to the 3:7 mixture of Ethiodol to ethanol have been explored. In general, permanent particulate embolics or liquid embolics can be used for AML embolization. Sole therapy with coils and vascular plugs should be avoided as collateral vessels can form distal to the site of occlusion to supply the AML.[41] However, coils may be employed in conjunction with particulate embolics in cases with large aneurysms.

One alternative is a less dilute form of Ethiodol/ethanol mixture. For example, Lee et al.[44] performed selective embolization of 21 symptomatic AMLs ranging in size from 6 to 15 cm using a 1:3 mixture of iodized oil and ethanol. All the lesions were successfully embolized, with only 2 patients requiring repeat embolization and without major complications.[44] Some investigators primarily use an Ethiodol/ethanol mixture and supplement with adjuncts such as polyvinyl alcohol (PVA) and coils.[45] Using a 1:2 mixture of Ethiodol/ethanol to treat 34 patients supplemented with PVA in 2 patients and coils in 3, Chick et al.[45] achieved a 97% radiologic success rate, with only one lesion growing by greater than 2 cm, and a clinical success rate of 85%, with 2 patients undergoing surgery and 2 having repeat embolization. PVA was used in 2 patients to reduce alcohol volumes and obtain effective embolization, whereas coils were used in 3 patients who had large aneurysms in the AML, which were felt to be unsuitable for alcohol or particle embolization techniques alone.[45]

Other centers use particulate embolization to treat AMLs, sometimes routinely mixed with alcohol and less commonly supplemented with coil embolization. PVA, which must be sized according to the size of aneurysms and vasculature within the AML (typically ranging between 200 and 700 μm), can be used alone or with adjuncts. One concern of using PVA alone is reports of a postembolization hemorrhage rate of 23% to 40%.[47] The addition of absolute ethanol to PVA appears to minimize the risk of postembolization hemorrhage observed with PVA alone.[48,49] Embolization with a mixture of 96% ethanol and PVA particles has a high initial technical success rate up to 94%.[48] Follow-up of AMLs treated with this technique have shown frequent reduction in tumor size (67%), preservation of renal function, and avoidance of surgical intervention to treat the AML.[48,49] Recurrence and need for retreatment may be slightly greater than the Ethiodol/ethanol mixture technique. Ramon et al. found 37% of cases treated with ethanol and PVA required repeat intervention to treat recanalized vessels or neovascularization of the tumor as compared to the 23% rate of retreatment in patients treated with Ethiodol/ethanol mixture.[40,49] Some interventionalists support the use of coils with PVA to reduce the postembolization hemorrhage, which can occur following PVA alone. This is based on a hypothesis that the hemorrhage occurs due to a highly pressurized aneurysm in the parent vessel supplying the AML.[4] Application of fibered coils in the parent vessel has been associated with lower postembolization hemorrhage rates than PVA alone.[47,50]

More recently, physicians have been investigating the use of trisacryl gelatin microspheres or calibrated microparticles (Embosphere Microspheres; BioSphere Medical, Inc., Rockland, Massachusetts) in conjunction with ethanol.[42] Typically, in these protocols, a 3-Fr high-flow microcatheter will be used coaxially to select vessels supplying the AML. Initially, a small volume of absolute alcohol, usually limited to 6 mL maximum volume for the entire procedure, will be injected to sclerose the tumor vessels. Periodically, between aliquots of ethanol, contrast will be injected to assess the embolization. After injection of alcohol has slowed blood flow to the tumor, embolization is completed using the calibrated microparticles, often 500 to 700 μm diameter. Some investigators also will place one or two coils in the feeding arterial pedicle if it is sufficiently long to allow safe placement.[42]

Regardless of the choice of permanent particulate embolic used, one important consideration is the size of embolic delivered. Smaller particles may be less effective than larger particles and more likely to be associated with acute pulmonary distress following therapy.[51,52] In a review of 66 embolization procedures in 48 patients to treat 72 AMLs, Villalta et al.[51] compared outcomes between patients embolized with particles less than 150 μm to those embolized with particles larger than 150 μm. No differences in reduction in tumor size existed between the two groups; however, repeat embolization of the same mass was almost sixfold more likely in those embolized with smaller agents.[51] Although complications were similar between the two groups, 2 of 3 patients who experienced acute respiratory distress following embolization had been treated with smaller particles. Given the increased rate of repeat embolization and the possible increased risk of acute respiratory distress following embolization with particles under 150 μm, the authors concluded embolization should only be performed with particles larger than 150 μm.[51,52]

POTENTIAL COMPLICATIONS

Transarterial embolization of AMLs is generally considered a safe procedure. Inadvertent nontarget embolization is the most feared complication as it can result in spine, lower extremity, and bowel infarction.[39] However, the actual incidence of spinal ischemia is difficult to estimate as no cases were reported in any of the series using Ethiodol/ethanol or ethanol with PVA discussed previously.[40,41,44,45,48,49] Additionally, reflux of embolics when using selective techniques can result in infarction of unaffected renal tissue and loss of renal function.[45,53] Incomplete embolization and vascular injury are rare, occurring in less than 2% of patients.[54] Incomplete embolization can be apparent on completion angiography and should be addressed with further embolization. However, repeat embolization is also occasionally required due to development of extrarenal collaterals or recanalization.[10,19] Overall, the incidence of infection related to renal artery embolization is very low.[53] Intrarenal gas on follow-up imaging does not necessarily indicate infection and may be a normal consequence of embolization with tissue infarction. Another uncommon complication following AML embolization is liquefactive necrosis of the tumor requiring percutaneous drainage.[46]

Postembolization syndrome (PES) is common after renal artery embolization for AML, occurring in up to 80% of treated patients.[44] Signs and symptoms of PES generally include mild flank pain, fever, nausea or vomiting, and leukocytosis, classically occurring 1 to 3 days post procedure. Treatment is supportive and generally on an outpatient basis, with the expectation of symptoms resolving within several days to 1 week. Increased severity or prolonged symptoms of PES should raise suspicion for a more serious complication and may necessitate further investigation and early posttreatment imaging.

TIPS AND TRICKS

- If 10- to 30-degree LAO projection fails to profile renal artery origins, a 30-degree right anterior oblique projection may be helpful.
- High-flow microcatheters will allow for selection of the arteries supplying the AML.
- Ethanol mixed with Ethiodol is an effective embolic agent.
- Patients with TSC are at risk for AML recurrence or new AML formation and therefore require active surveillance after embolization.

CONCLUSION

Embolization of renal AMLs is a safe and well-tolerated procedure, which can prevent life-threatening hemorrhage. Various techniques exist for embolization, with most relying on the use of ethanol as a liquid embolic to reach the small vessel level and induce sclerosis within the tumor itself. Additionally, some protocols add particulate or coil embolics to occlude the large vessels supplying, and the aneurysms within, the AML. Overall, recurrence occurs regardless of technique, with a greater preponderance in patients with TSC compared to sporadic AMLs. Thus, following embolization, continued surveillance is necessary to detect recurrence and detect new tumor formation.

REFERENCES

1. Eble JN. Angiomyolipoma of kidney. *Semin Diagn Pathol.* 1998;15(1):21–40.
2. Bissler JJ, Kingswood JC. Renal angiomyolipomata. *Kidney Int.* 2004;66(3):924–934. doi:10.1111/j.1523-1755.2004.00838.x.
3. Chatziioannou A, Gargas D, Malagari K, et al. Transcatheter arterial embolization as therapy of renal angiomyolipomas: the evolution in 15 years of experience. *Eur J Radiol.* 2012;81(9):2308–2312. doi:10.1016/j.ejrad.2011.06.003.
4. Halpenny D, Snow A, McNeill G, et al. The radiological diagnosis and treatment of renal angiomyolipoma-current status. *Clin Radiol.* 2010;65(2):99–108. doi:10.1016/j.crad.2009.09.014.
5. Hajdu SI, Foote FW. Angiomyolipoma of the kidney: report of 27 cases and review of the literature. *J Urol.* 1969;102(4):396–401.
6. Fujii Y, Ajima J, Oka K, et al. Benign renal tumors detected among healthy adults by abdominal ultrasonography. *Eur Urol.* 1995;27(2):124–127.
7. Henske EP, Ao X, Short MP, et al. Frequent progesterone receptor immunoreactivity in tuberous sclerosis-associated renal angiomyolipomas. *Mod Pathol.* 1998;11(7):665–668.
8. Bernstein J, Robbins TO, Kissane JM. The renal lesions of tuberous sclerosis. *Semin Diagn Pathol.* 1986;3(2):97–105.
9. Chesa Ponce N, Artiles Hernández JL, Ponce Socorro JM, et al. Wunderlich's syndrome as the first manifestation of a renal angiomyolipoma [in Spanish]. *Arch Esp Urol.* 1995;48(3): 305–308.
10. Schillinger F, Montagnac R. Chronic renal failure and its treatment in tuberous sclerosis. *Nephrol Dial Transplant.* 1996; 11(3):481–485.
11. Govednik-Horny C, Atkins M. Angiomyolipoma with vascular invasion during pregnancy. *Ann Vasc Surg.* 2011;25(8):1138. e9–e13. doi:10.1016/j.avsg.2011.05.023.
12. Castle SM, Gorbatiy V, Ekwenna O, et al. Radiofrequency ablation (RFA) therapy for renal angiomyolipoma (AML): an alternative to angio-embolization and nephron-sparing surgery. *BJU Int.* 2012;109(3):384–387. doi:10.1111/j.1464-410X .2011.10376.x.
13. Oesterling JE, Fishman EK, Goldman SM, et al. The management of renal angiomyolipoma. *J Urol.* 1986;135(6):1121–1124.
14. Yamakado K, Tanaka N, Nakagawa T, et al. Renal angiomyolipoma: relationships between tumor size, aneurysm formation, and rupture. *Radiology.* 2002;225(1):78–82.
15. Kessler OJ, Gillon G, Neuman M, et al. Management of renal angiomyolipoma: analysis of 15 cases. *Eur Urol.* 1998;33(6): 572–575.
16. Nelson CP, Sanda MG. Contemporary diagnosis and management of renal angiomyolipoma. *J Urol.* 2002;168(4, pt 1): 1315–1325. doi:10.1097/01.ju.0000028200.86216.b2.
17. Siegel CL, Middleton WD, Teefey SA, et al. Angiomyolipoma and renal cell carcinoma: US differentiation. *Radiology.* 1996; 198(3):789–793.
18. Kim JK, Park S-Y, Shon J-H, et al. Angiomyolipoma with minimal fat: differentiation from renal cell carcinoma at biphasic helical CT. *Radiology.* 2004;230(3):677–684. doi:10.1148 /radiol.2303030003.
19. Forman HP, Middleton WD, Melson GL, et al. Hyperechoic renal cell carcinomas: increase in detection at US. *Radiology.* 1993;188(2):431–434.
20. Jinzaki M, Ohkuma K, Tanimoto A, et al. Small solid renal lesions: usefulness of power Doppler US. *Radiology.* 1998; 209(2):543–550.
21. Sherman JL, Hartman DS, Friedman AC, et al. Angiomyolipoma: computed tomographic-pathologic correlation of 17 cases. *AJR Am J Roentgenol.* 1981;137(6):1221–1226. doi:10.2214/ajr .137.6.1221.
22. Simpson E, Patel U. Diagnosis of angiomyolipoma using computed tomography-region of interest. *Clin Radiol.* 2006;61(5):410–416. doi:10.1016/j.crad.2005.12.013.
23. Kurosaki Y, Tanaka Y, Kuramoto K, et al. Improved CT fat detection in small kidney angiomyolipomas using thin sections and single voxel measurements. *J Comput Assist Tomogr.* 1993;17(5):745–748.
24. Prando A, Prando P, Prando D. Urothelial cancer of the renal pelvicaliceal system: unusual imaging manifestations. *Radiographics.* 2010;30(6):1553–1566. doi:10.1148/rg.306105501.
25. Hélénon O, Merran S, Paraf F, et al. Unusual fat-containing tumors of the kidney: a diagnostic dilemma. *Radiographics.* 1997; 17(1):129–144.
26. Israel GM, Hindman N, Hecht E, et al. The use of opposed-phase chemical shift MRI in the diagnosis of renal angiomyolipomas. *AJR Am J Roentgenol.* 2005;184(6):1868–1872. doi:10.2214/ajr.184.6.01841868.
27. Kido T, Yamashita Y, Sumi S, et al. Chemical shift GRE MRI of renal angiomyolipoma. *J Comput Assist Tomogr.* 1997;21(2): 268–270.
28. Hafron J, Fogarty JD, Hoenig DM, et al. Imaging characteristics of minimal fat renal angiomyolipoma with histologic correlations. *Urology.* 2005;66(6):1155–1159. doi:10.1016/j .urology.2005.06.119.
29. Dickinson M, Ruckle H, Beaghler M, et al. Renal angiomyolipoma: optimal treatment based on size and symptoms. *Clin Nephrol.* 1998;49(5):281–286.
30. Steiner MS, Goldman SM, Fishman EK, et al. The natural history of renal angiomyolipoma. *J Urol.* 1993;150(6):1782–1786.
31. Sooriakumaran P, Gibbs P, Coughlin G, et al. Angiomyolipomata: challenges, solutions, and future prospects based on over 100 cases treated. *BJU Int.* 2010;105(1):101–106. doi:10.1111 /j.1464-410X.2009.08649.x.
32. Mues AC, Palacios JM, Haramis G, et al. Contemporary experience in the management of angiomyolipoma. *J Endourol.* 2010;24(11):1883–1886. doi:10.1089/end.2010.0223.
33. Lucas SM, Stern JM, Adibi M, et al. Renal function outcomes in patients treated for renal masses smaller than 4 cm by ablative and extirpative techniques. *J Urol.* 2008;179(1):75–79; discussion 79–80. doi:10.1016/j.juro.2007.08.156.
34. Berglund RK, Bernstein M, Manion MT, et al. Incidental angiomyolipoma resected during renal surgery for an enhancing renal mass. *BJU Int.* 2009;104(11):1650–1654. doi:10.1111 /j.1464-410X.2009.08677.x.
35. Msezane L, Chang A, Shikanov S, et al. Laparoscopic nephron-sparing surgery in the management of angiomyolipoma: a single center experience. *J Endourol.* 2010;24(4):583–587. doi:10.1089/end.2009.0330.
36. Faddegon S, So A. Treatment of angiomyolipoma at a tertiary care centre: the decision between surgery and angioembolization. *Can Urol Assoc J.* 2011;5(6):E138–E141. doi:10.5489 /cuaj.10028.

37. Cadeddu JA. Re: Radiofrequency ablation (RFA) therapy for renal angiomyolipoma (AML): an alternative to angioembolization and nephron-sparing surgery. *J Urol.* 2012;188(1):71. doi:10.1016/j.juro.2012.03.053.
38. Staehler M, Sauter M, Helck A, et al. Nephron-sparing resection of angiomyolipoma after sirolimus pretreatment in patients with tuberous sclerosis. *Int Urol Nephrol.* 2012;44(6):1657–1661. doi:10.1007/s11255-012-0292-z.
39. Sauk S, Zuckerman DA. Renal artery embolization. *Semin Intervent Radiol.* 2011;28(4):396–406. doi:10.1055/s-0031-1296082.
40. Kothary N, Soulen MC, Clark TWI, et al. Renal angiomyolipoma: long-term results after arterial embolization. *J Vasc Interv Radiol.* 2005;16(1):45–50. doi:10.1097/01.RVI.0000143769.79774.70.
41. Bishay VL, Crino PB, Wein AJ, et al. Embolization of giant renal angiomyolipomas: technique and results. *J Vasc Interv Radiol.* 2010;21(1):67–72. doi:10.1016/j.jvir.2009.09.020.
42. Planché O, Correas J-M, Mader B, et al. Prophylactic embolization of renal angiomyolipomas: evaluation of therapeutic response using CT 3D volume calculation and density histograms. *J Vasc Interv Radiol.* 2011;22(10):1388–1395. doi:10.1016/j.jvir.2011.05.016.
43. Han YM, Kim JK, Roh BS, et al. Renal angiomyolipoma: selective arterial embolization—effectiveness and changes in angiomyogenic components in long-term follow-up. *Radiology.* 1997;204(1):65–70.
44. Lee W, Kim TS, Chung JW, et al. Renal angiomyolipoma: embolotherapy with a mixture of alcohol and iodized oil. *J Vasc Interv Radiol.* 1998;9(2):255–261.
45. Chick CM, Tan B-S, Cheng C, et al. Long-term follow-up of the treatment of renal angiomyolipomas after selective arterial embolization with alcohol. *BJU Int.* 2010;105(3):390–394. doi:10.1111/j.1464-410X.2009.08813.x.
46. Soulen MC, Faykus MH, Shlansky-Goldberg RD, et al. Elective embolization for prevention of hemorrhage from renal angiomyolipomas. *J Vasc Interv Radiol.* 1994;5(4):587–591.
47. Lenton J, Kessel D, Watkinson AF. Embolization of renal angiomyolipoma: immediate complications and long-term outcomes. *Clin Radiol.* 2008;63(8):864–870. doi:10.1016/j.crad.2008.02.005.
48. Rimon U, Duvdevani M, Garniek A, et al. Ethanol and polyvinyl alcohol mixture for transcatheter embolization of renal angiomyolipoma. *AJR Am J Roentgenol.* 2006;187(3):762–768. doi:10.2214/AJR.05.0629.
49. Ramon J, Rimon U, Garniek A, et al. Renal angiomyolipoma: long-term results following selective arterial embolization. *Eur Urol.* 2009;55(5):1155–1161. doi:10.1016/j.eururo.2008.04.025.
50. Ewalt DH, Diamond N, Rees C, et al. Long-term outcome of transcatheter embolization of renal angiomyolipomas due to tuberous sclerosis complex. *J Urol.* 2005;174(5):1764–1766. doi:10.1097/01.ju.0000177497.31986.64.
51. Villalta JD, Sorensen MD, Durack JC, et al. Selective arterial embolization of angiomyolipomas: a comparison of smaller and larger embolic agents. *J Urol.* 2011;186(3):921–927. doi:10.1016/j.juro.2011.04.082.
52. Lee F, Aaronson DS, Blaschko S, et al. Selective arterial embolization of angiomyolipoma leading to pulmonary hypertension. *Can J Urol.* 2010;17(3):5232–5235.
53. Ginat DT, Saad WEA, Turba UC. Transcatheter renal artery embolization: clinical applications and techniques. *Tech Vasc Interv Radiol.* 2009;12(4):224–239.
54. Schwartz MJ, Smith EB, Trost DW. Renal artery embolization: clinical indications and experience from over 100 cases. *BJU Int.* 2007;99(4):881–886.

50

Intractable Hematuria

Romaric Loffroy

Intractable hematuria from the bladder is a potentially life-threatening event that raises major therapeutic challenges. Causes of severe hematuria include mainly unresectable bladder carcinoma, radiation cystitis, and cyclophosphamide-induced cystitis. In many patients, bleeding cannot be adequately controlled by conservative measures, such as irrigation with formalin, silver nitrate or alum (aluminum sulfate) solution, intravesical hydrostatic pressure, hyperbaric oxygen, or endoscopic diathermy.[1,2] Radical surgery is not always feasible because the operative risk is often high in this patient population. Angiography with embolization is a minimally invasive procedure that is emerging as a safe, and effective means to control bladder bleeding. Indeed, vesical artery embolization is occasionally indicated in these patients when all other measures have failed. Despite limited published experience with this procedure, success in 90% of patients is reported when the vesical arteries can be identified.[3–8]

DEVICE/MATERIAL DESCRIPTION

Conditioning of patients is important before embolization can be considered. Indeed, patients should be prepared appropriately before embolization, which should include patient resuscitation and optimum hydration, bladder irrigation with clot evacuation, and blood transfusion when indicated.

Pelvic endovascular procedures are usually performed using local anesthesia with a digital subtraction angiography unit. Unilateral or bilateral retrograde catheterization of the femoral artery is performed using a 5-Fr or 6-Fr sheath. Then, selective angiography of the internal iliac arteries is routinely performed using a 5-Fr Cobra or Simmons (Cordis Johnson&Johnson) type 2 catheter to delineate the pelvic arterial anatomy. The Simmons catheter tip is then placed as subselectively as possible into the anterior division of the internal iliac artery to opacify its branches. The vesical arteries can arise as discrete branches of the anterior division of the hypogastric artery and as branches from the pudendal and uterine arteries. Abnormal hypervascularity or even a mass may be seen at angiography, but visualization of extravasation is unusual. Based on angiographic findings, superselective catheterization of the vesical branches is routinely done using a 3-Fr coaxial microcatheter.

Flow-directed embolization is usually achieved using polyvinyl alcohol particles or trisacryl gelatin microspheres mixed with contrast medium (Fig. 50.1). Initially, 300- to 500-μm particles are typically used. As the distal branches fill, larger particles (usually 500- to 700-μm) are administered for a more proximal embolization (Fig. 50.2).

Occasionally when the vesical arteries cannot be selectively catheterized, coil blockade is performed. This technique consists of occluding a distal branch at its ostium while preserving flow in the vesical branches to steer the particles into these branches and protect the proximally embolized territory from distal particulate embolization. Coil blockade is performed using 0.018-in fibered or soft platinum microcoils of various lengths and diameters.[8]

When the main distal branches of the anterior division of the internal iliac artery cannot be selectively catheterized, the catheter tip is left in the anterior division of the internal iliac artery and embolization is performed from this position using 0.035-in steel coils of an appropriate size or mechanically disrupted absorbable gelatin sponge powder sheet regardless of whether or not bleeding was detected by angiography (Fig. 50.3).[5,6] Sometimes even when the bladder arteries were selectively catheterized and embolized, all anterior branches can be subsequently embolized. As needed, the same procedure is repeated on the opposite side via an ipsilateral or contralateral puncture. The main techniques of bladder embolization are described in Figure 50.4.

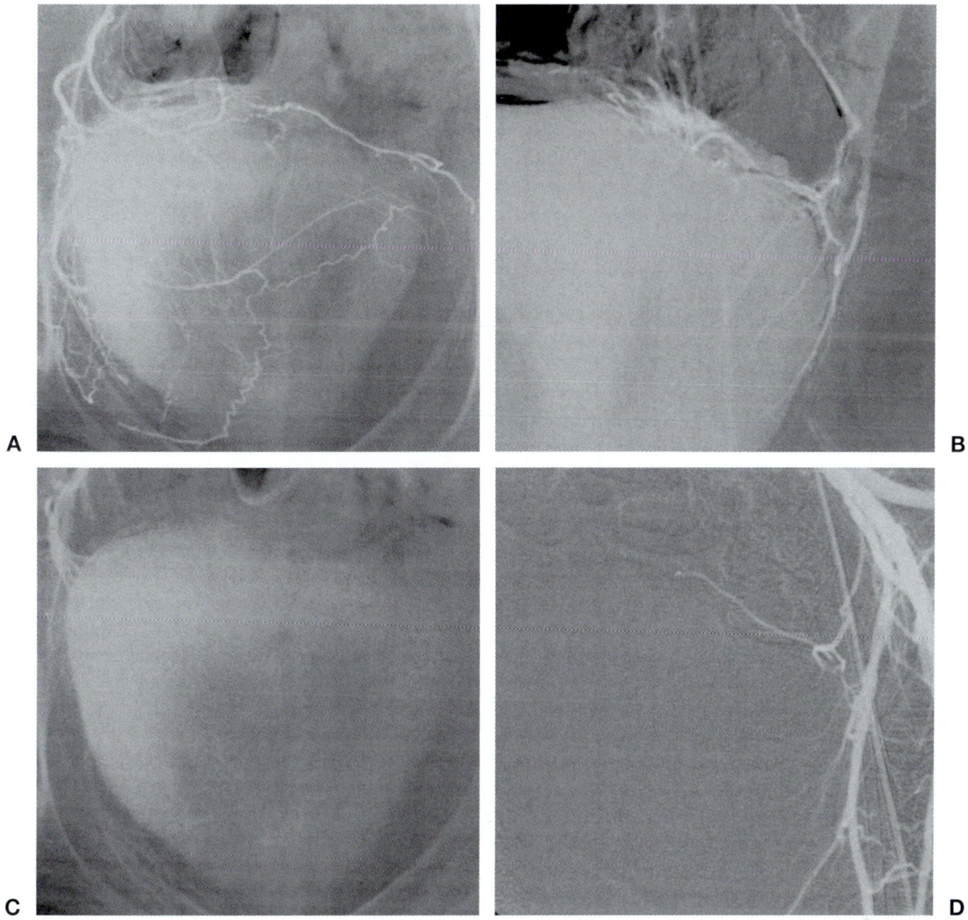

Figure 50.1 Right and left vesical arteriograms in an 18-year-old woman with cyclophosphamide-induced cystitis obtained before **(A,B)** and after **(C,D)** superselective embolization with 300- to 500-μm calibrated trisacryl gelatin microspheres. The bleeding was successfully controlled, and there were no complications.

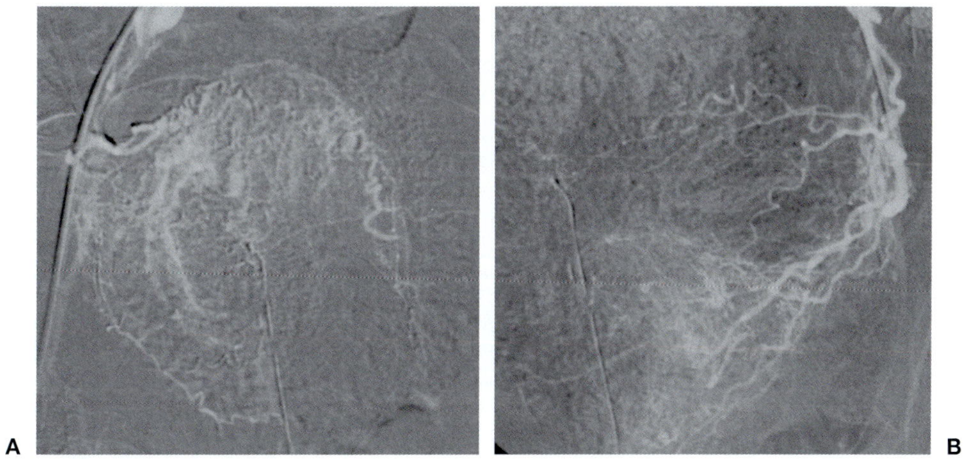

Figure 50.2 Preembolization right **(A)** and left **(B)** arteriograms in an 80-year-old man with bladder cancer showing increased vascularity of the bladder. Hematuria was controlled after bilateral superselective embolization of the superior and inferior vesical arteries with 500- to 700-μm permanent particles. Note the decrease in bladder vascularity **(C,D)**.

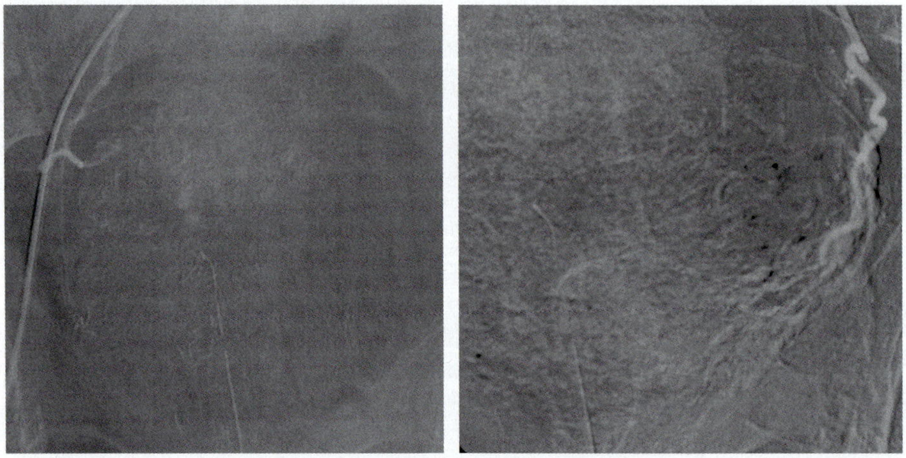

C D

Figure 50.2 *(Continued)*

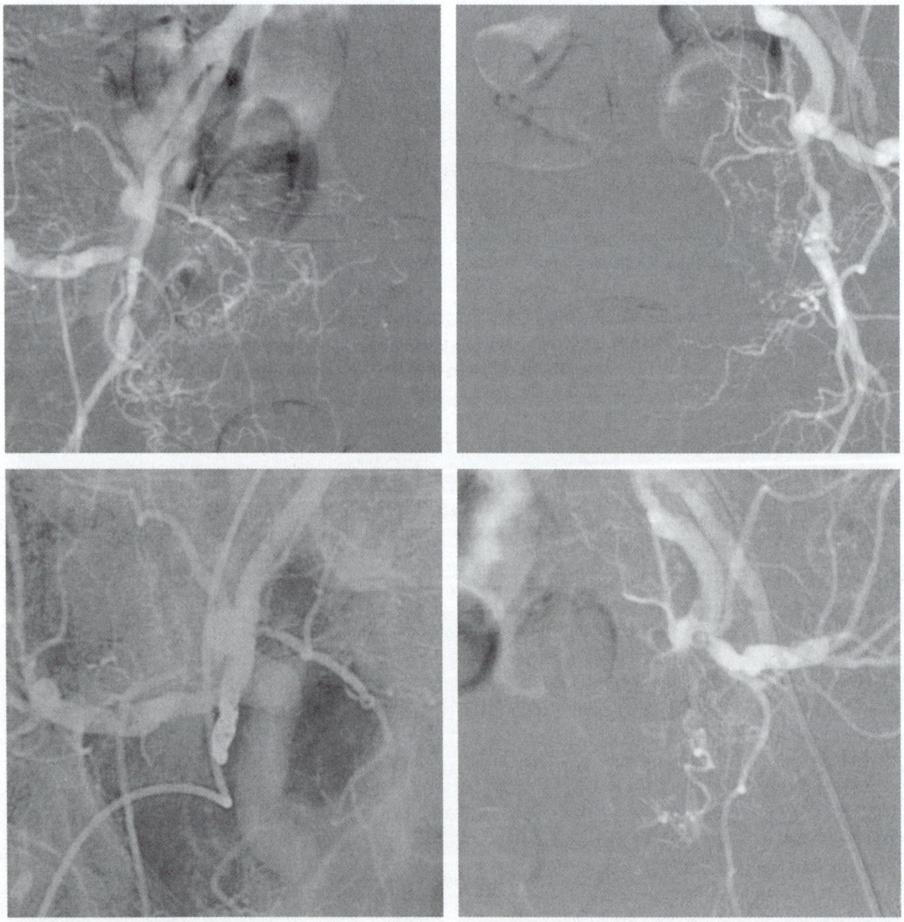

A B C D

Figure 50.3 Images from an 81-year-old man with bleeding caused by extensive prostate cancer. Selective right **(A)** and left **(B)** internal iliac arteriograms showing increased vascularity in the pelvic area from several small feeding arteries arising from the anterior division of the internal iliac arteries. Angiogram after bilateral proximal coil embolization: complete occlusion of the branches of both anterior divisions **(C,D)**. Flow to the posterior division is maintained despite coil migration on the left. The course was uneventful.

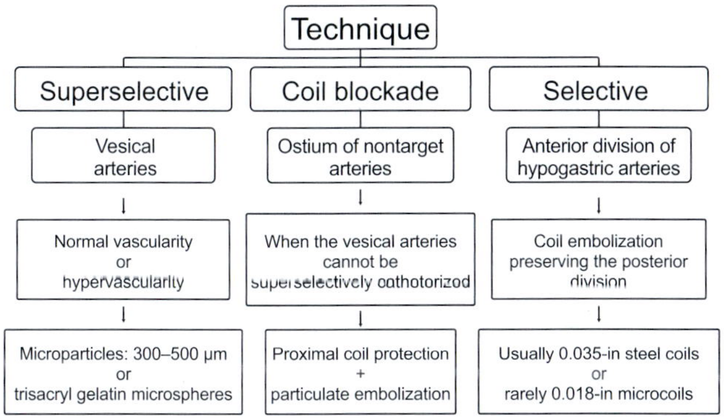

Figure 50.4 Techniques of bladder embolization.

TECHNIQUE

Earlier studies suggest a higher risk of rebleeding after unilateral embolization than after bilateral embolization.[9,10] Rebleeding after unilateral embolization is probably related to the rich collateral blood supply to the internal iliac artery from the contralateral internal iliac, inferior mesenteric, external iliac, and femoral arteries. To prevent rebleeding from these collateral vessels, the anterior division of the internal iliac artery should probably be embolized bilaterally regardless of whether the bleeding site is detectable on angiography.[6,7,11–13]

The influence of the type of embolic agent on clinical outcomes is controversial. In most previous series, the number of patients was too small to allow conclusions to be made about the best embolic agents for this indication.[5–8,14] Although authors have used various embolic materials with time, particulate embolic agents, such as calibrated trisacryl gelatin microspheres, are preferred currently. Recanalization may develop after 2 to 3 weeks when gelatin sponge particles are used.[15] When superselective catheterization is not possible, the distal arterial territory can be protected by placing coils immediately distal to the branches requiring embolization. This technique is helpful when a tumor has recruited several small collateral feeding vessels from the branches of the internal iliac artery. It can help prevent ischemic complications.

CLINICAL OUTCOMES

Severe hematuria that persists despite conventional treatment raises major therapeutic challenges. Patients are usually older and have radiation cystitis, cyclophosphamide-induced cystitis, or inoperable bladder or prostate cancer with bladder invasion and advanced disease. Prolonged or repeated hospitalization for bladder irrigation and multiple blood transfusions are not practical, and the risk of major morbidity associated with radical surgery is often unacceptably high. Endovascular embolization is a minimally invasive method that allows the patient to stay at home without catheters. Most studies of endovascular embolization for severe hematuria are small case series, but the technical success rate is high, ranging from 92.6% to 100%.[3–8,13] Embolotherapy can provide at least short-term success that is adequate to palliatively improve quality of life with few complications. Indeed, the initial clinical success can be very high, especially in the most recently published studies in which superselective embolization was performed in most patients, supporting the use of this technique in such a setting (Table 50.1).[7,8,13]

POTENTIAL COMPLICATIONS

Bladder embolization has been shown to be a safe procedure with a low risk of complications. In general, there is a small risk of bladder infarction due to the rich blood supply of the organ. A postembolization syndrome has been reported, but this is self-limited and can be treated with symptomatic medication. Other reported complications include buttock or perineal pain, Brown-Sequard syndrome because of the presence of anastomoses between the vesical arteries and the lateral sacral arteries which has to be checked during angiography, bladder necrosis, gluteal paresis, or skin necrosis.[4,5,12,16–19] The risk of bladder ischemia and infarction is unusual due to the rich blood supply of the organ. However, the ischemic complication rate has been reported to be as high as 68.5% when a superselective embolization is not performed.[12] This has led to the recommendation that superselective embolization of the bladder arteries should be performed whenever possible to minimize the risk of ischemic complications at other sites of the internal iliac territory. The changes in mean pressure, pulse volume, and blood flow noted even after bilateral internal iliac embolization decrease the risk of ischemic infarction.[20] In recent studies, superselective embolization was used preferentially, and complication rates were low at approximately 10% (Table 50.1).[7,8,13]

Of course, the mortality rate and follow-up after embolization are usually relatively high and short in most studies because the target population is composed chiefly of older individuals with advanced malignancy. However, the mortality is rarely due to rebleeding, and embolization obviates the need for radical surgery in more than 90% of patients. Furthermore, early rebleeding can be controlled by a repeat and more aggressive embolization.

TIPS AND TRICKS

- Causes of severe hematuria include mainly unresectable bladder carcinoma, radiation cystitis, cyclophosphamide-induced cystitis, or inoperable prostate cancer with bladder invasion.
- Bladder embolization should be considered early after failed conservative medical measures in the management of uncontrolled bladder hemorrhage.

Table 50.1 Outcomes of Bladder Embolization in Main Series over a 30-Year Period

Study Year	Patient No./Age (years)	Technical Success (%)	Superselective Embolization (%)	Bilateral Embolization (%)	Clinical Success (%)	Complication Rate (%)	30-Day Mortality (%)	Late Rebleeding (%)	Follow-up (months)
1979[3]	14/NA	100	14.3	100	85.7	NA	NA	14.3	7
1980[4]	9/70	100	0	100	88.9	55.5	0	22.2	10
1988[11]	17/72	100	NA	NA	76.5	NA	NA	NA	NA
1988[5]	10/71	100	0	40	70	20	30	20	NA
1989[12]	53/NA	92.6	0	100	76.8	68.5	NA	24.7	6
2003[6]	6/80	100	0	100	83.3	50	0	0	20
2008[7]	10/78	100	100	100	100	10	NA	10	20
2009[13]	11/76	100	90.9	90.9	90.9	9.1	NA	18.2	2
2010[19]	44/79	100	100	100	82	27	NA	50	10.5
2010[8]	20/73	90	88.9	72.2	100	10	20	28.6	16

- Patients should be adequately prepared before embolization. This includes resuscitation and optimum hydration, bladder irrigation with clot evacuation, and blood transfusion when indicated.
- Selective angiography of the anterior division of the internal iliac arteries must be done routinely using a 5-Fr Cobra or Simmons type 2 catheter to delineate the pelvic arterial anatomy.
- The presence of anastomoses between the vesical arteries and the lateral sacral arteries has to be checked during angiography to avoid Brown-Sequard syndrome.
- Every effort should be made to perform flow-directed embolization of the vesical arteries bilaterally and as selectively as possible using a microcatheter, with permanent calibrated particulate agents ranging from 300–500 μm in size.
- When the vesical arteries cannot be superselectively catheterized, coil embolization distal to the vesical artery can be performed. Particles can then be administered proximal to the vesical arteries; the coils will protect the proximally embolized territory from distal particulate embolization.
- When catheterization is technically difficult or impossible, selective embolization of the anterior division of the internal iliac arteries can be done using standard coils of an appropriate size.

CONCLUSION

Transcatheter arterial embolization is a feasible and safe way to control bleeding from the bladder after failure of conservative management. This applies regardless of the etiology of the bleeding. In most cases, embolization is a well-tolerated procedure that obviates the need for surgery. Embolization should be viewed as a minimally invasive palliative measure. It controls the immediate problem of life-threatening hemorrhage and provides sustained bleeding control, contributing to improve palliative care and quality of life by decreasing the need for blood transfusion, bladder irrigation, and repeat cystoscopy. Every effort should be made to perform embolization bilaterally and as selectively as possible with permanent embolic agents to increase the likelihood of success and to minimize the risk of complications.

REFERENCES

1. Choong S, Walkden M, Kirby R. The management of intractable haematuria. *BJU Int.* 2000;86:951–959.
2. Capelli-Schellpfeffer M, Gerber GS. The use of hyperbaric oxygen in urology. *J Urol.* 1999;162:647–654.
3. Lang EK, Deutsch JS, Goodman JR, et al. Transcatheter embolization of hypogastric branch arteries in the management of intractable bladder hemorrhage. *J Urol.* 1979;121:30–36.
4. Carmignani G, Belgrano E, Puppo P, et al. Transcatheter embolization of the hypogastric arteries in cases of bladder hemorrhage from advanced pelvic cancers: followup in 9 cases. *J Urol.* 1980;124:196–200.
5. Appleton DS, Sibley GN, Doyle PT. Internal iliac artery embolisation for the control of severe bladder and prostate haemorrhage. *Br J Urol.* 1988;61:45–47.
6. Nabi G, Sheikh N, Greene D, et al. Therapeutic transcatheter arterial embolization in the management of intractable haemorrhage from pelvic urological malignancies: preliminary experience and long-term follow-up. *BJU Int.* 2003;92: 245–247.
7. Rastinehad AR, Caplin DM, Ost MC, et al. Selective arterial prostatic embolization (SAPE) for refractory hematuria of prostatic origin. *Urology.* 2008;71:181–184.
8. Delgal A, Cercueil JP, Koutlidis N, et al. Outcome of transcatheter arterial embolization for bladder and prostate hemorrhage. *J Urol.* 2010;183:1947–1953.
9. Hald T, Mygind T. Control of life-threatening vesical hemorrhage by unilateral hypogastric artery muscle embolization. *J Urol.* 1974;112:60–63.
10. Hietala SO. Urinary bladder necrosis following selective embolization of the internal iliac artery. *Acta Radiol Diagn.* 1978;19:316–320.
11. Ozono S, Okajima E, Hirao Y, et al. Transcatheter arterial embolization of vesical artery in the treatment of invasive bladder cancer. *Eur Urol.* 1988;15:176–179.
12. Pisco JM, Martins JM, Correia MG. Internal iliac artery: embolization to control hemorrhage from pelvic neoplasms. *Radiology.* 1989;172:337–339.
13. Prasad V, Sacks BA, Kraus S, et al. Embolotherapy for lower urinary tract hemorrhage. *J Vasc Interv Radiol.* 2009;20:965–970.
14. Gujral S, Bell R, Kabala J, et al. Internal iliac artery embolisation for intractable bladder hemorrhage in the peri-operative phase. *Postgrad Med J.* 1999;75:167–168.
15. Loffroy R, Guiu B, Cercueil JP, et al. Endovascular therapeutic embolisation: an overview of occluding agents and their effects on embolised tissues. *Curr Vasc Pharmacol.* 2009;7:250–263.
16. Sieber PR. Bladder necrosis secondary to pelvic artery embolization: case report and literature review. *J Urol.* 1994;151:422.
17. Kobayashi T, Kusano S, Matsubayashi T, et al. Selective embolization of the vesical artery in the management of massive bladder hemorrhage. *Radiology.* 1980;136:345–348.
18. McIvor J, Williams G, Southcott RD. Control of severe vesical haemorrhage by therapeutic embolisation. *Clin Radiol.* 1982;33:561–567.
19. Liguori G, Amodeo A, Mucelli FP, et al. Intractable haematuria: long-term results after selective embolization of the internal iliac arteries. *BJU Int.* 2010;106:500–503.
20. Burchell RC. Physiology of internal artery ligation. *J Obstet Gynecol Br Commonw.* 1968;75:642–651.

51

Benign Prostatic Hyperplasia

Francisco Cesar Carnevale • Airton Mota Moreira

BACKGROUND

Benign Prostatic Hyperplasia

Symptomatic benign prostatic hyperplasia (BPH) typically occurs at the beginning of the sixth decade, with more than 40% of men aged 60 years and older presenting with clinical manifestations. As the world's population ages, the prevalence of BPH is expected to increase, calling for a therapy that minimizes the risk for adverse outcomes.[1–3]

The standard management of BPH is based on the overall health of the patient, on the severity of the lower urinary tract symptoms (LUTS), and on quality-of-life considerations. Voiding difficulties attributable to BPH can be quantified with the American Urological Association Symptom Index (AUA-SI) score or International Prostate Symptom Score (IPSS). Various medications can decrease the severity of voiding symptoms secondary to BPH. Impotence, decreased libido, and ejaculatory disorders are known side effects of these medications. Watchful waiting is a management strategy in which the patient is monitored by his physician but receives no active intervention for BPH; this is the preferred management strategy for patients with mild symptoms.[4]

The American Urological Association (AUA) guidelines indicate that patients with mild LUTS secondary to BPH (AUA-SI score <8) and patients with moderate or severe symptoms (AUA-SI score ≥ 8) who are not bothered by their LUTS should be managed using a strategy of watchful waiting. If the patient elects interventional therapy and there is sufficient evidence of obstruction, the patient and urologist should discuss the benefits and risks of the various available interventions.[4]

Many advances have been made in the medications and minimally invasive procedures used to treat BPH since the 1990s. Despite these advances, transurethral resection of the prostate (TURP), which was developed in the 1920s, remains the treatment of choice when medical management fails. TURP is still the gold standard of interventional treatment for small prostate glands (smaller than 80 to 100 g) and is performed under direct endoscopic visualization with an electrocautery tool to remove prostatic tissue. Although considered a safe technique with a mortality rate below 0.25%, it is not without adverse events. The most frequent complications are ejaculatory disorders (up to 50%), early urinary incontinence (30% to 40%), acute urinary retention caused by blood clots (2% to 5%), sexual impotence (up to 5%), and the need for blood transfusions (0.4% to 7%). Patients who have undergone TURP require surgical retreatment for LUTS symptoms in 3% to 14.5% of cases.[4–6]

Open prostatectomy involves the surgical removal (enucleation) of the inner portion of the prostate gland via a suprapubic or retropubic incision in the lower abdomen. Open prostatectomy is typically performed on patients with prostate volumes greater than 80 to 100 mL with a higher risk of blood loss and transfusion and a longer hospital stay than TURP. Open prostatectomies may only be needed for men with very enlarged prostate glands (it may be more effective than TURP in relieving the blockage of urine flow) and for men with bladder diverticula (pockets) or stones.[7,8]

The high prevalence rate of BPH has a tremendous impact on the health and quality of life of men. Increasingly, BPH therapy trends are moving away from the standard operations toward less invasive pharmacologic options and minimally invasive procedures provided in an outpatient setting. Minimally invasive techniques have been developed as alternative treatments for LUTS, such as transurethral microwave thermotherapy and laser ablations, but they involve introducing energy into the gland and all require access through the urethra. Nevertheless, complications from these procedures are similar to TURP.[9–11] Prostatic artery embolization (PAE) has emerged as a new minimally invasive alternative of treatment for symptomatic patients with enlarged prostates due to BPH.[12–14]

Prostatic Artery Embolization

The first animal study to evaluate the feasibility and safety of PAE was conducted in a canine model and demonstrated the promising potential of PAE to decrease prostate volume and urethral stenosis due to BPH. The success rate for identification and selective catheterization of the prostatic arteries was 100%. Initial computed tomography (CT) showed good distribution of particles in the embolized prostate with no evidence of nontarget embolization. CT after 1 month showed decreased perfusion, cavitary necrosis, and 40% prostate volume reduction. There was excellent radiologic–pathologic correlation.[15] Subsequently, the technical feasibility and safety of prostate embolization was evaluated in pigs[16] and dogs[17] with prostate volume reduction and without sexual or erectile complications.

Embolization of the prostatic arteries has been used for many years to control serious bleeding after biopsy or prostatectomy.[18–20] The first published case in which it was recognized that PAE could have a therapeutic effect on BPH was in 2000 by DeMeritt and colleagues.[12] The first intentional treatment of BPH with PAE in humans was done by Carnevale et al.[13] in June 2008 and was published in 2010. In this report, PAE was performed in two patients with acute urinary retention due to BPH who were refractory to treatment with selective α-blockers, were being managed with long-term indwelling catheters, and were waiting for surgery. The same investigators published midterm follow-up data for these two patients in 2011, confirming the efficacy of the procedure.[14]

TECHNICAL DETAILS

Preprocedure Imaging Evaluation

Ultrasound (US) is the most common method to evaluate the prostate and bladder. The prostate volume is measured by standard transabdominal view or transrectal US if prostate biopsy is necessary. Prostate vascularization can be visualized using Doppler, and transabdominal US can measure the postvoid residual urine volume. Bladder evaluation comprises measurement of wall thickness and an assessment of characteristics such as the presence of diverticula, trabeculations, and other possible findings such as polyps, calculus, or other lesions. Protrusion of the median lobe is measured using the prostate protrusion index and prostate volume is measured using three incidences.

Magnetic resonance imaging (MRI) of the prostate is very useful, giving more details than US mainly related to the central gland and peripheral zone. Prostate measurements (cephalocaudal, transverse, and anteroposterior) are obtained and volume is calculated by the ellipse formula. It is the best method to evaluate patients before and after PAE. CT with contrast can be useful to identify the characteristics of the main artery supplying the prostate and any arterial atherosclerotic lesion or obstruction that could contraindicate or make the intervention more difficult.[21]

Embolization Technique

BPH treatment with PAE requires a well-trained interventional radiologist because of the complex prostatic vascular anatomy and the potential for complications in elderly patients with atherosclerosis, very small prostatic arteries, and comorbidities. Intervention can be performed under local anesthesia on an outpatient basis. A 400 mg intravenous dose of ciprofloxacin is given before the procedure followed by 500 mg orally twice a day for 7 days after PAE. Patients also receive nonopioid analgesics and nonsteroidal anti-inflammatory medications after embolization. Intervention can be performed via a unilateral common femoral arterial approach. Femoral pulses should be examined before choosing which side will be used for access. To provide good orientation to the prostate site and related structures in the pelvis, we recommend that a Foley catheter be placed into the bladder and that the balloon be filled with a mixture of 30% iodinated contrast medium and 70% normal saline (Fig. 51.1). This is used during the procedure to give both a better image and understanding of the prostate, the internal iliac artery branches, and related structures (Fig. 51.2) to help avoid nontarget embolization complications. It is an excellent landmark during the procedure and we have not

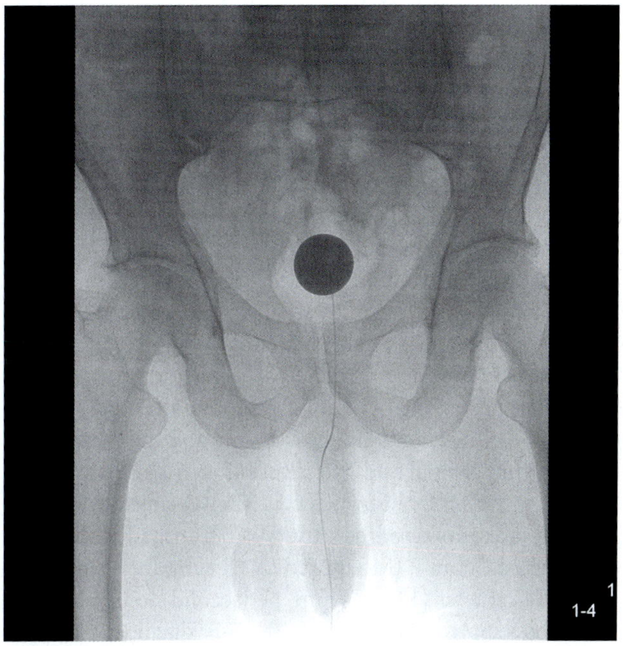

Figure 51.1 The Foley catheter introduced before the procedure filled with contrast medium gives a better understanding of the prostate position and related structures.

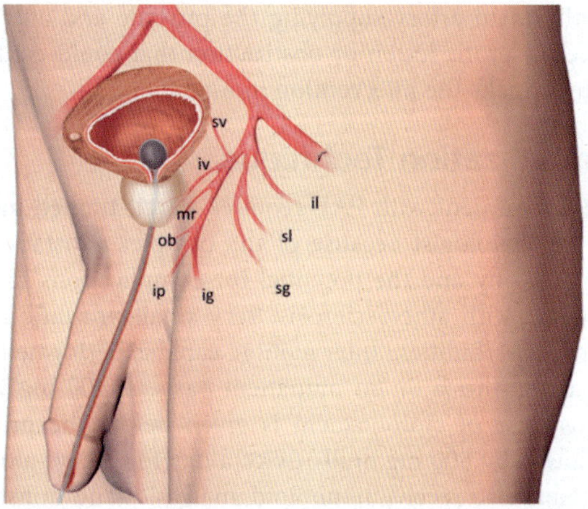

Figure 51.2 Illustration of the anterior and posterior branches of the internal iliac artery and the relationship with the Foley balloon filled with contrast medium. sv, superior vesical artery; iv, inferior vesical artery; mr, middle rectal artery; ob, obturator artery; ip, internal pudendal artery; ig, inferior gluteal artery; sg, superior gluteal artery; sl, lateral sacral artery; il, iliolumbar artery.

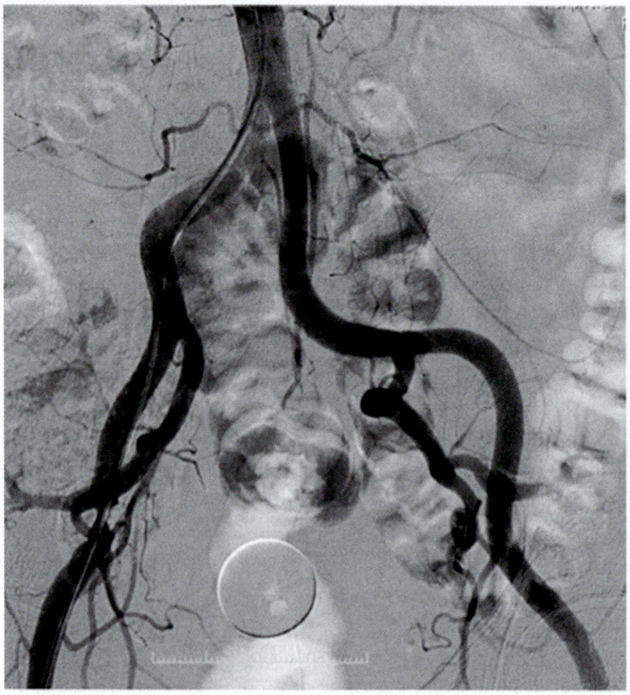

Figure 51.3 Digital subtraction arteriogram showing the tortuosity of the pelvic arteries under posteroanterior view.

observed any severe complications due to its use. It can also be a reference if using cone-beam CT and can help eliminate the patient's need to strain to void after the procedure.

Knowing the vascular anatomy of the prostate is essential for the successful performance of this procedure. Due to many arterial anastomoses and branches to related pelvic structures, various nomenclatures have been used for the arteries supplying the prostate. Names such as the inferior vesical artery (IVA), prostatovesical artery, vesicoprostatic artery, and prostatic artery have been used.[21,22] According to the urologists' nomenclature, the IVA has traditionally been considered the main prostatic artery. It usually arises as the second or third branch of the anterior trunk of the internal iliac artery. Generally, one main prostatic artery is found on each side in that position, but the main prostatic artery or additional prostatic branches arising from the superior vesical, internal pudendal, obturator, and middle rectal arteries can also be found in some patients.[23]

Initial pelvic angiography is performed (20 mL; 10 mL per second) to evaluate the iliac vessels and the prostate arteries during arterial and late phases (Fig. 51.3). After crossing the aortic bifurcation, selective digital subtraction arteriogram of the internal iliac artery is performed with a 5-Fr vertebral or Cobra 2 (Merit Medical System, Inc., South Jordan, UT) catheter (12 mL; 4 mL per second) to better assess the blood supply to the prostate. The 5-Fr diagnostic catheter should be placed at the common internal iliac trunk to avoid missing any branch arising from the anterior and posterior division. It is not uncommon to find an IVA arising as a common pedicle with the superior vesical artery (also called *umbilical artery*) as the first branch of the anterior division. The 5-Fr Roberts Uterine Catheter (RUC; Cook Medical, Inc., Bloomington, Indiana) can be used but, due to its long curve, we have observed less torquability and pushability with the microwire when using the coaxial system. For the ipsilateral internal iliac artery catheterization, a Simmons 1 or 2 catheter (Merit Medical System, Inc., South Jordan, UT) can be used, but we prefer to work with the same vertebral catheter making a Waltman loop because, if necessary, it can be used as a regular vertebral catheter to get more torquability and pushability.

The best projection in which to identify the IVA and all possible accessory branches to the prostate is the 25- to 55-degree ipsilateral oblique view. A caudal view (10 to 20 degrees) can help to identify some bladder branches. This perspective, with the help of the Foley balloon filled with dilute contrast, gives a better understanding of all five anterior branches and gives orientation to the prostatic arteries. After performing the internal iliac arteriogram, attention should be given to the arteries feeding the area immediately below the balloon. In this view, the branches of the anterior division will be straightened and the prostate branches and the rectal branches stay in the anterior and posterior position, respectively. The PROVISO acronym (internal **P**udendal, middle **R**ectal, **O**bturator, **V**esical **I**nferior, and **S**uperior under **O**blique view) is a very useful trick to remember the names of the arteries during arteriography (Fig. 51.4).

Catheterization of the IVA is performed using the same ipsilateral oblique perspective under the road map technique.

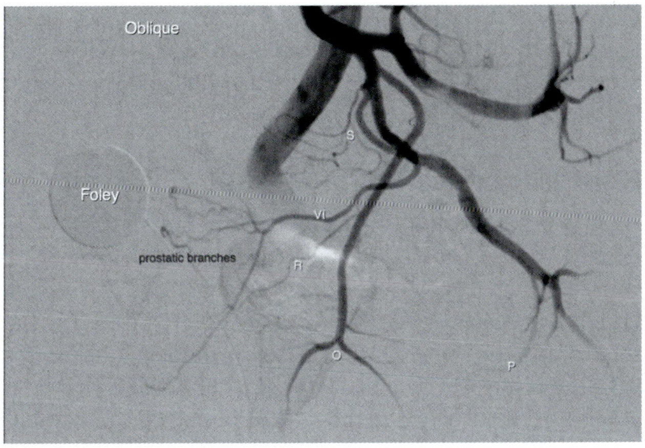

Figure 51.4 Digital subtraction arteriogram showing the anterior branches of the internal iliac arteries and the PROVISO branches (P, pudendal; R, rectal; O, obturator; VI, vesical inferior; S, superior vesical; O, oblique perspective). The intraprostatic arterial branches and the Foley balloon are observed.

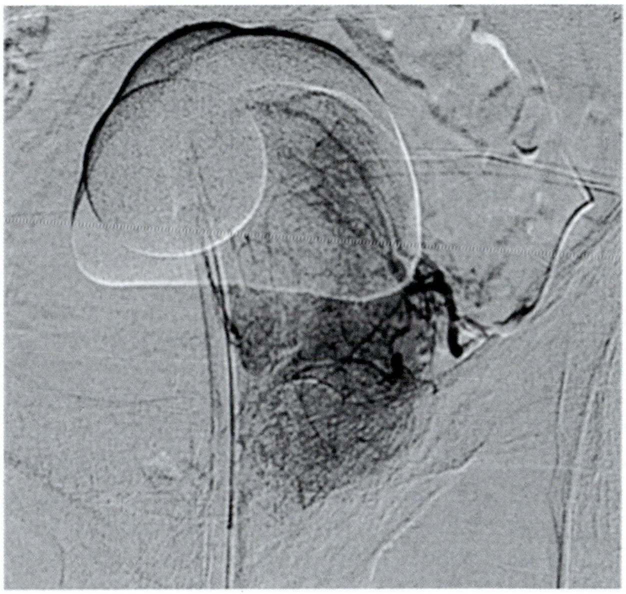

Figure 51.6 Digital subtraction arteriogram under posteroanterior view: IVA catheterization with microcatheter showing the Foley balloon and the protrusion of the left prostate lobe into the bladder.

With the microcatheter placed into the IVA, arteriography is performed by manually injecting 2 to 3 mL of contrast medium. The ipsilateral oblique view is useful for identifying any collateral branches, the small group of arteries feeding the urethra, the central gland, and the capsular arteries (Fig. 51.5). The posteroanterior view is more anatomical and helps to identify some contralateral prostate lobe branches and the parenchymal phase (Fig. 51.6). After checking both views, the microcatheter should be advanced well into the IVA at the ostium of the prostatic arteries and embolization is performed under direct fluoroscopic visualization. Care must be taken with the position of the tip of the microcatheter to avoid spasm or dissection of the tiny intraprostatic branches. Concerning the position of the microcatheter for embolization, we define it as distal embolization when the microcatheter tip is placed at the origin of the intraprostatic branches (Fig. 51.7), compared to proximal embolization when the microcatheter tip is at the origin or very proximal portion of the IVA. In this proximal position, there is a higher risk of nontarget embolization, especially to the rectum or bladder. Diagnostic arteriography performed in this position is very

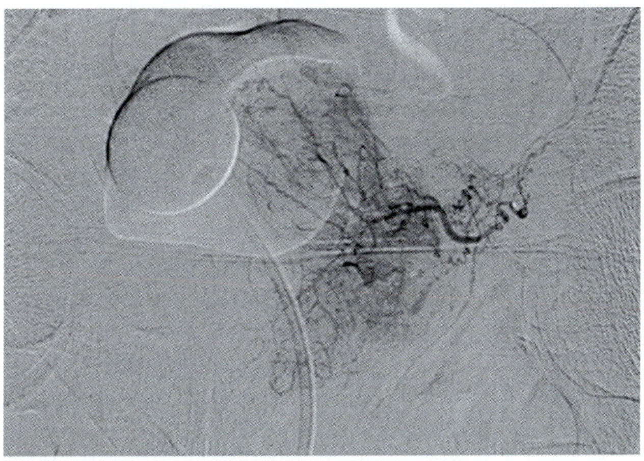

Figure 51.5 Digital subtraction arteriogram under ipsilateral oblique view. IVA catheterization with microcatheter showing the Foley balloon and the protrusion of the left prostate lobe into the bladder.

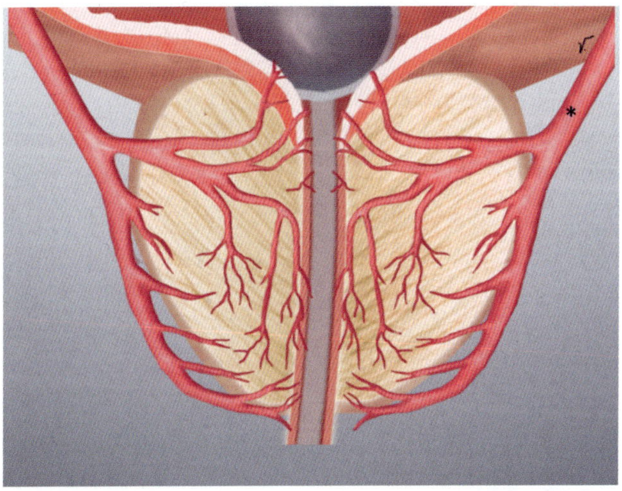

Figure 51.7 Illustration explaining the ideal positioning of the microcatheter tip (*asterisk*) for a safe embolization.

important to identify the prostatic branches, to avoid nontarget embolization, and to occlude any collaterals and shunts, if necessary. Cone-beam CT can be very useful to understand the pelvic anatomy and identify the bladder and rectal branches, thus avoiding complications.[24]

Atherosclerotic disease; thin, tortuous vessels; and lack of knowledge regarding the possible prostatic arterial vessels and sources for nontarget embolization can contribute to increased procedure time. The use of small-diameter hydrophilic microcatheters is mandatory and can facilitate the catheterization of the prostatic arteries, decreasing the procedure and fluoroscopy times. We have used microcatheters smaller than 2.4-Fr in combination with 0.014- or 0.016-in shapable hydrophilic microwires without continuous flushing. Road mapping is used for the catheterization of prostatic arteries. When vasospasm occurs, nitroglycerin can be used but has limited usefulness due to severe atherosclerosis in these arteries. Sometimes, proceeding to the contralateral side may be a good strategy while waiting for the relief of vasospasm.

Varying particulate embolic agents can be used. We have experienced 300- to 500-μm and 100- to 300-μm Embosphere Microspheres (BioSphere Medical, Inc., Roissy-en-France, France) with excellent technical and clinical results after more than 5 years of follow-up in the initial patients. At the end of the embolization, a venous phase blush can be observed, and we consider total stasis as the end point (Fig. 51.8). In general, one 2-mL syringe of microspheres has been enough for bilateral PAE. If any accessory prostatic branch is not embolized, poor long-term clinical results may occur, including reduced prostate shrinkage and return of LUTS. Embolization is performed on the contralateral side using the same technique. Bilateral inferior vesical arteries and any other prostatic branches should be embolized to achieve optimal prostate ischemia, resulting in volume reduction for better long-term results.

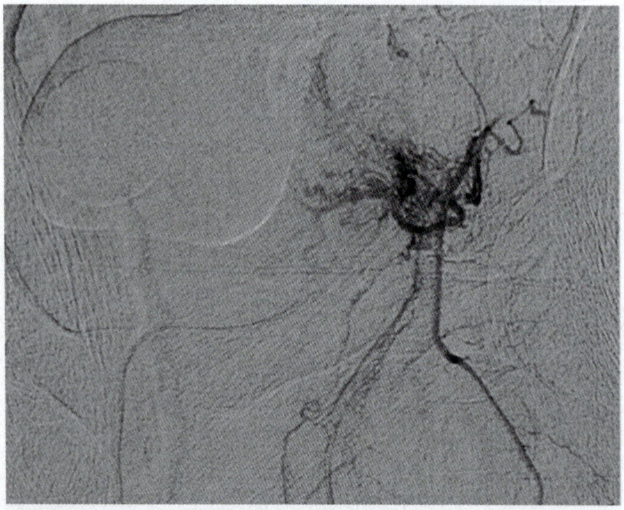

Figure 51.8 End point after left prostatic artery embolization with prostate devascularization, total stasis, and venous phase with contrast reflux into the proximal internal iliac branches.

Postprocedure Management

After the procedure, patients remain supine for 4 to 6 hours without moving the punctured leg to avoid bleeding complications from disrupting the vascular site. If a vascular closure device is used, bed rest can be reduced. During this resting time after PAE, the use of the Foley balloon is very important because patients can void normally without straining, which reduces the risk of puncture site complications. The Foley catheter is removed after 2 to 4 hours in patients without acute urinary retention and the patient can be discharged home. Patients with acute urinary retention are instructed to return 1 week later for removal of the Foley catheter to attempt spontaneous voiding. If the Foley catheter cannot be removed, another attempt is tried every week. We consider it a clinical failure if the patient cannot urinate spontaneously after 1 month.

PAE is not a painful procedure, and patients typically receive oral hydration, nonopioid pain relievers, antibiotics, and nonsteroidal anti-inflammatory drugs, if needed. Proton pump inhibitors for gastric and duodenal protection are indicated as well. Dysuria and frequent urination are the most common symptoms seen immediately after PAE and usually last for 3 to 5 days. Patients receiving oral medication to control LUTS continue this medication for 1 week after PAE. Telephone follow-up is recommended during the first week after the procedure. Patients return for office follow-up 1 month after the procedure.

Postprocedure Imaging

Both US and MRI are useful methods of measurements before and after PAE. Patients have demonstrated an average of greater than 30% to 40% reduction in the prostate volume after PAE as measured by US and MRI during follow-up. However, we have observed greater variations in the US results and prefer MRI for evaluating and following patients before and after this procedure. Volume decrease is most evident during the first 3 months after embolization and is sustained over time. We have seen a higher volume reduction rate (40%) in patients with large prostate glands (>90 g) compared to small prostate glands (30%). Progressive volume reduction of the prostate occurs after embolization and infarcts have been seen in 70% to 80% of the patients, exclusively in the prostatic central zone. On MRI, this is characterized by hyperintensity on T1 weighted images and predominant hypointensity on T2 weighted images; these areas demonstrate a progressive size reduction over time (Fig. 51.9). Prostate volume reduction has been observed in patients with and without infarcts, but the presence of infarcts is associated with a greater degree of volume reduction

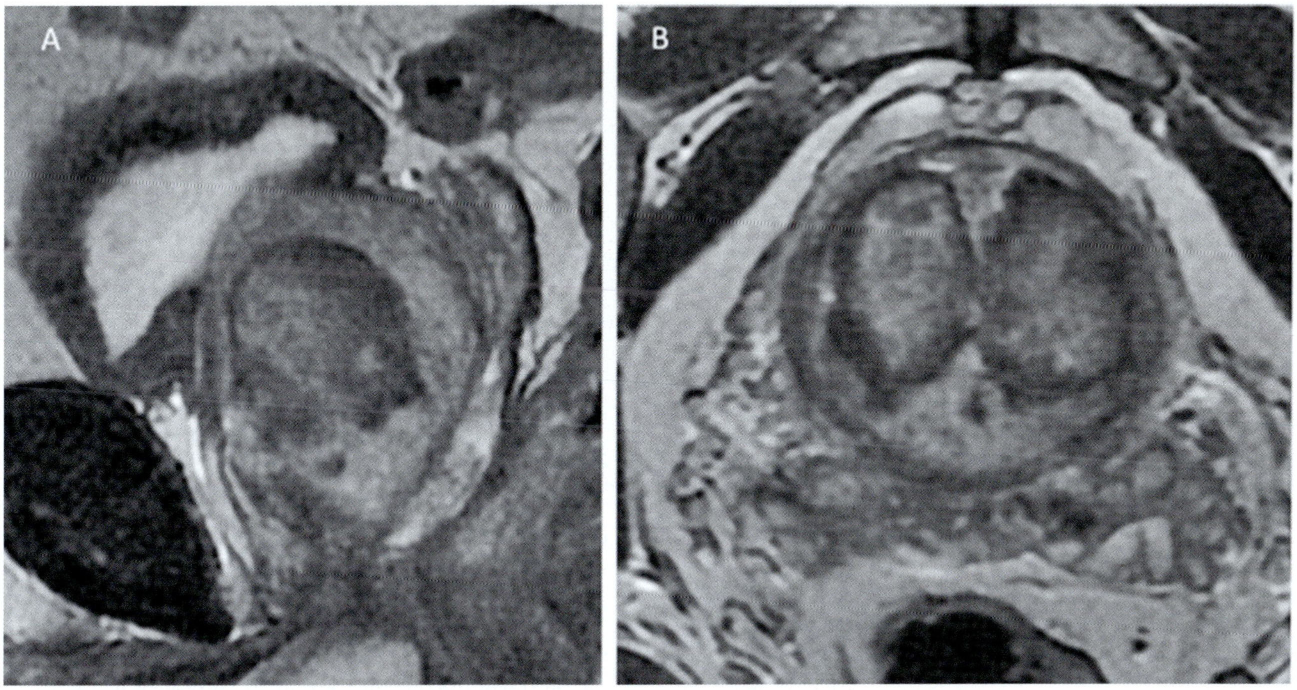

Figure 51.9 MRI after bilateral prostatic artery embolization with bilateral infarcted areas on sagittal **(A)** and axial **(B)** views.

after embolization. No significant changes have been found in the prostatic peripheral zone.[23]

After the PAE procedure, we suggest urodynamic studies every year; IPSS, International Index of Erectile Function questionnaires, quality-of-life questionnaires, prostate-specific antigen test, US, and MRI should be performed to assess effectiveness at 3 and 12 months and every year thereafter. Urodynamic findings after PAE have demonstrated that maximum bladder capacity and maximum flow rates improved significantly. Bladder tone also improves and patients obtained better maximum flow rate (Qmax) with reduction of the detrusor pressure (Pdet) and of the postvoid residual (PVR) urine volume. This means that patients void better without straining and with less residual urine in the bladder after voiding.[25,26]

OUTCOMES

The aim of PAE is to produce as much gland ischemia as possible because we have observed that better long-term clinical and urodynamic results are correlated with prostate ischemia.[23] Technical success is defined as the successful catheterization and embolization of the right and left main prostatic arteries. Clinical success is defined by multiple criteria including removal of the Foley catheter in patients with acute urinary retention, improvement in LUTS and quality of life, and no sexual disorders or serious adverse events from the procedure.

Since the initial case reports on PAE were published, there have been several other case series that have confirmed the technical and clinical success of this procedure. Pisco et al.[27] reported on 15 patients undergoing PAE for symptomatic BPH. In this series, the technical success rate for bilateral PAE was 86.7%, and it was 93.3% for unilateral or bilateral PAE with failures due to tortuosity and atherosclerotic change of the iliac arteries. After a mean follow-up of 7.9 months, improvements were noted in LUTS, quality of life, erectile function, and peak urinary flow. The clinical failure rate was 28.6%. On MRI, there was a mean prostate volume decrease of 28.9 mL. Bladder ischemia requiring surgical repair was the only complication reported in this series. Pisco et al.[28] followed this study with another report on 89 consecutive patients. In this study, 79/89 underwent a bilateral PAE (88.8%) and 7/89 patients underwent a unilateral PAE (7.9%), for a 96.7% technical success rate for unilateral or bilateral PAE. Ninety-one percent of the patients treated were discharged from the hospital 6 to 8 hours after the procedure, whereas the remaining patients were discharged the following morning. At 3 months, the clinical failure rate was 18.3%. The remaining patients reported improvements in LUTS and quality of life. Minor complications included urinary tract infections (19%), transient hematuria (10%), and transient hemospermia (7%). No other major complications were reported.

Bagla et al.[29] has reported early results from a U.S. trial. In this study, the technical success rate was 90%, with 18/20 undergoing bilateral PAE; 1 patient underwent a unilateral PAE. These patients demonstrated improvements in LUTS (AUA score improvement at 1, 3, and 6 months of 10.8, 12.1, and 9.8 points, respectively), quality of life, and sexual function. There was a mean prostate volume decrease of 18%. No minor or major complications were reported in this series.

Our group followed up our original case reports by publishing our experience with PAE in 11 patients with acute urinary retention caused by BPH.[25,26] Bilateral PAE was performed in 75% of procedures, with unilateral PAE performed in the remaining patients. Factors precluding performance of bilateral PAE included an IVA dissection, microcatheter tracking failure, and nonvisualization of the prostatic arteries. Ten of 11 patients were able to void spontaneously without catheterization after PAE. Improvements were also noted in quality of life and erectile function. The mean prostate volume reduction was 31.7% on MRI.

We continue to observe significant improvements in quality of life based on patient questionnaires; objective urodynamic data corroborate these self-reported assessments. This improvement appears to be sustained over time. With over 5 years of follow-up in some patients, we have observed initial clinical failure in only 3% and recurrence of LUTS in 8% after PAE in 100 treated patients. It is important to note that good clinical outcomes and improvements in urodynamic data, even in patients who underwent unilateral PAE, suggest that factors from PAE other than prostate reduction, such as prostate tissue change, can contribute to improving symptoms and better voiding. This suggests that some patients can benefit even when only unilateral embolization is possible.[24–30]

POTENTIAL COMPLICATIONS

The major complication rate after PAE is very low. As described earlier, Pisco et al.[27] reported one patient who required surgery for limited bladder ischemia. We have not experienced major complications in our series of patients. However, we have noted that there are expected symptoms that should constitute a postembolization syndrome (or post-PAE syndrome). These include nausea, vomiting, fever in the absence of infection, urethral burning, periprostatic or pelvic pain, and very small amounts of blood in urine and/or mixed in the stool with mucus for 2 to 3 days. Because this post-PAE syndrome is mild and the embolization is performed under local anesthesia, patients can be discharged on the same day of the procedure. In our experience, the presence of a small amount of blood in the urine or mixed in the stool (<10%) is likely to be the result of arterial communications between the prostate, bladder, and rectum. Further evaluation of one patient experiencing blood mixed in the stool demonstrated ischemic rectitis with rectal ulcers identified at day 4 by colonoscopy, which disappeared by day 16 without treatment.[31] Although no patient with these symptoms have required treatment, this does highlight the risk of nontarget embolization in association with this procedure.

TIPS AND TRICKS

- A multidisciplinary approach with urologists, diagnostic radiologists, and interventional radiologists is essential. Interventional radiologists should follow all patients after the procedure to document symptomatic improvement after PAE.
- Gain a complete understanding of BPH and typical presenting symptoms before engaging in PAE.
- Preembolization evaluation with MRI and urodynamic studies should be used for patient selection.
- Use the Foley balloon technique as a landmark during PAE and for patient comfort.
- Use a microcatheter in every case for distal intraprostatic artery positioning and prostate embolization.
- Embolize as much prostatic tissue as possible during PAE procedures.
- Try to perform bilateral PAE for better long-term clinical results.
- Remove the Foley balloon before patient discharge.
- Perform the intervention in an outpatient basis.
- Follow patients very closely during the first week after PAE; patients may often feel worse during this time but will then notice improvement in their symptoms.
- Stop BPH medication 1 week after PAE.
- Use MRI for follow-up.

CONCLUSION

BPH can be treated safely by PAE with low rates of side effects and can reduce prostate volume by an average of more than 30%. Overall clinical improvement in LUTS assessed by IPSS, quality of life, and urodynamic data is achieved without urinary incontinence, ejaculatory disorders, or erectile dysfunction. Nevertheless, a multidisciplinary approach with urologists, diagnostic radiologists, and interventional radiologists is essential.

REFERENCES

1. Wei JT, Calhoun E, Jacobsen SJ. Urologic disease in America project: benign prostatic hyperplasia. *J Urol.* 2005;173:1256–1261.
2. Emberton M, Andriole GL, de la Rosette J, et al. Benign prostatic hyperplasia. A progressive disease of aging men. *Urology.* 2003;61:267–273.
3. Ziada A, Rosenblum M, Crawford ED. Benign prostatic hyperplasia: an overview. *Urology.* 1999;53:1–6.
4. AUA Practice Guidelines Committee. AUA guideline on management of benign prostatic hyperplasia (2003). Chapter 1: diagnosis and treatment recommendations. *J Urol.* 2003;170:530–547.

5. Wasson J, Reda D, Bruskewitz R, et al. A comparison of transurethral surgery with watchful waiting for moderate symptoms of benign prostatic hyperplasia. The Veterans Affairs Cooperative Study Group on Transurethral Resection of the Prostate. *N Engl J Med.* 1995;332:75.
6. Rassweiler J, Teber D, Kuntz R, et al. Complications of transurethral resection of the prostate (TURP)—incidence, management, and prevention. *Eur Urol.* 2006;50:969–979.
7. Dall'Oglio M, Srougi M, Antunes A, et al. An improved technique for controlling bleeding during simple retropubic prostatectomy: a randomized controlled study. *BJU Int.* 2006;98:384.
8. Gacci M, Bartoletti R, Figlioli S, et al. Urinary symptoms, quality of life and sexual function in patients with benign prostatic hypertrophy before and after prostatectomy: a prospective study. *BJU Int.* 2003;91:196–200.
9. Rubenstein J, McVary KT. Transurethral microwave thermotherapy of the prostate (TUMT). http://www.usrf.org/news/TUMT/TUMThistory.htm. Accessed September 7, 2014.
10. Muruve NA, Steinbecker K. Transurethral needle ablation of the prostate (TUNA). http://emedicine.medscape.com/article/449477-overview. Accessed September 7, 2014.
11. Wheelahan J, Scott NA, Cartmill R, et al. Minimally invasive laser techniques for prostatectomy: a systematic review. *BJU Int.* 2000;86:805–815
12. DeMeritt JS, Elmasri FF, Esposito MP, et al. Relief of benign prostatic hyperplasia-related bladder outlet obstruction after transarterial polyvinyl alcohol prostate embolization. *J Vasc Interv Radiol.* 2000;11:767–700.
13. Carnevale FC, Antunes AA, da Motta Leal Filho JM, et al. Prostatic artery embolization as a primary treatment for benign prostatic hyperplasia: preliminary results in two patients. *Cardiovasc Intervent Radiol.* 2010;33:355–361.
14. Carnevale FC, da Motta-Leal-Filho JM, Antunes AA, et al. Midterm follow-up after prostate embolization in two patients with benign prostatic hyperplasia. *Cardiovasc Intervent Radiol.* 2011;34:1330–1333.
15. Faintuch S, Mostafa EM, Carnevale FC, et al. Prostatic artery embolization as a primary treatment for benign prostatic hyperplasia in a canine model. *J Vasc Interv Radiol.* 2008;19:S7.
16. Sun F, Sánchez FM, Crisostomo V, et al. Benign prostatic hyperplasia: transcatheter arterial embolization as potential treatment—preliminary study in pigs. *Radiology.* 2008;246:783–789.
17. Jeon GS, Won JH, Lee BM, et al. The effect of transarterial prostate embolization in hormone-induced benign prostatic hyperplasia in dogs: a pilot study. *J Vasc Interv Radiol.* 2009;20:384–390.
18. Appleton DS, Sibley GN, Doyle PT. Internal iliac artery embolisation for the control of severe bladder and prostate haemorrhage. *Br J Urol.* 1988;61:45–47.
19. Michel F, Dubruille T, Cercueil JP. Arterial embolization for massive hematuria following transurethral prostatectomy. *J Urol.* 2002;168:2550–2551.
20. Rastinehad AR, Caplin DM, Ost MC, et al. Selective arterial prostatic embolization (SAPE) for refractory hematuria of prostatic origin. *Urology.* 2008;71:181–118.
21. Bilhim T, Pisco JM, Furtado A, et al. Prostatic arterial supply: demonstration by multirow detector angio CT and catheter angiography. *Eur Radiol.* 2011;21:1119–1126.
22. Clegg EJ. The arterial supply of the human prostate and seminal vesicles. *J Anat.* 1955;89:209–216.
23. Carnevale FC, Antunes AA. Prostatic artery embolization for enlarged prostates due to benign prostate hyperplasia: how I do it. *Cardiovasc Intervent Radiol.* 2013;36:1452–1463.
24. Bagla S, Rholl KS, Sterling KM, et al. Utility of cone-beam CT imaging in prostatic artery embolization. *J Vasc Interv Radiol.* 2013;24:1603–1607.
25. Carnevale FC, da Motta-Leal-Filho JM, Antunes AA, et al. Quality of life and clinical symptoms improvement support prostatic artery embolization for patients with acute urinary retention due to benign prostatic hyperplasia. *J Vasc Interv Radiol.* 2013;24:535–542.
26. Antunes AA, Carnevale FC, da Motta-Leal-Filho JM, et al. Clinical, laboratorial and urodynamic findings of prostatic artery embolization for the treatment of urinary retention related to benign prostatic hyperplasia: a prospective single center pilot study. *Cardiovasc Intervent Radiol.* 2013;36:978–986.
27. Pisco JM, Pinheiro LC, Bilhim T, et al. Prostatic arterial embolization to treat benign prostatic hyperplasia. *J Vasc Interv Radiol.* 2011;22:11–19.
28. Pisco J, Pinheiro LC, Bilhim T, et al. Prostatic arterial embolization for benign prostatic hyperplasia: short- and intermediate-term results. *Radiology.* 2013;266:668–677.
29. Bagla S, Martin CP, van Breda A, et al. Early results from a United States trial of prostatic artery embolization in the treatment of benign prostatic hyperplasia. *J Vasc Interv Radiol.* 2014;25(1):47–52.
30. Bilhim T, Pisco J, Tinto HR, et al. Unilateral versus bilateral prostatic arterial embolization for lower urinary tract symptoms in patients with prostatic enlargement. *Cardiovasc Intervent Radiol.* 2013;36:403–411.
31. Moreira AM, Marques CFS, Antunes AA, et al. Transient ischemic rectitis as a potential complication after prostatic artery embolization: case report and review of the literature. *Cardiovasc Intervent Radiol.* 2013;36:1690–1694.

52

Priapism

Daniel Do • Marcelo Guimaraes

Priapism is defined as the state of tumescence in the absence of sexual stimulation persisting beyond 4 hours and can be divided into ischemic or low-flow and nonischemic or high-flow classifications.[1] Overall incidence of priapism is reported to be low within the general population (0.5 to 0.9 cases per 100,000 person-years).[2–4] Resolution of priapism while preserving erectile function remains the goal of treatment strategies.[1]

Ischemic priapism, also known as *veno-occlusive priapism*, represents approximately 95% of cases.[5] This stems from persisting cavernosal smooth muscle relaxation with resultant failure of contraction, which in turn causes compartment syndrome, increasing intracavernosal anoxia, and acidosis. Immediate treatment is required as tissue damage may begin in as little as 12 hours from onset.[6] Most patients suffering from ischemic priapism for duration greater than 24 hours experience complete erectile dysfunction.[7] Treatment includes pain control, intracavernosal injection of a sympathomimetic drug, aspiration of the corpora, and surgical shunting; endovascular intervention typically has no significant role in treating low-flow priapism. Sickle cell disease represents the most common cause of ischemic priapism in childhood and is found in 63% of cases. In adults, 23% of cases are attributable to sickle cell disease, with a reported lifetime probability of development in 29% to 42% of patients.[4,5,8,9] Given this, concomitant workup and treatment of underlying hematologic blood dyscrasias are often performed on presentation. As endovascular embolic therapy has a limited role in the treatment of ischemic priapism, this chapter will primarily focus on nonischemic priapism.

Nonischemic priapism, also known as *arterial priapism*, was first described by Burt et al.[10] in 1960 and represents a relatively rare phenomenon. It is most commonly a result of perineal or penile trauma, which results in an abnormal fistulous communication typically involving the cavernosal artery and adjacent penile sinusoidal spaces.[5,11] Additional causes related to metastatic disease and intracavernosal injections have been reported,[12,13] with spontaneous resolution rates of up to 62%.[1] High-flow priapism is not considered a urologic emergency as there is maintained arterial inflow through the fistula, allowing oxygenation of the cavernous tissue. Although not at risk for ischemic damage, long-term sequelae may occur from possible structural damage secondary to the increased and persistent arterial inflow.[13–15] Treatment strategies for managing nonischemic priapism include watchful waiting, application of ice packs, ultrasound-guided compression, surgical intervention, endovascular introduction of methylene blue, and endovascular embolization.[14,16,17]

Endovascular techniques have been described using both temporary and permanent embolic agents, including autologous blood clot and gelfoam as well as microcoils, acrylic glue, and particles, respectively.[1,4,18,19] Endovascular intervention, first reported by Wear et al.[19] in 1977, is considered the standard of care beyond conservative treatment, with reported success rates approaching 90%. The risk of erectile dysfunction has been reported to be as low as 5% with use of temporary embolic agents.[1]

Surgical options including shunting, penile exploration, and direct arterial fistulous ligation are considered a last resort treatment strategy.[1] Overall success rate of 20% for shunt surgery and 63% for ligation surgery have been reported.[1,13]

CLINICAL APPLICATIONS

Correct identification of priapism classification is critical as endovascular management plays a role only in cases of nonischemic priapism. A typical clinical history for nonischemic priapism includes an episode of trauma followed by a nonpainful, partially rigid erection. The onset of priapism may be delayed up to 2 to 3 weeks and can be secondary to arterial spasm or ischemia.[4] Physical examination will confirm a partially tumescent corpora carvernosa, and routine laboratory testing is performed to exclude anemia and possible hematologic abnormalities, none of which would be expected with nonischemic priapism.[4] Acquisition of cavernous blood gas analysis should reflect arterial blood color and normal levels of pO2, pC02, and pH.

Color duplex ultrasonography of both the penis and perineum is recommended. Visualization of normal or increased blood flow velocities within the cavernosal arteries confirms a diagnosis of nonischemic priapism.[16,20] Additionally, size of the cavernosal artery may demonstrate enlargement greater than reported upper normal limits of 0.7 mm.[21] Direct visualization of the causative fistula and/or pseudoaneurysm is often encountered and can assist in localization and preprocedural planning.[1,4,20,22] Initial treatment strategy can encompass observation in conjunction with ice packs and site-specific perineal compression. Spontaneous resolution of nonischemic priapism has been reported in up to 62% of cases.[1] However, observation alone can pose a theoretical risk of secondary tissue fibrosis due to excessive, constant arterial inflow resulting in erectile dysfunction.[13–15,23] Timing of definitive therapy remains institution and patient dependent.

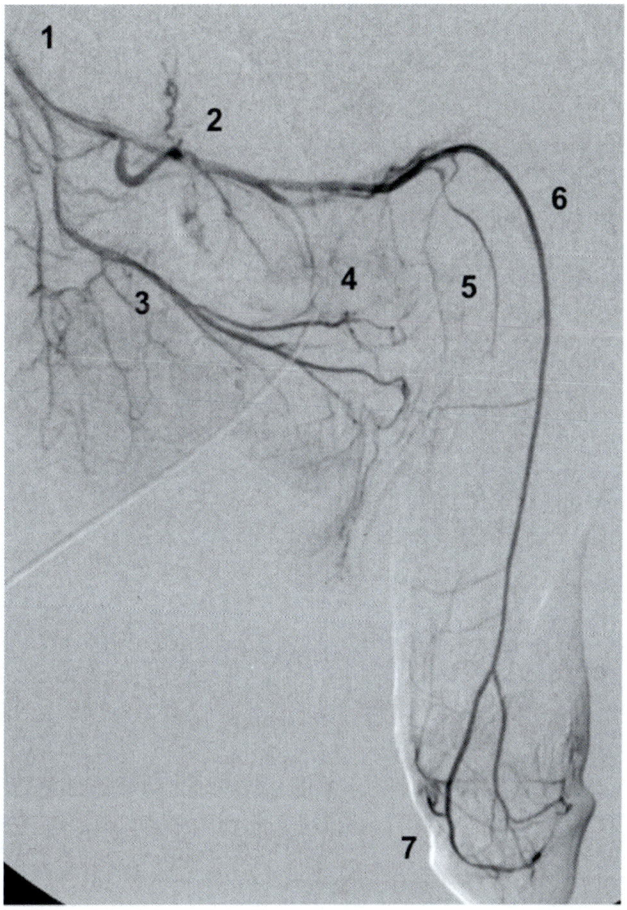

Figure 52.1 The main branches of the IPA (*1*) include the penile artery (*2*), scrotal branch (*3*), penile bulbar artery (*4*), deep penile (cavernous) artery (*5*), the dorsal penile artery (*6*), and the coronal arch artery (*7*).

TECHNIQUE

Before diagnostic angiography, diagnosis should be confirmed with corporal blood gas analysis and ultrasound. Because the arterial inflow is maintained, there should be adequate time for scheduling and planning before intervention. Foley catheter placement should be considered to improve visualization of the pelvic arteries, especially of the internal pudendal artery (IPA) origin. The IPA is typically the smallest branch of the anterior trunk of the internal iliac artery and is responsible for the external genitalia blood supply. Branches of the IPA include the perineal artery, penile artery, penile bulbar artery, deep penile (cavernous) artery, and the dorsal penile artery (Fig. 52.1). It is important to keep in mind that the right and left sided circulations may communicate through branches at the level of the bulb of the penis and between the obturator and IPA.

Standard femoral artery access and angiographic techniques are used. The angiogram should not be the initial imaging modality, and location of the offending lesion can be ascertained from the diagnostic ultrasound. A contralateral femoral artery puncture is typically performed. Following this, a diagnostic pelvic angiogram (Fig 52.2A–C) with selection of the internal iliac artery or its anterior division on the affected side is performed; a Cobra (Cook Medical, Inc., Bloomington, Indiana) or Roberts Uterine Catheter (RUC) (Cook Medical Inc., Bloomington, Indiana) can be used for this angiogram. The Waltman loop technique may be used to form a loop in the 5-Fr diagnostic catheter, which facilitates ipsilateral or contralateral internal iliac arteries catheterization. Interrogation of the unaffected internal iliac artery should be performed to exclude the presence of undetected lesions. Most fistulas will be supplied by the distal IPA. Superselective catheterization of the IPA can be gained through use of standard microcatheter and microwire, introduced coaxially, and advanced just proximal to the fistula.[13]

The most common abnormal angiographic findings are distal IPA pseudoaneurysm (Fig. 52.2B) or arteriovenous fistula (Fig. 52.3). However, the abnormal contrast blush related a vascular lesion identified at the base of the penis (arrow) should not be confused with a normal blush in the bulb of the corpus spongiosum (Fig. 52.4A,B).

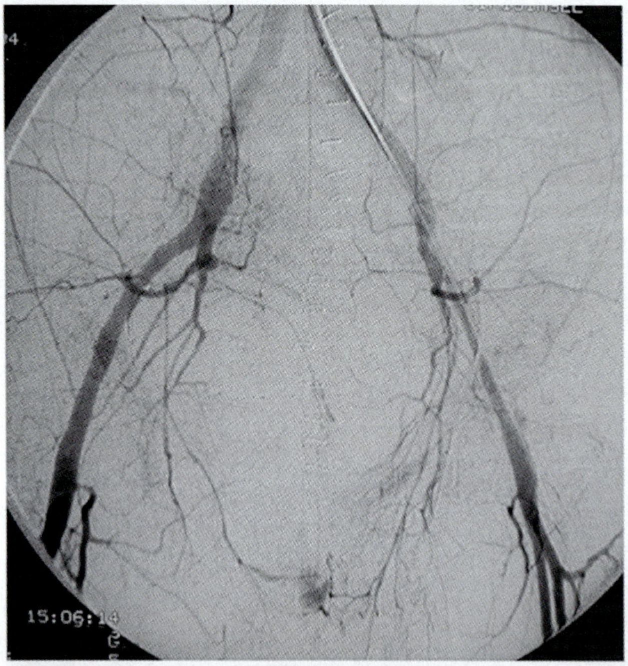

A

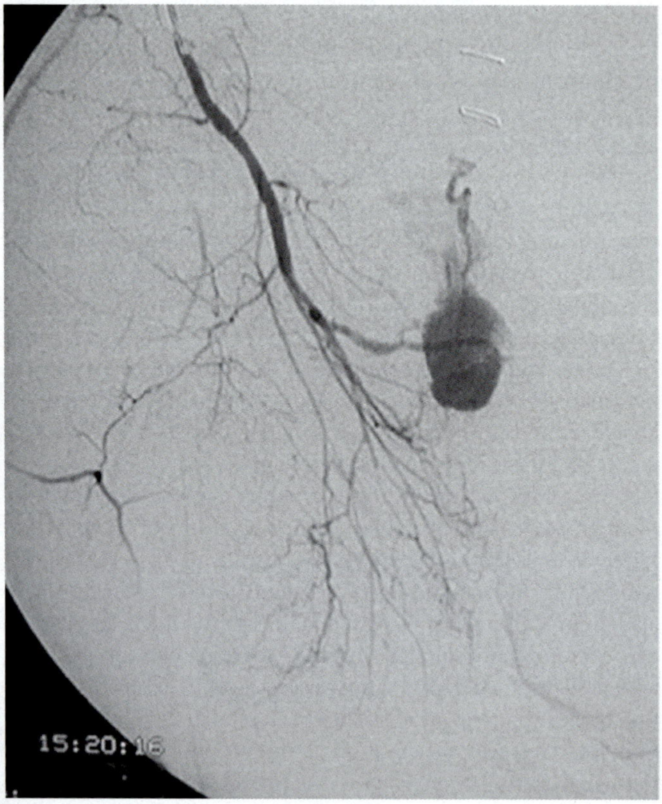

B

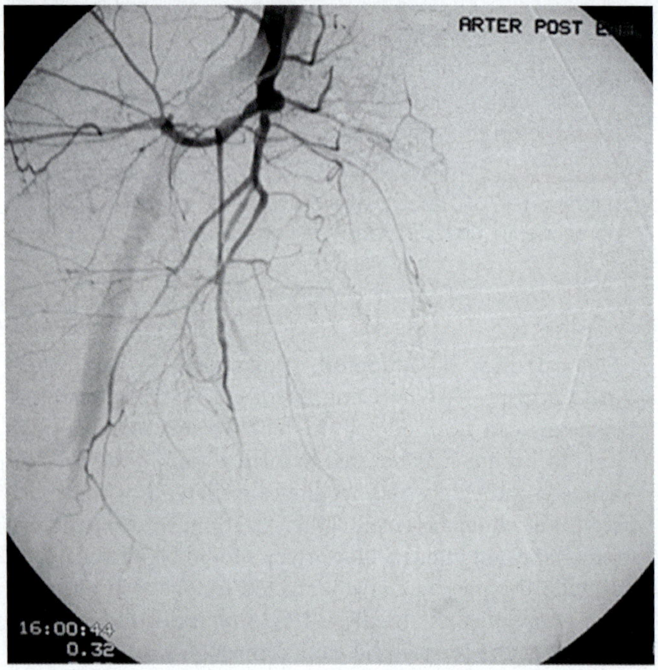

C

Figure 52.2 **A:** Initial pelvic angiogram is always performed to map out the pelvic anatomy. Abnormal arterial blush is identified at the base of the penis. Frequently, it may be difficult to assess in the initial pelvic angiogram which side has the arterial lesion feeding vessel. **B:** Selective internal pudendal angiogram is important to reveal the side that should be embolized. Brisk contrast extravasation is detected from a distal branch of the right internal pudendal artery. **C:** After gelfoam embolization, control right hypogastric angiogram demonstrates adequate treatment of the pseudoaneurysm.

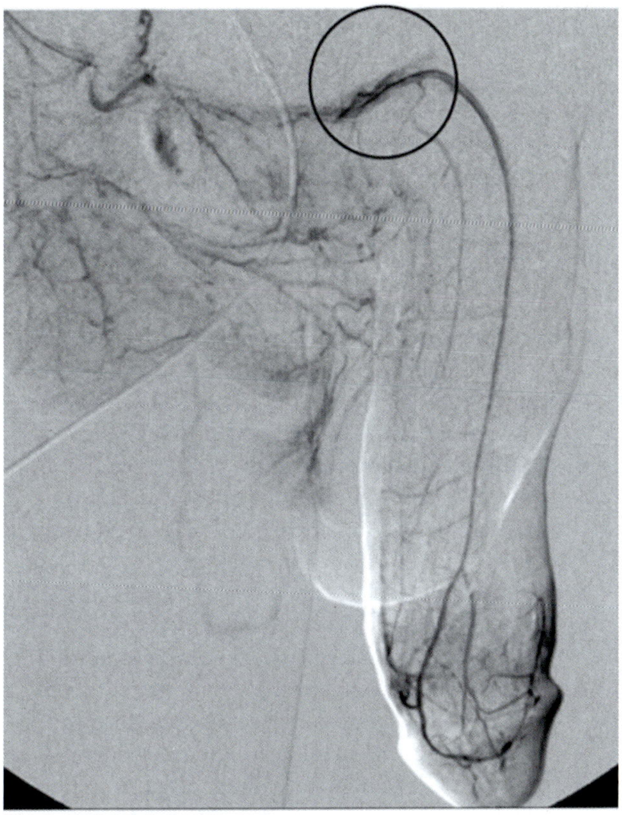

Figure 52.3 Selective right IPA arteriogram, late arterial phase, demonstrates early venous drainage *(circled)*. Arteriovenous fistula from a branch of the penile artery was superselectively catheterized and treated with a single drop of glue (70% glue).

Most lesions involve the distal IPA itself or a distal branch including the common penile artery and the cavernous, dorsal penile, and bulbourethral end arteries.[13,24] Successful vascular occlusion has been achieved with various embolic agents including autologous blood clot, gelatin sponge, polyvinyl alcohol (PVA), *N*-butyl cyanoacrylate (NBCA), and microcoils.[1,4,18,25,26] Permanent embolic agents pose a theoretical increased risk of subsequent development of erectile dysfunction, whereas temporary embolic agents pose an increased risk of recurrence.[1,14] The ultimate choice of embolic agent should depend on angiographic anatomy, clinical presentation, and operator's experience. We always discuss with the patient the risks and benefits of the embolic agents and also include the decision about which embolic material will be used.

In our practice, occlusion with small microcoils is expected to be safer than using liquid embolic agents in high-flow arteriovenous fistulas. However, embolic material should be delivered as close to the point of fistulization as possible. In slow-flow arteriovenous fistulas or in pseudoaneurysms, very small gelfoam torpedo(es) pushed through (not injected) a microcatheter may be used. Alternatively, a small microcoil or a very small amount of glue may be used. Glue requires an experienced operator to prepare an adequate glue/Ethiodol concentration (70% glue, 30% Ethiodol) and to have precise delivery. A lower concentration of glue may favor distal nontarget embolization.

COMPLICATIONS

Regarding endovascular treatment of nonischemic priapism, success rates have been reported as high as 80% to 90% with

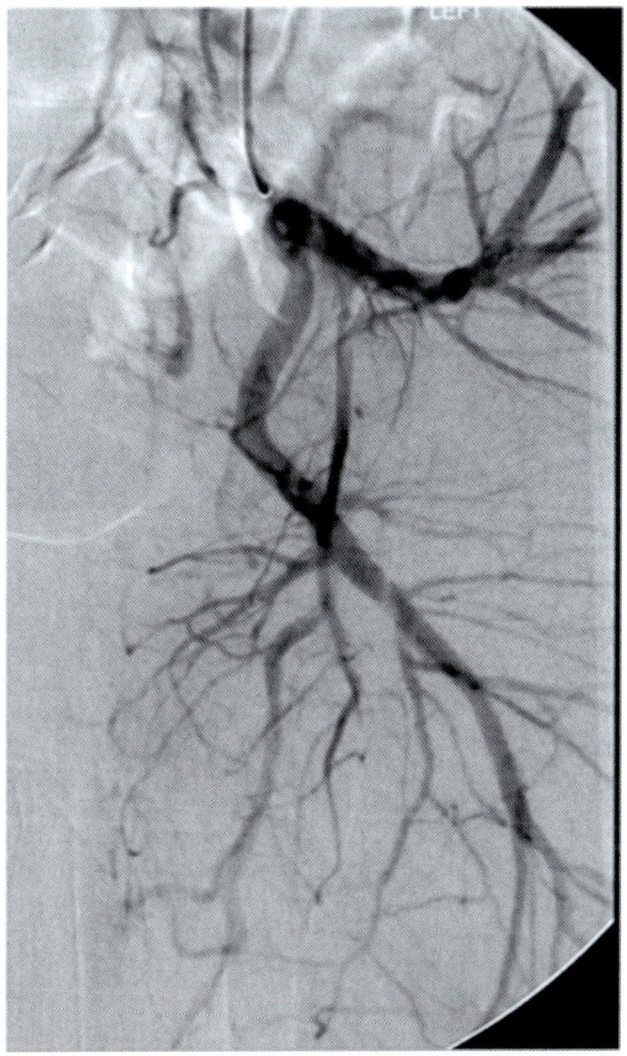

A

Figure 52.4 **A,B:** The normal contrast blush related to the bulb of the corpus spongiosum is identified at the base of the penis (*arrow*), especially in the venous phase. This finding should not be confused with a vascular lesion. *(Continued)*

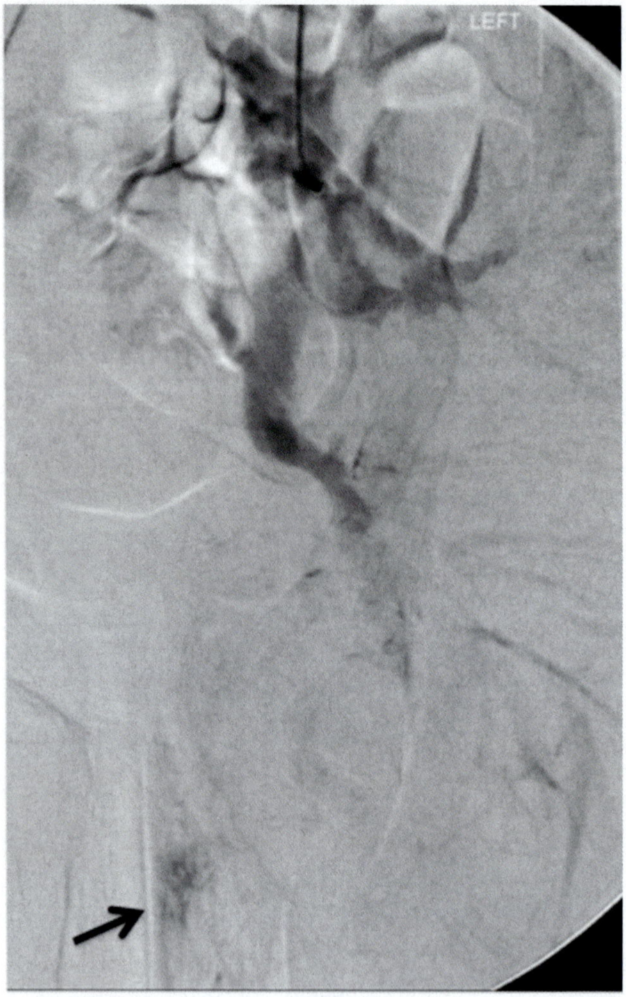

B

Figure 52.4 (Continued)

a maximum of three endovascular sessions.[13] Reported recurrence rates vary from 7% to 40% without specific mention of embolotherapy used.[4,11,15] Erectile dysfunction remains the most significant complication; it has been reported in as many as 39% with the use of permanent embolic agents and in as few as 5% with the use of temporary embolic agents.[1] Rare complications of abscess formation within the corpus cavernosum, penile curving, and gluteal ischemia have also been reported.[16,18,23]

CONCLUSION

In conclusion, embolization is an important tool in the management of high-flow or nonischemic priapism with high success and low complications rates. If technically feasible, preference should be given to temporary embolic agents. On the other hand, permanent embolic agents may be used by experienced interventionists.

TIPS AND TRICKS

- It is crucial that the correct diagnosis of nonischemic priapism be made through careful history, physical examination, cavernous blood gas analysis, and supporting ultrasound findings.
- Misdiagnosis can lead to an unwarranted endovascular procedure in addition to permanent erectile dysfunction if the correct treatment is delayed.
- Ultrasound should be performed in all cases and used to examine the penis, confirming the diagnosis. Examination of the perineum should be performed especially in cases involving saddle injuries as fistulas involving the IPA may be visualized.
- Ultrasound identification of the causative lesion allows for preprocedural angiographic imaging expectations and anticipated contralateral puncture to assist endovascular cannulation.
- Placement of a Foley catheter helps visualize distal pelvic branches
- Perform bilateral internal pudendal arteriograms to understand the vascularization of the external genitalia and penis before embolization is performed.
- On initial endovascular intervention, consider primary use of temporary embolic agents if technically feasible to minimize potential complications involving erectile dysfunction.
- Use of permanent embolic agents may be considered as a primary embolic agent for recurring/persisting lesions and potentially large arteriovenous fistulas.

REFERENCES

1. Montague DK, Jarow J, Broderick GA, et al; Members of the Erectile Dysfunction Guideline Update Panel; American Urological Association. American Urological Association guideline on the management of priapism. *J Urol.* 2003;170(4, pt 1):1318–1324.
2. Kulmala RV, Lehtonen TA, Tammela TL. Priapism, its incidence and seasonal distribution in Finland. *Scand J Urol Nephrol.* 1995; 29(1):93–96.
3. Eland IA, van der Lei J, Stricker BH, et al. Incidence of priapism in the general population. *Urology.* 2001;57(5):970–972.
4. Salonia A, Eardley I, Giuliano F, et al. European Association of Urology guidelines on priapism. *Eur Urol.* 2014;65(2):480–489.
5. Broderick GA, Kadioglu A, Bivalacqua TJ, et al. Priapism: pathogenesis, epidemiology, and management. *J Sex Med.* 2010; 7(1, pt 2):476–500.
6. Pryor J, Akkus E, Alter G, et al. Priapism. *J Sex Med.* 2004; 1(1):116–120.
7. Pryor JP, Hehir M. The management of priapism. *Br J Urol.* 1982; 54(6):751–754.
8. Nelson JH III, Winter CC. Priapism: evolution of management in 48 patients in a 22-year series. *J Urol.* 1977;117(4):455–458.

9. Bivalacqua TJ, Musicki B, Kutlu O, et al. New insights into the pathophysiology of sickle cell disease-associated priapism. *J Sex Med.* 2012;9(1):79–87.
10. Burt FB, Schirmer HK, Scott WW. A new concept in the management of priapism. *J Urol.* 1960;83:60–61.
11. O'Sullivan P, Browne R, McEniff N, et al. Treatment of "high-flow" priapism with superselective transcatheter embolization: a useful alternative to surgery. *Cardiovasc Intervent Radiol.* 2006;29(2):198–201.
12. Dubocq FM, Tefilli MV, Grignon DJ, et al. High flow malignant priapism with isolated metastasis to the corpora cavernosa. *Urology.* 1998;51(2):324–326.
13. Kuefer R, Bartsch G Jr, Herkommer K, et al. Changing diagnostic and therapeutic concepts in high-flow priapism. *Int J Impot Res.* 2005;17(2):109–113.
14. Cantasdemir M, Gulsen F, Solak S, et al. Posttraumatic high-flow priapism in children treated with autologous blood clot embolization: long-term results and review of the literature. *Pediatr Radiol.* 2011;41(5):627–632.
15. Ciampalini S, Savoca G, Buttazzi L, et al. High-flow priapism: treatment and long-term follow-up. *Urology.* 2002;59(1):110–113.
16. Zhao S, Zhou J, Zhang YF, et al. Therapeutic embolization of high-flow priapism 1 year follow up with color Doppler sonography. *Eur J Radiol.* 2013;82(12):e769–e774.
17. Steers WD, Selby JB Jr. Use of methylene blue and selective embolization of the pudendal artery for high flow priapism refractory to medical and surgical treatments. *J Urol.* 1991;146(5):1361–1363.
18. Song PH, Moon KH. Priapism: current updates in clinical management. *Korean J Urol.* 2013;54(12):816–823.
19. Wear JB Jr, Crummy AB, Munson BO. A new approach to the treatment of priapism. *J Urol.* 1977;117(2):252–254.
20. Kang BC, Lee DY, Byun JY, et al. Post-traumatic arterial priapism: colour Doppler examination and superselective arterial embolization. *Clin Radiol.* 1998;53(11):830–834.
21. Wahl SI, Rubin MB, Bakal CW. Radiologic evaluation of penile arterial anatomy in arteriogenic impotence. *Int J Impot Res.* 1997;9(2):93–97.
22. Bartsch G Jr, Kuefer R, Engel O, et al. High-flow priapism: colour-Doppler ultrasound-guided supraselective embolization therapy. *World J Urol.* 2004;22(5):368–370.
23. Hatzichristou D, Salpiggidis G, Hatzimouratidis K, et al. Management strategy for arterial priapism: therapeutic dilemmas. *J Urol.* 2002;168(5):2074–2077.
24. Volkmer BG, Nesslauer T, Kraemer SC, et al. Prepubertal high flow priapism: incidence, diagnosis and treatment. *J Urol.* 2001;166(3):1018–1023.
25. Rados M, Sunjara V, Sjekavica I, et al. Post-traumatic high-flow priapism treated by endovascular embolization using N-butyl-cyanoacrylate. *Radiol Oncol.* 2010;44(2):103–106.
26. Kim KR, Shin JH, Song HY, et al. Treatment of high-flow priapism with superselective transcatheter embolization in 27 patients: a multicenter study. *J Vasc Interv Radiol.* 2007;18(10):1222–1226.

53

Varicocele

Raj Ayyagari • Jeffrey S. Pollak

BACKGROUND

Pathophysiology

By far the most common genitourinary venous pathologic entity that lends itself to embolization therapy is the varicocele, an abnormal and often symptomatic tortuous dilation of the pampiniform venous plexus in the male scrotum. Varicoceles are thought to be caused by acquired incompetence or congenital lack of one-way valves in the gonadal vein (also known as the internal spermatic vein), resulting in abnormal retrograde reflux of venous blood from the inferior vena cava or renal vein, down the gonadal vein, and into the pampiniform plexus surrounding the testicle. Prolonged and repetitive reflux of flow results in abnormal dilation of the venous plexus, manifesting as an often palpable and sometimes painful nest of tortuous and dilated veins in the scrotum, giving a so-called "bag of worms" appearance (Fig. 53.1). The pathophysiology is similar to that seen in lower extremity varicose veins.

The prevalence of varicoceles in the general male population is estimated to be 15% to 17%, increasing in incidence with age from less than 1% of boys younger than 10 years of age up to approximately 15% of boys in late adolescence.[1] Approximately 90% of patients have left-sided varicoceles, and about 10% of patients' varicoceles are bilateral.[2] Right-sided varicoceles are rare and found in less than 1% of patients.[1] However, most varicoceles are asymptomatic.

There are multiple theories about the left-sided predominance of varicoceles, and indeed, the pathophysiology is likely multifactorial. These theories are best understood when considering the normal anatomy of the gonadal veins (Fig. 53.2). The left gonadal vein is one of the longest veins in the body, ascending from the scrotum out of the inguinal canal and up through the retroperitoneum to join the left renal vein at a perpendicular angle in 80% to 90% of the population (the remainder generally join the inferior vena cava directly).[3] The right gonadal vein follows the same general course in the pelvis but then commonly joins the inferior vena cava directly at an oblique angle. The intravascular pressure within the left renal vein is often increased compared to that of the right renal vein because the left renal vein is compressed between the aorta and the superior mesenteric artery, the so-called "nutcracker" effect. This elevated left renal vein pressure and perhaps the anatomical configuration of the venous junction itself are thought to contribute to higher resistance outflow of the left gonadal vein and thus to abnormal reflux of venous blood down the left gonadal vein.[4] This pathophysiology is thought to be further exacerbated by situations that increase intra-abdominal pressure, such as repetitive heavy lifting, coughing, playing certain musical instruments, and even prolonged standing. Some authors believe that there may even be a heritable component that predisposes people to venous incompetency in general and to varicoceles in particular.[5] For these reasons, left-sided and bilateral varicoceles seldom need further workup, whereas an isolated right-sided varicocele or the sudden onset of any varicocele should prompt further investigation with cross-sectional imaging to look for (1) conditions that would cause venous outflow obstruction, such as caval or renal vein thrombosis; (2) conditions that would cause obstruction of the right gonadal vein, such as malignant retroperitoneal lymphadenopathy; or, rarely (3), situs inversus. By

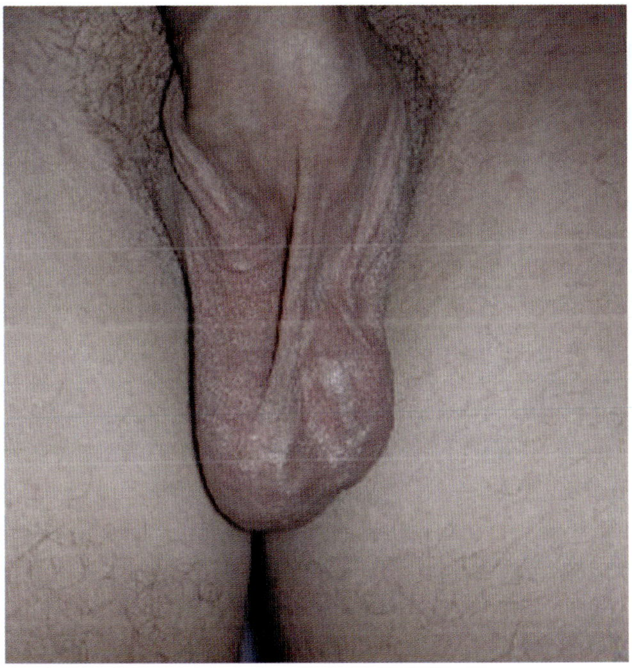

Figure 53.1 Photograph of a left-sided scrotal varicocele, which results from abnormal gonadal venous reflux causing dilation of the pampiniform venous plexus surrounding the testicle. (Adapted from Commons. Wikimedia.org, a public domain repository for images.)

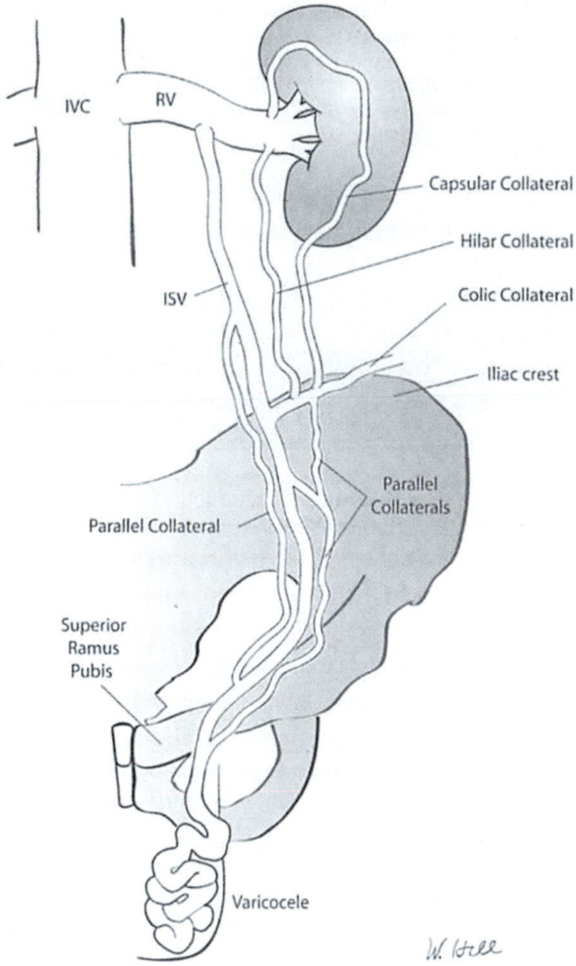

Figure 53.2 Diagram of left-sided male gonadal venous anatomy demonstrating capsular, hilar, colic, and parallel collateral venous channels. The left gonadal vein (internal spermatic vein [*ISV*]) joins the renal vein (*RV*) at a right angle. Abnormal reflux down the gonadal vein results in pathologic dilation of the pampiniform plexus, resulting in a varicocele. IVC, inferior vena cava. (Adapted from Kandarpa K, Machan L. *Handbook of Interventional Radiologic Procedures*. 4th ed. Philadelphia, PA: Lippincott Williams & Wilkins; 2011.)

the time the problem has become evident, normal antegrade venous flow through the gonadal vein may be completely absent, with the venous drainage of the affected hemiscrotum occurring via other collateral scrotal veins such as the external pudendal, cremasteric, and deferential veins. The external pudendal vein drains into the greater saphenous vein, the cremasteric vein drains via the inferior epigastric vein into the external iliac vein, and the deferential vein drains via the superior vesicular vein into the internal iliac vein.

Diagnosis

Varicoceles are usually diagnosed clinically, with patients presenting with palpable and often painful scrotal varicosities. A physical examination should be performed with the patient standing, with careful palpation of both sides of the scrotum done with and without the patient performing a Valsalva maneuver. A grading system for varicocele severity proposed by Dubin and Amelar[6] is frequently used, with grade 0 describing a varicocele that is nonpalpable but visible on ultrasound; grade 1 describing a small varicocele palpable only with Valsalva maneuver; grade 2 describing a moderate-sized varicocele palpable without Valsalva maneuver but not visible; and grade 3 describing a large varicocele that is visible without Valsalva maneuver.

Real-time grayscale scrotal ultrasound with color-flow Doppler is used to confirm the presence of a varicocele or to detect a small varicocele not evident on physical exam (Fig. 53.3). Images are obtained both during rest and Valsalva maneuver to identify abnormal reflux. Prolonged Valsalva-augmented venous reflux longer than 1 second is considered diagnostic of a varicocele.[7] Pampiniform plexus vessel diameter of 3 mm or greater, indicative of abnormal venous distension, is also considered diagnostic.[7] These findings will often be present with the patient supine, but if there is a question, visualizing the scrotal vessels with the patient upright will often augment the findings. Gonadal venography generally does not play a role in diagnosis and is performed only during the actual endovascular treatment of a varicocele.

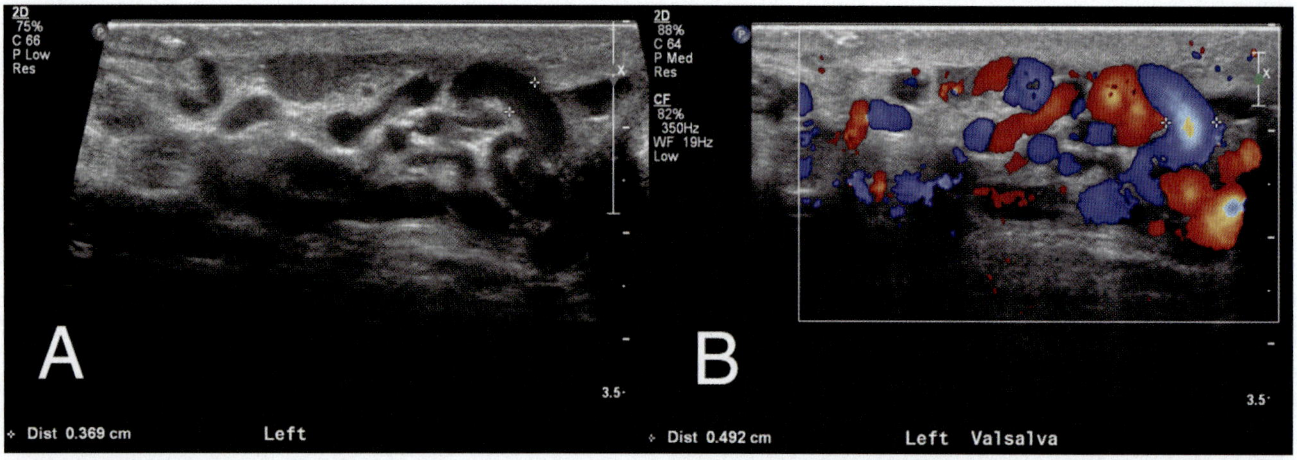

Figure 53.3 **A,B:** Grayscale ultrasound and color Doppler images of the left scrotum showing abnormally dilated and tortuous veins in the left pampiniform plexus. The gray-scale image on the left shows vessels dilated greater than 3 mm. The right image demonstrates significant refluxing vascular flow with Valsalva maneuver, confirming abnormal reflux into the pampiniform plexus.

Indications for Treatment

Any symptomatic varicocele found either on physical exam or with ultrasound merits treatment. However, special consideration should be given to those patients who present with coexisting problems such as inguinal hernias or complex pain syndromes including chronic postoperative groin pain. Such patients should be counseled that treatment of the varicocele may only partially treat their pain at best, and it is appropriate to also refer such patients to a general surgeon or urologist for more complete evaluation of their symptoms before formulating a treatment plan.

Varicoceles are sometimes discovered in boys being evaluated for hypogonadism, and indeed, testicular atrophy can sometimes be reversed or prevented if effective treatment of the varicocele is performed in a timely fashion. [8-10] Varicoceles are also frequently discovered in adult males undergoing workup for infertility, with a prevalence of 30% to 40% in such patients.[11,12] Infertile men with varicocele are often found to have decreased sperm motility, decreased sperm count, and increased abnormal sperm morphology. The detrimental effect of a varicocele in both situations of hypogonadism and infertility is thought to be related to the elevated ambient temperature around the affected testicle brought on by the surrounding abnormally engorged veins. In the case of infertility, the abnormally elevated scrotal temperature is thought to affect sperm production in both testicles, even when the varicocele is unilateral.[13] This phenomenon would tend to undermine other theories that invoke etiologies such as the reflux of toxic metabolites or hypoxia due to venous stasis, as such insults would seemingly affect sperm production on the affected side only given the sparse cross-collateral venous flow between the left and right scrotum. Obliteration of the abnormally engorged veins is reasoned to restore a normal ambient scrotal temperature and to eliminate any reversible detriment on testicular size and sperm production. Indeed, a growing number of studies support a causal relationship between varicoceles and decreased sperm quality by demonstrating positive effects on semen quality after varicocele treatment.[14,15] However, varicoceles have only been shown to be associated with infertility when they are palpable.[16] Furthermore, the positive impact of varicocele treatment on actual fertility remains controversial.[17]

The workup for patients with hypogonadism centers on longitudinal ultrasonographic evaluation of testicular size and growth, whereas workup for patients with infertility should include at least two longitudinal preprocedural semen analyses. Monitoring and treatment recommendations for patients with varicocele and hypogonadism or infertility have been delineated by the Practice Committee of the American Society for Reproductive Medicine and are summarized in the following table (Table 53.1).[18]

Thus, in summary, the treatment of varicoceles is warranted for indications including scrotal pain, male infertility in the presence a palpable varicocele, and persistent hypogonadism in adolescent patients. Treatment is also appropriate for any patient who is uncomfortable with the cosmetic appearance of the varicocele, and indeed, some varicoceles can become quite large. Furthermore, varicocele embolization is warranted for any of the conditions mentioned earlier in the setting of recurrence after prior surgical attempt at varicocele ligation.

Once the diagnosis of varicocele has been confidently made and there is an appropriate indication for treatment, further preprocedural evaluation for a percutaneous embolization procedure is straightforward. Laboratory analysis to ensure appropriate clotting parameters (international normalized ratio and platelet level) and renal function (serum creatinine level or estimated glomerular filtration rate) is

Table 53.1 Recommended Indications for Varicocele Embolization Proposed by the Practice Committee of the American Society for Reproductive Medicine

- Adolescents with varicocele and reduced ipsilateral testicular size should be offered varicocele repair. Adolescents with varicocele but normal ipsilateral testicular size should be monitored with annual measurements of testicular size and/or semen analysis.
- Adult men with asymptomatic varicocele and normal semen analysis should be followed with semen analysis every 1–2 years.
- Adult men with palpable or symptomatic varicocele with either normal or abnormal semen analysis should be offered varicocele repair.
- Varicocele treatment should be offered to the male partner of a couple attempting to conceive when (1) a varicocele is palpable, (2) the couple has documented infertility, and (3) the female has normal fertility or potentially correctable infertility and the male partner has one or more abnormal semen parameters.
- After treatment of a varicocele, semen analysis should be performed at approximately 3-month intervals for at least 1 year or until pregnancy occurs.

Adapted from The Male Infertility Best Practice Policy Committee of the American Urological Association, the Practice Committee of the American Society for Reproductive Medicine. Report on varicocele and infertility. *Fertil Steril*. 2008;90(suppl 5):S247–S249.

performed. If the patient is young and healthy with no other significant medical history, some authors will forgo such analysis. Clotting diatheses often can be effectively managed in the periprocedural setting with transfusions of blood products. Patients with borderline renal function can also be cautiously considered for embolization, given the relatively small amount of intravenous contrast used for the procedure. The only real contraindication to percutaneous varicocele embolization is a severe reaction to intravenous contrast, in which case surgical repair should be considered.

TECHNICAL DETAILS

There is no effective medical treatment for varicoceles. Treatment options for varicocele repair include surgical ligation and percutaneous embolization. Both treatments work by eliminating abnormal retrograde blood flow through the gonadal vein and down into the pampiniform plexus. Patients often wonder why occluding the main vessel that is supposed to drain the testicle is not harmful, or how blood flow will return from the testicle once this vessel is occluded. It is helpful to explain that by the time the diagnosis has been made, the gonadal vein has already effectively been "broken" and that there are other collateral scrotal veins such as the external pudendal, cremasteric, and deferential veins that have since been providing venous drainage for the testicle and will continue to do so after embolization.

Embolization Materials

Various embolization materials have been used for varicocele embolization and can broadly be categorized into mechanical occlusion devices, such as vascular coils and detachable balloons, and sclerosing agents, such as sodium tetradecyl sulfate (Sotradecol; AngioDynamics, Latham, New York). Coils and Sotradecol comprise the mainstay of embolization materials used in modern-day practice, although cyanoacrylate-based glue is a liquid embolic agent commonly used for this application in European centers. Polidocanol is another sclerosant agent used by some, although this agent is not available within the United States. Many of the remaining materials described in the following discussion are for historical interest only.

Platinum-based or nickel-chromium alloy coils are the most commonly used embolic agent and are deposited within the gonadal vein at various levels to provide a macrovascular-level mechanical occlusion and thus prevent reflux of venous blood down into the scrotum. These coils serve as thrombogenic agents, thus proper occlusion with such coils depends on the body's ability to form clot effectively. These coils are manufactured in various shapes and sizes and come in both 0.035-in/0.038-in and 0.018-in varieties for use with either standard size 4-Fr or 5-Fr catheters or smaller microcatheters, respectively. Modern embolization coils are inert, magnetic resonance imaging–compatible, and have not been significantly associated with any adverse side effects. These points should routinely be mentioned to patients, who will often have concerns about having foreign objects implanted within them for the rest of their lives.

Recently developed detachable vascular occlusion plugs are highly effective devices that allow for greater precision of placement and more efficient occlusion, with one such device often providing an occlusion equivalent to several coils. However, such advantages usually have little practical significance in the low-flow, relatively peripheral gonadal vein and do not justify the current higher cost of such devices. In the past, tungsten coils and detachable balloons were used; however, these devices have been removed from the market due to unfavorable cost and efficacy profiles.

Many authors advocate the use of a chemical sclerosing agent for varicocele embolization, often in conjunction with vascular coil placement. [19-21] The most commonly used agents are sodium tetradecyl sulfate (Sotradecol) and sodium morrhuate, which are anionic surfactant detergents that act by causing an inflammatory disruption of the endothelial linings of the treated vessels and triggering the aggregation of platelets and granulocytes.[22] Previously, application of these agents had been limited to the gonadal vein itself due to concerns for scrotal thrombophlebitis if the sclerosing agent passed below the level of the inguinal canal. Indeed, manual compression of the inguinal canal and balloon occlusion of the inferior gonadal vein during sclerosant injection used to be standard. However, reports of investigators injecting sclerosing agents directly into the pampiniform plexus with good results began to emerge, and now some authors advocate deliberate transvenous catheter injection of sclerosant into the pampiniform plexus itself, in conjunction with coil embolization.[23] There is evidence that this combined technique provides better results, owing to the complementary macrovascular coil-mediated gonadal vein occlusion and the microvascular sclerosant-mediated pampiniform plexus sclerosis.[19–21] Indeed, the sclerosant liquid foam can pass into and treat small parallel channels not occluded mechanically by coils. The combined coil embolization and Sotradecol sclerosing technique is described in detail in the following discussion. In the past, other agents such as heated contrast, hypertonic glucose with monoethanolamine, and absolute ethanol were used, but these agents have fallen out of favor due to unfavorable pain and efficacy profiles.

Technique

Transvenous varicocele embolization can be performed as an outpatient procedure under intravenous moderate sedation using standard medications such as fentanyl and midazolam. The patient needs to be arousable and cooperative during the procedure to perform the Valsalva maneuver at times during the embolization. It is helpful to perform the procedure on a table that can be tilted to facilitate identification and cannulation of vessels that have competent valves and thus may not be immediately recognized. Vascular access can be obtained from either the right common femoral vein or right internal jugular vein, depending on operator preference. Jugular access can be ergonomically advantageous when bilateral or right-sided varicocele embolization is planned. Such access also eliminates the need to have the patient lay flat after the procedure and the small but slightly increased hematoma risk with femoral vein access. However, femoral vein access often proves more convenient when a unilateral left-sided varicocele embolization is planned.

With either jugular or femoral access, the vein is accessed with ultrasound guidance and a 6-Fr or 7-Fr vascular sheath is placed. If treating the left side, the left renal vein is then easily selected with a 5-Fr hockey stick–shaped catheter (Terumo Medical Corporation, Somerset, New Jersey) from the jugular approach or with a 7-Fr Hopkins-customized gonadal guiding catheter (Cordis Corporation, Miami Lakes, Florida) from the femoral approach (Fig. 53.4). Either catheter can then be easily manipulated into the left gonadal vein using contrast injections to guide catheter positioning. If the 7-Fr gonadal catheter is used to select the left gonadal vein, a coaxial 5-Fr glide catheter is then used to navigate further down into the left gonadal vein. Renal venography done while the patient performs a Valsalva maneuver is sometimes necessary to identify the left gonadal vein, and tilting the patient feet-down can help with this, especially if there is a competent valve in the gonadal vein. If treating the right side, the right gonadal vein can be selected from the jugular approach with a 5-Fr hockey stick–shaped catheter or with a Simmons-1 catheter from the femoral approach. Sometimes, the use of a coaxially placed microcatheter is necessary to navigate through diffi-

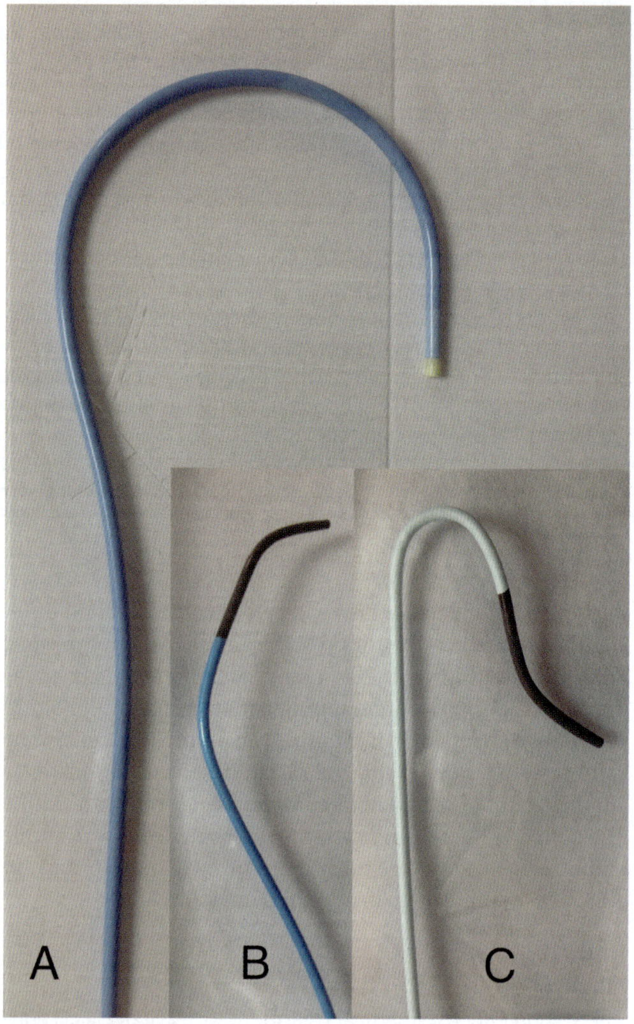

Figure 53.4 Angiographic catheters commonly used for varicocele embolization. **A:** A 7-Fr gonadal guiding catheter used to select the left gonadal vein from a common femoral access. **B:** A 5-Fr hockey-stick catheter used for selecting right and left gonadal veins from internal jugular access. **C:** Simmons-1 catheter used to select the right gonadal vein from a common femoral access. (Photos taken by Dr. Raj Ayyagari.)

cult angles, narrowed or ectopic veins, or competent venous valves and is certainly necessary if treating the right gonadal vein via a femorally placed Simmons-1 catheter.

When selecting the gonadal veins, one must be cognizant of their classic anatomy and common variants. The left gonadal vein drains into the left renal vein approximately 80% to 90% of the time, with multiple gonadal branches seen draining into the renal vein about 10% to 20% of the time and a rare branch even seen draining directly into the vena cava on occasion.[2] The right gonadal vein drains directly into the vena cava at an anterolateral position just below the right renal vein about 80% of the time, while the right gonadal vein will drain into the right renal vein about 10% of the time, and multiple branches draining into the vena cava and right renal vein may be seen 10% to 15% of the time.[2]

Once the targeted gonadal vein is selected, gentle gonadal venography is performed while the patient performs a robust Valsalva maneuver. If the gonadal venous valves are incompetent or absent, contrast will reflux all the way down the gonadal vein and into an often prominent scrotal varicocele (Fig. 53.5). At this point, it is important to map out the entire gonadal venous system, noting commonly present parallel collateral gonadal venous channels as well as any collaterals from capsular, hilar, colic, and lumbar branches. Any or all of these vessels may contribute to reflux and need to be factored into a strategic embolization plan. These branches will often coalesce into one or two gonadal vein channels in the region between the lower sacroiliac joint and the internal ring of the inguinal canal, and thorough occlusion of these more inferior channels will result in successful treatment. If not treated thoroughly, such branches can contribute to later varicocele recurrence.

The catheter is then manipulated to the first coil deposition location, generally at the level of the internal ring of the inguinal canal (Figs. 53.6, 53.7, 53.9, 53.10). This location is selected to allow for coil placement as low as possible, without having the coils pass through the external ring into the scrotum where they may become palpable. The catheter tip can usually be advanced easily using gentle contrast puffing, but if needed, a glide wire can be used to help navigate down the gonadal vein. If a guide wire is used, care should be taken to minimize the potential for vasospasm or perforation and subsequent contrast extravasation. If vasospasm is encountered, the operator will often find spontaneous resolution after waiting several minutes. If vessel perforation and contrast extravasation is encountered, this is of little clinical consequence, although sometimes the venous anatomy can become obscured and make it necessary to abort the procedure and reattempt at a later time once the contrast has dissipated.

If embolization will be done with coils only and no sclerosant will be used, then the vessel diameter is measured and an appropriately oversized coil (usually 20% oversizing

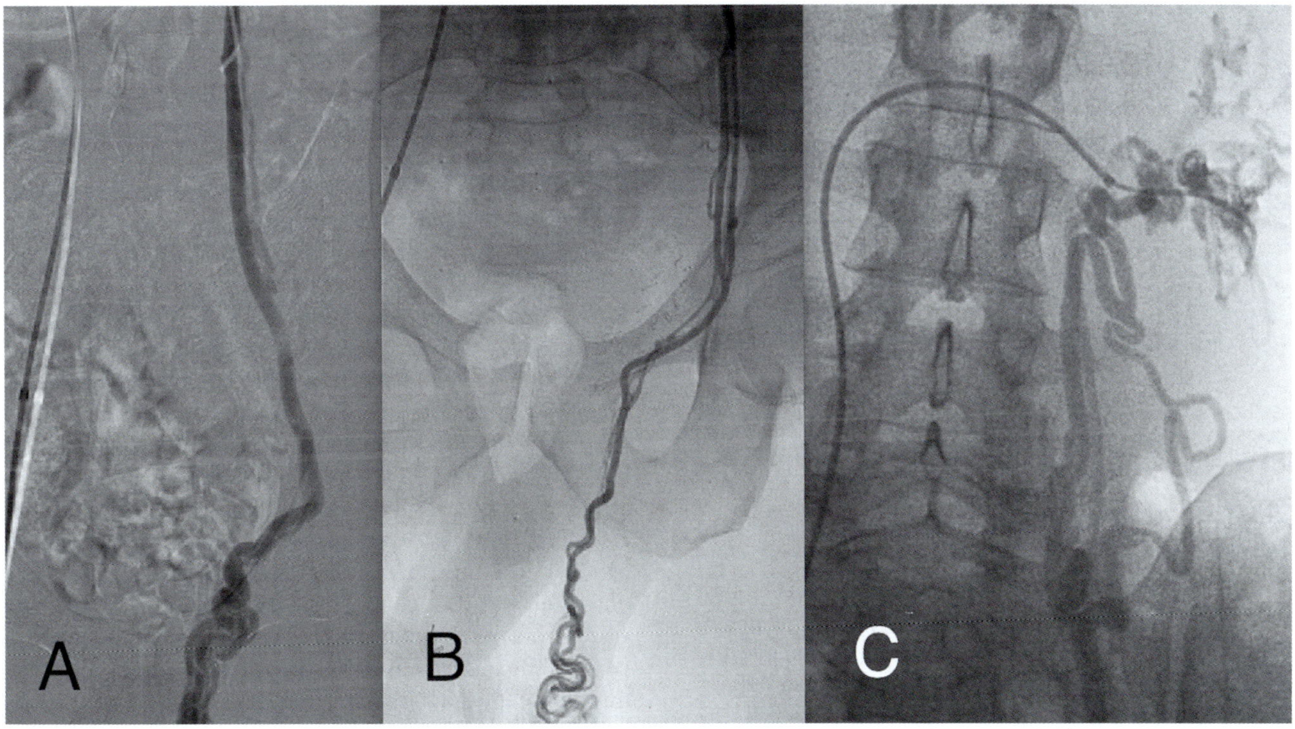

Figure 53.5 Left-sided gonadal venograms in three different patients. **A:** Classic anatomy with a single gonadal vein in the lower pelvis with reflux into a dilated left varicocele. **B:** Multiple parallel gonadal venous channels passing into the scrotum, which would need to be embolized effectively. **C:** A complex configuration of hilar and colic collateral channels connecting to the gonadal vein, any of which could contribute to varicocele recurrence after embolization.

is sufficient) is selected. The initial coil is deployed during Valsalva maneuver to ensure proper positioning and expansion of the coil to its full diameter (the diameter of the vein can dilate with increased intra-abdominal pressure). Additional appropriately sized coils are then deposited sequentially up the gonadal vein, commonly up to a level above the upper sacroiliac joint (Figs. 53.6 and 53.7). Care must be taken to selectively catheterize and coil-embolize any contributing collateral channels along the way to help prevent recurrence. Sometimes, such collaterals will only become visible once the gonadal vein has been occluded more distally. Care must also be taken to deploy the final coil

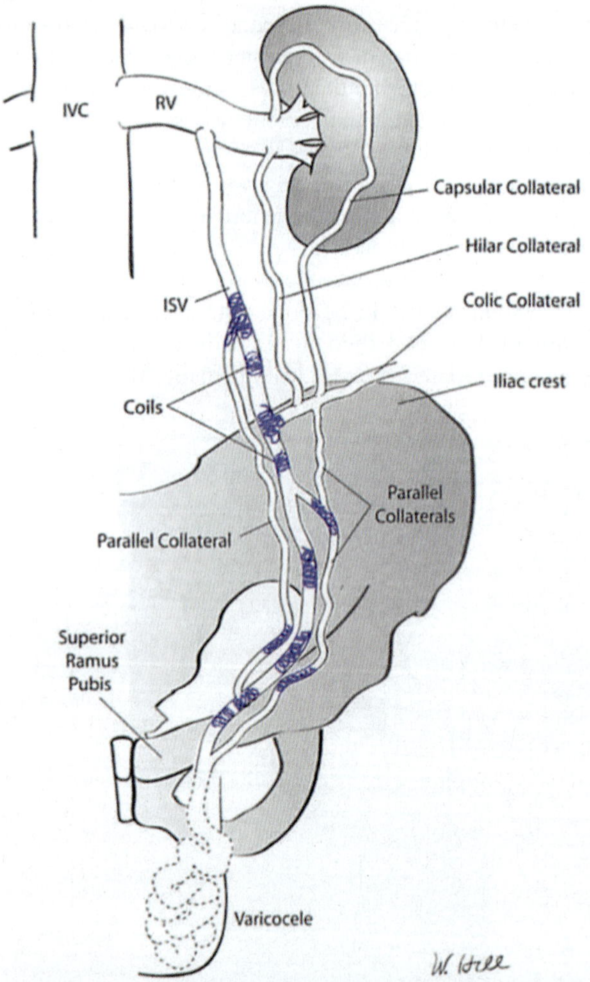

Figure 53.6 Embolization of the left gonadal vein and collaterals using coils only. Coils (*blue*) are placed from the level of the inguinal ring up to the mid-to-upper gonadal vein but safely away from the renal vein. Coils may also need to be placed in parallel collateral channels to avoid recurrence. IVC, inferior vena cava; RV, renal vein; ISV, internal spermatic vein. (Adapted from Kandarpa K, Machan L. *Handbook of Interventional Radiologic Procedures*. 4th ed. Philadelphia, PA: Lippincott Williams & Wilkins; 2011.)

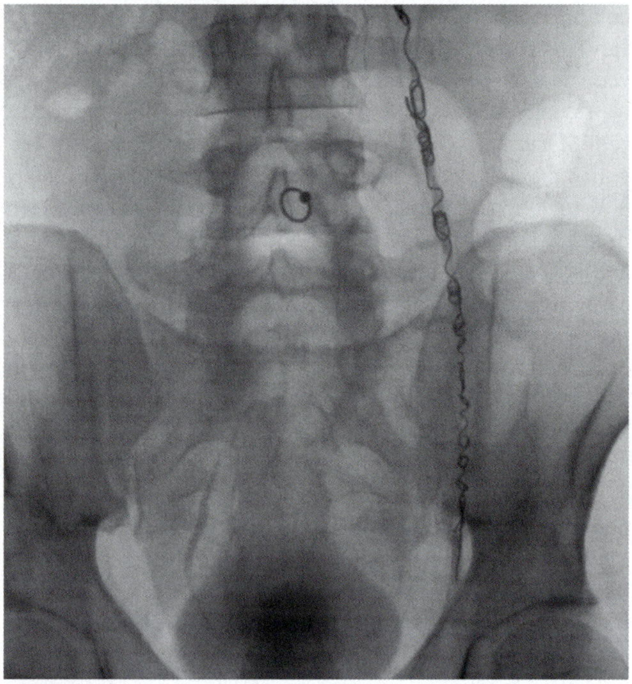

Figure 53.7 Radiograph taken after embolization of the left gonadal vein using coils only.

sufficiently far away from the gonadal–renal venous confluence (Figs. 53.6 and 53.7) so as to avoid migration and nontarget embolization of coils to the heart and lungs.

If sclerosant therapy will be combined with coils, which these authors recommend, then the sclerosant is prepared before deployment of the first coil. These authors use 2% Sotradecol foam, prepared by combining 2 mL of 3% Sotradecol solution with 1 mL of sterile saline and then aggressively mixing the solution with an equal volume of air to form about 6 mL of 2% Sotradecol foam (Fig. 53.8).[19–21]

The first coil is then deployed at the level of the internal inguinal ring as described earlier, and the catheter tip is then gently maneuvered past the coil once it is deployed (Fig. 53.9). While the patient performs a sustained Valsalva maneuver, an aliquot of contrast is injected into the pampiniform plexus to measure the approximate volume of sclerosant needed to fill the targeted vessels (usually ≤3 mL). This is then quickly followed by injection of an appropriate volume of Sotradecol foam that is seen to displace the contrast. The catheter is then cleared with a small aliquot of saline. Using this contrast displacement method, one can easily avoid overinjecting the sclerosant foam into nontarget vessels. The injection is performed distal to the coil to help minimize reflux of sclerosant up toward the renal vein and to help direct it down into the pampiniform plexus, where stasis of the sclerosant is enhanced by the presence of the coil. After a dwell time of a few minutes, often, a second aliquot of sclerosant is injected into the pampiniform plexus using the same contrast displacement technique. The catheter tip

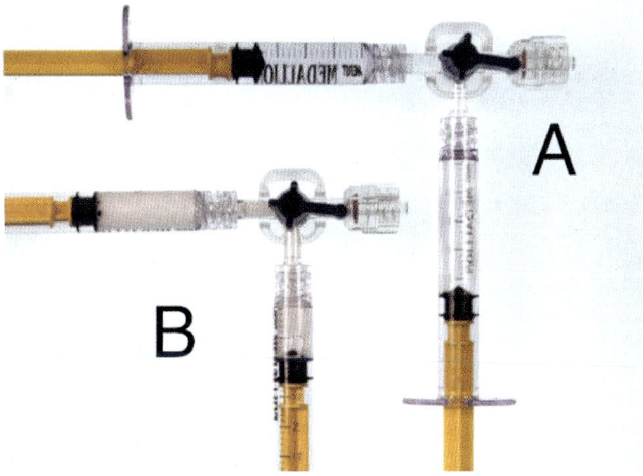

Figure 53.8 Preparation of 2% Sotradecol foam. Assembly **A** shows a syringe containing 2 mL of 3% Sotradecol solution combined with 1 mL of saline connected to a syringe with 3 mL of air. After vigorous mixing, assembly **B** shows approximately 6 mL of 2% Sotradecol foam ready for injection. (Photograph taken by and used with permission from Dr. Robert White.)

is then gently withdrawn back through the coil, and another appropriately sized coil is deposited within the first one. A few minutes later, repeat venogram is performed during Valsalva maneuver to confirm occlusion of the distal gonadal vein. Additional coils can be placed if needed to complete the occlusion, although two coils are often sufficient if appropriate time is given for thrombosis to occur. The catheter is then withdrawn back to the region of the sacroiliac joint, and the entire process is repeated. An appropriately oversized coil is deployed, and then the segment between the two coiled areas is treated with one or two aliquots of Sotradecol foam. An additional coil is then placed within the most recently placed coil, and afterward, a follow-up venogram is performed to confirm occlusion, with additional coils placed if necessary (Figs. 53.9 and 53.10). Again, care must be taken to adequately treat any contributing collateral channels found along the way to help prevent recurrence. A major benefit of using a fluid sclerosant is that it will often percolate into such channels and treat them, avoiding the need to selectively catheterize and coil these vessels. Once embolization is complete, all catheters and sheaths are removed and hemostasis at the venous access site is generally achieved with 5 minutes of manual compression. Patients are usually given 30 mg of intravenous ketorolac during the embolization, which effectively treats sclerosant-related inflammatory pain in the left scrotum and pelvis.

Overall, this combined technique seems to provide a more thorough embolization and can also be cost-effective because it uses significantly fewer coils. Additionally, noncontributory gonadal and collateral venous segments closer to the kidney are left patent to facilitate easier access to them if follow-up treatment is needed in the rare case of recurrence.[19–21]

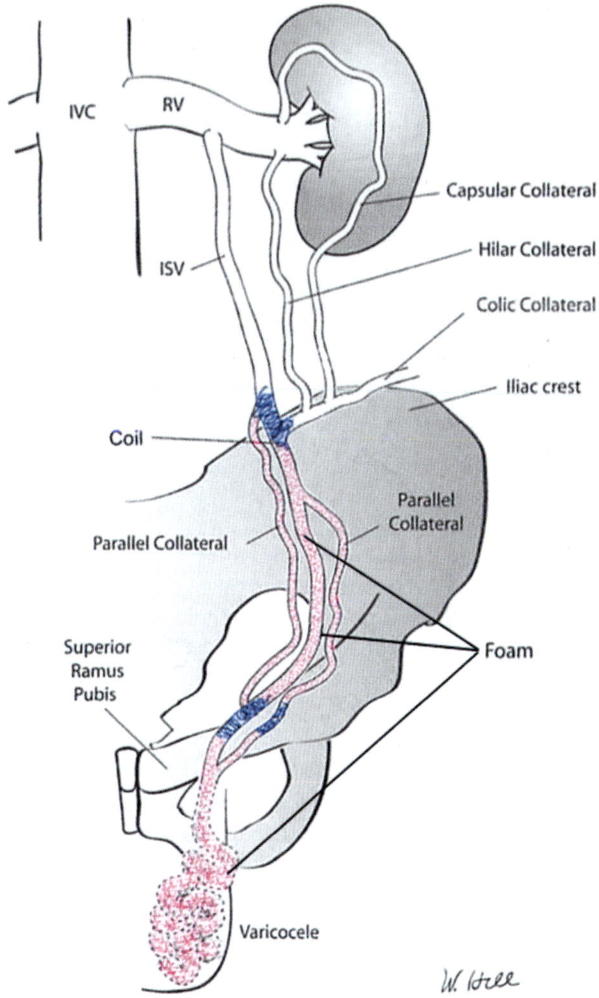

Figure 53.9 Embolization of the left gonadal vein and its collaterals using the combined coil and Sotradecol embolization technique. Coils (*blue*) are placed at the level of the inguinal ring and then strategically higher up in the region of the sacroiliac joint. Two percent Sotradecol foam (*purple*) is also injected into the dilated pampiniform plexus and pelvic gonadal vein as well into any collateral branches. Parallel collateral channels are treated to avoid recurrence. Note that significantly fewer coils are used with this technique. IVC, inferior vena cava; RV, renal vein; ISV, internal spermatic vein. (Adapted from Kandarpa K, Machan L. *Handbook of Interventional Radiologic Procedures*. 4th ed. Philadelphia, PA: Lippincott Williams & Wilkins; 2011.)

Postprocedure Management

As described, transvenous varicocele embolization is a well-tolerated outpatient procedure that entails minimal

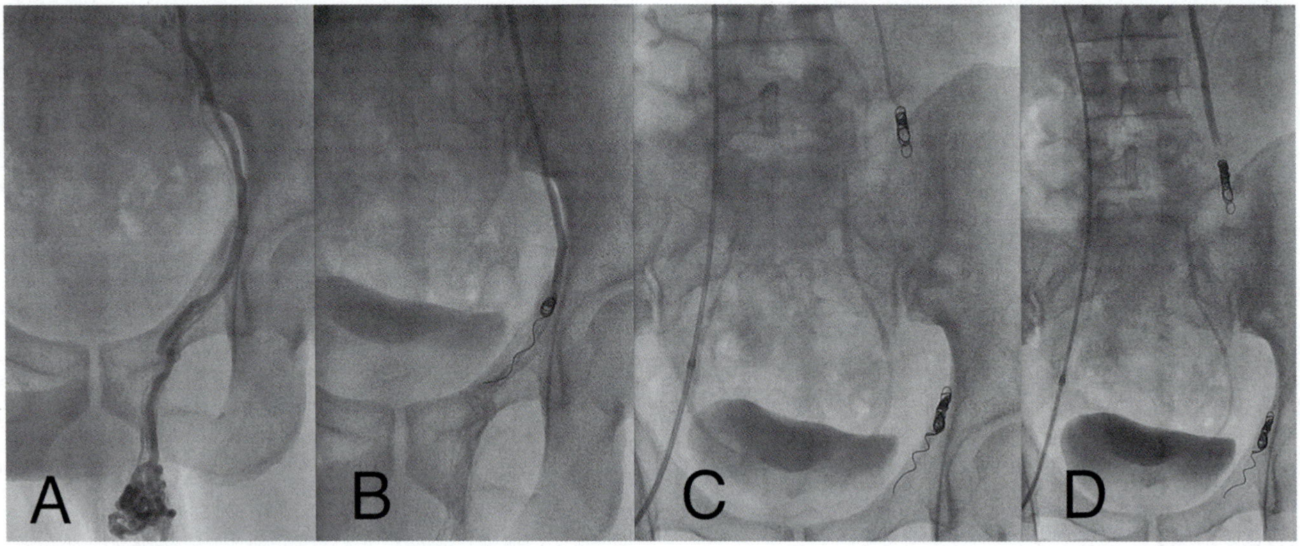

Figure 53.10 **A–D:** Radiographs taken during and after embolization of the left gonadal vein using the combined coil and 2% Sotradecol foam technique. Coils are placed strategically at the level of the inguinal ring and higher up in the region of the sacroiliac joint. Injected Sotradecol foam is not radiopaque and thus not visible on these images.

recovery time and postprocedure care. Following the procedure, patients are observed in a recovery area for 2 to 3 hours. If right femoral vein access is used, two of those hours are spent lying flat, with the right hip joint immobile. Patients are able to eat as soon as they desire. Minimal postprocedure pain in the left scrotum is usually well treated with nonprescription oral ibuprofen, as is minor pain at the venous access site.

Patients are discharged home with instructions to rest for 1 day and to refrain from strenuous activity or heavy lifting for 2 days, mainly to prevent venous access site hematomas. They are permitted to return to normal nonstrenuous activity the day after the procedure. Patients will often have residual left scrotal pain for a few days after the sclerosant therapy, which is expected and normal. Such pain is easily treated with nonprescription doses of ibuprofen and is not an indication for any restriction on activity. In the rare case that ibuprofen is insufficient, a short 2- to 3-day course of oral ketorolac can be prescribed. Patients can remove their dressings usually after 48 hours. Patients are counseled that sometimes they may subsequently feel a palpable bump or "cord" in the groin on the embolized side, which corresponds to the temporarily palpable thrombosed gonadal vein running out of the external ring of the inguinal canal. Patients may also feel palpable thrombosed varices in the scrotum, depending on the size of the varicocele. Patients will sometimes worry that such bumps are coils that have migrated, and supportive reassurance helps to allay such concerns.

Patients can be seen in follow-up with a postprocedure scrotal ultrasound after 3 months, by which time scrotal varices should have thrombosed completely and any palpable thrombosed vessels should have reduced in prominence (Fig. 53.11). For patients who had varicocele embolization in the setting of infertility, semen analysis should not be done until at least 3 months after embolization as any beneficial effects on sperm quality may not be seen before then. Another semen analysis 6 months after embolization may reveal further improvement. Recurrence rates are generally less than 10% and seem to be lower when combined sclerotherapy is used.[19–21] For the rare patient who has persistent or recurrent symptomatic scrotal varices after treatment, repeat venography and embolization can be offered to search for and treat a recanalized gonadal vein or newly prominent collateral veins that are refluxing into the pampiniform plexus.

OUTCOMES

When treating varicoceles for pain, the success rate of percutaneous embolization ranges from 90% to 97%; this is similar to the success rate reported after surgical ligation.[24,25] When treating varicoceles in the setting of male infertility, both approaches also yield similar rates of improvement in semen parameters such as sperm count and motility (27% to 78% of cases after embolization and 24% to 84% of cases after surgical ligation).[12,26] As stated previously, improvements in sperm parameters generally take at least 3 months. Many studies indicate that recurrence rates after percutaneous embolization compare favorably to those of surgical repair.[27]

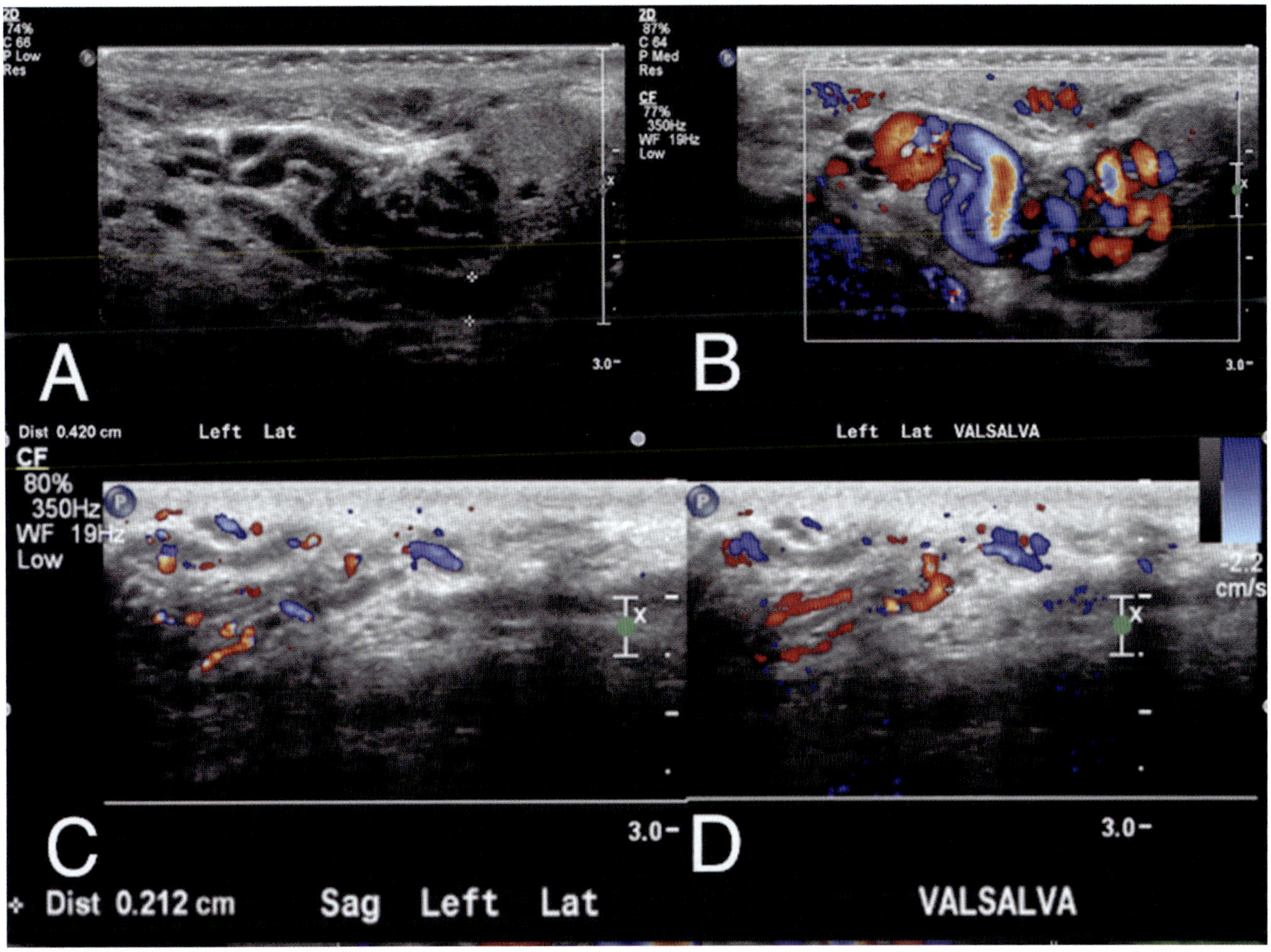

Figure 53.11 Grayscale ultrasound and color Doppler images of the left scrotum before **(A, B)** and 3 months after varicocele embolization **(C, D)** using the combined coil–Sotradecol embolization technique. The upper preembolization images show abnormally dilated and tortuous veins in the left pampiniform plexus with significant refluxing vascular flow with Valsalva maneuver. The lower images obtained 3 months after embolization show normal caliber veins, some thrombosed, with no reflux seen during Valsalva maneuver.

Although both procedures are done on an outpatient basis, surgical ligation requires general anesthesia, whereas percutaneous embolization requires only intravenous moderate sedation medications. Furthermore, embolization is superior to surgical ligation when considering posttreatment recovery time. Percutaneous embolization involves a single small percutaneous venous access site and, on average, 1 day of recovery time, with most patients being able to return to their normal daily activities the following day. Surgical ligation, on the other hand, involves a larger incision that requires, on average, 6 days of recovery time (Fig. 53.12), depending on the surgical approach and location of the incision (inguinal, retroperitoneal, or infrainguinal).[28,29] Additionally, although the risks of surgical repair are low, they are higher than percutaneous embolization, owing primarily to the risks of hematoma and

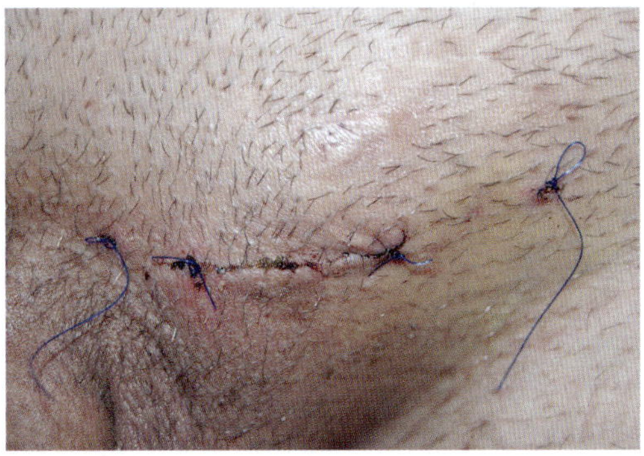

Figure 53.12 Left-sided inguinal incision following surgical varicocele ligation. (Adapted from Commons.Wikimedia.org, a public domain repository for images.)

infection at the incision site and postoperative hydrocele formation, although rare neurovascular injuries to the testicle resulting in atrophy or chronic pain have also been reported.[25] Hydrocele formation is particularly common after surgical ligation in the pediatric population, with incidence as high as 32%, although this is less common when microsurgical techniques are employed.[30] However, hydrocele formation is rare after percutaneous embolization.[31–33] The one theoretical disadvantage of percutaneous embolization compared to surgical ligation is the radiation exposure involved with the image guidance for the procedure. So long as routine care is taken to use fluoroscopy sparingly, optimize x-ray beam collimation, use gonadal shielding when possible, and avoid digital subtraction imaging in favor of low-dose pulsed fluoroscopy, the radiation dose for this procedure is minimal.[34]

POTENTIAL COMPLICATIONS

Complications of transvenous varicocele embolization are rare (<5%), seldom serious, and easily managed.[2] With any percutaneous venous access, there is a small risk of bleeding, usually manifesting as an access site groin hematoma for this procedure. If this occurs before the patient has been discharged, additional manual compression and further immobilization are often all that is needed. If a patient calls from home with concerns for a hematoma, it is generally prudent to have the patient return to the office or the emergency department for further evaluation. Other rare complications include access site infections that can be treated with oral antibiotics, femoral deep venous thrombosis, allergic contrast reactions, contrast nephropathy, and coil migration.

TIPS AND TRICKS

- Use a tilt table to help identify gonadal venous channels with competent valves.
- Microcatheters can also be used to access veins with competent valves.
- Initial coil placement should be done during Valsalva maneuver to ensure proper coil deployment in the desired location.
- Treat the pampiniform plexus and distal gonadal vein with 2% Sotradecol foam using the contrast displacement method.
- Search for and consider treating hilar, capsular, colic, and parallel gonadal vein channels as needed to prevent recurrence.
- Recurrent varicoceles may result from reflux via the cremasteric, deferential, or external pudendal veins.

REFERENCES

1. Diamond DA. Adolescent varicocele: emerging understanding. *BJU Int.* 2003;92(suppl 1):48–51.
2. Mauro MA, Murphy KP, Thomson KR, et al, eds. *Image-Guided Interventions.* Philadelphia, PA: Saunders-Elsevier; 2008.
3. Lechter A, Lopez G, Martinez C, et al. Anatomy of the gonadal veins: a reappraisal. *Surgery.* 1991;109:735–739.
4. Mali WP, Oei HY, Arndt JW, et al. Hemodynamics of the varicocele, part II. Correlation among the results of renocaval pressure measurements, varicocele scintigraphy, and phlebography. *J Urol.* 1986;135:489–493.
5. Gökçe A, Davarci M, Yalçinkaya FR, et al. Hereditary behavior of varicocele. *J Androl.* 2010;31(3):288–290.
6. Dubin L, Amelar R. Varicocele. *Urol Clin North Am.* 1978;5:567.
7. Middleton WD, Kurtz AB, Hertzberg BS. *Ultrasound: The Requisites.* St. Louis, MO: Mosby; 2004.
8. Reyes BL, Trerotola SO, Venbrux AC, et al. Percutaneous embolotherapy of adolescent varicocele: results and long-term follow-up. *J Vasc Interv Radiol.* 1994;5:131–134.
9. Kass EJ, Reitelman C. Adolescent varicocele. *Urol Clin North Am.* 1995;22:151–158.
10. Laven JS, Hanns LG, Mali WP, et al. Effects of varicocele treatment in adolescents: a randomized study. *Fertil Steril.* 1992;58:756–762.
11. Shlansky-Galdberg RD, VanArsdalen KI, Rutter CM, et al. Percutaneous varicocele embolization versus surgical ligation for the treatment of infertility: changes in seminal parameters and pregnancy outcomes. *J Vasc Interv Radiol.* 1997;8:759–767.
12. Schlesinger MH, Wilets IF, Nagler HM. Treatment outcome after varicocelectomy. A critical analysis. *Urol Clin North Am.* 1994;21:517–529.
13. Zorgniotti A, MacLeod J. Studies in temperature, human semen quality, and varicocele. *Fertil Steril.* 1973;24:854–863.
14. Gat Y, Bachar GN, Everacrt K, et al. Induction of spermatogenesis in azoospermic men after internal spermatic vein embolization for treatment of varicocele. *Hum Reprod.* 2005;20:1013–1017.
15. Jarow JP. Effects of varicocele on male infertility. *Hum Reprod Update.* 2001;7:59–64.
16. The Male Infertility Best Practice Policy Committee of the American Urological Association, the Practice Committee of the American Society for Reproductive Medicine. Report on varicocele and infertility. *Fertil Steril.* 2004;82(suppl 1):S142–S145.
17. Marsman WP. Clinical versus subclinical varicocele: venographic findings and improvement of fertility after embolization. *Radiology.* 1985;155:635–638.
18. The Male Infertility Best Practice Policy Committee of the American Urological Association, the Practice Committee of the American Society for Reproductive Medicine. Report on varicocele and infertility. *Fertil Steril.* 2008;90(suppl 5):S247–S249.
19. Kandarpa K, Machan L. *Handbook of Interventional Radiologic Procedures.* 4th ed. Philadelphia, PA: Lippincott Williams & Wilkins; 2011.
20. Reiner E, Pollak JS, White RI, et al. Initial experience with 3% sodium tetradecyl sulfate foam and fibered coils for management of adolescent varicocele. *J Vasc Interv Radiol.* 2008;19:207–210.

21. Arici M, Reiner E, Kirsch J, et al. Results of varicocele embolization using sotradecol foam and fibered coils. *J Vasc Interv Radiol.* 2010;21:S79.
22. Stroncek DF, Hutton SW, Silvis SE, et al. Sodium morrhuate stimulates granulocytes and damages erythrocytes and endothelial cells: probable mechanism of an adverse reaction during sclerotherapy. *J Lab Clin Med.* 1985;106(5):498–504.
23. Gandini R, Konda D, Reale C, et al. Male varicocele: transcatheter foam sclerotherapy with sodium tetradecyl sulfate—outcome in 244 patients. *Radiology.* 2008;246:612–618.
24. Evers JLH, Collins JA. Assessment of efficacy of varicocele repair for male subfertility: a systematic review. *Lancet.* 2003;361:1849–1852.
25. Alqahtani A, Yazbeck J, Garel L. Percutaneous embolization of varicocele in children: a Canadian experience. *J Pediatr Surg.* 2002;37:783–785.
26. Zuckcrman AM, Michell SE, Venbrux AC. Percutaneous varicocele occlusion: long-term follow-up. *J Vasc Interv Radiol.* 1994;5:315–319.
27. Venbrux AC, Trerotola SO. Transcatheter embolotherapy of varicoceles. *Semin Intervent Radiol.* 1994;11:305–311.
28. Sayfan J, Soffer Y, Orda R. Varicocele treatment: prospective randomized trial of 3 methods. *J Urol.* 1992;148:1477–1449.
29. Enquist E, Stein BS, Sieman M. Subinguinal varicocelectomy: a comparative study. *Fertil Steril.* 1994;6:1092.
30. Diamond DA, Xuewu J, Cilento BG Jr, et al. Varicocele surgery: a decade's experience at a children's hospital. *BJU Int.* 2009;104: 246–249.
31. Fayad F, Sellier N, Chabaud M, et al. Percutaneous retrograde endovascular occlusion for pediatric varicocele. *J Pediatr Surg.* 2011;46:525–529.
32. Storm DW, Hogan MJ, Jayanthi VR. Initial experience with percutaneous selective embolization: a truly minimally invasive treatment of the adolescent varicocele with no risk of hydrocele development. *J Pediatr Urol.* 2010;6:567–571.
33. Granata C, Oddone M, Toma P, et al. Retrograde percutaneous sclerotherapy of left idiopathic varicocele in children: results and follow-up. *Pediatr Surg Int.* 2008;24:583–587.
34. Chalmers N, Hufton AP, Jackson RW. Radiation risk estimation in varicocele embolization. *Br J Radiol.* 2000;73:293–297.

54

Uterine Fibroids

James B. Spies

Uterine fibroid embolization (UFE) is now well established as an effective treatment for uterine fibroids, with substantial evidence of its efficacy. Since the first published small case series reported by Ravina et al.[1] in 1995, there have been hundreds of publications on the procedure, including several randomized trials. The accumulated evidence led the American College of Obstetricians and Gynecologists[2] in 2008 to recognize UFE as a safe and effective alternative to hysterectomy in women who have completed childbearing.

This chapter reviews the indications for UFE, the technical details of the procedure, periprocedural care, and anticipated outcomes, with the intent of summarizing this treatment option and its place in current fibroid management.

BACKGROUND

Leiomyomas are the most common tumor of the female reproductive tract, affecting a large proportion of women of reproductive age, with a cumulative incidence of 80% in African American women and nearly 70% in Caucasians by age 50 years in the United States.[3] The prevalence is even higher if hysterectomy specimens are examined using serial thin uterine sections, with leiomyomas found in 77% of uteri in one study.[4]

Fibroids are a condition of women of reproductive age, typically arising in a patient's 30s and regressing after menopause. The natural history of fibroids is typically progressive growth until menopause, with the greatest growth most likely in medium to large fibroids that are intramural.[5] The growth rate is variable between patients and for individual fibroids within a single uterus.

Of those women with fibroids, a substantial proportion will develop symptoms during the course of their reproductive lives.[6] The most common symptom is menorrhagia, which is often accompanied by cramping, pelvic pain, pressure, and increased urinary frequency. Less commonly, patients may have dyspareunia, urinary incontinence, urinary retention, or hydronephrosis. For many women, symptoms are of sufficient severity to warrant treatment.

TECHNICAL DETAILS

Patient Selection

To properly select patients for UFE, it is important that they be properly assessed with a gynecologic history and physical examination, including a pelvic examination by a medical provider experienced in gynecologic care. Often, this will be the patient's gynecologist before referral for UFE evaluation. The diagnosis must be confirmed with imaging. The choice of imaging modality depends on available resources. Ultrasound certainly can confirm the diagnosis of fibroids and exclude other gynecologic pathology in most cases. However, the findings should be confirmed by personal review of the images rather than relying on the report alone. The quality of ultrasound examinations is very variable, and very poor quality or limited examinations should be repeated to ensure that other significant gynecologic pathology is not present.

Ideally, magnetic resonance imaging (MRI) would be the modality of choice for imaging fibroids and the uterus. It provides better spatial resolution and anatomic detail of the architecture of the uterus than ultrasound, and it also provides excellent assessment of adnexal structures. Some uterine conditions, such as adenomyosis, are much more reliably identified with MRI, and in one study, the management of patients was altered based on MRI findings in 22% of cases.[7] Based on the MRI findings, UFE was not performed in 19% of women in whom the procedure was initially planned.

There are no clearly established criteria for who should or should not be treated with embolization. The evidence to date has not been definitive in establishing selection criteria. Some exclusion criteria have been suggested based primarily on a concern that some specific subtypes of fibroids or patients with certain clinical conditions might not do as well.[8] The uterine-specific factors include uteri greater than 20 to 24 weeks size (potentially poorer outcomes), submucosal fibroids greater than 10 cm (due to potential increased risk of fibroid expulsion and infection), and pedunculated fibroids (either submucosal or serosal) that have an attachment to the uterine wall less than 50% the diameter of the fibroid (due to potential for detachment). Unfortunately, there is little evidence to support any of these suppositions, at least to the extent that the evidence makes these "contraindications." For example, although there is some evidence that very large uteri may not have as much shrinkage as smaller uteri and patient satisfaction may trend lower,[9] there are other studies suggesting this is not the case.[10] Similarly, there is little evidence that narrow-based pedunculated fibroids are unsafe to treat.[11,12]

Other nonuterine factors that have been considered contraindications include large hydrosalpinx (due to perceived increased risk of infection), prior pelvic surgery, or procedure that might alter pelvic arterial anatomy, such as salpingo-oophorectomy or surgery for ectopic pregnancy or pelvic radiation. There is essentially no evidence to support these views.

Thus, there are few absolute contraindications and few proven relative contraindications. Clearly, current pregnancy or known or suspected uterine or adnexal malignancy are contraindications. Most anatomic limitations related to fibroids themselves are really in the context of considering the other treatment options for the patient. Large intracavitary fibroids may be more prone to expulsion, and in some cases, other treatments such as myomectomy or hysterectomy may be preferred. Similarly, a small pedunculated serosal fibroid in a multifibroid uterus may be best treated by UFE, whereas a large pedunculated single serosal fibroid might be better approached surgically with myomectomy.

Further, the question of future fertility must always be considered. Although the fertility outcomes are reviewed later in this chapter, the question of whether the patient is interested in future childbearing must be answered. The limited data available from randomized trials currently suggest that myomectomy should be the first consideration in a patient who would like to become pregnant in the subsequent 2 years.

When evaluating patients for UFE, the anatomy of the uterus, the presence or absence of adnexal abnormalities, the patient's age, her interest in pregnancy, and her willingness to consider hysterectomy or other surgical alternatives all should be considered before making a recommendation for the patient. UFE is suitable for most patients with symptomatic fibroids, but so are other fibroid treatments. The patient should understand the range of the options for her in order for her to make an informed choice.

Technique

UFE is an angiographic procedure usually performed via femoral arterial access. Most practitioners use unilateral femoral access, usually on the right side. There is an alternate method, that of bilateral femoral access, which has been used by some groups. Because each UFE usually requires embolization of both uterine arteries, bilateral approach allows for simultaneous embolization. This results in shorter fluoroscopy times and shorter procedure times.[13]

Regardless of whether unilateral or bilateral access is used, UFE requires selective catheterization of the uterine arteries before embolization. There is some controversy regarding placement of the catheter tip within the vessel. Early in the development of UFE, a case report was published on a patient who experienced sexual dysfunction after UFE, and the authors speculated it could be from occlusion of the cervical vaginal branch of the uterine artery.[14] This lead to the belief that embolization should only be done with the catheter tip distal to that branch. This can be difficult as it often arises from the mid transverse portion of the uterine artery and is distal to multiple looping segments of the vessel. Even with the use of a microcatheter, placement of the catheter tip at that level can be very difficult. This degree of manipulation of the catheter can also cause significant spasm in the vessel. Because successful embolization of the fibroids depends on the free flow of the embolic material to the fibroid vessels, it is important to avoid spasm that might impede that flow. Thus, our approach is to place the catheter tip distal to that branch if feasible without causing spasm, but if not, then more proximal position would be acceptable.

Spasm both limits the flow to the fibroids but can also lead to a false end point, with the appearance that there has been adequate reduction in flow when in fact a part of the apparent reduction in flow is due to flow restriction from spasm. One means of trying to avoid or relieve spasm is the use of a microcatheter. Some interventionalists use them routinely for just that reason, whereas others use them selectively. Use of a microcatheter should be the first consideration in relieving spasm. Antispasm medications, such as nitroglycerin, may also be used to help relieve spasm.

Once the catheter(s) is (are) in appropriate position, most interventionalists will perform a preembolization arteriogram to verify anatomy, assess for communications with the ovarian arteries, and ensure there are no abnormal arteriovenous communications before embolization. There

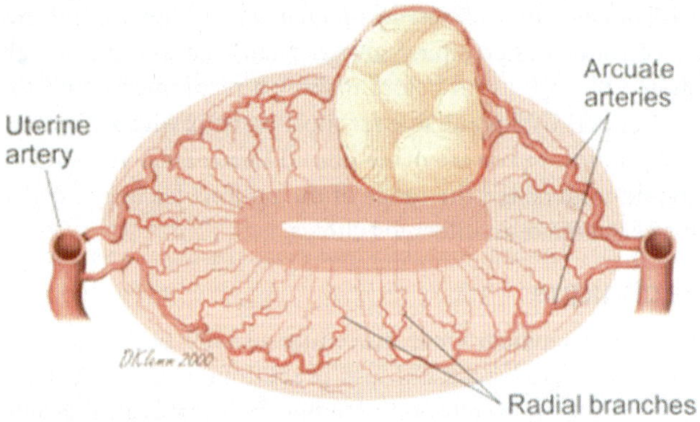

Figure 54.1 Schematic of the vascular supply to a typical leiomyoma, with enlarged end vessels supplying the fibroid, with separate supply to the normal myometrium.

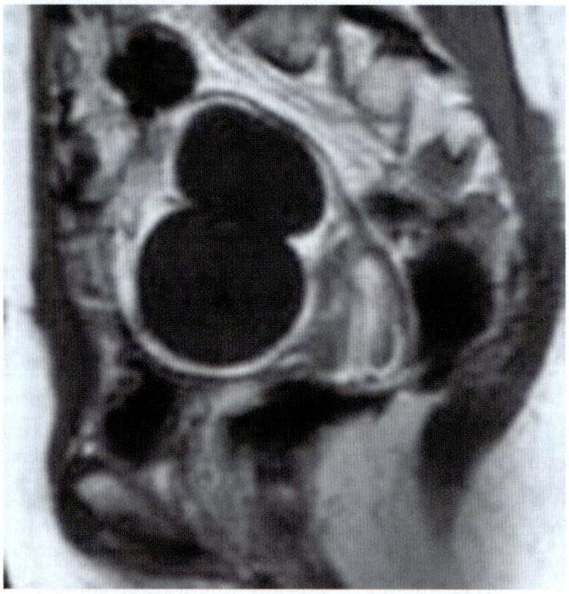

Figure 54.2 Contrast-enhanced MRI sagittal image 48 hours after uterine embolization demonstrating normal myometrial perfusion (enhancement) and no perfusion of the two fibroids.

is at least one reported case of misembolization of embolic material due to a uterine arteriovenous fistula, with embolic material passing through a patent foramen ovale into the heart, brain, and other organs.[15]

Embolic material is injected in small aliquots, with the flow within the uterine arteries carrying the embolic to the fibroid vessels. The vessels feeding fibroids are very large compared to normal myometrial branches (Fig. 54.1). As a result, the flow to them is greatest initially. There is therefore preferential flow to the fibroids. Fibroids are supplied by a limited number of end vessels, and if these are occluded, collaterals cannot reperfuse the fibroid. Because fibroids are very sensitive to ischemia, the occlusion of the feeding vessels typically results in the complete or near complete infarction of the fibroid without injury to adjacent normal myometrium (Fig. 54.2). The extent of fibroid occlusion can vary depending on the embolic material chosen and the end point of embolization. These two topics are discussed further in the following sections.

Although most patients will have uterine and fibroid supply from both uterine arteries, there are some variations. First, occasionally there is only one or perhaps two fibroids that are supplied by one vessel only, with the opposite uterine artery normal. These may be treated by unilateral embolization if certain conditions can be met. First, MRI should be used to clearly define the number and location of the fibroids and to confirm that they are only on one side of the uterus. Unilateral embolization of major fibroids and nontreatment of smaller fibroids on the opposite side will only hasten the recurrence of fibroids and should be avoided. With unilateral fibroids, angiography at the time of embolization must confirm supply to the fibroids from the one uterine artery only. The uterine artery that is to be considered for nonembolization must be normal, perfusing normal myometrium only. If these criteria are met, there is evidence that fibroid infarction rates will match those of bilateral embolization, and it is likely the patient will have diminished pain after embolization when compared to bilateral UFE.[16,17]

There are also variations of the uterine arteries or additional supply to the uterus or fibroids from other vessels, most commonly the ovarian arteries. Several studies have evaluated the frequency of ovarian artery supply to the uterus and it occurs in approximately 5% of cases.[18–20] Most interventionalists will perform an aortogram after embolization if ovarian supply from the uterus is suspected. Pelage et al.[21] recommended performing an aortogram in those cases in which there is a large uterus, a large fundal fibroid, prior myomectomy, or tubal surgery; a study should also be done in cases in which one uterine artery is diminutive or absent.

Currently, most experts recommend that if ovarian artery embolization is to be performed as an adjunct to UFE, a microcatheter should be used for selective catheterization of the vessel and that the tip of the microcatheter be advanced about a third of the distance from the origin to the level of the ovary. Embolization is typically performed with particulate embolics, and usually, only a small amount of embolic is needed, with an end point of near stasis regardless of embolic. In most cases of ovarian embolization, only one ovarian artery requires embolization. Although data are not extensive, it does not appear that embolization of the ovarian arteries increases the risk of ovarian failure after embolization.[22–24] Rarely, other sources of supply, such as the round ligament artery[25] or the inferior mesenteric artery,[26] can provide the uterus or fibroids and should be considered when neither the uterine or the ovarian arteries appear to provide all the vascular supply to the fibroids.

Embolic Material

There are several embolic materials currently available for embolization and also a considerable amount of literature regarding the relative effectiveness of these different products.

There are three embolic materials currently cleared by the U.S. Food and Drug Administration (FDA) specifically for UFE. These are trisacryl gelatin microspheres (TAGM, Embosphere Microspheres; Merit Medical Systems, Inc., South Jordan, Utah), polyvinyl alcohol (PVA) particles (Contour; Boston Scientific Corporation, Natick, Massachusetts), and spherical polyvinyl alcohol (sPVA, Contour SE; Boston Scientific Corporation, Natick, Massachusetts). There are additional materials that are cleared for use for hypervascularized tumors and that are regularly used for fibroid embolization. These are acrylamido PVA microspheres (Bead Block; Biocompatibles, Inc., Oxford, Connecticut), Polyzene-F–coated PVA hydrogel spheres (Embozene Microspheres; CeloNova BioSciences, Inc., San Antonio, Texas), and PVA particles (Cook Medical, Inc., Bloomington, Indiana). In addition, gelatin sponge is used in some settings, although it does not have FDA clearance for use as an embolic agent.

There have been several studies comparing the outcomes of embolization from different embolics. Based on the outcomes from some long-term studies, it has become clear that the best measure of an embolic's efficacy for UFE is the extent to which the fibroids are infarcted.[27] This has been measured by estimating the fibroid infarction rate, usually the estimated percentage of the visible fibroid tissue no longer perfused on a contrast-enhanced MRI.[28]

The first randomized comparative study of embolics for UFE was by Spies et al.,[29] in which the outcomes of UFE using TAGM and PVA particles were compared. Surprisingly, there were few differences between the materials. Before that study, it was widely believed that the use of TAGM caused less postprocedural pain than PVA, but no difference was found. The fibroid infarction rates were nearly identical, with 77% of TAGM and 76% of PVA patients with complete fibroid infarction. This study set the benchmark by which other embolics would be subsequently be compared.

The same group initiated a second study comparing sPVA to Embospheres for UFE and surprisingly did find a significant difference between the two materials.[30] There was a large difference in fibroid infarction rate, with sPVA having a mean residual perfused fibroid volume of 44% versus 9.6% for TAGM. The TAGM group also noted a greater improvement in quality of life scores at 3 months after treatment. Siskin et al.[31] published a similar comparative study and had similar findings: treatment failure in 29.6% of the sPVA group and 3.8% for TAGM, with less fibroid infarction in the sPVA group. Additional studies have confirmed that for UFE, spherical PVA is not as effective as conventional PVA and TAGM for this procedure.

A single randomized trial has compared acrylamido PVA microspheres to TAGM. No difference in fibroid infarction rates was noted, although there was a better quality of life outcome for TAGM.[32] Unfortunately, there were only 44 patients in this study, a small number to compare the embolic efficacy. There have been other nonrandomized trials that have found poorer outcomes with acrylamido PVA, and at this time, the question remains unsettled.

There are case series supporting the efficacy of Polyzene-F–coated PVA hydrogel spheres (Embozene),[33,34] with preliminary evidence suggesting excellent clinical outcomes and high rates of fibroid infarction. There are no comparative studies published to date with the product, although a randomized trial is ongoing currently.

There is relatively little published experience on the use of gelatin sponge for UFE in Western countries, but it has been the standard used in Japan for many years. Katsumori[35–37] has reported extensively on both the short- and long-term outcomes using this material, finding very similar short-, mid-, and long-term outcomes. Whereas in the West gelatin sponge is commonly used as a slurry or as large pledgets, in Japan, it is cut into very small particles of between 500 and 1,000 μm in size. It is not known whether this preparation is critical in obtaining good results.

End Points of Embolization

There has been much discussion over the years regarding the extent to which the uterine arteries need to be occluded to result in fibroid ischemia sufficient to infarct the fibroids. These discussions have been hampered by the lack of tools to objectively measure the end point. Most articles reporting results have used a descriptive end point that can be subject to variation in interpretation.

Initially, UFE was performed with PVA, with either a gelatin sponge plug or a coil used at the end of the embolization to completely occlude the uterine artery, leaving just a stump of a vessel.[38,39] Although the initial results suggested this was successful in causing fibroid shrinkage and presumably fibroid infarction, it also resulted in very significant ischemic pain immediately after the procedure. This technique has been largely abandoned.

When TAGM was first tested in the United States, a descriptive end point was created, with complete occlusion of the fibroid flow but with remaining slow flow in the uterine arteries.[40] This has subsequently been described as the pruned-tree appearance, with complete distal occlusion of the uterine artery branches to the fibroids, but the main trunk of the uterine artery still patent with sluggish flow (Fig. 54.3). This has become the standard end point of embolization, and complete occlusion of the vessel by TAGM results in more severe ischemia and therefore should be avoided as TAGM packs tightly in vessels.

PVA particle, acrylamido PVA, and Polyzene-F-coated PVA hydrogel all are used with a similar end point—with near stasis. This is described as very sluggish residual flow, often with to-and-fro flow in the angled segments of the

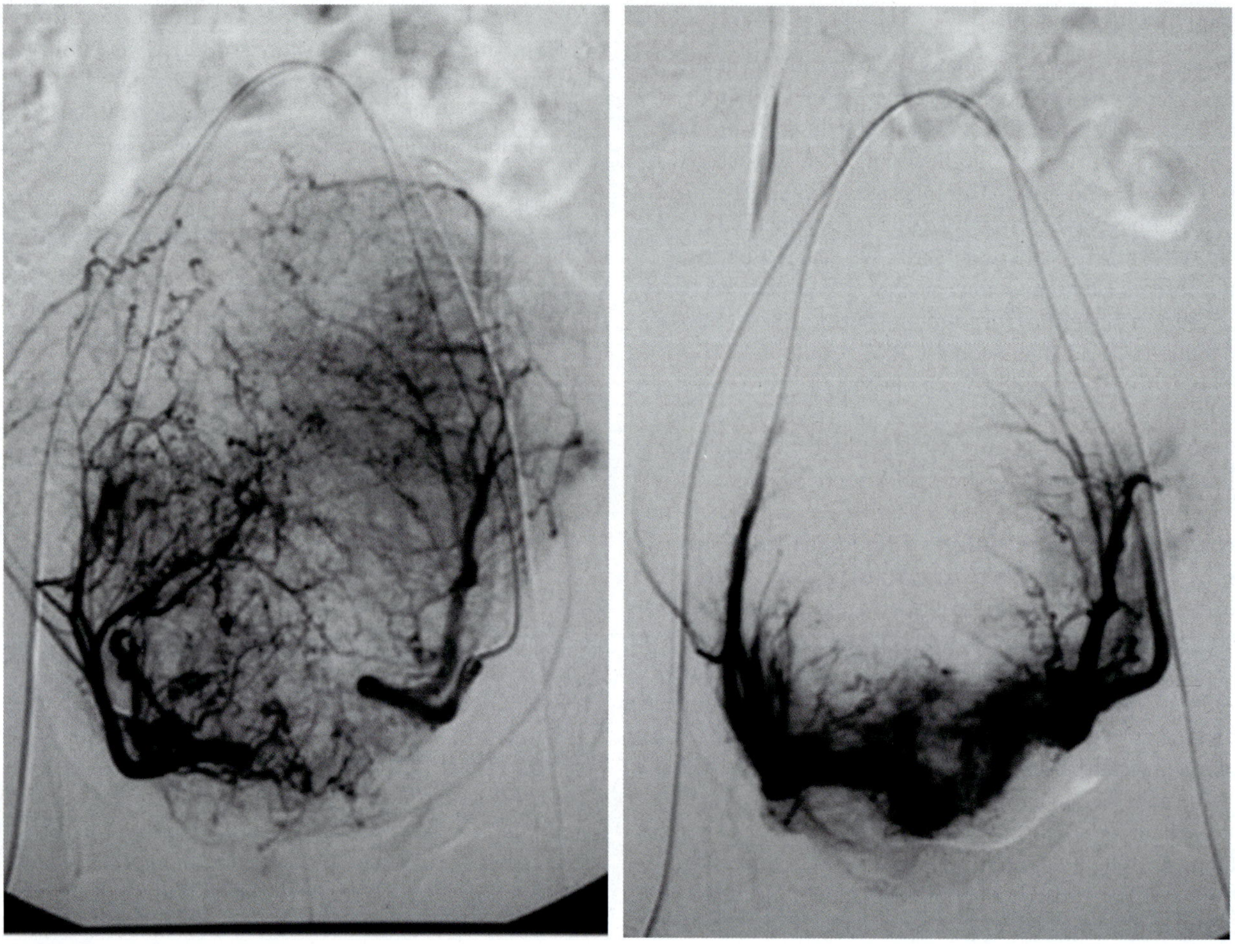

A B

Figure 54.3 Typical angiographic images using TAGM as the embolic material. **A:** Bilateral uterine arteriogram demonstrating multiple enlarged vessels feeding fibroids. **B:** Bilateral uterine arteriogram after embolization demonstrating limited embolization with a pruned-tree appearance, with the distal portions of the fibroid vessels occluded but their proximal portions patent and the main uterine arteries patent.

vessel and essentially complete occlusion of all portions of the fibroid feeding branches angiographically (Fig. 54.4). This more aggressive end point is suggested to ensure that these materials, which are believed to not pack as densely as TAGM, do not recanalize early after the completion of the embolization.

Periprocedural Management

Preprocedure Considerations

Beyond the usual evaluation and preparation of any patient who is to undergo a sedated angiographic procedure, there are a few potential problems that should be considered. These are important because they can help address the common issues that patients are likely to experience after embolization.

Because there is typically significant ischemic pain that occurs immediately after embolization, it is important to have a pain protocol, including patient-controlled analgesia (PCA) pump, ready for start in the angiography suite immediately after the procedure. Although a patient can be treated with intermittent dosing of intravenous narcotics during the transition to the recovery area, there can be delays in nursing response or in the initiation of the PCA pump if left to the recovery area. In any case, it is important for the interventionalist to plan the pain management protocol carefully and instruct nursing staff on the plan and orders to ensure a smooth transition of care.

Many interventionalists routinely use prophylactic antibiotics for UFE. Although there is little evidence to support their use as the risk of periprocedure infection is low, a single preoperative dose has little risk. There is no clear preference of antibiotics defined in the literature. The most important point is for the antibiotic to be given intravenously 30 to 60 minutes before the procedure. There is no evidence for continued use beyond that single preprocedure dose and there is potential harm, therefore it is not recommended.

A Foley catheter is helpful as the uterine arteries can become obscured by the contrast filling the bladder if the

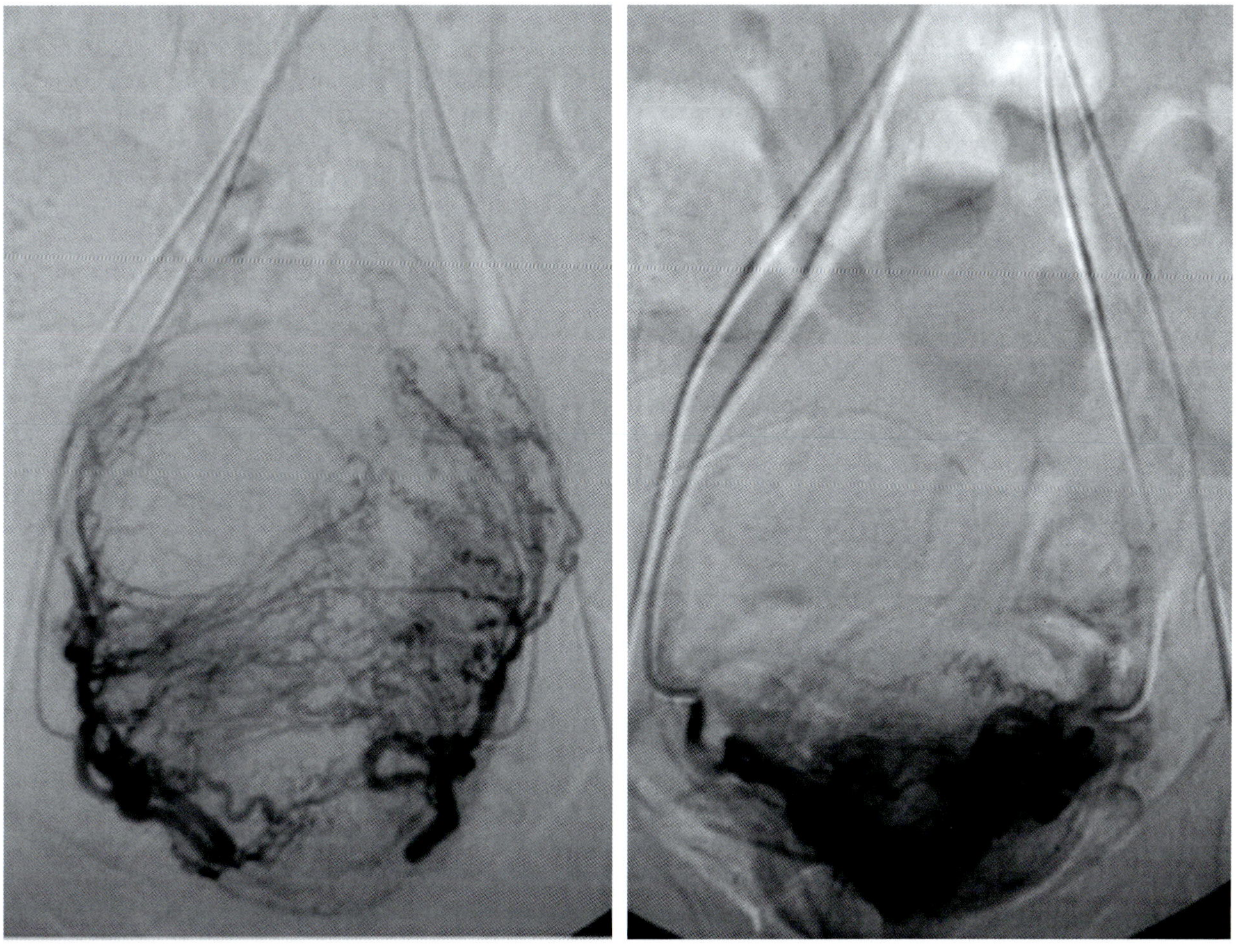

Figure 54.4 Uterine arteriographic end points using particle PVA. **A:** Bilateral uterine arteriogram before embolization showing enlarged vessels feeding fibroids. **B:** Bilateral uterine arteriogram after embolization, with a "near stasis" end point, essentially complete occlusion of all portions of the fibroid feeding branches, but the main uterine arteries remaining patent.

procedure is prolonged. It also is helpful for the first several hours while the patient is at bedrest after the procedure. Some operators choose not to use Foley catheters to reduce the chance of urinary tract infection. If used, it should be discontinued at the earliest time possible, typically within several hours after the procedure when the patient first ambulates.

There is a risk of venous thromboembolism, as will be discussed in a later section. This risk can be potentially reduced by the routine use of pneumatic compression devices and the prophylactic use of low-molecular-weight heparin in patients at high risk.

Postprocedure Pain Management

The key to a successful recovery is proper anticipation of patient problems and planning to manage them. The recovery process can be divided into two phases: in hospital and postdischarge.

Typically, patients will experience moderate to severe pain for several hours after the procedure. This is ischemic pain in the uterus and is caused at least in part by myometrial ischemia. It is known that there is occlusion of some normal uterine branches after UFE, and this results in nonperfusion temporarily to much of the deep myometrium.[41] The degree of myometrial ischemia may be end point driven, although to date, there has been little study on that question. The significant ischemic pain that occurs for several hours after UFE is the first management priority.

There has been a detailed analysis of recovery after uterine embolization published by Bruno et al.[42] Using data from a randomized trial comparing PVA particle and TAGM, the two most commonly used embolics currently and the end points as described in the earlier section, using a 10-point pain scale, the mean peak pain score was 3.03 in the first 24 hours, a relatively modest pain level. Eleven of 99 patients had a peak pain score of greater than 7 on that scale. This level of pain control may be attributed to the use of a standardized pain management regimen, with patients maintained on a PCA pump (in this study primarily morphine) and while being given regular intravenous doses of ketorolac every 6 hours. Supplemental doses of intravenous narcotics, either morphine or fentanyl, were used as needed. In this study, all patients were observed overnight. Nausea was a frequent additional issue, either due to the narcotics or from the procedure itself, and was managed with doses of ondansetron or promethazine as needed.

Pain management also is important after discharge home. Typically, this is a combination of around-the-clock oral nonsteroidal anti-inflammatory medications at a prescription dose and a combination oral narcotic/acetaminophen tablet taken as needed. Anti-inflammatories may be tapered after 4 to 5 days or sooner if cramping is well controlled. Typically, patients will experience cramping for 2 to 3 days and will need to limit activity during that time and for several days thereafter. Fatigue, loss of appetite, and malaise are common, and a third of patients will develop a low-grade temperature in the first week after embolization.[42] These symptoms usually are self-limited and only require supportive care.

OUTCOMES

Clinical Outcomes

A substantial literature now exists documenting treatment outcomes after UFE. A PubMed search of UFE yields over 1,000 references, suggesting that the number of studies related to this topic is large. Given the limitations of space, this review of outcomes will to center on the pivotal randomized trials.

As of October 2013, there have been 37 published papers from randomized trials comparing technical aspects of UFE or comparing other therapies for fibroids with UFE. We will focus on two studies, the REST and EMMY Trials, that compare UFE primarily to hysterectomy and two that compare outcomes to myomectomy (the Fibroids of the Uterus: Myomectomy versus Embolization [FUME] Trial and a trial by Mara and coworkers from Prague). There are 9 publications from the EMMY Trial from the Netherlands, 4 from the REST Trial from the United Kingdom, 2 publications from the study of Mara and coworkers comparing UFE to myomectomy, and 1 from the FUME Trial. We will concentrate on the key publications from these studies comparing hysterectomy or myomectomy to UFE.

The EMMY Trial was a multicenter study completed in the Netherlands. There are several related publications, but two are key—the short-term results[43] and the 2-year results[44]—and these will be reviewed here. The study included 177 patients randomly assigned to UFE (n = 88) or hysterectomy (n = 89). Short-term length of stay was shorter for UFE and there were no differences in major complications. Minor complications were more frequent with uterine embolization. There were higher readmission rates for UFE (11.1% vs. 0%, $P = .003$). To determine longer term outcomes, the EMMY Trial was designed to determine if uterine embolization was "not inferior" to hysterectomy, defined as at least 75% of UFE patients avoiding hysterectomy at 2 years after treatment. By the end of the initial 2 years after treatment, 24% of patients had undergone hysterectomy and the conclusion was that UFE was not inferior to hysterectomy. Both groups had similar improvements in health-related quality of life after treatment and had similar satisfaction levels with the outcomes from treatment.

The REST Trial was a multicenter study from the United Kingdom that randomized patients to either surgery (hysterectomy or myomectomy) or embolization in a ratio of 2 embolization patients to each surgery patient.[45] The primary outcome measure was health-related quality of life after treatment using the SF-36. In the periprocedure period, the study found that UFE is less painful than surgery and has a shorter length of stay and a faster return to work. They found no differences in complications between the two groups. The median follow-up in the REST Trial was 32 months. They found no differences in the quality of life scores at 12 months. Both groups had significant improvement and there was no difference in satisfaction levels. Having said that, reintervention rates were much higher in UFE patients (21 for UFE vs. 1 for surgery, $P < .001$). Ten of these interventions occurred in the first year, presumably due to failure of symptom control, and 11 during subsequent follow-up.

The FUME Trial[46] provides the best evidence of the relative effectiveness of embolization and myomectomy for controlling symptoms. One hundred sixty-three women were randomized to either myomectomy or embolization. Symptom status and quality of life were measured using the Uterine Fibroid Symptom and Health-Related Quality of Life (UFS QOL) questionnaire, a validated fibroid-specific questionnaire,[47] and were compared at 1 and 2 years. Initial symptom control was excellent for both groups, although the myomectomy patients had lower mean symptom scores (fewer symptoms) at 3 months compared to the mean scores for UFE patients. The health-related quality of life scores were also poorer for the UFE group. Reinterventions trended toward greater frequency in the UFE group (14.8% vs. 4%, $P = .067$).

Thus, there are similar outcomes in terms of symptoms and quality of life when comparing surgery to UFE, but most studies have shown higher reintervention rates for UFE. This is balanced by the shorter recovery time, lower overall pain during recovery after UFE, and the minimally invasive nature of the procedure.

Reproductive Outcomes

Mara and coworkers from Prague[48] are the only ones to date to review comparative reproductive outcomes in a randomized trial to date. In this study, 121 patients with a mean age of 32 years were randomly assigned to either myomectomy or uterine embolization. The patients were followed for 2 years and the reproductive outcomes were reported. Overall, the reproductive outcomes were better for the myomectomy group. The pregnancy rate after myomectomy was 78%, the delivery rate was 48%, and the abortion rate was 23% (compared to a pregnancy rate of 50%, delivery rate of 19%, and abortion rate of 64% for UFE). All of these differences were statistically significant. The study had some limitations in that myomectomy was recommended and performed after UFE in a third of the patients (19 of 58 patients), which delayed a trial of pregnancy in those patients and may also have imparted additional reproductive risk due to a second intervention. Regardless, based on this single trial, there appears likely that myomectomy may provide better reproductive outcomes than UFE in the short term.

A systematic review by Homer and Saridogan[49] of reproductive outcomes after UFE provides additional insight. Its focus was on whether UFE imparts additional risk of early and late pregnancy complications when compared to women with fibroids that are untreated. This review summarizes all the reported pregnancies after UFE in the literature (N = 227), with controls identified from various studies. The results of this analysis demonstrate that there are increased rates of miscarriage (odds ratio [OR] = 2.8), cesarean section (OR =2.1), and postpartum hemorrhage (OR = 6.4) after UFE compared to controls. These results need to be interpreted with caution as the control groups were likely dissimilar in extent of disease, prior interventions, and age. Well-designed prospective registries might provide additional insights into pregnancy outcomes.

These studies suggest that although patients may become pregnant after UFE, the reproductive outcomes after myomectomy may be better for many patients. This presumes that the patient has not had prior interventions for fibroids and that she is at an age in which she is likely to become pregnant. Myomectomy also should be the first choice in those patients being considered for assisted reproductive technologies. On the other hand, the reproductive outcomes after a second myomectomy are uncertain and many women have extensive or large fibroids, and it often is not clear if myomectomy is feasible. For these patients, embolization may be a better choice. Each patient's circumstance needs to be individually considered, including patient's reproductive plans, her preferences, the extent of the fibroids, patient age, and feasibility of other therapies.

COMPLICATIONS

Overall, UFE is safe in the short-term and complications are infrequent. Due to space limitations, the focus here will be on complications specifically associated with UFE, with the assumption that the angiographic risks of this type of procedure are well-known.

Embolization-Related Complications

The embolization-related complications are rare. If the catheters or microcatheters are safely placed within the uterine arteries, then there is little likelihood that there will be a complication. Having said that, there are case reports of significant complications related to injury of adjacent structures, such as the vaginal wall, labia, bladder, and even the buttock.[50–55] There are several case reports in the literature reporting ischemic myometrial injury after embolization,[56–58] and this may result in the need for hysterectomy. However, this type of complication is rare as it was not reported in the FIBROID Registry or other large studies of complications.[59,60]

Ovarian dysfunction is a special case of embolization-related complication. The frequency of true ischemic injury to the ovaries is not known, but we know the frequency of amenorrhea after embolization in the FIBROID Registry was reported at 7.3%, 86% of whom were aged 45 years or older. A recent review of the impact of ovarian dysfunction by Kaump et al.[61] showed that most reports of ovarian dysfunction occurred in patients older than the age of 45 years and that there was little evidence of ovarian dysfunction in those younger than 40 years of age.

Fibroid Passage and Infection

The most common late complication that occurs after uterine embolization is fibroid passage, often associated with infection.[59] Although both fibroid passage and fibroid infection can occur as isolated events, often, there is a combination of both, with a spectrum of presentations ranging from minor episodes of tissue passage without infection to chronic low-grade infection and discharge to major tissue passage with substantial pain, bleeding, or infection.

In 2011, Shlansky-Goldberg reviewed his institution's experience with fibroid expulsion and that report provides new insights into this complication.[62] Of 759 patients treated, 37 (5%) had either bulk passage of a fibroid or sloughing over period of time. The mean time of fibroid expulsion was 14.8 weeks after treatment, with the range from 1.6 to 105.9 weeks. The most common presentation of women with symptomatic expulsion was bulk passage of either an entire fibroid or a major fragment, occurring in 89% (31 patients) in this series. Outcomes were generally good, with half the patients requiring no operative intervention. However, in the others, intervention was required, and in 16% (6 of 37) of those with symptomatic expulsion, hysterectomy was required.

Systemic Complications

Malaise, fatigue, and fever are common accompaniments to recovery after uterine embolization, and these are not considered complications.[42] Rarely, pain can be severe and persisting and may require readmission. In this circumstance, if pain does not immediately respond to intravenous medications, a contrast-enhanced MRI should be obtained to assess for possible myometrial injury.

Venous thromboembolism is potentially among the most serious of UFE complications. This is a rare event, but pulmonary embolus has been reported in approximately 1 in

400 patients.[63] It has been established that patients become temporarily hypercoagulable after UFE, similar although not as severe as the hypercoagulability that occurs after surgery.[64] This predisposes to venous thrombosis. There has been one case report of death from pulmonary embolism after UFE,[65] and interventionalists should consider prophylactic measures, particularly in high-risk patients, to prevent these serious outcomes.

TIPS AND TRICKS

Tips

- Complete occlusion of the uterine arteries is not necessary. Embolization should be continued until there is distal occlusion of the fibroid branches, with slow flow in the uterine arteries.
- The likelihood of fibroid expulsion can be estimated to some degree. The greater the fibroid size that has a submucosal component, the more likely it is to be expelled after embolization.
- Although it has often been said that the presence of an intrauterine device increases the risk of infection after UFE and therefore they should be removed, there is no evidence to confirm that belief and some evidence to the contrary.
- Controlling the radiation dose is important; the easiest ways to reduce are to reduce fluoroscopy frame rate to 7.5 per second or less and reduce the rate of filming to 0.5 or 1 per second. Collimation is also important.
- There is no clear advantage of trisacryl gelatin microspheres over PVA particles, the two most frequently used products that have specific clearance by the FDA.
- It is important to look for causes other than fibroids when the bleeding or pain pattern is atypical.
- Understanding the other treatments for fibroids is key to appropriately counseling patients, including the advantages and disadvantages they may have compared to UFE for that patient.
- Cervical fibroids are the one class of fibroids that are regularly not well treated with embolization.

Tricks

- If you have an assistant, bilateral femoral access with simultaneous embolization decreases procedure time and radiation exposure.
- Even when one's routine is unilateral femoral access, consider a second femoral access when the ipsilateral femoral catheterization is difficult.
- Use microcatheters whenever there is uterine artery spasm.
- Retracting the microcatheter a centimeter or two within the uterine artery to above a kink often will relieve spasm.
- Never embolize unless the catheter tip is within the uterine artery; nonselective embolization with particulate embolic will result in injury to other pelvic structures. Also, the catheter should be well within the uterine artery and care should be taken to avoid reflux.
- It is helpful to wait several minutes at the apparent conclusion of the embolization to be sure the end point is stable.
- If an abdominal aortogram is done, it should be done at the end of the embolization. Ovarian arteries that provide supply to the fibroids at the beginning of the embolization often do not at the end of the uterine embolization.

CONCLUSION

UFE should be considered a first-line therapy for women with symptomatic uterine fibroids, with an extensive literature demonstrating its effectiveness and safety. With appropriate patient selection, technique, and periprocedural care, patients can anticipate a rapid recovery and routine to normal activity, with excellent clinical outcomes.

REFERENCES

1. Ravina J, Herbreteau D, Ciraru-Vigneron N, et al. Arterial embolisation to treat uterine myomata. *Lancet*. 1995;346:671–672.
2. American College of Obstetricians and Gynecologists. ACOG practice bulletin. Alternatives to hysterectomy in the management of leiomyomas. *Obstet Gynecol*. 2008;112:387–400.
3. Day Baird D, Dunson D, Hill M, et al. High cumulative incidence of uterine leiomyoma in black and white women: ultrasound evidence. *Am J Obstet Gynecol*. 2003;188:100–107.
4. Cramer SF, Patel A. The frequency of uterine leiomyomas. *Am J Clin Pathol*. 1990;94:435–438.
5. DeWaay DJ, Syrop CH, Nygaard IE, et al. Natural history of uterine polyps and leiomyomata. *Obstet Gynecol*. 2002;100:3–7.
6. Parker WH. Etiology, symptomatology, and diagnosis of uterine myomas. *Fertil Steril*. 2007;87:725–736.
7. Omary R, Vasireddy S, Chrisman H, et al. The effect of pelvic MR imaging on the diagnoisis and treatment of women with presumed symptomatic uterine fibroids. *J Vasc Interv Radiol*. 2002;13:1149–1153.
8. Stokes L, Wallace M, Godwin R, et al. Quality improvement guidelines for uterine artery embolization for symptomatic leiomyomas. *J Vasc Interv Radiol*. 2010;21:1153–1163.
9. Spies J, Roth A, Jha R, et al. Uterine artery embolization for leiomyomata: factors associated with successful symptomatic and imaging outcome. *Radiology*. 2002;222:45–52.
10. Smeets AJ, Nijenhuis RJ, van Rooij WJ, et al. Uterine artery embolization in patients with a large fibroid burden: long-term clinical and MR follow-up. *Cardiovasc Intervent Radiol*. 2010;33:943–948.
11. Katsumori T, Akazawa K, Mihara T. Uterine artery embolization for pedunculated subserosal fibroids. *AJR Am J Roentgenol*. 2005;184:399–402.

12. Smeets AJ, Nijenhuis RJ, Boekkooi PF, et al. Safety and effectiveness of uterine artery embolization in patients with pedunculated fibroids. *J Vasc Interv Radiol.* 2009;20:1172–1175.
13. Costantino M, Lee J, McCullough M, et al. Bilateral versus unilateral femoral access for uterine artery embolization: results of a randomized comparative trial. *J Vasc Interv Radiol.* 2010;21:829–835; quiz 835.
14. Lai A, Goodwin S, Bonilla S, et al. Sexual dysfunction after uterine artery embolization. *J Vasc Interv Radiol.* 2000;11:755–758.
15. Anonymous. Fatal non-target embolization via an intra-fibroid arterial venous fistula during uterine fibroid embolization. *J Vasc Interv Radiol.* 2008;12:419–420.
16. Bratby MJ, Hussain FF, Walker WJ. Outcomes after unilateral uterine artery embolization: a retrospective review. *Cardiovasc Intervent Radiol.* 2008;31(2):254–259.
17. Stall L, Lee J, McCullough M, et al. Effectiveness of elective unilateral uterine artery embolization: a case-control study. *J Vasc Interv Radiol.* 2011;22:716–722.
18. Abbara S, Nikolic B, Pelage JP, et al. Frequency and extent of uterine perfusion via ovarian arteries observed during uterine artery embolization for leiomyomas. *AJR Am J Roentgenol.* 2007;188:1558–1563.
19. Binkert CA, Andrews RT, Kaufman JA. Utility of nonselective abdominal aortography in demonstrating ovarian artery collaterals in patients undergoing uterine artery embolization for fibroids. *J Vasc Interv Radiol.* 2001;12:841–845.
20. Pelage JP, Le Dref O, Jacob D, et al. Ovarian artery supply of uterine fibroid. *J Vasc Interv Radiol.* 2000;11:535.
21. Pelage JP, Walker WJ, Le Dref O, et al. Ovarian artery: angiographic appearance, embolization and relevance to uterine fibroid embolization. *Cardiovasc Intervent Radiol.* 2003;26: 227–233.
22. Hu N, Kaw D, McCullough M, et al. Menopause and menopausal symptoms after ovarian artery embolization: a comparison with uterine artery embolization controls. *J Vasc Interv Radiol.* 2011;22:710–715.
23. Kim HS, Tsai J, Lee JM, et al. Effects of utero-ovarian anastomoses on basal follicle-stimulating hormone level change after uterine artery embolization with tris-acryl gelatin microspheres. *J Vasc Intervent Radiol.* 2006;17:965–971.
24. Kroencke T, Scheurig-Muenkler C. Safety and efficacy of ovarian artery embolization for symptomatic uterine leiomyomata. Presented at: Cardiovascular and Interventional Radiology Society of Europe Annual Scientific Meeting; October 6, 2010; Valencia, Spain.
25. Saraiya PV, Chang TC, Pelage JP, et al. Uterine artery replacement by the round ligament artery: an anatomic variant discovered during uterine artery embolization for leiomyomata. *J Vasc Interv Radiol.* 2002;13:939–941.
26. Chang S, Lee MS, Kim MD, et al. Inferior mesenteric artery collaterals to the uterus during uterine artery embolization: prevalence, risk factors, and clinical outcomes. *J Vasc Intervent Radiol.* 2013;24:1353–1360.
27. Pelage J, Guaou Guaou N, Jha R, et al. Long-term imaging outcome after embolization for uterine fibroid tumors. *Radiology.* 2004;230:803–809.
28. Banovac F, Ascher S, Jones D, et al. MR imaging outcome after uterine artery embolization for leiomyomata using tris-acryl gelatin microspheres. *J Vasc Interv Radiol.* 2002;13:681–687.
29. Spies J, Allison S, Sterbis K, et al. Polyvinyl alcohol particles and tris acryl gelatin microspheres for uterine artery embolization for leiomyomas: results of a randomized comparative study. *J Vasc Interv Radiol.* 2004;15:793–800.
30. Spies JB, Allison S, Flick P, et al. Spherical polyvinyl alcohol versus tris-acryl gelatin microspheres for uterine artery embolization for leiomyomas: results of a limited randomized comparative study. *J Vasc Interv Radiol.* 2005;16:1431–1437.
31. Siskin GP, Beck A, Schuster M, et al. Leiomyoma infarction after uterine artery embolization: a prospective randomized study comparing tris-acryl gelatin microspheres versus polyvinyl alcohol microspheres. *J Vasc Interv Radiol.* 2008;19: 58–65.
32. Worthington-Kirsch RL, Siskin GP, Hegener P, et al. Comparison of the efficacy of the embolic agents acrylamido polyvinyl alcohol microspheres and tris-acryl gelatin microspheres for uterine artery embolization for leiomyomas: a prospective randomized controlled trial. *Cardiovasc Intervent Radiol.* 2011;34:493–501.
33. Smeets AJ, Nijenhuis RJ, van Rooij WJ, et al. Embolization of uterine leiomyomas with polyzene F-coated hydrogel microspheres: initial experience. *J Vasc Intervent Radiol.* 2010;21: 1830–1834.
34. Stampfl U, Radeleff B, Sommer C, et al. Midterm results of uterine artery embolization using narrow-size calibrated embozene microspheres. *Cardiovasc Intervent Radiol.* 2011;34:295–305.
35. Katsumori T, Bamba M, Kobayashi TK, et al. Uterine leiomyoma after embolization by means of gelatin sponge particles alone: report of a case with histopathologic features. *Ann Diagn Pathol.* 2002;6:307–311.
36. Katsumori T, Kasahara T, Akazawa K. Long-term outcomes of uterine artery embolization using gelatin sponge particles alone for symptomatic fibroids. *AJR Am J Roentgenol.* 2006;186: 847–853.
37. Katsumori T, Nakajima K, Mihara T, et al. Uterine artery embolization using gelatin sponge particles alone for symptomatic uterine fibroids; midterm results. *AJR Am J Roentgenol.* 2002;178:135–139.
38. Goodwin S, Vedantham S, McLucas B, et al. Preliminary experience with uterine artery embolization for uterine fibroids. *J Vasc Interv Radiol.* 1997;8:517–826.
39. Walker W. Uterine embolization for leiomyomata: midterm results. *Min Invas Ther Alied Technol.* 1999;8:449–454.
40. Spies J, Bennati J, Worthington-Kirsch R, et al. Initial U.S. Experience using tris-acryl gelatin microspheres for uterine artery embolization for leiomyomata. *J Vasc Intervent Radiol.* 2001;12: 1059–1063.
41. Scheurig-Muenkler C, Wagner M, Franiel T, et al. Effect of uterine artery embolization on uterine and leiomyoma perfusion: evidence of transient myometrial ischemia on magnetic resonance imaging. *J Vasc Interv Radiol.* 2010;21(9):1347–1353.
42. Bruno J, Allison S, McCullough M, et al. Recovery after uterine artery embolization for leiomyomas: a detailed analysis of its duration and severity. *J Vasc Interv Radiol.* 2004;15:801–807.
43. Hehenkamp WJ, Volkers N, Donderwinkel P, et al. Uterine artery embolization versus hysterectomy in the treatment of symptomatic uterine fibroids (EMMY trial): peri- and postprocedural results from a randomized controlled trial. *Am J Obstet Gynecol.* 2005;193:1618–1629.

44. Hehenkamp WJ, Volkers NA, Birnie E, et al. Symptomatic uterine fibroids: treatment with uterine artery embolization or hysterectomy—results from the randomized clinical Embolisation versus Hysterectomy (EMMY) Trial. *Radiology*. 2008;246: 823–832.
45. Edwards RD, Moss JG, Lumsden MA, et al. Uterine-artery embolization versus surgery for symptomatic uterine fibroids. *N Engl J Med*. 2007;356:360–370.
46. Manyonda IT, Bratby M, Horst JS, et al. Uterine artery embolization versus myomectomy: impact on quality of life—results of the FUME (Fibroids of the Uterus: Myomectomy versus Embolization) Trial. *Cardiovasc Intervent Radiol*. 2012;35:530–536.
47. Spies J, Coyne K, Guaou Guaou N, et al. The UFS-QOL, a new disease-specific symptom and health-related quality of life questionnaire for leiomyomata. *Obstet Gynecol*. 2002;99:290–300.
48. Mara M, Maskova J, Fucikova Z, et al. Midterm clinical and first reproductive results of a randomized controlled trial comparing uterine fibroid embolization and myomectomy. *Cardiovasc Intervent Radiol*. 2008;31:73–85.
49. Homer H, Saridogan E. Uterine artery embolization for fibroids is associated with an increased risk of miscarriage. *Fertil Steril*. 2010;94:324–330.
50. Dietz DM, Stahlfeld KR, Bansal SK, et al. Buttock necrosis after uterine artery embolization. *Obstet Gynecol*. 2004;104:1159–1161.
51. El-Shalakany AH, Nasr El-Din MH, Wafa GA, et al. Massive vault necrosis with bladder fistula after uterine artery embolisation. *BJOG*. 2003;110:215–216.
52. Lowenstein L, Solt I, Siegler E. Focal cervical and vaginal necrosis following uterine artery embolization. *Eur J Obstet Gynecol Reprod Biol*. 2004;116:250–251.
53. Payne JF, Haney AF. Serious complications of uterine artery embolization for conservative treatment of fibroids. *Fertil Steril*. 2003;79:128–131.
54. Sultana CJ, Goldberg J, Aizenman L, et al. Vesicouterine fistula after uterine artery embolization: a case report. *Am J Obstet Gynecol*. 2002;187:1726–1727.
55. Yeagley TJ, Goldberg J, Klein TA, et al. Labial necrosis after uterine artery embolization for leiomyomata. *Obstet Gynecol*. 2002;100:881–882.
56. Godfrey CD, Zbella EA. Uterine necrosis after uterine artery embolization for leiomyoma. *Obstet Gynecol*. 2001;98:950–952.
57. McLucas B, Sostrin S. Uterine necrosis after uterine artery embolization for leiomyoma. *Obstet Gynecol*. 2002;100:1357–1358.
58. Pelage JP, Walker WJ, Dref OL. Uterine necrosis after uterine artery embolization for leiomyoma. *Obstet Gynecol*. 2002;99: 676–677; author reply 7.
59. Spies J, Spector A, Roth A, et al. Complications after uterine artery embolization for leiomyomata. *Obstet and Gynecol*. 2002;100: 873–880.
60. Worthington-Kirsch R, Spies J, Myers E, et al. The Fibroid Registry for Outcomes Data (FIBROID) for uterine artery embolization: short-term outcomes. *Obstet Gynecol*. 2005;106:52–59.
61. Kaump GR, Spies JB. The impact of uterine artery embolization on ovarian function. *J Vasc Intervent Radiol*. 2013;24:459–467.
62. Shlansky-Goldberg RD, Coryell L, Stavropoulos SW, et al. Outcomes following fibroid expulsion after uterine artery embolization. *J Vasc Intervent Radiol*. 2011;22:1586–1593.
63. Czeyda-Pommersheim F, Magee ST, Cooper C, et al. Venous thromboembolism after uterine fibroid embolization. *Cardiovasc Intervent Radiol*. 2006;29:1136–1140.
64. Nikolic B, Kessler CM, Jacobs HM, et al. Changes in blood coagulation markers associated with uterine artery embolization for leiomyomata. *J Vasc Interv Radiol*. 2003;14:1147–1153.
65. Hamoda H, Tait P, Edmonds DK. Fatal pulmonary embolus after uterine artery fibroid embolisation. *Cardiovasc Intervent Radiol*. 2009;32:1080–1082.

55

Adenomyosis

Paul N. M. Lohle

BACKGROUND

In the pathophysiology of heavy menstrual bleeding (HMB), two groups may be distinguished: HMB based on anatomic or organic abnormalities (fibroids, adenomyosis, clotting disorders) and essential HMB.[1] There is relatively little knowledge about the exact pathophysiology of HMB in relation to fibroids, polyps, and adenomyosis.

Adenomyosis, associated with HMB, is a benign invasion of endometrium into the myometrium that results in a diffusely enlarged uterus that microscopically exhibits ectopic nonneoplastic endometrial glands and stroma surrounded by the hypertrophic and hyperplastic myometrium.[2] The prevalence of adenomyosis is estimated to be 5% to 8% and up to 40% to 70%.[2–4] This range may be explained by the different study designs, the random testing described in studies, the lack of a gold standard for identifying adenomyosis, and the use of different transvaginal ultrasound (TVUS), magnetic resonance imaging (MRI), and pathologic anatomical criteria for adenomyosis. Adenomyosis has either a focal or diffuse distribution in the uterine wall. Another problem regarding the relation between HMB and adenomyosis is the fact that in 60% to 80% of the cases, the uterus with adenomyosis is accompanied with other pathology, mostly fibroids, sometimes even in large numbers, small and/or large.[3] Risk factors for adenomyosis are caesarean section, induced abortion or curettage, multiparity, miscarriage, endometriosis, and smoking.[5]

The clinical diagnosis of adenomyosis is sometimes difficult because the presenting symptoms overlap with common uterine disorders such as uterine fibroids.[4,6] Therefore, adenomyosis is frequently a so-called forgotten diagnosis because of its noncharacteristic clinical appearance.[7] Adenomyosis may be the cause of disabling symptoms such as, in particular, HMB; abdominal, pelvic, low back, and heavy menstrual pain, with or without bulk-related symptoms; and fertility issues in premenopausal women.[8]

The information on the occurrence of uterine adenomyosis varies considerably. The prevalence of adenomyosis in the specimen obtained from hysterectomy is reported between 8.8% and 31%.[9,10] With broad criteria for the diagnosis of adenomyosis, a prevalence as high as 70% in women between 40 and 50 years of age is suggested.[4] The incidence of adenomyosis in the population at risk is estimated at 8.1% to 16.7%, with symptomatology in approximately two-thirds of women. Of women with clinical manifestations of adenomyosis, about one-fifth are younger than 40 years of age, but most are between 40 and 50 years of age.[11–13]

Imaging of Adenomyosis

The first-line imaging technique, in women with suspected symptomatic adenomyosis, is usually TVUS, which is inexpensive and readily available. Fundamental TVUS signs to diagnose adenomyosis are an increased myometrial echogenicity or linear hyperechoic bands extending deep into the myometrium, indicating the presence of islets of ectopic endometrial tissue; hypoechoic areas in the myometrium compatible with hyperplasia of the muscle tissue surrounding the ectopic tissue; anechoic areas due to glandular dilatation or myometrial cysts; poor definition of the junctional zone; and an enlargement of the uterus with asymmetrical thickening of one of the walls. The presence of at least three of these signs is highly suggestive of adenomyosis.[14]

Particularly useful both in doubtful TVUS cases and in providing a complete evaluation of the disease with its panoramic views is MRI. The T2 weighted images with contrast-enhanced T1 weighted MRI provide the thickness of the junctional zone, which can be measured reliably; a thickness over 12 mm is considered diagnostic of adenomyosis

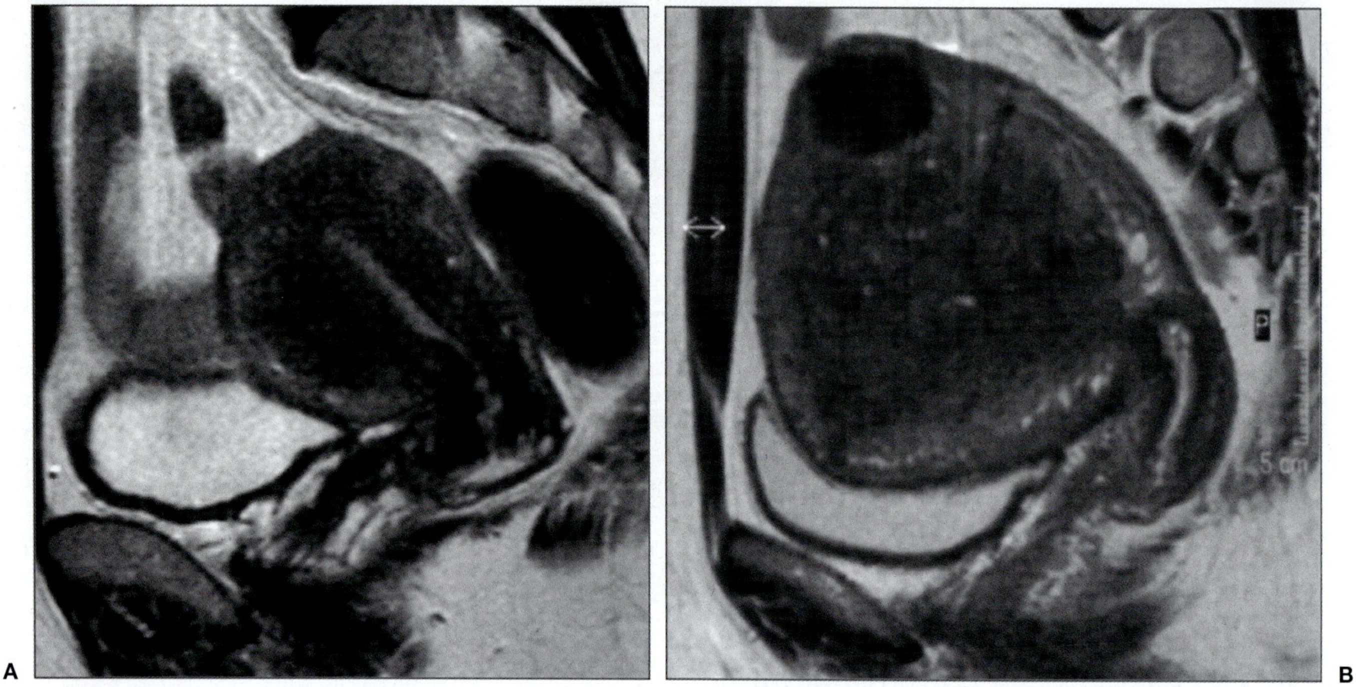

Figure 55.1 **A:** Sagittal T2 weighted magnetic resonance (MR) image of pure diffuse adenomyosis with broadening of the junction zone exceeding 12-mm thickness. **B:** Sagittal T2 weighted MR image of diffuse adenomyosis dominance mixed with one small fibroid. There is broadening of the junction zone exceeding 12-mm thickness, with small high-intensity foci and an enlarged uterus.

(Fig. 55.1A). The occurrence of foci of high signal intensity within the myometrium of the uterus forms an additional but not an obligatory criterion (Fig. 55.1B). MRI can label adenomyosis as focal or diffuse and can be repeated in time to assess the effect of treatment. To assess the diagnostic power of MRI versus TVUS in women with adenomyosis, several studies have been conducted and published. A meta-analysis including six diagnostic accuracy studies of high quality compared TVUS and MRI with histologic proven adenomyosis.[15] Champaneria et al.[15] demonstrated that the correct diagnosis of the occurrence of adenomyosis was provided more often with MRI (sensitivity 0.77/specificity 0.89) than with TVUS (sensitivity 0.72/specificity 0.81), although without statistically significant difference. Another meta-analysis with the study of 1,898 women comparing the TVUS results with the histologic outcome of a symptomatic population of women showed similar sensitivity and specificity results as the meta-analysis of Champaneria et al.: TVUS sensitivity 0.83/specificity 0.85.[16] In terms of accuracy, TVUS and MRI seem comparable for diagnosing adenomyosis. Regarding diagnostic imaging before uterine artery embolization, TVUS may very well identify fibroids and adenomyosis. Whether additional imaging such as MRI is needed in all cases is debatable. Nevertheless, in daily practice and from personal experience, MRI is less operator-dependent and therefore very useful and often better compared to TVUS in detecting adenomyosis and determining the vascularization and, thus, the infarction grade after embolization. The combination of both modalities in daily practice provides the best accuracy of ±90%.[7,17]

Treatment Option for Adenomyosis

Conservative Treatment for Adenomyosis

Women with symptomatic adenomyosis may receive medical treatment, which ranges from local treatment with the release of medications by an intrauterine device (IUD) to systemically administered treatment. IUD-released progestogens are used to reduce HMBs in women with adenomyosis. These medications, such as a Mirena coil, cause the decidualization of the endometrium of the uterus and, consequently, atrophic changes to decrease the amount of blood loss in these women with symptomatic adenomyosis.[18]

Existing medications for systemic administration include gonadotropin-releasing hormone (GnRH) agonists. GnRH agonists induce menopause by reducing the release of pituitary gonadotropins. The levels of estrogen are lowered, producing atrophy and reduced volume of the uterus with reduction of symptoms, because adenomyosis is an estrogen-dependent disease. If the therapy is stopped, the effect is reversible and symptoms will return.[19]

Surgical Treatment for Adenomyosis

The usual and preferred surgical approach for focal adenomyosis is excision or enucleation, but the kind of therapy is very much dependent on the type of lesion and the degree of myometrial involvement.[19] The preferred surgical treatment for women with symptomatic adenomyosis and deep involvement of the myometrium is hysterectomy. The different surgical options and techniques for the treatment of symptomatic adenomyosis have their advantages and disadvantages. When hysterectomy is being considered for diffuse adenomyosis, transvaginal access is preferable to transabdominal access due to the lower morbidity and shorter hospital stay of the former. Concerning the complications of transvaginal hysterectomy, a study on two groups of patients with fibroids versus adenomyosis reported a higher risk of lesions to the urinary bladder in patients from the latter group.[20] The reason is probably the greater complexity in identifying the vesicovaginal septum due to the presence of adhesions, which is explained by the frequent presence of pelvic adherences and endometriosis accompanying adenomyosis.[8] Hysterectomy is regularly indicated as a definitive treatment. Rates of complication after hysterectomy range between 1.5% and 29.3%. Hysterectomy is associated with complications such as blood loss, bowel and general urogenital injury, pain, and infection. The recovery time ranges from 6 to 8 weeks,[19,21,22] and health care–related expenses and lost time at work[23] render hysterectomy an option associated with high costs.

Magnetic Resonance Imaging–Guided High-Intensity Focused Ultrasound for Adenomyosis

Magnetic resonance imaging–guided high-intensity focused ultrasound (MRI-HIFU) is a noninvasive image-guided technique that facilitates treatment of tumors by thermoablation with ultrasound waves. The applications are still under research. The therapy is entirely guided by MRI, providing therapy planning, monitoring, and visualization of the treatment result. MRI-HIFU has a broad spectrum of applications, including ablation of uterine fibroids.[24] The advantage of the noninvasive character of the treatment is that it can be performed on an outpatient basis and that recovery is fast. MRI-HIFU has been used in adenomyosis with varying results. Therefore, although the technique seems to be a useful alternative, further studies are needed to clarify its effective role.[25]

TECHNIQUE

The gynecologist Ravina and interventional neuroradiologist Merland were the first to report the uterine artery embolization (UAE) treatment for symptomatic uterine fibroids in Paris.[26] UAE has emerged as an effective therapy in the treatment of uterine pathology and, in particular, uterine fibroids. The clinical success rate of UAE for uterine fibroids with respect to symptomatic improvement of associated menorrhagia and pelvic pain ranges from 85% to 95% to 80% to 90%.[27,28] This minimally invasive therapeutic alternative to surgery is reported to be associated with a high patient satisfaction.[29–33] There is about 25% chance of failure of symptom control or recurrence after UAE for uterine fibroids at 5-year follow-up.[34,35]

The most common indication for selective uterine artery angiography is for embolizing symptomatic fibroids. Based on the resemblance of symptoms caused by fibroids and adenomyosis and the positive results after UAE for fibroids, this intervention has been investigated as an option to treat adenomyosis. Successful infarction of symptomatic fibroids with UAE has been obtained in women suffering from focal or diffuse adenomyosis with or without fibroids. The basic principle is selective infarction of the adenomyosis with particulate embolic materials delivered directly into the uterine arteries and/or uterine artery branches toward the adenomatous tissue in the uterus.

On the day of the UAE procedure, patients are prepared with or without intravenous antibiotic prophylaxis, sedation with 2.5 to 5 mg midazolam when required, and a urinary bladder catheter. Concerning the right moment to perform the UAE procedure in women with adenomyosis, Chen et al.[36] evaluated UAE during the menstrual cycle in terms of differences in treatment efficacy. Patients were scheduled for UAE during the proliferative or luteal phase of menstruation. Their data showed that the difference in timing of UAE did not have a significant effect on efficacy in the treatment of adenomyosis.[36]

An applicable and accepted approach of UAE for adenomyosis is the bilateral UAE carried out after establishing arterial access to the common femoral artery. Selective catheterization of both uterine arteries is performed under fluoroscopic imaging. Bilateral embolization is mandatory. This is usually accomplished by a femoral artery puncture on one side followed by contralateral uterine artery catheterization and after the Waltman loop maneuver embolization of the ipsilateral uterine artery (Fig. 55.2). One may also favor a puncture of both femoral arteries, selecting the ipsilateral internal iliac artery with a recurved "hockey stick–like" catheter.

The UAE catheterization technique for symptomatic adenomyosis is in principle no different from the technique for symptomatic fibroids, apart maybe from the angiographic embolization end point and maybe the embolic agent size. It is reported by some authors that the angiographic embolization end point should be complete stasis at the level of the ascending distal part of both uterine arteries in case of adenomyosis.[37,38]

When performing UAE, the uterine arteries can be catheterized using a hydrophilic Terumo guidewire with a short-angled tip (Terumo, Tokyo, Japan) and an angled 5-Fr catheter (such as a catheter with a Cobra-2 configuration), but spasm can be a problem so 4-Fr hydrophilic catheters or even 3-Fr microcatheters may be necessary. Once the tip of the (micro)catheter has a stable position in the horizontal part of the uterine artery, a diagnostic angiographic image is obtained. Some experienced interventional radiologists claim to know when dealing with adenomyosis based on the diagnostic angiographic vessel pattern of the uterine branches (Fig. 55.3). Once the "free-flow situation for embolization" with

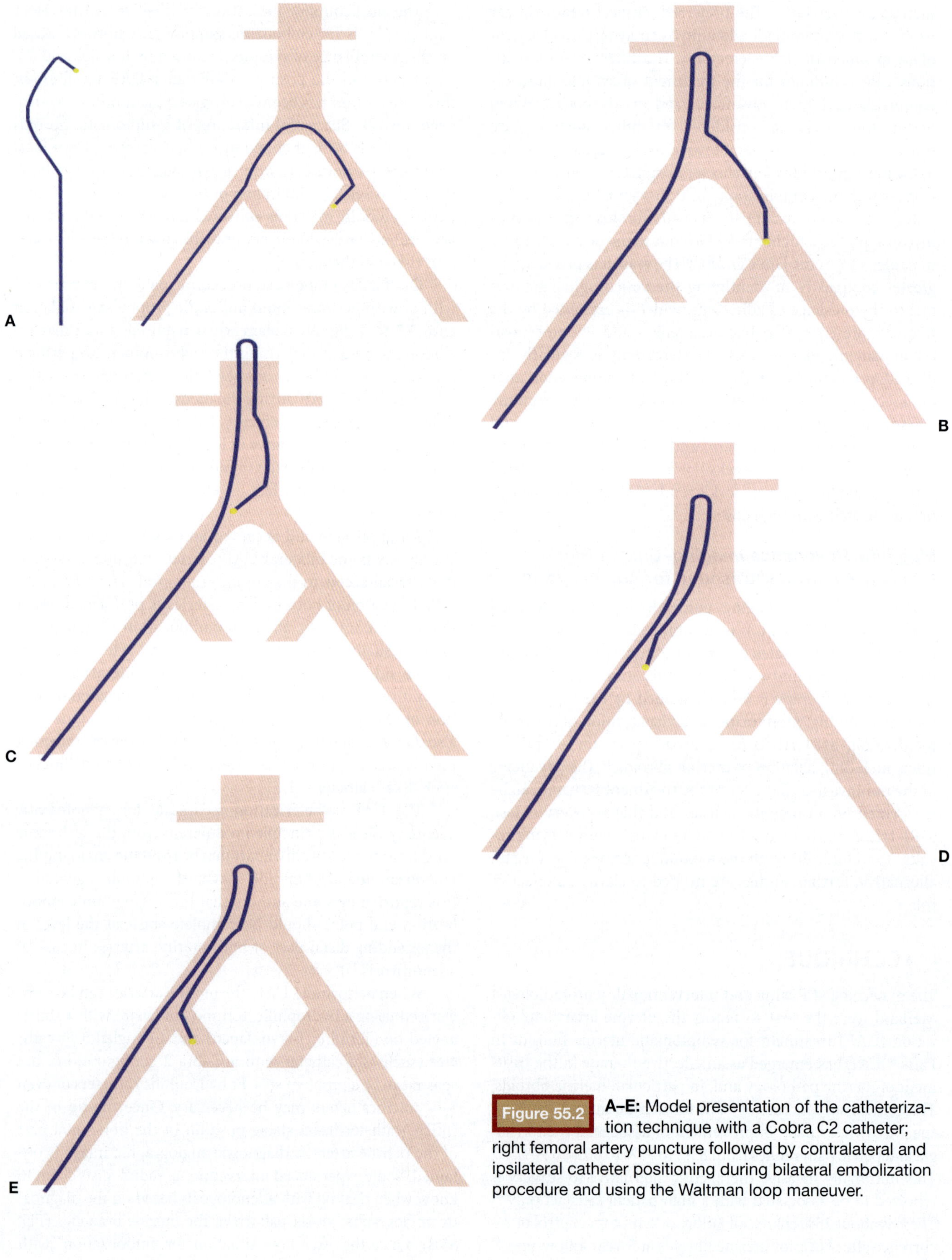

Figure 55.2 **A–E:** Model presentation of the catheterization technique with a Cobra C2 catheter; right femoral artery puncture followed by contralateral and ipsilateral catheter positioning during bilateral embolization procedure and using the Waltman loop maneuver.

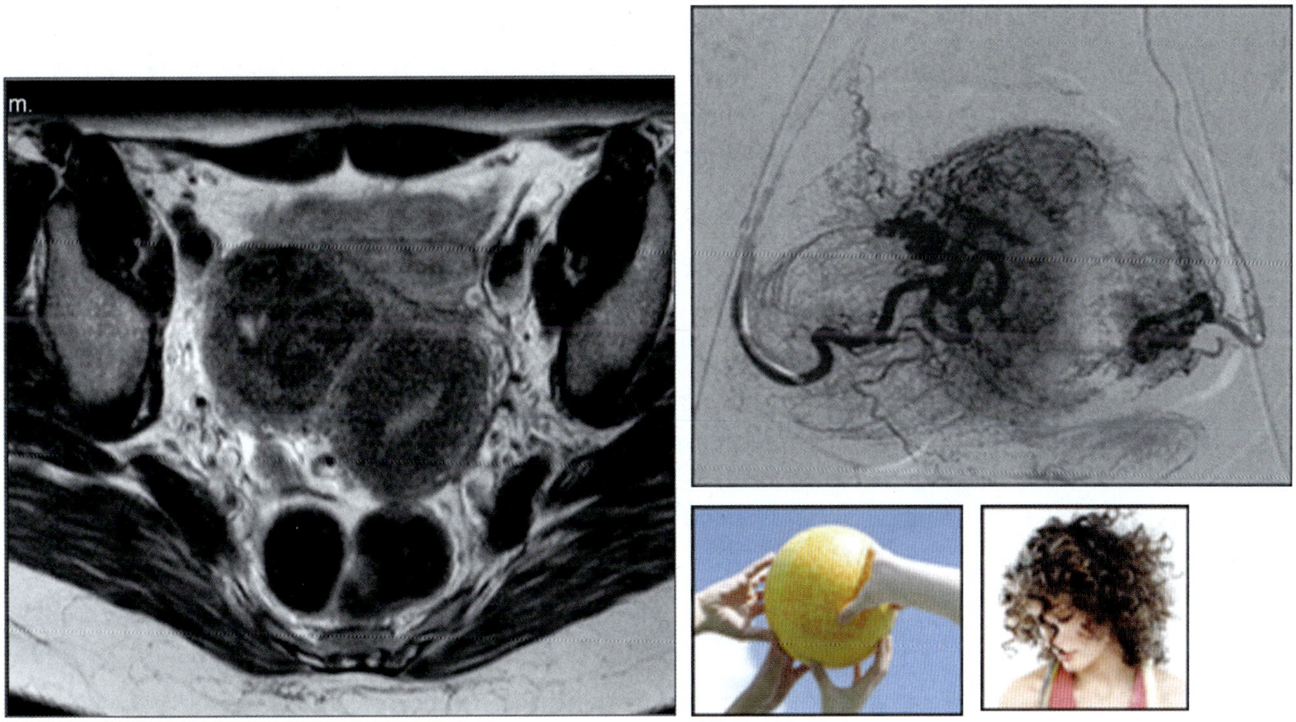

A

B

Figure 55.3 **A:** Transverse T2 weighted MR image of a patient with a uterine fibroid (*right*) and adenomyosis surrounding the uterine cavity (*left*) inside the uterus. **B:** Digital subtraction angiographic image demonstrating a uterine fibroid (*right*) and adenomyosis surrounding the uterine cavity (*left*) inside the uterus. The vessel pattern from the perifibroid plexus resembles fingers surrounding a ball, whereas deep penetrating adenomyosis vessel branches often resemble curly hair.

the catheter tip in the horizontal part of the uterine artery is secured, a small syringe containing the embolic material mixed with contrast is attached to the catheter. The embolic agent is administered and gently injected through the catheter into the uterine artery, creating a blockage of the uterine artery branches toward the adenomatous tissue.

The angiographic end point of embolization is the elimination of the adenomatous tissue blush with complete stasis of flow of contrast at the distal end of the ascending segment of both uterine arteries. The stability of the end point is regularly checked after 5 minutes and additional particles injected if the end point is not reached. In the author's experience, a somewhat more aggressive embolization until complete stasis of contrast at the distal end of the ascending segment of both uterine arteries in women with adenomyosis (as opposed to fibroids) provides better infarction rates and durable clinical results. This is in contrast to the angiographic end point of embolization until near stasis, which seems to be sufficient for treating symptomatic fibroids.[34]

Failures can be due to incomplete embolization, when the operator fails to catheterize both uterine arteries, or vasospasm of the uterine arteries causing no free-flow embolization; clumping of embolic material; no proper embolization end point; or collateral supply from the ovarian or accessory uterine arteries (Fig. 55.4).

After UAE, patients experience severe pelvic cramping for 12 to 24 hours, followed by gradually decreasing cramping for about 7 days. Approximately 80% of the patients suffer from postembolization syndrome, which includes pain, fever, nausea and/or vomiting, and leukocytosis lasting for a few hours or a few days. Therefore, during and after embolization, intravenous narcotics (with or without the use of a patient-controlled analgesia [PCA] pump) and nonsteroidal anti-inflammatory drugs are administered for adequate pain control and to reduce the previously mentioned symptoms.[39] Most patients are managed overnight in the hospital for pain but can be sent home the next day with oral pain medication for 2 weeks. Severe complications are rare (permanent amenorrhea 2% to 5%, expulsion of a coexisting uterine fibroid <2%, sepsis <1%, emergent hysterectomy <1%, death <1%), but uterine infection may require hysterectomy. Young patients who suffer from adenomyosis who desire pregnancy should be properly counselled that there is an incidence of at least 2% to 5% of premature menopause, that is, ovarian failure causing permanent amenorrhea and infertility. Fluoroscopy should be kept to a minimum in all cases, especially in young women. Simultaneous UAE, that is, embolization of both uterine arteries at the same time, reduces the radiation dosage and, in particular, the radiation exposure to the ovaries.

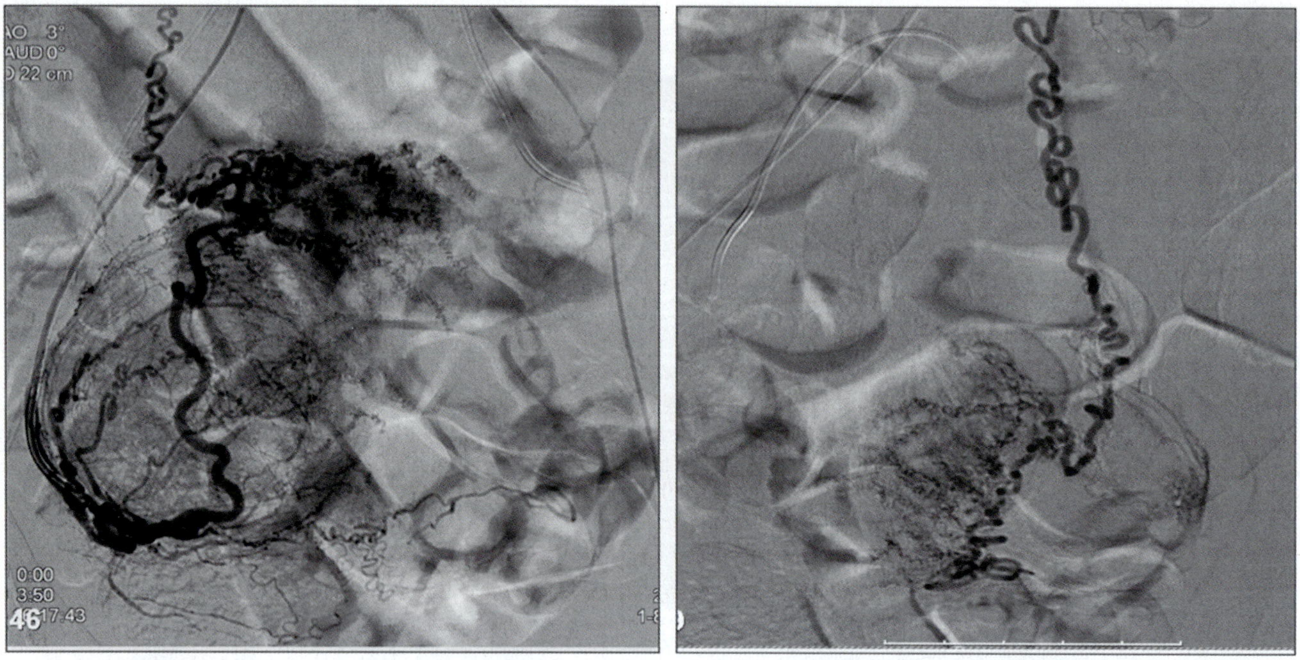

A B

Figure 55.4 Digital subtraction angiographic image during contrast injection to demonstrate the possibility of additional blood supply: right ovarian artery blood supply to the uterine fibroid and adenomyosis **(A)** or left ovarian artery blood supply to uterine adenomatous tissue **(B)**.

EMBOLIC AGENT

The choice of embolic material is a matter of operator preference, but permanent particulate embolic materials are generally used. Coil occlusion of the uterine artery is not necessary and actually discouraged. The most widely used embolic agent is nonspherical polyvinyl alcohol (PVA) particles ranging from 255 to 900 μm in size.[40] Examples of nonspherical PVA particles are Contour (Boston Scientific Corporation, Natick, Massachusetts) and Ivalon (Cook Medical, Inc., Bloomington, Indiana). More recently, however, more and more interventional radiologists prefer the use of spherical embolics, the calibrated microspheres (the preferred size 500 or 700 μm), to facilitate deep penetration into the small afferent arterioles of adenomyosis, creating enough deep infarction (Fig. 55.5). Examples of spherical calibrated microspheres are Embozene (CeloNova BioSciences, Inc., San Antonio, Texas), Embosphere (Merit Medical Systems, Inc., South Jordan, Utah), Contour SE (Boston Scientific Corporation, Natick, Massachusetts), and Bead Block microspheres (Biocompatibles, Inc., Oxford, Connecticutt). In contrast to the perifibroid vascularization pattern of uterine fibroids, adenomyosis has a deep and more diffuse distribution of parallel afferent arterioles throughout the myometrium. The difference in vascularization might explain the reports in the past of higher failure rates in women with adenomyosis compared to UAE for fibroids.

The currently available data do not seem to indicate a preferred embolic agent for use in women with symptomatic adenomyosis. Although in part based on speculation and the author's experience, deep penetration with the embolic agent seems to be needed for optimal infarction of areas with adenomyosis. Calibrated microspheres are able to selectively occlude the tiny arterial branches of the adenomatous tissue deep in the uterine stroma and thus create adequate tissue infarction. It has been demonstrated that calibrated microspheres have a more predictable behavior. Their uniform size and shape and their constant compressibility and elasticity result in deeper penetration into the small arterioles than nonspherical PVA particles.[37,38,41]

OUTCOMES

Many studies have documented the treatment of adenomyosis with UAE.[37–39,42–49] Although the first results of UAE for adenomyosis were disappointing, later reports showed significant clinical improvement in most of the treated women with adenomyosis.

To this day, however, there is no randomized controlled trial (RCT) assessing the efficacy of UAE for adenomyosis in comparison to surgery or other treatment options. Although there are critical commentaries by physicians on the published data available,[50] the current facts with level 2 evidence demonstrate that UAE for symptomatic adenomyosis is an attractive, sensible, and valuable treatment option.

A meta-analysis has been published on UAE for the treatment of adenomyosis, including 15 studies with a total of 511 patients, published between 1999 and 2010.[40] Clinical improvement of bleeding, pain, and bulk-related symptoms were reported by three-quarters of included women with a median follow-up of 26.9 months. In this review, a distinction was made between pure adenomyosis and adenomyosis with uterine fibroids and short-, mid-, and long-term results were described (Table 55.1). Short-term follow-up after UAE in pure adenomyosis resulted in improvement of symptoms in 83% of women with a median follow-up of 9.4 months. The uterine volumes decreased by 25% to 32%. Mid- and long-term results, after a median follow-up of 40.6 months, showed sustained improvement in the vast majority. The short-term results in patients with adenomyosis and fibroids demonstrate clinical improvement in 93% of women with a median follow-up of 10.7 months. Long-term follow-up (34.2 months) showed that 82.4% of women reported

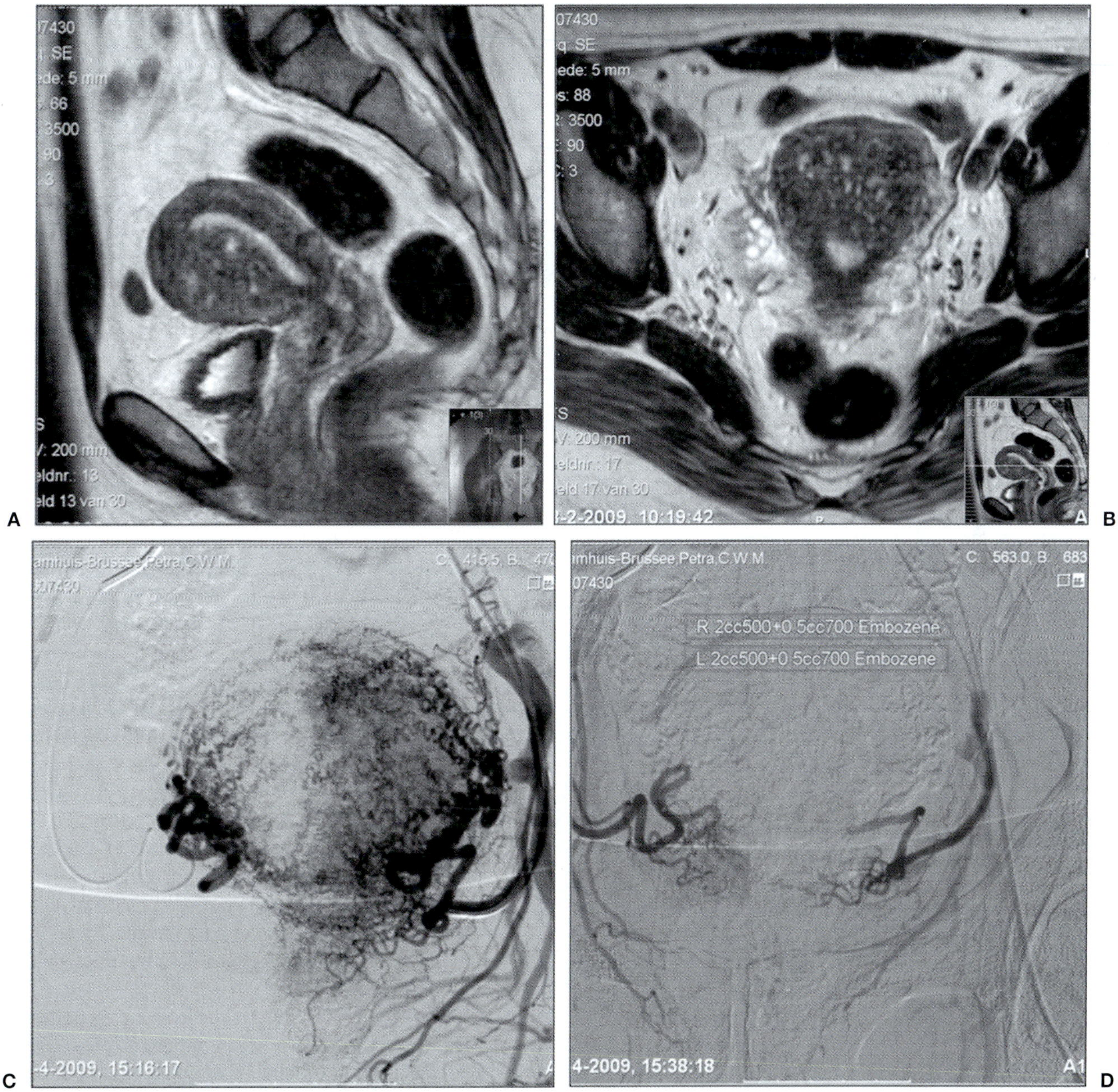

Figure 55.5 **A,B:** Sagittal **(A)** and transverse **(B)** T2 weighted MR image of a patient with pure adenomyosis. There is broadening of the junction zone exceeding 12-mm thickness, with small high-intensity foci and a slightly enlarged uterus. **C,D:** Digital subtraction angiographic image during contrast injection of the patient with pure adenomyosis before **(C)** and after **(D)** targeted embolization with calibrated microspheres. *(Continued)*

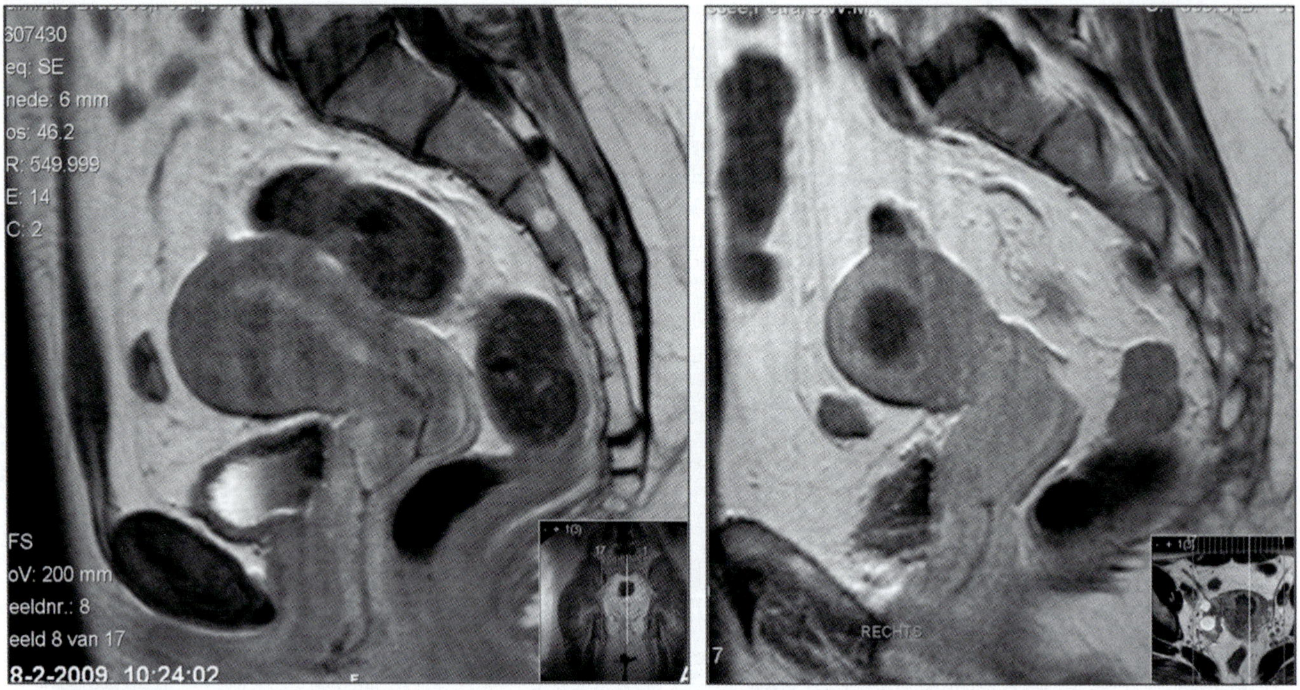

E F

Figure 55.5 *(Continued)* **E,F:** Sagittal T1 weighted MR image with contrast before and after the embolization procedure in this patient with pure adenomyosis. The MR images demonstrate enhancement of the adenomyosis before embolization **(E)** and infarcted adenomyosis with shrinkage after UAE **(F)**.

sustained significant improvement of symptoms after UAE. The meta-analysis indicated that hysterectomy after UAE was needed in 13% of women with adenomyosis, mostly around 12 months after UAE. Most patients experienced some form of mild postembolization syndrome. The risk of permanent amenorrhea was approximately 21%, occurring 3 to 6 months after UAE. However, permanent amenorrhea occurred only in women older than 45 years of age at the time of UAE. No deaths or serious adverse events related to UAE for adenomyosis were reported.

Table 55.1 Short- and Long-term Clinical Success Rate after Selective Uterine Artery Embolization in Women with Symptomatic Pure Adenomyosis or Accompanied with Fibroids

Average Clinical Success after Uterine Artery Embolization	Pure Adenomyosis	Adenomyosis Mixed with Fibroids
Short term (±1 y)	83%	93%
Long term (63 y)	65%	82%

TIPS AND TRICKS

- Adenomyosis should be remembered as a potential cause of disabling symptoms such as HMB, heavy menstrual pain with or without bulk-related symptoms, and fertility issues in premenopausal women.
- A junctional zone thickness over 12 mm as measured on T2 weighted images with contrast-enhanced T1 weighted MRI is considered diagnostic of adenomyosis.
- Differences in the timing of when UAE is performed during the menstrual cycle does not have a significant effect on efficacy for adenomyosis.
- The angiographic end point of embolization recommended in patients with adenomyosis is the elimination of the adenomatous tissue blush with complete stasis of flow of contrast at the distal end of the ascending segment of both uterine arteries. This likely provides better infarction rates and durable clinical results.
- Calibrated microspheres are the embolic agent of choice for adenomyosis because they can provide the deep penetration needed for optimal infarction of adenomatous tissue. The use of agents that result in a more proximal embolization may explain the higher failure rates reported in adenomyosis patients.

CONCLUSIONS

During the last decade, the UAE technique has undergone several refinements and extended its application beyond the embolization of uterine fibroids. Nowadays, women with pure adenomyosis or adenomyosis with fibroids are potential candidates for UAE. Many studies have reported the success of UAE with a long-lasting positive effect of adenomyosis-related symptoms with improvement or elimination of HMB, pelvic pain, and bulk-related symptoms. With the level of evidence available, UAE has proven to be an attractive treatment option and a valuable alternative to hysterectomy for women with symptomatic adenomyosis.

REFERENCES

1. Rybo G. Population studies on menorrhagia. *Res Clin Forums.* 1983;5:77–81.
2. Bird CC, McElin TW, Manalo-Estrella P. The elusive adenomyosis of the uterus—revisited. *Am J Obstet Gynecol.* 1972;112: 583–593.
3. Levgur M, Abadi M, Tucker A. Adenomyosis: symptoms, histology and pregnancy terminations. *Obstet Gynecol.* 2000;95: 688–691.
4. Azziz, R. Adenomyosis: current perspectives. *Obstet Gynecol Clin North Am.* 1989;16:221–235.
5. Vercellini P, Viganò P, Somigliana, E, et al. Adenomyosis: epidemiological factors. *Best Pract Res Clin Obstet Gynaecol.* 2006;20:465–477.
6. Vercellini P, Ragni G, Trespidi L, et al. Adenomyosis: a déjà vu? *Obstet Gynecol Surv.* 1993;48:789–794.
7. Levgur M. Therapeutic options for adenomyosis: a review. *Arch Gynecol Obstet.* 2007;276:1–15.
8. Valentini AL, Speca S, Gui B, et al. Adenomyosis: from the sign to the diagnosis. Imaging, diagnostic pitfalls and differential diagnosis: a pictorial review. *Radiol Med.* 2011;116: 1267–1287.
9. Benson RC, Sneeden VD. Adenomyosis: a reappraisal of symptomatology. *Am J Obstet Gynecol.* 1958;76:1044–1057.
10. Owolabi TO, Strickler RC. Adenomyosis: a neglected diagnosis. *Obstet Gynecol.* 1977;50:424–427.
11. Utsunomiya D, Notsute S, Hayashida Y, et al. Endometrial carcinoma in adenomyosis: assessment of myometrial invasion on T2-weighted spin-echo and gadolinium-enhanced T1-weighted images. *AJR Am J Roentgenol.* 2004;182:399–404.
12. Bergeron C, Amant F, Ferency A. A pathology and physiopathology of adenomyosis. *Best Pract Res Clin Obstet Gynaecol.* 2006; 20:511–521.
13. Peric H, Fraser IS. The symptomatology of adenomyosis. *Best Pract Res Clin Obstet Gynaecol.* 2006;20:547–555.
14. Dueholm M. Transvaginal ultrasound for diagnosis of adenomyosis: a review. *Best Pract Res Clin Obstet Gynaecol.* 2006;20: 569–682.
15. Champaneria R, Abedin P, Daniels J, et al. Ultrasound scan and magnetic resonance imaging for the diagnosis of adenomyosis: systematic review comparing test accuracy. *Acta Obstet Gynecol Scand.* 2010;89;1374–1384.
16. Meredith SM, Sanchez-Ramos L, Kaunitz AM. Diagnostic accuracy of transvaginal sonography for the diagnosis of adenomyosis: systematic review and metaanalysis. *Am J Obstet Gynecol.* 2009;201:e1–e6.
17. Mijatovic V, van Waesberghe JH, Schats R, et al. Adenomyose in historisch perspectief met focus op moderne beeldvorming en behandeling. *NTOG.* 2010;123:335–343.
18. Fedele L, Bianchi E, Raffaelli R, et al. Treatment of adenomyosis associated menorrhagia with levonorgestrel releasing intrauterine device. *Fertil Steril.* 1997;68:426–429.
19. Faquhar C, Brosens I. Medical and surgical management of adenomyosis. *Best Pract Res Clin Obstet Gynaecol.* 2006;20: 603–616.
20. Furuhashy M, Miyabe M, Katsumata Y, et al. Comparison of complication of vaginal hysterectomy in patients with leiomyomas and in patients with adenomyosis. *Arch Gynecol Obstet.* 1998;262:69–73.
21. Meyers ER, Steege JF. Risk adjustment for complications of hysterectomy: utility of routinely collected administrative data. *Prim Care Update Ob Gyns.* 1998;5:202–203.
22. Dembek CJ, Pelletier EM, Isaacson KB, et al. Payer costs in patients undergoing uterine artery embolization, hysterectomy, or myomectomy for treatment of uterine fibroids. *J Vasc Interv Radiol.* 2007;18:1207–1213.
23. Volkers NA, Hehenkamp WJ, Smit P, et al. Economic evaluation of uterine artery embolization versus hysterectomy in the treatment of symptomatic uterine fibroids: results from the randomized EMMY trial. *J Vasc Interv Radiol.* 2008;19:1007–1016.
24. Voogt MJ, van Stralen M, Ikink ME, et al. Targeted vessel ablation for more efficient magnetic resonance-guided high-intensity focused ultrasound ablation of uterine fibroids. *Cardiovasc Intervent Radiol.* 2012;35:1205–1210.
25. Rabinovici J, Stewart EA. New interventional techniques for adenomyosis. *Best Pract Res Clin Obstet Gynaecol.* 2006;20:617–636.
26. Ravina JH, Aymard A, Ciraru N, et al. Treatment by embolization of small uterine myomata. *Bull Acad Natl Med.* 2004;188: 1173–1181.
27. Katsumori T, Kasahara T, Kin, Y et al. Magnetic resonance angiography of uterine artery: changes with embolization using gelatin sponge particles alone for fibroids. *Cardiovasc Intervent Radiol.* 2007;30:398–404.
28. Goodwin SC, Spies JB. Uterine fibroid embolization. *N Engl J Med.* 2009;361:690–697.
29. Worthington-Kirsch RL, Popky GL, Hutchins FL Jr. Uterine arterial embolization for the management of leiomyomas: quality-of-life assessment and clinical response. *Radiology.* 1998; 208:625–629.
30. Spies JB, Roth AR, Jha RC, et al. Leiomyomata treated with uterine artery embolization: factors associated with successful symptom and imaging outcome. *Radiology.* 2002;222:45–52.
31. Hehenkamp WJ, Volkers NA, Birnie E, et al. Symptomatic uterine fibroids: treatment with uterine artery embolization or hysterectomy-results from the randomized clinical Embolisation versus Hysterectomy (EMMY) Trial. *Radiology.* 2008;246:823–832.
32. Hirst A, Dutton S, Wu O, et al. A multi-centre retrospective cohort study comparing the efficacy, safety and cost-effectiveness of hysterectomy and uterine artery embolisation for the treatment of symptomatic uterine fibroids. The HOPEFUL study. *Health Technol Assess.* 2008;12:1–248.

33. Kroencke TJ, Scheurig C, Poellinger, et al. Uterine artery embolization for leiomyomas: percentage of infarction predicts clinical outcome. *Radiology*. 2010;255:834–841.
34. Spies JB, Bruno J, Czeyda-Pommersheim F, et al. Long term outcome of uterine artery embolization of leiomyomata. *Obstet Gynecol*. 2005;106:933–939.
35. Lohle PN, Voogt MJ, De Vries J, et al. Long-term outcome of uterine artery embolization for symptomatic uterine leiomyomas. *J Vasc Interv Radiol*. 2008;19:319–326.
36. Chen CL, Li FJ, Liu P, et al. The relevance between the effect on dysmenorrhea and the time of surgery of artery embolization in the treatment of adenomyosis. *Zhonghua Fu Chan Ke Za Zhi*. 2008;43:884–887.
37. Lohle PN, De Vries J, Klazen CA, et al. Uterine artery embolization for symptomatic adenomyosis with or without uterine leiomyomas with the use of calibrated tris-acryl gelatin microspheres: midterm clinical and MR imaging follow-up. *J Vasc Interv Radiol*. 2007;18:835–841.
38. Smeets AJ, Nijenhuis RJ, Boekkooi PF, et al. Long-term follow-up of uterine artery embolization for symptomatic adenomyosis. *Cardiovasc Intervent Radiol*. 2012;35:815–819.
39. Froeling V, Scheurig-Muenkler C, Hamm B, et al. Uterine artery embolization to treat uterine adenomyosis with or without uterine leiomyomata: results of symptom control and health-related quality of life 40 months after treatment. *Cardiovasc Intervent Radiol*. 2012;35:523–529.
40. Popovic M, Puchner S, Berzaczy D, et al. Uterine artery embolization for the treatment of adenomyosis: a review. *J Vasc Interv Radiol*. 2011;22:901–909.
41. Chua GC, Wilsher M, Young MP, et al. Comparison of particle penetration with non-spherical polyvinyl alcohol versus tris-acryl gelatin microspheres in women undergoing premyomectomy uterine artery embolization. *Clin Radiol*. 2005;60:116–122.
42. Smith SJ, Sewall LE, Handelsman A. A clinical failure of uterine fibroid embolization due to adenomyosis. *J Vasc Interv Radiol*. 1999;10:1171–1174.
43. Goodwin SC, McLucas B, Lee M, et al. Uterine artery embolization for the treatment of uterine leiomyomata midterm results. *J Vasc Interv Radiol*. 1999;10:1159–1165.
44. Siskin GP, Tublin ME, Stainken BF, et al. Uterine artery embolization for the treatment of adenomyosis: clinical response and evaluation with MR imaging. *Am J Roentgenol*. 2001;177:297–302.
45. Kim MD, Won JW, Lee DY, et al. Uterine artery embolization for adenomyosis without fibroids. *Clin Radiol*. 2004;59:520–526.
46. Pelage JP, Jacob D, Fazel A, et al. Midterm results of uterine artery embolization for symptomatic adenomyosis: initial experience. *Radiology*. 2005;234:948–953.
47. Kitamura Y, Allison SJ, Jha RC, et al. MRI of adenomyosis: changes with uterine artery embolization. *AJR Am J Roentgenol*. 2006;186:855–864.
48. Kim MD, Kim S, Kim NK, et al. Long-term results of uterine artery embolization for symptomatic adenomyosis. *AJR Am J Roentgenol*. 2007;188:176–181.
49. Bratby MJ, Walker WJ. Uterine artery embolisation for symptomatic adenomyosis-midterm results. *Eur J Radiol*. 2009;70:128–132.
50. Lei Yu, Wu T, Spain J, et al. Uterine artery embolization for the treatment of adenomyosis: questions for long-term efficacy. *J Vasc Interv Radiol*. 2012;23:430–432.

56

Gynecologic Malignancies

Theresa M. Caridi • Richard Shlansky-Goldberg

BACKGROUND

In the United States in 2010, 83,745 women were diagnosed and 28,770 died from a gynecologic cancer.[1] These include cervical, ovarian, uterine, vaginal, and vulvar cancers and the rare fallopian tube malignancy. In addition, these structures may be involved in metastatic disease from nongynecologic sources. Survival rates for nearly all cancers have improved significantly since the 1970s due largely to earlier detection and/or advances in treatment. Many gynecologic cancers are curable, and the mainstay of treatment remains a combination of surgery, radiation therapy, and chemotherapy. Staging and pathology ultimately determine the treatment type and whether individual or combination therapy is needed. In rare circumstances, embolization of gynecologic malignancies may be employed. These include the setting of life-threatening hemorrhage, preoperatively when there is a predisposition for massive bleeding, and rarely as a treatment of the cancer itself. Treatment of nonhemorrhagic gynecologic malignancy by endovascular methods is infrequent, not only because cure is often achieved by other methods but also because prior treatment with pelvic irradiation increases the risk for uterine necrosis after embolization. Regarding significant bleeding from primary or metastatic disease or as a complication of surgical or radiation therapy, endovascular treatment decreases morbidity and mortality as it is minimally invasive and generally more effective at rapidly achieving cessation of bleeding than surgery (Figs. 56.1 and 56.2).[2]

Cervical Cancer

The American Cancer Society estimates approximately 12,340 new cases and 4,030 deaths from invasive cervical cancer in 2013.[3] Historically, cervical cancer was once one of the most common causes of cancer death for women; however, between 1955 and 1992, the cervical cancer death rate declined by almost 70% owing to the increased use of the Pap test. Cervical cancer is now highly preventable in most Western countries because of both Pap screening and more recently availability of a vaccine to prevent human papillomavirus infections. When found early, cervical cancer is highly treatable and associated with long survival and good quality of life. Treatment usually consists of surgery, radiation therapy, and chemotherapy. The role of embolization is limited due to early detection and curable disease, but it can be useful in the setting of advanced disease with chemoinfusion/embolization, hemorrhage, and also bleeding from a cone biopsy.

Ovarian Cancer

Ovarian cancer accounts for about 3% of cancers among women, but it causes more deaths than any other cancer of the female reproductive system.[1] The American Cancer Society estimates approximately 22,240 new cases and 14,230 deaths from ovarian cancer in 2013.[3] A woman's risk of getting ovarian cancer during her lifetime is approximately 1 in 72, and her lifetime chance of dying from ovarian cancer is about 1 in 100, not including low malignant potential ovarian tumors. However, the rate at which women are diagnosed with ovarian cancer has been slowly falling over the past 20 years. The primary treatments for ovarian cancer include surgery, chemotherapy, hormone therapy, targeted therapy (such as bevacizumab), and radiation therapy. Often, a combination of treatments is enlisted. The role for embolization is limited, as combination therapy is often curative, or at least aimed at cure. Additionally, ovarian cancer historically has a low propensity to result in life-threatening hemorrhage.

Uterine Malignancy

The American Cancer Society estimates approximately 49,560 new cases and 8,190 deaths from cancer of the uterus

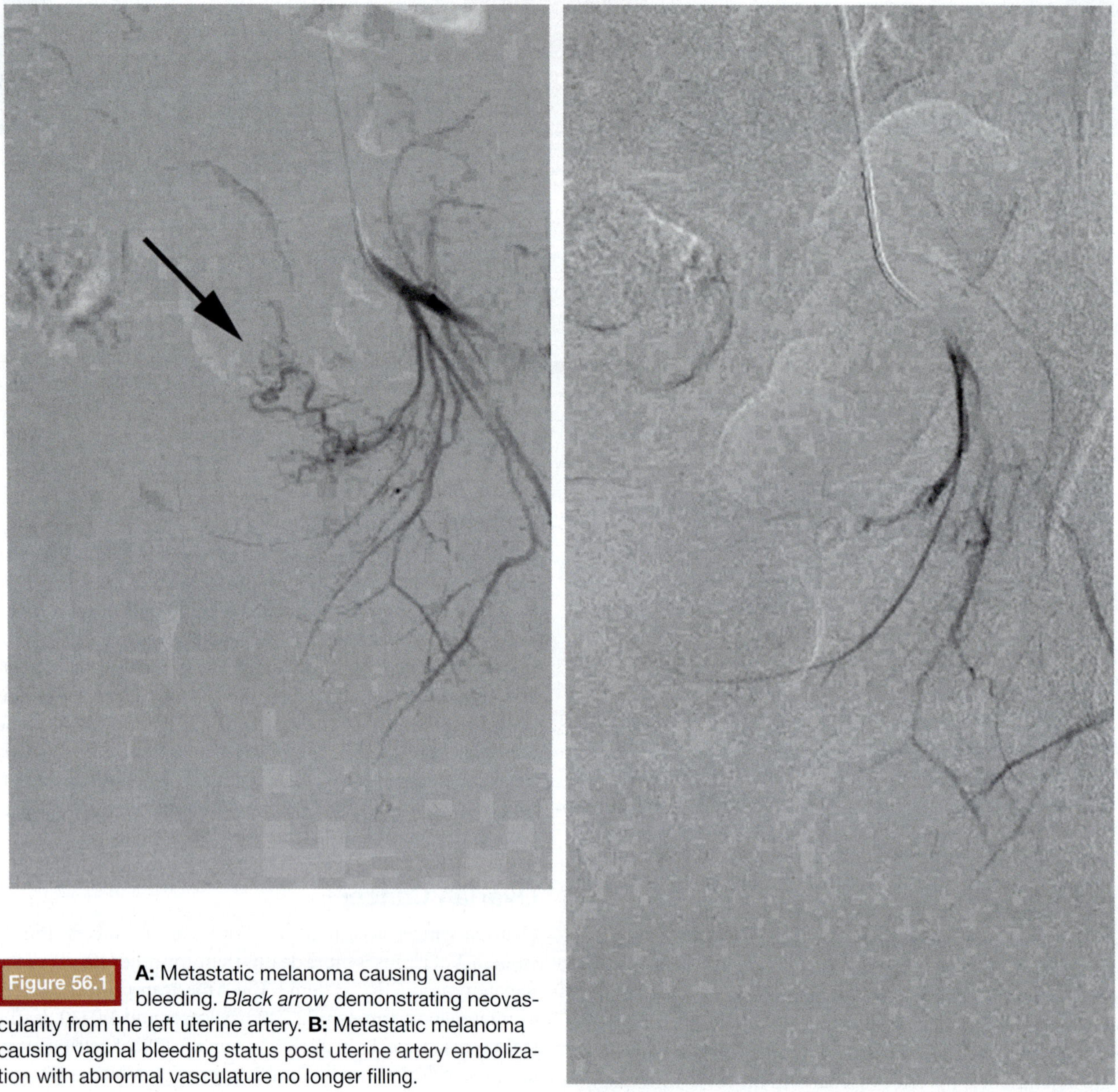

A

B

Figure 56.1 **A:** Metastatic melanoma causing vaginal bleeding. *Black arrow* demonstrating neovascularity from the left uterine artery. **B:** Metastatic melanoma causing vaginal bleeding status post uterine artery embolization with abnormal vasculature no longer filling.

in 2013.[3] The death rate for uterine cancer, which was the leading cause of cancer death in the early 20th century, declined from 1930 to 1997 but has since been nearly stable. The grouping of uterine cancer includes both endometrial cancers and uterine sarcomas, with only 2% being uterine sarcoma. The four established methods of treatment for women with endometrial cancer are surgery, radiation therapy, hormonal therapy, and chemotherapy. Again, there is a limited role for embolization except in the setting of hemorrhage. Similarly, a malignancy involving but not originating from the uterus is gestational trophoblastic disease. Like those neoplasms noted earlier, these lesions may also cause uncontrollable bleeding.[4]

Vaginal and Vulvar Cancer

In 2010, there were 1,211 women in the United States diagnosed with vaginal cancer and 4,305 women with vulvar cancer.[1] Vaginal and vulvar cancers are rare, accounting together for approximately 6% to 7% of all gynecologic cancers diagnosed in the United States. Deaths are also low in number, with 423 women in the United States in 2010 who died from vaginal cancer and 942 who died from vulvar cancer. Invasive vaginal and vulvar cancers are treated mainly with radiation therapy and surgery. Chemotherapy in combination with radiation may be used to treat advanced disease. As in other gynecologic malignancies aforementioned, embolization is not a mainstay of treatment apart from the setting of hemorrhage.

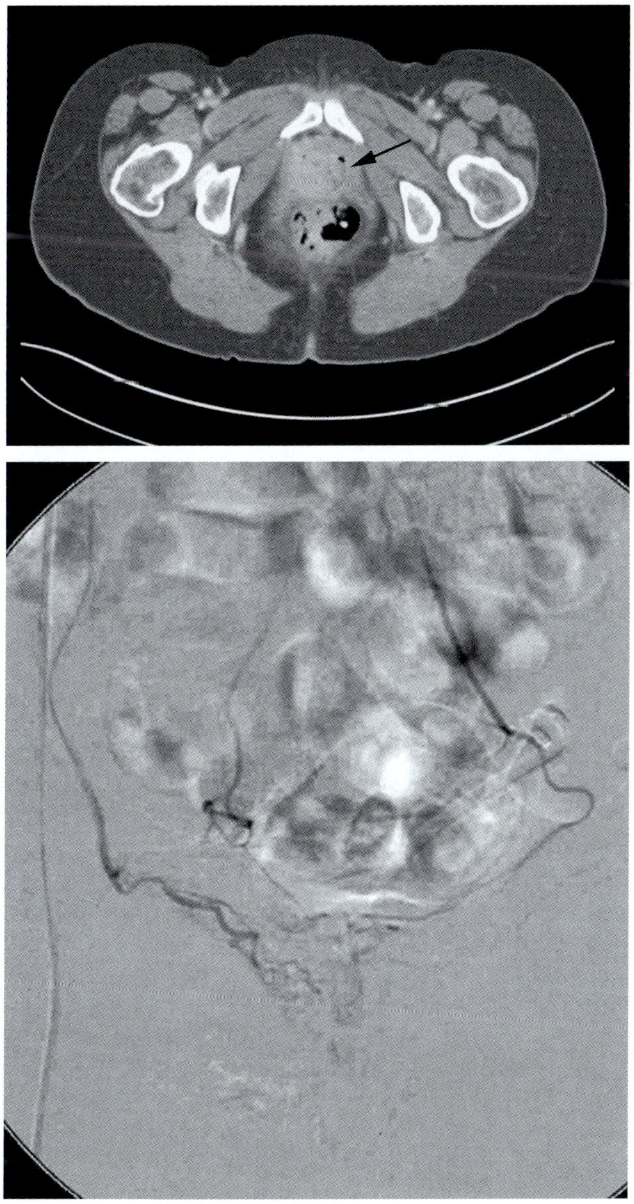

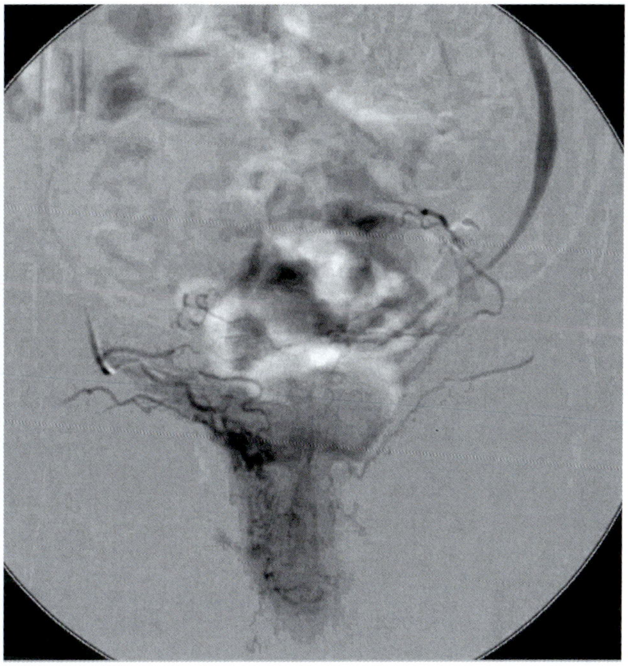

Figure 56.2 **A:** CT scan from patient with leiomyosarcoma involving extension into vagina with bleeding. *Arrow* depicts mass in region of the vagina. **B:** Angiogram of right uterine artery from a patient with leiomyosarcoma with extension into vagina. Note the neovascularity involving the vaginal branches. **C:** Angiogram of right vaginal artery from a patient with leiomyosarcoma involving extension into vagina following embolization causing devascularization of the vaginal branches. Note collateral filling of the hemorrhoidal vessels probably due to spasm.

In the 1970s, early reports of transarterial embolization for gynecologic malignancy were published. Schwartz et al. reported seven patients, two of whom were bleeding from their malignancy itself and five from bleeding related to therapy.[5,6] Four out of the seven patients had bleeding controlled with autologous clot embolization or balloon tamponade, whereas three failed who had bleeding treated with vasopressin. Following this, Athanasoulis et al.[7] published the use of gelatin sponge to successfully treat bleeding from radiation used as therapy for two cases of cervical carcinoma. Miller et al.[8] also published two cases with gelatin sponge to treat radiation-induced bleeding associated with gynecologic malignancies using a femoral approach in one and a brachial in another. Kelemen et al.[9] along with Smith and Wyatt[10] demonstrated the technique of bilateral anterior division internal iliac embolization with gelatin sponge for massive vaginal bleeding from pelvic malignancies. In the 1980s, embolization was described as a technique to control bleeding from gestational trophoblastic disease and as a preoperative technique to reduce intraoperative bleeding.[11,12]

More recently, with the use of microcatheters and permanent embolics such as coils and particles, embolization has become easier and safer; chemotherapy can be added to embolization procedures as well. Arterial infusion with or without embolics is being used to treat ovarian and cervical cancer. In the 1990s, embolization with intra-arterial infusion of chemotherapeutic agents was described.[13] Twenty-two patients with advanced gynecologic cancer underwent embolization and infusion of cisplatin with a 73% response rate, allowing a large portion of patients to be surgically resected.

More recent reports with larger numbers of patients with advanced gynecologic cancers have been published, demonstrating the advantage of embolization over surgery in palliative care of patients with bleeding complications from their malignancy.[2] Advances in the care of patients with cervical cancer with transuterine arterial chemotherapy have allowed for fertility-sparing management using arterial cisplatin and intravenous nedaplatin or irinotecan and vaginal trachelectomy.[14] In addition, a phase II study of 22 patients using transuterine embolotherapy with cisplatin and Gelfoam sponges with intravenous chemotherapy demonstrated 5-year progression-free and overall survival rates in stages IB2 to IIB to be 70.0% and 69.5%, respectively. The 2 patients with stage IVA tumors were alive without recurrence for 72 and 84 months after enrollment.[15]

TECHNIQUE

The most likely use of embolization for gynecologic malignancies is in life-threatening hemorrhage and typically involves embolization of the hypogastric or uterine arteries and, less commonly but occasionally, the ovarian arteries. As with treatment of benign disease, there is variation in operator approach to embolization of the pelvic vessels. All are performed in an angiography suite equipped for digital subtraction angiography or in an operating room with similar equipment. The standard approach is right common femoral artery access followed by aortography with a nonselective flush catheter, particularly in the setting of hemorrhage. The flush catheter is positioned at approximately the L1 vertebral body level to allow for imaging of the ovarian arterial origins in addition to the pelvic flow. Selective and superselective catheterization can be performed with any of several 4-Fr or 5-Fr catheters, such as a Cobra, VS, Simmons, or Roberts Uterine Catheter (RUC) (Table 56.1). Many operators will switch to a microcatheter to select the uterine artery for embolization because it will allow greater flow and reduce the incidence of spasm. Others perform bilateral femoral punctures to reduce procedure and radiation time.[16] Regardless of the suspected source of hemorrhage, bilateral angiography as well as embolization is often performed owing to the vast pelvic blood supply in uterine disease.

Ipsilateral catheterization is commonly performed with use of the Waltman loop technique but again can be performed by accessing the contralateral common femoral artery in a bilateral puncture approach. Waltman et al.[17] described looping of a catheter back over itself by selecting a suitable visceral vessel and pushing the catheter up into the aorta, with attention given to avoid damage to the visceral vessel of choice. Historically, this technique worked well with braided catheters; however, some operators suggest the newer hydrophilically coated 4-Fr and 5-Fr catheters are more susceptible to kinking while the Waltman loop is being formed. Also, these catheters have the tendency to uncoil while the loop is withdrawn into the ipsilateral iliac artery and risk dissecting a vessel while reforming the reverse shape.

Noting these limitations, Cope[18] in 1986 described the catheter reversal maneuver with a suture, which eliminated the need to select a vessel to form a loop, thereby reducing the risk of dissection and atheroemboli. The technique was further refined for uterine artery embolization using a 4-Fr non–tapered angled glide catheter (Boston Scientific Corporation, Natick, Massachusetts) and more recently with the RUC.[19] The suture technique involves threading 2 to 3 cm of 4-0 Tevdek II suture into the end of a catheter. Then, a 0.035-in wire is back-loaded into the catheter so that approximately 3 to 4 cm of wire remains outside the tip of

Table 56.1 Authors' Preferences for Uterine Artery Embolization

Femoral artery access	5-Fr/15 cm Transitionless Micropuncture Push Plus Introducer Set (Cook Medical, Inc., Bloomington, Indiana)
Main catheter	5-Fr Roberts Uterine Catheter, Beacon Tip (Cook Medical, Inc., Bloomington, Indiana); other catheters: Roche inferior mesenteric catheter (Cook Medical, Inc., Bloomington, Indiana), tight-curve Binkert catheter (Cook Medical, Inc., Bloomington, Indiana), internal mammary catheter (Boston Scientific Corporation, Natick, Massachusetts)
Wire	0.035 in × 145 cm, 15 mm tip, TFE Coated Newton Cerebral LLT curved, fixed core, Safe-T-J Guidewire (Cook Medical, Inc., Bloomington, Indiana)
Suture	Tevdek II (Teleflex Medical, Research Triangle Park, NC)
Microcatheter	140 cm, 8 cm FasTracker 325 Infusion Guiding Catheter with Hydrolene (Boston Scientific Corporation, Natick, Massachusetts)
Embolization material	500–700 μm Embosphere 2-mL prefilled syringe (Merit Medical Systems, Inc., South Jordan, Utah); 355–500 μm polyvinyl alcohol particles (Boston Scientific Corporation, Natick, Massachusetts)

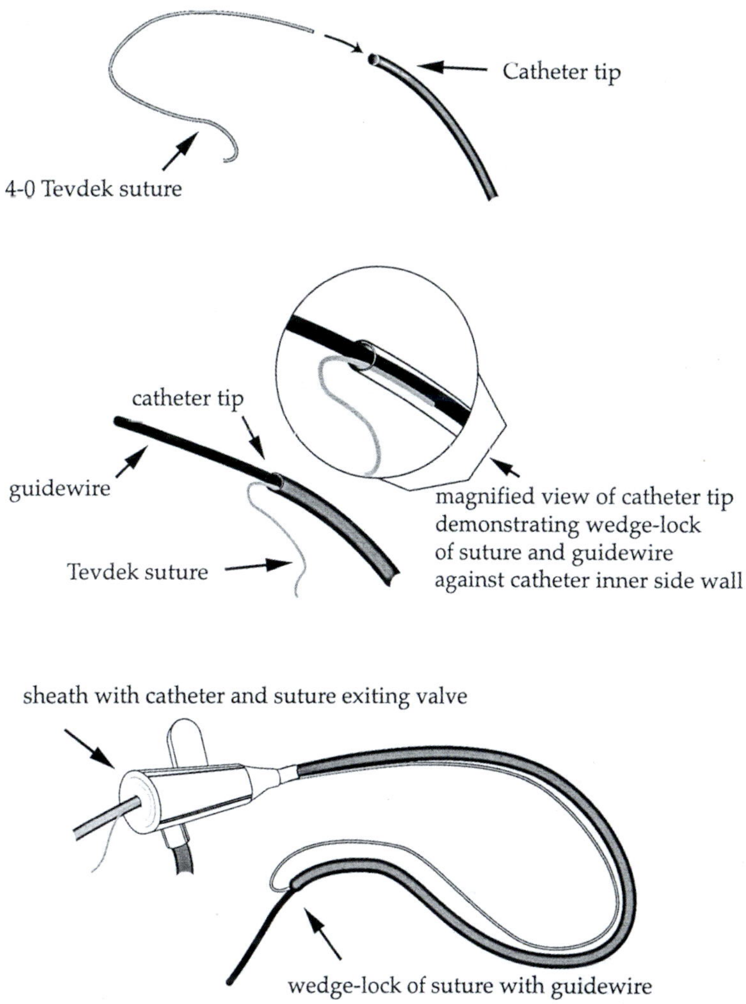

a.

b.

c.

Figure 56.3 Preparation of catheter with the Tevdek suture. **A:** A 4-0 Tevdek II suture is introduced 2 to 3 cm into the tip of the catheter. **B:** The 0.035-in Teflon-coated LLT 15-mm wire is back-loaded into the tip of the 4-Fr catheter, creating a friction lock to pull the tip of the catheter into a reverse configuration. **C:** Demonstration of the suture locked to the tip of the catheter with the trailing end exiting the sheath so it may be pulled to reverse the catheter in the aorta. Only the floppy portion of the LLT wire is protruding from the tip of the catheter to enable minimal tension to reverse the catheter. (Adapted from Waltman AC, Courey WR, Athanasoulis C, et al. Technique for left gastric artery catheterization. *Radiology*. 1973;109(3):732–734.)

the catheter. The friction of the suture and wire against the inner sidewall of the catheter allow the suture to remain tightly fixed to the tip of the catheter. The unit as a whole can then be introduced through a 5-Fr sheath (Fig. 56.3). The tip of the wire/suture/catheter combination is advanced high within the abdominal aorta, with the opposite end of the suture lying outside of the sheath. As the catheter is pushed into the sheath and the trailing end of the suture is simultaneously pulled, the catheter folds back on itself to form (Fig. 56.4). The wire can then be withdrawn, releasing the suture, which is simply withdrawn from the sheath. The catheter is withdrawn from the sheath to engage the ipsilateral common iliac, internal iliac, and ultimately the uterine artery if desired (Fig. 56.5). A coaxial microcatheter can be advanced into the horizontal segment of the uterine artery if indicated. Following ipsilateral embolization, the catheter is advanced into the aorta and pulled down into the contralateral iliac artery for treatment of the other side.

Both temporary and permanent embolic materials are available for occlusion. Permanent embolic agents such as particulate agents, metallic coils, plugs, and liquid embolics are typically required for hemorrhage from progressive malignant disease.[20] Oftentimes, however, temporary agents such as absorbable gelatin sponge are used in conjunction with a permanent embolic. Vessel size, type of hemorrhage (focal or diffuse), end organ, and collateral supply dictate the embolic chosen. For example, particles are useful in diffuse arterial hemorrhage and coils are more effective for a focal arterial abnormality. With regard to particles, the level of vascular occlusion is controlled by the size selected. The particulates are not radiopaque and therefore are injected as a mixture with contrast material. Embolization should occur until marked pruning of the arterial tree is seen on postembolization angiography.

New liquid polymers are approved by the U.S. Food and Drug Administration for use in the central nervous system and are used infrequently in an off-label fashion in the pelvic vessels.[20] Some authors do report durable occlusion of both small pelvic arteries and major inflow arteries with liquid embolics.

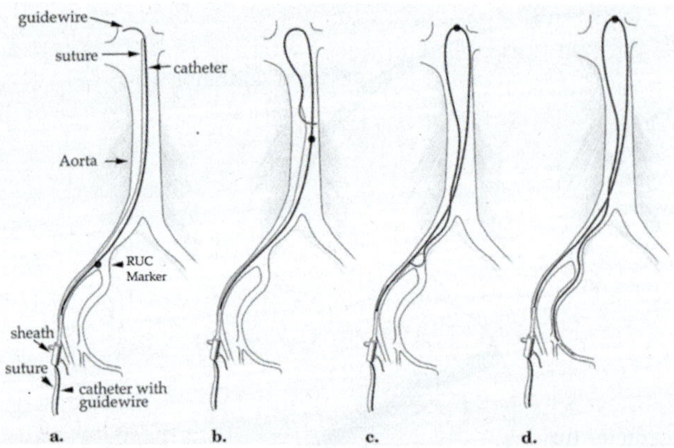

Figure 56.4 Formation of a Waltman loop with the 4-0 Tevdek II suture. **A:** The catheter with the Tevdek suture friction-locked to its tip with the floppy portion of the guidewire extending 2 to 3 cm from the catheter tip is introduced into the aorta. **B:** The trailing end of the suture is pulled as the catheter is advanced, resulting in the catheter reversing on itself. **C:** The suture is continued to be withdrawn, which pulls the tip of the catheter into the ipsilateral common iliac artery, near the origin of the internal iliac artery. When using an RUC, the catheter is fully formed when the radiopaque marker at the bend reaches the apex of the loop. **D:** The wire is removed so as to release the suture, which is pulled out of the sheath. The catheter is then withdrawn, which advances it into the internal iliac artery to select the uterine artery. (Adapted from Cope C. Suture technique to reshapet the "Sidewinder" catheter curve. J *Intervent Radiol*. 1986;1:63–64.)

To deliver these embolics, the authors' preference is single puncture access into the right common femoral artery, followed by advancement of the preloaded 5-Fr Roberts catheter with Tevdek suture. A microcatheter is typically used to access the horizontal segment of the uterine artery if desired before embolization is performed. Strategies and tips regarding this technique are discussed in the "Tips and Tricks" section.

CLINICAL APPLICATIONS

As previously mentioned, the most likely use of embolization for gynecologic malignancies is in the setting of massive genital bleeding related to uncontrolled tumor growth of advanced uterine cancer (whether cervical cancer, endometrial cancer, or uterine sarcoma) with parametrial and fornix infiltration.[2] Massive genital bleeding is a serious complication, allowing for deterioration of the patient's clinical status and a worse prognosis. In some cases, packing the vaginal canal is sufficient to tamponade the tumoral bleeding. These patients then go on to external radiotherapy. When this type of conservative approach is unsuccessful, endovascular or surgical therapy is needed. Embolization often involves hypogastric or uterine artery embolization, whereas surgical treatment can involve arterial ligation or hysterectomy.

Studies show pelvic uterine embolization is nearly bloodless, atraumatic, and more efficient when compared to surgery for massive bleeding. An additional benefit of

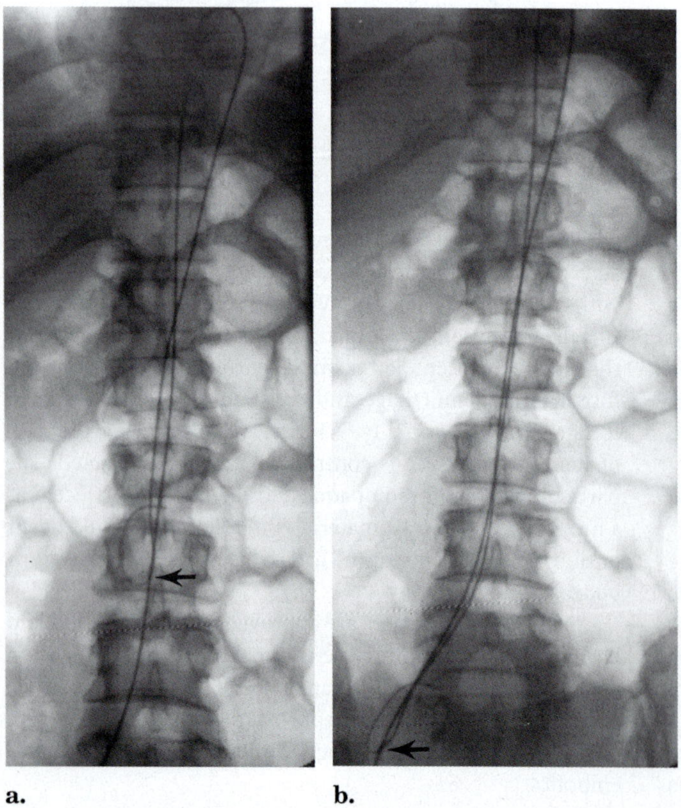

Figure 56.5 Suture reversing the direction of a tapered angled catheter for selecting the ipsilateral uterine artery. **A:** Initially, the catheter is inserted into the aorta with the suture and guidewire together. Only 2 to 3 cm of the guidewire, the floppy portion, extends beyond the catheter tip. The suture is then pulled to fold the catheter back on itself (*arrow*) and form a large loop that prevents the catheter from kinking. **B:** The suture continues to be withdrawn from the sheath, pulling the catheter tip (*arrow*) into the common iliac artery and preventing it from unfolding or inadvertently selecting other vessels. (Adapted from Shlansky-Goldberg R, Cope C. A new twist on the Waltman loop for uterine fibroid embolization. *J Vasc Interv Radiol*. 2001;12(8):997–1000.)

endovascular treatment in the setting of bleeding gynecologic malignancy is it enables continuation of external radiotherapy without delay. Surgical management on the other hand is associated with significant morbidity and oftentimes a longer recovery without the ability to continue external radiotherapy. Surgery can also compromise desired fertility because of hysterectomy or oophorectomy. Furthermore, the reported efficacy of embolization for massive genital bleeding is as high as 90% and, if unsuccessful, does not preclude additional surgical intervention.

Two primary techniques are performed, depending on the patient's clinical status. In the scenario of poor patient status and diffuse massive hemorrhage, embolization of the bilateral internal iliac arteries may be warranted.[2] This can be accomplished rapidly by deploying coils within both internal iliac arteries. Another option is delivering permanent particles into the anterior division after protecting the posterior division with coil blockade. Recognizing that arterial branches not contributing to the hemorrhage may be sacrificed, some authors suggest proximal internal iliac artery coil occlusion with the premise that it will aid to quickly stop hemorrhage while releasing the distal microcirculation for eventual revascularization. This, however, may lead to failure due to collateralization and inability to offer any other endovascular solution. Rarely, access into the uterine arteries provides such difficulty that proximal embolization within the internal iliac arteries is necessary. This is sometimes seen with severe hypotension or shock and rarely with difficult arterial anatomy. In the alternate scenario where a patient's clinical status is stable, superselective microcatheterization of the bilateral uterine arteries with superselective embolization can be performed.

There are no absolute contraindications to embolization for life-threatening pelvic hemorrhage in the background of gynecologic malignancy, whereas elective embolization should be avoided in those with previous pelvic irradiation, chronic kidney disease, pelvic infection, refractory coagulopathy, use of gonadotropin-releasing hormone analogues (due to uterine artery constriction), or intrauterine pregnancy with normal placental implantation.[20]

POTENTIAL COMPLICATIONS

Fortunately, complications of embolization for gynecologic malignancies are rare, with an incidence estimated at 6% to 9%.[20] Complications can be separated into five major categories: those related to angiography, ischemia, thromboembolism, radiation, and drugs. Complications of basic angiography include access site bleeding/hematoma, vascular damage, and contrast reaction or nephrotoxicity. In the setting of uterine artery catheterization in particular, spasm of the uterine arteries can occur, requiring intra-arterial nitroglycerin to complete the planned embolization.

Although the intended result of embolization is ischemia, complications can occur from ischemic damage to the uterus and/or ovaries.[20] Fortunately, they often have the capacity to recover. Pelvic pain is not uncommon following uterine artery embolization and is also related to ischemia. Fever and nausea are not uncommon and along with pain are part of a spectrum of postembolization syndrome. Nontarget embolization can occur as with any embolization procedure. The ovary is the organ most frequently affected due to the utero-ovarian vascular anastomoses. Premature menopause can also ensue when the ovarian supply is embolized, particularly if the patient is in the premenopausal state. Fertility following uterine artery embolization for gynecologic malignancy has not been discussed in the literature except for uterine fibroid embolization, in part because the procedure is performed rarely except in life-threatening hemorrhage and also fertility is unlikely to be a point of concern in women with advanced malignancy. Other nontarget embolization can occur with occlusion of adjacent branch vessels to the bladder or rectum, resulting in bladder/rectal necrosis or sexual dysfunction.

Deep venous thrombosis (DVT) and pulmonary embolism have been reported after uterine artery embolization, with one thought being stagnation and clotting of the venous drainage at least in part from blockage of the arterial inflow. Additionally, development of thrombus is common in the setting of malignancy due to hypercoagulable state, and if there is bulky pelvic disease, direct pressure can further result in compromised venous flow and the propensity to form DVT. Finally, patients with gynecologic malignancy are at times treated with hormonal therapy, also increasing the risk for DVT.

Angiography and embolization is performed under fluoroscopy, therefore women are exposed to radiation. Theoretically, prolonged angiography and embolization can lead to radiation burn to the skin, although no known cases have been found in the literature regarding uterine artery embolization. The amount of radiation to the ovaries varies widely depending on anatomy and operator experience; however, it is not expected to affect fertility and again is not usually of concern in advanced malignant disease.

Most embolization procedures are performed using moderate sedation with use of a short-acting intravenous narcotic and sedative, typically fentanyl and Versed. Allergic reactions can occur, although are atypical, and more common side effects include dry mouth and urinary retention. Medications can also result in oversedation; however, care is taken to administer sedation in small doses as needed. Reversal medications can also be employed if indicated. As with any procedure, there is always a risk of death related to one of the previously mentioned complications. In the setting of uterine artery embolization, the most likely cause of immediate death of those mentioned is pulmonary embolism.

TIPS AND TRICKS

For embolization of gynecologic malignancies via the uterine arteries, there are a few basic suggestions made by the authors to promote technical success and efficiency. An RUC with its long reversed curve tip makes catheterization rather quick and simple, especially when combined with the Cope suture technique (Fig. 56.6). A list of recommended materials can be seen in Table 56.1. A very basic suggestion is the use of a 5-Fr/15 cm transitionless sheath, which eliminates the conversion from micropuncture to 0.035-in system if a micropuncture system is used. Additionally, when the use of the authors' technique is employed, this sheath allows for easy advancement of the Tevdek wire–loaded Roberts catheter. Otherwise, the RUC would need to be reshaped over the bifurcation.

Numerous other catheters can be used such as the cobra shape, but the RUC represents the authors' preferences. In terms of selection of the common iliac artery, followed by internal iliac artery, anterior division of the internal iliac artery, and ultimately the uterine artery, we recommend specific positioning of the tip of the catheter to achieve easy, rapid, and safe catheterization. Initially, lateralizing the tip of the RUC to achieve catheterization of the common iliac artery followed by quickly changing to a posterior and medial tip position to select the internal iliac artery is standard opening technique. As the RUC is retracted (bringing the tip down deeper into the pelvis), the tip of the catheter should be turned in an anterolateral position in parallel to the external iliac artery to catheterize the anterior division of the internal iliac artery and subsequently the uterine artery. One gets accustomed to the deflected tip appearance as the RUC enters the origin of the uterine artery.

It may be difficult to catheterize the uterine arteries when they originate at an upgoing angle greater than 90 degrees relative to the inferior gluteal artery as the terminal branch of the anterior division. Useful catheters in this setting are the Roche inferior mesenteric (RIM), the tight-curve Binkert (TC-BNK), and the internal mammary (IM) catheter, all of which have a distal J curve to engage the upgoing vessel (Figs. 56.7 and 56.8). Also, ipsilateral catheterization with these catheters may be difficult to perform with the distal curve so a contralateral access may be needed. Alternatively, a J-curved microcatheter through a non–J-curved main catheter can also be used.

In addition to evaluating the uterine arteries, aortography at the level of the ovarian arteries should be performed if there is any concern for ovarian supply.

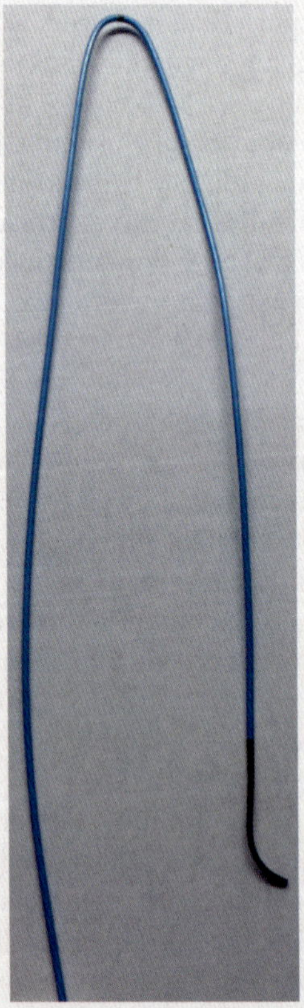

Figure 56.6 RUC designed for ipsilateral and contralateral uterine arteriography with its long reverse curve. The radiopaque marker band at the apex of the catheter aids in reforming the reverse curve.

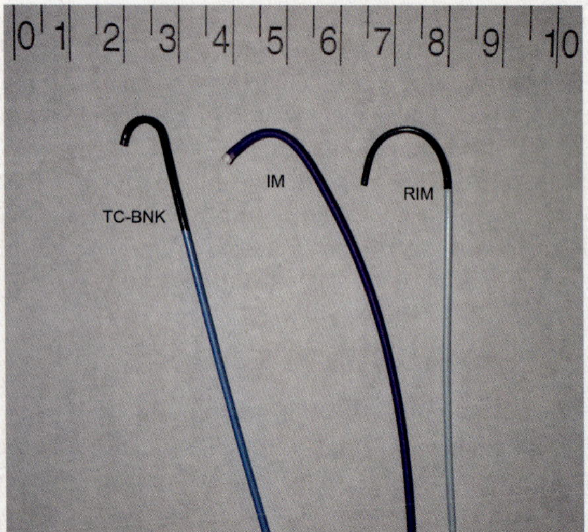

Figure 56.7 Useful J-curved catheters for catheterizing upgoing uterine arteries. Tight-curve Binkert (*TC-BNK*), internal mammary (*IM*), and Roche inferior mesenteric (*RIM*).

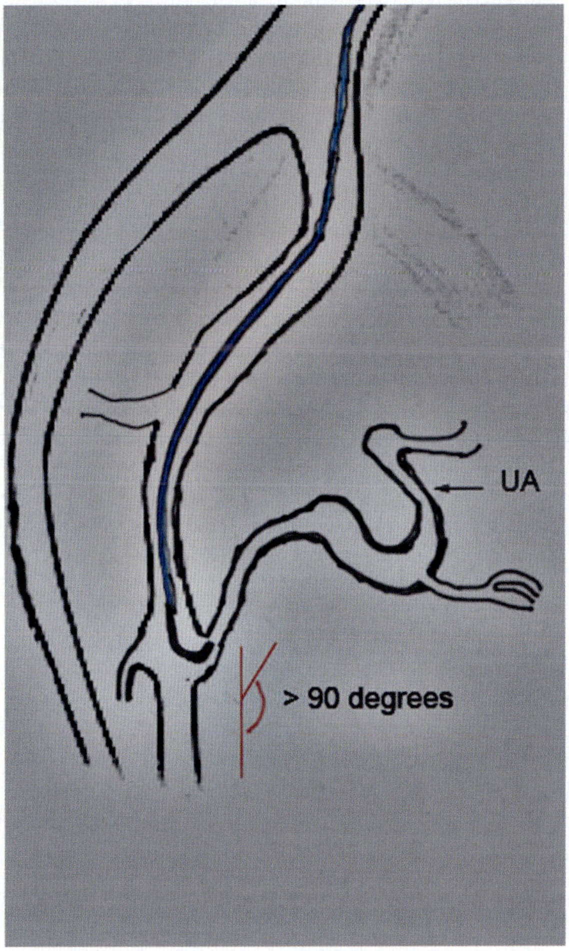

Figure 56.8 Use of a J-curved catheter to engage an upgoing uterine artery (*UA*). Ideal catheters for this are the RIM, the Binkert, and the IM catheters.

Tips

- *Always* use a microcatheter coaxial to the diagnostic catheter to prevent spasm.
- Ensure that there is pulsatility in the uterine artery during embolization; otherwise, there is spasm which may lead to nontarget embolization.
- The internal iliac artery comes off posteriorly, whereas the anterior division of the internal iliac and uterine arteries come off anteriorly.
- Once the internal iliac is selected, keep the nose of the catheter parallel to the external iliac and positioned anteriorly to guide the tip into the uterine artery.
- Study the ovarian arteries with a flush aortogram. Include the renal arteries because the ovarian arteries can originate off the renal arteries.
- Parasitized collaterals from a malignancy may involve visceral vessels so perform an adequate diagnostic study.
- Look for neovascularity because active bleeding will probably not be seen.

Tricks

- Use Tevdek maneuver to reshape your reversed curve catheter such as the RUC.
- Use BNK or RIM catheter for contralateral catheterization of an upgoing uterine artery.
- Use a curved microcatheter for ipsilateral upgoing uterine arteries because making a reverse curve with a BNK or RIM is difficult.
- Use dry embolic such as PVA with 100% contrast when there is difficulty imaging patients due to large body habitus.
- Use 1-mL polycarbonate syringes to infuse embolic via a three-way stopcock to prevent catheter clogging. One-mL syringe develops higher infusion pressures.
- Use five cardiac beat rule for PVA. No forward progression of contrast within the horizontal segment of the uterine for five beats for general embolization of the uterine artery. Can use the same end point for trisacryl gelatin microsphere but prune tree embolization is adequate.

REFERENCES

1. Centers for Disease Control and Prevention. United States cancer statistics: 1999–2010 cancer incidence and mortality data. 2013. http://www.cdc.gov/uscs. Accessed September 29, 2014.
2. Tinelli A, Prudenzano R, Malvasi A, et al. Emergency endovascular nanopharmacologic treatment in advanced gynecological cancers. *Int J Gynecol Cancer*. 2010;20(7):1250–1255.
3. Siegel R, Naishadham D, Jemal A. Cancer statistics, 2013. *CA Cancer J Clin*. 2013;63(1):11–30.
4. Moodley M, Moodley J. Transcatheter angiographic embolization for the control of massive pelvic hemorrhage due to gestational trophoblastic disease: a case series and review of the literature. *Int J Gynecol Cancer*. 2003;13(1):94–97.
5. Goldstein HM, Medellin H, Ben-Menachem Y, et al. Transcatheter arterial embolization in the management of bleeding in the cancer patient. *Radiology*. 1975;115(3):603–608.
6. Schwartz PE, Goldstein HM, Wallace S, et al. Control of arterial hemorrhage using percutaneous arterial catheter techniques in patients with gynecologic malignancies. *Gynecol Oncol*. 1975; 3(4):276–288.
7. Athanasoulis CA, Waltman AC, Barnes AB, et al. Angiographic control of pelvic bleeding from treated carcinoma of the cervix. *Gynecol Oncol*. 1976;4(2):144–150.
8. Miller FJ Jr, Mortel R, Mann WJ, et al. Selective arterial embolization for control of hemorrhage in pelvic malignancy: femoral and brachial catheter approaches. *AJR Am J Roentgenol*. 1976;126(5):1028–1032.

9. Kelemen J, Scultety S, Nemeth A, et al. Embolization of the arteria iliaca interna as treatment of life-endangering haemorrhages caused by intrapelvic malignant tumours. *Diagn Imaging.* 1979;48(5):275–285.
10. Smith DC, Wyatt JF. Embolization of the hypogastric arteries in the control of massive vaginal hemorrhage. *Obstet Gynecol.* 1977;49(3):317–322.
11. Takemura M, Yamasaki M, Tanaka F, et al. Transcatheter arterial embolization in the management of gynecological neoplasms. *Gynecol Oncol.* 1989;34(1):38–42.
12. Vujic I, Lutz MH, Curry N, et al. Angiographic management of bleeding in gestational trophoblastic malignancy. *Am J Obstet Gynecol.* 1984;149(1):90–92.
13. Yamada T, Ohsugi F, Irie T, et al. Extended intraarterial cisplatin infusion for treatment of gynecologic cancer after alteration of intrapelvic blood flow and implantation of a vascular access device. *Cardiovasc Intervent Radiol.* 1996;19(3):139–145.
14. Tsubamoto H, Kanazawa R, Inoue K, et al. Fertility-sparing management for bulky cervical cancer using neoadjuvant transuterine arterial chemotherapy followed by vaginal trachelectomy. *Int J Gynecol Cancer.* 2012;22(6):1057–1062.
15. Tsubamoto H, Maeda H, Kanazawa R, et al. Phase II trial on neoadjuvant intravenous and trans-uterine arterial chemotherapy for locally advanced bulky cervical adenocarcinoma. *Gynecol Oncol.* 2013;129(1):129–134.
16. Costantino M, Lee J, McCullough M, et al. Bilateral versus unilateral femoral access for uterine artery embolization: results of a randomized comparative trial. *J Vasc Interv Radiol.* 2010;21(6):829–835.
17. Waltman AC, Courey WR, Athanasoulis C, et al. Technique for left gastric artery catheterization. *Radiology.* 1973;109(3):732–734.
18. Cope C. Suture technique to reshapet the "Sidewinder" catheter curve. *J Intervent Radiol.* 1986;1:63–64.
19. Shlansky-Goldberg R, Cope C. A new twist on the Waltman loop for uterine fibroid embolization. *J Vasc Interv Radiol.* 2001;12(8):997–1000.
20. Katz MD, Sugay SB, Walker DK, et al. Beyond hemostasis: spectrum of gynecologic and obstetric indications for transcatheter embolization. *Radiographics.* 2012;32(6):1713–1731.

57

Pelvic Arteriovenous Malformations

Patricia E. Burrows

BACKGROUND

An arteriovenous malformation (AVM) is characterized by the presence of direct arteriovenous connections leading to arteriovenous shunting. Several genetic mutations affecting the transforming growth factor-beta superfamily and the Ras signaling pathway are known to cause familial AVM, but most AVMs are sporadic. In the female pelvis, two sites account for the most AVMs: the pelvic wall and the uterus. These are often referred to as *congenital* and *acquired AVMs*, respectively, but neither is seen in early childhood.

Pelvic Wall Arteriovenous Malformation

Pelvic wall AVMs primarily involve the bone and soft tissue of the pelvic wall and drain into branches of the internal iliac veins. As they enlarge, arteries and veins from the pelvic viscera can be recruited. An AVM of the pelvic wall is typically supplied by *numerous* branches of the pudendal, obturator, and gluteal arteries, as well as collaterals from adjacent visceral branches, and can achieve massive size and flow. Although some asymptomatic patients are diagnosed by cross-sectional imaging of the pelvis for other indications, the majority present with pain, bleeding, dyspnea due to high-output heart failure, or combinations of these symptoms.[1] Footdrop due to nerve compression and lower extremity edema due to associated proximal iliac vein compression have also been described.[2] Ligation or proximal embolization of the internal iliac arteries is frequently performed but is always ineffective because of the rapid reperfusion of the AVM through collaterals.[3]

Uterine Arteriovenous Malformation

Uterine AVMs typically result from uterine trauma, such as pregnancy or curettage, or in association with trophoblastic malignancy and typically present with vaginal bleeding, sometimes years after the trauma. Uterine AVMs arise in the muscle of the uterus and typically are supplied by uterine and ovarian arteries and drain into gonadal and internal iliac veins. Extensive lesions can involve vessels from the adjacent bladder and vagina. Color Doppler ultrasonography is diagnostic. Retained products of conception should be ruled out.

TECHNIQUES

One suggested technique for embolization of arteriolovenous fistula or AVM with single venous outflow is as follows:

1. Perform a pelvic aortogram to delineate arterial and venous anatomy.
2. Perform a selective internal iliac angiogram to better define the vascular anatomy, as needed.
3. Identify the point at which all of the feeding arteries connect to the same segment of draining vein.
4. Access the immediate draining vein (transvenous or percutaneous). Percutaneous access is achieved with ultrasound guidance or fluoroscopic guidance with or without road map.
5. Deliver a detachable framing coil or other large occlusive device into the immediate draining vein and continue packing the varix with coils. When the coil mass is stable and has slowed the blood flow, ethanol or *N*-butyl cyanoacrylate (NBCA) can be injected into the coil mass or additional coils can be placed to reach occlusion. If the draining vein is massive, outflow control can be assisted by transjugular positioning of an occlusion balloon or partly deployed inferior vena cava (IVC) filter. These can

be removed after the coil mass has been created and deemed to be stable.

6. Repeat internal iliac arterial or aortic contrast injections to monitor the occlusion of the venous outflow.
7. Small residual shunts can be occluded by transarterial microcatheter embolization or percutaneous direct puncture technique.

Techniques for embolization of uterine AVM:

1. Perform abdominal aortogram to identify arterial supply and angioarchitecture.
2. Perform selective, bilateral uterine artery catheterization.
3. For an AVM with small arteriovenous shunts, bilateral uterine artery embolization with large particles and/or Gelfoam (Pfizer, New York, New York) is carried out.
4. For an AVM with large arteriovenous shunts, superselective or percutaneous embolization using permanent occlusive agents such as NBCA, Onyx (Covidien, Irvine, California), or coils is used.
5. Ultrasound-guided percutaneous cannulation of nidus, or immediate draining vein, followed by intranidal embolization with ethanol, glue, or Onyx is also effective in achieving obliteration of the shunt.
6. Perform postembolization angiography.
7. Clinical follow-up supplemented with color Doppler ultrasonography.

OUTCOMES

Pelvic Wall Arteriovenous Malformation

When treating pelvic wall AVMs, arterial embolization using acrylic embolization material, coils, or particles can result in symptomatic improvement but is rarely curative because of the large number of feeding arteries involved.[4–6] Jacobowitz and colleagues[5] reported a retrospective review of 35 patients undergoing arterial embolization, using acrylic polymer (glue), of pelvic vascular malformations; most were AVMs. Presenting problems included pain (59%), a visible or palpable lesion (62%), pulsation or thrill (44%), hemorrhage (27%), congestive heart failure (18%), and symptoms due to mass effect (35%). One-third of patients had undergone previous, unsuccessful attempted surgical treatment of the lesion. Patients underwent a mean of 2.4 embolization procedures over an average period of 23.3 months. Five patients went on to have adjunctive surgical procedures. Eighty-three percent of patients were asymptomatic or significantly improved at mean follow-up of 84 months, although none were cured, and symptomatic recurrences occurred frequently. Ethylene vinyl alcohol copolymer (Onyx) has been effective in a few cases because of the characteristic of this agent to progressively penetrate anastomotic feeding channels as well as the draining vein.[7]

Because most pelvic AVMs have single outflow venous anatomy, they are best treated by outflow venous occlusion.[1,3,4] In this technique, the outflow vein is packed with embolic material, usually coils, but also potentially ethanol or a polymerizing agent (NBCA, Onyx) (Fig. 57.1). This obviates, or markedly reduces, the need for and risks associated with superselective embolization of the pelvic arteries. The procedure involves careful review of arteriographic images to identify the *common immediate draining vein*. The immediate draining vein can be catheterized from the contralateral femoral vein, the internal jugular vein, or percutaneously using a micropuncture system or catheter introduced directly through the pelvic wall. My preference is to use the direct percutaneous approach because it is the quickest and most accurate method of catheterizing the immediate draining vein. Retrograde catheterization from the contralateral femoral vein is the most difficult because the draining pelvic veins are usually tortuous. Complications of venous embolization include pulmonary embolism and pelvic bleeding from residual arterialized, partly occluded veins. Migration of coils or thrombus can be controlled by proximal venous balloon occlusion, although this can be difficult because of the extremely large size of the draining vein. Placement of an IVC filter or other tethering device in the internal iliac vein can be effective in preventing dislodgment of coils.[4] Fortunately, there are now many detachable coils available in large diameters. These can be used to create a frame or basket to which pushable, large-diameter coils can be added. My approach to the massive draining vein involves initial placement of coils into the varix, followed by injection of NBCA into the coil mass. Additional arterial or percutaneous embolization may be needed to complete the occlusion. In the largest published series of venous outflow occlusion for pelvic AVM, 12 patients underwent coil embolization of the dilated draining vein followed by transarterial ethanol embolization. Eighty-three percent of patients were cured with one major complication (focal bladder necrosis).[1]

Uterine Arteriovenous Malformation

In one series of 265 women with premenopausal uterine bleeding who underwent transvaginal sonography, 3.4% were found to have a uterine AVM. In 6, or two-thirds, of these patients, the AVM resolved spontaneously, and two additional lesions resolved after chemotherapy for an associated hydatidiform mole. One patient required embolization and 5 patients had uneventful pregnancies after resolution of the AVM.[8] In 1993, a series of 15 patients with uterine AVM was reported from the University of Toronto.[9] Twenty-five embolization procedures were carried out using a combination of glue, particles, coils, and Gelfoam. Bleeding was controlled in 14 of 15 patients, and a total of five uneventful intrauterine pregnancies were carried to term. Lim and colleagues[10] reported 14 patients who were embolized for a uterine AVM that persisted after treatment of trophoblastic tumors. Uterine arterial embolization was effective in controlling bleeding in 11 patients, and 3 went on to have normal pregnancies. Wang and colleagues[11] report 42 patients with uterine vascular malformation who underwent 49 embolization procedures. The authors used coils to occlude

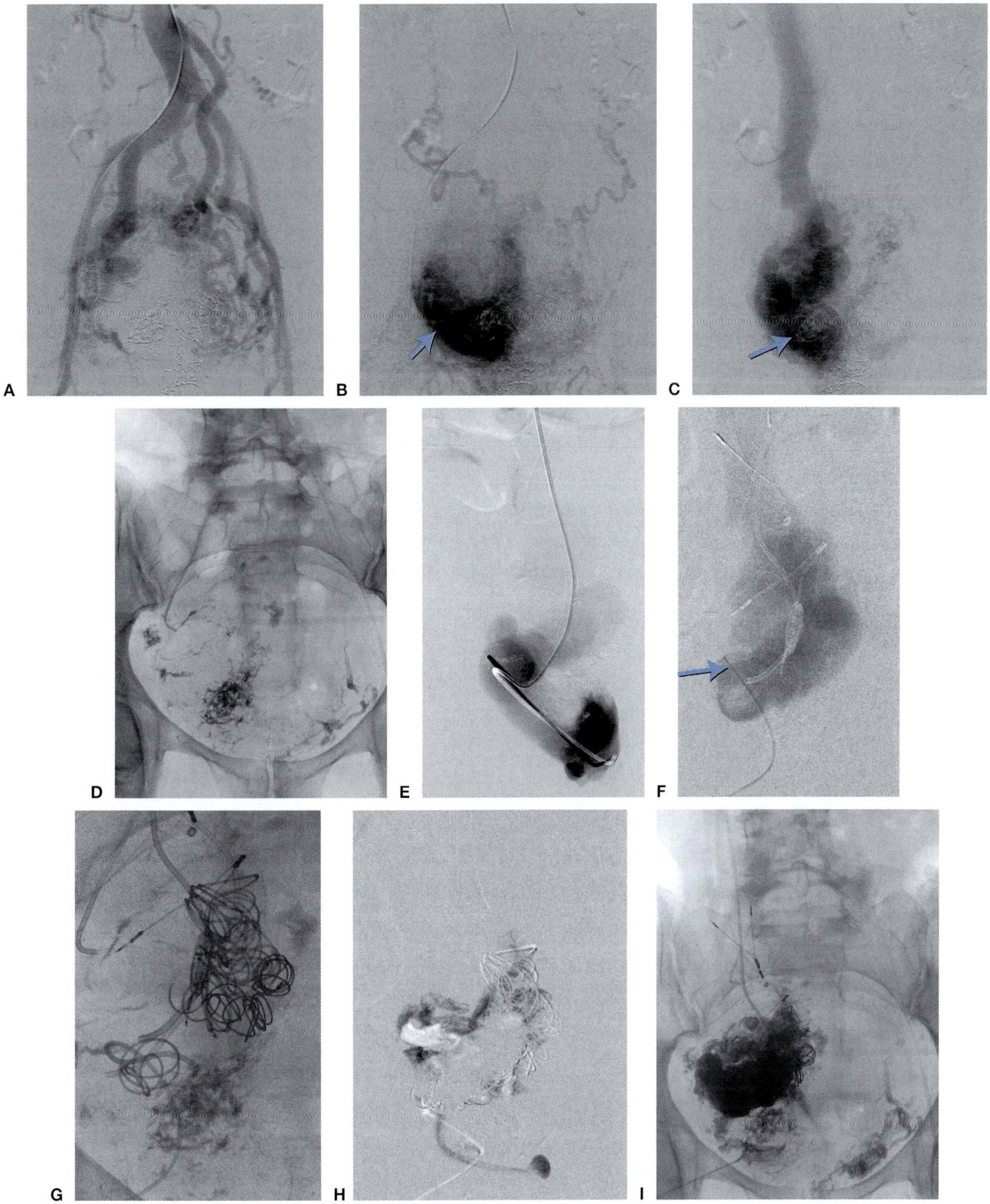

Figure 57.1 Venous outflow embolization for large pelvic AVM. Transarterial embolization with NBCA had been performed on multiple occasions. Patient had recurrent hemorrhage. **A–C:** Images from an abdominal aortogram show a large AVM supplied by internal iliac branches bilaterally and inferior mesenteric artery but draining to a common varix of internal pudendal vein (*arrow*). **D:** Unsubtracted image demonstrates previously injected transarterial NBCA. **E:** Image from a retrograde venogram performed via the internal jugular vein. A bird's nest filter was subsequently placed to prevent pulmonary embolization of embolic material. **F:** Road map image after percutaneous catheterization (*arrow*) of the immediate draining vein. IVC filter is in place. **G:** Fluoroscopic image after placement of Nester coils (Cook Medical, Inc., Bloomington, Indiana) in the varix. **H:** Road map image during injection of NBCA around the coils. **I:** Fluoroscopic image after packing the varix with coils and NBCA. *(Continued)*

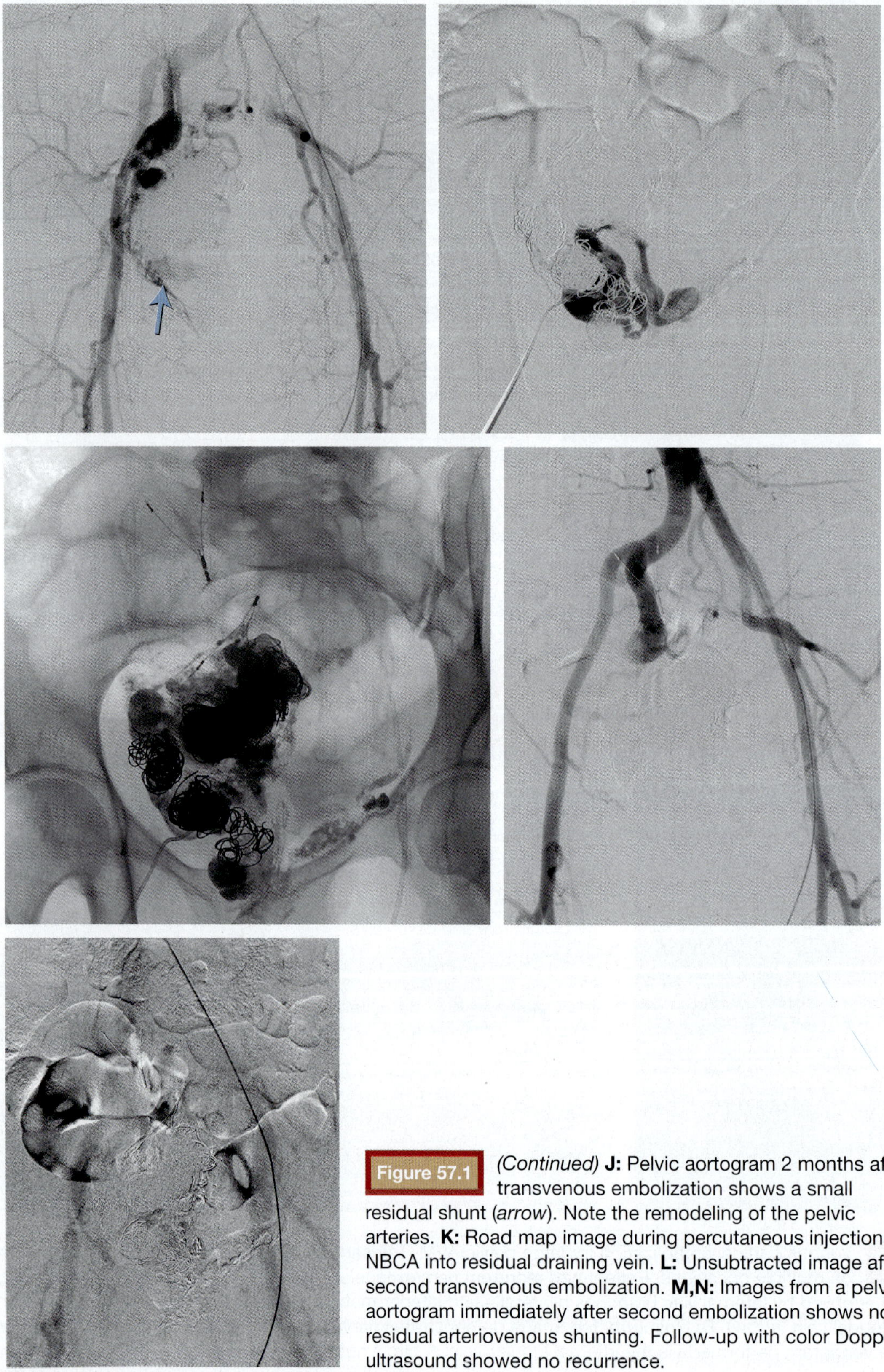

J K L M N

Figure 57.1 *(Continued)* **J:** Pelvic aortogram 2 months after transvenous embolization shows a small residual shunt (*arrow*). Note the remodeling of the pelvic arteries. **K:** Road map image during percutaneous injection of NBCA into residual draining vein. **L:** Unsubtracted image after second transvenous embolization. **M,N:** Images from a pelvic aortogram immediately after second embolization shows no residual arteriovenous shunting. Follow-up with color Doppler ultrasound showed no recurrence.

arteriovenous fistulae and Gelfoam as embolic material and recommended bilateral embolization in most cases. Seven patients required repeat embolization for recurrence of bleeding. Eight patients conceived after embolization and 5 delivered normal infants. In a review of the literature between 2000 and 2011, it was reported that 32% of patients undergoing embolization required a repeat procedure, but the final success rate was 89%.[12] From this brief review of published experience, it would appear that embolization is effective regardless of which embolic agent is used. However, the extent and flow characteristics of uterine AVMs are variable. Small lesions can probably be observed and followed by color Doppler ultrasound. Extensive lesions should be embolized like any other AVM. Intranidal embolization with permanent occlusive agents such as NBCA, Onyx, or ethanol are the optimal techniques, in my opinion (Fig. 57.2). Percutaneous embolization through the anterior pelvic wall is feasible and effective.[3]

TIPS AND TRICKS

- Place a Foley catheter and administer steroids and antibiotics.
- Use high-volume pelvic aortogram to assess arterial supply and venous drainage and monitor result.
- Avoid proximal occlusion of feeding arteries.
- Use permanent occlusive agents.
- Deliver liquid embolic agents only into the AVM nidus or immediate draining vein.
- To occlude a single outflow varix, start with long, detachable 0.035-in coils of the approximate diameter of the varix to create a frame. Once the frame is stable, add less expensive pushable coils.
- Consider placing a temporary IVC filter to prevent pulmonary embolism.

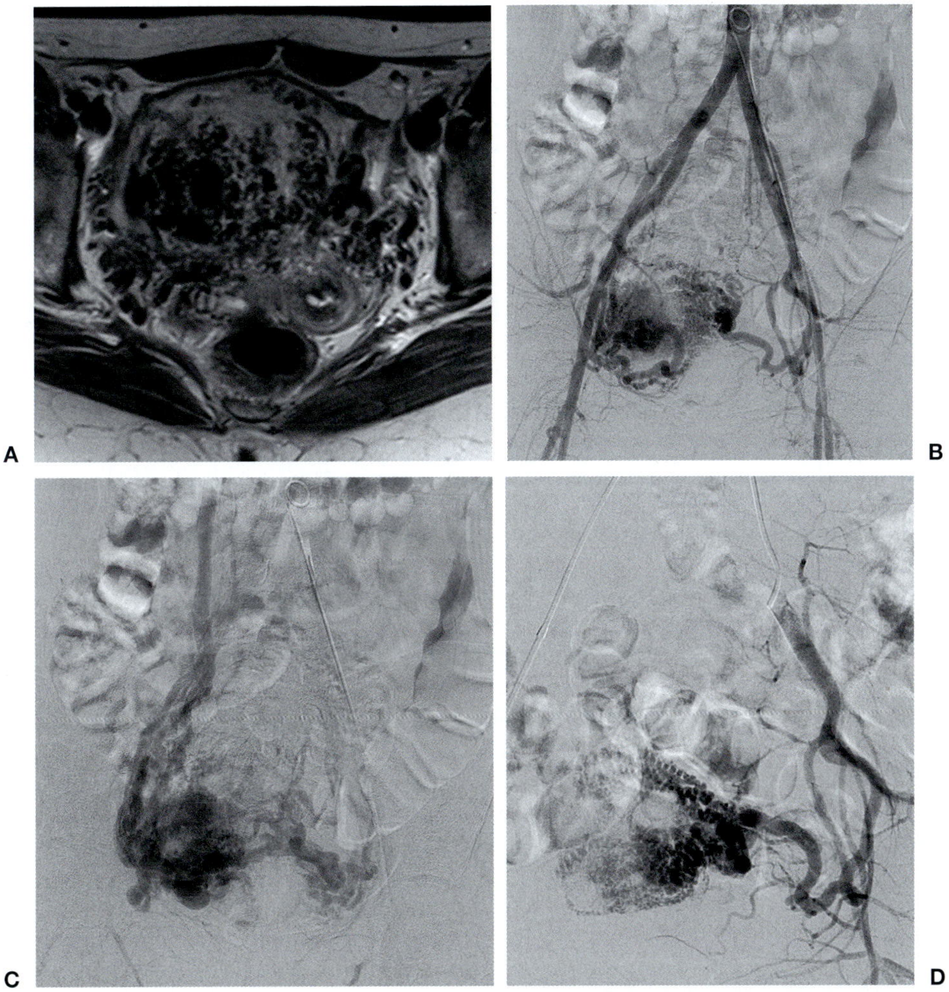

Figure 57.2 Symptomatic uterine AVM in a 30-year-old woman. Vaginal bleeding recurred after two previous embolizations with PVA particles. **A:** T1 weighted axial magnetic resonance image of the pelvis shows numerous flow voids within the muscle of the uterus. Percutaneous access is straightforward through an anterior approach. **B,C:** Images from a pelvic aortogram shows an extensive uterine AVM draining mainly to the iliac veins. **D:** A left internal iliac arteriogram shows normal uterine arteries apparently not supplying the AVM. *(Continued)*

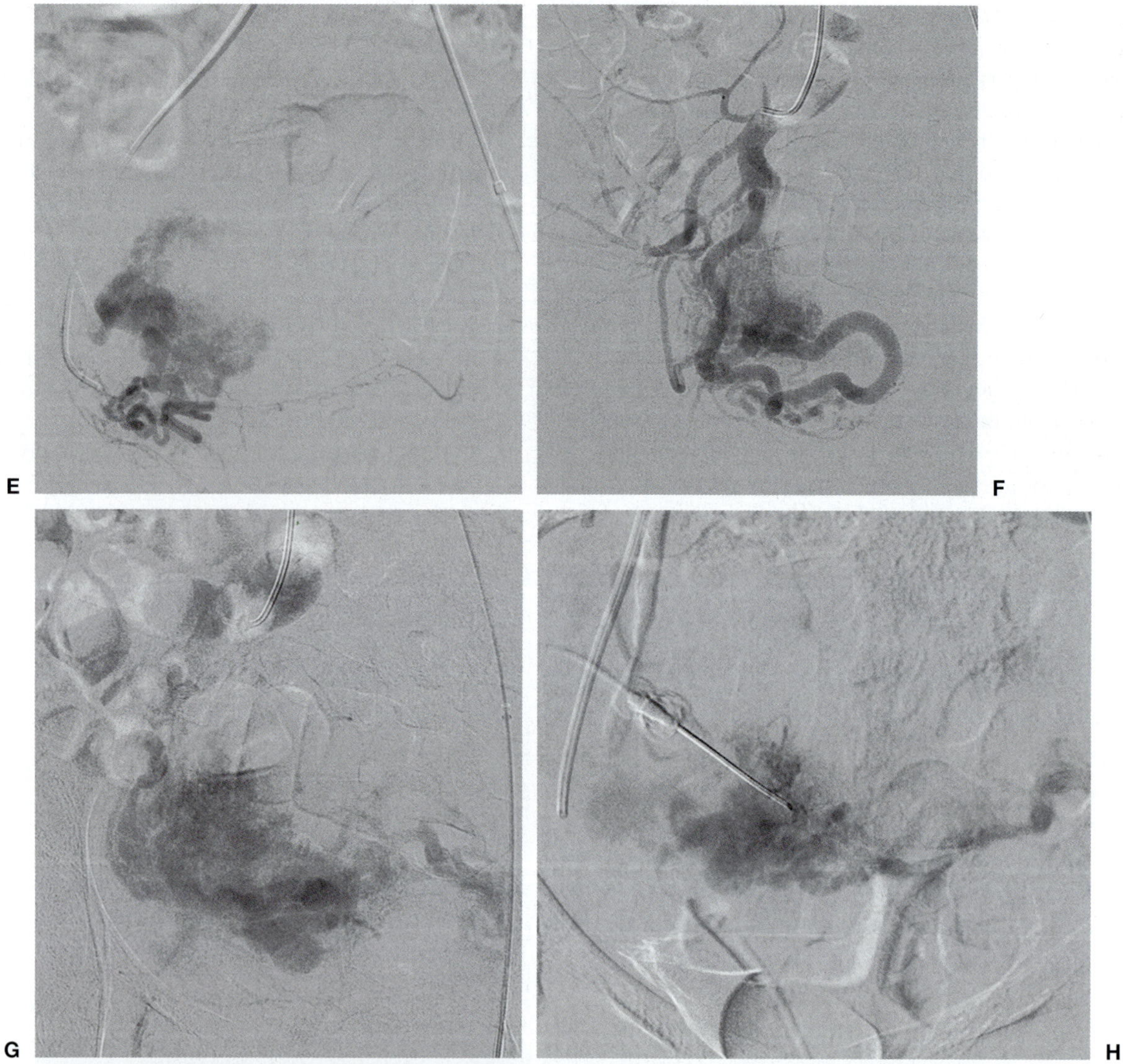

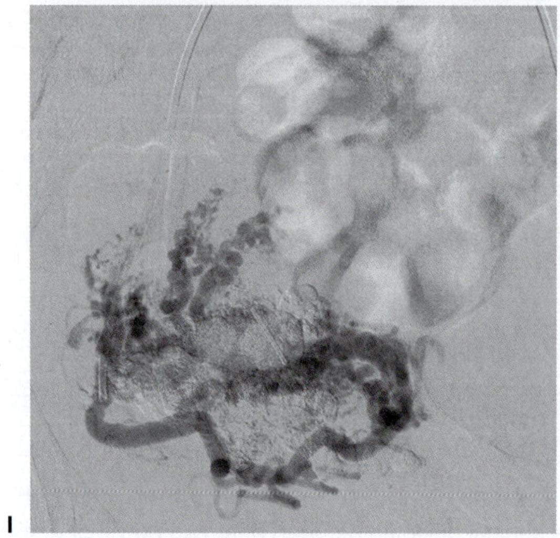

Figure 57.2 *(Continued)* **E:** Right vesicular arteriogram shows secondary supply to the AVM. This should not be embolized. **F,G:** Right internal iliac arteriogram shows supply from the right uterine artery. Tortuosity of the uterine artery makes intranidal catheterization technically difficult. **H:** Percutaneous angiogram of the AVM after direct puncture shows opacification of the nidus and draining veins. This was embolized with ethanol and NBCA. **I:** Right uterine arteriogram following percutaneous embolization shows obliteration of much of the AVM with preservation of the muscular arteries. The patient will be followed by ultrasonography.

REFERENCES

1. Do YS, Kim YW, Park KB, et al. Endovascular treatment combined with emboloscleorotherapy for pelvic arteriovenous malformations. *J Vasc Surg*. 2012;55(2):465–471.
2. Choi SY, Do YS, Lee do Y, et al. Treatment of a pelvic arteriovenous malformation by stent graft placement combined with sclerotherapy. *J Vasc Surg*. 2010;51(4):1006–1009.
3. Burrows PE. Endovascular treatment of fast-flow vascular anomalies. In: Mulliken JB, Burrows PE, Fishman SJ, eds. *Mulliken and Young's Vascular Anomalies Hemangiomas and Malformations*. 2nd ed. New York, NY: Oxford University Press; 2013:710–765.
4. Burrows PE. Vascular malformations involving the female pelvis. *Semin Intervent Radiol*. 2008;25(4):347–360.
5. Jacobowitz GR, Rosen RJ, Rockman CB, et al. Transcatheter embolization of complex pelvic vascular malformations: results and long-term follow-up. *J Vasc Surg*. 2001;33(1):51–55.
6. Takaya N, Iwase T, Maehara A, et al. Transcatheter embolization of arteriovenous malformations in Cowden disease. *Jpn Circ J*. 1999;63(4):326–329.
7. Castaneda F, Goodwin SC, Swischuk JL, et al. Treatment of pelvic arteriovenous malformations with ethylene vinyl alcohol copolymer (Onyx). *J Vasc Interv Radiol*. 2002;13(5):513–516.
8. Timmerman D, Van den Bosch T, Peeraer K, et al. Vascular malformations in the uterus: ultrasonographic diagnosis and conservative management. *Eur J Obstet Gynecol Reprod Biol*. 2000;92(1):171–178.
9. Ghai S, Rajan DK, Asch MR, et al. Efficacy of embolization in traumatic uterine vascular malformations. *J Vasc Interv Radiol*. 2003;14(11):1401–1408.
10. Lim AK, Agarwal R, Seckl MJ, et al. Embolization of bleeding residual uterine vascular malformations in patients with treated gestational trophoblastic tumors. *Radiology*. 2002;222(3):640–644.
11. Wang Z, Chen J, Shi H, et al. Efficacy and safety of embolization in iatrogenic traumatic uterine vascular malformations. *Clin Radiol*. 2012;67(6):541–545.
12. Sanguin S, Lanta-Delmas S, Le Blanche A, et al. Uterine arteriovenous malformations: diagnosis and treatment in 2011 [in French]. *Gynecol Obstet Fertil*. 2011;39(12):722–727.

58

Postpartum Hemorrhage

Omid Kohannim • Justin McWilliams

BACKGROUND

Epidemiology and Risk Factors

Postpartum hemorrhage (PPH), defined as blood loss exceeding 500 mL after vaginal delivery or 1,000 mL after a cesarean section, has an incidence of 5% to 8% and is among the leading causes of maternal mortality across the world. Approximately 140,000 women die from the condition every year. Mortality from PPH has decreased in Western countries; nonetheless, it remains one of the top causes of death from pregnancy in the United States, United Kingdom, and France. In addition to causing mortality, PPH also leads to morbidities, such as coagulopathy, shock, renal failure, and acute respiratory distress syndrome.[1–3]

The most consistent risk factors for PPH are fetal macrosomia, retained placenta or prolonged third stage of labor, prolonged labor in general, delivery via cesarean section, trauma to the genital tract, and the avoidance of uterotonic agents in the third stage of labor.[1] Several other risk factors, such as placenta accreta, instrumental delivery, and hypertensive disorders have also been reported.[4] Demographic factors, such as Hispanic and non-Hispanic white ethnicity have also been found to increase risk for PPH.[5] Unfortunately, however, PPH remains relatively unpredictable from a clinical standpoint.

Etiology and Diagnosis

Etiologies of PPH can be divided into six categories: uterine atony, trauma to the genital tract, retained products of conception, coagulopathy, uterine inversion, and abnormal placentation. Uterine atony accounts for most causes, as normal uterine contraction and subsequent compression of large vessels between muscle fibers are the prime mechanisms of preventing hemorrhage. Each of the previously mentioned etiologies can be further subcategorized. Uterine atony, for instance, can be related to labor (e.g., induction, prolonged labor, infection), uterine overdistension, or anesthetics. Similarly, coagulopathy can be subdivided into disseminated intravascular coagulation, thrombocytopenia, anticoagulation, and inherited disorders.[1]

There are two categories of PPH: early or primary PPH refers to excessive bleeding that occurs within 24 hours after delivery, whereas late or secondary PPH occurs between 24 hours and 6 to 12 weeks after delivery.[6,7] Primary and secondary PPH have incidence rates of 4% to 6% and 1%, respectively. Causes of primary and secondary PPH vary. Primary PPH is usually due to the so-called four Ts, which refer to tone (i.e., lack thereof, or atony), trauma, tissue (i.e., retained products of conception), and thrombosis. These account for approximately 70% to 80%, 28%, 11%, and 1% of causes, respectively. Secondary PPH is usually caused by retained products of conception, subinvolution of placental site, infection, and coagulopathy.[2,8,9] Etiologies of primary and secondary PPH are summarized in Table 58.1.

As mentioned earlier, most cases of PPH are due to uterine atony, which is often a clinical diagnosis. There are occasions, however, when clinical diagnosis is difficult, and imaging may become helpful. Although ultrasonography is the first-line imaging modality in patients with PPH due to its safety and low cost, it may be limited by pain and bowel gas and cannot typically pinpoint the source of acute hemorrhage. Computed tomography (CT) imaging may be more useful in certain cases. In PPH, CT may identify severe arterial bleeding in the arterial phase, and smaller hemorrhage in the delayed phase, by visualization of contrast extravasation into the uterine cavity. This cannot only be diagnostically valuable when clinical evidence is unreliable but also guide subsequent interventions by pinpointing the site of bleeding. CT can also delineate other causes of PPH, such as concealed or puerperal genital hematomas.[2] In particular, if a patient has signs of PPH

Table 58.1 Causes of Primary and Secondary Postpartum Hemorrhage

Primary (early)	Secondary (late)
Uterine atony	Abnormal placentation
Labor-related	Subinvolution of placental site
Overdistension of uterus	Placenta accreta
Anesthesia	Retained products of conception
Pelvic trauma	Infection
Iatrogenic	Endometritis
Spontaneous	Infection of cesarean section scar
Retained products of conception	Coagulopathy
Coagulopathy	Uterine pathology
DIC	Fibroids
Thrombocytopenia	Cervical cancer
Inherited disorders	
Uterine inversion	
Abnormal placentation	
Placenta previa	
Placenta accreta	

DIC, disseminated intravascular coagulation
Adapted from Neill A, Thornton S. Secondary postpartum haemorrhage. *J Obstet Gynaecol*. 2002;22(2):119–122; Oyelese Y, Ananth CV. Postpartum hemorrhage: epidemiology, risk factors, and causes. *Clin Obstet Gynecol*. 2010;53(1):147–156.

without direct vaginal bleeding, CT is indicated[7]. Uterine rupture, which has a hypoattenuating appearance within the highly enhancing myometrium, may also be diagnosed with CT. When retained products of conception are suspected as the etiology of PPH, an echogenic, intracavitary, endometrial mass on ultrasonography or T2-hyperintense lesions on magnetic resonance imaging (MRI) can also be used for diagnosis.[2]

Management

The management of PPH requires a multidisciplinary approach, often involving the obstetricians, nurses, anesthesiologists, laboratory specialists, and radiologists. Management always begins with resuscitative and conservative measures, necessitating close attention to airway, breathing, and circulation. Close monitoring, large-bore intravenous lines, blood cross-typing, and transfusion are often needed. Pharmacologic treatment predominantly entails the use of uterotonic agents to control bleeding and is typically the next step in management. Uterotonic agents include oxytocin, prostaglandins, and ergot derivatives such as methylergonovine. Administration of uterotonic agents addresses the most common cause of primary PPH, which is uterine atony. Minor procedures such as repair of lacerations, uterine compression, massage, and tamponade are also important components of the management, particularly when uterotonic agents do not suffice. One particular tamponade technique involves the use of a Bakri balloon (Cook Medical, Bloomington, Indiana),[9] which has been shown to be effective in several case studies.[10,11] This is a 24-Fr, 58-cm silicone device with two drainage holes at the tip of its shaft and a balloon, which can be inflated up to 800 mL, although usually no more than 500 mL. Bleeding control may be achieved by inserting this device through the cervical opening and pulling it from the vagina during cesarean section or inserting it through the vagina during a vaginal delivery, both of which are then followed by vaginal packing, balloon inflation, and drainage.[9] In addition to these procedural measures, the uterus should be closely inspected for any retained products or clots.

When medical and conservative measures fail, PPH may then be surgically managed with arterial ligation and placement of a brace suture. Hysterectomy is typically the last resort. The management steps partly depend on the mode of delivery. If the patient is bleeding after cesarean section, surgical management may be more plausible. Alternative causes for bleeding should also be explored in refractory cases. In patients with coagulopathy, for instance, plasma components need to be replaced. As we will discuss later, it has become increasingly apparent that interventional radiology can play an important role in the management of PPH through arterial embolization and balloon catheterization, ideally replacing the need for surgery. Various approaches in the management of PPH are listed in Table 58.2.[3,6]

Table 58.2 Management Approaches in Postpartum Hemorrhage

Approaches
Medical
Pharmacologic
Oxytocin
Misoprostol
Ergot alkaloids
Nonpharmacologic
Fluid resuscitation
Blood typing and crossmatching
Blood transfusion
Examination of uterus, perineum, and vagina
Inspection of the placenta
Uterine compression and massage
Uterine packing or tamponade (e.g., with Bakri balloon)
Laceration repair
Curettage
Exclusion of coagulation disorders, pseudoaneurysms, AVFs
Surgical
Pressure on aorta
Arterial ligation
B-Lynch brace suture
Hysterectomy (last resort)
Interventional
Arterial embolization
Balloon catheterization

AVFs, arteriovenous fistulas.

TECHNICAL DETAILS

In 1979, Brown et al.[12] introduced angiographic arterial embolization as an alternative technique to control PPH, offering advantages over surgery, including specific identification of bleeding sites and potential preservation of fertility. In their paper, Brown et al.[12] described the case of a 22-year-old woman with preeclampsia who underwent labor augmentation and subsequently developed primary PPH refractory to conservative management. When her bleeding continued despite evacuation of a large posterior hematoma and total hysterectomy, she was transferred to a radiology suite, where angiography revealed bleeding from an internal pudendal artery branch. Embolization with Gelfoam (Pharmacia & Upjohn, Kalamazoo, Michigan) was performed, which led to control of bleeding and stabilization of the patient (Fig. 58.1). Soon after, Pais et al.[13] reported two cases of arterial embolization for achieving hemostasis in PPH. Since the Brown et al.[12] and Pais et al.[13] cases, arterial embolization has been extensively studied for PPH and its value has been increasingly recognized despite the fact that several questions still remain unanswered in the field.[14]

Anatomy

The uterine artery, which is the predominant supply to the uterus, originates from the anterior division of the internal iliac (hypogastric) artery. This artery divides into a large ascending branch and a small descending branch. The descending branch is also called the *cervicovaginal artery* and supplies the cervix and vagina. The ascending branch gives off multiple arcuate vessels to the body and fundus of the uterus then divides into the tubal and ovarian terminal branches. The vaginal artery can either originate from the

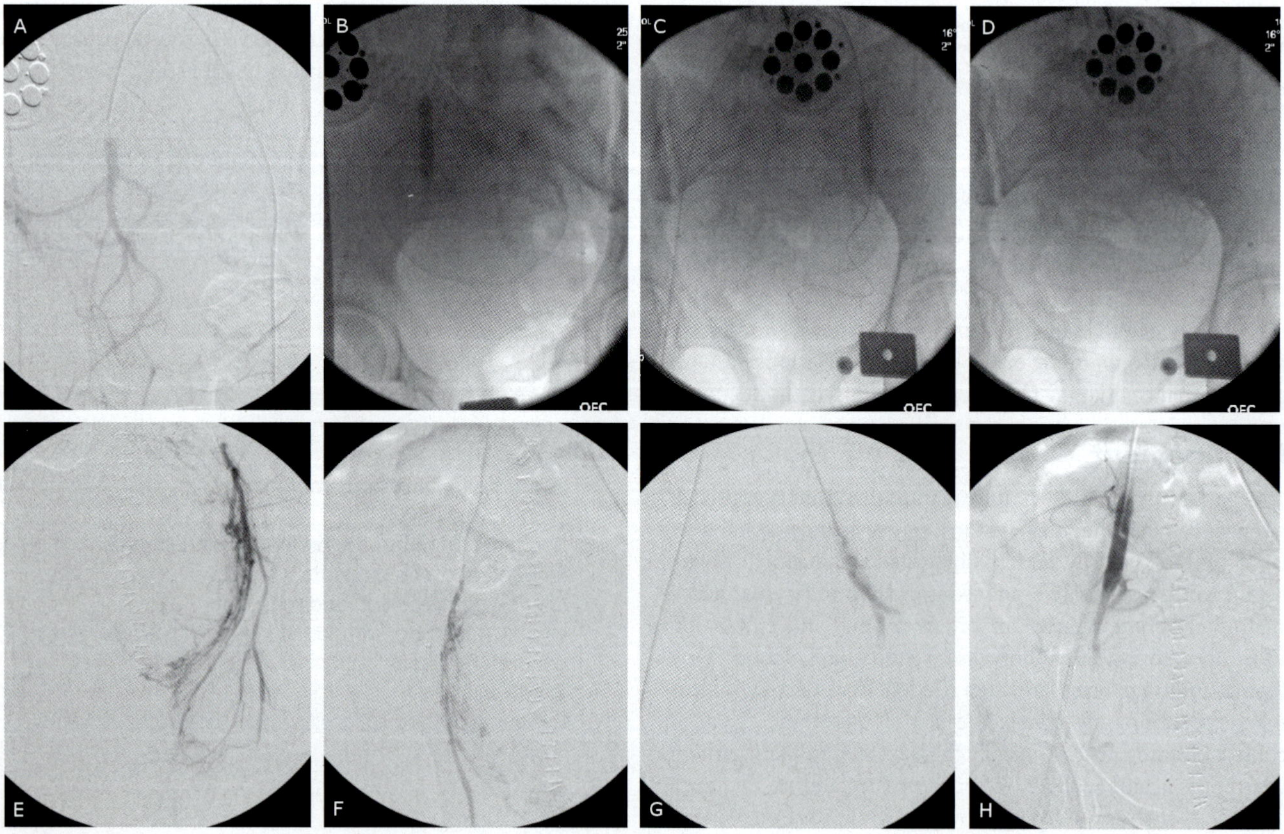

Figure 58.1 A 25-year-old female with placenta percreta and increta. Prophylactic balloon occlusion with provisional embolization was requested before cesarean delivery. **A:** Internal iliac angiography is performed to determine ideal position and sizing of the occlusion balloon. **B:** Occlusion balloon in place in the right internal iliac artery. Contrast can be injected through the inflated balloon catheter to confirm sluggish distal flow. **C:** The procedure is repeated on the left side. **D:** The occlusion balloons are secured in position and deflated until the fetus is delivered to prevent fetal hypoxia. Position is reconfirmed with fluoroscopy at the time of inflation. **E,F:** Angiography through the balloon catheters following fetal delivery demonstrates persistent placental opacification secondary to retained placental components. **G,H:** Angiography following Gelfoam embolization demonstrates stasis in the anterior divisions of the internal iliac arteries bilaterally.

anterior division of the internal iliac artery or arise from the uterine artery. The ovarian artery, which supplies about 10% of the uterine fundus, originates from the aorta and makes anastomoses with uterine artery branches.[2,12] Knowledge of pelvic arterial anatomy, in addition to the anatomical variations in the anterior division of the internal iliac artery,[15] can help improve treatment success and safety of arterial embolization in PPH.

Technique

The technique of arterial embolization in the setting of PPH has not greatly changed since the first reported case by Brown et al.[12] After local anesthesia, arterial access is achieved with a catheter through the common femoral artery, typically unilaterally, although a bilateral approach has also been espoused due to its rapidity.[16] Diagnostic angiography of the internal iliac arteries, particularly of the anterior division, is performed to study the anatomy and detect extravasation. Embolization of both uterine arteries under fluoroscopic guidance is typically attempted next, most often empirically. Unilateral embolization is not usually done as recanalization of collateral vessels may lead to more bleeding. Internal iliac and abdominal angiography may also be performed as the source of bleeding may not be the uterine artery.[3,7,17] The anterior division of the internal iliac arteries may be embolized when access to the uterine arteries or identification of the exact source of hemorrhage is difficult.[3] Postembolization angiography is conducted to ensure extravasation has stopped. In cases of recurrent PPH, there may be other sources of bleeding such as the ovarian artery, which is why juxtarenal angiography may also be done in refractory cases.[16,17]

Embolization is most frequently performed using absorbable gelatin sponge to provide temporary occlusion.[18] Blood flow typically returns after a few weeks as the surrounding tissues absorb the material. This transient blockage followed by recanalization of the artery has been observed to be adequate for control of the hemorrhage. Very small particles (i.e., microparticles) may cause uterine necrosis[19] and are thus generally avoided. Nonabsorbable materials (e.g., polyvinyl alcohol particles) can be used to occlude distal vessels. Absorbable particles, on the other hand, block arterial flow more proximally.[20] As in the original case by Brown et al.,[12] Gelfoam has been the material of choice for these procedures and was the most common material used in the literature, as reviewed by Vedantham et al.,[21] often in form of pledgets. Because the gravid uterus comprises a system of collateral vessels as opposed to a single, predominant vessel, coil embolization is not typically used.[22] Large vessel lacerations may, however, necessitate the use of metal coils in a fraction of cases.[23] Despite its higher cost and difficulty of use, embolization with *N*-butyl cyanoacrylate (NBCA) has also shown promise in patients with PPH, particularly in those who are at risk for or have already developed disseminated intravascular coagulation[24] or at times of severe hemodynamic instability (Fig. 58.2).[22]

OUTCOMES

Emergency Embolization

Most interventions in PPH are performed in an emergent setting due to the unpredictability of bleeding. Despite the lack of randomized trials on the topic, several retrospective and prospective cohort studies have examined the effectiveness of embolization in the emergency management of PPH.[23,25–38] These studies have generally found the technique to be effective, with success rates ranging from 73% to 100%. Table 58.3 lists the studies since 1998 with at least 15 patients for emergency treatment of PPH with

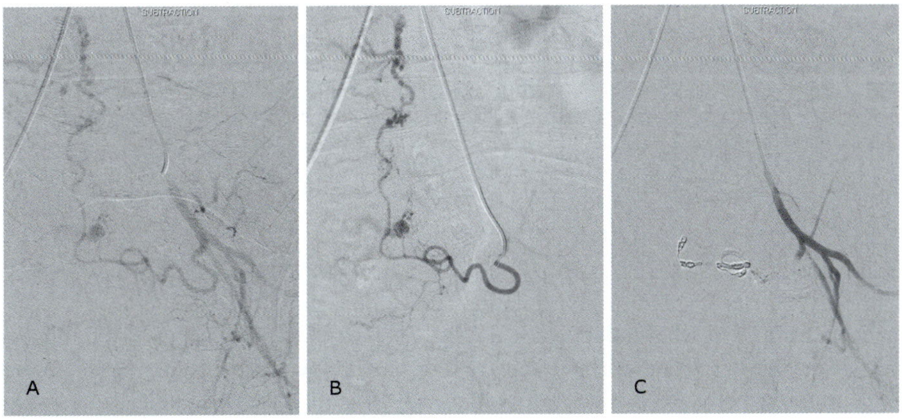

Figure 58.2 A 25-year-old female with PPH after dilation and evacuation of a 23-week pregnancy. **A:** Internal iliac angiography demonstrates a pseudoaneurysm arising from the vertical segment of the left uterine artery. **B:** Selective uterine angiography confirms this finding and also demonstrates active extravasation from the ruptured pseudoaneurysm. **C:** Following coil and Onyx (Covidien, Irvine, California) embolization, stasis is achieved in the left uterine artery. The patient recovered uneventfully.

Table 58.3 Summary of Reported Success Rates and Complications of Arterial Embolization in Emergency Postpartum Hemorrhage Based on Cohort Studies (N ≥15)

Study	N	Success Rate	Complications (number of patients)
Boulleret et al.[25]	36	100%	Puncture site false aneurysm (1), lower limb paresthesia (2), femoral vein thrombosis (1), minor puncture site hematoma (7)
Chauleur et al.[26]	46	89%	Iodine allergy (1), pulmonary edema (1), puncture site hematoma (1), hemoperitoneum related to epigastric artery dissection (1)
Choi et al.[27]	40	90%	Fever (5), pulmonary edema (2), colitis (1), ischemic sciatic neuropathy (1)
Deux et al.[28]	25	96%	Blood transfusions after procedure (3)
Eriksson et al.[29]	20	100%	Low-grade febrile reaction (7), endometrial infection (1), transient pelvic pain (2), transient leg numbness (2), reduced sensation to touch in thigh (1)
Ganguli et al.[30]	66	95%	Deep vein thrombosis in lower extremity (1), postprocedural pancreatitis (1), likely endometritis (1)
Kirby et al.[23]	43	79%	Groin hematoma (1), left obturator artery perforation (1), bleeding, necrotic fibroid tumor, requiring myomectomy after 2 mo (1), likely endometritis (1)
Lee et al.[31]	251	87%	Uterine artery dissection (2), transient lower extremity numbness (2), lower extremity edema (1), puncture site hematoma (3)
Ojala et al.[32]	22	77%	Cervical and vaginal necrosis (1), popliteal artery thrombosis, iatrogenic (1), sciatic nerve ischemia (1)
Ornan et al.[33]	28	96%	Technical error (1), light rebleeding in patient with vWD (1), bowel necrosis (1), and buttock claudication (1) in patients with internal iliac artery ligation before embolization
Pelage et al.[34]	27	100%	Delayed hysterectomy in patient with placenta accreta (1)
Pelage et al.[34]	35	100%	Foot ischemia (1), recurrent hemorrhage after 5 d necessitating hysterectomy (1)
Soncini et al.	16	93%	Pain (1), transient fever (1)
Touboul et al.[37]	102	73%	Pulmonary edema (5), renal failure (7); myocardial ischemia (3), lumbar plexus ischemia (1), gluteal pain (1)
Vegas et al.[38]	27	96%	Vaginocutaneous fistula (1)

WD, von Willebrand disease.

embolization. Lee et al.[31] conducted the largest study to date on this topic. The authors performed a retrospective analysis of 251 women at their institution who underwent arterial embolization due to medically or surgically refractory primary PPH. Most commonly, both uterine arteries were embolized. Anterior divisions of the internal iliac arteries were embolized in cases of failure of response to uterine embolization or poor arterial access. They found the clinical and technical success rates of the embolization procedure to be 86.5% and 89.6%, respectively. Before these, there were also smaller reports of success with embolization in the literature.[38–41] Several studies have, in fact, argued that embolization is underused.[18,22,42,43]

One of the challenges in the interpretation of the studies mentioned earlier is that PPH is clinically heterogeneous, which is difficult to standardize across reports.[23,39] Patients often vary in the degree of severity of their bleeding. Touboul et al.[37] for instance, included only severe PPH in their study, which may account for their low success rate of 73%. Primary and secondary PPH with various etiologies have also been intermixed in studies. Furthermore, Kirby et al.[23] argued that clinical success has also not been uniform across different studies, as some have, for instance, included patients with postembolization rebleeding under clinical success. The efficacy of arterial embolization appears high, but large standardized studies, if not randomized trials, are needed to better assess its role in management of PPH (Table 58.3)

A debated topic in the field has been whether embolization should precede surgery or follow failed surgical attempts. In a systematic review of 46 studies, Doumouchtsis et al.[39] compared the success rates of arterial embolization, balloon tamponade, uterine compression sutures, and iliac artery ligation or uterine devascularization and found all of these to be similar: 90.7%, 84.0%, 91.7%, and 84.6%, respectively. Embolization has been shown to be effective when done after surgery,[40] but most studies conclude that embolization should be considered before surgical alternatives. In a small retrospective study, Bloom et al.[41] directly compared embolization performed before versus after surgery and reported that the former may be preferred. When interventional radiology resources are available, embolization before surgery cannot only reduce rates of complications, intensive care unit admission, and blood transfusion requirements but also preserve fertility. More obvious advantages of embolization before surgery include avoidance of laparotomy and anesthesia.[41] The recommendations by the American College of Obstetricians and Gynecologists (ACOG) state that women can undergo embolization either due to excessive bleeding after hysterectomy or as an alternative to hysterectomy,[42] but no definitive guidelines are present. Another related and open question regarding management of PPH with embolization is whether a patient should undergo embolization or surgery when hemodynamically unstable. ACOG recommends arterial embolization only in stable patients.[42] Investigators speculate, nonetheless, that its role may become more important in time-sensitive cases with unstable patients[23] and may be considered with close monitoring.[31]

Prophylactic Interventions in Abnormal Placentation

Interventional procedures play an important role not only in the emergency management of PPH but also in the prophylaxis of PPH in patients with high risk, particularly in the settings of abnormal placentation. Abnormal placentation has been rising in incidence due to higher rates of cesarean sections. There are various types of abnormal placentation. Placenta accreta occurs when the placenta is abnormally attached to the uterus. Invasion of the uterine musculature is termed *placenta increta* and that of the musculature, serosa, and sometimes neighboring structures is called *placenta percreta*.[43] Patients with placenta previa, that is, a placenta located abnormally close to the cervix, are at higher risk for developing placenta accreta.

Abnormal placentation can be diagnosed during prenatal visits through assessment of risk factors and application of ultrasonography and MRI.[44,45] On ultrasound, several findings can point to the diagnosis of placenta accreta. These include the presence of lacunae in the placental parenchyma with turbulent flow on color Doppler—the most reliable finding—placenta previa, reduced thickness of myometrium, and absence of a hypoechoic, retroplacental line (i.e., absence of clear space). The most consistent findings on MRI are bulging of the uterus, a heterogeneous placenta, and placental bands, which are dark on T2.[46] Early prenatal diagnosis of abnormal placentation has allowed for the notion of prophylactic interventions for these high-risk pregnancies. The coordination of early diagnosis and preventive management requires a multidisciplinary approach between obstetricians and interventional radiologists at equipped facilities.

In 1992, Alvarez et al.[47] studied prophylactic embolization in five patients, all of whom except one had placenta previa. Their study composed of a mixture of patients who underwent embolization either following failed medical and surgical management of PPH or following prophylactic placement of arterial catheters. The authors found that the prophylactic approach allowed for selective embolization of the affected internal iliac artery. Additionally, patients in the prophylactic group had reduced hospital stay and blood transfusion requirement when compared to the curative group.[47] A more recent prospective study of 11 patients found prophylactic embolization to not only reduce risk of PPH but also increase fertility and decrease mortality and morbidity.[48] In this study, embolization in women with placenta accreta was performed before placenta removal; in the case of placenta increta or percreta, the placenta was not removed. Due to the paucity of large comparison studies, it is difficult to conclude whether prophylactic embolization is always necessary and the procedure remains controversial. Soyer et al.,[49] for instance, did not recommend this as they found emergency embolization in their cohort of 10 women to be sufficient and effective despite severe bleeding from abnormal placentation. Diop et al.[50] compared the cases of emergency and preventive embolization in a mixed cohort of 17 patients and found reduced blood loss and delay time to embolization in the prophylactic group. The success rate of embolization, however, was 100% in both cases.

An alternative to the preoperative placement of catheters for embolization is the placement of occlusive balloon catheters for PPH prophylaxis, which may or may not precede arterial embolization (Fig. 58.3). This approach was introduced in 1997 by Dubois et al.,[51] where internal iliac artery balloon catheterization and embolization during cesarean delivery and hysterectomy led to decreased blood loss. Since then, several cohort studies have investigated the role of prophylactic balloon catheterization in preventing PPH. The most recent and largest study in this area is a retrospective, case-control study by Ballas et al.,[52] where preoperative, internal iliac artery balloon placement was compared to no intervention in 117 women with a diagnosis of placenta accreta confirmed by pathology. The

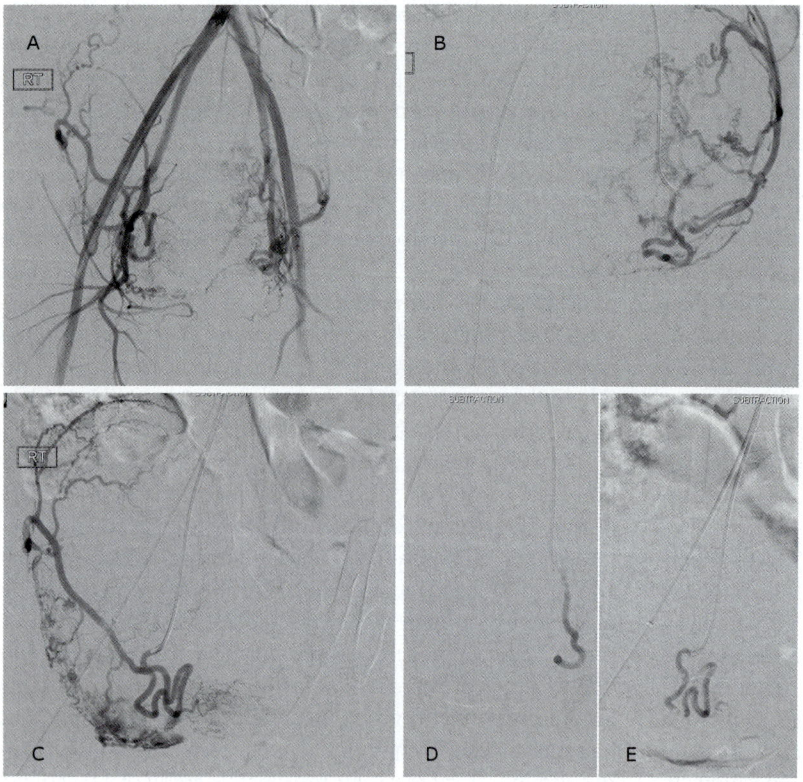

Figure 58.3 A 32-year-old female with clinical evidence of PPH. **A:** Pelvic aortogram demonstrates the hypervascular postgravid uterus without definite active extravasation. **B,C:** Bilateral uterine artery angiography demonstrates the expected appearance of the postgravid uterus. **D,E:** Following bilateral uterine artery embolization with Gelfoam, postembolization angiography demonstrates stasis in the uterine arteries. The patient experienced no further hemorrhage.

investigators of this study compared several outcomes between the two groups, including estimated blood loss, blood transfusion units, massive transfusions, operative time, hospitalization duration, and complications. They found that patients with prophylactic balloon catheters experienced less blood loss and required less massive transfusions. The authors, therefore, concluded that the preventive procedure is safe and effective. Despite its large size, however, the study was not randomized, and it could not differentiate between the effects of balloon placement and prenatal placenta accreta diagnosis, which were highly correlated.

Before the Ballas et al.[52] report, there were several smaller studies, reviewed by Dilauro et al.,[45] with less definitive results. As in the Ballas et al.[52] study, several of these explored balloon catheterization without subsequent arterial embolization. In agreement with Ballas et al.,[52] the researchers in three of these studies found that the procedure reduced blood loss.[53–55] Two controlled studies, however, reported no effect on blood loss from prophylactic balloon catheterization.[56,57] Shrivastava et al.,[56] in particular, compared patients with balloon catheter placement and hysterectomy to those with hysterectomy alone in a relatively large cohort (N = 69) and detected no difference between operative duration, estimated blood loss, units of blood transfusions, and hospital stay between the two groups.[56] Three of their patients with interventions also had complications, including arterial thrombosis and dissection. Several studies have also investigated prophylactic balloon catheterization followed by arterial embolization in the setting of abnormal placentation.[32,58,59] Here, again, the results have been mixed regarding whether intervention reduces blood loss. Cohort studies on prophylactic interventions for abnormal placentation have been summarized in Table 58.4.

As discussed previously, there is significant variation in the internal iliac artery anatomy among patients. Most studies have reported the placement of balloon catheters in the anterior division of the internal iliac arteries. Shih et al.,[60] however, implemented a different technique in a single case report, where catheters were positioned more proximally in the common iliac artery. They argued that this approach allows for easier lodging of the balloon catheter, particularly in cases where the patient's anatomy varies from the norm. Additionally, there are several collateral vessels in the pelvic region during pregnancy (e.g., external iliac and femoral arteries), which may cause failure of internal iliac artery balloon occlusion. Shih et al.[60] claimed that their technique reduced hemorrhage by preventing collateral flow, albeit with a risk of thrombosis, embolism, and reperfusion injury to the lower extremities with a prolonged common iliac artery occlusion. An even simpler approach using a single large balloon to temporarily occlude the pelvic aorta has also been condoned by several authors based on success in case reports.[61–63] This technique is typically performed in the settings of pelvic fracture or abdominal trauma. By impeding blood flow from external iliac, sacral, lumbar, and potentially inferior mesenteric

Table 58.4 Summary of Case Studies on Prophylactic Interventional Procedures for Abnormal Placentation

Study	N	Control group	Interventional Technique	Effective in Reducing Blood Loss	Intervention-Related Complications (N)
Ballas et al.[52]	117	Yes	BC	Yes	Femoral artery thrombosis (1), superficial catheter site hematoma (1)
Bodner et al.[58]	28	Yes	BC and TAE	No	DIC (2), cystostomy and bladder repair (2)
Carnevale et al.[53]	21	No	BC	Yes	Femoral artery thrombosis (1), external iliac artery thrombosis (1)
Levine et al.[57]	9	Yes	BC	No	Fever (2), bilateral injury to ureters and pulmonary edema (1)
Ojala et al.[32]	7	No	BC and TAE	Yes	None
Sadashivaiah et al.[54]	13	No	BC	Yes	Groin hematoma (1)
Shrivastava et al.[56]	69	Yes	BC	No	Internal iliac thrombosis and groin hematoma (1), internal iliac dissection (1), femoral artery thrombosis (1)
Sivan et al.[59]	25	No	BC and TAE	Yes	None
Tan et al.[55]	25	Yes	BC	Yes	None

BC, balloon catheterization; TAE, transarterial embolization; DIC, disseminated intravascular coagulation.

arteries, aortic balloon occlusion can also provide effective and rapid hemostasis in cases of abnormal placentation and PPH, albeit at the risk of aortic rupture, severe hemodynamic changes, reperfusion injury, and thrombosis.[62,64]

The Royal College of Obstetricians and Gynaecologists recommended in their 2007 guidelines that in the setting of suspected abnormalities of the placenta, balloon catheter inflation of internal iliac or uterine arteries can be done prophylactically, with embolization if hemorrhage is refractory to balloon inflation.[65] To date, studies have been limited to cohorts and case reports and have not always been controlled. Future randomized controlled studies may be able to provide more definite answers (Table 58.4).

Fertility

Preservation of the uterus is a key potential advantage of arterial embolization in the management of PPH. However, no clinical trials have investigated fertility following the use of embolization for PPH. Several small-scale studies have, however, reported encouraging results. Several of these cohort studies, primarily aimed at evaluating the efficacy of embolization, have also followed patients for fertility and found at least one successful pregnancy and normal menstruation in those not requiring hysterectomy.[34,35,66,67] Single case reports have also documented successful postembolization pregnancies.[68] In a larger, more detailed telephone follow-up study of patients who underwent embolization for severe PPH, Salomon et al.[69] found that nearly a fourth of the women later delivered healthy babies, although early miscarriage and recurrence of PPH were also observed.[69] In a similarly designed study, Fiori et al.[70] reported normal and spontaneous pregnancies in 60% and 40% of their cohort, respectively. Miscarriages, recurrence of PPH, and unplanned pregnancies have been found in a fraction of women in other similar studies.[71,72] A detailed review of literature by Delotte et al.[73] found that 71% of pregnancies after embolization resulted in deliveries, 18% in miscarriages, and 11% in voluntary terminations.[73] The authors discussed that the miscarriage rate was not higher than that of typical first-trimester miscarriage but that the elective termination rate was high, most likely due to the psychological effects of PPH on the patient.[73] Generally, studies conclude that women with PPH who undergo arterial embolization almost always resume normal menses and can usually become pregnant with healthy babies. It is, however, crucial for pregnancies occurring after embolization procedures to be closely followed, particularly with serial ultrasonography.[74]

POTENTIAL COMPLICATIONS

The potential complications of arterial embolization for PPH are estimated to occur in 5% to 9% of cases.[36,41] We list complications reported in several cohort studies for emergency and prophylactic interventions in Table 58.3. In their systematic review, Doumouchtsis et al.[39] also summarize several complications of arterial embolization, including buttock, small bowel, and foot ischemia; leg and buttock numbness; uterine and bladder necrosis; puncture site hematomas and false aneurysms; as well as popliteal artery thrombosis.[39] The most common complication of the procedure is a transient postembolization fever.[44] Clinical findings suggestive of endometritis have also been reported.[23,30] Most of these complications are minor and self-limited. There are, nonetheless, case reports of major complications in the literature. Coulange et al.[20] reported two unusual cases of uterine necrosis, which they attributed to lack of collateral vasculature and the use of very fine and emulsified gelatin particles, which can occlude too distally. Massive uterine necrosis with histopathologic evidence was also reported in another patient, whose complication was also a likely result of small particle embolization.[19] In a recent study of 44 women, Pellerin et al.[75] advocated that a superselective Gelfoam slurry embolization in the uterine arteries may be safer to the myometrium than more standard techniques, as they observed no evidence of uterine necrosis in follow-up 1-month MRI scans. Nontrivial complications are, therefore, mostly technical, and it has been argued that most of these can be avoided by using appropriate tools and techniques.[41] Nonetheless, skilled nursing care after the procedure is critical to look for complications. This is often done in the labor and delivery unit, although the patient's hemodynamic status may call for intensive care unit monitoring.[74]

As discussed earlier, embolization is close to 90% effective in cases of PPH. A natural question that arises in the field is why the remaining cases fail. Earlier studies predominantly consisted of too few patients to assess risk factors for embolization failure. More recently, however, there has been an interest in thorough analysis of such predictive factors in larger cohorts. A retrospective study (N = 117) in 2009 identified severe bleeding (>1,500 mL) and requirement of at least 6 blood transfusion units to be the sole predictor for embolization failure among many factors that they studied.[76] In addition to massive blood transfusion, disseminated intravascular coagulation and cesarean delivery were found to be associated with embolization failure in the study by Lee et al.[31] (N = 251), although the latter factor did not remain significant in multivariate analysis. Disseminated intravascular coagulation was noted to be the only significant predictor in multivariate analysis of 257 patients in another recent retrospective study.[77] A fourth retrospective study (N = 98) reported blood transfusion, placenta accreta, and certain laboratory abnormalities (including hemoglobin, fibrinogen, and prothrombin time) as predictive factors.[78] Placenta accreta has frequently been reported to be associated with unsuccessful embolization due to persistent hemorrhage,[35,79,80] with a failure rate estimated as 23%,[81] which is why early diagnosis and prophylactic measures are more important in this setting. A summary of predictive findings from the previously mentioned studies and others[27,37,82] are shown in Table 58.5. Overall, the largest studies find that failure of embolization in PPH is related to the severity of bleeding and disseminated intravascular coagulation. Arterial embolization can be repeated in cases of failure. Lee et al.[31] observed 34 failures in their 251 patients, 12 of whom underwent repeat embolization. In 9 of the 12 patients, hemostasis was achieved. The authors recommended that patients who failed embolization undergo repeat embolization before hysterectomy, mainly to preserve fertility (Table 58.5).

Prophylactic balloon occlusion is also not devoid of complications, some of which we list in Table 58.4. The overall complication rate of this procedure falls within the range of 3% to 16%,[52,56] although this rate is difficult to estimate. Complications likely occur due to operator-dependent

Table 58.5 Statistically Significant Predictive Factors of Embolization Failure in Postpartum Hemorrhage

Factor	Source(s) of Evidence (N)
PPH etiology	
Placenta accreta	Poujade et al.[78]
PPH severity	
High transfusion requirement	Sentilhes et al.[76] (117), Poujade et al.[78] (98), Lee et al.[31] (251)
Massive blood loss	Sentilhes et al.[76] (117), Choi et al.[27] (40), Touboul et al.[37] (102)
Anatomical factors	
Embolization of non-UA	Choi et al.[27] (40)
Uterine arterial vasculature variant	Bros et al.[82] (12)
Gynecologic factors	
Primiparity	Bros et al.[82] (12)
Laboratory abnormalities	
Hemoglobin	Poujade et al.[78] (98)
Prothrombin	Poujade et al.[78] (98)
Fibrinogen	Poujade et al.[78] (98)
Other factors	
Cesarean section	Choi et al.[27] (40), Touboul et al.[37] (102)
Coagulation disorders	Bros et al.[82] (12)
DIC	Lee et al.[31] (251), Kim et al.[77] (257)

Massive blood loss may also be reflected in hemoglobin levels.
Number of patients in each study (N) are shown in corresponding parentheses.
PPH, postpartum hemorrhage; UA, uterine artery; DIC, disseminated intravascular coagulation.

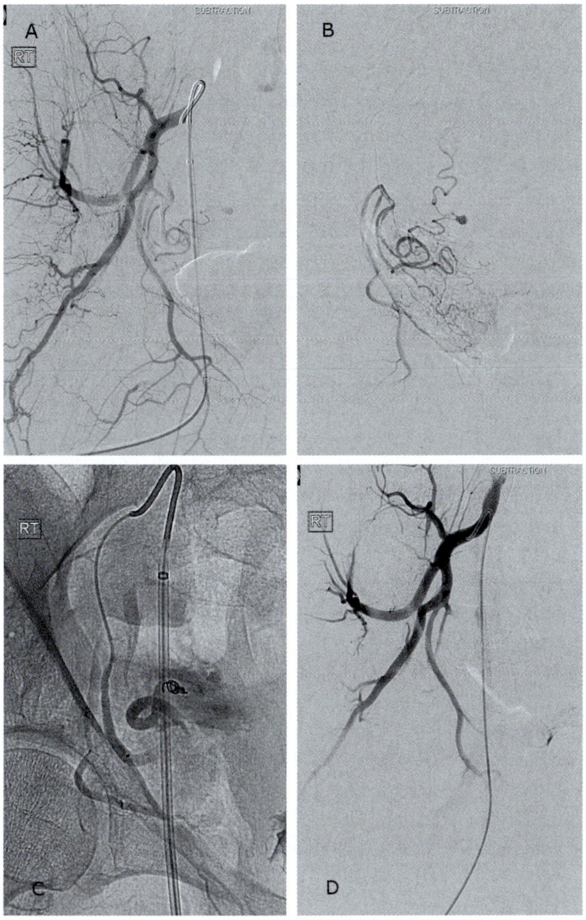

Figure 58.4 A 42-year-old female status post caesarian section and subsequent hysterectomy for persistent vaginal bleeding. Despite hysterectomy, the patient has had intermittent severe vaginal bleeding requiring blood transfusions over the course of several weeks. **A:** Initial internal iliac angiography demonstrates late filling of a small pseudoaneurysm of the right uterine artery. **B:** Right uterine artery angiography confirms this finding. The supplying artery is small and tortuous. **C:** Angiography following superselective particle and coil embolization demonstrates stasis in the uterine artery. **D:** Postembolization internal iliac angiography confirms occlusion of the pseudoaneurysm and maintenance of flow in nontarget branches. Following the procedure, bleeding did not recur.

factors, such as experience, technique, number of attempts, and procedure duration,[45,56] but this also is difficult to assess. Arterial thrombosis is one of the most common and serious complications, reported in three of the cohort studies we summarized earlier.[52,53,56] Two earlier case reports also described women with abnormal placentation who underwent prophylactic balloon placement and subsequently experienced iliac and popliteal artery thrombosis with limb ischemia, both of which resolved after surgical thrombectomy.[83,84] Carnevale et al.[53] attributed femoral and external iliac arterial thromboses in 2 of their 21 patients to extended surgical time.[53] Most other complications of balloon occlusion relate to the placement of the catheters and occurs in 6% to 16% of cases.[45] Catheter site hematomas[52,54,56] and arterial dissection[56] have, for instance, been reported. Other such complications include pseudoaneurysms, air embolization from lines, and hypotension[45] (Fig. 58.4).

Radiation Exposure

An important safety concern for patients undergoing arterial embolization in the context of PPH is radiation exposure. Unlike the case of embolization for fibroids, the fetus is also exposed to radiation during interventional management of PPH. Although the teratogenic and carcinogenic effects of radiation from interventional procedures are not entirely clear, it is recognized that pregnant women should be exposed to as little radiation as possible.[7] General guidelines including fluoroscopy time, shielding, magnification, table position, beam geometry, and others exist for an interventional radiology suite to minimize radiation to a pregnant patient; these are feasible particularly when practiced by an experienced radiologist.[85] Andrews and Brown[86] studied uterine artery embolization in over 30 patients performed by one interventional radiologist at a single institution and found that careful technique led to a reduction from 77.8 to 11.3 mSv of radiation. This amount of ionizing radiation, they concluded, is analogous to that of diagnostic imaging studies. Radiation below 50 mSv has indeed not been associated with any harm to the fetus.[87]

RARE CAUSES OF POSTPARTUM HEMORRHAGE TREATED BY EMBOLIZATION

As discussed earlier, PPH can have various causes, the most common of which is uterine atony. There are uncommon, albeit important, causes of PPH that particularly illustrate the value of arterial embolization. Rupture of pseudoaneurysms is one such rare cause. Cases of pseudoaneurysms have been sporadically reported in several mixed cohorts of PPH,[28,88] which reported treatment with embolization. Soyer et al.[89] specifically studied seven cases of ruptured pseudoaneurysms in uterine and vaginal arteries, which they also managed successfully with arterial embolization. Importantly in these cases, angiography with anatomical expertise can help in both diagnosis and treatment, whereas uterine artery ligation and hysterectomy can actually fail to stop bleeding.[89] The authors mostly used gelatin sponge for their embolization, which they argued was efficient in ruptured pseudoaneurysms and less costly than coils. Ganguli et al.,[30] however, used metal coils in their cases of pseudoaneurysms, which they also found to be effective. An extension of the study by Soyer et al. analyzed 588 patients with PPH and found the incidence of pseudoaneurysms to be nearly 3%.[90] All 18 patients with pseudoaneurysms in their retrospective study were treated with embolization, only 1 of whom required reembolization. Like the Soyer et al. study, they reported that metal coils provide no additional benefit to gelatin sponge in these cases. Pseudoaneurysms should be suspected when there is delayed hemorrhage after cesarean section.[30,89] Absence of uterine atony, lack of response to prostaglandin analogues, and refractory vaginal tears also point to likely pseudoaneurysms.[89,91] In these cases, Soyer et al.[89] argued arterial embolization should be the treatment of choice.

Arteriovenous fistulas represent another rare cause of major PPH, which may often be concealed. As in the case of pseudoaneurysms, angiography can help not only in diagnosis but also in treatment. A CT angiogram can also be highly sensitive and specific in these cases. Po et al.[92] reported a case of occult PPH, where angiography revealed a traumatic vaginal arteriovenous fistula. Embolization with gelatin pledgets and microcoils in the pudendal artery led to control of bleeding without any complications. A case of arteriovenous malformation as a cause of secondary PPH was reported by Kelly et al.,[93] where ultrasound was used to make the diagnosis and unilateral embolization of the uterine artery stopped the bleeding, with no complications other than transient fever and discomfort.[93] Pelage et al.[34] also diagnosed one of the patients in their cohort to have an arteriovenous fistula, who successfully underwent unilateral embolization of the uterine artery.

TIPS AND TRICKS

- Have a low threshold for requesting anesthesiologist assistance in patients with severe PPH.
- The Roberts Uterine Catheter (RUC) (Cook Medical, Bloomington, Indiana) allows rapid selection of the internal iliac arteries and uterine arteries.
- Achieve a catheter position in the distal uterine artery, often in the horizontal portion, to avoid non-target embolization.
- Gelfoam pledgets and/or slurry and calibrated particles of medium to large size (e.g., trisacryl gelatin microspheres 700–900 μm) enable rapid and effective uterine artery embolization.
- Avoid very small particles (e.g., Gelfoam powder or small microspheres) to reduce risk of uterine necrosis.
- When microcatheterization is needed, use a high-flow microcatheter to allow high flow rate injections and use of large particles and Gelfoam.
- Both uterine arteries should usually be embolized to stasis in cases of severe PPH, even when no definite extravasation is detected on angiography.
- In case of recurrent or continued bleeding after initial internal iliac or uterine artery embolization, ovarian angiography and complete iliac angiography should be performed, with provisional embolization.
- Over-the-wire Fogarty balloons (Edwards Lifesciences, Irvine, California) or compliant angioplasty balloons can be used for balloon occlusion. Use low-pressure inflation and minimal oversizing to prevent arterial damage.

CONCLUSION

Refractory PPH requires a multidisciplinary approach. Interventional techniques for preventing and treating PPH, including balloon occlusion and arterial embolization, are associated with high likelihood of success and a low rate of major complications. Although the data supporting their use remain sparse, these techniques are likely underused.

REFERENCES

1. Oyelese Y, Ananth CV. Postpartum hemorrhage: epidemiology, risk factors, and causes. *Clin Obstet Gynecol.* 2010;53(1):147–156.
2. Lee NK, Kim S, Lee JW, et al. Postpartum hemorrhage: clinical and radiologic aspects. *Eur J Radiol.* 2010;74(1):50–59.
3. Winograd RH. Uterine artery embolization for postpartum hemorrhage. *Best Pract Res Clin Obstet Gynaecol.* 2008;22(6): 1119–1132.
4. Sheiner E, Sarid L, Levy A, et al. Obstetric risk factors and outcome of pregnancies complicated with early postpartum hemorrhage: a population-based study. *J Matern Fetal Neonatal Med.* 2005;18(3):149–154.
5. Wetta LA, Szychowski JM, Seals S, et al. Risk factors for uterine atony/postpartum hemorrhage requiring treatment after vaginal delivery. *Am J Obstet Gynecol.* 2013;209:51.e1–51.e6.
6. Poggi SB. Postpartum hemorrhage & the abnormal puerperium. In: DeCherney AH, Nathan L, Laufer N, et al, eds. *Current Diagnosis & Treatment: Obstetrics & Gynecology.* 11th ed. New York, NY: McGraw-Hill; 2013:349–368.
7. Thabet A, Kalva SP, Liu B, et al. Interventional radiology in pregnancy complications: indications, technique, and methods for minimizing radiation exposure. *Radiographics.* 2012;32(1):255–274.
8. Neill A, Thornton S. Secondary postpartum haemorrhage. *J Obstet Gynaecol.* 2002;22(2):119–122.
9. Bakri YN, Amri A, Abdul Jabbar F. Tamponade-balloon for obstetrical bleeding. *Int J Gynaecol Obstet.* 2001;74(2):139–142.
10. Gronvall M, Tikkanen M, Tallberg E, et al. Use of Bakri balloon tamponade in the treatment of postpartum hemorrhage: a series of 50 cases from a tertiary teaching hospital. *Acta Obstet Gynecol Scand.* 2013;92(4):433–438.
11. Vitthala S, Tsoumpou I, Anjum ZK, et al. Use of Bakri balloon in post-partum haemorrhage: a series of 15 cases. *Aust N Z J Obstet Gynaecol.* 2009;49(2):191–194.
12. Brown BJ, Heaston DK, Poulson AM, et al. Uncontrollable postpartum bleeding: a new approach to hemostasis through angiographic arterial embolization. *Obstet Gynecol.* 1979;54(3): 361–365.
13. Pais SO, Glickman M, Schwartz P, et al. Embolization of pelvic arteries for control of postpartum hemorrhage. *Obstet Gynecol.* 1980;55(6):754–758.
14. Veille J-C, Siskin, GP. Applications of pelvic embolization beyond uterine fibroid embolization. In: Siskin GP, ed. *Interventional Radiology in Women's Health.* New York, NY: Thieme; 2009:77–89.
15. Pelage JP, Le Dref O, Soyer P, et al. Arterial anatomy of the female genital tract: variations and relevance to transcatheter embolization of the uterus. *AJR Am J Roentgenol.* 1999;172(4): 989–994.

16. Oei PL, Chua S, Tan L, et al. Arterial embolization for bleeding following hysterectomy for intractable postpartum hemorrhage. *Int J Gynaecol Obstet*. 1998;62(1):83–86.
17. Maassen MS, Lambers MD, Tutein Nolthenius RP, et al. Complications and failure of uterine artery embolisation for intractable postpartum haemorrhage. *BJOG*. 2009;116(1):55–61.
18. Corr P. Arterial embolization for haemorrhage in the obstetric patient. *Best Pract Res Clin Obstet Gynaecol*. 2001;15(4):557–561.
19. Cottier JP, Fignon A, Tranquart F, et al. Uterine necrosis after arterial embolization for postpartum hemorrhage. *Obstet Gynecol*. 2002;100(5, pt 2):1074–1077.
20. Coulange L, Butori N, Loffroy R, et al. Uterine necrosis following selective embolization for postpartum hemorrhage using absorbable material. *Acta Obstet Gynecol Scand*. 2009;88(2):238–240.
21. Vedantham S, Goodwin SC, McLucas B, et al. Uterine artery embolization: an underused method of controlling pelvic hemorrhage. *Am J Obstet Gynecol*. 1997;176(4):938–948.
22. Lee JS, Shepherd SM. Endovascular treatment of postpartum hemorrhage. *Clin Obstet Gynecol*. 2010;53(1):209–218.
23. Kirby JM, Kachura JR, Rajan DK, et al. Arterial embolization for primary postpartum hemorrhage. *J Vasc Interv Radiol*. 2009;20(8):1036–1045.
24. Kanematsu M, Watanabe H, Kondo H, et al. Postpartum hemorrhage in coagulopathic patients: preliminary experience with uterine arterial embolization with N-butyl cyanoacrylate. *J Vasc Interv Radiol*. 2011;22(12):1773–1776.
25. Boulleret C, Chahid T, Gallot D, et al. Hypogastric arterial selective and superselective embolization for severe postpartum hemorrhage: a retrospective review of 36 cases. *Cardiovasc Intervent Radiol*. 2004;27(4):344–348.
26. Chauleur C, Fanget C, Tourne G, et al. Serious primary post-partum hemorrhage, arterial embolization and future fertility: a retrospective study of 46 cases. *Hum Reprod*. 2008;23(7):1553–1559.
27. Choi YH, Baba Y, Ikeda S, et al. Efficacy of uterine artery embolization for patients with postpartum hemorrhage. *OJRad*. 2013;3:51–55.
28. Deux JF, Bazot M, Le Blanche AF, et al. Is selective embolization of uterine arteries a safe alternative to hysterectomy in patients with postpartum hemorrhage? *AJR Am J Roentgenol*. 2001;177(1):145–149.
29. Eriksson LG, Mulic-Lutvica A, Jangland L, et al. Massive postpartum hemorrhage treated with transcatheter arterial embolization: technical aspects and long-term effects on fertility and menstrual cycle. *Acta Radiol*. 2007;48(6):635–642.
30. Ganguli S, Stecker MS, Pyne D, et al. Uterine artery embolization in the treatment of postpartum uterine hemorrhage. *J Vasc Interv Radiol*. 2011;22(2):169–176.
31. Lee HY, Shin JH, Kim J, et al. Primary postpartum hemorrhage: outcome of pelvic arterial embolization in 251 patients at a single institution. *Radiology*. 2012;264(3):903–909.
32. Ojala K, Perala J, Kariniemi J, et al. Arterial embolization and prophylactic catheterization for the treatment for severe obstetric hemorrhage*. *Acta Obstet Gynecol Scand*. 2005;84(11):1075–1080.
33. Ornan D, White R, Pollak J, et al. Pelvic embolization for intractable postpartum hemorrhage: long-term follow-up and implications for fertility. *Obstet Gynecol*. 2003;102(5, pt 1):904–910.
34. Pelage JP, Le Dref O, Jacob D, et al. Selective arterial embolization of the uterine arteries in the management of intractable post-partum hemorrhage. *Acta Obstet Gynecol Scand*. 1999;78(8):698–703.
35. Pelage JP, Le Dref O, Mateo J, et al. Life-threatening primary postpartum hemorrhage: treatment with emergency selective arterial embolization. *Radiology*. 1998;208(2):359–362.
36. Soncini E, Pelicelli A, Larini P, et al. Uterine artery embolization in the treatment and prevention of postpartum hemorrhage. *Int J Gynaecol Obstet*. 2007;96(3):181–185.
37. Touboul C, Badiou W, Saada J, et al. Efficacy of selective arterial embolisation for the treatment of life-threatening post-partum haemorrhage in a large population. *PLoS One*. 2008;3(11):e3819.
38. Vegas G, Illescas T, Munoz M, et al. Selective pelvic arterial embolization in the management of obstetric hemorrhage. *Eur J Obstet Gynecol Reprod Biol*. 2006;127(1):68–72.
39. Doumouchtsis SK, Papageorghiou AT, Arulkumaran S. Systematic review of conservative management of postpartum hemorrhage: what to do when medical treatment fails. *Obstet Gynecol Surv*. 2007;62(8):540–547.
40. Collins CD, Jackson JE. Pelvic arterial embolization following hysterectomy and bilateral internal iliac artery ligation for intractable primary post partum haemorrhage. *Clin Radiol*. 1995;50(10):710–713; discussion 713–714.
41. Bloom AI, Verstandig A, Gielchinsky Y, et al. Arterial embolisation for persistent primary postpartum haemorrhage: before or after hysterectomy? *BJOG*. 2004;111(8):880–884.
42. American College of Obstetricians and Gynecologists. ACOG practice bulletin: clinical management guidelines for obstetrician-gynecologists number 76, October 2006: postpartum hemorrhage. *Obstet Gynecol*. 2006;108(4):1039–1047.
43. Oyelese Y, Smulian JC. Placenta previa, placenta accreta, and vasa previa. *Obstet Gynecol*. 2006;107(4):927–941.
44. Hansch E, Chitkara U, McAlpine J, et al. Pelvic arterial embolization for control of obstetric hemorrhage: a five-year experience. *Am J Obstet Gynecol*. 1999;180(6, pt 1):1454–1460.
45. Dilauro MD, Dason S, Athreya S. Prophylactic balloon occlusion of internal iliac arteries in women with placenta accreta: literature review and analysis. *Clin Radiol*. 2012;67(6):515–520.
46. Baughman WC, Corteville JE, Shah RR. Placenta accreta: spectrum of US and MR imaging findings. *Radiographics*. 2008;28(7):1905–1916.
47. Alvarez M, Lockwood CJ, Ghidini A, et al. Prophylactic and emergent arterial catheterization for selective embolization in obstetric hemorrhage. *Am J Perinatol*. 1992;9(5–6):441–444.
48. Yu PC, Ou HY, Tsang LL, et al. Prophylactic intraoperative uterine artery embolization to control hemorrhage in abnormal placentation during late gestation. *Fertil Steril*. 2009;91(5):1951–1955.
49. Soyer P, Morel O, Fargeaudou Y, et al. Value of pelvic embolization in the management of severe postpartum hemorrhage due to placenta accreta, increta or percreta. *Eur J Radiol*. 2011;80(3):729–735.
50. Diop AN, Chabrot P, Bertrand A, et al. Placenta accreta: management with uterine artery embolization in 17 cases. *J Vasc Interv Radiol*. 2010;21(5):644–648.
51. Dubois J, Garel L, Grignon A, et al. Placenta percreta: balloon occlusion and embolization of the internal iliac arteries to reduce intraoperative blood losses. *Am J Obstet Gynecol*. 1997;176(3):723–726.

52. Ballas J, Hull AD, Saenz C, et al. Preoperative intravascular balloon catheters and surgical outcomes in pregnancies complicated by placenta accreta: a management paradox. *Am J Obstet Gynecol.* 2012;207(3):216.e1–216.e5.
53. Carnevale FC, Kondo MM, de Oliveira Sousa W Jr, et al. Perioperative temporary occlusion of the internal iliac arteries as prophylaxis in cesarean section at risk of hemorrhage in placenta accreta. *Cardiovasc Intervent Radiol.* 2011;34(4):758–764.
54. Sadashivaiah J, Wilson R, Thein A, et al. Role of prophylactic uterine artery balloon catheters in the management of women with suspected placenta accreta. *Int J Obstet Anesth.* 2011;20(4):282–287.
55. Tan CH, Tay KH, Sheah K, et al. Perioperative endovascular internal iliac artery occlusion balloon placement in management of placenta accreta. *AJR Am J Roentgenol.* 2007;189(5):1158–1163.
56. Shrivastava V, Nageotte M, Major C, et al. Case-control comparison of cesarean hysterectomy with and without prophylactic placement of intravascular balloon catheters for placenta accreta. *Am J Obstet Gynecol.* 2007;197(4):402.e1–402.e5.
57. Levine AB, Kuhlman K, Bonn J. Placenta accreta: comparison of cases managed with and without pelvic artery balloon catheters. *J Matern Fetal Med.* 1999;8(4):173–176.
58. Bodner LJ, Nosher JL, Gribbin C, et al. Balloon-assisted occlusion of the internal iliac arteries in patients with placenta accreta/percreta. *Cardiovasc Intervent Radiol.* 2006;29(3):354–361.
59. Sivan E, Spira M, Achiron R, et al. Prophylactic pelvic artery catheterization and embolization in women with placenta accreta: can it prevent cesarean hysterectomy? *Am J Perinatol.* 2010;27(6):455–461.
60. Shih JC, Liu KL, Shyu MK. Temporary balloon occlusion of the common iliac artery: new approach to bleeding control during cesarean hysterectomy for placenta percreta. *Am J Obstet Gynecol.* 2005;193(5):1756–1758.
61. Bell-Thomas SM, Penketh RJ, Lord RH, et al. Emergency use of a transfemoral aortic occlusion catheter to control massive haemorrhage at caesarean hysterectomy. *BJOG.* 2003;110(12):1120–1122.
62. Masamoto H, Uehara H, Gibo M, et al. Elective use of aortic balloon occlusion in cesarean hysterectomy for placenta previa percreta. *Gynecol Obstet Invest.* 2009;67(2):92–95.
63. Paull JD, Smith J, Williams L, et al. Balloon occlusion of the abdominal aorta during caesarean hysterectomy for placenta percreta. *Anaesth Intensive Care.* 1995;23(6):731–734.
64. Clausen C, Stensballe J, Albrechtsen CK, et al. Balloon occlusion of the internal iliac arteries in the multidisciplinary management of placenta percreta. *Acta Obstet Gynecol Scand.* 2013;92(4):386–391.
65. Royal College of Obstetricians and Gynaecologists, Royal College of Radiologists, British Society of Interventional Radiology. The role of emergency and elective interventional radiology in postpartum haemorrhage. http://www.rcog.org.uk/files/rcog-corp/uploaded-files/GoodPractice6RoleEmergency2007.pdf. Accessed date was 08/12/2013 .
66. Greenwood LH, Glickman MG, Schwartz PE, et al. Obstetric and nonmalignant gynecologic bleeding: treatment with angiographic embolization. *Radiology.* 1987;164(1):155–159.
67. Hong TM, Tseng HS, Lee RC, et al. Uterine artery embolization: an effective treatment for intractable obstetric haemorrhage. *Clin Radiol.* 2004;59(1):96–101.
68. Wang H, Garmel S. Successful term pregnancy after bilateral uterine artery embolization for postpartum hemorrhage. *Obstet Gynecol.* 2003;102(3):603–604.
69. Salomon LJ, deTayrac R, Castaigne-Meary V, et al. Fertility and pregnancy outcome following pelvic arterial embolization for severe post-partum haemorrhage. A cohort study. *Hum Reprod.* 2003;18(4):849–852.
70. Fiori O, Deux JF, Kambale JC, et al. Impact of pelvic arterial embolization for intractable postpartum hemorrhage on fertility. *Am J Obstet Gynecol.* 2009;200(4):384.e1–384.e4.
71. Descargues G, Mauger Tinlot F, Douvrin F, et al. Menses, fertility and pregnancy after arterial embolization for the control of postpartum haemorrhage. *Hum Reprod.* 2004;19(2):339–343.
72. Gaia G, Chabrot P, Cassagnes L, et al. Menses recovery and fertility after artery embolization for PPH: a single-center retrospective observational study. *Eur Radiol.* 2009;19(2):481–487.
73. Delotte J, Novellas S, Koh C, et al. Obstetrical prognosis and pregnancy outcome following pelvic arterial embolisation for post-partum hemorrhage. *Eur J Obstet Gynecol Reprod Biol.* 2009;145(2):129–132.
74. Hunter LA. Exploring the role of uterine artery embolization in the management of postpartum hemorrhage. *J Perinat Neonatal Nurs.* 2010;24(3):207–214.
75. Pellerin O, Bats AS, Di Primio M, et al. Postpartum hemorrhage treated with gelfoam slurry embolization using the superselective technique: immediate results and 1-month MRI follow-up. *Cardiovasc Intervent Radiol.* 2013;36(1):98–104.
76. Sentilhes L, Gromez A, Clavier E, et al. Predictors of failed pelvic arterial embolization for severe postpartum hemorrhage. *Obstet Gynecol.* 2009;113(5):992–999.
77. Kim YJ, Yoon CJ, Seong NJ, et al. Failed pelvic arterial embolization for postpartum hemorrhage: clinical outcomes and predictive factors. *J Vasc Interv Radiol.* 2013;24(5):703–709.
78. Poujade O, Zappa M, Letendre I, et al. Predictive factors for failure of pelvic arterial embolization for postpartum hemorrhage. *Int J Gynaecol Obstet.* 2012;117(2):119–123.
79. Chou YJ, Cheng YF, Shen CC, et al. Failure of uterine arterial embolization: placenta accreta with profuse postpartum hemorrhage. *Acta Obstet Gynecol Scand.* 2004;83(7):688–690.
80. Descargues G, Douvrin F, Degre S, et al. Abnormal placentation and selective embolization of the uterine arteries. *Eur J Obstet Gynecol Reprod Biol.* 2001;99(1):47–52.
81. Alanis M, Hurst BS, Marshburn PB, et al. Conservative management of placenta increta with selective arterial embolization preserves future fertility and results in a favorable outcome in subsequent pregnancies. *Fertil Steril.* 2006;86(5):1514.e3–1514.e7.
82. Bros S, Chabrot P, Kastler A, et al. Recurrent bleeding within 24 hours after uterine artery embolization for severe postpartum hemorrhage: are there predictive factors? *Cardiovasc Intervent Radiol.* 2012;35(3):508–514.
83. Greenberg JI, Suliman A, Iranpour P, et al. Prophylactic balloon occlusion of the internal iliac arteries to treat abnormal placentation: a cautionary case. *Am J Obstet Gynecol.* 2007;197(5):470.e1–470.e4.
84. Sewell MF, Rosenblum D, Ehrenberg H. Arterial embolus during common iliac balloon catheterization at cesarean hysterectomy. *Obstet Gynecol.* 2006;108(3, pt 2):746–748.
85. Marx MV. Interventional radiology: management of the pregnant patient. *Tech Vasc Interv Radiol.* 2010;13(3):154–157.

86. Andrews RT, Brown PH. Uterine arterial embolization: factors influencing patient radiation exposure. *Radiology*. 2000; 217(3):713–722.
87. ACOG Committee on Obstetric Practice. ACOG Committee Opinion. Number 299, September 2004 (replaces No. 158, September 1995). Guidelines for diagnostic imaging during pregnancy. *Obstet Gynecol*. 2004;104(3):647–651.
88. Pelage JP, Soyer P, Repiquet D, et al. Secondary postpartum hemorrhage: treatment with selective arterial embolization. *Radiology*. 1999;212(2):385–389.
89. Soyer P, Fargeaudou Y, Morel O, et al. Severe postpartum haemorrhage from ruptured pseudoaneurysm: successful treatment with transcatheter arterial embolization. *Eur Radiol*. 2008;18(6):1181–1187.
90. Dohan A, Soyer P, Subhani A, et al. Postpartum hemorrhage resulting from pelvic pseudoaneurysm: a retrospective analysis of 588 consecutive cases treated by arterial embolization. *Cardiovasc Intervent Radiol*. 2013;36:1247–1255.
91. Nagayama C, Gibo M, Nitta H, et al. Rupture of pseudoaneurysm after vaginal delivery successfully treated by selective arterial embolization. *Arch Gynecol Obstet*. 2011;283(1): 37–40.
92. Po LK, Simons ME, Levinsky ES. Concealed postpartum hemorrhage treated with transcatheter arterial embolization. *Obstet Gynecol*. 2012;120(2, pt 2):461–464.
93. Kelly SM, Belli AM, Campbell S. Arteriovenous malformation of the uterus associated with secondary postpartum hemorrhage. *Ultrasound Obstet Gynecol*. 2003;21(6):602–605.

59

Pelvic Congestion Syndrome

Howard Richard

Pelvic pain can be divided into acute pain, recurrent pelvic pain, and chronic pelvic pain. Acute pain rarely lasts more than 1 month. It typically resolves of its own accord. Recurrent pain is pain that occurs on a regular basis such as the cyclic pain of dysmenorrhea or the episodic pain of dyspareunia. Chronic pelvic pain is defined as pain located primarily in the pelvis that lasts more than 3 to 6 months.[1–3] There are many different causes of chronic pelvic pain, and textbooks have been written delineating the differential diagnosis. It is important to note that although chronic pelvic pain often originates with a biologic underpinning, patients will develop psychological and sociologic components with the passage of time.[4] The psychological aspects such as depression and sociologic aspects such as interpersonal relationship dysfunction should be considered in the management of these problems.

Chronic pelvic pain can be attributed to gynecologic, uterine or extrauterine, urologic, gastrointestinal, musculoskeletal, or multiple causes. With the discussion of chronic pain based on pelvic venous congestion, we are chiefly concerned about extrauterine gynecologic pain. Richet[5] first described pelvic venous varicosities in 1857. Grossly dilated or varicose veins with marked venous incompetence can be noted in women, particularly following pregnancy. Taylor[6] reported a connection between the varicosities and pelvic pain in 1949. These varices can extend to the perineal tissues and even to the buttocks and the upper legs.[7,8] Dilated ovarian intrauterine vascular plexus can be identified at laparoscopy (Fig. 59.1). This can be challenging secondary to the positive pressure used in laparoscopy. In fact, up to 90% of patients with negative laparoscopy potentially have pelvic congestion syndrome (PCS).[9]

The clinical features of PCS consist of a deep-seated pelvic pain, classically seen in multiparous women. The pain worsens with prolonged standing or walking and classically improves when in a recumbent position. The patients can have a congestive dysmenorrhea with symptoms worsening before menses. Patients can suffer deep dyspareunia with a postcoital ache, which may last for several days.[10,11] This can be accompanied by emotional disturbance such as depression and sociologic turmoil in the patient's interpersonal relationships.

The clinical signs of PCS include external varices involving the external genitalia and superficial vulvar and perivulvar tissue (Fig. 59.2).[12,13] Patients may have pain to palpation over the ovarian point, which is two-thirds of the distance from the anterior superior iliac spine to the umbilicus. When evaluating the cervix in these patients, there may be excess clear mucoid discharge. The cervix may be blue secondary to venous engorgement. On bimanual examination, cervical motion tenderness may be found.[10,14]

Ovarian vein anatomy contributes to the pathogenesis of PCS. In normal patients, ovarian venous return is aided by spontaneous contractility. In some women, the ovarian vein smooth muscle undergoes age-related thinning.[15] When this is associated with an increase in venous diameter during pregnancy, the valves are no longer able to function properly. This can result in venous insufficiency. The vascular endothelium is known to contain estrogen receptors, which are related to the trophic response of vascular smooth muscle. In addition, nerves are identified within layers of the veins. The vascular filling and engorgement is also capable of generating pain signals in some patients by releasing pain mediators

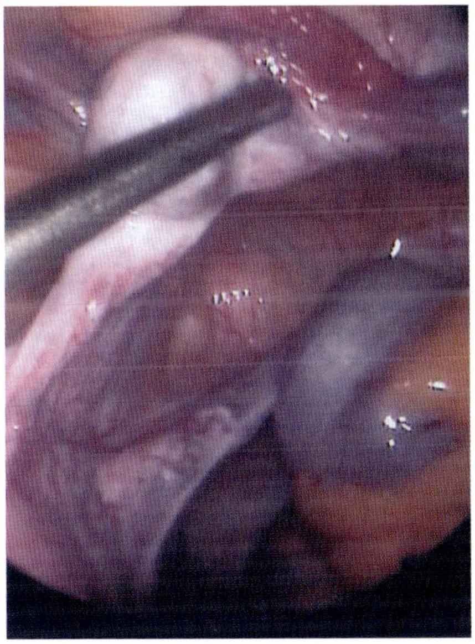

Figure 59.1 Dilated varices seen at laparoscopy.

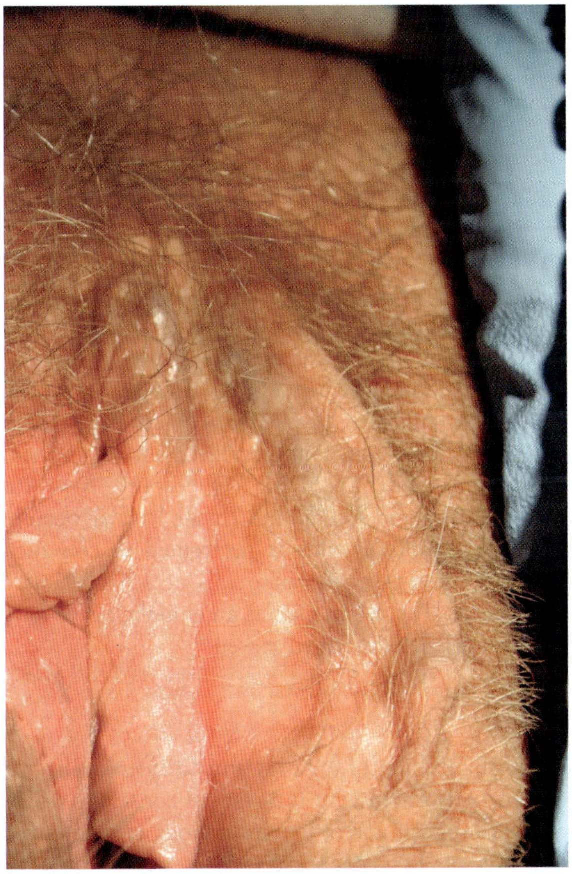

Figure 59.2 This image demonstrates labial varices.

such as substance P.[16] The internal iliac vein can also convey pressure to the periovarian and periuterine vascular plexus. These veins have valves in approximately 10% of patients, and this represents a potential pathway for reflux into the periuterine and periovarian vascular plexus in the event of valvular dysfunction.

Varicose vein development may also be related to genetic structural vein wall anomalies.[17] This can be exacerbated by hormonal and hemodynamic factors related to pregnancy. The combination of genetic predisposition and pregnancy can combine to create the environment for the formation of pelvic varicosities. These venous structures can generate pain signals upon distention in some, but not all, women. Therefore, in some patients, the combination of incompetent distended veins with the ability of the veins to generate pain signals with distention results in the syndrome of pelvic venous congestion.

In evaluating patients for the diagnosis of pelvic venous congestion, various imaging modalities have demonstrated dilated veins in asymptomatic women. Ultrasound, computed tomography (CT), and magnetic resonance imaging scans are able to clearly define dilated ovarian veins. However studies have failed to demonstrate any correlation between the presence of dilated veins and the presence of symptomatic pelvic venous congestion.[18–20] On imaging examination, patients with pelvic venous congestion can have polycystic-appearing ovaries. When evaluating patients with PCS and polycystic-appearing ovaries, patients with PCS demonstrate an increased number of a atrophic follicles consistent with follicular atresia.[21] This is a distinct difference from patients with polycystic ovary disease and normal patients. Although both patients with pelvic venous congestion and polycystic ovary disease can demonstrate elevated androstenedione content, patients with pelvic congestion demonstrated a decreased response of estradiol to follicle-stimulating hormone (FSH) as contrasted with the normal response of estradiol to FSH in patients with polycystic ovary disease and normal patients.[22,23]

Functional imaging can be performed with catheter venography. Selective catheterization and retrograde venography of the left renal vein only allows visualization of ovarian vein in patients with incompetent valves. However, in some patients, the proximal valve may be competent. Therefore, selective ovarian venography is required to allow passive reflux to extend all the way down the ovarian vein into the pelvic veins. In some patients, the reflux can extend to the perivulvar or upper lower extremity veins. Sometimes, this reflux can be seen extending into the periuterine venous plexus and then ascending in the internal iliac veins (Fig. 59.3). It is possible to perform direct transuterine venography with injection of contrast directly into the uterus (Fig. 59.4). Beard et al.[14] first described this technique in the mid-1980s. A grading schema was developed to define the abnormalities on transuterine venography, taking the following factors into account: an ovarian vein diameter greater than 8 mm, a tortuous venous plexus with flow from

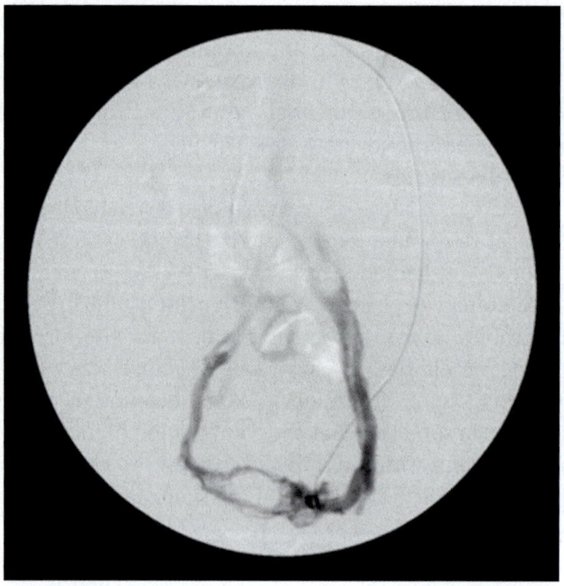

Figure 59.3 Retrograde left ovarian venogram demonstrates reflux into the periuterine venous plexus. In addition, there is drainage into the internal iliac veins.

side to side, and a delay in washout of contrast from the pelvis. The scoring system was devised in which a score of 5 or more gives a diagnostic sensitivity of 91% and specificity of 89% on the diagnosis of pelvic venous congestion syndrome.

Treatment options for pelvic venous congestion syndrome include hysterectomy and bilateral oophorectomy. This surgery is often used in patients with chronic pelvic pain because some of these patients will have a working diagnosis of adenomyosis, endometriosis, or uterine fibroids. Beard et al.[10] reported a study of 36 patients who were diagnosed with PCS and treated with hysterectomy and bilateral oophorectomy. At 1-year follow-up, 12 of the 36 patients had some residual pain, and 1 patient had no significant change in her pain. Therefore, two-thirds of the patients were cured with removal of uterus and ovaries, which can likely be attributed to ligation of the periuterine periovarian venous plexus. Unfortunately, this also shows us that one-third of the patients had persistent pain despite the surgery. Patients with persistent pelvic venous congestion after hysterectomy may benefit from transvenous embolization.

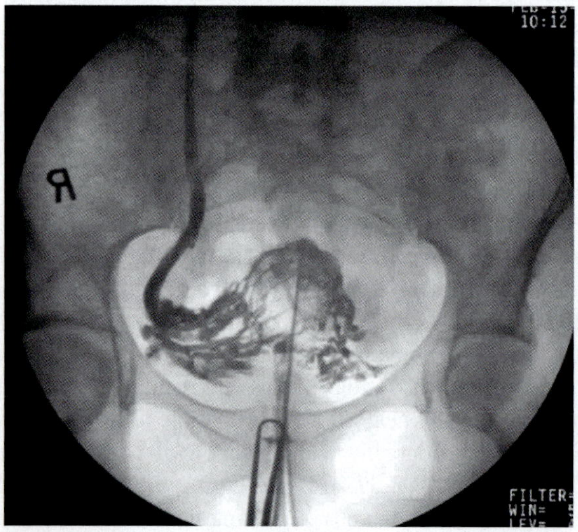

Figure 59.4 A transuterine venogram demonstrates the periuterine vascular plexus. Outflow is predominately via the left ovarian vein.

DEVICE/MATERIAL DESCRIPTION

Venous embolization for PCS can be performed via the internal jugular or femoral venous approach. When the procedure is performed via the internal jugular venous approach, a 6-Fr 55 cm straight vascular sheath is used. This allows for stable access to the inferior vena cava. The left renal vein can be catheterized with a vertebral curve or Cobra catheter (Cook Bloomington, Indiana). Both of these catheters will usually allow access to the left ovarian vein. In some cases, the sheath can be advanced into the left renal vein and a reverse curve catheter such as a Roush inferior mesentric (RIM) (Cook Bloomington, Indiana) can be used to gain access to the left ovarian vein. Catheterization of the right ovarian vein is often accomplished with either an multi purpose B (MPB) (Cook Bloomington, Indiana) curve or a Cobra catheter. Evaluation of the pelvic veins is often accomplished with a Berenstein (Cordis Bridgewater, New Jersey) or vertebral curve catheter.

When the procedure is performed via the femoral venous access, a reverse curve sheath such as the Hopkins curve sheath (Cook Bloomington, Indiana) can be used in the left renal vein. Reverse curve catheters such as Simmons-type catheters (Cook Bloomington, Indiana) can be used to gain access to the right ovarian vein.

Embolization can be performed with a sclerosant slurry. Various sclerosants have been used. Hypertonic saline mix with Gelfoam (Ethicon, Sommerville, New Jersey) slurry, Sotradecol (Angiodynamics Inc., Quensbury, New York), Sotradecol foam, and sodium morrhuate have all been used with success. Typically, this is performed in conjunction with embolization using pushable coils, detachable coils, and vascular plugs. The use of glue as an embolic agent for this indication has been described as well.[24]

TECHNIQUE

Venous embolization of the ovarian and internal iliac veins is typically performed with intravenous conscious sedation. The internal jugular and or femoral venous access routes can be employed based on operator preference. Left ovarian veins classically arise from the left renal vein (Fig. 59.5). Left renal venography can demonstrate reflux into an incompetent left ovarian vein. However, some patients will have a competent

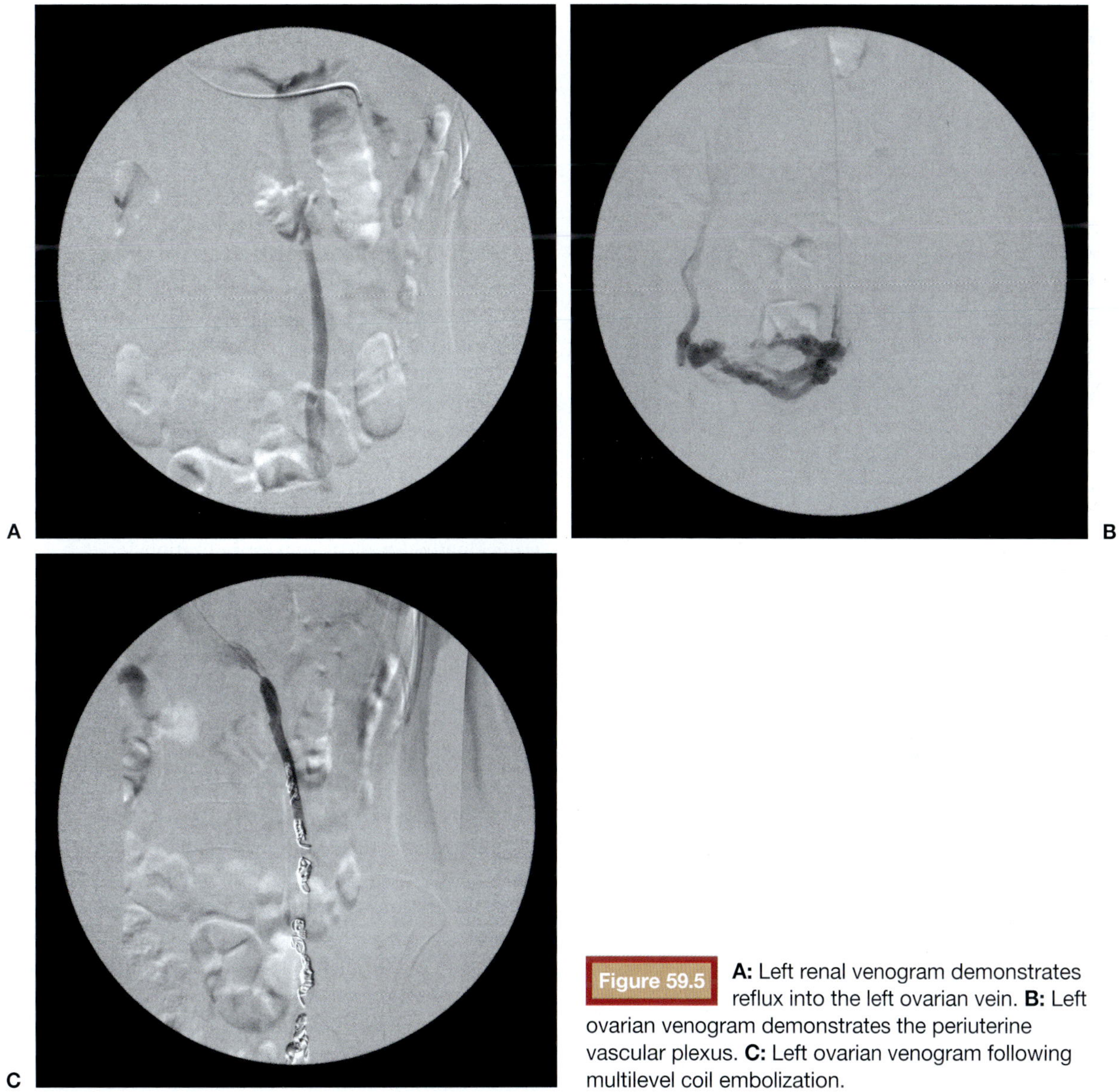

Figure 59.5 **A:** Left renal venogram demonstrates reflux into the left ovarian vein. **B:** Left ovarian venogram demonstrates the periuterine vascular plexus. **C:** Left ovarian venogram following multilevel coil embolization.

cephalad left ovarian vein valve, and in these patients, selective left ovarian venography is required to confirm the diagnosis of ovarian reflux. Following catheterization of the left ovarian vein, the catheter can be advanced into the pelvis, whereupon venography can demonstrate the periuterine and periovarian venous plexus. Marked stasis of contrast and accumulation and pooling of contrast in the pelvis is consistent with the diagnosis of pelvic venous congestion. Embolization is then performed using a combination of sclerosant slurry and coils or vascular plugs. The embolization is performed at several levels throughout the course of the ovarian vein. This is important because reflux into patent tributaries of the ovarian vein can lead to treatment failure via collateral pathways that circumvent coils placed distally in the target vein. In addition, it is not uncommon to find parallel channels and these should be selectively catheterized and embolized independently.

Catheterization of the right ovarian vein is often challenging. Classically, a right renal venogram will demonstrate a landmark for the right ovarian vein. The right ovarian vein is classically located immediately caudal to the confluence of the right renal vein and the inferior vena cava. Variant anatomy exists, and on occasion, the right ovarian vein can be identified as a branch of the right renal vein (Fig. 59.6). Alternatively, the right ovarian vein may enter the inferior vena cava caudal to the confluence of the right renal vein and the inferior vena cava (Table 59.1). Following catheterization of the right ovarian vein, catheterization and embolization is performed in a similar fashion to that of the left ovarian vein.

For most patients, performance of ovarian venography and embolization without an assessment of the internal iliac veins represents an incomplete evaluation of PCS. Selective internal iliac venography is performed to identify persistently

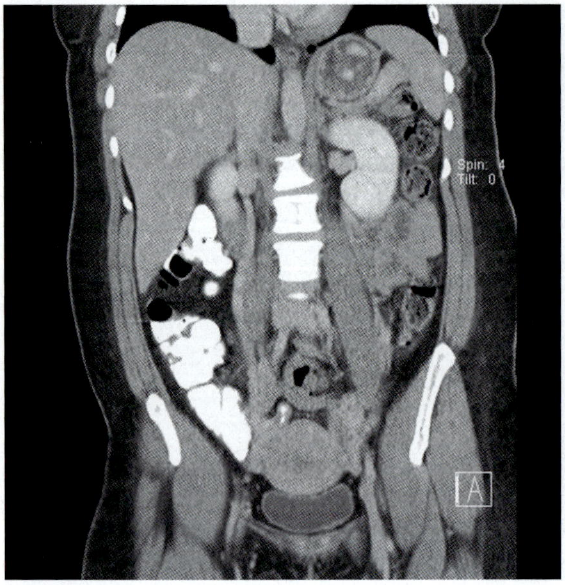

Figure 59.6 This reformatted CT image demonstrates the right ovarian vein entering the right renal vein.

abnormal periovarian and periuterine vascular plexus. Balloon occlusion venography can be helpful in challenging anatomy. Once these venous plexus are identified, they can be embolized with sclerosants alone or with sclerosants and coils. If using coils, care must be taken to ensure the coils do not migrate and/or embolize to the lungs; coils can be placed via an over-the-wire Fogarty occlusion balloon catheter (Cook Bloomington, Indiana) to minimize this risk. As outlined in an earlier chapter, introducing the leading aspect of a coil into side branches can help anchor the coil nest and minimize the risk of migration. Following embolization of the right internal iliac venous plexus, the left internal iliac venous plexus can be catheterized and embolized in a similar fashion.

CLINICAL APPLICATIONS

In patients with pelvic venous congestion, ovarian and internal iliac venous embolization can provide significant clinical relief. The first report of transcatheter embolization of the ovarian veins was described by Edwards et al. in 1993.[25] Since that time, several studies have been published demonstrating the success of embolization at addressing the pain associated with PCS. Most of the studies published to date involve performance of a unilateral or bilateral ovarian vein coil embolization without embolization of one or both internal iliac veins. These data, however, demonstrate the shortcomings of this approach. For example, Capasso et al.[26] reported on ovarian vein embolization in 19 patients (13 underwent unilateral ovarian vein embolization and 6 underwent bilateral ovarian vein embolization). After a mean of 15.4 months follow-up, significant relief was experienced in 57.9%, partial relief in 15.8%, and no relief in 26.3% of patients. Similarly, Kwon et al.[27] described their experience with ovarian vein embolization in 67 patients (unilateral embolization in 65 patients, unilateral embolization in 2 patients). They found significant relief in 82%, no relief in 15%, and worsening symptoms in the remaining 3% of patients. Other studies evaluating ovarian vein embolization for PCS have had similar findings.[28,29] Although the use of isolated ovarian vein embolization can still provide most patients with significant symptomatic improvement, the failure rate seen in these studies supports the addition of internal iliac venography and embolization to a treatment protocol. Interestingly, Gandini et al.[30] reported their experience with bilateral ovarian vein embolization using a sclerosant in 38 patients and found significant relief in 100% of patients after a mean follow-up period of 12 months.[30]

In general, the addition of internal iliac venography and embolization as well as the addition of sclerosants to the embolization technique has improved the results of this procedure. Venbrux et al.[31] described their experience in 56 patients, with all patients undergoing bilateral ovarian vein embolization and 43 patients undergoing internal iliac vein embolization. Procedures in this study were performed with coils and a sclerosant. After a mean follow-up period of 22.1 months, significant or partial relief was seen in 96% of patients, whereas 4% of patients experienced no improvement in their symptoms. Similarly, Kim et al.[32] reported their experience with 127 patients (106 undergoing bilateral ovarian vein embolization, 20 undergoing unilateral ovarian vein embolization, and 108 undergoing internal iliac vein embolization) treated with coils and sclerosants.[32] They found significant relief in 85%, no relief in 12%, and worsening symptoms in 3% of their patients after a mean follow-up of 45 months. In 2013, Laborda et al.[33] published the largest study evaluating ovarian and internal iliac vein embolization for PCS. There were 202 patients with chronic pelvic pain who were treated with coil embolization, leading to clinical success in 93.9% of patients after 5 years (179 patients completed the 5-year follow-up period); 33.5% of patients reported complete disappearance of their symptoms after embolization.[33]

Chung and Huh[34] published a randomized study supporting the use of embolization in the treatment of PCS in 2003. They evaluated 106 patients with PCS and pelvic

Table 59.1 Ovarian Vein Locations

Vein Confluence	Expected Location	Alternate Location
Left ovarian	Left renal vein	IVC Left renal vein branch Circumaortic left renal vein
Right ovarian	IVC and right renal vein confluence	Right renal vein branch Caudal IVC Right renal vein

IVC, inferior vena cava.

pain who were initially treated unsuccessfully with medroxyprogesterone. These patients were randomly assigned to three treatment groups: ovarian vein embolization with coils (n = 52), hysterectomy with bilateral salpingo-oophorectomy and hormone replacement therapy (n = 27), and hysterectomy with a unilateral salpingo-oophorectomy on the affected side (n = 27). All patients underwent venography before treatment to confirm the diagnosis of PCS. Based on the use of a visual analog scale to assess pain, embolization was significantly more effective at reducing pelvic pain compared to the other methods of treatment.

POTENTIAL COMPLICATIONS

Complications include access site injury such as a hematoma. This can manifest as pain at the catheter insertion site. As this is a venous procedure, these are typically self-limited. Nontarget embolization is always a concern, particularly with coil embolization. Migration of coils into the heart and pulmonary circulation has been reported.[31,35] This can be minimized by either (1) not using coils in the internal iliac veins or (2) only placing coils into the internal iliac veins following ipsilateral ovarian vein embolization and behind an over-the-wire Fogarty balloon occlusion catheter to allow for safe controlled formation of a stable coil mass. Cardiac arrhythmias have also been reported after this embolization for PCS.[36] Future fertility remains a question after embolization for PCS. However, Kim et al.[32] reported that there were no significant changes in FSH, luteinizing hormone, or estradiol levels. In addition, they reported a 50% pregnancy rate in premenopausal women undergoing this procedure.

TIPS AND TRICKS

- Counsel patients that they should not expect improvement until 2–6 wk after the procedure.
- Counsel patients that they may set off airport metal detectors because of the embolization coils. Tell them to simply state that they have an implanted medical device.
- Start with a left ovarian vein. When performing the left ovarian venogram, image the reflux through the right ovarian vein to identify the right ovarian vein origin from the inferior vena cava.
- Balloon occlusion venography can demonstrate reflux into the periuterine venous plexus and facilitate catheterization.
- If you only embolize the ovarian veins, you may have patients experience an early relapse; these patients should be brought back to have the internal iliac veins embolized.
- In patients with PCS and hematuria, consider the nutcracker syndrome and measure a pressure gradient across the left renal vein.

SUMMARY

Ovarian and internal iliac vein embolization has been shown to be an effective treatment for the symptoms associated with PCS. Although prospective randomized trials comparing embolization with medical and/or surgical therapy need to be performed to gain a more comprehensive understanding of this procedure, available data suggest that this is a safe and effective minimally invasive treatment option for these patients.

REFERENCES

1. Santosh A, Liaquat HB, Fatima N, et al. Chronic pelvic pain: a dilemma. *J Pak Med Assoc.* 2010;60:257–260.
2. Freedman J, Ganeshan A, Crowe PM. Pelvic congestion syndrome: the role of interventional radiology in the treatment of chronic pelvic pain. *Postgrad Med J.* 2010;86:704–710.
3. Black CM, Thorpe K, Venbrux A, et al. Research reporting standards for endovascular treatment of pelvic venous insufficiency. *J Vasc Interv Radiol.* 2010;21:796–803.
4. Farquhar CM, Rogers V, Franks S, et al. A randomized controlled trial of medroxyprogesterone acetate and psychotherapy for the treatment of pelvic congestion. *Br J Obstet Gynaecol.* 1989;96(10):1153–1162.
5. Richet MA. *Traite Pratique d'Anatomie Medico-Chirurgicale.* Paris, France: Chamerot Libraire Editeur; 1857.
6. Taylor HC. Vascular congestion and hyperemia; their effects on structure and function in the female reproductive system. *Am J Obstet Gynecol.* 1949;57:637–653.
7. van der Vleuten CJ, van Kempen JA, Schultze-Kool LJ. Embolization to treat pelvic congestion syndrome and vulval varicose veins. *Int J Gynaecol Obstet.* 2012;118:227–230.
8. Meneses L, Fava M, Diaz P, et al. Embolization of incompetent pelvic veins for the treatment of recurrent varicose veins in lower limbs and pelvic congestion syndrome. *Cardiovasc Intervent Radiol.* 2013;36:128–132.
9. Sharma D, Dahiya K, Duhan N, et al. Diagnostic laparoscopy in chronic pelvic pain. *Arch Gynecol Obstet.* 2011;283:295–297.
10. Beard RW, Reginald PW, Wadsworth J. Clinical features of women with chronic lower abdominal pain and pelvic congestion. *Br J Obstet Gynaecol.* 1988;95(2):153–161.
11. Hobbs JT. The pelvic congestion syndrome. *Br J Hosp Med.* 1990;43(3):200–206.
12. Castenmiller PH, de Leur K, de Jong TE, et al. Clinical results after coil embolization of the ovarian vein in patients with primary and recurrent lower-limb varices with respect to vulval varices. *Phlebology.* 2013;28(5):234–238.
13. Paraskevas P. Successful ultrasound-guided foam sclerotherapy for vulval and leg varicosities secondary to ovarian vein reflux: a case study. *Phlebology.* 2011;26(1):29–31.
14. Beard RW, Highman JH, Pearce S, et al. Diagnosis of pelvic varicosities in women with chronic pelvic pain. *Lancet.* 1984;2:946–949.
15. Stones RW, Turmaine M, Beard RW, et al. The fine structure of the human ovarian vein. *J Anat.* 1994;185(pt 2):285–294.
16. Stones RW, Loesch A, Beard RW, et al. Endothelial localization and pharmacology in the human ovarian vein. *Obstet Gynecol.* 1995;85(2):273–278.

17. Raffetto JD, Khalil RA. Mechanisms of varicose vein formation: valve dysfunction and wall dilation. *Phlebology.* 2008;23(2): 85–98.
18. Park SJ, Lim JW, Ko YT, et al. Diagnosis of pelvic congestion syndrome using transabdominal and transvaginal sonography. *AJR Am J Roentgenol.* 2004;182(3):683–688.
19. Rozenblit AM, Ricci ZJ, Tuvia J, et al. Incompetent and dilated ovarian veins: a common CT finding in asymptomatic parous women. *AJR Am J Roentgenol.* 2001;176(1):119–122.
20. Nascimento AB, Mitchell DG, Holland G. Ovarian veins: magnetic resonance imaging findings in an asymptomatic population. *J Magn Reson Imaging.* 2002;15(5):551–556.
21. Bonney RC, Watson H, Beesley JS, et al. Endometrial phospholipases A2, polycystic ovaries and pelvic pain. *Br J Obstet Gynaecol.* 1992;99(6):486–491.
22. Adams J, Reginald PW, Franks S, et al. Uterine size and endometrial thickness and the significance of cystic ovaries in women with pelvic pain due to congestion. *Br J Obstet Gynaecol.* 1990; 97(7):583–587.
23. Gilling-Smith C, Mason H, Willis D, et al. In-vitro ovarian steroidogenesis in women with pelvic congestion. *Hum Reprod.* 2000;15(12):2570–2576.
24. Maleux G, Stockx L, Wilms G, et al. Ovarian vein embolization for the treatment of pelvic congestion syndrome: long-term technical and clinical results. *J Vasc Interv Radiol.* 2000;11: 859–864.
25. Edwards RD, Robertson JR, MacLean AB, et al. Case report: pelvic pain syndrome—successful treatment of a case by ovarian vein embolization. *Clin Radiol.* 1993;47:429–431.
26. Capasso P, Simons C, Trotteur G, et al. Treatment of symptomatic pelvic varices by ovarian vein embolization. *Cardiovasc Intervent Radiol.* 1997;20:107–111.
27. Kwon SH, Oh JH, Ko KR, et al. Transcatheter ovarian vein embolization using coils for the treatment of pelvic congestion syndrome. *Cardiovasc Intervent Radiol.* 2007;3:655–661.
28. Cordts PR, Eclavea A, Buckley PJ, et al. Pelvic congestion syndrome: early clinical results after transcatheter ovarian vein embolization. *J Vasc Surg.* 1998;28:862–868.
29. Tarazov PG, Prozorovskij KV, Ryzhkov VK. Pelvic pain syndrome caused by ovarian varices. Treatment by transcatheter embolization. *Acta Radiol.* 1997;38:1023–1025.
30. Gandini R, Chiocchi M, Konda D, et al. Transcatheter foam sclerotherapy of symptomatic female varicocele with sodium-tetradecyl-sulfate foam. *Cardiovasc Intervent Radiol.* 2008;31: 778–784.
31. Venbrux AC, Chang AH, Kim HS, et al. Pelvic congestion syndrome (pelvic venous incompetence): impact of ovarian and internal iliac vein embolotherapy on menstrual cycle and chronic pelvic pain. *J Vasc Interv Radiol.* 2002;13: 171–178.
32. Kim HS, Malhotra AD, Rowe PC, et al. Embolotherapy for pelvic congestion syndrome: long-term results. *J Vasc Interv Radiol.* 2006;17:289–297.
33. Laborda A, Medrano J, de Blas I, et al. Endovascular treatment of pelvic congestion syndrome: visual analog scale (VAS) long-term follow-up clinical evaluation in 202 patients. *Cardiovasc Intervent Radiol.* 2013;36(4):1006–1014.
34. Chung MH, Huh CY. Comparison of treatments for pelvic congestion syndrome. *Tohoku J Exp Med.* 2003;201:131–138.
35. Rastogi N, Kabutey NK, Kim D. Unintended coil migration into the right ventricle during the right ovarian vein coil embolization. *Vasc Endovascular Surg.* 2011;45(7):660–664.
36. Coakley FV, Varghese SI, Hricak H. CT and MRI of pelvic varices in women. *J Comput Assist Tomogr.* 1999;23:429–434.

60

Pediatric Embolization

Sergio Sierre

BACKGROUND

Endovascular techniques used in children for diagnostic and therapeutic purposes are relatively similar compared to those used for adults. Most of these procedures performed in the pediatric population have been extrapolated from the adult experience. However, vascular interventional radiology in pediatrics differs from adult vascular interventions in several aspects, and we frequently face the need for miniaturization of equipment for appropriate use in the pediatric population. Despite anatomical and technical issues, significant clinical and technical success rates have been achieved with endovascular techniques in the pediatric population.[1]

Furthermore, when the patient is evaluated for moderate sedation or general anesthesia, it is important to consider the maintenance of body temperature control, fluid balance, iodine contrast dose, radiation safety, and equipment selection. Also, technique standardization of any angiographic/vascular procedure is limited due to the fact that different devices are necessary to perform procedures safely in patients with a large range of body size. Children have both advantages and disadvantages and may require alternative techniques. Complications may be similar to those reported in adults, but specific problems may be seen with different prevalence (i.e., vessel thrombosis).[1,2]

There has been tremendous growth in pediatric vascular interventions, and most recently, pediatric embolotherapy has become technically feasible mainly due to the availability of smaller diagnostic catheters and microcatheters. This chapter will focus on some specific indications for embolotherapy in pediatrics, emphasizing particular issues to be considered in this age group.[1–3]

Patient Preparation

For all procedures, informed consent is obtained from the parent, guardian, or the patient if they are of legal age to consent. In these forms, the procedure is described, therapeutic alternatives are discussed, and procedure-related complications are mentioned. Routine blood work and coagulation studies are requested. For therapeutic procedures, the coagulation references are platelet count over 50,000/μL, prothrombin time less than 18 seconds, partial thromboplastin time less than 32 seconds, and international normalized ratio less than 1.2. If the blood tests are abnormal, coagulation has to be optimized to avoid procedural bleeding, and a consultation with a hematologist is recommended. Patients are not routinely blood matched, except for those procedures when a possibility of significant blood loss exists, such as transarterial or transjugular intrahepatic portosystemic shunt procedures in coagulopathic patients.[4]

Patient's diet is held for an appropriate time as determined by age, alimentary requirements, type of sedation, and need for general anesthesia. Regarding diet, solids may be consumed until 8 hours before sedation or general anesthesia in 6 months of age or older patients. In younger patients, breast milk and formula are permitted until 4 hours before the procedure. Also, patients are able to take clear fluids by mouth up to 2 hours before the procedure. Antibiotics are not routinely prescribed before the embolization procedure, with particular exception for splenic embolization and patients with congenital heart defects. For the former, we usually use a recommended broad-spectrum antibiotic regimen (ceftriaxone/clindamycin) just before and for 5 days after the embolization procedure. For the latter, we use a prophylactic single dose of cefazolin or cefotaxime, 50 mg/kg.[2,4]

In all cases, the angiography room must be warm, particularly when procedures are performed in newborns and infants. Patients must be at a constant body temperature, and covers, hat, Bair Hugger (Arizant Healthcare, Inc., St Paul, Minnesota), heat lamp, and warming blanket are frequently necessary. Also, any solutions used including the contrast medium should be slightly heated. In pediatrics, the amount of contrast media is a limiting factor. The accepted dose of nonionic contrast should not exceed 5 mL/kg.[1–4]

Sedation/Anesthesia

A sedation protocol is essential to establish a successful pediatric interventional practice. The choice of whether to use conscious sedation or general anesthesia is influenced by many factors, but for embolization procedures, general anesthesia is preferred.[3,5]

When planning for sedation, special consideration should be given to children who are very ill, especially those with hepatic and/or renal failure. These patients are at greater risk for acute drug toxicity, hypotension, respiratory depression, and prolonged sedation because of their inability to metabolize and excrete most sedation drugs. Therefore, general anesthesia is often preferred for this group.[2–4] General anesthesia is also preferred when the procedure is expected to be lengthy or painful, when there is a history of failed or difficult sedation, or when there are contraindications or unacceptable risks to sedation.[3] Hence, general anesthesia is usually indicated for embolization procedures.[1–5]

Radiation Safety

Children are more radiation-sensitive than adults and have a longer lifespan during which to manifest radiation-induced cancers. Therefore, it is prudent and important to use appropriate radiation safety techniques when performing pediatric interventional procedures.[6] Radiologists, radiologic technologists, and all supervising physicians have a responsibility to minimize the radiation dose to individual patients and to staff while maintaining the necessary diagnostic image quality, following the "as low as reasonably achievable (ALARA)" principle. Vascular procedures might be associated with a moderate radiation dose. Also, lengthy or repeated procedures may result in significant radiation exposure, making it extremely necessary to respect and follow the radiation safety protocols. Examination protocols should vary, taking into account patient body habitus, such as height and/or weight, body mass index, or lateral width. The dose reduction devices that are available on imaging equipment should be active; if not, manual techniques should be used to moderate the exposure while maintaining the necessary diagnostic image quality.[7]

Some techniques for decreasing patient radiation dose should be considered, using reduced-dose protocols, the last-image-hold feature, pulsed fluoroscopy, tightly collimating to the area of interest, and minimizing the use of magnification. Periodically, radiation exposures should be measured and patient radiation doses estimated by a medical physicist in accordance with the appropriate technical standards.[5–7]

Vascular Access

Vascular access in children based on palpation and anatomic landmarks can be challenging. Ultrasound (US) guidance for the arterial puncture may increase the chances of successfully gaining access to these small-caliber arteries.[5,8] In children weighing more than 30 kg, femoral access is obtained with use of an 18-gauge needle, and a 4-Fr or 5-Fr catheter is inserted. In children weighing between 10 and 30 kg, a 20-gauge needle might be used for arterial puncture and a 4-Fr catheter is used.

Arterial puncture in children weighing less than 10 kg can be technically challenging and should not be done with anything larger than a 20-gauge needle. For smaller children, the use of 3-Fr devices is recommended.[4,5] Vascular sheaths are placed in all patients because these procedures are often lengthy and can require catheter exchanges. To prevent vessel thrombosis, an initial bolus of heparin is given (75 to 100 units/kg). In case of lengthy procedures, a subsequent heparin injection should follow. Arterial spasm is frequent in this population and may be treated with intra-arterial injection of papaverine (1 mg/kg) or nitroglycerin (2 to 3 units/kg).[1,2,4,5]

Embolic Agents

Embolic agents used in pediatric embolotherapy are the same as those used in adult patients. Cautions should be considered in case of alcohol use. A maximum dose of 1 mL/kg (or 60 mL) per session should never be exceeded.[1,2] Microcatheters allow practitioners to perform many of these pediatric embolization procedures, and coaxial systems (guide catheter/microcatheters) are ideal for this purpose.

Indications

Diagnostic arteriography is gradually being replaced with noninvasive imaging. Indications for diagnostic vascular studies still occur, but frequently, these diagnostic studies are done in conjunction with a therapeutic intervention (i.e., embolization).

Transcatheter embolization is currently a common procedure in pediatric tertiary centers performed by physicians trained in endovascular procedures and aware of technical modifications and alternatives needed for this age group of patients.[1,4,5]

It is important to ensure the relevance of the procedure and decision must be taken based on a multidisciplinary approach. This chapter will focus on some particular entities almost exclusively found in pediatric patients, such as vascular tumors and congenital shunts and fistulas. Vascular malformations, a pathology very frequently found in pediatric interventional radiology practice, will not be discussed in this chapter (see Chapter 13).

VASCULAR ANOMALIES

In 1982, Drs. Mulliken and Glowacki proposed a classification of vascular congenital anomalies based on the clinical, biologic, and cytologic findings. According to this classification, vascular anomalies were divided into either vascular tumors (hemangioma, hemangioendothelioma, and other vascular tumors) or vascular malformations (capillary, venous, lymphatic, arteriovenous, and combined lesions).[9,10]

Vascular malformations are composed of irregularly dilated, malformed, or dysplastic vessels, with variably thickened vascular channels lined with mature endothelial cells. These lesions are usually present at birth and do not regress. Vascular malformations exhibit a predictable group of clinical patterns that vary in severity and rate of progression. These vascular malformations were named and classified based on the affected vascular channel (arterial, capillary, venous, or lymphatic or in combination).[9–11] Later, a complementary hemodynamic classification was described in 1993, dividing vascular malformations into high-flow and low-flow lesions.[12]

Sclerotherapy is the technique used to treat low-flow vascular malformations. High-flow lesions are treated with superselective transarterial, direct, and transvenous access, with flow reduction techniques, to deliver an adequate dose of sclerosant and embolic agents to the malformation nidus.[9–11,13]

Vascular tumors demonstrate rapid neonatal growth, endothelial hypercellularity, increased cellular turnover, and in the case of infantile hemangiomas, a later involutive phase. Hemangiomas are the most frequent tumors in infancy.[10,11,13,14]

Main indications of embolotherapy in vascular tumors are hemangiomas refractory to medical treatment, hemangioendotheliomas with Kasabach-Merritt phenomenon, and liver hemangioma with cardiac failure.[1,2,10,11,14]

Vascular Tumors

The most frequent vascular tumors in infancy are infantile hemangiomas. Congenital hemangiomas (noninvoluting congenital hemangiomas [NICH] or rapidly involuting congenital hemangiomas [RICH]), hemangioendotheliomas, tufted angiomas, and sarcomas are other vascular tumors seen in children.[10,11,14]

Hemangiomas

Hemangiomas are the most common tumors in infancy, with predominance in the females (3:1). Generally, they appear in the first week of life, and 60% of the cases are located at the head and neck. As mentioned, the classic infantile hemangioma presents a first stage of rapid proliferation of approximately 3 to 12 months of duration, with a period of stability and a stage of slow regression lasting from 2 to 10 years. Frequently, nearly 80% of these tumors do not need treatment.

The diagnosis of the hemangiomas is mainly clinical. Doppler US and magnetic resonance imaging are useful diagnostic imaging methods, demonstrating the hypervascularity and extension of these tumors. Angiography and the endovascular techniques are only reserved for therapeutic purposes.[2,10,11,14]

Hemangiomas Refractory to Treatment

Hemangiomas will only need treatment in 10% to 20% of cases, such as periocular hemangiomas with orbital compromise and/or vision impairment; visceral hemangiomas associated with cardiac insufficiency; hemangiomas with persistent ulceration; hemangiomas compromising the airway; facial hemangiomas with rapid growth and distortion, with presumption of important sequels; symptomatic muscular hemangiomas; and in the presence of Kasabach-Merritt phenomenon.

In case a hemangioma needs treatment, medical treatment is usually the first option. The most common first-line therapy is propranolol (2 to 3 mg/kg/day) that typically has excellent results. Other treatments include steroids, interferon, and vincristine.[10,14–16]

Embolization and/or surgery are required when medical alternatives are ineffective, mostly in cases of liver hemangiomas with cardiac failure, hemangioendothelioma complicated by Kasabach-Merritt phenomenon, and uncontrolled proliferative hemangioma with functional disorder that do not respond to pharmacologic treatment.[10,17,18] Embolization of hemangiomas imposes a precise, distal, intratumoral occlusion. Particulated agents (gelfoam and 300 μm microparticles of polyvinyl alcohol or acrylic microspheres) are usually employed for this purpose.[17,19]

Patients' weight is a bounding factor in the use of contrast media in these procedures. Therefore, in some cases, a first procedure will be focused on the embolization of main tumor-feeding vessels. If symptoms persist, this procedure can be repeated.[1,2,5,17]

Kaposiform Hemangioendothelioma

The Kasabach-Merritt phenomenon (KMP) consists of severe thrombocytopenia, microangiopathic hemolytic anemia, and localized consumption coagulopathy, in association with a rapid tumor growth, with reported death rates of 20% to 30%. KMP is actually related to another type of vascular tumor (kaposiform hemangioendothelioma, tufted angioma) and not to the "classic" hemangioma. These tumors present a more invasive and aggressive behavior. Hence, the KMP phenomenon, due to the associated high death rate, needs to be treated.[2,11,17,18] Medical treatment is recommended. Steroids are the first-choice treatment, keeping interferon and vincristine for steroid-refractory treatment. Embolization is needed if medical treatment fails and is always associated with medical treatment.[2,10,14,18] Embolization, performed by arterial approach, aims at reducing the high flow. In cases of KMP, a distal intratumoral occlusion (Fig. 60.1A–D) is also necessary; therefore, particles are also frequently used in these cases.[2,10,15,17,18]

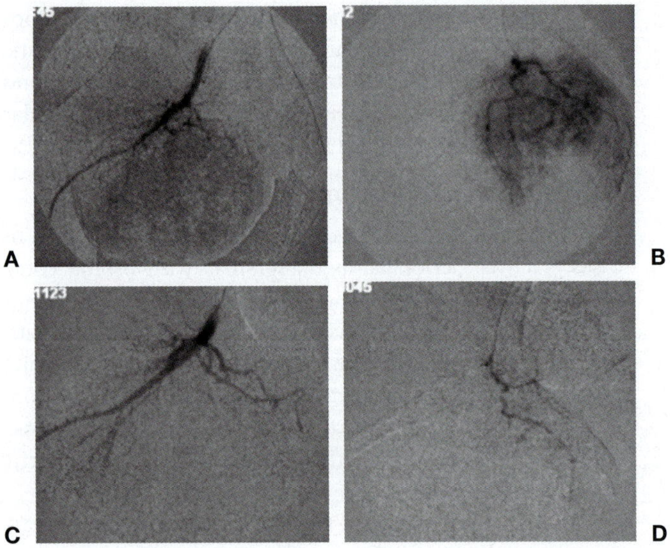

Figure 60.1 Hemangioendothelioma. **A,B:** Hemangioendothelioma in a 10-day-old patient with associated KMP. Hypervascular lesion at the proximal right thigh. **C,D:** Postembolization control angiogram: complete devascularization was achieved after embolization with acrylic microparticles.

Hepatic Hemangiomas

No treatment is required in case of asymptomatic hepatic hemangiomas, but these cases should be closely followed. The main indications for treatment of hepatic hemangiomas are congestive heart failure or KMP.[15–17,19] Again, if treatment is needed, medical treatment with propranolol is a first-line therapy. Other treatments include steroids, interferon, and vincristine.[10,14–16]

In nonresponding patients or in cases where an emergent endovascular treatment is indicated due to a rapid and deleterious progression, embolization is indicated.[17] When a hepatic hemangioma needs treatment, a complete vascular mapping is necessary, identifying the arterial vascularization of the tumor (hepatic and extrahepatic feeders) and the patency of the portal vein.[19] Different patterns of angiographic findings have been described for hepatic hemangiomas.[19] Embolic material is selected depending on the vascular pattern. The most classical appearance is an early filling of abnormal vascular channels without evidence of direct shunting. Others may show high-flow nodules without direct shunts. Embolization is performed by arterial approach for these types, and large particles ($\geq$500 μm) can be used for this purpose. Fatal complications have been reported with the use of small-caliber particles in such cases due to migration to the pulmonary circulation. Hepatic necrosis has also been described with small particles ($<$300 μm).[17,19,20] The choice of the embolic agent is based on the size of the shunts. Also, in small and ill patients, the amount of fluid needed for the delivery of the embolic agent should be minimized. There are no specific recommendations about "contrast:saline solution" for particles infusion; this solution should maintain enough radiopacity to be clearly seen under fluoroscopy. We usually use a 70% contrast/30% saline solution for this purpose.

Hemodynamic patterns including arteriovenous shunts, portovenous shunts, or both arteriovenous and portovenous shunts have been described. Embolization with platinum microcoils are generally safe in such cases and permit the occlusion of the shunts. Glue (*N*-butyl cyanoacrylate) is also an effective material in patients with direct arteriovenous and arterioportal shunting arising from multiple sources.[17,19,20] Glue dilution is based on shunt flow. For shunts involving arterial feeders, a 50:50 (glue:Ethiodol) or greater solution is preferred. Whenever possible, flow reduction techniques might be considered.

Staged procedures are prudent to minimize the appearance of complications such hepatic ischemia, hepatic necrosis, or death.[17]

Knowing the portal involvement in tumor supply is extremely important for embolization planning. Arterial embolization in cases of portovenous fistulas might be ineffective in reducing the cardiac symptoms and may induce hepatic necrosis. In such cases, embolization of portovenous fistulas from transhepatic or transvenous approach is advocated. If necessary, after the venous occlusion, the arterial embolization may be considered. Clinical treatment (propanolol, steroids, and or vincristine) should be maintained after embolization until nearly complete regression of the lesions.[2,17,19,20] The differential diagnosis of liver hemangiomas includes mesenchymal hamartoma, hepatic angiosarcoma, hepatic epithelioid hemangioendothelioma, or metastatic disease, such as neuroblastoma.[10,17,20]

CONGENITAL PORTOSYSTEMIC SHUNTS

Congenital portosystemic shunts are rarely seen. These abnormal communications can be congenital or acquired, asymptomatic (frequently diagnosed incidentally), or diagnosed due to the presence of shunt complications. Most of them occur in infants.[21,22] These shunts are related to the lack of complete involution of one or several fetal vessels, establishing abnormal vascular communications between any vein of the portal system and any vein of the inferior vena cava system. They may exist inside or outside the liver, may be single or multiple, and vary in size. These anomalous communications can cause a partial or complete diversion of the portal flow to a systemic vessel.[23] Some small intrahepatic portosystemic shunts located between the portal branches and hepatic veins may resolve spontaneously by age 1 to 2 years; others, mostly the large shunts, such as extrahepatic, persistent ductus venosus, or still patent intrahepatic shunts, persist throughout life and carry risks of complications. They differ from the acquired intrahepatic and extrahepatic portosystemic shunts occurring as a consequence of portal hypertension.[24]

Associated risks of severe complications exist including neonatal cholestasis, benign and malignant liver tumors, hepatopulmonary syndrome, portopulmonary hypertension, and encephalopathy. The presence of an anomalous portosystemic shunt should be considered in patients with central, not cardiogenic, cyanosis and normal thoracic imaging results (radiography and/or computed tomography [CT]). Hence, the severity of some of these complications and the potential reversibility after shunt occlusion make necessary the treatment of these abnormal communications.[23–29]

The diagnosis of these entities may be obtained with US and Doppler US imaging, allowing identification of the anomalous communication.

Once a congenital portosystemic shunt is found in a child, either during the investigation of a complication during the neonatal period or later as a fortuitous finding, the first step is to be sure that the shunt is not the consequence of portal hypertension or, during early infancy, of a liver hemangioma that would require a specific treatment.[23,24]

Congenital portosystemic venous shunts are best classified into intrahepatic and extrahepatic varieties. In the former, the connections are created between branches of the portal vein, after its division, and the hepatic veins or inferior vena cava. In extrahepatic shunts, the anastomoses are established between the portomesenteric vasculature, before division of the portal vein, and a systemic vein.[21–24,30,31] Therefore, these shunts are divided into two broad types: (1) intrahepatic shunts located between the portal vein or one or several of its branches on one side and the inferior vena cava or a hepatic vein on the other, including the ductus venosus (Fig. 60.2A–D), and (2) extrahepatic shunts, which

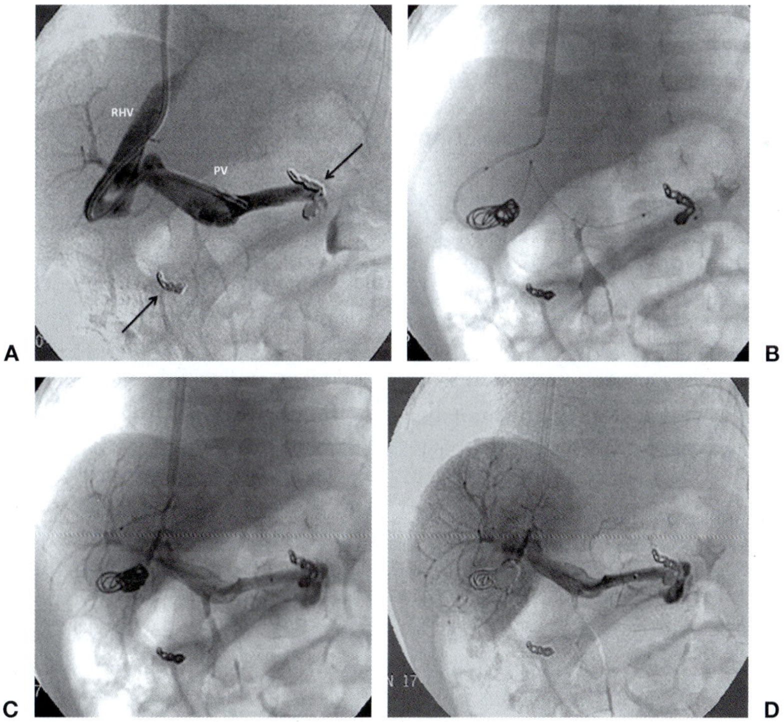

Figure 60.2 Congenital intrahepatic portovenous shunt. **A:** Portography demonstrating an intrahepatic venous shunt. The catheter was advanced into the portal vein from a transjugular approach and the hepatic vein through the communication. Microcoils are seen (*black arrows*) after previous occlusion of two arteriovenous fistulas (from splenic and gastroduodenal artery feeders to splenic and pancreatic veins/image not shown). RHV, right hepatic vein; PV, portal vein. **B:** Microcoil (4 mm and 6 mm Axium microcoils [Covidien, Mansfield, Massachusetts]) embolization of the venovenous communication. **C,D:** Final angiogram, without **(C)** and with digital subtraction **(D)**. After embolization, patency of the portal vein is seen, with proper filling of the intrahepatic portal branches and no further opacification of the portohepatic vein fistula.

join directly the portal trunk or one of its branches of origin to the inferior vena cava or one of its branches.[24]

As far as the time of closure is concerned, there is no doubt that closure should be carried out when one of the complications is present, with the exception of neonatal cholestasis, which resolves spontaneously. Symptomatic or complicated portosystemic shunts must be closed and this can be performed in one or two steps—by endovascular techniques or surgically—depending on the level of portal pressure during an occlusion test.[23,24,26]

Imaging studies sometimes fail to show a patent intrahepatic portal system, and there are reports of extreme hypoplasia of the portal trunk, even suggesting that the portal vein and its intrahepatic branches are lacking, a condition known in the literature as *congenital absence of the portal vein* or *Abernethy malformation*. In such cases, acute closure of the shunt may have devastating consequences, including acute portal hypertension, gastrointestinal bleeding, and severe damage to the gut. However, it is also suggested that the hypoplastic portal vein and/or branches are able to expand after closure of the shunt and that revascularization of these "disconnected" intrahepatic portal branches may occur.[23,24,32,33]

Indications for Shunt Closure

With the exception of neonatal cholestasis, which resolves spontaneously, closure of the shunt is mandatory whenever a complication is present. When no complication is detected, closure of the shunt can be delayed in cases of a small intrahepatic shunt found in early infancy because there is a reasonable hope of spontaneous shunt regression during the first year. In all other cases, closure of the shunt should be considered early, to prevent complications, for different reasons:

a. Hepatopulmonary syndrome and pulmonary hypertension may be present during the very first years of life.
b. The regression of pulmonary hypertension cannot be ascertained once irreversible lesions of the pulmonary arteries are present.
c. Chronic hyperammonemia and high blood levels of manganese have adverse effects on the developing brain.
d. The plasticity of the intrahepatic portal system may be better in younger children.

The plasticity of the intrahepatic portal system allows revascularization of the liver after shunt closure, even when no intrahepatic portal structures can be detected on imaging studies. This leaves little or no place for liver transplantation in the management of these children.[23,24,26,29,32,34]

Closure of congenital shunts in children should start by measuring portal pressure while transiently occluding the shunt during catheterization with an occlusion balloon (Fig. 60.3A–E). Depending on the shunt anatomy, whether attempting to treat the shunt with endovascular techniques or surgically, if the portal pressure is too high to allow shunt closure, then a two-step surgical treatment is indicated. In such cases, surgical banding of the shunt is recommended to maintain portal pressure around 20 mm Hg, followed by closure of the shunt a few months later, after checking by imaging studies that the intrahepatic portal branches have developed satisfactorily.[23,24,26,35]

Embolization of this kind of communications with different conventional embolic agents (i.e., stainless-steel and platinum coils, acrylate) has been described; however, this might be complicated or even impossible as a result of the diameter of the fistula.[25,36,37] The anatomic characteristics of the vascular malformations (large communications) are amenable to be treated with the Amplatzer occlusion devices. Several reports exist in the literature of closure of these portosystemic shunts with Amplatzer plugs. When possible, the endovascular treatment with this device to occlude large communications is highly recommended as it can obviate complex surgeries. A patent ductus venosus can be successfully managed in this way, except when it is too wide or short to safely block the device in its lumen (Fig. 60.3A–E), in which case surgery must be undertaken.[23,25,38–41]

End-to-side shunts such as those joining a splenic or mesenteric vein to an affluent of the inferior vena cava such as a renal vein or an iliac vein can be easily closed percutaneously. On the other hand, when the shunt is side-to-side, surgery is certainly preferable, at least in young children, to the placement of a covered stent that would require lifelong anticoagulation treatment and would probably become inadequate in size with growth.[23–26,33] Side-to-side shunts between the main portal vein and the inferior vena cava are frequently indications for surgery, usually performed in one step. However, in some cases, depending on the anatomy and location of the communication, the endovascular techniques may be useful for resolution of this type of shunt.[25] On the contrary, end-to-side shunts between the main portal vein and the inferior vena cava usually require a two-step surgical procedure to avoid acute severe portal hypertension.[23,24,33,34]

A major complication related to vascular embolization in such cases is portal vein thrombosis, generally related to improper location or migration of the embolic agent. This serious complication is different from the portal vein thrombosis that may occur after occlusion of arterioportal fistulas, which will be discussed later. Neither anticoagulation nor antiaggregation is indicated after endovascular treatment of such portosystemic shunts.[23–25] Follow-up control imaging is usually performed with Doppler US and demonstrates redirection of portal flow with no filling of the anomalous communication and subsequent regression of symptoms.

Interventional radiology techniques have an important role in the diagnosis and management of these congenital shunts involving the portal vein. The appropriate decision about the optimal treatment timing and approach, surgical

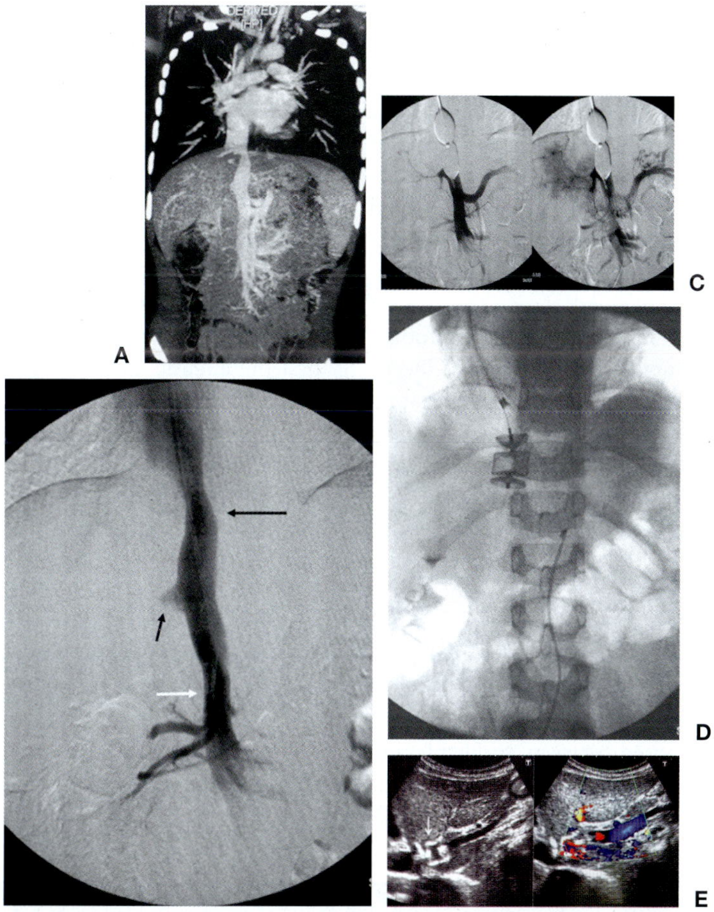

Figure 60.3 Congenital extrahepatic portovenous shunt. **A:** Abdominal multislice CT, coronal view. A portosystemic (portal vein to inferior vena cava) shunt is present. **B:** Venogram from a transjugular approach. The catheter tip (*white arrow*) is placed in the mesenteric vein. The origin of a hypoplastic portal vein (*short black arrow*) is seen. The shunt is opacified (*long black arrow*), communicating the mesenteric vein to the distal portion of the inferior vena cava. **C:** Angiogram during shunt balloon occlusion demonstrating the presence of a hypoplastic portal vein. **D:** Shunt embolization with an Amplatzer device. The plug is placed at the abnormal conduit. **E:** US and Color Doppler US control. Complete occlusion of the portosystemic shunt. The device is clearly seen (*arrow*).

or endovascular, should be taken based on a multidisciplinary management of such patients.

CONGENITAL ARTERIOPORTAL FISTULAS

Arterioportal fistulas (APFs) are a rare but treatable cause of portal hypertension associated with gastrointestinal hemorrhage in early childhood. APF may be primary (congenital) or secondary (acquired). Congenital APFs are defined as an intrahepatic communication between the hepatic artery and the portal venous system, without any connection with the systemic venous circulation or a clear secondary cause, and with onset before 18 years of age.[17,22,42] Less than 10% of APFs involving the hepatic artery are congenital. The presence of multiple or diffuse feeding vessels to the fistula is a frequent and characteristic feature of congenital lesions.[43] Among the most commonly reported causes of acquired APF are blunt abdominal trauma, surgical procedures such as the Kasai procedure and segmental liver transplantation, hepatic artery aneurysm, cirrhosis, biliary atresia, and tumors.[42,44]

Endovascular treatment of this entity aims at permanent occlusion of the fistula and restoration of normal liver hemodynamics. Transarterial embolization is a minimally invasive, effective, and safe therapy that allows resolution of the pathology with a shorter hospital stay and decreased morbidity. It is the treatment of choice among other options, such as surgical ligation of the involved hepatic artery, partial hepatectomy, portocaval shunt, and liver transplantation.[43–45]

In most patients with APF, clinical symptoms are related to the development of portal hypertension that appears in the first year of life. The severity of the symptoms is proportional to the size of the fistula and the flow within it. The fistula progressively decreases and then reverses the normal antegrade flow in the portal vein while the hepatic artery flow, and diameter, increase due to the fact that arterial flow directly communicates with a territory of low pressure.[42,43,46]

The hepatic artery is usually enlarged in all patients. This hemodynamic alteration also produces a decrease in blood flow distal to the fistula in the abdominal aorta beyond the celiac trunk (aortic tapering). Some authors have suggested that this steal effect compromises perfusion of the superior and inferior mesenteric circulations, producing bowel hypoxia, thus worsening intestinal edema.[43]

In a review of the largest series, the most commonly found clinical features were upper gastrointestinal bleeding, failure to thrive, chronic diarrhea with steatorrhea, and protein-losing enteropathy. In these same series, the most important findings on physical examination at diagnosis were splenomegaly, hepatomegaly, ascites, and edema. The variable clinical presentation might be related to variations in the angioarchitecture, size of the fistula, flow within the malformation, and, consequently, the degree of portal hypertension.[43,44]

In contrast to patients with arteriovenous fistulas in other locations, congestive heart failure is rare in patients with APF. This seems to be related to the protective effect of the hepatic sinusoids interposed between the fistula and the right heart cavities. The typical symptoms of chronic malabsorption, diarrhea, and abdominal pain are likely associated with mesenteric vascular congestion. Protein-losing enteropathy, steatorrhea, and malabsorption contribute to patient malnutrition and may be due to edema and dilation of the lymphatic system and pancreatic hypoperfusion.[46]

Treatment

No cases of spontaneous closure of an APF have been reported; therefore, intervention is warranted in all symptomatic patients. Transcatheter embolization of the fistula by means of endovascular techniques has been proposed as the first therapeutic option with a high success rate in patients with unilateral lesions or in those with few feeding arteries. Congenital APF may have a single feeding artery or multiple or diffuse feeding vessels (Fig. 60.4A–F).[43–45,47] The presence of the former characteristic thus increases the chance of successful occlusion of an APF via endovascular procedures. However, in many series, more than one intervention has been necessary to achieve occlusion. Occasionally, after an apparently technically successful procedure, new collateral feeders not seen during the first intervention might appear and act as persistent anomalous arterial to portal connections keeping the fistula patent. In these patients, nonsurgical treatment is preferable because the success rate is not higher with surgery.[43,44] A differential diagnosis might be established with

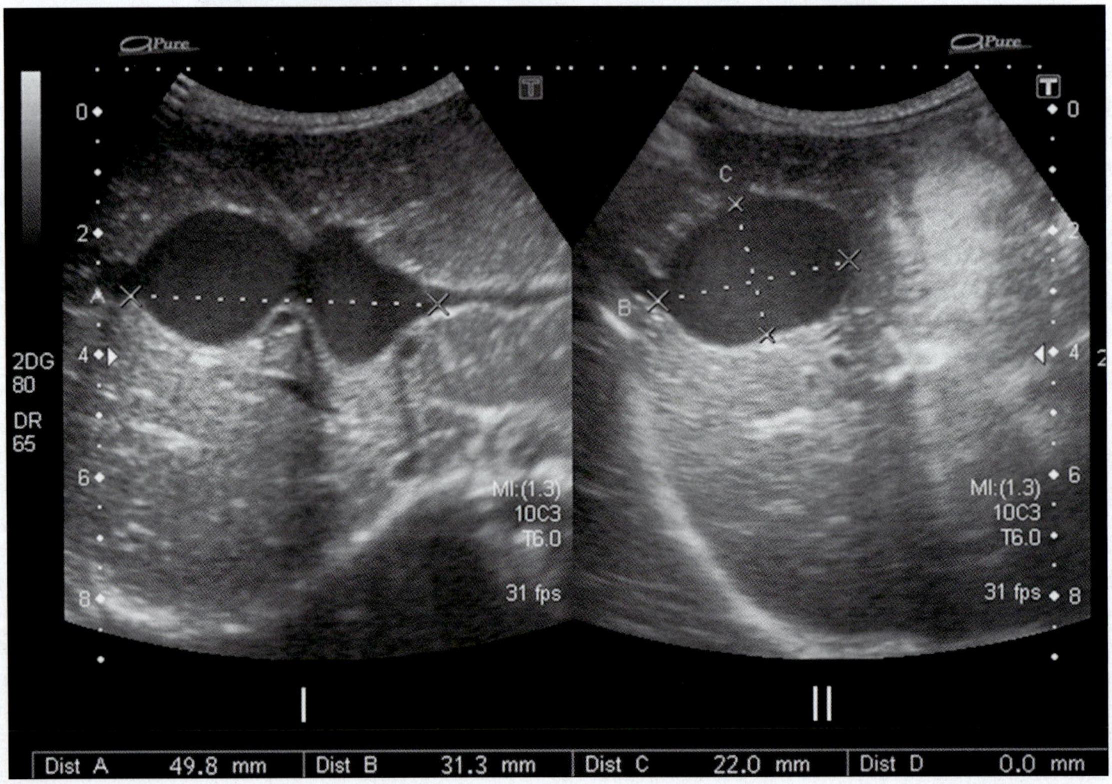

Figure 60.4 Congenital APF. **A:** US images show an anechoic bilobulated structure between the left hepatic artery and the portal vein. *(Continued)*

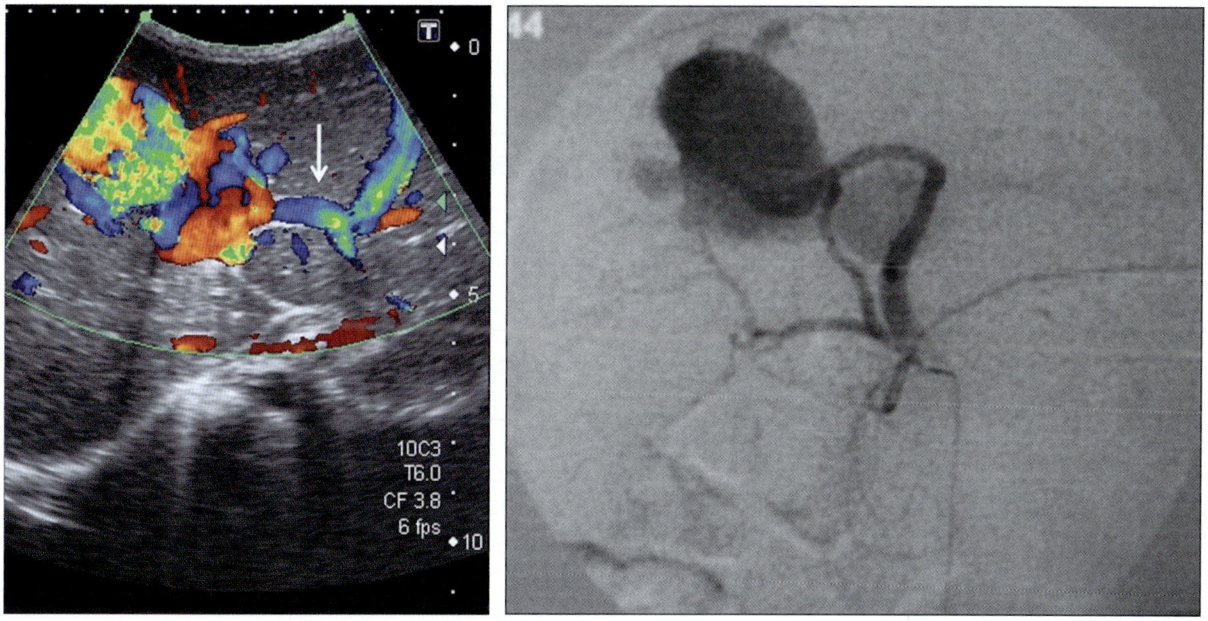

B C

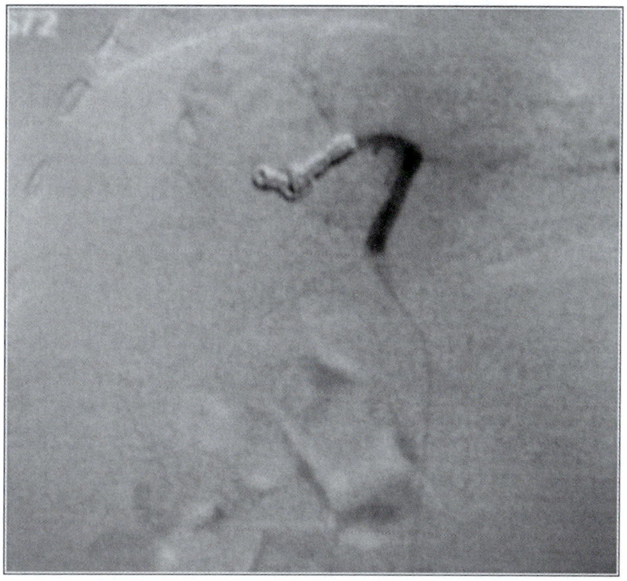

E

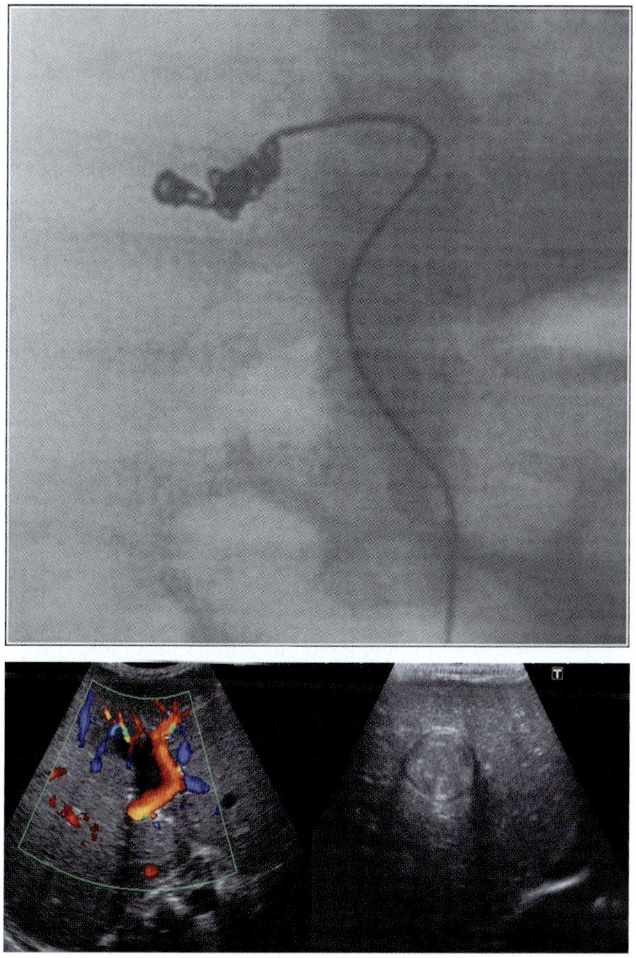

D F

Figure 60.4 *(Continued)* **B:** Color Doppler US mapping demonstrating high flow inside the APF. A communication can be observed between the ectatic left hepatic artery (*arrow*) and the portal vein. **C:** Selective left hepatic arteriogram: arteriovenous fistula between the left hepatic artery and the portal vein. **D:** Transarterial microcoil (4-mm MicroNester coils [Cook Medical, Inc., Bloomington, Indiana]) embolization of the feeding artery. **E:** Postembolization angiogram: the feeding vessel is occluded. **F:** Color Doppler US and US images after embolization: the color Doppler signal within the malformation has disappeared, with complete occlusion of the malformation.

hepatic arteriovenous malformations, a fast-flow vascular malformation. This entity may present a single or several arterial feeders and show a characteristic nidus not seen in APF. Hepatic arteriovenous malformations may be focal or diffuse, and embolization is usually, but not always, an option due to the risk of hepatic ischemia and necrosis.[17] Metallic coils are the recommended agents for permanent arterial embolization of APF. The use of Amplatzer plugs has also been reported for this indication. Acrylic or polyvinyl alcohol microspheres have also been described in case small feeders are present. Microspheres larger than 500 μm should be used based on that this caliber is large enough to occlude the arterioportal connection, avoiding the risks of migration to the portal system and hepatic ischemia. There are no reports about the use of liquid embolic agents, such as Onyx (Covidien, Irvine, California) and/or acrylate for APF embolization.[17,43–45,47]

Portal vein thrombosis is a major complication during the embolization procedure and in the early posttreatment period. This complication may be related to nontarget embolization, directly locating the embolic agent at the wrong site, or the material moving from the original site to the portal system because of high flow in the fistula. Another reason for this severe complication is related to sudden flow changes after embolization of the fistula. Therefore, immediately after the procedure, heparinization is recommended. In our experience, after the intervention, for thrombosis prophylaxis, subcutaneous low-molecular-weight heparin was administered for 3 days once the end point (anti-Xa = 0.5 to 1 IU/mL) had been achieved. The Doppler US follow-up in the early posttreatment period is crucial to detect this vascular complication.[17,43,45]

TIPS AND TRICKS

Tips

- Attention should always be drawn to the maintenance of patient body temperature control, fluid balance, and total dose of iodine contrast used.
- Appropriate radiation safety techniques when performing pediatric interventional procedures must be considered, following the ALARA principle.
- For transarterial embolization procedures, general anesthesia is preferred.
- US guidance for the arterial puncture increases the chances of a successful access in small patients.
- Vascular sheaths should always be placed at the access site.
- Microcatheters and coaxial systems are ideal for embolization in pediatrics.
- Percutaneous sclerotherapy is the technique used to treat low-flow vascular malformations. On the other hand, high-flow lesions are treated with superselective transarterial, direct, and transvenous access.
- The diagnosis of the hemangiomas is mainly clinical. Angiography and further endovascular techniques are only reserved for therapeutic purposes when medical treatment fails.
- The presence of an anomalous portosystemic shunt should be considered in patients with central, not cardiogenic, cyanosis and normal thoracic imaging.
- In pediatric interventional radiology, optimal clinical results are obtained as a result of a multidisciplinary discussion, management, and patients' follow-up.

Tricks

- The accepted dose of nonionic contrast should not exceed 5 mL/kg. Usually, we use undiluted contrast material; however, in patients weighing less than 10 kg, we often dilute 1:1 with saline.
- Radiation safety tricks may include reduced-dose protocols, the last-image-hold feature, pulsed fluoroscopy, tight collimation, and minimizing the use of magnification.
- Arterial puncture in children weighing less than 10 kg should not be done with anything larger than a 20-gauge needle.
- Arterial spasm, frequent in this population, may be treated with intra-arterial injection of papaverine (1 mg/kg) or nitroglycerin (2–3 units/kg).
- Considering patients' weight and the use of contrast media for embolization procedures, in some cases, a first procedure will be focused on the embolization of main tumor-feeding vessels. If symptoms persist, this procedure can be repeated.
- Embolization of hemangiomas imposes a precise, distal, intratumoral occlusion. Particulated agents (gelfoam and ≥300 μm microparticles) are usually employed for this purpose.
- Regarding treatment of hepatic vascular tumors, staged procedures are prudent to minimize the appearance of complications such as hepatic ischemia or necrosis.
- Treatment of portosystemic shunts should be considered when a complication is present (with the exception of neonatal cholestasis, which may resolve spontaneously).
- If treatment is needed, an occlusion test for portal pressure assessment should be performed. Then, endovascular or surgical treatment can be carried out, in one or two steps, depending on the test result.
- Metallic coils are the recommended agents for permanent arterial embolization of congenital APFs. Vascular plugs may also be useful for this purpose.
- Immediately after the embolization of congenital APF, heparinization is recommended to avoid portal vein thrombosis.

CONCLUSION

Embolotherapy has demonstrated its effectiveness with current available materials and equipment in a wide range of indications in pediatric patients. These techniques should be performed by specifically trained physicians, with knowledge of the pediatric pathology and experience in the management of the specific considerations related to this age group. A multidisciplinary discussion, management, and follow-up are essential for the continuous evolution of endovascular techniques in pediatrics.

REFERENCES

1. Dubois J, Garel L, Culham G. Pediatric Interventional angiography. In: Baum S, Pentecost MJ, eds. *Abram's Angiography Interventional Radiology*. Philadelphia, PA: Lippincott Williams & Wilkins; 2006:1046–1067.
2. Dubois J, Garel L. Embolotherapy in pediatrics. In: Golzarian J, Sun S, Sharafuddin MJ, eds. *Vascular Embolotherapy*. Berlin, Germany: Springer-Verlag; 2006:297–320.
3. Kaye RD, Sane SS, Towbin RB. Pediatric intervention: an update—part I. *J Vasc Interv Radiol*. 2000;11:683–697.
4. Kaye RD, Sane SS, Towbin RB. Pediatric intervention: an update—part II. *J Vasc Interv Radiol*. 2000;11:807–822.
5. Donaldson JS. Pediatric vascular procedures: arterial and venous. In: Slovis T, ed. *Caffey's Pediatric Diagnostic Imaging*. Philadelphia, PA: Mosby Elsevier; 2008:3100–3116.
6. Sidhu M, Strauss KJ, Connolly MB, et al. Radiation safety in pediatric interventional radiology. *Tech Vasc Interv Radiol*. 2010; 13:158–166.
7. Connolly B, Racadio J, Towbin R. Practice of ALARA in the pediatric interventional suite. *Pediatr Radiol*. 2006;36:163–167.
8. Jaques PF, Mauro MA, Keefe B. US guidance for vascular access. Technical note. *J Vasc Interv Radiol*. 1992;3:427–430.
9. Legiehn GM, Heran MK. *A step-by-step practical approach to imaging diagnosis and interventional radiologic therapy in vascular malformations. Semin Intervent Radiol*. 2010;27:209–231.
10. Dubois J, Alison M. Vascular anomalies: what a radiologist needs to know. *Pediatr Radiol*. 2010;40:895–905.
11. Ernemann U, Kramer U, Miller S, et al. Current concepts in the classification, diagnosis and treatment of vascular anomalies. *Eur J Radiol*. 2010;75:2–11.
12. Jackson IT, Carreno R, Potparic Z, et al. Hemangiomas, vascular malformations, and lymphovenous malformations: classification and methods of treatment. *Plast Reconstr Surg*. 1993; 91:1216–1230.
13. Legiehn GM, Heran MK. Classification, diagnosis, and interventional radiologic management of vascular malformations. *Orthop Clin North Am*. 2006;37:435–474.
14. Chen TS, MD, Eichenfield LF, Friedlander SF. *Infantile hemangiomas: an update on pathogenesis and therapy. Pediatrics*. 2013;131:99–108.
15. Sans V, de la Roque ED, Berge J, et al. Propranolol for severe infantile hemangiomas: follow-up report. *Pediatrics*. 2009;124:423–431.
16. Leaute-Labreze C, Dumas de la Roque E, Hubiche T, et al. Propranolol for severe hemangiomas of infancy. *N Engl J Med*. 2008;358:2649–2651.
17. Burrows PE, Dubois J, Kassarjian A. Pediatric hepatic vascular anomalies. *Pediatr Radiol*. 2001;31:533–545.
18. Garcia-Monaco R, Giachetti A, Peralta O, et al. Kaposiform hemangioendothelioma with Kasabach-Merritt phenomenon: successful treatment with embolization and vincristine in two newborns. *J Vasc Interv Radiol*. 2012;23:417–422.
19. Kassarjian A, Dubois J, Burrows PE. Angiographic classification of hepatic hemangiomas in infants. *Radiology*. 2002;222: 693–698.
20. Christison-Lagay ER, Burrows PE, Alomari A, et al. Hepatic hemangiomas: subtype classification and development of a clinical practice algorithm and registry. *J Pediatr Surg*. 2007;42:62–67.
21. Alonso-Gamarra E, Parrón M, Pérez A, et al. Clinical and radiologic manifestations of congenital extrahepatic portosystemic shunts: a comprehensive review. *Radiographics*. 2011;31: 707–722.
22. Gallego C, Miralles M, Marín C, et al. Congenital hepatic shunts. *Radiographics*. 2004;24:755–772.
23. Bernard O, Franchi-Abella S, Branchereau S, et al. Congenital portosystemic shunts in children: recognition, evaluation, and management. *Semin Liver Dis*. 2012;32:273–287.
24. Franchi-Abella S, Branchereau S, Lambert V, et al. Complications of congenital portosystemic shunts in children: therapeutic options and outcomes. *J Pediatr Gastroenterol Nutr*. 2010; 51:322–330.
25. Alonso J, Sierre S, Lipsich J, et al. Endovascular treatment of congenital portal vein fistulas with the Amplatzer occlusion device. *J Vasc Interv Radiol*. 2004;15:989–993.
26. Stringer MD. The clinical anatomy of congenital portosystemic venous shunts. *Clin Anat*. 2008;21:147–157.
27. Eroglu Y, Donaldson J, Sorensen LG, et al. Improved neurocognitive function after radiologic closure of congenital portosystemic shunts. *J Pediatr Gastroenterol Nutr*. 2004;39:410–417.
28. Kim T, Murakami T, Sugihara E, et al. Hepatic nodular lesions associated with abnormal development of the portal vein. *AJR Am J Roentgenol*. 2004;183:1333–1338.
29. Morikawa N, Honna T, Kuroda T, et al. Resolution of hepatopulmonary syndrome after ligation of a portosystemic shunt in a pediatric patient with an Abernethy malformation. *J Pediatr Surg*. 2008;43:e35–e38.
30. Howard ER, Davenport M. Congenital extrahepatic portocaval shunts—the Abernethy malformation. *J Pediatr Surg*. 1997; 32:494–497.
31. Murray CP, Yoo SJ, Babyn PS. Congenital extrahepatic portosystemic shunts. *Pediatr Radiol*. 2003;33:614–620.
32. Barsky MF, Rankin RN, Wall WJ, et al. Patent ductus venosus: problems in assessment and management. *Can J Surg*. 1989;32: 271–275.
33. Takehara Y, Mori K, Edagawa T, et al. Presumed hypoplastic intrahepatic portal system due to patent ductus venosus: importance of direct occlusion test of ductus venosus under open laparotomy. *Pediatr Int*. 2004;46:484–486.
34. Yoshimoto Y, Shimizu R, Saeki T, et al. Patent ductus venosus in children: a case report and review of the literature. *J Pediatr Surg*. 2004;39:E1–E5.
35. Yagi H, Takada Y, Fujimoto Y, et al. Successful surgical ligation under intraoperative portal vein pressure monitoring of a large portosystemic shunt presenting as an intrapulmonary shunt: report of a case. *Surg Today*. 2004;34:1049–1052.

36. Gupta V, Kalra N, Vyas S, et al. Embolization of congenital intrahepatic porto-systemic shunt by n-butyl cyanoacrylate. *Indian J Pediatr.* 2009;76:1059–1060.
37. Yamagami T, Yoshimatsu R, Matsumoto T, et al. Successful embolization using interlocking detachable coils for a congenital extrahepatic portosystemic venous shunt in a child. *J Pediatr Surg.* 2007;42:1949–1952.
38. Gillespie MJ, Golden A, Sivarajan VB, et al. Transcatheter closure of patent ductus venosus with the Amplatzer vascular plug in twin brothers. *Pediatr Cardiol.* 2006;27:142–145.
39. Chiu SN, Chien YH, Wu MH, et al. Transcatheter closure of portal-systemic shunt combining congenital double extrahepatic inferior vena cava with vascular plug. *J Pediatr.* 2008;153:723.
40. Cho YK, Chang NK, Ma JS. Successful transcatheter closure of a large patent ductus venosus with the Amplatzer vascular plug II. *Pediatr Cardiol.* 2009;30:540–542.
41. Evans WN, Galindo A, Acherman RJ, et al. Congenital portosystemic shunts and AMPLATZER vascular plug occlusion in newborns. *Pediatr Cardiol.* 2009;30:1083–1088.
42. Norton SP, Jacobson K, Moroz SP, et al. The congenital intrahepatic arterioportal fistula syndrome: elucidation and proposed classification. *J Pediatr Gastroenterol Nutr.* 2006;43:248–255.
43. Teplisky D, Tincani EU, Lipsich J, et al. Congenital arterioportal fistulas: radiological treatment and color Doppler US follow-up. *Pediatr Radiol.* 2012;42:1326–1332.
44. Vauthey JN, Tomczak RJ, Helmberger T, et al. The arterioportal fistula syndrome: clinicopathologic features, diagnosis, and therapy. *Gastroenterology.* 1997;113:1390–1401.
45. Kumar N, de Goyet JV, Sharif K, et al. Congenital, solitary, large, intrahepatic arterioportal fistula in a child: management and review of the literature. *Pediatr Radiol.* 2003;33:20–23.
46. Iñon AE, D'Agostino D. Portal hypertension secondary to congenital arterioportal fistula. *J Pediatr Gastroenterol Nutr.* 1987;6:471–473.
47. Raghuram L, Korah IP, Jaya V, et al. Coil embolization of a solitary congenital intrahepatic hepatoportal fistula. *Abdom Imaging.* 2001;26:194–196.

III

Practice Development and the Future of Embolotherapy

61

Strategies for the Development of an Embolotherapy Service

Gary P. Siskin • John C. Dalfino

The growing role that embolotherapy has been playing in medical care should be apparent to all practicing interventionalists. As embolization procedures continue to either replace or play an adjunctive role to existing medical and surgical therapy, it becomes incumbent on those performing these procedures to assume the role of a treating physician and to assume significant responsibility for the care of these patients. This is the cornerstone of a true embolization service.

Physicians participating in an embolization service must have a complete working knowledge of the indications and contraindications for these procedures, the applicable vascular anatomy, the technical steps of the procedure, the embolic agent(s) and other equipment being used, the expected outcomes, and the potential complications and how these complications are best managed. This is a big task because embolization procedures are performed for various conditions falling under the domain of so many different medical specialties. In other words, the individual specializing in interventional oncology and spending much of his or her time performing procedures such as chemoembolization or radioembolization may not have the same degree of knowledge in the neuro or gynecologic applications of embolotherapy. The physicians performing these procedures must recognize these limitations if they are seeking to grow their practice into different areas. The technical skill-set and familiarity with embolic agents may be there, but a commitment must be made to the additional work required to claim the same degree of expertise as those regularly performing these procedures.

The knowledge base is only one part of this, though. For a successful embolization service to be in place within a hospital, interventionalists must make a true commitment to the care of these patients and the development of these procedures. Although it has been said frequently in recent years, no physician understands the role of and potential issues surrounding embolization procedures better than the person performing the embolization procedure. It is unreasonable to expect a gynecologist caring for a patient with fibroids undergoing a uterine artery embolization procedure, an oncologist caring for a patient undergoing chemoembolization, or a pulmonologist caring for a patient with a pulmonary arteriovenous malformation (AVM) undergoing embolization to understand the technical challenges, expected outcomes, and potential complications of the procedure better than an interventionalist. This fact alone should provide the justification for any interventionalist performing embolization procedures to be actively engaged in the longitudinal care of his or her patients.[1]

But there is more. Embolization has become the primary therapeutic options for so many different conditions, and as such, it is just inappropriate for the physician providing a therapeutic service to not be a part of the preprocedure and postprocedure care of his or her patient. This continuity of care is of course good for patients because the person with the most expertise with the procedure is keeping an eye on them. It is, however, also good for the physician. It is not possible to have a preprocedure conversation with a patient regarding expected outcomes and potential risks if one does not personally provide follow-up care. Without a suitable amount of postprocedure experience, one can never gain the familiarity with outcomes and complications to enable this type of conversation to take place. Therefore, this becomes inappropriate care and will likely form the basis for others to become actively engaged in embolotherapy.

All of this lends support to what is now becoming a mandatory clinical practice model for interventionalists performing embolization procedures. Interventional radiologists continue to be the specialists performing the largest volume of embolization procedures, but like so many areas under the heading of endovascular care, this is changing. A growing number of vascular surgeons, neurosurgeons, neurologists, and nephrologists are incorporating embolization into their procedural skill-set, and managing an entire episode of care is fundamental to their respective clinical practices. Although this is being increasingly recognized by interventional radiologists, there are some physicians who continue to either disagree with this model of practice or are not given the resources and/or support from their diagnostic radiology colleagues to become actively engaged in direct patient care. At some point, these physicians will have to make a decision regarding whether or not it is appropriate for them to continue performing these procedures. Longitudinal patient care is that important.

THE OUTPATIENT OFFICE

For most procedural specialists, the outpatient office forms the core of their practices. An increasing number of procedures are originating in the outpatient setting; therefore, an office must be available for an episode of care involving embolization to begin. The office is where patients are initially assessed and counseled, where arrangements are made for office or hospital-based procedures, where billing originates from, and where patients are seen in follow-up after procedures are performed.[2] One need only take a quick look at this markedly consolidated list to understand that these items are difficult to administer from the confines of a fluoroscopy suite. Therefore, the core of an embolization service must take place in a dedicated office space in the community or hospital setting.

The physical space for an outpatient office represents only one part of this effort when establishing an embolization service. Successful practices are built around practitioners and staff who fully understand and appreciate the nuances of these procedures. Nurse practitioners[3] and physician assistants[4] have been playing an integral role within interventional practices for the past several years and will continue to do so. In the authors' experience, these individuals are able to provide not only procedural assistance but also can truly be a valuable link between patients and the practice as they go through their procedural recovery. It always helps patients to know that they have points of contact within a medical practice should they have questions or concerns, and physicians who are able to share this responsibility with others are more likely to bring success to their entire practice in this area. Additional aspects of an outpatient office range from the office staff such as nurses, receptionists, and billing personnel to the computer-based electronic medical records that are prevalent today. These services need to be in place to ensure appropriate communication with referring physicians, consulting services, hospitals, and third-party payers.

PREPROCEDURE ASSESSMENT

Despite the different specialty backgrounds of physicians performing embolization procedures, these individuals are all asked in one manner or another to consult on a patient with a medical problem that may benefit from the procedures they offer. Keeping in mind the earlier point about who actually has the expertise about embolization procedures, it becomes the consultant's responsibility to answer the referring physician's questions and to determine if a patient is or is not a candidate for an embolization procedure. This commonly involves reviewing medical records, radiologic images, lab work, and the notes from previous procedures. An infrastructure must therefore be in place to ensure that this information is available for review at the time of an initial consultation. This information is often enough to determine a patient's candidacy for embolization.

A discussion must then take place to review the decision-making process for determining why a patient is a candidate for embolization and why that procedure is being recommended. The procedure should be reviewed in its entirety with the patient, especially if they may be only minimally sedated; they will likely be more comfortable if they know what is happening. Almost more importantly, expectations for recovery should be reviewed as well. Patients undergoing embolization often have the idea that a "procedure" such as embolization cannot possibly be associated with a difficult recovery period ("it is not surgery"). Although this may be true in some instances, the various chapters in this textbook clearly demonstrate that the recovery after some embolization procedures may be difficult for these patients and the families caring for them. The expected postprocedure symptoms, the duration of this recovery, and the ways to get in touch with staff at all hours of the day need to be reviewed with patients and their families.

The final step in this preprocedure consultation is to be certain that patients understand not only the procedure but also the role that this procedure is playing in the overall management of their condition. For some patients, surgery may follow an embolization procedure, whereas for others, particularly in the area of interventional oncology, liver-directed therapy may be followed by surgical or medical therapy. Patients need to understand when embolization is a stand-alone treatment and when it is one step in a long process involving many treatment strategies offered by many different physicians. The same conversation should be had with the physician referring the patient to your service because they should also understand when additional therapy may or may not be required after embolization. This is important in both the inpatient and outpatient setting.

PROCEDURAL CARE

The base of knowledge required for successful performance of embolization procedures has been extensively reviewed throughout this textbook. It should be said here, though, that patients must feel that they are being treated by physicians who have and are comfortable with the knowledge and technical skill required to treat their condition successfully. Ensuring that patients have this type of confidence in their physician goes a long way toward increasing their comfort as they enter a procedure suite for their embolization procedure.

No matter how confident patients are with their physicians, and no matter how eager they are to have this procedure performed, most patients will prefer to be adequately sedated throughout the course of an embolization procedure. Therefore, physicians actively participating in an embolization service and regularly performing these procedures must have a good understanding of the sedation needs in association with the procedure being performed and the sedation demands of the individual patient. This should be a point of discussion during a preprocedure consultation. For some embolization procedures, general anesthesia may be required, but in the author's experience, most embolization procedures can be performed successfully with moderate sedation using drugs such as midazolam and fentanyl. Use of these medications will require appropriate monitoring of patients during and after the performance of the procedure.

The risk of transient bacteremia after embolization has been historically demonstrated,[5] which is why interventionalists participating in an embolization service should have an understanding regarding the use of prophylactic antibiotics before these procedures. Practice guidelines from the Society of Interventional Radiology have recommended the use of prophylactic antibiotics targeted against skin pathogens before solid organ embolization procedures involving the liver, kidney, or spleen, especially when there is a high likelihood of infarction; this includes chemoembolization procedures.[6] Prophylaxis is also recommended before uterine fibroid embolization procedures, although there is no consensus regarding antibiotic use when embolization is being performed to control bleeding from a viscus or solid organ.[6]

POSTPROCEDURE MANAGEMENT

The recovery period after embolization is the greatest area of opportunity for physicians participating in an embolization service. It is here that patients will judge the care that they received. Remember that there is rarely any visible manifestation of the procedure that was just performed. Most patients leave an interventional procedure area with nothing more than a Band-Aid as evidence that they underwent a procedure. There is no surgical incision closed with obvious attention on cosmetic healing to confirm the technical proficiency of the surgeon. Therefore, patients are left assuming that the job was done and was done well. Managing patients after an embolization procedure represents the real opportunity physicians have to demonstrate their caring and their expertise; it is what the patients will remember. Therefore, physicians must be certain that patients and their families are adequately counseled regarding the expected symptoms after embolization. In addition, an easy means of communication between patients and the physician practice must be established to address questions and/or concerns during this recovery period.

Postembolization Syndrome

The different applications of embolization are each associated with a unique set of postprocedural issues that need to be recognized and addressed by the treating physician. These are all specifically discussed in previous chapters of this textbook. However, patients undergoing solid organ or solid tumor embolization typically experience a postembolization syndrome that has been well described in the literature. For any patient undergoing procedures such as chemoembolization, splenic artery embolization, uterine artery embolization for fibroids, and renal artery embolization for an angiomyolipoma (to name a few), patients should be appropriately counseled regarding the symptoms that make up the postembolization syndrome. Interestingly, some consider postembolization syndrome to be a complication of an embolization procedure, but these authors disagree. The postembolization syndrome is an expected consequence or side effect of solid organ or solid tumor embolization, and patients should expect to experience the associated symptoms with variable degrees of intensity.[7] Symptoms severe enough to require readmission to the hospital after discharge should be considered a complication.[7]

The clinical manifestations of postembolization syndrome include pain, fever, nausea and vomiting, loss of appetite, and generalized malaise. These symptoms generally occur within 1 to 3 days after embolization and are believed to be a consequence of the tissue ischemia induced by the procedure. Tissue breakdown products may induce an inflammatory response and the production of cytokines. It has been suggested that it may be mediated by interleukins 1 and 6 and by tumor necrosis factor-alpha.[8,9] They may be responsible for the pain, fever, and nausea commonly seen after embolization. Leukocytosis in the first 24 hours after embolization is common as well. This needs to always be considered if evaluating patients shortly after embolization because a failure to recognize this may cause one to be overly concerned about early infection.[10] Experience suggests that even though these symptoms occur in most patients undergoing solid organ or solid tumor embolization, they can be more severe in patients in whom a large tumor volume was embolized or a large volume of normal tissue was embolized.

The symptoms associated with the postembolization syndrome are typically self-limited for most patients. However, effective management can improve patient comfort and lead to a more rapid recovery after embolization. The medications used can be directed toward which symptoms the patient is actually experiencing, including anti-inflammatory, antipyretic, and antinausea medication. Pain medication should be an important part of the medication regimen for patients experiencing pain after embolization. Generally speaking, the efficacy of a pain regimen is often enhanced by the additive effect of two analgesics that relieve pain by different mechanisms.[11] Although prophylactic medication may be appropriate in some settings, it is important to remember that medications have their own side effects that can actually prolong the recovery period. For example, opioid analgesics are effective at addressing pain after embolization but can contribute to both nausea and constipation that many patients experience. These symptoms can make a recovery period more difficult, so careful use of these medications is recommended, but if needed, additional medications can be offered to address their side effects.

Infection

Prolonged symptoms after embolization should always raise the possibility of an infection. In general, fever starting or worsening after postprocedure days 5 to 7 should increase one's suspicion for infection. Other symptoms may lead one toward a diagnosis of infection as well, including a foul-smelling discharge after uterine artery embolization for fibroids.[12] Cultures should be obtained and antibiotic therapy can be initiated at that time. Imaging may be challenging to interpret because gas may be present within a solid organ after embolization; it does not necessarily mean that an infection or abscess is present.

It is also possible for infections to take place after embolization due to colonization of coils, which can act as a foreign body nidus.[13] An infection can be attributed to coil colonization if there is a short time interval between coil placement and the onset of the infectious event, if the causative organism is a part of normal human flora, if the infection is found to be located around the coils, and if other concurrent infections are not present.[14] If this should occur, the causative agent can penetrate through the wall of the artery and cause a parenchymal infection. This can cause a significant inflammatory response and edema, which can predispose the patient to formation of an abscess.[13] If this occurs, removal of the infected coil is the chosen treatment, but if this is not possible, then prolonged high-dose intravenous (IV) antibiotics is a suitable alternative.

Neurologic Issues

Headache

Headache is a fairly frequent complaint following cerebral angiography and interventions. Baron et al.[15] found postprocedural headaches to be common after coil embolization (72%), glue embolization (33%), and stent placement (14%). In this series, 118 urgent diagnostic studies were performed to further evaluate these headaches, all of which were negative.[15] Although there is no robust data supporting any particular criteria for imaging for the workup of postangiography headache, it is probably prudent to consider imaging in patients who complain of severe headache that is not relieved by a dose of narcotics or when accompanied by abnormal neurologic findings. The use of glucocorticoids can be considered prophylactically or posttreatment in patients undergoing embolization of AVMs or tumors to avoid headaches due to cerebral edema.

Cranial Nerve Palsies

Cranial nerve palsies can occur after both intracranial and extracranial embolization procedures. During extracranial embolizations, such as for glomus jugulare tumors, cranial nerve palsies are usually caused by inadvertent embolization of the vasa vasorum of the cranial nerves.[16] These injuries can occur with both particulate and liquid embolic agents, although they tend to be transient when particulate agents are used and more permanent when liquid agents are used.[17] Although these injuries are probably not completely avoidable, positioning the catheter tip as close as possible to the target lesion will reduce the risk of embolizing, noninvolved vessels. Embolization with liquid embolic agents carries the additional risk of traction injuries to adjacent cranial nerves during catheter removal. For instance, transient facial and V3 palsies have been reported after catheter extraction from Onyx (Covidien, Irvine, California). casts in the middle meningeal and internal maxillary arteries after embolization of dural arteriovenous fistulas (dAVFs) and AVMs.[18]

Ischemic Stroke

Ischemic stroke can occur from any intravascular procedure in which the aortic arch, precerebral, or cerebral vessels are accessed. Most strokes related to diagnostic or interventional angiographic procedures occur during the procedure itself. Less commonly, a stroke can occur in the postprocedure period. In either case, prompt recognition of ischemic complications is essential so that corrective action can be taken as soon as possible.

Immediately following arch or cerebral angiography, it is advisable to check the patient for evidence of stroke by performing a neurologic exam. The Cincinnati Prehospital Stroke Scale (CPSS) is a validated tool for identifying stroke in both the inpatient and outpatient setting. The patient is assessed for facial droop, upper extremity drift, and aphasia. A positive score on any of these items will identify nearly 90% of anterior circulation strokes.[19] If a stroke is suspected, the patient should have a noncontrast CT scan performed to rule out intracranial hemorrhage. Unless otherwise contraindicated, IV tissue plasminogen activator can be administered. Depending on the severity and suspected cause of the stroke, consideration should be made for acute endovascular clot thrombolysis.

QUALITY IMPROVEMENT

A quality improvement program should be an important component of an embolization service. Specifically, interventionalists should collect and evaluate data to determine the appropriateness of the indications they use for embolization, the degree of success they are achieving after these procedures, and the incidence of complications after embolization.[20] This enables interventionalists to identify problems and to put corrective measures in place with the goal of improving the quality of care.[21] Ultimately, this type of effort can demonstrate the ongoing value of embolotherapy to the patients being served and can help ensure the growth of this area of medicine.[22]

ONGOING DEVELOPMENT OF AN EMBOLIZATION SERVICE

Even with all of the previously described pieces in place, ongoing work is required to manage and grow an embolization service. At the specialty level, research is continuously required to understand the place of embolization in the care of the many patients described throughout this textbook. Comparative effectiveness studies simply have to get done to best understand the role of embolization as opposed to hysterectomy for fibroids, chemotherapy or radiation for cancer, or surgery for trauma. Without an organized effort to carry out this type of research, questions will always linger about the superiority, equivalence, or inferiority of embolization as treatment for many of the conditions described in this textbook.

At the local level, efforts should always be made by those participating in an embolization service to educate everyone involved in patient care. Direct outreach to patients is an appropriate way to make them as well as advocacy groups aware of these procedures as treatment options that should be discussed with physicians. Referring physicians should know about all treatment options available to their patients and not just the ones offered by members of their own specialty. Finally, hospital administrators and third-party payers should always be enlightened regarding the benefits of these procedures from a cost-savings perspective and from the potential growth and attention they can bring to an institution.

CONCLUSION

Embolization has progressed to the point where dedicated expertise is required for success. The expertise that the interventionalist brings to the care of patients requiring embolization is significant and should be treated as such. Physicians with this expertise are encouraged to develop and participate in an embolization service. This can help ensure that patients being served by these physicians and these procedures are receiving care that exceeds expectations.

REFERENCES

1. American College of Radiology, American Society of Interventional and Therapeutic Neuroradiology, Society of Interventional Radiology. Practice guideline for interventional clinical practice. *J Vasc Interv Radiol.* 2005;16:149–155.
2. Siskin GP, Bagla S, Sansivero GE, et al. The interventional radiology clinic: what you need to know. *Semin Interv Radiol.* 2005;22:39–44.
3. Taylor K, Sansivero GE, Ray CE. The role of the nurse practitioner in interventional radiology. *J Vasc Interv Radiol.* 2012; 23:347–350.
4. Rosenberg SM, Rosenthal DA, Rajan DK, et al. Position statement: the role of physician assistants in interventional radiology. *J Vasc Interv Radiol.* 2008;19:1685–1689.
5. Meyer P, Reizine D, Aymard A, et al. Septic complications in interventional radiology: evaluation of risk and preventive measures: preliminary studies. *J Vasc Interv Radiol.* 1988;3: 73–75.
6. Venkatesan AM, Kundu S, Sacks D, et al. Practice guideline for adult antibiotic prophylaxis during vascular and interventional radiology procedures. *J Vasc Interv Radiol.* 2010;21:1611–1630.
7. Hovsepian DM, Siskin GP, Bonn J, et al. Quality improvement guidelines for uterine artery embolization for symptomatic leiomyomata. *J Vasc Interv Radiol.* 2004;15:535–541.
8. Rysava R, Hruskova Z, Tesar V, et al. Can adequate treatment influence the postembolization syndrome and cytokine release in patients undergoing iatrogenic renal artery embolization? *Prague Med Rep.* 2011;112:253–262.
9. Bissler JJ, Racadio J, Donnelly LF, et al. Reduction of postembolization syndrome after ablation of renal angiomyolipoma. *Am J Kidney Dis.* 2002;39:966–971.
10. Ganguli S, Faintuch S, Salazar GM, et al. Postembolization syndrome: changes in white blood cell counts immediately after uterine artery embolization. *J Vasc Interv Radiol.* 2008;19: 443–445.
11. Wideman GL, Keffer, Morris E, et al. Analgesic efficacy of a combination of hydrocodone with ibuprofen in postoperative pain. *Clin Pharmacol Ther.* 1999;65:66–76.
12. Rajan DK, Beecroft JR, Clark TW, et al. Risk of intrauterine infectious complications after uterine artery embolization. *J Vasc Interv Radiol.* 2004;15:1415–1421.
13. Falagas ME, Nikou SA, Siempos II. Infections related to coils used for embolization of arteries: review of the published evidence. *J Vasc Interv Radiol.* 2007;18:697–701.
14. Jenkinson MD, Javadpour M, Nixon T, et al. Intracerebral abscess formation following embolization of an internal carotid artery aneurysm using Gugliemi detachable coils. *Acta Neurochir (Wien).* 2003;145:703–705.
15. Baron EP, Moskowitz SI, Tepper SJ, et al. Headache following intracranial neuroendovascular procedures. *Headache.* 2012: 52(5);739–748.

16. Gaynor BG, Elhammady MS, Jethanamest DM, et al. Incidence of cranial nerve palsy after preoperative embolization of glomus jugulare tumors using Onyx. *J Neurosurg*. 2014;120:377–381.
17. Gartrell BC, Hansen MR, Gantz BJ, et al. Facial and lower cranial neuropathies after preoperative embolization of jugular foramen lesions with ethylene vinyl alcohol. *Otol Neurotol*. 2012;33:1270–1275.
18. Nyberg EM, Chaudry MI, Turk AS, et al. Transient cranial neuropathies as sequelae on Onyx embolization of arteriovenous shunt lesions near the skull base: possible axonotmetic traction injuries. *J Neurointerv Surg*. 2013;5:e21.
19. Kothari RU, Pancioli A, Liu T, et al. Cincinnati Prehospital Stroke Scale: reproducibility and validity. *Ann Emerg Med*. 1999;33:373–378.
20. Angle JF, Siddiqi NH, Wallace MJ, et al. Quality improvement guidelines for percutaneous transcatheter embolization. *J Vasc Interv Radiol*. 2010;21:1479–1486.
21. Salazar GM, Abudjudeh H. Quality assurance in interventional radiology. *AJR Am J Roentgenol*. 2012;199:W441–W443.
22. Steele JR, Wallace MJ, Hovsepian DM, et al. Guidelines for establishing a quality improvement program in interventional radiology. *J Vasc Interv Radiol*. 2010;21:617–625.

INDEX

Page numbers followed by *f* and *t* indicated figures and tables, respectively.

J

K

L

M

N

O

Q

R

S